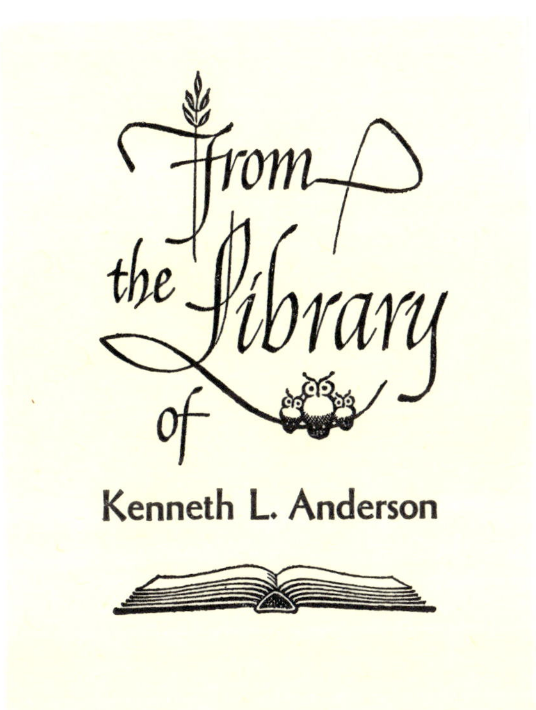

From
the Library
of
Kenneth L. Anderson

METHODOLOGY OF IMMUNOCHEMICAL AND IMMUNOLOGICAL RESEARCH

METHODOLOGY OF IMMUNOCHEMICAL AND IMMUNOLOGICAL RESEARCH

J. B. G. KWAPINSKI, M.B., D.M., Ph.D., FAAM,

Professor, Department of Medical Microbiology
The University of Manitoba
Winnipeg, Canada.

WILEY-INTERSCIENCE, a Division of John Wiley & Sons, Inc.
New York · London · Sydney · Toronto

Library of Congress Cataloging in Publication Data:

Kwapinski, Jerzy B   G   1920-
Methodology of immunochemical and immunological research.

First published in 1965 under title: Methods of serological research.
Bibliography: p.
1. Immunology—Technique. 2. Serology—Technique.
3. Immunochemistry—Technique. I. Title.

QR183.K85   1972   574.2′9′028   72–3977
ISBN 0–471–51111–0

Printed in the United States of America

10 9 8 7 6 5 4 3 2 1

PREFACE

Research methodology may be described as both a science based on theoretical principles and an art of experimentation. As new ideas and theories appear, their validity and consequences are investigated by appropriate experiments. Thus, the methodology not only provides means for examining the theories but also it promotes new ideas and leads to further discoveries. Therefore, both the theory and the methodology are essential for discovery of the truth, and are mutually complementary. These important objectives of the methodolgy of immunochemical and serological research are achieved by the investigation, evaluation and categorization of immunochemical and serological procedures, and by designing new methods of experimentation and serological practice.

Since the publication of Methods of Serological Research in 1965, a considerable progress has been made in the immunochemical and serological methodology, culminating in an increasing number of automatic and semi-automatic apparatus and procedures for immunochemical examinations of antigens and immunoglobulins.

Application of the automated or semi-automated procedures has greatly facilitated and increased the precision and reproducibility of immunochemical and serological research. There exists a great need for purification and standardization of immunological and immunochemical reactants. Perhaps not far away is the time when various immunological reagents, such as immunoglobulins, antigens and complement, will be prepared synthetically, as our knowledge on the immunochemical properties and synthesis of these polymers improves.

After all, the immunological and immunochemical methodology and research greatly rely on utilization of the physico-chemical procedures and reagents; and it is increasingly evident that immunoglobulins and complex antigens are active chemical entities, possessing certain specific conformations which make them most readily definable by immunochemical methods. But in the very essence, the conformation of these entities results from a quantum and a distribution of kinetic energy existing in, and between the constituting molecules, electrons, protons and neutrons; and the immunological and immunochemical reactions essentially depend on an exchange of the energy quanta between conformationally fitting partners of an im-

munological system and reaction. I envisage that before long the immunochemical and serological methodology will employ quantum biophysical
and quantum biochemical procedures with their armament suited for a
precise and logical study of the origin and synthesis of antibodies and antigens and of interactions between the mutually conforming molecules endowed with what is conventionally termed as the immunological specificity
or selectivity.

J. B. G. KWAPINSKI

Winnipeg, Manitoba
January 1972

CONTENTS

Page

METHODOLOGY OF IMMUNOCHEMICAL AND IMMUNOLOGICAL RESEARCH

Chapter One

THE EVOLUTION OF IMMUNOLOGICAL RESEARCH

The foundation of immunological research was laid by Bordet in 1895 with his classical work on the properties of "immune sera," or "antisera," of immunized animals. This fundamental publication was preceded by Landois' observations (1875) on the clumping of red blood cells of one animal in a serum sample of another species; Nutall's (1888), Büchner's (1889), and Pfeiffer's (1893, 1894) reports on the bactericidal or bacteriolytic power of the blood serum; and von Behring and Kitasato's (1890) observations on the neutralization of bacterial exotoxins by the sera of animals injected repeatedly with nonlethal doses of toxins.

The term "antigen" was introduced by Landsteiner (1900), who also differentiated various classes of antigenic substances. Antibodies were first identified as electrophoretically distinct globulins by Tiselius (1936) and Tiselius and Kabat (1939), but a precise elucidation of the immunochemical and molecular structure of these immunoglobulins has been achieved much later (Edelman, 1959, Putnam et al., 1962, Fleischman, 1966). The mechanism of immunological reaction has been the subject of a number of theories. The side chains (Ehrlich, 1900), mass action (Arrhenius and Madsen, 1904), adsorption (Bordet, 1920), and the lattice hypothesis (Marrack, 1938), as well as a "quantitative" modification of the hypothesis (Heidelberger, 1939) were proposed, but the forces and basic stereophysical mechanism of the antigen-antibody reactions were elucidated by Pauling (1945) and Valentine and Green (1967).

Immunochemical research in various areas has been initiated by Heidelberger and his co-workers (1925), Haurowitz (1938), Kabat (1939), Salton (1952), Morgan (1960), Kwapinski (1954), Westphal (1962), and others, who introduced immunochemical methods for extraction, purification, and identification of immunologically active substances. Rapid progress in immunochemical research has been due to the application of the procedures for preparation, purification, and measurement of antigens and antibodies, based on (a) electrophoresis (free-boundary electrophoresis, Tiselius, 1930; electrofocusing, Svensson, 1962; disk electrophoresis,

Ornstein, 1964 and Davis, 1964; continuous particle electrophoresis, Hanning, 1964); (b) chromatography (Peterson and Sober, 1956); (c) differential ultracentrifugation and gradient centrifugation (Svedberg, 1940, Brakke, 1951); (d) the countercurrent distribution method (Craig, 1960).

Immunochemical methods for the purification and identification of immunoglobulins have improved greatly the knowledge about antibodies and have contributed to the elucidation of mechanisms involved in the antigen-antibody reactions.

Bacteriolysis and the *bacteriolytic test* were probably the first immunological phenomenon and assay described. Early observations by Pfeiffer (1893, 1894) and by Pfeiffer and Issaeff (1894) on the lysis of *Vibrio comma* in vivo were followed by Bordet's discovery (1895, 1898) of two different substances, one thermolabile, the other relatively heat-stable, involved in the phenomenon of lysis of bacterial cells and animal blood cells. These observations led directly to the designs of various immune lytic tests, for example, *complement fixation* and *complement absorption* (Bordet and Gengou, 1901).

The complement-fixation reaction was applied independently to the diagnosis of typhoid fever by both Widal (1896) and Lesaurd (1896). Since the introduction of the complement-fixation reaction to the immunology of syphilis (Wassermann et al., 1906), this test has become very popular and has been modified by many investigators to suit different antigens, antibodies, and other experimental conditions. The term "reagin" (the substance that reacts) was applied by Citrol (1907) to the reactive substances of syphilitic serum. The first quantitative complement fixation test was introduced by Wadsworth et al. (1931); a microtechnique was described by Fulton and Dumbell in 1949, and an indirect complement fixation test was designed in 1948 by Rice.

The method of *complement determination* in human sera was introduced by Ecker et al. (1943), the *properdin assay* by Pillemer et al. (1956), and the *passive hemolytic test* by Fisher (1951). Other less popular immune lytic tests were described a few decades after the early reports of Pfeiffer (1894) and Bordet (1895). The *immune leukolysis* test was published in 1920 by Mauriac and Moureau, and the immune platelet test as late as 1953 by Cruz.

Agglutination or aggregation of bacteria was first observed in 1896 by Gruber and Durham. The difference between flagellar and somatic types of agglutination was shown by Smith and Reagh (1903), Beyer and Reagh (1904), and in a more extensive study by Weil and Felix (1916). The test-tube agglutination was used in those early investigations. The capillary-tube agglutination test was introduced by Hudson and Mudd (1935), and the technique of slide agglutination by Castañeda and Silva (1942). The first chromatoagglutination test was devised by Spalding and Metcalf (1954), and a growth-agglutination test was described by Wynne et al. in 1953. The agglutination tests with collodion particles as carriers of antigens were first described by Loeb (1922) and by Freund (1930). Other inert particles were subsequently introduced as antigen carriers, for example, oil droplets (Boroff, 1938), resin (Evans and Haines, 1954), polysterene latex (Plotz and Singer, 1956), bentonite (Bloch and Bunim, 1959), and acryl (Winblad, 1961).

The *precipitation reaction* was first described by Kraus in 1897 in a system consisting of a culture filtrate of *Pasteurella pestis* or *Vibrio comma* and a homologous antiserum. Similar experiments on the precipitation of various antigens added to an antibody-containing serum in test tubes were conducted by Bordet as early as 1899. The ring precipitation test was introduced by Ascoli (1902). This interfacial precipitin test was greatly improved by the introduction of the gel media, at first in the form of gelatin (Bechhold, 1905) and later as purified agar gels (Reiner and Kopp, 1927) or solid nutrient media (Petrie and Steabben, 1943). Convenient techniques of the diffusion precipitation test were devised by Oudin (1946), Elek (1948), and Ouchterlony (1948), and the immunoelectrophoresis method was introduced by Grabar and Williams (1953). The first chromatoprecipitation technique was described in 1950 by Castañeda.

Flocculation occurring in the nearly neutral antigen-antibody (ricin-antiricin) mixtures was noticed as early as 1902 by Danysz. The flocculation test, however, was introduced much later by Ramon (1922) and was used for the observation in vitro of the serological reactions between toxins and antitoxins. An important contribution to the flocculation test was provided by the studies of Dean and Webb (1926) on the optimal antigen-antibody ratio. This test, with emulsified antigens, was introduced into the serology of syphilis by Sachs and Georgi (1918) and by Kline (1930).

Hemagglutination tests, which involve reactions between antisera and antigen-coated erythrocytes, were made a few decades after the isohemagglutination test described in 1900 by Landsteiner, and the conglutination reaction was reported independently in 1906 by Bordet and Gay and by Muir and Browning.

The isohemagglutination reaction has been widely applied in studies of blood groups and blood factors, using tube, slide, or capillary technique (Chown, 1944). The cold hemagglutination reaction was described in detail by Landsteiner as early as 1903, but it was 1918 when cold agglutinins were associated with bronchopneumonia by Clough and Richter and as late as 1943 when they were associated with primary interstitial pneumonia by Peterson et al.

The *conglutination test* was thoroughly studied by Bordet and Gay (1906) and by Muir and Browning (1906), but was first employed diagnostically in 1947 by Hole and Coombs for the detection of antibodies in the sera of ponies convalescent from glanders. The conglutination test was developed into a conglutinating complement-absorption test by Streng (1910). The T-hemagglutination was first described by Thomsen in 1922, and an appropriate T-hemagglutination test was devised by Friedenreich in 1930. Bacteriogenic hemagglutination was reported in 1940 by Davidsohn and Toharsky. The first serological test based on a reaction of the cell-adsorbed antigens with the homologous antibodies was reported in 1941 by Roberts and Jones.

A *hemagglutination reaction* involving erythrocytes artificially modified by the diazotization and a homologous antibody was demonstrated in 1942 by Pressman et al. The idea of using red blood cells as a medium for the antibody absorption was suggested by Landsteiner (1945); but the first hemagglutination test with antigen-coated red blood cells and a corresponding antibody was introduced in 1947 by Keogh et al. This test was adjusted to various types of antigens by treating the erythrocytes with viruses (Burnet, 1946), tannic acid (Boyden, 1951), or proteolytic enzymes (Stulberg et al., 1956).

The *neutralization reaction* was first employed by Sternberg (1892) in a study on vaccinia. Various modifications of the neutralization test were described much later, for example, a neutralization technique in the chick embryo (Hilleman and Horsfall, 1950) or in the tissue culture (Kaplan, 1955).

The first *immunoinhibition test* described was probably the agglutination-inhibition reaction, reported in 1902 by Castellani. The precipitation-inhibition test was published much later by Culbertson (1932), and the first active hemagglutination-inhibition test published was the inhibition of the virus hemagglutination by a homologous antibody (Salk et al., 1940). Similar inhibition tests with bacterial hemagglutinins were devised by Dolby (1958) and Kwapinski (1958). Other serobiochemical inhibition tests were also described, for example, the virus-hemolysis inhibition test (Hirst, 1941), antistreptolysin test (Todd, 1932), antistreptokinase test (Garner and Tillett, 1934), anticoagulase test (Smith and Hall, 1944), antihyaluronidase test (McCarty, 1949, Hazlehurst, 1950), and the immobilization test (Nelson and Mayer, 1949).

Specific structural immunoreactions, involving certain anatomical structures of bacteria and a corresponding antibody, were first observed by Roger (1896) and described later by Neufeld (1903) and Ettinger-Tulczynska (1933). Other specific structural reactions were devised later by Tomcsik et al., (1958, 1959).

Physical tests which reveal the antibody-antigen reactions by the determination of certain physical changes include the viscosity test (Loiseleur, 1946), the optical-rotation test (Ishizaka and Campbell, 1959), the alteration of the thickness of an antigen-antibody monolayer (Chambers et al., 1941), and the long-chain reaction (Stollerman and Ekstedt, 1957). The phenomenon of immune adherence was described as early as 1917 by Rieckenberg, but it was applied by Nelson to a definite immunological test as late as 1953.

Several tests were designed for the detection of incomplete or "weak" antibodies, for example, the anti-gamma-globulin test (Moreschi, 1908; Coombs and Mourant, 1947), the augmentation test (Coombs et al., 1945), the albumin agglutination test (Diamond and Denton, 1945), and the precipitation adherence test (Vaughan, 1956).

Immunohistochemical procedures for the detection of antigens in the tissues were first described by Creech and Jones (1941) and greatly developed by Coons et al. (1942). The radioisotope technique was introduced to the serological investigations in 1942 by Stanley.

The *opsonophagocytic test* originated from the early observations by Metchnikoff (1883, 1897) and Denys and LeClef (1895) on the phagocytosis of bacteria and leukocytes promoted by an action of blood serum. More thorough studies on the opsonins were conducted by Wright and Douglas (1904). Modification of the phagocytosis test by the use of the tissue culture cells was described in 1960 by Shepard, and the phagocytosis-inhibition test was introduced by Merchant and Chamberlain in 1952. *Bacteriotropins* were detected during the investigation of Neufeld and Rimpau (1904) on a thermostable serum substance that promotes phagocytosis. A more accurate bacteriotropin test was devised in 1933 by Hughes.

Early observations on *immunohistiotropic reactions* were made by Jenner (1798) during his studies on revaccination against smallpox. The phenomenon of anaphylaxis was first discovered by Magendie (1839), and was rediscovered and elucidated by Richet et al. (1902). A test for the anaphylactic reaction in vivo was devised by Richet (1911), and an anaphylactic test in vitro was described by Schultz (1910) and Dale (1913).

Contributions to the development and improvement of the serological and immunochemical methods made by many investigators during 80 years of the history of immunology are presented in subsequent chapters of this book.

Chapter Two

PREPARATION OF ANTIGENS

The two essential components of every immunological reaction are the antigen and the antibody. The role of all other constituents of serological tests is to reveal the antigen-antibody complex thus formed.

Complete or functional antigens are immunogenic molecules (conformational subunits) capable of eliciting in a genetically competent host the synthesis of antibodies and of reacting with them in an observable way. Complex haptens (partial antigens) are substances capable of reacting specifically with the corresponding antibodies, forming visible products of the reaction, but unable to induce antibody synthesis unless complexed with, or adsorbed onto, carrier molecules or particles that have converted them into complete antigens. Haptens are ligands that often conjugate spontaneously with a native, natural carrier. The capability of a hapten to elicit antibody production under suitable circumstances appears to be directly dependent on its capacity to conjugate *in vivo* with the carrier molecules of an immunologically compatible host. Haptens are capable of provoking delayed hypersensitivity reactions. Simple haptens (haptids), which have low molecular weight and are monovalent, neither elicit the antibody response nor are able to participate in any observable direct immunological reaction; but they absorb homologous antibodies thus causing a blocking effect and rendering these specific molecules inert for reactions with the immunnologically related complete antigens or complex haptens.

Immunogenicity is a function of a certain minimal complexity and molecular size of an antigen, irrespective of the nature of the substance. Thus materials with a molecular weight of less than 5,000 are usually nonimmunogenic and nonantigenic. Substances possessing a slightly higher molecular weight are weak antigens; for example, the lysozyme possessing a molecular weight of 15,000 is a weak antigen. Functional antigens are more highly organized and complex bodies with a higher molecular weight than the complex haptens (Table 1). The molecular weights of antigenic proteins vary between 34,500 and 5,000,000. Complete antigens are predominantly proteins, but some polysaccharides and nucleic acids may display full antigenic properties under certain conditions.

Table 1. Classification of Antigens

Antigens

Complete antigens — Incomplete antigens

Proteins Lipopolysaccharides Polysaccharides

Nucleoproteins

Complex haptens — Simple haptens

Poly-peptides	Lipids Phosphatides Steroids	Nucleic acids	Disaccharides Monoses
		Nucleosides Nucleotides	Simple organic compounds
Polysaccharides			Peptides

The immunological specificity of antigens is described by antigenic determinants, representing certain discrete areas on macromolecules or conformational submits that impair the immunological specificity. Antigenic determinants (antigenic determinant sites) apparently have spherical shape and the size ranging from 200 to 700 $Å^2$; however, the determinant sphere on a protein macromolecule has a radius of about 6 Å (Kabat, 1966). A part of the sphere is exposed for reaction with a complementary site on the antibody macromolecule. Immunological character of protein antigens is determined by the arrangement of amino acids on the surface of antigen molecules. Antigenic determinants of polysaccharides and mucopolysaccharides seem to consist of combinations of hexose units, arranged in a certain sequence. The antigenic determinant in molecules of teichoic acids seems to be glycosidically linked sugars. Antigenic determinants on the macromolecules of nucleic acids are nucleotide bases. If a potential immunogenic site is hidden within a molecule, it is unaccessible for biosynthesis and it cannot elicit immune response.

Antigens are multivalent (possess several determinants per molecule) and multispecific. An antigen molecule can carry 5 to 23 reactive groups and several types of antigenic determinants which may be repeated along a polypeptide or polysaccharide chain. Particulate antigens may possess a large number of antibody receptors. For example, there are 200 to 5000 Rh-receptors on a single red cell (Grubb, 1955). The number of receptors can be computed from the formula $(W \times N)/(M \times R)$ where W = weight, in grams, of the adsorbed antibody; N = Avogadros' number

(6.02×10^{23}); M = molecular weight of the antibody; R = number of cells.

Antigenic potency of the polypeptide and protein macromolecules appears to depend on the presence of tyrosine and, to a lesser extent, of glutamic acid, tryptophan, and phenylalanine, which greatly enhance the antigenic power of synthetic polypeptides. Serological activity and specificity of polypeptides and proteins appear to be related to the tyrosine content. Antigenicity of proteins and polypeptides does not seem to depend on the $R\text{-}NH_3$ or phenolic groups. Deamination and guadination do not affect the capacity of protein molecules to react with their antibodies.

Nucleic acids are complex haptens. The DNA strands, denaturated by boiling, cooled rapidly so that the strands of the double helix remain separated, and mixed with methylated bovine serum albumin, form a complex which gives rise to anti-DNA antibodies. Antibodies to ribonucleic acid may be obtained by intravenous injections of a ribosome suspension. Sera from *lupus erythematosus* contain specific antibodies against single-stranded DNA, and sera from some bacterial infections react with the double- and single-stranded DNA molecules. Purine and pyrimidine bases are simple haptens and can induce antibody production when coupled chemically to a protein.

Natural antigen molecules possess multiple surface reaction sites (antigen-determinant sites), composed of different physical configurations. Several antigenic determinants of diverse immunological specificity may exist in a single molecule of a pure substance, whereas an antigenic grouping (determinant) can elicit the synthesis of different antibodies. Molecules of a single antigen usually display immunological microheterogeneity in an ostensibly homogeneous antigen preparation. A large protein molecule frequently possesses multiple determinancy which refers to specific chains or fragment antigens.

Antigen preparations, obtained by different methods or extracted from individual, serologically related strains or species, usually vary in the amount of a common antigenic determinant. The specificity of antigens, and particularly of the protein antigens, is altered by heating at temperatures over 60°,* or by exposing them to other denaturing agents, enzymatic digestion, oxidation, iodination, nitration, or diazotization. Reducing substances, acids and alkali, cause considerable alterations of the antigenic potency and specificity.

The panels and quantities of antigens appearing in the cell tissues and organs of an animal vary during different developmental stages, but the immunological difference is most easily observable between the early development and senescence. There are some indications that antigenic pat-

---

* Temperatures in this book are expressed in terms of the centigrade scale.

terns and amounts of different antigens vary in developmental stages of microorganisms although precise data on the ontogenic development in microorganisms for lacking. Since the genetic information in the embryo is incompletely expressed, the synthesis of antigens in kind and amount, and the complexity of macromolecules thus formed are restricted as compared to the full panel and amount of different antigens found in a normal, mature individual when the genetic information has been fully expressed. Thus organ-specific antigens in man appear before the fifth fetal month but they reach the maximum concentration at about 10 years of age and subsequently diminish throughout the remainder of life.

Isoantigens are representatives of certain inheritable, species-specific antigens. Allotypes represent an important class of isoantigenic differences occurring among the γG immunoglobulins of various animal species. Human erythrocytes contain one of the two known allotypes, the Gm and Inv factors. The allotype differences depend on small discrepancies in the amino acid sequence of the γG globulin molecule.

Isoantigens are restricted to a species of animals, whereas the heterophile (Forssman's) haptens occur in a number of different species. The heterophile Forssman's haptens are probably globosides, and some of them consist of N-acylsphingosine, galactose, and N-acetylglucosamine. Another class of glycosphingolipids, the gangliosides, are constituents of neuronal membranes; they contain N-acetyl neuraminic acid residues attached to the backbone of ceramide-glucose-galactose-N-acetylgalactosamine-galactose.

Antigenic similarities between species and between individuals of a species are found most commonly among the antigens that have specialized functions or occur in certain specialized tissues or organs (tissue- or organ-specific antigens). For example, serum albumin, brain and lens proteins of closely related animal species, show the presence of common antigenic components. Antigens in microorganisms possess different range of immunological activity; the immunochemically characterizable type-specific antigens, which occur among one, two, or three strains of a species, whereas group- or species-specific antigens are shared by larger groups of microorganisms. Tracing of the distribution of the group-, species-, and genus-specific antigens among morphologically and biochemically similar microorganisms provides suitable immunochemical tools for the determination of probable phylogenetic connections and evolutionary patterns of microorganisms (Kwapinski, 1972).

B.   PATTERN FOR IMMUNOCHEMICAL ANALYSIS OF ANTIGENS

Immunochemical analysis of antigens consists in the following parts.

1. Selection of the antigen source and cultivation of microorganisms.

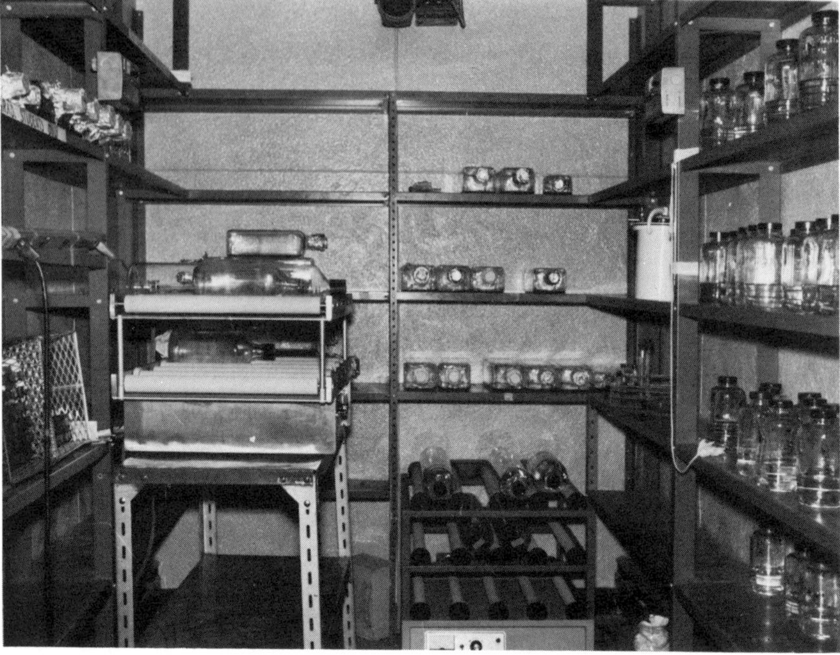

Figure 1. The inner view of a walk-in incubator. Cultures of microorganisms are grown in a liquid medium, maintained in the screw-capped bottles (left). Viruses are propagated in tissue cultures, kept statically in test tubes or moved gently on a roll-a-cell tissue culture apparatus (right).

2. Harvesting of the materials to be used for antigen preparations (Fig. 1), and determination of their morphological, cultural, anatomical, and biochemical identity and purity by microscopic, cytological, cultural, and biochemical tests.

3. Separation of particulate and nonparticulate matter by physico-chemical method.

4. Purification of particulate and nonparticulate antigens, and determination of physicochemical and serological homogeneity of the purified materials.

5. Determination of the qualitative and quantitative chemical composition of the preparations.

6. Determination of the range of the immunological activity and specificity of the antigen preparations.

7. Statistical computation-analysis of data.

Data obtained from various experiments and research projects, notes on observations performed during the investigations, ideas formed, and bibliographic notes can be collected and stored most efficiently by means of punch card systems. Very convenient punch card systems or modern handling of data has been designed by Harris (1961), and a detailed information may be obtained by consulting this paper.

The immunochemical analysis is performed by the following successive steps.

1. Physicochemical screening and identification of categories of polymers present in an antigen source.
2. Separation and purification of different classes of polymers.
3. Determination of the physicochemical homogeneity of the purified polymers.
4. Qualitative chemical determination of the polymers.
5. Quantitative chemical analysis of the polymers.
6. Examination of the immunological activity and specificity of polymers.

Approximately 1 g of dry weight of the material is required for a thorough immunochemical analysis. The total mass is usually divided into two portions, one of which is lyophilized, whereas the other portion is dried to the constant weight in a vacuum oven at $70°$ for 4 to 6 hours or at $45°$ for 1 to 2 days if the sample is to be saved. Quicker drying is attained in the Aberhalden drying pistol, attached to a high vacuum pump. The lyophilized material is used for immunological studies, whereas the material dried *in vacuo* is suitable for chemical and physicochemical studies.

I. SOURCES OF ANTIGENS

Antigen preparations employed in various immunological tests have either a particulate or a nonparticulate form, are insoluble or soluble, crude or purified. Particulate antigen preparations are represented by bacteria, rickettsiae, microfungi, spores of bacteria and fungi, and different animal and plant cells. Cell walls, mycelial walls, cytoplasmic and spore membranes, mitochondria, and ribosomes also belong to the category of particulate antigens. Nonparticulate antigens occur in the form of crude or purified preparations, which are soluble or insoluble in water, ether, alcohol, or cholorform. The crude, nonparticulate antigen preparations, such as extracts from bacterial cells and from infected tissues and cells, culture filtrates, exudates, blood plasma, and spinal fluid contain a number of different antigens. Individual materials or fractions can be separated from these sources and purified by appropriate immunochemical procedures.

Preparations of microbial antigens are made from the microorganisms grown in a suitable culture medium or in animal tissues if the microorganism is not reproducible at present in any synthetic or semisynthetic culture medium. Microorganisms which do not grow in the artificial culture media should be cultivated in either body cavities or organs of susceptible animals or tissue cultures. The gross cultivation of microorganisms must be preceded by the determination of their morphological, biochemical, and biological activities (pathogenicity, virulence, or saprophytism) according to the conventional methods. Sources for animal or plant antigens are provided by individual organs, tissues, cells, or secretions obtained by biopsy or autopsy of animals or by the dissection of plants.

The composition of a suitable culture medium for the growth of microorganisms depends largely on the metabolic requirements of the species under investigation. The culture medium should contain only the vitally indispensable ingredients, and it must be free from polymerized, nondialyzable substances which might stimulate antibody formation in animals. The vast majority of bacteria and microfungi can be cultivated in Kwapinski's et al. (1965, 1969, 1970, 1971) semisynthetic or synthetic culture media (Table 2). Kwapinski's (1965) synthetic culture media have the following composition:

Medium I: 4.0 g sodium chloride, 5.0 g sodium biphosphate 12 H_2O, 0.005 g zinc sulfate, 5.0 g asparagine, 2.5 mg histidine, 2.5 mg leucine, 2.5 mg proline, 10.0 mg alanine, 10.0 mg glycine, and 10 mg tryptophan, distilled water 985 ml.

Table 2. Compositions of Kwapinski's Semisynthetic Culture Media

Kwapinski's Actinomyces Medium	KAM	KPM	KNM	KSM
Casamino acids	5.0[a]	5.0	3.0	3.0
Asparagine				2.5
Sodium pyruvate	1.0	1.0	1.0	1.0
Magnesium citrate		0.1	0.1	0.1
K_2HPO	1.5	1.5	1.0	1.0
NaH_2PO_4				.05
L(+) cysteine hydrochloride	0.5	0.5		
Thioglycollate		1.0		
Distilled water	900	985	900	890

Autoclave at 121° for 15 minutes, adjust to pH 6.8–7.1 and add the following solution, sterilized by membrane filtration:

	KAM	KPM	KNM	KSM
Dextrose	5.0	5.0	10.0	
Maltose	3.0			
Lactose	2.0			
Mannitol				1.0
Inositol			1.0	
Sorbitol				1.0
Fructose		1.0		
Raffinose		1.0		
Distilled water	100	985	100	100

[a] Quantities expressed in grams.

Medium II: 0.25% arabinose, 0.25% xylose, 1% galactose, 2% glucose, 0.5% mannose, 0.25% rhamnose, 0.5% asparagine, and 0.2% ammonium chloride, dissolved in a 0.1 M, pH 6.5, phosphate buffer.

Medium II is especially suitable for culturing fungi and higher bacteria. These culture media are adjusted to the optimal pH for an individual species, and they can be enriched by increasing the concentrations of sugars or amino acids, or by supplementing them with a specific growth factor, if required.

For fastidious bacteria, the Williams' (1955) culture medium modified by Mickelson (1964) is recommended (Table 3).

Slime and capsule formation is very satisfactory in Gaudy and Wolfe's (1962) medium which consists of 0.5% glucose, 0.02% $MgSO_4 \cdot 7H_2O$, 0.005% $CaCl_2$, and 0.001% $FeCl \cdot 6H_2O$ made in a potassium phosphate buffer, pH 7.1, added to a final concentration of 0.01 M.

Spore production is attained by cultivating spore-forming bacteria on one of the following culture media: (a) the Stewart and Halvorson's (1953) medium consisting of 1.0 g K_2HPO_4, 4.0 g $(NH_4)_2SO_4$, 2.0 g yeast extract, 0.1 g $MnSO_4 \cdot H_2O$, 0.8 g $MgSO_4 \cdot 7H_2O$, 10 mg $ZnSO_4 \cdot 7H_2O$, 10 mg $CuSO_4 \cdot 5H_2O$, 100 mg $CaCl_2$, 1 mg $FeSO_4$, 4.0 g glucose, and 20.0 g agar per liter of distilled water; (b) Halvorson's (1957) medium which contains 5 g Trypticase, 5 g yeast extract, 5 g sodium chloride, and 20 g agar per 1000 ml of water. The agar plates should be incubated at 28 to 35° for 4 to 7 days, until at least 95% of the cells have produced spores. The remaining vegetative cells can be autolyzed by leaving the plate at 4° for 24 hours, preferably in the presence of Merthiolate (Thiomersal) (Walker et al., 1961). Alternatively, spores may be purified either by the use of a bacteriolytic agent present in the cultures of *Bacillus cereus* (Norris, 1957) or by lysozyme (Walker, 1959).

For cultivation of fungi, Mayer's sporulation medium, as modified by Kwapinski (1965), is recommended. This medium contains per 1 liter of distilled water: 165.0 g glucose, 2.0 g asparagine, 0.05 g magnesium sulfate, 0.06 g potassium phosphate (KH_2PO_4), 0.5 g potassium nitrate, 0.02 g sodium potassium titrate, 0.02 g ferric citrate, and 0.25 g agar. An alternative medium (Salvin, 1969) has the following composition:

L-Asparagine	7.0 g
Ammonium chloride	7.0 g
Dipotassium phosphate	1.31 g
Sodium citrate $\cdot 5\frac{1}{2}H_2O$	0.9 g
Magnesium sulfate	1.5 g
Ferric citrate	0.3 g
Dextrose	10.0 g
Glycerin	25.0 g
Water to make	1000.0 ml

Table 3. Composition of the Modified Williams' Medium (Mickelson, 1964)

L-Alanine	0.1[a]
L-Arginine	0.1
L-Asparagine	0.1
L-Aspartic acid	0.1
L-Cysteine HCl	0.05
L-Cystine	0.05
L-Glutamic acid	0.5
Glycine	0.2
L-Histidine HCl	0.2
L-Hydroxyproline	0.1
L-Isoleucine	0.1
L-Leucine	0.1
L-Lysine HCl	0.1
L-Methionine	0.1
L-Norleucine	0.1
L-Phenylalanine	0.1
L-Proline	0.1
L-Serine	0.1
L-Threonine	0.1
L-Tryptophan	0.1
L-Tyrosine	0.1
L-Valine	0.1
L-Glutamine	0.05
Adenine	0.01
Guanine	0.01
Uracil	0.01
Folic acid	0.005
Biotin	0.0025
p-Aminobenzoic acid	0.1
Thiamine	0.5
Riboflavine	0.5
Pyridoxal·HCl	1.0
Pyridoxamine	1.0
Ca-pentothenate	0.5
Niacin	1.0
K_2HPO_4	0.5
KH_2PO_4	0.5
Na_2HPO_4	—
$MgSO_4 \cdot 7H_2O$	0.2
$FeSO_4 \cdot 7H_2O$	0.01
$MnSO_4 \cdot 4H_2O$	0.01
$ZnSO_4 \cdot 7H_2O$	—
NaCl	0.01
$Na(C_2H_2O_2)_2 \cdot 3H_2O$	10.0
$NH_4C_2H_2O_2$	0.1
Glucose	10.0
pH	7.0

[a] Quantities expressed in grams.

Protozoa, cultivable outside animal cells and tissues, such as amoebae, may be grown in Phillips' (1950), Miller's (1953), or Stoll's (1957) medium. It is recommended to adapt the amoebae to monobacterial cultures of *Aerobacter aerogenes* or to another species of nonpathogenic bacteria. Phillips' (1950) medium is composed of sodium thioglycollate, horse serum, and a suspension of *Trypanosoma* or a suitable bacterium culture, for example, *Aerobacter aerogenes*. The amoebae can also be grown in a medium containing a suspension of penicillin-inhibited *Streptobacillus* in a liquid thioglycollate serum medium. Rich cultures of amoebae are produced in 48 hours and are transplanted into a new batch of the medium.

Microcultures of the amoebae are initiated from single trophozoites, washed free from components of the medium in a sterile Locke's solution, and transferred by microisolation to microtubes containing the medium above, enriched with dead or live trypanosomas. The amoebae grow equally well in the presence of live and dead trypanosomas. The trypanosomas are killed by the exposure to the temperature of 46° for 1 hour and 15 minutes in a water bath before being added to the other components of a culture medium. The advantage of utilizing trypanosomas for complete media for growing amoeba is that trypanosoma may be inactivated at temperatures only a little higher than 37°, unlike the bacteria which require a much higher temperature. Therefore, there is no deleterious effect on proteins and enzyme systems which is caused by higher temperatures.

Microorganisms uncultivable outside living tissues or cells are propagated in either the cells of tissue cultures, allantoic and amnion fluids, yolk sac of hen or duck embryos, or the peritoneal or pleural cavities, *humor vitreous*, spinal fluid, or organs of susceptible animals.

The most adequate procedure for mass propagation of viruses is the suspended (Spinner) cell-culture technique (Fig. 2). Dispersion of the tissue cells is best attained in a continuous automatic trypsinizing flask (Rappaport, 1956). Alternatively, a simplified technique of an overnight extraction by Bodian (1956) may be followed. Tissue cells dispersed by prewarmed trypsin (alternatively, by the chelating action of sodium versenate) are harvested by centrifugation at $100 \times g$ for 30 minutes. The cell sediment should be washed several times in a phosphate-buffered saline, resuspended in a synthetic medium, filtered through a layer of cheese cloth, and diluted to 350,000 cells/ml of a growth medium. Rappaport's (1956) or Waymouth's (1959) synthetic TC-media are recommended (Tables 4 and 5), although the No. 199 (Morgan et al., 1950) and Eagle's (1955) media are also satisfactory.

Table 4. Rappaport's Tissue Culture Media

Contents per Liter of Tris(Hydroxymethyl Aminomethane) Buffer,
8×10^{-3} M, at pH 7.6

NaCl	8.0[a]	$ZnSO_4$	3.0[b]
KCl	0.4	$Fe(NO_3)_3$	2.0
$MgSO_4 \cdot 7H_2O$	0.1	$CoCl_2$	0.2
$MgCl_2 \cdot 6H_2O$	0.1	$MnCl_2$	0.5
Na_2HPO_4	0.08	$CuSO_4$	0.4
NaH_2PO_4	0.02	*l*-Histidine·HCl	10.0
$CaCl_2$	0.42	*l*-Arginine·HCl	7.0
$NaHCO_3$	0.78	*l*-Lysine·HCl	8.0
Glucose	20.0[b]	*l*-Methionine	6.0
l-Cysteine·HCl	30.0	*l*-Threonine	14.0
l-Isoleucine	60.0		
d-Ribose	30.0		

[a] Quantities measured in grams.

[b] Quantities measured in milligrams.

Table 5. Selected Tissue-Culture Media
(Concentrations in Milligrams per Liter)

Medium	Morgan, Morton, Parker, 1950	Eagle, 1955	Waymouth, 1959
Amino acids			
L-Alanine	50	—	—
L-Arginine HCl	70	105	75
L-Aspartic	60	—	60
L-Cysteine HCl	0.1	—	90
L-Cystine	20	24	15
L-Glutamic acid	150	—	150
L-Glutamine	100	292	350
Glycine	50	—	50
L-Histidine HCl	20	31	150
L-Hydroxyproline	10	—	—
L-Isoleucine	40	52	25
L-Leucine	120	52	50
L-Lysine HCl	70	58	240
L-Methionine	30	15	50
L-Phenylalanine	50	32	50
L-Proline	40	—	50
L-Serine	50	—	—
L-Threonine	60	48	75
L-Tryptophan	20	10	40
L-Tyrosine	40	36	40
L-Valine	50	46	65

(*Continued*)

Table 5—(Continued)

Medium	Morgan, Morton, Parker, 1950	Eagle, 1955	Waymouth, 1959
Vitamins			
Ascorbic acid	0.05	—	17.5
Biotin	0.01	1.0	0.02
Calciferol	0.1	—	—
Calcium pantothenate	0.01	1.0	1.0
Choline chloride	0.50	1.0	250
Folic acid	0.01	1.0	0.4
i-Inositol	0.05	2.0	1.0
Menadione	0.01	—	—
Niacinamide	0.025	1.0	1.0
Nicotinic acid	0.025	1.0	—
p-Aminobenzoate	0.05	—	—
Pyridoxal HCl	0.025	1.0	—
Pyridoxine HCl	0.025	—	1.0
Riboflavin	0.01	0.1	1.0
Thiamine HCl	0.01	1.0	1.0
α-Tocopherol phosphate	0.01	—	—
Vitamin A	0.1	—	—
Vitamin B_{12}	—	—	0.2
Coenzymes			
Adenosine triphosphate	10	—	—
Nucleic acid derivatives			
Adenine	10	—	—
Guanine HCl	0.3	—	—
Hypoxanthine	0.3	—	25
Thymine	0.3	—	—
Uracil	0.3	—	—
Xanthine	0.3	—	—
Miscellaneous			
Cholesterol	0.2	—	—
Deoxyribose	0.5	—	—
Glucose	1000	1000	5000
Glutathione	0.05	—	15
Oleic acid	5.0	—	—
Ribose	0.5	—	—
Sodium Acetate	50	—	—
Antibiotics	+	+	+
Balanced salt solution	+	+	+
Trace elements	+	+	+

II. HARVESTING OF MATERIALS FOR ANTIGEN PREPARATION

Microorganisms grown in a culture medium, as well as blood cells may be harvested easily by centrifugation of the cell suspensions at low speed, followed by thorough washing of deposited cells, with the centrifugation at about $1000 \times g$.*

Microorganisms propagated in body cavities are collected by aspirating the exudates and passing them through bacterial candles or 0.47-μ porosity filters, which allow the bacteria and viruses, but not the host cells, to pass. The same procedure is applied to the infected allantoic or amnion fluid, vitreous humor, and spinal fluid. Samples of noninfected tissues, *humor vitreous,* the artificially induced peritoneal and pleural exudates, or the pulp of organs must be collected as control material.

Infected tissue cultures or animal organs are suspended in buffered saline and disintegrated with fine glass beads in an electric high-speed homogenizer, or by a short 2 to 3 minute sonication at 9 kHz. The microorganisms are separated from the debris of animal cells by fractional centrifugation, filtration through membranes of graduated porosity, according to the size of particular microorganisms, or by absorption on resins with subsequent elution.

Soluble antigens released from the microorganisms during the cultivation and separated by filtration or centrifugation of the culture fluids; pleural and peritoneal exudates or spinal fluid can be concentrated by one of the concentration methods presented on pp. 223 and 224.

Bacteria, rickettsiae, and viruses that cannot be propagated in any artificial culture medium but only in the living host or tissue cultures can be separated from the host material by differential centrifugation, membrane and gel filtration, filtration, electrophoresis, or a selective absorption. Antigens that have been liberated from the microorganisms or dissipated in the host tissues can be recovered only by direct extraction of infected tissues, followed by a selective absorption, column filtration, electrophoresis, electrofocusing, or density-gradient centrifugation (see pp. 99-130). Alternatively, the bacterial antigens present in the host tissues can be detected and studied by immunohisto-chemical methods.

* The acceleration imparted by a centrifuge ($\times g$) is calculated from the formulas:

$$\times g = \frac{0.0109 \cdot r \cdot n^2}{981} = 1.11 \times 10^{-5} \cdot r \cdot n^2$$

or

$$\text{R.C.F.} = \frac{4(3.1416)^2 r \, n^2}{32.2}$$

where r = radius (in feet), n = revolutions per second $\left(\dfrac{\text{rpm}}{60}\right)$

1. Harvesting of bacteria and fungi

Once the full growth of microorganisms is obtained, the identity and purity of cultures must be checked by subculturing samples of the cultures on solid media and incubating them in aerobic and anaerobic condition. Morphological characteristics and biochemical, immunological, and biological activities of the cultured strains should also be determined. Microorganisms are then separated from the culture fluid by the centrifugation at 10,000 $\times$ g for 10 minutes, or by filtration through a 0.47-μ porosity membrane, or a Schott G4 or G5 glass pad. The sedimented cells or those collected on the filter are washed with saline solution or with distilled water. Cells to be fractionated by immunochemical methods must be rinsed repeatedly until no protein, nucleic acid or sugar is detected in the washings when examined at 280- and 254-nm wavelength, or when tested with Millon-, Molisch-, or Korson-reagent.

Constituents of microbial L cultures can be partitioned by means of a differential centrifugation (Weibull and Beckman, 1961).

Bacterial spores are cleansed in the manner described by Walker et al. (1961). Spores are first washed seven or eight times with acidified distilled water, pH 2.0 to 2.5, and are then exposed to a 35% Dioxane solution for 5 minutes to remove residual vegetative matter. The spores are then washed three times with distilled water, treated with lysozyme (0.5 mg/ml spore suspension) at 37° for 30 minutes, and washed with alkaline distilled water, pH 10.5 to 11.0. Finally, the spores are washed in deionized distilled water and stored at 4°.

Separation of the hyphae from other anatomical constituents of certain fungi, for example, aspergilli, may be attained by growing them in the modified sporulation medium (p. 13). During a 2- to 4-day incubation at 25°, the hyphae detach from a thick pellicle, which contains conidia and conidiophores, and they can be collected in a pure form from the liquid phase (Kwapinski, 1965). The conidia may be washed off from the pellicle with an 0.01% solution of Tween 80.

2. Isolation of Bacteria from Hosts, Organs, and Fluids

Bacteria grown in, or released into, the host cavities or body fluids, such as the pleural and peritoneal cavities, vitreous humor, and spinal fluid, can be relatively easily separated from the host matter by means of differential centrifugation or filtration.

Isolation and purification of bacteria from tissues and cells is more difficult. Some microorganisms, for example, treponemas, may be released from organs by Magnuson et al. (1948) method. In this procedure, the organ is cut into fine pieces, ground in a mortar, and suspended in a buffer for 5 to 15 hours to eluate the microorganisms. The eluate is centrifuged at 150–200 $\times$g for 10 to 20 minutes to remove host cells, and the supernatant is recentrifuged at 3000–5000 × g for 50 to 60 minutes to concentrate the bacteria.

A refined technique, suitable for the isolation of bacteria from tissues and cells, has been designed by Kwapinski (1972). According to this method, the tissues are first immersed in 1.0% formalin overnight, and then are washed thoroughly in distilled water, cut to pieces (on an automatic tissue cutting machine, and homogenized in a high-speed electric mixer (Fig. 3) at 2°. The homogenate is suspended in distilled water and dialyzed against distilled water until all formalin has been removed. The dialyzed material is suspended in 4 volumes of an 0.01 M, pH 7.4 Tris-phosphate buffer and sonicated at 9 kHz for 10 minutes or at 20 kHz for 3 minutes. The suspension of disrupted tissues and cells is adjusted to pH 7.2 with the aid of a pH meter (Fig. 4) and exposed at 37° to hyaluronidase (3 units/ml) for 2 hours. The mixture is then adjusted to pH 7.8–8.3 and digested with trypsin (1 mg/ml) at 37° for 3 hours, on a shaking water bath.

After the trypsinization, the tissue suspension is adjusted to pH 6.0, and the mixture is diluted with distilled water (1:4) and homogenized on a high-speed omnimixer for 2 minutes.

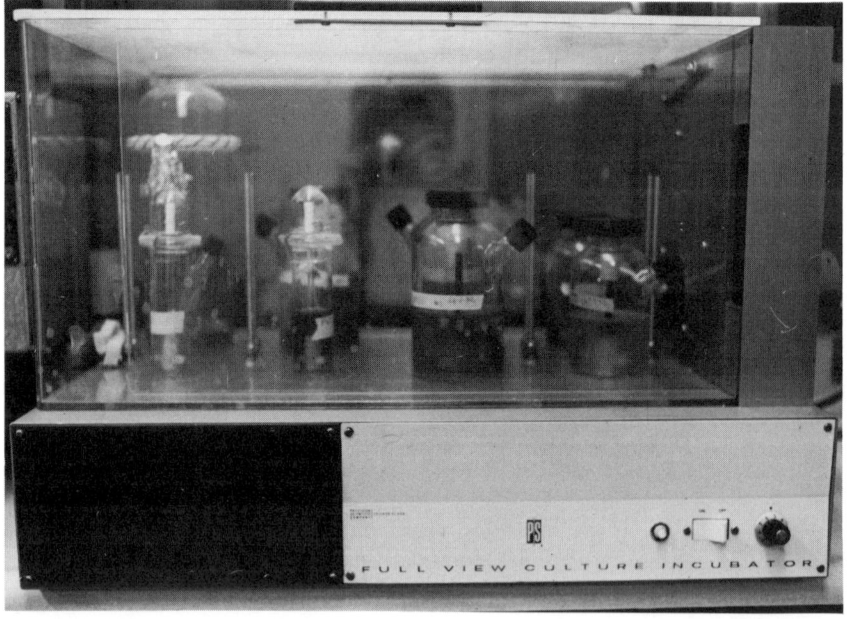

Figure 2.   Replication of viruses in suspended cell cultures, incubated in a CO_2-incubator.

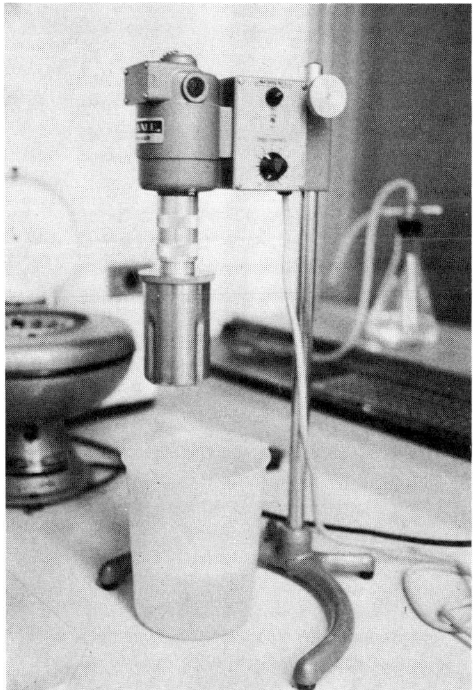

Figure 3. A high-speed electric homogenizer, used to disrupt tissues and homogenize cells and bacteria. The material to be homogenized is placed in the steel chamber equipped with a stirrer and kept on ice for the homogenization period.

The bacteria are recovered and purified by two or three series of centrifugation in a sucrose gradient, consisting of 20:10:5% (12:9:5 ml) or 30:10:5% (7:5:5 ml) of sucrose. The tissue homogenates (3–4 ml) is layered over the upper, 5% sucrose layer. The gradient is centrifuged at 6000–7000 $\times$ g for 1 hour. During this time, one or two bands are formed on the gradient interphases, whereas the bacteria-free tissue is sedimented (Fig. 5). The interphase band(s) contain bacteria, which are further purified by a repeated gradient of the same type, or in a sucrose gradient consisting of 30, 20, and 10% sucrose (5:5:5 ml). Additional purification of the bacteria is obtained by the continuous particle electrophoresis, electrofocusing or polyacrylamide-gel electrophoresis.

3. Harvesting of Cultivable Protozoa

Protozoa may be separated from the bacteria and culture medium by the centrifugation at 177 $\times$ g for 5 minutes, followed by repeated washing of the deposited protozoa with saline and recentrifugation. To release the

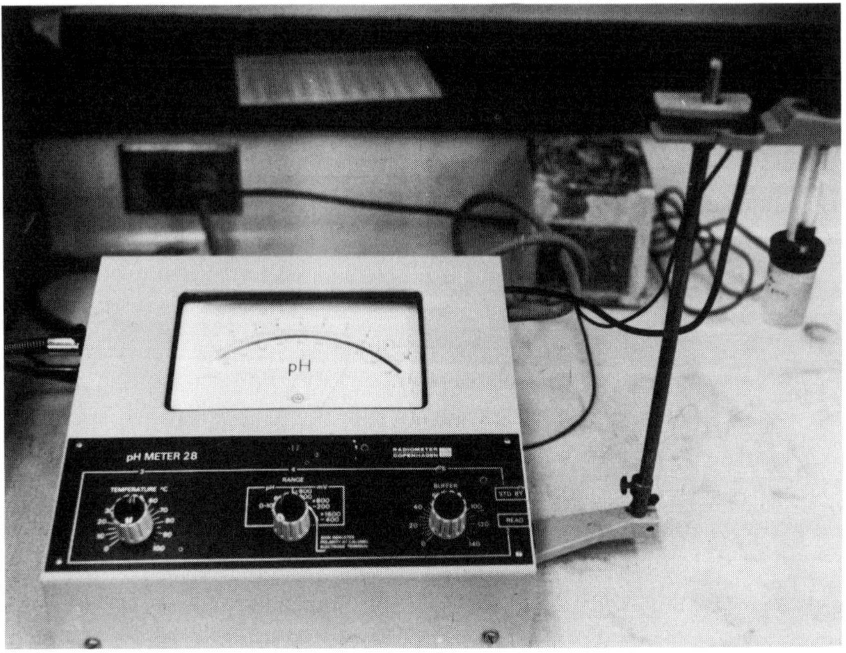

Figure 4. Automatic pH meter.

inner content of amoebae, the amoebae are suspended in chilled, distilled water and ruptured by vigorous passage through a 20-gauge needle. The mixture is left at 4° overnight and then the mixture is adjusted to isotonicity by adding 1.7% soduim chloride, and is clarified by high-speed centrifugation in the cold.

The protozoa grown in the peritoneal cavity of sensitive animals may be harvested according to Fulton and Spooner's (1957) method. The exudates, formed in the peritoneal cavity in response to the infection with protozoa, are collected by means of a syringe and filtered through cotton wool to remove debris. The filtrate is centrifuged at 2000 × g for 15 minutes. The supernatant is discarded, and the sediment containing protozoa and white cells is resuspended in 0.2% glucose dissolved in a mixture of 1 part horse serum and 9 parts of phosphate-buffered saline, pH 7.4. The protozoa are freed from white blood cells by shaking the mixture with glass beads for 5 minutes. Intact white blood cells are removed by passing the suspension through a sintered glass filter with a porosity of 15 to 40 μ. Residual erythrocytes are removed by the addition of specific agglutinins. The protozoa are collected with the filtrate and are killed with formaldehyde added to the 1% final concentration, and left at room temperature for 24 hours.

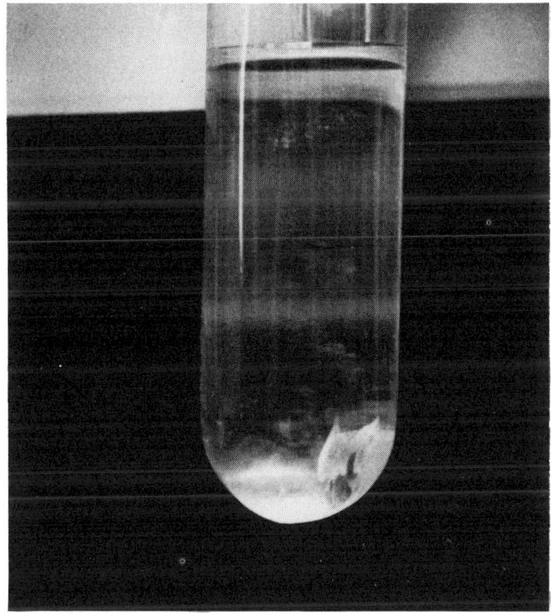

Figure 5. Different density bands formed on the gradient interphase, containing bacteria in the upper band and disrupted mammalian cells in the lower band.

The organisms are then centrifuged and resuspended in saline and adjusted to a desired optical density.

4. Harvesting of Blood Cells

According to Amos and Peacocke's (1963) method, a sample of blood is mixed with 5% polyvinyl pyrrolidine and sodium ethylene diaminotetra-acetic acid (EDTA), 10:2:1, held in a silicone treated test tube. The mixture is allowed to stand at room temperature for 30 minutes. The pink plasma containing leukocytes, platelets, and many erythrocytes is collected and centrifuged at $100 \times g$ for 10 minutes. The supernatant containing platelets is pipetted off, whereas the sediment containing leukocytes and erythrocytes is resuspended in 0.1 ml of the original supernatant fluid. The suspension is allowed to stand at room temperature until erythrocytes have formed rouleaux and have settled. The leukocyte-rich supernatant fluid is collected, whereas the erythrocytes may be recovered from the deposit. The supernatant is layered on 0.2 ml of the platelet-free plasma, which may be obtained by the centrifugation of the platelet containing supernatant fluid at $4000 \times g$ for 10 minutes. The leukocytes are spun down to the plasma at $100 \times g$ for 1 minute whereas the platelets remain in suspension.

Cells may be enumerated accurately by the aid of an electronic cell counter and pulse-height analyser (Miller and Phillips, 1969). Viability of cells can be determined by the measurement of the uptake of fluorescein diacetate according to Rotman and Papermaster's (1966) technique. Cell density is measured most conveniently in a microhematocrit by comparison to the density of a mixture of dimethyl- and di-*n*-butyl phthalate, as described by Danon and Markovsky (1964).

5. *Isolation and Preparation of Rickettsial Antigens*

Rickettsiae grown in cells of the chorioallantoic or amniotic membrane and in the tissue cultures of infected embryos and released into the fluids or the tissue culture medium can relatively easily be separated and isolated by employing four cycles of high- and low-speed differential centrifugation at $0°$ (Colon and Moulder, 1960). In each cycle, the microorganisms are sedimented at $5000 \times g$ for 30 minutes, resuspended in 0.1 *M*, pH 7.4, phosphate buffer, and clarified at $8000 \times g$ for 10 minutes. The low-speed pellet is discarded each time. The number of rickettsiae present in the final material can be determined by Sharp's (1959) sedimentation method, as modified by Litwin (1959).

To release the rickettsiae from cells, the cells are suspended in distilled water, a formolized $M/1$ KCl solution or in 0.15 *M* phosphate buffer, pH 7.4, diluted 1:1 with saline, or in 0.0004 *M* phosphate-citrate buffer, pH 7.4, and homogenized in an electric homogenizer or disrupted in an ultrasonic generator at 40 kHz. Rickettsiae are then separated from the host cell debris by differential centrifugation at $800 \times g$ and $23,000 \times g$ for 30 to 60 minutes.

Other techniques for the isolation of the rickettsiae from crude preparations and concentrations employ absorption on Celite (Wissemann et al., 1951), column chromatography, density gradient fractionation (Ribi and Hoyer, 1960), continuous-flow centrifugation at a flow rate of 150 ml/hour, (Ormsbee, 1962), and continuous particle electrophoresis. The differential centrifugation is conducted in 1 *M* KCl and can be followed by centrifugation in a linear glycerin density gradient. Alternatively, the differential centrifugation in 1 *M* KCl may be followed by several washes with decreasing concentrations of KCl and finally with water (Anacker et al., 1962). Differential centrifugation can be preceded by precipitation, following which the supernatant is centrifuged at 30,000 rpm for 1 hour. The absorption procedure, as described by Colter et al. (1956), employs 1 g of washed Celite for every 6 g of the yolk sac culture. This mixture is homogenized and centrifuged immediately at $100–150 \times g$ for 30 minutes. The supernatant is then removed and recentrifuged at $2000–3000 \times g$ for 45 minutes. The pellet is resuspended in the medium of Bovarnick et al. (1950), and the cycle of differential centrifugation with Celite is repeated. The sediment of this partially purified suspension of rickettsiae is resuspended in $M/50$ potassium phosphate buffer, pH 7.2, layered over 2 volumes of 8% KCl, and centrifuged for 1 hour at 3000 × g. The last part of the procedure should be repeated.

Purification of rickettsiae by density-gradient sedimentation (Ribi and Hoyer, 1960) is conducted by means of a centrifugation linear density-gradient centrifugation. Use 40% sucrose in $M/1$ KCl and 40% glycerin solution in distilled water to prepare a blue gradient. This suspension made from washed rickettsiae is then carefully layered over the gradient and centrifuged 90 minutes at 1600 × g at 20°. After centrifugation, the rickettsiae are found in the central turbid band. This layer can be collected selectively with a syringe fitted with a 14-gauge cannula.

For a further purification, the separated layer is diluted with about 30 ml of $M/1$ KCl and centrifuged 15 minutes at 15,000 × g. One turbid band now appears at a similar position as before.

With larger volumes of a suspension of rickettsiae, a larger, for example, 250-ml volume, gradient is used, and the centrifugation at 1200 × g is prolonged to 4 hours.

Cell walls that surround the protoplasm in the rickettsiae can be obtained by rupturing the purified rickettsiae and placing the material on the glycerin or sucrose gradient. The cell walls are found in the upper band. According to the method of Schaechter et al. (1957), purified rickettsiae are frozen and thawed twice, then suspended in an aqueous solution of 1% sodium desoxycholate at pH 7.0 and incubated at 45° under constant agitation for 4 hours. The suspensions should then be centrifuged at 24,000 × g for 30 minutes and the sediment washed three times with distilled water. The purified cell walls of rickettsiae occur as translucent, slightly shruken structures of ovoid shape. They consist of twelve amino acids, polysaccharides, and small amounts of ribonucleic acid.

Soluble antigens of rickettsiae can be obtained by the technique described by Colter et al. (1956), in which the rickettsiae are subjected to ultrasonic vibrations at a frequency of 287,000 Hz, for a total period of 10 minutes at 0°. The disintegrated organisms are then centrifuged at 8000 and 12,000 rpm at 0° for 1 hour to obtain different antigen fractions. The supernatant fluid is passed through a sterilizing Seitz pad or a 0.45-μ porosity membrane yielding in the filtrate a partially purified preparation of rickettsial antigens.

6. Isolation and Preparation of Virus Antigens

Tissue cells infected with viruses are first harvested together with the liquid medium, rapidly frozen and thawed several times, and centrifuged at about $400 \times g$ for 10 minutes to remove cellular debris. This is followed by the ultracentrifugation at $40,000 \times g$ for 1 hour at 4° (Fig. 6).

Virus particles can be freed from components of host tissues by such methods as the differential gradient centrifugation, ultrafiltration, continuous particle electrophoresis, column chromatography with selective adsorption on the aluminum-phosphate, calcium-phosphate gel, DEAE cellulose, diatomaceous silica (Celite), Sephadex G-150 and G-200, agarose, or acrylamide gel columns. Plant viruses are harvested from the diseased parts and homogenized at 3° in 0.5-M boric acid buffer, pH 7.5, containing 0.1% thioglycollic acid. Approximately 1.5 ml of buffer is used per 1.0 g of plant tissue.

Owing to the low mobility of virus particles in an electrical field, they can be easily separated from the descending limb of the Tiselius cell upon the completion of electrophoresis (Schwerdt and Schaffer, 1956). The electrophoresis is run in an $M/15$ buffer, pH 7, with a field strength of 4.5 to 4.8 V/cm, at 0° for 5 hours. Electrophoresis, the density gradient, and ultracentrifugation are the most efficient purification methods for viruses, although adsorption-elution techniques are sometimes effective.

The density gradient fractionation, according to Schwerdt and Schaffer (1956), is carried out as follows: 0.7 ml volumes of 45, 37, 29, 20, and 11% sucrose solutions made in 0.14 M NaCl are introduced in that order

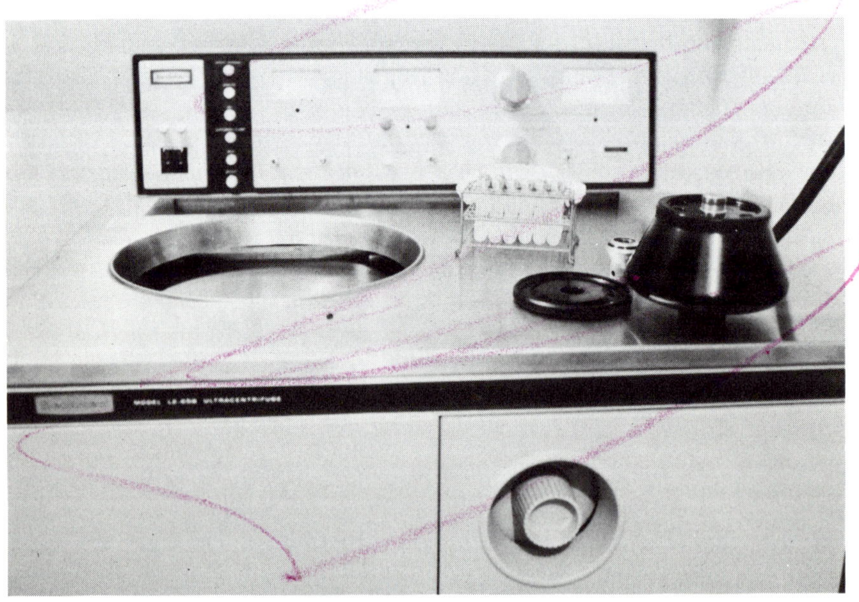

Figure 6.   The preparative ultracentrifuge.

into a 5-ml Lusteroid tube. After standing overnight at 0.5° to obtain a continuous gradient, 0.5 ml of a virus preparation isolated in the Tiselius apparatus is layered on the surface of each of three sucrose density gradients prepared in that manner. These are then centrifuged in a Spinco Model L centrifuge with the swinging cup rotor (SW 39) at 70,000 × *g* until the various components are resolved, which usually occurs in 2 hours. Individual fractions are removed using a syringe and hypodermic needle. Withdrawal of individual zones is facilitated by the use of perforated Perspex discs clamped by a central stainless steel rod and placed in the centrifuge tube. Sucrose can be removed from virus particles by repeated washing in 0.004 *M* McIlvaine buffer (pH 7.8) with centrifugation at 35,000 × *g* for 30 minutes for each wash (Zwartouw et al., 1962).

Larger viruses, the chlamydiae, and the rickettsiae are contained within a rigid envelope or cell wall. The virus and chlamydial envelope, and cell walls of rickettsiae can be separated from the cytoplasmic material by the following procedure published by Schaechter et al. (1957) and adapted by Jenkin (1960): purified virus particles suspended in 0.01 *M*, pH 7.4, phosphate buffer containing 1% sodium deoxycholate are shaken for 4 hours at 45°, then cooled to 0°, and centrifuged at 8000 × *g* for 20 minutes. The sediment is washed three times in distilled water, yielding the final preparation of envelopes.

The complement-fixing virus antigens can be concentrated and purified by the following procedure of adsorption and elution (Suggs et al., 1961): the infected tissue culture is first dialyzed against 0.1 and 0.01 *M* Tris (hydroxy-methyl)-aminoethane buffer, pH 8.2. Washed DEAE cellulose is then added to the dialyzate at a concentration of 1.0 g for 0.1 g of protein. The mixture should be agitated for 1 to 2 hours at 4°, then filtered through a coarse sintered glass filter. The antigen adsorbed onto DEAE-cellulose is eluted by agitation for 1 hour with a 2-*M* NaCl Tris buffer, pH 8.2. The slurry should be passed through a coarse sintered glass filter. The filtrate-containing antigen is finally dialyzed overnight to remove most of the salt.

Concentration and Purification of Virus Particles by Gradient Resolubilization. Small viruses may be concentrated and purified by the technique of gradient resolubilization (Anderson, 1966) more efficiently than by a continuous flow centrifugation. In this technique, particles are flocculated in the cold with ethanol, ammonium sulfate, or by heavy metals. The suspension is then run through B-IX rotor which contains a positive density gradient and a negative gradient of the precipitating agent.

A very good purification and concentration of certain virus particles is attained by a single-tube isopycnic separation over cesium chloride density gradients (Anderson et al., 1966). Various viruses have been successfully purified by chromatography on strongly basic resins, such as Dowex 1 and Amberlight IRA-400 and on the anion exchanger Ecteola-cellulose. A very fine separation of different types of viruses have been obtained by the absorption chromatography on aluminum hydroxide (Woods and Robbins, 1961), calcium phosphate, counter-current distribution (Bengtsson and Philipson, 1963), and by zonal-rate gradient centrifugation.

A good separation and purification of viruses may be obtained on molecular sieve columns packed with agarose, agar, dextran, polyacrylamide, or porous glass particles.

The adsorbent used by Riley (1950) consists of 95% silicon dioxide suspension with a particle size 5 to 40 μ in diameter. Celite 501 or 503 is equally efficient. The adsorbent in the form of 10% aqueous suspension is introduced into 10×250 mm chromatographic tubes. The solvent consists of aqueous sodium chloride of varying molar concentration. A slight negative pressure is employed to regulate the flow, and the whole process of adsorption-elution is completed in 30 minutes. Some viruses, for example, influenza viruses, can be efficiently purified by absorption onto human erythrocytes, followed by elution with sterile physiological saline (Sheffield et al., 1954). A standardized method of bacteriophage concentration and purification in an aqueous polymer two-phase system was described by Frick (1960).

Virus particles can be disrupted with 1% sodium dodecyl sulfate. Crude viral antigens can be satsfactorily prepared by Barwell's (1952) or Rondle and Dumbell's (1962) techniques. In the Barwell method, partially purified viruses are extracted with 0.02 N hydrochloric acid at 37° for 20 minutes. The extract is neutralized, and the resulting precipitate is discarded. The supernatant contains a crude antigen preparation. In the technique by Rondle and Dumbell, infected membranes are harvested and suspended either in 0.004-M phosphate-citrate buffer, pH 7.4, or in 0.15-M phosphate buffer, pH 7.4, mixed with an equal volume of isotonic saline. The suspensions are shaken at 20° for 5 minutes, and left at 4° for 16 hours, then centrifuged at 500–700 $\times$ g for 10 minutes to remove debris of infected membranes. Extractions in a buffer can be repeated several times if required. All extracts are pooled and centrifuged at 6500 $\times$ g for 10 minutes to sediment virus particles. Antigenic fractions of viruses can be prepared by the method of Benedict and O'Brien (1956), as presented diagrammatically in Table 6, or by the method of Ross and Gogolak (1957). In the latter technique, viruses disrupted in the Raytheon magnetoconstriction oscillator for 3 hours at 5° and lyophilized are extracted three times with anhydrous ethyl ether at room temperature. The ether extract should be clarified by centrifugation and the pellet evaporated to dryness. The dried material may be subsequently extracted with acetone and methanol to obtain an acetone and a methanol-soluble fraction.

Table 6. Preparation of Virus Antigens by the Method of Benedict and O'Brien

Virus in $M/5$, pH 8, phosphate buffer
___

2.5% SLS[a] to 0.5% concentration
centrifugation at 35,000 × g

Supernatant	Pellet

5% BaCl₂, centrifuged at 500 −700 × g

Pellet	Supernatant

Centrifuged at 30,000 × g

Precipitate	Supernatant

Dissolved, centrifuged
at 20,000 × g

Supernatant
___

5% phenol,
centrifuged at 35,000 × g

Precipitate	Supernatant

Methanol, chloroform	Chiefly protein

| Residue | Lipid fraction |
| (insoluble) | |

[a] SLS = sodium lauryl sulfate. All centrifugations may be carried out for 30 minutes.

The ether-insoluble material is suspended in a small volume of distilled water and rehydrated for 18 hours at 5°. A normal NaOH solution is then added to give a final 20-N concentration, and this mixture is heated at 56° for 15 minutes, then partially neutralized with 0.5 ml of $N/2$ HCl. The mixture should now be centrifuged at 25,000 × g for 30 minutes at 5°. The sediment is extracted two more times with alkali and treated as described above; all extracts are pooled and dialyzed against distilled water for 3 days at 5°. The alkali-insoluble material is stored as a separate fraction. Fractions thus obtained contain either crude particulate antigens or crude soluble antigens. All antigen preparations can be preserved with 0.01% Merthiolate or Thiomersal (sodium ethyl mercurithiosalicylate) or 0.5% phenol, 0.1% sodium azide, or ethylene oxide. Soluble antigens can be sterilized, lipid and polysaccharide fractions, by heating, protein fractions, by filtration through an 0.45-μ porosity membrane filter, or through a Seitz or Berkefeld filter.

Preparation and Purification of Bacteriophage Antigens. Bacteriophages are propagated by inoculating a culture of sensitive microorganisms at the beginning of the logarithmic phase with a bacteriophage suspension. It is recommended to provide an input multiplicity of three phages per microbial cell (Romig, 1962). The cultures are incubated at a suitable temperature until the suspension becomes clear. At this time chloroform is added in a ratio of 1:50 and the mixture is stirred 15 minutes, and then allowed to settle out. The lyzate is decanted and clarified by centrifugation at 12,000–15,000 $\times$ g through a continuous flow device.

The bacteriophages are freed from bacterial products by digestion with the following enzymes: 0.01 μg/ml of deoxyribonuclease, 0.05 μg/ml of ribonuclease, and 0.2 μg/ml of egg white lysozyme. These enzymes are allowed to react for 2 to 3 hours at room temperature. The phages are then centrifuged at 45,000–55,000 $\times$ g for 45 minutes and resuspended in a $\mu/15$, pH 7.0, phosphate buffer containing 1 g of sodium citrate $\cdot$ 2H$_2$O and 0.2 g of MgSO$_4$ $\cdot$ 7H$_2$O per liter. They can be washed in this buffer and recentrifuged several times if required. Protein- and nucleic acid-antigens may be obtained from bacteriophages by Kwapinski's (1969) method.

7. Recovery of Soluble Microbial and Tissue Antigens from Host

Antigens released from microorganisms in host tissues, as a result of an autolysis, or lysis by host enzymes, can either remain free or be bound by certain tissue components to form autoantigens.

Autoantigens can be regarded as complex tissue components of a host which are able to react specifically with some globulins of its blood serum. An autoimmune state emerges from a biological association of microbial antigens and hereditary factors in the host tissues which are responsible for the occurrence of "forbidden clones" of the immunologically competent lymphocytic and plasma cells (Burnet, 1961). These clones are resistant to the immunological homeostatic control and give rise to a variety of sub-clones and specific reactivities. Their multiplication is stimulated by contact with the host tissue, giving rise to an increased concentration of the immunologically competent cells or antibodies which are responsible for pathological changes and symptoms of autoimmune diseases.

Soluble microbial antigens, autoantigens, or tissue antigens can be extracted by the procedures designed by Watson et al. (1947), Larson (1957), or Kwapinski (1965, 1972).

In Larson's method, infected tissues are ground with sterile sand and suspended in three to five volumes of 0.85% solution of sodium chloride, then mixed with two volumes of cold ether, and agitated overnight at 37°. The aqueous phase should be separated from the etheric extract and centrifuged at 2000 to 3000 $\times$ g for 30 minutes. The clear supernatant represents a crude antigen solution.

Kwapinski's method for the extraction of autoantigens and bacterial antigens from the host tissue is diagrammatically presented in Tables 7 and

8. It is recommended that the autoantigen preparations be absorbed with the antisera versus fractions isolated from the noninfected tissues to remove "normal" tissue antigens.

Table 7. Flow-Diagram of Chemical Preparation of Autoantigens and Antigens of Bacteria (Kwapinski, 1965)

Disintegrated cells
____

0.5 N ammonium hydroxide
Extract
____

5% TCA

| Precipitate (chiefly protein) | Supernatant (chiefly polysaccharide) |

1 Na acetate, pH 6.5

| Precipitate | Extract |

5% TCA

| Precipitate | Supernatant |

| 0.1 M NaOH Centrifugation Extract | Acetone/alcohol 3:1 Precipitate |

| 5% TCA | 2% TCA 100° 2 minutes |

| Precipitate | Extract |

| Dialysis lyophilization Fraction N | Dialysis lyophilization Fraction P |

| (nucleo) protein | (polysaccharide) |

Chemical Fractionation of Tissue Extracts. According to Watson's et al. technique (1947), tissues are first frozen and then partially thawed and minced, and extracted with 0.85% saline at 5° for 24 hours, with frequent agitation. The extract is filtered through a filter, adjusted to pH 7.0, using a 1 M phosphate buffer, and added to a volume of 1 M calcium chloride, pH 9.7, in the ratio of 100 ml of extract per 1.2 ml of the calcium chloride solution. The mixture is maintained at pH 7.0 for 2 to $2\frac{1}{2}$ hours in the refrigerator. The resulting precipitate is removed by centrifugation. The supernatant should be retreated with 1 M calcium chloride, as above. Both precipitates thus obtained are washed with 0.05 M phosphate buffer at pH 7.0, pooled, suspended in 1.0 M citrate buffer at pH 6.0, and dialyzed against 0.1 M citrate buffer, pH 6.0, until the precipitate dissolves completely, and then against distilled water, and lyophilized.

Table 8. Recovery and Fractionation of Particulate and Nonparticulate Antigens from Infected Tissues (Kwapinski, 1972)

Tissue

Cut to pieces, suspended in **HBSS*** (1:15, homogenized). Adjust to pH 7.2. Add hyaluronidase (3.0 units/ml), 37° for 1 hour.

Digestate

Sonicate 10 minutes. Centrifuge 15 minutes at 6000 $\times$ g.

Supernatant

Filtration at 0.45-μ. porosity.

Sediment (cell debris)

Suspend in **HBSS**, pH 7.2. Disruption in French press. Centrifuge 15 minutes at 6000 $\times$ g

Filtrate

Ultracentrifugation 107,000 $\times$ g for 1 hour

Supernatant

Recentrifuge 15 minutes at 25,000 $\times$ g.

Pellet / **Supernatant**

Sediment / **Sediment**

Supernatant (subviral)

Combined sediment

Resuspend in **HBSS** (1 ml/g). Centrifuge 5 minutes at 3000 $\times$ g.

Continuous particle electrophoresis or ultrafiltration.

Wash in **PBS**, 3$\times$; centrifuge at 5000 $\times$ g for 15 minutes.

Supernatant (particulate matter) / **Sediment** (discarded)

Fractions with different electric charge or molecular size.

Washed sediment

Dialyse at 4° against water. Concentrate partly by lyophilization

Separation and purification by: electro-focusing, acrylamide-electrophoresis, or Sephadex-gel filtration.

Concentrate particulate matter

Examine in electron microscope. Purify by differential sucrose gradient at 37,000 $\times$ g for 12 hours.

Suspend in 3 volumes of 1 M KCl, homogenize for 5 minutes in a high-speed stirrer. Add 3 volumes of distilled water. Centrifuge at 10,000 $\times$ g for 30 minutes.

Collect bands (layers)

Sediment (cell debris)

Interphase (nucleic acid)

Upper layer (phospholipids)

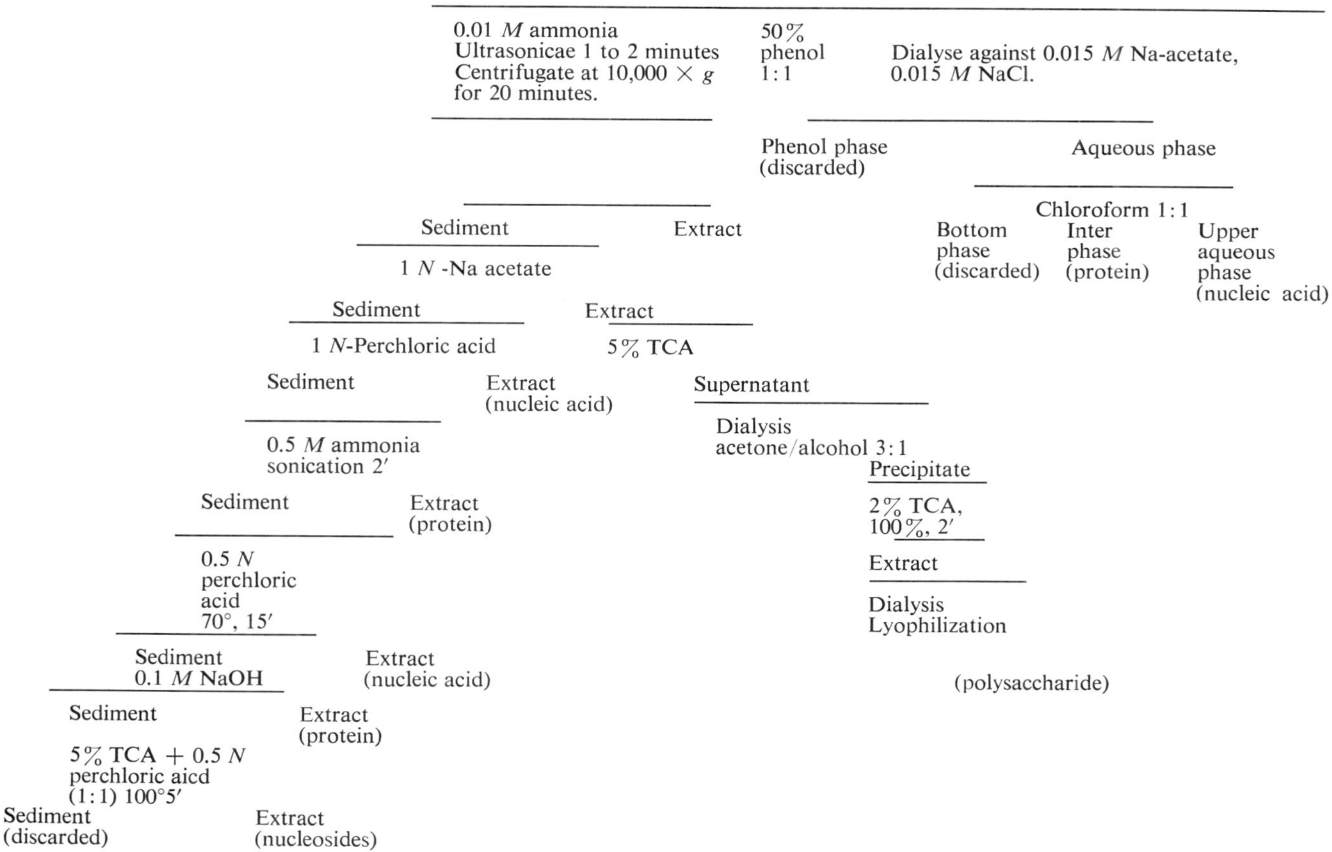

0.01 M ammonia
Ultrasonicae 1 to 2 minutes
Centrifugate at 10,000 $\times$ g
for 20 minutes.

50% phenol 1:1

Dialyse against 0.015 M Na-acetate, 0.015 M NaCl.

Phenol phase (discarded)

Aqueous phase

Sediment — Extract

1 N -Na acetate

Chloroform 1:1

Bottom phase (discarded)

Inter phase (protein)

Upper aqueous phase (nucleic acid)

Sediment — Extract

1 N-Perchloric acid — 5% TCA

Sediment — Extract (nucleic acid)

Supernatant

0.5 M ammonia sonication 2′

Dialysis acetone/alcohol 3:1

Precipitate

Sediment — Extract (protein)

2% TCA, 100%, 2′

0.5 N perchloric acid 70°, 15′

Extract

Dialysis Lyophilization

Sediment 0.1 M NaOH — Extract (nucleic acid)

(polysaccharide)

Sediment — Extract (protein)

5% TCA + 0.5 N perchloric aicd (1:1) 100°5′

Sediment (discarded) — Extract (nucleosides)

*Hank's Buffered Salt Solution

33

Fractionation of protein extracts can be attained by electrophoresis in the Tiselius macrocell, adapted for separating serum proteins (Blix et al., 1941). The limitation of this technique is an appreciable absorption of antigens on the walls of the macrocell.

Alternatively, the extract may be fractionated by chemical precipitation. In this procedure, the extract is first concentrated by ultrafiltration, and then dialyzed against sodium acetate-sodium chloride buffer to give final pH 6.85 and 0.1 M salt concentration. All other operations are conducted at $-5°$. To obtain the first fraction, an acetate, pH 5.8, buffered alcohol solution is added to the dialyzate to final concentration of 25% alcohol. After 48 hours, the precipitate should be centrifuged, washed with 25% buffered alcohol solution, and dialyzed against 2 M sodium chloride and distilled water for 3 hours each time. The first fraction is recovered from the dialyzate by centrifugation.

The second fraction is obtained by increasing the amount of the acetate-buffered ethanol in the original dialyzed extract to 40% alcohol concentration. The resulting precipitate must be collected by centrifugation, washed with 40% ethanol, buffered at pH 6.2, redissolved and dialyzed against 2 M sodium chloride for 12 hours, then against distilled water, and finally lyophilized.

Specific polysaccharide antigens can be obtained from tissues according to Felton's et al. (1956) technique by extracting tissues homogenized in a Waring blender with 0.5 N NaOH for 18 to 24 hours at room temperature. The mixture is then adjusted to pH 7.0 with glacial acetic acid and centrifuged. The supernatant is treated with two volumes of cold 95% ethyl alcohol and left at 4° for 18 hours, and centrifuged. The precipitate should be dissolved in a small amount of water and mixed with an equal volume of 15% trichloracetic acid to remove the protein. After centrifugation, the polysaccharide fraction is precipitated from the supernatant with three volumes of cold alcohol, left at 4° overnight, and then centrifuged. The precipitate is dissolved at pH 7.0, reprecipitated with two volumes of alcohol and a one-fourth volume of ether, washed with acetone and ether, and dried in a vacuum desiccator.

Preparation of lipid antigens from tissues by Pangborn's technique (1942, 1944) is frequently used for extraction and purification of the cardiolipin. In this procedure, the tissue (beef heart) is extracted with ethyl alcohol, and the phosphatides are precipitated with barium chloride. Methods of extraction of blood group substances from human saliva, the ovarian cyst fluid, or animal stomach tissues were published by Beiser and Kabat (1952) and Baer et al. (1954).

III. PREPARATION OF CELLULAR ANTIGENS

The following antigens may be found in intact bacterial cells: the superficially situated capsular antigen, the lid antigen K, the flagellar antigen H, the virulence antigen Vi, which is predominantly situated on the surface of cells, and the somatic antigen O. The "somatic antigen" is anatomically and chemically complex. It contains the following anatomical units: the cell wall, cytoplasmic membrane, protoplast, ribosomes, chromatinic bodies, and intracellular inclusions, chromophores, and vacuoles. Anatomical structure of the cell wall consists of a microfibrillar network, onto which a homogenous filling material is superimposed. The fibrillar network is built up of mucocomplexes containing muramic acid, N-acetyl-D-glucosamine, and some amino acids. The filling material contains proteins, polysaccharides, and lipids.

Some particulate antigens can be morphologically differentiated by a phase-contrast, interference-contrast, or electron microscope, whereas other antigens may only be identified by their physical properties, such as the degree of heat-alcohol tolerance, or by chemical characteristics.

Capsules produced in suitable media by certain bacteria and fungi predominantly consist of either homopolysaccharides, heteropolysaccharides containing glucose, mannose, xylose and glucuronic acid residues, or of peptides and exceptionally of nucleic acids. The homopolysaccharides occur in the capsules in the form of starch, dextrans, levans, or seldom cellulose. The capsular heteropolysaccharides frequently contain glucose and hyaluronic acid. Capsules composed of polypeptides or proteins are formed by *Bacillus anthracis* and *Pasteurella pestis*. Nucleotide capsules are produced by *Halobacterium*. The polysaccharide and nucleotide capsules are heat-resistant whereas protein capsules are heat-labile.

Capsules can easily be released from the bacterial cell surface by extraction with dilute acids, alkalis, or with phosphate buffer and a calcium chloride solution. Microorganisms which ordinarily produce capsules may be decapsulated by repeated daily transfers in the culture media containing 10% autogenous immune serum, or by treatment with appropriate enzymes. For example, hyaluronate capsules or capsular gel can be removed from the surface of streptococcal cells by adding bovine testis hyaluronidase to a suspension of the bacteria, in a ratio of 1 TRU* (0.1 ml) of the enzyme per 7.4 of bacterial suspension and incubating this mixture at 37° for 12 minutes. The bacteria should then be centrifuged and washed. Decapsulated microorganisms reveal antigens located normally beneath the capsules and can be used as preparations of the lid antigen K. Some bacteria, for example, *Mycococcus,* form capsules (Fig. 7) in Gaudy and Wolfe's (1962)

* TRU = turbidity reducing unit.

medium, but not in Kwapinski's semisynthetic, liquid media; thus two different batches of the cells, one encapsulated and the other uncapsulated, may easily be obtained. The flagellar antigen (H) consists of approximately 70% protein (flagellin), 20% lipid, and 10% polysaccharide. It undergoes denaturation by heat and alcohol. Formalized 0.5% suspensions of flagellated bacteria are commonly used as crude preparations of the H antigen. Similar preparations of formalized or living bacteria are used for the Vi agglutination.

Destruction of the flagellar antigen by alcohol or heating at 100° for 30 minutes uncovers the somatic antigen O in flagellated bacteria. Thus suspensions of bacteria are heated at 100° for 60 to 90 minutes in a boiling water bath, and then centrifuged at 1400 × g for 30 minutes. The sediment is collected and resuspended in 0.3% formalinized saline. These suspensions are commonly used as crude preparations of the O antigen for the agglutination test.

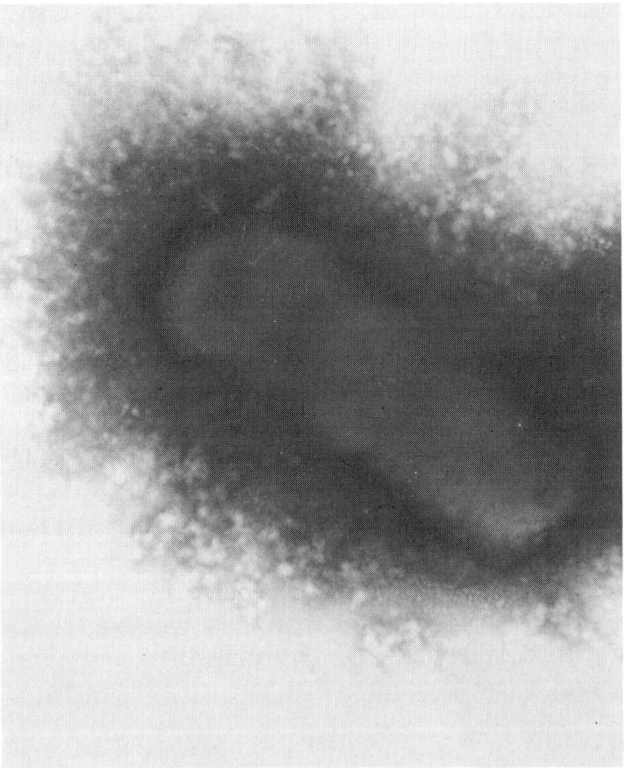

Figure 7.   A large capsule surrounding a bacterium (25,000×).

Principal categories of bacterial antigens can be distinguished as diagrammatically presented in Table 9. Cellular organelles of higher microorganisms may be separated as shown in Table 10.

Table 9. The Division of Principal Categories of Bacterial Antigens

Culture
of bacteria
———————

Centrifugation

Supernatant	Sediment
Extracellular antigens	Cellular antigens

pH 6.5 buffer
centrifugation

Supernatant	Sediment
Capsular antigens	Somatic antigens

Disintegration
centrifugation

Sediment	Supernatant
Cell walls	Cytoplasm

1. Preparation of Flagellar Antigens

Bacterial flagella constitute approximately 2% of the dry weight of flagellated bacteria. Flagella grow more abundantly at temperatures between 22 and 25° than at 37°. It is therefore recommended that the strain of bacteria for testing be adapted to growth at lower temperatures prior to the preparation of flagellar antigens. The bacteria are incubated 24 to 36 hours at 22 to 26° and are removed from the culture medium by centrifugation at $2000 \times g$ for 20 minutes. Flagella may be separated from cells either by vigorous shaking and differential centrifugation (Weibull, 1948; Koffler and Kobayashi, 1957) or by blending the flagella and precipitating with ammonium sulfate (Uchida et al., 1952).

In Weibull's technique a saline suspension of flagellated bacteria is agitated in a shaking machine for 1 hour. Bacterial cells are removed by centrifugation at $3000 \times g$ for 10 minutes, and the flagella are precipitated from the supernatant by half saturation with ammonium sulfate adjusted to pH 7. After centrifugation, the flagella are resuspended and large aggregates are removed by bringing the centrifuge to about $30,000 \times g$ a moment. The deposit is then washed and resedimented at $40,000 g$ for 1

Table 10. Separation of Cellular Organelles
(Kwapinski, 1970, unpublished)

Yeast suspension
in 10^{-5} M EDTA, pH 7.15
____
Disrupted in a sonicator
or in Mickle disintegrator
centrifuged at
$1200 \times g$, 10 minutes
____

Cell walls and cell debris	Supernatant
$5{:}20\%$ sucrose gradient, $177 \times g$, 15 minutes	$8000 \times g$, 15 minutes

Upper band:	Sediment: cell debris	Cytoplasmic	Supernatant
Cell Walls		Membranes	$12,000 \times g$, 30 minutes

Mitochondria

Supernatant

$100,000 \times g$, 1 hour

Ribosomes	Soluble material

hour. The flagella are now washed three times in a dilute aqueous borate buffer, pH 8.5, by centrifugation, each time at 40,000 g for 1 hour. Finally, this sediment is resuspended and centrifuged at 19,000 rpm to remove aggregated material. The supernatant contains purified flagella.

In the method described by Uchida et al. (1952), the bacteria harvested from an agar culture and suspended in a small quantity of saline solution are shaken in a Waring blender for 1 minute to detach the flagella. The bacterial bodies are spun down at $4000 \times g$. The supernatant containing the flagella is treated twice with ethanol added to a final concentration of 19%, at pH 5.8 and $-5°$, first in the presence of 0.04 M Na and again in the presence of 0.02 M Zn. Alternatively, the flagella may be precipitated at a half saturation of ammonium sulfate at pH 7.0 to 7.2, twice repeated. The precipitate is then dialyzed against water. Further purification may be attained by differential centrifugation with the cycle of $44,000 \times g$ for 30 minutes and $4000 \times g$ for 20 minutes. Masses of flagella obtained by either method appear as a water-clear pellet. Tested with the Molisch reagent, this suspension must give no reaction. Preparations of this material, stained by the Bailey or Leifson method and examined microscopically, should show only strands of flagella and not cells or small particles. Viewed in the electron microscope, the flagella appear in a thread-like form.

In Ada's et al. (1964) technique, the flagella may be detached from bacteria either by the shearing action of rotating blades in a blender rotating at low voltage for 10 minutes repeated twice, or by vigorous shaking. The bacteria are then sedimented at 4000 × g in 20 minutes. The flagella containing supernatant is collected and freed from the cell debris by four cycles of differential centrifugation-clarification in a swing-out head, at 5000 × g, 25 minutes, and 40,000 × g, 45 minutes. The flagella sedimented at 40,000 × g are resuspended in distilled water containing 1/100,000 parts of Merthiolate.

2. Preparation of Capsular Antigens

Capsular antigens are found in morphologically distinct bacterial capsules or in apparently nonorganized slime layers which are more or less loosely attached to the cell walls of certain bacteria. This superficially located material can be separated by differential centrifugation, followed by cold ethanol precipitation in the presence of 1 to 2% sodium acetate and dialysis (Thorne et al., 1954; Henriksen and Eriksen, 1961). Techniques of Baker et al. (1952), Guex-Holzer and Tomcsik (1956), Dolby (1958), and Kwapinski (1958) were devised predominantly for the bacteria and Kligman's method (1948) was used originally for preparing the capsules of microfungi. The potassium thiocyanate technique of Amies (1957) and the method of Landy and Trapani (1954) are used for the isolation and purification of the protein capsular antigens. Suitable methods for obtaining slime-layer materials were designed by Gaudy and Wolfe (1962) and Doggott et al. (1965). The recommended techniques are presented below.

Preparation of Capsular Polysaccharide Antigens by Kwapinski's Technique. Bacterial cells are gently rinsed with distilled water and resuspended in a 0.15 M, pH 6.5, phosphate buffer containing 0.9% sodium chloride. This mixture is agitated for 6 hours on an electric shaker at 2°, and centrifuged for 10 minutes at 10,000 × g. The sediment is washed with a small volume of phosphate buffer, centrifuged, and the washings are combined with the original supernatant. The combined supernatant fluids, containing the material released from the surface of bacteria, filtered through a 0.22- or 0.45-μ membrane filter, dialyzed against distilled water and lyophilized. Controls for capsular material consist of dialyzed samples of the culture medium.

Capsular material can be used for serological tests in the crude state or in a purified form. Capsular polysaccharides are isolated in the following manner. The lyophilized, crude material is dissolved in 50 to 100 ml of distilled water, adjusted to pH 6.5, boiled for 2 minutes at 100°, and filtered. The filtrate is treated with four volumes of a 3:1 mixture of acetone and ethyl alcohol, and left overnight at 2°. The flocculent precipitate should be collected by centrifugation. To liberate the polysaccharide fraction from protein impurities, the sediment is dissolved in 50 ml of 5% acetc acid, boiled for 2 to 3 minutes, and centrifuged at 14,000 rpm for 5 minutes. The purified fraction is precipitated from the clear supernatant fluid with four volumes of a 3:1 mixture of acetone and alcohol. The precipitate is collected by centrifugation, dissolved in water, dialyzed, and lyophilized.

The Guex-Holzer and Tomcsik Technique for Preparation of Capsular Antigens. The bacteria are first shaken with chloroform (10 ml/1200 ml of aqueous suspension of microorganisms), left overnight at room temperature, then heated in a boiling water bath for 4 hours, and centrifuged. The supernatant, which contains the capsular material, is collected and concentrated at 60° in vacuo, then cleared by centrifugation. Two and a half volumes of 96% ethanol is added to the clear supernatant to precipitate the capsular material. The precipitate should be further purified by dissolving in distilled water and reprecipitating with 0.7 volume of ethanol.

Water-insoluble materials in the precipitates are discarded by centrifugation. The supernatant may yield two or more fractions under fractional precipitation, for example, at 1.1 to 2.5 volumes of ethanol. Any protein contaminate attached to these fractions can be removed by digestion with trypsin and dialysis.

Kligman's Technique for Capsular Materials. The microorganisms, washed with distilled water, are suspended in 0.5 *N* HCl, and heated for 35 minutes at 75°. The mixture is cooled and centrifuged to discard the cells. The supernatant must be neutralized with 0.5 *N* NaOH and treated with three volumes of ethyl alcohol in the presence of 10% sodium acetate. The mixture is left overnight at 2°. The precipitate is collected and dissolved in water, producing an opalescent solution. Three volumes of ethyl alcohol and 10% sodium acetate are added to this solution in the cold. The resulting precipitate must be collected, dissolved in distilled water, and repurified by precipitation with ethanol.

Dolby's Method (1958) for Preparation of Superficial Antigens. The superficially located antigens of bacteria are prepared by a 12-hour extraction at 4° with 0.05 *M* cacium chloride. Bacterial cells are suspended in this solution in the proportion of 25 to 30 $\times$ 10^{13} cells/100 ml. The extract, filtered through a bacteriological candle, is fractionated at 0° with methyl alcohol added gradually to 10 to 15%, 40%, and 44% (*v/v*) concentration.

The Slime Layer Isolation (Gaudy and Wolfe, 1962). Harvested bacteria are freed from the medium by centrifugation for 45 minutes at 12,000 $\times$ g and washed twice with deionized water. The third or subsequent washing with deionized water releases a viscous material from the slime layer. This should be homogenized for 2 minutes and centrifuged for 40 minutes at 18,000 $\times$ g to remove remaining bacterial cells.

The supernatant is now brought to pH 1 or 2 with 6 M HCl, mixed with three volumes of 95% ethyl alcohol, and left for 15 minutes with frequent stirring, then centrifuged at 12,000 $\times$ g for 20 minutes. The precipitate containing cell debris should be discarded, and the supernatant is neutralized with 1 M NaOH. After standing at room temperature for 10 to 12 hours, the precipitate formed is collected by centrifugation at 12,000 $\times$ g.

The gel-like sediment can be dissolved in a small amount of distilled water and recentrifuged to remove any debris. The supernatant should be dialyzed against four changes of deionized water for 24 hours at 4°. Purification of the slime material is attained by precipitation with 95% ethyl alcohol at $\frac{1}{2}$, 1, 2, 3, 4, and 5 volumes; a few drops of dilute NaCl solution are added to initiate precipitation. The gelatinous precipitates are collected and washed with 95% ethanol, acetone, and ether, and air-dried.

This material can be dissolved in deionized water, and centrifuged at 13,000 rpm for 45 minutes to remove insoluble residues. The supernatant is made strongly alkaline by addition of one fifth volume of 5 M NaOH, and treated with one volume of 95% ethyl alcohol at 4°. This gelatinous precipitate is washed with 95% ethanol, acetone, and ether, and air-dried.

According to Doggott et al. (1965), the extracellular slime may be separated from the cells by forcing a suspension in water of bacteria, grown on a solid medium and covered with a dialyzing membrane, through a 20-gauge needle. The solution is then centrifuged at 18,000 $\times$ g for 30 minutes. The supernatant contains the slime, which may be precipitated with 9 volumes of a 1:1 mixture of ethanol and benzene.

According to Brown's et al. (1969) technique, the slime layer is detached from bacteria either by stirring the cells for 30 seconds in an electric, high-speed homogenizer or by shaking for 30 minutes with 10% (v/v) ethylene glycol, at 37°. The cells are sedimented at 2000 $\times$ g for 2 hours. The supernatant is collected, and the slime is precipitated with ethanol, added in an equal volume, and left at 4° for 24 hours. The supernatant is then decanted, and the slime deposit is redissolved in a small volume of hot (60°) 0.1% KOH. The slime solution is cooled to 18° and reprecipitated with an equal volume of ethanol, and left at 4° overnight. The supernatant fluid is then decanted, and the slime is washed with 90% (v/v) ethanol, ethanol and finally ether. The slime is dried over phosphorus pentoxide and potassium hydroxide *in vacuo* and stored in a desiccator over P_2O_5.

3. Preparation of Exoantigens

Filtrates from cultures of microorganisms contain various products of microbial metabolism, including some macromolecular substances, enzymes, and sometimes toxins secreted by, or released from, the bacteria. Apart from these substances, the filtrate may contain small amounts of capsular or somatic antigens released from the aged, autolyzed cells.

Comprehensive techniques for chemical separation of the extracellular antigens were described by Kwapinski (1970) and Strange and Thorne (1958). Individual groups of polymers present in culture filtrates can be isolated by preparative gel electrophoresis, column gel-chromatography differential gradient centrifugation, or ultrafiltration (pp. 90, 102, 125). These methods have largely replaced chemical fractionation techniques. Chemical procedures for the isolation of polysaccharide fractions were published by Wadsworth and Brown (1937), Dingle and Fothergill (1939), Boyden and Sorkin (1955, see Table 11) and Kwapinski (1965). The Seibert (1941) and Landy and Trapani (1954) methods are suitable for the isolation from culture filtrates of both the polysaccharide and protein fractions.

Seibert's Method of Preparing Protein Exoantigens.   This method has been used specifically for obtaining the protein derivate, PPD, from culture filtrates of mycobacteria. In this technique, the culture filtrate passes through a bacterial filter, for example, such as a $0.45\text{-}\mu$ porosity-membrane, is mixed at the ratio of 3:1 with phosphate buffer, pH 7.3, containing 8 ml of toluol per liter, and concentrated by ultrafiltration. The ultrafiltrate is passed through a membrane filter and lyophilized. The dry material is then redissolved in the buffer and mixed at 5 to 6° with an equal volume of saturated ammonium sulfate, previously neutralized to phenol red with solid disodium phosphate.

The resultant precipitates should be centrifuged, dissolved in the phosphate buffer, and reprecipitated at a half saturation with neutral ammonium sulfate, centrifuged, and redissolved in the buffer. This procedure must be repeated six times. The final solution is passed through a Mandler filter, ultrafiltered, and washed to free from sulfate with a buffer containing 2 ml of toluol per liter. The concentrated solution is then filtered through a Mandler candle or a $0.45\text{-}\mu$ porosity membrane filter and lyophilized.

Chromatographic Separation of Extracellular Antigens.   Many antigens occurring in culture filtrates can be isolated by anion or cation exchange-column chromatography or by filtration on a Sephadex G-100 column (Kwapinski, 1970, unpublished; Peterson and Sober, 1956; Hanson and Holm, 1961; Thomson, 1963).

Table 11. Chemical Fractionation of Culture Filtrates According to
Boyden and Sorkin (1955)

Filtrate + 10% acetic acid to pH 4.1

Centrifuged

Supernatant		Sediment
Adjusted to pH 6.5 + 96% ethyl alcohol 1/volume		Dissolved in sodium bicarbonate solution, recprecipitated, washed with 96% alcohol and ether

Supernatant	Sediment
+ 2.2 volume of 96% alcohol	Washed with 48% alcohol, dried with 96% alcohol and ether

Fraction 1

Fraction 2

Supernatant	Sediment
+ 96% alcohol to 76% final concentration	Washed with 70% alcohol, dissolved in water, a half saturated ammonium sulfate added

Supernatant	Precipitate	Supernatant	Precipitate
Dialyzed, concentrated by ultrafiltration + 36% alcohol 1/1		Dialyzed, precipitated with alcohol Fraction 3a	Dialyzed, washed with alcohol Fraction 3b

Sediment, Fraction 4

The anion exchange chromatography is run on DEAE-cellulose or carboxy-methyl-cellulose (CM 70, Whatman). Columns, 2.4 cm in diameter, are filled up to a height of about 6 cm, with the exchange suspension in an initial buffer. The filtrate is then loaded on the column. The various fractions are eluted under gravity flow with phosphate buffers, pH 6.8, using stepwise increased ionic strengths ranging from 0.001 to 0.1 M buffer, containing 0.005 to 0.1 M sodium chloride. Each eluate collected as 5- to 25-ml fractions should be dialyzed against tap water in the cold and concentrated by lyophilization or pervaporation.

Separation of extracellular antigens on a Sephadex G-100 column is performed by layering a dialyzed and 20× concentrated culture filtrate on the column equilibrated with 0.05 M Tris, 0.2 M NaCl, pH 7.0 buffer. The fractions are eluted first with 0.05 M Tris, 0.02 M NaCl, pH 6.0 buffer and then with a pH 8.7 buffer, and collected in a refrigerated, automatic fraction collector. The fractions are screened at 254 and 280 nm, and tested with Molisch's reagent for the presence of carbohydrates.

Preparation of Extracellular Enzymes. Extracellular enzymes can readily be obtained by precipitation of the culture filtrates with ammonium sulfate or sodium acetate in the cold. For example, a lecithinase preparation may be precipitated from a culture filtrate adjusted to pH 6.9 at 75% saturation with solid ammonium sulfate (Costlow, 1958). After standing 2 hours, the liquid should be centrifuged. The sediment is dissolved in cold distilled water and diluted with one half volume of saturated ammonium sulfate. The fluid is left in the cold for 1 hour, then centrifuged at 12,000 $\times$ g for 15 minutes. The supernatant should be collected and dialyzed against tap water in the cold for 24 hours and against distilled water until free of ammonium sulfate; the dialyzate can be lyophilized. Individual enzymes may be recovered at different concentrations of ammonium sulfate. In this process, fractionation of the crude filtrate must be controlled by appropriate biochemical tests for individual activity.

4. Preparation of Toxic Antigens

Toxic antigens present in culture filtrates can be precipitated with aluminum (Wright et al., 1954) or trichloracetic acid (Jacobs and Behan, 1950), and isolated in a more purified form by different fractionation procedures (Lepow and Pillemer, 1952; Pope and Stevens, 1953; Pentz and Shigemura, 1955; Largier, 1957; Duff et al., 1957; Fiock et al., 1961). A measure of the effectiveness of preparation can be expressed by the purification factor (Tasman and Van Waasbergen, 1932), which is calculated from the formula:

$$\text{purification factor} = \frac{\text{Lf/mg } N \text{ in purified toxoid}}{\text{Lf/mg } N \text{ in crude toxoid}}$$

The Wright et al. Technique. Culture filtrates are mixed with aluminum potassium sulfate to give 0.1% concentration (in terms of the anhydrous salt). This mixture is adjusted to pH 5.9 with $N/1$ hydrochloric acid, and left overnight at 2 to 4°. The precipitate is centrifuged, and washed twice in sterile 0.9% solution of sodium chloride. The washed precipitate may be either resuspended in saline and preserved with Merthiolate (sodium mercury-ethyl-thiosalicylate) added to a concentration of 1:10,000 or dissolved in 2% solution of potassium sodium tartrate (Ando et al., 1936).

Concentration of Toxoids (Jacobs and Behan, 1950). The toxoid, or a toxic culture filtrate, is treated with a 1 N trichloracetic acid (163.5 g of TCA dissolved in water added to the 1-liter volume) to adjust the pH to about 3.5 to 4.0. The flocculent precipitate is collected by centrifugation and can be used as a crude concentrated toxoid if dissolved in a 1/15 molar phosphate buffer, pH 8.0. The toxoid may be purified by respectively washing the precipitate with 0.1 N trichloracetic acid, then dissolving in 10 ml of a pH 8.0 phosphate buffer, diluting to 400 ml with water, and reprecipitating with 2 N trichloracetic acid. A simple and effective concentration method is partial lyophilizaton and absorption of water on acrylamide gels.

Fractionation and Purification of Toxins. Although a modern procedure for the fractionation and purification of toxins employs the preparative polyacrylamide electrophoresis or electrofusing (see pp. 90, 122), the ammonium sulfate precipitation and tryptic digestion methods still maintain their usefulness. Lepow and Pillemer's (1952) technique for toxin purification employs a volume of 105 ml of toxic filtrate saturated at pH 7.0 with 49.7 g of ammonium sulfate, left overnight at 5°, then centrifuged. The sediment is dissolved in 79.6 ml of water and mixed with 318 ml of saturated ammonium sulfate, adjusting the liquid to pH 7.0. The mixtures are left overnight at 0°, then filtered. The filtrate is mixed with 790 ml of saturated ammonium sulfate at pH 7.0, left overnight at 0°, and filtered or centrifuged. The sediment is dissolved in water added up to 267 ml. To 260 ml of this solution, a volume of 96 ml of saturated ammonium sulfate is added and adjusted to pH 7.0. This mixture is left for 1 hour at 25°, and centrifuged. The supernatant is now treated with 260 ml of saturate ammonium sulfate at pH 7.0, left overnight at 25°, and centrifuged. The precipitate is dissolved in water added up to 374 ml, and absorbed for 1 hour at 25° with 75 ml of alumina cream. The purification may be continued by the multimembrane electrodecantation method of Largier (1957).

The Fiock et al. (1961) Technique for Purification of Toxins. The culture of toxigenic microorganisms is first adjusted to pH 6.0 and incubated for 2 hours at 37° in the presence of trypsin added to 0.1% concentration. (The trypsin digestion activates certain toxins.) The toxin is then concentrated by precipitation at approximately 60% saturation of ammonium sulfate. The precipitate is now diluted to three-fourths culture volume with distilled water and extracted at pH 6.0 with calcium chloride, added to a final concentration of 0.075 M (using a 1.0 M $CaCl_2$ solution) for 1 hour at room temperature. The solution is then filtered through a paper filter pulp, adjusted to pH 5.0 and 0.075 M concentration of calcium chloride, and cooled to −5°; 95% ethanol is added to give a final concentration of 25%, and the mixture is left overnight at −5°. The resulting precipitate should be collected by centrifugation at about 2000 × g for 30 minutes at −5°, dissolved in 0.2 M succinate buffer, pH 5.5, and dialyzed against this buffer to remove nonprotein nitrogen.

Crystallization of toxins from purified preparations can be attempted by the following procedure (Pillemer et al., 1948). A solution of purified toxin containing about 1% protein is adjusted to a suitable hydrogen-ion concentration, which for some toxins is between pH 5.5 and 6.5. Methanol is then added to a 20 or 30% concentration at $-5°$. Crystallization occurs at this temperature in a few days.

5. *Preparation of the Vi Antigen*

The Vi antigen, which consists of a polysaccharide composed of glucose, fructose, and *N*-acetylamino-hexuronic acid, may be isolated and purified by Webster's et al. (1952) Baker's et al. (1954) method.

The Webster et al. Method. The acetone dried bacteria are suspended in 0.9% solution of sodium chloride and shaken for 30 minutes, then sedimented for 30 minutes in an angle centrifuge. The supernatant is withdrawn and dialyzed in running tap water for 12 to 16 hours. Sodium chloride is then added to the dialyzate to 0.9% concentration, and this solution is precipitated with ethanol added slowly to the final 0.1, 0.2, and 0.3 *M*. Precipitates formed at each of these alcohol concentrations are collected by centrifugation and dissolved in distilled water. Acetic acid is then added to 0.1 *M,* followed by ethanol at 0.1, 0.2, and 0.3 *M*. The purified precipitates thus obtained should be redissolved in distilled water and treated with acetic acid added to 1 *M* concentration. These solutions are refluxed for 24 hours, then dialyzed, and reprecipitated with ethyl alcohol. Precipitates can be lyophilized.

The Baker et al. Technique (1954). Microorganisms are dried with acetone and suspended in 0.15 *M* sodium chloride, left for 2 hours at room temperature, and treated with two volumes of 95% ethyl alcohol. The precipitate, which consists of dissolved Vi and O antigens and some bacterial cells, is collected by centrifugation and extracted with 60% ethanol diluted in 0.15 *M* NaCl, at 37°, for 18 to 24 hours. This procedure should be repeated several times, and the extracts combined. Extracts contain most of the Vi antigen. This method was slightly modified by Baker and Whiteside (1960).

6. *Preparation of Somatic Antigens*

Somatic antigens are immunologically active compounds occurring in the cell walls, protoplasts, spheroplasts, chromoplasts, and other anatomical constituents of microbial cells. Substances present in the cytoplasmic inclusions are also cell components that may prove to be active antigenically. Micromanipulation and microsection techniques used for the separation of different anatomical structural components of microbial cells, including cell walls, require further improvement. Modern immunochemical analysis of microbial cells should take into account the origin and location of isolated fractions in the particular structural elements, but some antigens isolated from nondissected cells may often be useful for the serological classification of types or groups of microorganisms.

Physical methods for disrupting bacteria and other cells may be divided in solid shear and liquid shear methods, the latter one being preferred. The technique for liquid shear depends on the forcing of a suspension of cells to a small orifice under high pressure, for example, in the French press, or shaking the suspension with small glass beads in a Mickle disintegrator. Another physical method is disruption of cells by sonic or ultrasonic vibration. Ultrasonic treatment disrupts microorganisms by causing cavitation in the suspension. Unbroken organisms and cell debris are removed by centrifugation at about $5000 \times g$. Fragments of cytoplasmic membranes can be separated by a centrifugal force of about $20,000 \times g$ for 30 minutes, while ribosomes are sedimented at $100,000 \times g$ (in 1 to 3 hours) in an analytical ultracentrifuge.

A comprehensive preparation of somatic antigens consists of a stepwise extraction of various fractions from the cell walls and the cytoplasm of disrupted microbial cells. A technique used by Kwapinski and his associates for investigations on the antigenic structure of microorganisms is presented diagrammatically in Table 12. Prior to the extraction, washed microbial cells are suspended in distilled water and disintegrated with No. 12 "Ballotini" glass beads in the Mickle electromagnetic vibrator, at $2°$ in 1 to 2 hours, depending on the species, or in a Raytheon sonicator (Fig. 8), for 20 to 30 minutes, and then centrifuged at $10,000 \times g$ for 10 to 15 minutes. The supernatant fluid is collected, passed through a sintered glass filter No. 5, and recentrifuged for 10 minutes at $15,000 \times g$. The supernatant, containing cytoplasmic materials, is collected, and its purity is checked macroscopically in a phase-contrast microscope and in smears stained by Gram's method. Pure cytoplasm occurs in the form of homogenous masses which are colored pink by the Gram staining. The efficiency of cell disintegration is checked by a culture test, by observations in the phase-contrast or electron microscope (Fig. 9), and by examining Gram-stained smears under a light microscope. The disintegrated cells occur as pink-colored particles.

Cell walls present in the sediment are freed from any cytoplasmic material by washing repeatedly with distilled water until no traces of protein, nuclcic acid, or sugar are detectable at the 280- and 254-nm wavelength. To separate cell walls from any partially disrupted or intact cells, the washed sediment should be resuspended in distilled water and centrifuged for 3 minutes at 480 to $755 \times g$. The supernatant is carefully collected so as to be free of any sediment and recentrifuged in the same manner. The purity of cell wall preparations is checked in a phase-contrast microscope, or in an electron microscope. Cell walls and cytoplasmic material are fractionated as shown diagrammatically in Table 12.

Table 12. Kwapinski's (1965) Technique for Preparation of Nonparticulate Antigens

Disintegrated bacteria

Cell walls   Cytoplasm

Alcohol-ether   25% acetic acid
Residue   Extract   Supernatant   Sediment

1 M sodium acetate L_1 $N/2$ sodium acetate
Residue   Extract   Extract   Sediment

$N/5$ NaOH   Dialysis + acetone   Dialysis + acetone $N/1$ NaOH
Residue   Extract C_2 C_1 Filtrate

80% phenol   Dialysis + 25% acetic acid   Dialysis
Residue   Extract   Supernatant N_1

7.5% Sulfo-   Dialysis
salicylic   Supernatant   Sediment
acid
                  acetone $N/2$ NaOH
                  C_4 Extract

Residue   Extract   dialysis
                                                   N_2

Formamide   Dialysis
100°C, 15 minutes Extract C_s

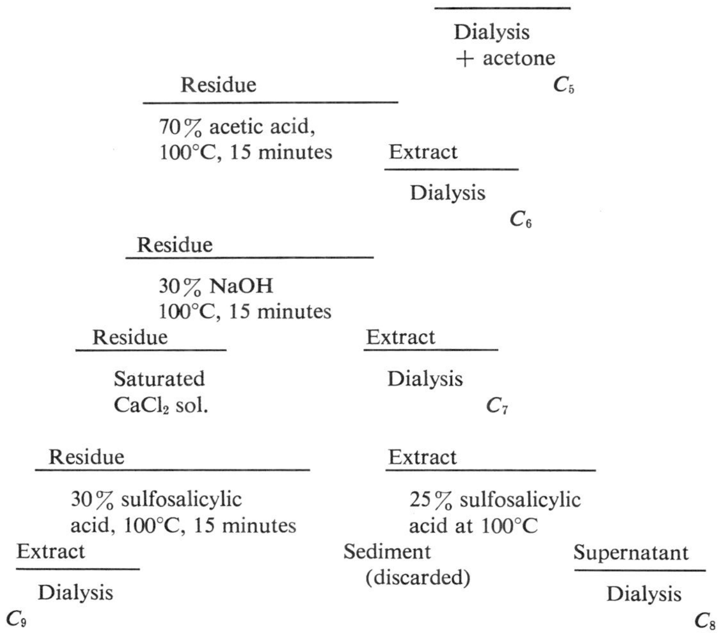

Residue
—————————————————————————————
70% acetic acid,
100°C, 15 minutes

Dialysis
+ acetone
C_5

Extract
—————————
Dialysis
C_6

Residue
—————————————————————————————
30% NaOH
100°C, 15 minutes

Extract
—————————
Dialysis
C_7

Residue
—————————
Saturated
$CaCl_2$ sol.

Residue
—————————————————————————————
30% sulfosalicylic
acid, 100°C, 15 minutes

Extract
—————————
Dialysis
C_9

Extract
—————————————————————————————
25% sulfosalicylic
acid at 100°C

Sediment
(discarded)

Supernatant
—————————————
Dialysis
C_8

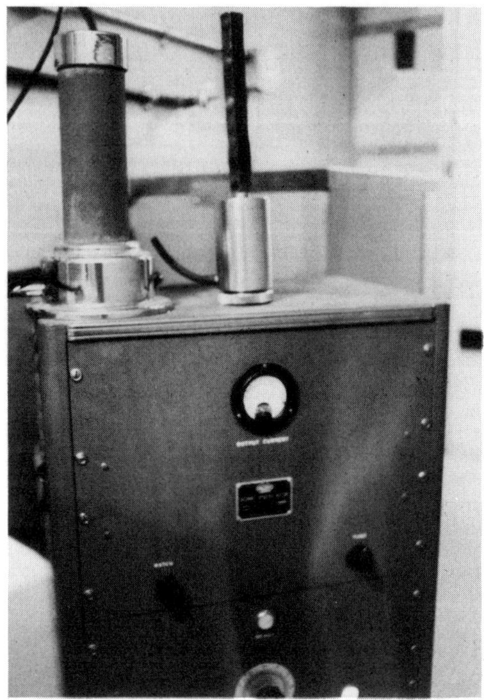

Figure 8. The Raytheon Magnetoconstrictive Oscillator.

The latter method was used in the original or a slightly modified form by various investigators, for example, Merkel (1961), Jungerman (1962), Krzywy (1963), Tubylewicz (1963), and Mordarska (1966).

According to the Munoz and Bestekin method, bacterial cells dried with acetone are ruptured in the Ribi pressure cell and extracted for 1 to 2 hours with saline at pH 8.5 in the cold, with constant stirring, then left overnight at 2 to 5°. This suspension is then centrifuged at 27,000 × *g* in a refrigerated centrifuge, and the supernatant is dialyzed against cold distilled water. Antigens present in the dialyzate can be purified by the use of curtain electrophoresis, cellulose column chromatography, or starch block electrophoresis, the last technique giving the best separation of antigenic materials.

7. Preparation of Cell Walls

Cell-Wall Preparation. Cell walls represent about 20% of the total mass of bacterial and rickettsiae cells. They consist of a complex network of immunochemical compounds, incorporated in the cell-wall structural network, which usually consists of two to three physically distinguishable layers. The cell wall can be separated from other anatomical structures by means of physical or chemical disintegration. Chemical methods for the cell-wall preparation depend on treatment of microbial cells with enzymes, such as carbohydrases, proteinases, or nucleases, or with chemical reagents to break up structural linkages between components of the cell walls. This treatment must not alter or destroy the original antigenic properties of the macromolecular cell-wall constituents. Cell walls obtained by the disintegration of viable bacteria should be washed with 0.1% aqueous formalin to prevent the action of autolytic enzymes. The following physical procedures are widely applied for the disintegration of microbial cells:

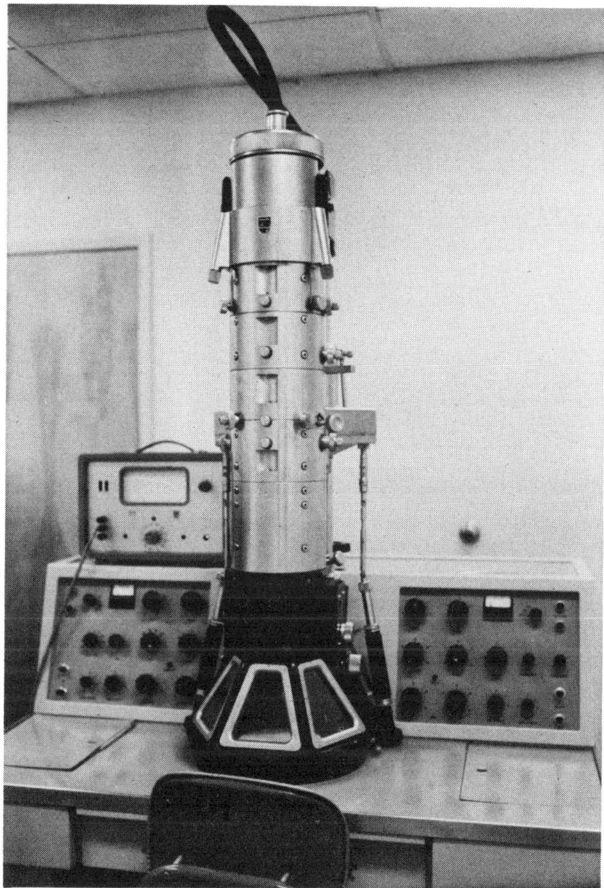

Figure 9. The electron microscope.

i. Cryolysis. This procedure consists of cycles of alternative freezing and thawing (D'Allessandro and Dardanoni, 1953; Hofsten and Tjeder, 1961). It should be noted, however, that some antigenic complexes break down under this treatment.

ii. Mechanical Disintegration. Cells are disrupted mechanically by grinding them with glass beads (0.01 to 0.20 mm diameter) in a high-speed homogenizer, cooled with liquid CO_2, metal ball mills, the Hughes or Edebo X press, the electromagnetic vibrator, the T-type bacterial disintegrator, or in centrifuge shaker.

iii. Osmotic Cell Rupture. The microorganisms are disrupted by a shearing force when a high hydraulic pressure is suddenly released, in a French pressure cell or another decompression chamber (Foster et al., 1962).

iv. Sonic Disintegration. Cells are broken by sonic waves in the Raytheon Magnetoconstrictive Oscillator (Fig. 8) by vibrating the cells in liquid at a frequency of approximately 10 kHz. The magnetoconstrictive effect is utilized by attaching a sample cup on a diaphragm resting on a magnetic rod and placing the rod within a coil of wire connected to an electronic oscillator.

v. Ultrasonic Disintegration of Cells. The disruption of cells by ultrasound depends on the "cavitation" induced by the ultrasound of an intensity maintained above a critical value. The cavitation is a phenomenon in which the sound waves cause very rapid alternations of pressure, resulting in the formation of large masses of minute gas-filled bubbles. The bubbles grow and pulsate through several sound cycles until at a critical size they disintegrate implosively giving rise to intense local shock waves and to microstreaming of the liquid around the points of collapse. The streaming around bubbles produces high shear gradients leading to the disruption of cells. The high frequency vibrations at the top of the titanium probe of an ultrasonic disintegrator transmit the ultrasound pressures to the cell suspensions. The cells are effectively disrupted at the frequency of the sound (11 μ for 20 kHz) within 5 to 15 minutes, depending on the source and physicochemical resistance of the cells.

Selected Techniques of the Cell-Wall Preparation by Physical Means: The Cryolysis Technique. According to the Hofsten and Tjeder technique, small pieces of dry ice (solid carbon dioxide) are first homogenized to form a fine powder. The microorganisms are then added to the powdered ice and homogenized for a few minutes or longer, as required. The homogenized material is left to thaw in a beaker placed in running cold water. The process of freezing, homogenization, and thawing can be repeated if required.

Sonic and Ultrasonic Disintegration. Cell breakage is obtained very efficiently by sonic or ultrasonic oscillation at 9 or 20 kHz, respectively, in a water-cooled Raytheon magnetoconstriction oscillator (Fig. 8) or in a

Biosonik III (Fig. 10). If a sonic oscillator is used, a relatively thick cell suspension, containing approximately 20 to 30 mg of wet mass per ml of a 0.02 *M,* pH 7.0, phosphate buffer or 0.1 *M* borate buffer, is subjected to the oscillation at 9 to 10 kHz with an audiofrequency current of about 1.1 to 1.2 A and 250 W, for 10 to 15 minutes, or longer, if required. The cell suspension must be cooled down below 5° before and during this operation. Slightly less dense cell suspensions are employed for the ultrasonicator, where the cells, held on ice, are subjected to the 20 kHz oscillations for 5 to 10 minutes.

Disruption of Bacteria in the Mickle Electromagnetic Vibrator. Washed bacteria are suspended in distilled water or in a pH 7.0 buffer to contain 20 to 30 mg of wet mass per ml and mixed with an equal volume of fine (0.01 to 0.2 mm diameter) glass beads (e.g., No. 12 "Ballotini") in the glass containers of this apparatus. The vibrator is run at 2 to 4° for 30 to 60 minutes, or for a few hours if required. After disintegration of the cells, the glass beads are removed by passing the suspension through a No. 1 sintered glass filter. Intact cells remaining in the filtrate are removed by centrifugation at 100 × *g* for 10 minutes, and the cell walls are then deposited at 8,000 × *g* in 10 minutes. Cell walls are washed with distilled

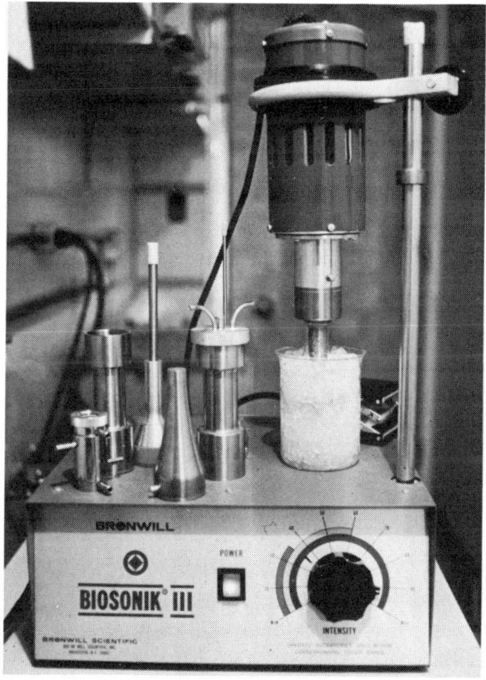

Figure 10. The Biosonik III ultrasonicator and different probes.

water and recentrifuged. A more rapid and efficient removal of contaminating cytoplasmic debris from the cell walls is obtained by washing with 1 *M* NaCl before washing with distilled water (Salton, 1953).

Separation of the cell walls from remaining intact cells is greatly facilitated by a linear glycerol or sucrose gradient centrifugation (Ribi and Hoyer, 1960, Kwapinski, 1972).

The Pressure-Cell Method.   The bacteria are suspended in 0.25 *M* sucrose buffer and subjected to a hydraulic pressure of 13,000 psi in a French pressure cell, when the high pressure is suddenly released (Ribi et al., 1958). A convenient automatic apparatus for disruption of cells by shearing is Ribi's fractionator. A simlar method, based on the rapid release of gas pressure, was devised by Fraser (1951).

Disintegration of microorganisms in Waring blender type homogenizer is less efficient than the methods relying on sonication, ultrasonication, and high hydraulic pressure. According to Lamanna and Mallette (1954), washed cells are suspended in 0.25 *M* sucrose in 0.01 phosphate buffer, mixed with glass powder, and agitated at a high speed in an electric homogenizer. The disintegration temperature should be kept around 3° by placing the container in a metal cylindrical case containing a mixture of ethylene glycolmonoethyl ether and dry ice (Kanai and Youmans, 1960).

Between 70 and 99% of microbial cells can be disrupted by physical means, depending on their structure and the method of disintegration. The nondisrupted cells are removed by the centrifugation at 64 to 114 $\times$ *g* for 3 to 4 minutes. Disintegrated cells are separated from the cytoplasmic material by centrifugation of the supernatant at 5000 to 8000 $\times$ *g* for 40 to 60 minutes. The exterior and interior of disrupted cells can be freed from the adhering cytoplasmic material and small particles by washing the sediment repeatedly with distilled water or saline until no protein, sugar, or nucleic acid can be detected in the washings, by the Millon (Sagakushi), Molisch, or Konsor tests, respectively. Finally, the cell walls are collected by centrifugation at 20,000 $\times$ *g* and observed in the phase-contrast microscope, or in the electron microscope.

Cell walls can be cleaned efficiently with a detergent like Tween 80. In the procedure of Kanai and Youmans (1960), the crude material containing cell walls is sedimented by centrifugation, resuspended in a large volume of 0.5% solution of Tween 80 and recentrifuged at 3000–4000 $\times$ *g* for 10 minutes. The sediment is collected and washed repeatedly with 0.5% Tween 80 solution, 1 *M* sodium chloride, and finally with distilled water.

Preparation of Cell Walls by Enzyme and Chemical Treatment.   Chemical methods of cell wall preparation on the treatment of microbial cells or mycelia with enzymes, or other chemical compounds that break up some structural linkages between different components of the cell walls.

Enzymes used for the cell-wall preparation are polysaccharidases such as lysozyme, proteolytic enzymes (trypsin and pepsin), nucleases (ribonuclease and deoxyribonuclease), crude autolytic or heterolytic culture filtrates, leukoenzymes, extracts from monocytes supported by glycine, and bacteriophages. Enzyme treatment is often preceded by mechanical agitation of the bacteria in various mills or vibrators. Lysozyme and microbial lytic filtrates are used in most procedures as the only lytic agents, whereas purified proteolytic enzymes, trypsin and pepsin, are more often applied in succession to each other, or even supplemented by the treatment of partially digested cells with ribonuclease and deoxyribonuclease.

The following chemical compounds are capable of dissolving cells of some bacteria: sodium taurocholate (Avery and Goebel, 1933; Casper, 1937), sodium deoxycholate (Jenkin, 1960), sodium lauryl sulfate, sodium dodecyl sulfate (Salton, 1957), a mixture of sulfosalicylic acid and ether or Elkosin (Kwapinski, 1965), and penicillin at a high concentration exceeding 100,000 U/ml (Kawata et al., 1960). A number of other chemical substances, for example, picric acid or formamide (Fuller, 1938), cause the disintegration of bacteria with the release of cytoplasm, when applied at a temperature over 100°. Considerable alterations of the chemical and antigenic properties of cell walls can be caused by such a drastic treatment. Here are some additional details concerning the preparation of cell walls by enzymic and chemical treatments.

The Lysozyme Technique. Lysozyme selectively depolymerizes cell walls of many species of bacteria and microfungi, leaving the cytoplasm intact and enclosed in the cytoplasmic membrane. The cytoplasm occurs in the form of spherical bodies, protoplasts or spheroplasts, as the result of the high surface tension exerted on their small volumes (Tomcsik and Guex-Holzer, 1952). At a further stage of the lysozyme activity, the turbidity of isolated cell-wall structures decreases, and reducing groups and acetylamino sugar complexes are liberated.

Either a crude source of lysozyme, for example, egg white, or purified and crystalline preparation of this polysaccharidase can be used for the isolation of cell walls. Crude preparations of the enzyme are used in 1:100 dilution, while a crystalline lysozyme is added in the concentration of 0.01 to 0.1 mg/ml of a suspension of live bacteria. Higher concentrations of this enzyme are less effective. These mixtures are left for 10 to 15 hours at room temperature. A solution of 1 *M* sodium chloride is then added dropwise until lysis of the bacteria occurs (Peterson and Hartsell, 1955; Elliott, 1960).

The technique of *isolation and purification of lysozyme* (Alderton et al., 1945) is as follows. One liter of egg white and 150 ml of a 10% suspension of bentonite in 1% potassium chloride are stirred 3 to 5 minutes to adsorb the lysozyme onto bentonite particles. The bentonite is then separated by centrifugation, and washed with 0.5 M phosphate buffer, pH 7.5, and with a 5% aqueous solution of pyridine three times, to remove adsorbed inactive proteins. Lysozyme is eluted from the bentonite by washing twice with 5% aqueous solution of pyridine, adjusted to pH 5.0 with sulfuric acid. The eluate can be lyophilized. The purification of lysozyme preparations may be attempted by treating a solution of lysozyme, adjusted to pH 5 and 7, with ammonium sulfate. The salt should be added at increments of 0.2 M by dialysis through a rotating membrane at 1°.

Crystalline egg-white lysozyme is produced commercially, for example, by the Nutritional Biochemical Corporation of the United States.

The Autolysis Technique. Certain enzymes of aged cultures of bacteria, for example, of *Diplococcus pneumoniae,* cause the autolysis of homologous bacteria at 30 to 37°. In the autolysis procedure (Eisler, 1941) the bacteria grown in the original culture medium or suspended in saline under a toluol layer added as a preservative are left for 48 hours at this temperature. Autolysis is expedited by the addition of 10% sodium dioxycholate.

The Lysis of Bacteria by Heterolytic Filtrates. The most active bacteriolytic factor known is produced by *Streptomyces albus* (Maxted, 1948). This microorganism can be cultivated on a 1.25% agar medium in Roux bottles at 30 to 37° for 4 days. The cultures are placed at −20° for 12 hours and are then thawed out. The fluid should be passed through a Seitz filter. The lytic complex can be precipitated from a semisynthetic culture filtrate of *Streptomyces albus* at 0.7 saturation of ammonium sulfate, by adding 472 g of solid ammonium sulfate per 1 liter of the fluid (McCarty, 1952). The precipitate is then dissolved in $M/15$ phosphate buffer, pH 8.0, in the presence of filter cell, and filtered. The supernatant is dialyzed against distilled water and finally against 0.0001 N hydrochloric acid. A brown precipitate is formed during the dialysis. After the centrifugation, the sediment and supernatant (p) are collected separately. The sediment should be dissolved in a phosphate buffer and mixed with 0.1 volume of 10% calcium chloride to remove the pigment. The precipitate is then collected by centrifugation and washed. It contains most of the cell-wall lytic enzyme.

The supernatant (p), which ordinarily shows a high proteolytic activity, is concentrated by reprecipitation at 0.7 saturation of ammonium sulfate followed by dialysis against a phosphate buffer. This proteolytic enzyme can be combined with the major part of the cell-wall lytic enzyme. Active lytic enzymes, produced by *Bacillus cereus,* can be isolated from the filtrates by a procedure described by Strange and Dark (1957).

Lysis by Bacteriophage. The following technique, based on the method of Schachman et al. (1952), is effective for the bacteriophage disruption of average bacteria. Microbial cells in the logarithmic phase of growth are harvested, washed, and mixed with an excess of a specific bacteriophage. After 10 to 60 minutes, the cells are centrifuged and resuspended in five times their volume of a 0.2% solution of casamino acids. This mixture is then aerated for 30 minutes, during which time massive lysis occurs. After the lysis, the bacteriophage and some other contaminating material can be removed by centrifugation at 25,000 to 40,000 rpm for 1 to 2 hours. Lysis of bacteria by bacteriophage can cause considerable changes in the antigenic structure of microorganisms.

The Cummins and Harris Method (1956) of Cell-Wall Preparation. The bacteria are first disintegrated at 4° with "Ballotini" glass beads No. 12 or 13 in a Mickle electromagnetic vibrator, using 4 g of glass beads and 6 ml of bacterial suspension per cup. (Rubber stoppers should be protected with cellophane.) After centrifugation at 1000 rpm for 5 to 10 minutes, the supernatant is decanted. The glass beads are washed three times with distilled water, and the washings are added to the original supernatant. This fluid is centrifuged at 1000 rpm for a few minutes to remove glass beads, and then at 4000 rpm to deposit the crude cell-wall fraction. Alternatively, glass beads can be removed by filtration through a No. 1 sintered glass filter. The sediment is then washed in distilled water, resuspended in 0.05 M phosphate buffer, pH 7.6, and digested at 37° for 3 hours with crystalline trypsin and ribonuclease used at 0.5 mg/ml. (Crystalline ribonuclease can be prepared by the method described by Kunitz, 1940.) The digested material is then centrifuged, the sediment washed twice in distilled water, resuspended in 0.02 N HCl, and treated with crystalline pepsin (1 mg/ml) at 37° for 18 to 24 hours. The mixture is finally centrifuged and washed several times in distilled water. Yamaguchi (1965) has modified the technique above, and his procedure is presented in Table 13.

Kwapinski's (1965, 1971) Method for Cell-Wall Preparation. Bacterial cells grown in a Kwapinski's (1969, 1970) semisynthetic culture medium are treated with 1% formalin and harvested by centrifugation at 12,000 $\times$ g for 10 minutes. The cells are then washed six times in a large volume of distilled water and finally suspended in 5 volumes of 10^{-3} EDTA, pH 7.15, containing Merthiolate (Thimerosal) and disrupted in the Biosonik III Ultrasonicator at 20 kHz for 15 minutes. The disrupted cells are collected by centrifugation at 23,500 $\times$ g for 10 minutes, and washed repeatedly with distilled water, until no protein and nucleic acid are detectable in the washings, as examined at 280- and 254-nm wavelengths. The cell walls are separated from nondisrupted cells by the centrifugation at 80 to 100 $\times$ g for 15 minutes in a sucrose gradient consisting of 5 and 20% or 5, 10, and 20% (5 to 7 ml) sucrose solutions. The cell walls are collected with the upper band occurring in the 5% layer of sucrose on centrifugation at 177–200 $\times$ g for 15 to 20 minutes. The cell walls are purified on a 5:10:20%

Table 13.　Yamaguchi's (1965) Technique for Cell-Wall Preparation

Bacteria

Suspended in water
Disrupted at 10 kHz (10 to 40 minutes)
centrifuged (1000 $\times$ g, 20 minutes)

Sediment
(discarded)

Supernatant

centrifuged (4000–7500 $\times$ g, 30 minutes)

Supernatant
(discarded)

Sediment

Washed with water, 1 M, NaCl, and
water centrifuged

1 part
crude
cell walls

2nd part

0.5% KOH in ethanol, 37°, 48 hour centrifuged	In 0.05 M phosphate buffer and chloroform Trypsin (0.5 ml/ml), 37° overnight, centrifuged

Supernatant (discarded)

Sediment　　　　　　　　　　　　　　　Sediment

Washed with alkaline ethanol and water　　　0.02 NHCl
+ trypsin + pepsin　　　　　　　　　　　Pepsin (1 mg/ml), overnight
　　　　　　　　　　　　　　　　　　　centrifuged

Supernatant (discarded)

Sediment

Washed

Purified
cell walls

Purified
cell walls

(5:5:5 ml) gradient and finally dialyzed against distilled water, at 0° for 20 hours, and checked for identity by a phase-contrast or interference-contrast microscopy. The cell walls are then purified by trypsinization. For this purpose, the suspension of cell walls is adjusted to pH 7.4 using 0.05–0.1 M phosphate buffer, and trypsin is added (1 mg/ml of the suspension). The mixture is incubated at 37° for 2 hours. A few drops of chloroform are added to prevent bacterial contamination. After the digestion, the cell walls are centrifuged and washed 3 times with 0.05 M phosphate buffer. The preparation may be further treated with ribonuclease (1 mg/ml) at 37° for 2 hours. After the digestion, the cell walls are washed several times with distilled water until no protein and nucleic acid is detectable in the washings at 280- and 254-nm wavelength.

The effectiveness of any physical or chemical method of cell-wall preparation must be checked by viewing or photographing the samples of disintegrated material in a phase-contrast or dark-field microscope or in an electron microscope, by studying the Gram-stained preparation under a light microscope, by applying a viable count-culture technique, or by studying the decrease of turbidity. For observation in an electron microscope, the cell-wall preparation should be suspended either in distilled water or in a volatile ammonium acetate, deposited on the formvar coated grids directly, by sedimenting or spraying. The preparations are then dried in air and shadowed with chromium. Alternatively, a "negative" staining with sodium phosphotungstate may be employed. In the phase-contrast or electron microscope, satisfactory cell-wall preparations appear in the form of homogenous, transparent membranes, 250 to 1000 nm in diameter (Fig. 11). Isolated cell walls or intact cells in unsatisfactory preparations are nontranslucent, dense, opaque, and granular. Viewed by dark-field illumination, the disintegrated cells are much less refractile than are the nonbroken cells. Gram-stained cell walls of disintegrated bacteria are only faintly colored.

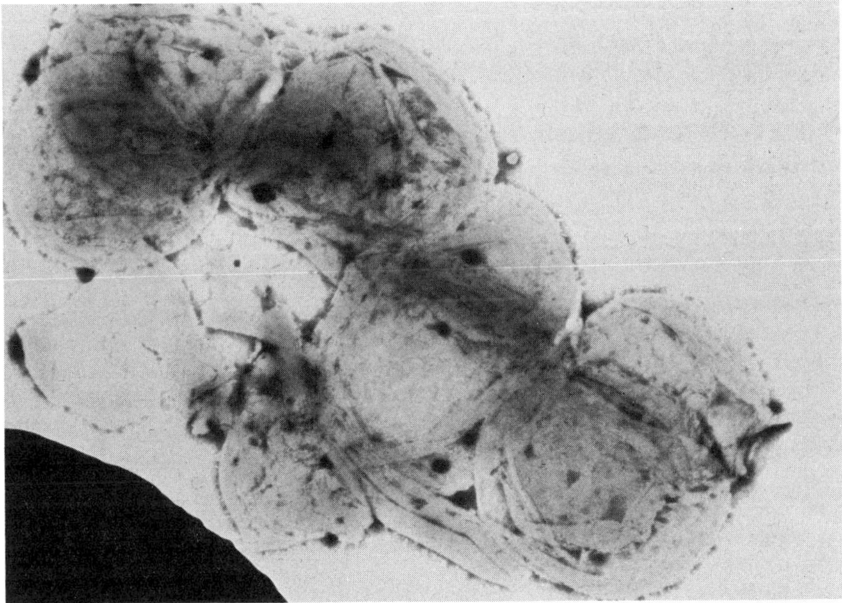

Figure 11.   Cell walls of a bacterium (25,920×).

Samples of the prepared microorganisms seeded onto suitable media will not yield any growth if the disintegration has been complete.

The decrease in turbidity is checked by withdrawing samples of the bacterial suspension undergoing disruption and making turbidimetric readings in a nephelometer or photometer. If a Klett-Summerson colorimeter is used it must be equipped with a 660-nm filter. The percentage of initial turbidity remaining after a time interval (IT%), which corresponds to the percentage of remaining intact cells, is calculated from the following equation (Ralston et al., 1961):

$$IT\% = U_t \cdot U_0 \times 100$$

where U_0 and U_t are Klett units at the beginning and at a time after the exposure of bacteria to a chemical or physical treatment.

8. *Preparation of Anatomical Components of Cytoplasm*

The cytoplasm consists of a structural network (endoplasmic reticulum) and a liquid portion, which in bacteria represent approximately one-third and two-thirds of the whole cytoplasm, respectively.

The cytoplasmic membrane represents between 10 and 15% of the dry weight of the bacterium, and it consists of protein (50 to 75%) and lipid (25 to 35%). Lipids contain triglycerides and phosphatides. The bacterial cytoplasmic membranes contain predominantly branched chain fatty acids. Occasionally, cytoplasmic membranes contain glucose and mannose and ribonucleic acid.

The liquid portion carries various granules, to include ribosomes, lysozymes, and nuclear bodies which are the chromatin-containing bodies in bacteria. Chromatin material is made of DNA in combination with protein. The DNA in bacteria represents up to 1 to 2% of the total dry weight of the bacteria. The RNA occurs mainly in a complex with protein, forming small particles or ribosomes. Ribosomal particles consist of 40 to 60% of RNA and 60 to 40% protein. Photosynthetic microorganisms possess chromoplasts in the cytoplasm, which consist of 40 to 50% protein and 20 to 30% lipid. Granules occurring in the cytoplasm may be either of lipid, or polymetaphosphate or polysaccharide in nature.

The liquid or soluble fraction or cell sap contains a considerable amount of protein, which may amount to 60 to 65% of the total dry weight of the liquid portion of cytoplasm, polysaccharides, and sometimes lipids. The cytoplasm also contains pools of low molecular weight compounds such as amino acids and nucleotides.

Mitochondria occurring in the microorganisms except bacteria and blue-green algae have the size ranging from 0.5×0.7 to $4.0\ \mu$ and they contain a high proportion of lipid and protein.

Particulate microcompounds of the plasm of animal and bacterial cells are separated most efficiently by a differential-gradient centrifugation.

The cytoplasmic or protoplast membrane may be separated by the technique of Vennes and Gerhardt (1956), and the protoplasts or spheroplasts by the method of Weibull (1953), Lederberg (1956), Smith et al. (1960), Freeman et al. (1963), or by other techniques cited on pp. 61–63. Techniques of the isolation of nuclear bodies and intracellular granules were published by Spiegelman et al. (1958) and Vennes and Gerhardt (1959), respectively, and a comprehensive method for the isolation of particulate cytoplasm constituents is presented on p. 38.

i. The Isolation of Cytoplasmic (Protoplast) Membrane. According to Vennes and Gerhardt (1956), a suspension of protoplasts, released from the cell walls by one of the methods described below and maintained in a phosphate-sucrose buffer, is treated with Versene (sodium-ethylene-diaminotetraacetic acid) at 0.01 M and with approximately 10 μg of deoxyribonuclease per milliliter. Protoplasts are disrupted in Versene during 30 minutes incubation at 37°, leaving intact protoplast membranes. The suspension should be centrifuged at 12,800 $\times$ *g* for 10 minutes; the pellet is washed once in saline solution and five times in distilled water. A similar method has been published by Carey and Baron (1959).

Viewed using a phase microscope, the protoplast membranes appear as delicate membranous structures. They can be lyzed by lipase. Preparations of cytoplasmic membranes from *Bacillus megaterium* contain 11% ribonucleic acid but no deoxyribonucleic acid.

ii. The Preparation of Protoplasts and Spheroplasts. Photoplasts can be formed in a culture medium containing an adequate concentration of penicillin or glycine (Jeynes, 1957). Alternatively, they may be released from cell walls by digestion of cells with muramidase (lysozyme) (Weibull, 1953), a fungal acetyl-hexosaminidase (Hash et al., 1964), or the snail gut juice (Svihla et al., 1961), or by complement lysis in the presence of a specific antiserum (Freeman et al., 1963). Protoplasts of certain bacteria are prepared more readily by the combined action of lysozyme and ethylenediaminotetraacetic acid (EDTA).

Protoplasts are osmotically fragile bodies, and they should be stabilized by addition of sucrose at a hypertonic concentration. An adequate protoplast-stabilizing solution contains 0.5 *M* sucrose, 0.6 *M* KCl, and 0.04 *M* sodium phosphate. Protoplasts are disintegrated by distilled water, sonic vibrations, or the ultraviolet irradiation.

Protoplast formation in the presence of penicillin is ascribed to inhibition of the biosynthesis of the cell wall. Crystalline penicillin should be added in a concentration of approximately 1000 units/ml to a culture of bacteria in 10 to 20% sucrose broth. The addition of 0.2% magnesium sulfate is sometimes advantageous. Gram-negative bacteria yield 100% protoplasts in 4 hours under these conditions (Welsch and Osterrieth, 1958). Protoplasts of certain bacteria can be obtained at a lower concentration of penicillin, for example, 50 units/ml, dissolved in a culture medium containing sucrose at 0.32 to 0.48 M (Hahn and Ciak, 1957). Protoplasts of various gram-negative bacteria are formed in the presence of $M/2$ to $M/1$ or 3% glycine in the culture media containing 0.2 M sucrose. More sensitive bacteria lose their cell walls in a few hours' incubation at 34° (Jeynes, 1957).

Techniques for the preparation of spheroplasts were devised by Mitchell and Moyle (1951), Weibull (1953), Lederberg (1956), Zinder and Arndt (1956), Dark and Strange (1957), Smith et al. (1960), Snoke (1961), Svihla et al. (1961), Freeman et al. (1963), Hash et al. (1964), and Kakefuda et al. (1967).

Weibull's Technique. A mature population of bacteria is centrifuged, washed with saline, resuspended in a sucrose-phosphate buffer, and treated with 0.1 mg/ml of lysozyme until a complete conversion of bacterial cells to spherical forms occurs. The protoplast formation can be observed under a cover glass using a dark-phase contrast microscope and a 1000 magnification. The protoplasts are then centrifuged for 20 minutes at 1000 × g and carefully washed twice in a sucrose-phosphate buffer.

Zinder's Technique, Modified by Smith et al. (1960). Washed bacteria are suspended in 1.0 M Tris-hydroxymethylamino-methane buffer, pH 9.0, containing 20% sucrose and 0.2% magnesium sulfate. After 20 minutes standing at room temperature, 0.5 mg/ml of lysozyme is added, and the mixture is left for a further 10 minutes. The yield and extent of conversion to spheres is checked periodically by withdrawing 1-ml samples of the material, diluting with three volumes of distilled water, and examining under the phase-contrast or interference microscope.

The extent of conversion to protoplasts can also be estimated by measuring a change in the optical density after lysis, using the modified technique of Hurwitz et al. (1958). In this procedure, a 1-ml sample of prepared cell suspension is added to 3 ml of distilled water, then further diluted with another 3 ml of water at 56°, and heated at 56° for 4 minutes to lyse the protoplasts; the nonchanged cells remain intact. The optical density of the lyzates measured at 660 nm is compared with a control suspension that has not been treated with lysozyme. If the yield of spheroplasts proves to be sufficient, the whole mixture is diluted with three volumes of distilled water.

The Freeman et al. Technique. The conversion of bacteria (*Vibrio comma*) to protoplasts in this technique depends on the presence of a specific antibody and complement. Thus the bacteria are suspended in a pH 8.0 physiological saline to a concentration of 1×10^9 cells/ml; 1 ml of complement and 1 ml of a specific hyperimmune serum, diluted 1:5 and 1:5000, respectively, and 2 ml of saline are added to 1 ml of the suspension of bacteria. (It is advisable to add sucrose to 0.5 M concentration for osmotic protection of protoplasts.) This mixture is incubated at 37° for 2 hours. Samples are withdrawn at 5- to 10-minute intervals, and protoplasts are observed in wet mounts under oil immersion by medium-dark phase microscopy, using a green filter. Conversion of bacterial cells to protoplasts starts in about 30 minutes and is complete in 60 to 90 minutes.

According to Kakefuda's et al. (1967) technique, the bacterial cells obtained from an early experimental phase of culture growth are incubated at 37° with muranidase (lysozyme) in 0.03 M Tris (hydroxymethyl)-aminomethane chloride (pH 6.3) containing 0.8 M sucrose (using 10 μg of the enzyme per 1 mg of cells). After 60 to 70 minutes of the incubation, the mixture is centrifuged successively at 300 × g, 1150 × g, and 14,000 × g. The spheroplasts are sedimented at 14,000 × g. The spheroplasts may be stabilized for electron-microscopic studies with 0.5% osmic acid in 0.8 M sucrose containing 0.03 M Tris (pH 6.3) and 0.01 N $CaCl_2$. The spheroplasts are treated with this solution in the cold for 2 minutes, and then centrifuged at 900 × g. The pellet is resuspended in the sucrose-osmic acid fixative and left at 4° overnight. The cells are then washed and treated with 0.5% solution of uranyl acetate for 2 hours. The material is finally centrifuged, dehydrated with graded acetone and propylene glycol and embedded in epoxy resin for sectioning.

Selection of a protoplast or spheroplast-preparation technique is greatly influenced by the physiocochemical structure of microorganisms. The Kakefuda's et al. and Smith's et al. techniques are generally the most efficient.

iii. *The Isolation of Nuclear Bodies.* Nuclear bodies are isolated according to the Spiegelman et al. (1958) method by treating protoplasts suspended in a succinate buffer with a commercial preparation of lipase, purified from contaminating enzymes by extraction with 10% sodium chloride and saturation with magnesium sulfate at 0°. Lipase should be added to the protoplast suspension at a final concentration of 40 to 50 μg/ml of protein. The nuclear bodies are separated from the lyzate by centrifugation at 10,000 × g for 5 minutes. The nonchromatinic center or core of nuclear bodies may be isolated from this material by washing the nuclear bodies twice with 10% sodium chloride which disperses the deoxyribonucleic acid, surrounding the nonchromatinic core.

Ribosome Isolation. Whole ribosomes may be isolated from animal cells by Wettstein's et al. (1963) method, and purified by precipitation with 0.05 M Mg^{++} as described by Takanami (1960). The ribosome protein may be separated from nucleic acid by urea and LiCl according to Spitnik-Elson's (1965) technique.

Ribosome Preparation. According to Wettstein's et al. (1963) method, the initial step is the homogenization of the cells in Hoagland's et al. (1958) medium. The medium consists of 0.005 M magnesium chloride, and 0.25 M sucrose. The homogenate is centrifuged at 15,000 $\times$ g at 0° for 10 minutes to remove mitochondria, nuclei, and cell debris (Korner, 1961); 1.3% sodium deoxycholate is added to the supernatant fluid. The supernatant is layered on a sucrose gradient, consisting of 3 ml or more of concentrated 1.5 or 1.8 M sucrose solution, overlayered with 4 ml of 0.5 M sucrose. The tubes are centrifuged at 105,000 $\times$ g for 4 hours. The transparent pellet containing ribosomes is then collected, dissolved in Hoagland's medium containing no sucrose, and clarified by low-speed centrifugation.

iv. *The Isolation of Intracellular Granules.* Intracellular granules present within the protoplasts can be isolated according to the technique of Vennes and Gerhardt (1959) by treating the protoplasts suspended in a sucrose-phosphate buffer with Versene and deoxyribonuclease. Versene used in a 0.01 M solution fixes membranes, and deoxyribonuclease prevents the resulting suspension from becoming viscous. The treated material is left overnight at 5°, then centrifuged at 12,800 $\times$ g for 30 minutes to remove membranes and lipid granules. The supernatant should be recentrifuged at 21,700 $\times$ g for 30 minutes. The pellet of small particles is suspended in saline. The isolation of chromatophores, large spherical molecules, about 600 Å in diameter, which seem to carry pigments of microorganisms can be attempted by an ultracentrifugal method (Schachman et al., 1952, 1954). The sedimentation constant of chromatophores of *Rhodospirillum* was estimated at 200 S.

v. *Isolation of Cytoplasmic Constituents of Mammalian Cells.* The cytoplasm, released from cells by physical disintegration and removal of cell debris on centrifugation, is placed in a Tris HCl buffer, pH 7.2, with sucrose added to a final concentration of 0.25 M (8.5% w/w) to maintain isotonicity and with 0.01 M $MgCl_2$ added to preserve ribosomes. This material is layered over a sucrose gradient which starts at 10% (w/w), 1.04 g/ml density. (If the sample has been prepared without sucrose, the sucrose gradient may start at 5% sucrose.) The gradient is formed using sucrose concentration ranging from 10 to 40% or preferably the 10 to 40% sucrose gradient is placed above a cushion of 50% sucrose to prevent pelleting of most substances on the rotor wall.

The moving-zone procedure is often preceded by a few steps of differential centrifugation to pellet successfully lower and lower S-rate classes. The resuspended pellet is contaminated with all the other components, but is found useful to concentrate certain classes of particles prior to the moving-zone centrifugation.

Nuclei are obtained by moving-zone centrifugation in a dextran gradient extending from 0 to 30% *w/w* dextran in 0.25 *M* sucrose and 0.006 *M* CaCl$_2$.

Soluble proteins, microsomes, polysomes, and ribosomes are obtained by a moving-zone procedure in 10 to 30% sucrose gradient in the presence of MG^{++} which preserve the ribosomes on the microsomes. Polysomes and ribosomes are obtained by moving-zone centrifugation in a shallow sucrose gradient extending from 13 to 20% at 240,000 × *g*.

9. *Isolation of Endospores and Endospore membranes*

Endospores of bacteria may be obtained by leaving the fully grown spore-forming bacteria at room temperature for several weeks. Vegetative cells in these circumstances undergo autolysis, leaving free endospores. The process of sporulation is quicker in Stewart and Halvorson's (1953) "G" medium (see p. 13). Spores are harvested by foam separation or centrifugation, washed repeatedly with distilled water, stained by Dorner's method, and examined in a light microscope, or observed unstained in a phase-contrast microscope. Only endospores, spherical, or ellipsoidal in shape, should be found.

Endospores may be released from the sporangia of certain bacteria by mechanical disintegration, with subsequent selective centrifugation and filtration (Izumi, 1959). In this technique, bacterial cells disintegrated in a T-1 or T-2 type bacterial cell disintegrator are first centrifuged at 200 × *g* for 5 to 8 minutes. The supernatant is then centrifuged at 500–700 × *g* rpm for 10 minutes and passed through a glass filter No. 3 and recentrifuged first at 700–1000 × *g* for 10 minutes, and finally at 3000–5000 × *g* for 30 minutes. The sediment obtained from this final centrifugation contains endospores, which should be washed in a phosphate buffer, pH 7.2, and recentrifuged at 5000 × *g* for 30 minutes.

The Separation of Endospore Membranes.   The contents of spores can be released by sonic disruption in a Raytheon 10-kHz sonic oscillator at 0 to 8° in a gaseous atmosphere of hydrogen (Berger and Marr, 1960). Spores should be suspended in 0.05 *M* phosphate buffer, pH 6.8, at an approximate concentration of 3 × 10^9 spores/ml. The disintegration of spores may be judged by testing the sedimentation ability of the treated material at 10,000 × *g* for 15 minutes. Under these circumstances, the residual spore sediment and the disrupted spores remain in suspension.

Endospore membranes can be separated from the internal contents of spores by disintegration in a sonic oscillator, a Mickle disintegrator, or a reciprocating shaker at 0°. Alternatively, a T-1 or T-2 bacterial cell disintegrator at 800 cycles in 50 minutes, followed by selective centrifugation (Yoshida et al., 1957; Salton and Marshall, 1959; Izumi, 1959), may be used. The speed of centrifugation is gradually increased from 150 $\times$ g for 10 minutes to 1500 $\times$ g for 15 minutes and to 15,000 $\times$ g for 20 minutes. The supernatant obtained at this stage contains the endospore cytoplasm while the sediment contains endospore membrane. The endospore membranes are then washed, first in a phosphate buffer, pH 7.2, and twice in distilled water with the centrifugation at 15,000 $\times$ g and 30,000 $\times$ g, respectively.

The Salton and Marshall (1959) Technique. Spores, washed three times with distilled water, are crushed by shaking for 2 hours with "Ballotini" beads (0.13-mm diameter) on a reciprocating shaker at 0°. The spore membranes are washed with distilled water and centrifuged. The spore walls are then digested for 2 hours at 37° with trypsin (1 mg of trypsin is used per milliliter of a spore membrane suspension in 0.1 M phosphate buffer, pH 8.0).

The Strange and Dark (1956) Technique. Spore suspensions are disintegrated with "Ballotini" beads No. 12 in a Mickle disintegrator for 15 to 30 minutes. Three drops of capryl alcohol are added to each vessel. The effectiveness of the disintegration procedure is monitored by the examination of stained films. When all the spores are ruptured, the suspension is centrifuged in an angle centrifuge at 1400 $\times$ g for 15 minutes. The sediment is washed three times in 1 M NaHCO$_3$, twice in water, three times in 1 N HCl, and three times in water to remove any material adhering to the coats. The washed spore membranes should be dried over sulfuric acid in a vacuum desiccator.

Electron microscope studies reveal that the endospore membrane is a complex morphological structure consisting of exosporium, outer coat, and inner coat (Izumi, 1959). Precise study of the antigenic structure of the endospore membrane will not be possible, until microtechniques for the separation of these individual anatomical constituents are devised.

The spore-coat material represents 20 to 35% of the total dried weight of spores. Spores isolated from various species of bacilli by Strange and Dark (1956) contained 13.0% nitrogen, 2 to 15% hexosamine, and 1.0 to 2.8% ash.

10. Isolation of Mitochondria

The following two methods are very suitable for the preparation of mitochondria.

According to the procedure described by Krawiec and Eisenstadt (1970), the mitochondria are obtained through the disruption of cells in a French pressure cell at less than 1200 psi, and by differential centrifugation, which finally yields the 10,000 $\times$ g pellet as a source of crude mitochondria. The mitochondria are purified in gradients of Renograsin (Squibb, New York).

Renograsin is substituted for sucrose since it does not adversely affect biochemical activities of materials, which are sometimes destroyed by sucrose. Linear, continuous, 20 to 50% Renograsin gradients containing 0.01 M Tris HCl (pH 7.4) and 0.1 mM EDTA are layered above the sample. The preparations are centrifuged at 20,000 to 22,000 rpm for 2 to 7 hours at 2°. Fractions are collected by piercing the nitrocellulose tube.

According to the method of Stutz and Noll (1967), the mitochondria are obtained from plant leaves in the following manner: The leaves are first washed in cold distilled water and homogenized for 30 seconds in a Waring Blender in a cold sucrose buffer consisting of 0.7 M sucrose, 0.1 M Tris HCl, pH 7.4, 0.005 M $MgCl_2$, 0.05 M KCl, and 0.005 M 2-mercaptoethanol. The homogenate is filtered through several layers of gauze and the filtrate is centrifuged at 600 $\times$ g for 2 minutes to remove nuclei and cell debris. Centrifugation at 1100 $\times$ g for 12 minutes results in pelleting chloroplasts whereas the supernatant contains cytoplasmic ribosomes and mitochondria. The chloroplasts are washed several times in the buffer above and centrifuged. The mitochondria are obtained from the supernatant that remained after the pelleting of crude mitochondria, by the centrifugation at 26,000 $\times$ g for 30 minutes. In the supernatant are present ribosomes and polysomes which must be purified by a sucrose gradient centrifugation. For this purpose, the supernatant containing ribosomes and polysomes is layered over 1 M sucrose in a hypotonic buffer consisting of 0.01 M Tris HCl, pH 7.5, enriched with 0.005 M $MgCl_2$, 0.05 M KCl, and 0.005 M 2-mercaptoethanol. The gradient is centrifuged in a Spinco-40 rotor at 40 Krpm for $2\frac{1}{2}$ hours at 2°, and ribosomes are recovered from a yellowish pellet.

IV. EXTRACTION OF SOLUBLE ANTIGENS FROM CELLS AND TISSUES

Non-particulate antigens are either secreted by cells into the environment, are released upon cell disintegration, or may be extracted from cells, tissues and organs and their particulate constituents.

1. Extraction of Cell-Wall Antigens

Methods for the isolation of antigenic components occurring in the microbial cell walls were published by Webster et al. (1955), Vennes and Gerhardt (1959), Kwapinski (1960, 1965), and Kwapinski and Snyder (1961).

Amino acids and monoses obtained from the cell walls and whole cells of different groups of microorganisms have shown distinctive chromatographic patterns (Kwapinski and Merkel, 1957; Cummins and Harris, 1958). Various types of microbial species were differentiated by the chromatographic patterns of polysaccharide fractions, isolated from whole or disintegrated mycelia (Kwapinski and Merkel, 1957). Microorganisms can also be chemically differentiated by relative proportions of higher carboxylic acids, as separated by the gas chromatography (Abel et al., 1963).

Webster's technique for isolation of the polysaccharide component depends on extraction of the cell walls with 0.5 M trichloracetic acid for 2 hours at 5°. The extract is then fractionated with ethyl alcohol.

Vennes and Gerhardt's technique is used to obtain polypeptides from cells walls or cells. The cell walls are solubilized with lysozyme added in the concentration of 0.1 mg/ml of 0.03 M phosphate buffer, pH 7.0. After incubation, the particulate material is removed by centrifugation. The supernatant should be dialyzed against distilled water. The phase, containing protein, is separated from the benzene phase in a separatory funnel, and the protein is precipitated with 10% trichloracetic or acetic acid. Purified lipids can be recovered from the benzene phase by evaporation of the solvent. This treatment can be repeated if necessary.

Polysaccharides may be detached from the lipids in the following manner. The fraction is dissolved in ether and mixed with an equal volume of 10% acetic acid. The mixture is shaken in a separatory funnel for 4 hours and left to separate into two layers. Polysaccharides are precipitated from the aqueous phase with a 3:1 mixture of acetone and ethyl alcohol, whereas the purified lipids are recovered from the etheric layer.

In an alternative procedure for the isolation of polysaccharides from lipid fractions (Geiger and Anderson, 1939), a benzene-insoluble fraction is suspended in water, acidified with acetic acid, and extracted with ether. The ether-soluble extract is then washed with water until the washing becomes neutral against litmus. The aqueous solution and washings are now combined and concentrated in vacuo to a syrupy consistency, then treated with 95% ethyl alcohol. The sedimented gum-like mass containing carbohydrates should be collected by centrifugation, washed with alcohol, and evaporated in vacuo.

Most bacterial or fungal pigments are dissolved in the organic solvents with the lipid fractions. Some pigments remain attached to the nucleoprotein or polysaccharide fractions of the cell or mycelial walls, and these can sometimes polypeptide is precipitated from the dialyzate by saturation with ammonium sulfate at pH 7.0, which is maintained by the addition of 1.0 M potassium pyrophosphate. The precipitate is collected by centrifugation, resuspended in 0.03 M phosphate buffer at pH 7.0, and dialyzed against a buffer until the test for sulfates is negative.

Kwapinski's Technique for Preparing Cell-Wall Antigens. The cell walls are extracted with a 1.5:1 mixture of ether and ethyl alcohol, and finally with chloroform to separate the lipids (Table 14). The extraction can be conducted either on an electric shaker at 2° for 12 to 24 hours or in a

Table 14. Diagram of the Preparation of Somatic Antigen Fractions (Kwapinski, 1965)

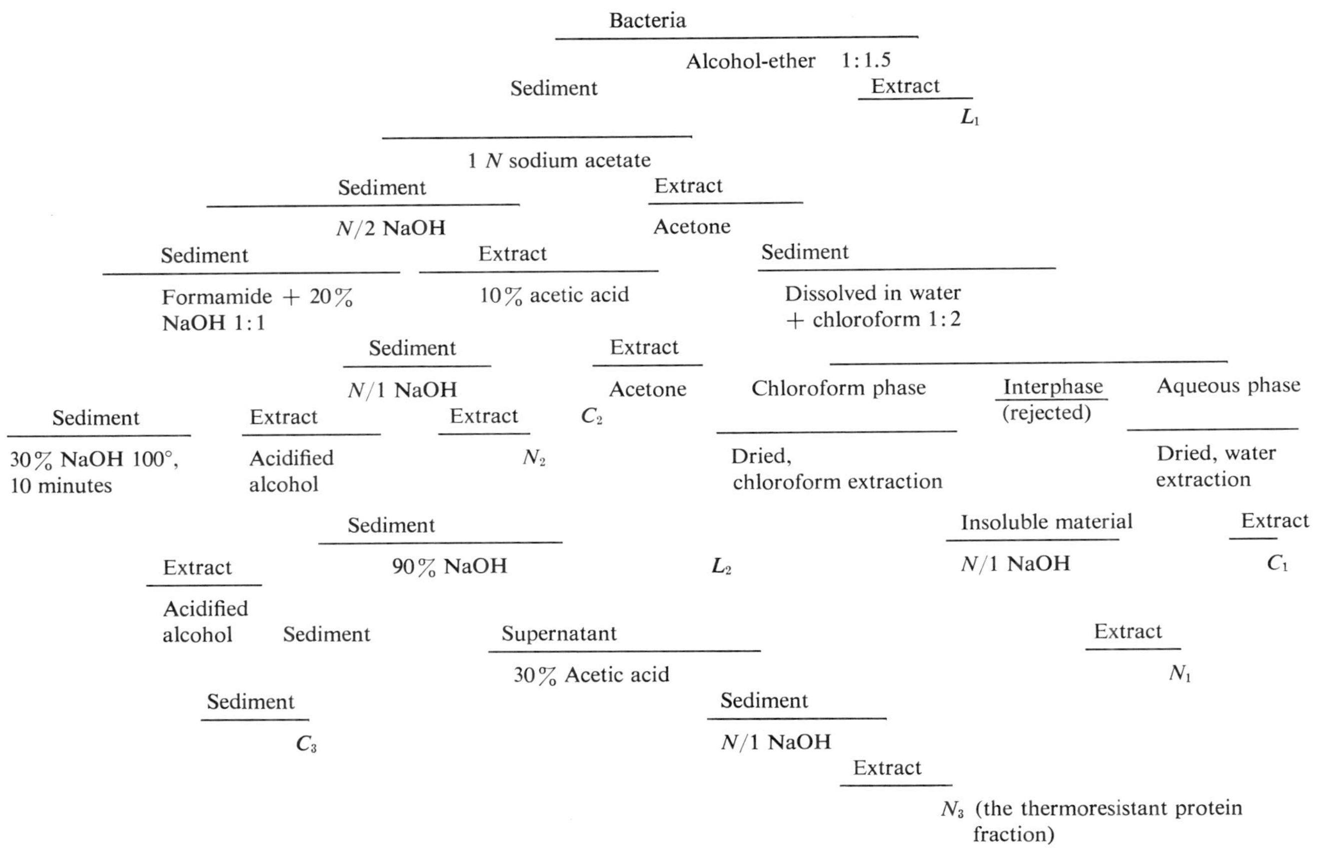

Bacteria
Alcohol-ether 1:1.5
Sediment | Extract
L_1

1 N sodium acetate
Sediment | Extract
$N/2$ NaOH | Acetone
Sediment | Extract | Sediment
Formamide + 20% NaOH 1:1 | 10% acetic acid | Dissolved in water + chloroform 1:2

Sediment | Extract
$N/1$ NaOH | Acetone | Chloroform phase | Interphase (rejected) | Aqueous phase
Sediment | Extract | Extract | C_2
30% NaOH 100°, 10 minutes | Acidified alcohol | N_2 | Dried, chloroform extraction | Dried, water extraction
Insoluble material | Extract
Extract | Sediment | $N/1$ NaOH | C_1
Acidified alcohol | 90% NaOH | L_2

Acidified alcohol | Sediment | Supernatant | Extract
30% Acetic acid | N_1
Sediment | Sediment
C_3 | $N/1$ NaOH
Extract
N_3 (the thermoresistant protein fraction)

Soxhlet apparatus in a 50° water bath for 4 to 5 hours. The extract is separated from the residual material by filtration through a Schott G5 filter, and the residue is washed with ether. The extract containing lipids should be concentrated and dried by blowing off the solvents with a stream of nitrogen or by distillation at 50° under reduced atmospheric pressure.

Lipid fractions obtained from the ether-alcohol extracts may have the consistency of stearin, wax, or petroleum jelly, and colors varying from white to yellow, orange, brown, pink, and reddish-brown, depending on the presence and quantity of pigments bound with the lipids. Pure lipid fractions, however, are usually in the form of white stearin flakes. Protein, polysaccharide, or pigment impurities can be removed from the lipids in the following manner. To detach proteins from the lipids, the isolated fraction is first dissolved in benzene and extracted for 6 hours with an equal volume of 0.5 N solution of sodium hydroxide in 45% ethyl alcohol. The alcohol be separated by repeated extractions with ether and alcohol and then precipitated by diluting the extracts with water. Other firmly bound pigments can be separated only after treatment with concentrated acids at temperatures exceeding 50°, which may cause deterioration of the antigenic potency of the fractions. As molecules of known bacterial pigments are small it seems unlikely that they are antigenic, but this question still remains open for study. Methods for partition of certain pigments was described by Mathews and Sistrom (1959) and Starr and Stephens (1964); see pp. 82 and 83.

The next stage in the immunochemical preparation, after the delipidization of cell or mycelial walls, consists of a stepwise isolation of polysaccharide fractions with sodium acetate or acetic acid, the extraction of proteins and nucleoproteins, and the isolation of firmly bound polysaccharide fractions with alkali or formamide. Details of this part of the preparation are as follows.

The delipidized cell or mycelial walls are first extracted with 1 M sodium acetate for 12 hours. The extract is separated from the residue by centrifugation, filtered, and treated with four volumes of cold acetone. The precipitate containing a crude polysaccharide fraction (C_2) is liberated from the protein impurities by boiling for 5 minutes with 5% acetic acid, followed by filtration and reprecipitation of the purified polysaccharide with cold acetone. The material, from which fraction C_2 has been isolated, is now extracted in the cold with 0.5 N NaOH for 6 hours. The extract containing a polysaccharide-protein complex or a crude protein fraction is filtered and mixed with four volumes of cold acetone. The precipitate is collected, re-extracted in 0.5 N NaOH, and the extract is treated with 10% TCA. The resultant precipitate should be purified by extraction in 1 M sodium acetate. The polysaccharide then dissolves, but impurities remain in suspension and are removed by centrifugation at 7000 $\times$ g. The supernatant is dialyzed and lyophilized (Fig. 12) to yield the fraction C_3.

The residue of cell or mycelial walls is now extracted in 90% phenol, in which certain proteins and polysaccharides dissolve. The extract separated by centrifugation is filtered and treated with 1% cold solution of hydrochloric acid in acetone, added in twofold or threefold volume. The resulting light brown precipitate should be centrifugel or separated by filtration, and dialyzed to remove phenol and other micromolecular substances. If the sediment has dissolved during the dialysis, it should be precipitated with 1% solution of hydrochloric acid in acetone. According to the species of microorganisms, these complexes consist predominantly of either a protein or a polysaccharide. Crude preparations of these "amphoteric" complexes behave characteristically in the solubility tests. They produce turbid or opalescent suspensions in water. The turbidity decreases following the drop-wise addition of 0.5 N NaOH up to about pH 11, but above this pH level the turbidity returns. The latter can be prevented by stepwise addition of 25% acetic acid, as the "amphoteric complexes" seem to dissolve at a higher ionic concentration. Separation of the constituents of these complexes is difficult. However, it can be accomplished by repeated extraction of the sediment containing the crude "amphoteric complex," using 1 N NaOH alternating with 50% acetic acid. The alkaline extract is treated with 10% TCA, yielding a precipitate of crude (nucleo)protein fraction which is purified by another extraction in 1 N NaOH, precipitation with 10% TCA, and dialysis. In this way, the (nucleo) protein fraction of the cell or mycelial walls of certain bacteria can be obtained. The extract of "amphoteric complexes" in 50% hot acetic acid should be cooled and centrifuged, and the supernatant fluid treated with three volumes of acetone. A crude polysaccharide fraction then precipitates; this fraction must be purified by boiling 5 minutes in 10% acetic acid at 100°. The fluid is liberated from any solid particles by centrifugation at 15,000 $\times$ g for 10 minutes, then dialyzed, and lyophilized to yield polysaccharide fraction C_4.

Polysaccharides and some proteins or polypeptides occurring in the cell walls of the *Eubacteriales* can be extracted rather easily by the solvents presented, and with this the fractionation is usually concluded. In contrast, cell walls of the *Actinomycetales* and mycelial walls of microfungi include some resistant polysaccharides containing nitrogen and sulfur; and these carbohydrates can be extracted only by more drastic means, which often may reduce or intefere with the antigenic potency of the isolated fractions.

In this final stage of fractionation, the residual material of cell or mycelial walls is extracted for 30 minutes in 30% sodium hydroxide at 100° and centrifuged. The sediment is left for further fractionation. The extract is dialyzed and treated with four volumes of a 1:1 mixture of acetone and

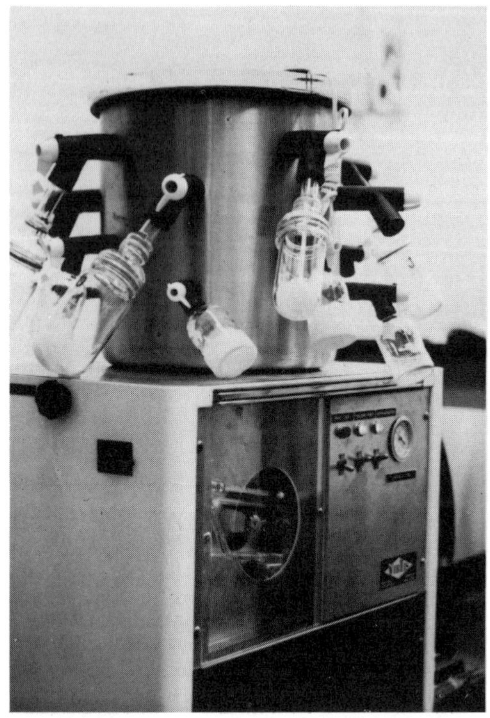

Figure 12. Lyophilizer (freeze-drier), consisting of a vacuum pump unit and a manifold to which the frozen sample containers are attached.

alcohol, and left overnight at 2°. A flocculant precipitate appears which is centrifuged, dissolved in 100 ml of distilled water, acidified if required, filtered, dialyzed, and lyophilized to yield the polysaccharide fractions C_5. The residual material of cell or mycelial walls is extracted for 15 minutes with formamide at 100 to 120° in a paraffin oil bath. The extract is filtered and mixed with three volumes of acetone to precipitate a polysaccharide fraction C_6.

The cell- and mycelial walls of almost all bacteria are completely fractionated at this stage, but some fungi still contain a residual cell-wall material resistant to the foregoing extractions. The polymerized substances which cannot be extracted with strong, concentrated solutions of alkali or acids show physicochemical properties similar to those of cellulose or chitin. Some of them, for example, those occurring in the mycelia of *Trichophyton gypseum,* can be extracted with Schweitzer's reagent and precipitated with concentrated hydrochloric acid. The copper ion originating from the reagent, which is responsible for a greenish blue coloration of extracted material, can be removed by saturation of the fraction suspended in 10% solution of sodium hydroxide with hydrogen sulfite. The chitin is not entirely soluble, but it may be purified when suspended in 2 *N* NaOH and boiled at 100° for 15 minutes. After centrifugation, the supernatant fluid containing negligible impurities should be discarded, and the sediment dialyzed and lyophilized.

Soluble antigen preparations may be separated either from the whole cytoplasm or from individual anatomical components such as cytoplasmic membrane, protoplast, nuclear bodies, intracellular granules, structural cystoplasmic network, cytoplasmic inclusions, and vacuoles. Some of the structural cell components may appear at a specific stage of the individual development of microbial cells; and investigations on these components may provide interesting data on immunoontogenesis of bacteria.

2. Preparation of Cytoplasm Antigens.

The first step in preparing cytoplasmic antigens is to release the cytoplasm from the cell walls and possibly from the cytoplasmic membrane. This can be achieved by (a) mechanical rupture of cells and subsequent removal of the cell-wall fragments, (b) the isolation of protoplasts, and (c) the cultivation of microorganisms in the presence of substances, such as penicillin, which inhibit or prevent the development of cell walls (Lederberg, 1956; Park and Strominger, 1957; Hahn and Ciak, 1957).

According to Kwapinski and Alcasid's (1970) technique, bacterial cells, treated with 1% formalin at 25° for 16 hours, are collected by centrifugation at 10,000 × *g* for 15 minutes in the model B-20 International Refrigerated Centrifuge. The bacteria are washed six times with distilled water, and then resuspended in a five times larger volume of a 10^{-3}-*M* solution of EDTA, pH 7.15, containing 1:100,000 Thimerosal, and disrupted in the Raytheon oscillator at 9 kHz or in the Biosonik III ultrasonicator at 20 kHz for 15 minutes. After the disintegration, the cell debris is removed by centrifugation at 5000 × *g* for 10 minutes. The supernatant is collected and recentrifuged at the same speed for 10 minutes one or more times, until no particulate material is found microscopically in smears prepared from the supernatant. The supernatant collected after the last centrifugation is adjusted approximately to the transmittance of 0.5 as measured at 350-nm wavelength in a spectrophotometer. This material represents a cytoplasm preparation and is used for the antiserum production and the immunodiffusion test.

Preparation of Endotoxic Complexes. The technique by Ribi et al. (1959), used originally for the extraction of endotoxin (antigen O) of the *Enterobacteriaceae,* is applied as follows. Bacterial cells, washed with saline, are suspended in 0.15 *M* NaCl and extracted with ethyl ether for 12 to

16 hours, and left in a separatory funnel. The aqueous phase should be collected and the residual ether removed by bubbling air through the suspension. The aqueous phase is then dialyzed against distilled water or treated directly at 4° with 71% alcohol by volume. The precipitate is separated by centrifugation at 2000 × g for 45 minutes, washed with alcohol, and dried in vacuo. The endotoxin can also be precipitated and purified by adding ammonium sulfate to full saturation at 4°.

3. Preparation of Boivin-Type Antigens

Boivin-type antigens are lipopolysaccharide-protein-lipid complexes. These substances can be isolated from various bacteria by the extraction with trichloracetic acid (Freeman et al., 1940), diethylene glycol (Davies et al., 1954), or by tryptic digestion (Topley et al., 1937).

In the first type of procedure, dried bacteria are suspended in five times their weight of cold distilled water and shaken at 0° for 3 hours with an equal volume of ice-cold 0.1 to 0.5 N trichloracetic acid. After centrifugation at 12,000 to 16,000 × g, the supernatant is dialyzed against running water, then centrifuged, and filtered through an L2 Chamberland candle. The filtrate is concentrated in vacuo and treated with ethyl alcohol added to the 68% concentration. The precipitate should be washed with ethyl alcohol and ether and dried *in vacuo* over phosphorus pentoxide.

The Isolation and Purification of Immunochemical Components of Cytoplasm (Kwapinski et al., 1971). The cytoplasm material obtained by Kwapinski and Alcasid's (1971) method is divided into two parts, the particulate and nonparticulate material by centrifugation at 104,000 × g for 15 minutes. The particulate material, containing ribosomes, chromatophores, cytoplasmic inclusions, the cytoplasmic fibrillar network, and the debris of the cytoplasmic membrane are collected with the sediment. Chemical and antigenic components may be extracted from these structural materials by the methods described on pp. 67–73.

The liquid portion of cytoplasm contains a number of heteropolymers that are separated by a successive application of the electrofocusing and polyacrylamide electrophoresis or a gel chromatography on Sephadex G-100 or G-150 and polyacrylamide electrophoresis. Usually the initial separation of different polymers is attained by the application of the electrofocusing using ampholytes in the range of pH 3 to 10. The fractions are collected and monitored at 280, 254 nm and 210 nm by a Duall-Beam UV Analyzer equipped with a built-in recorder to detect peptide linkages, nucleic-acid-cytosine, and aromatic proteins, respectively.

The materials collected from peak zones (Fig. 13) are dialyzed at 4° against distilled water for 48 to 72 hours, concentrated by lyophilization (Fig. 12) and purified by a preparative polyacrylamide-gel electrophoresis (p. 90). Normally, a 7.5% acrylamide gel in 6 M urea, pH 9.5 is

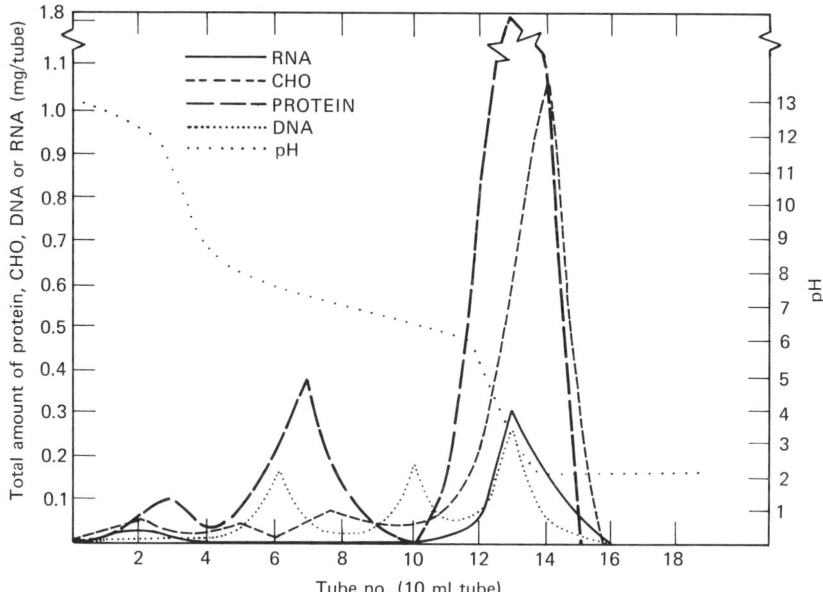

Figure 13.   A graph presenting the separation of different polymer categories by the isoelectrofocusing procedure.

used, and a current of 30 mA, increased to 80 mA after 1 hour, is applied. Fractions are again collected in an automatic fraction collector, monitored, and recorded automatically as above. The fractions, dialyzed at 4° against distilled water for 48 hours and concentrated 10 to 20 times by lyophilization, are also examined for the presence of carbohydrates with an alpha-naphthol reagent (Dische, 1955) and measured at 480 nm in a spectro-photometer equipped with an automatic recorder.

The phospholipids, if present in a cytoplasm preparation, are extracted with a 3:9:1 mixture of ether, acetone and ethyl alcohol, at 70° for 10 hours.

The process of separation and purification of different polymer categories present in the cytoplasm is controlled by Kwapinski's (1972) comprehensive polyacrylamide disk electrophoresis (p. 138), applying similar quantities of the initial material and of fractions separated at peak zones (Fig. 14). The chemical identity and homogeneity of the polymers thus obtained are revealed by specific staining methods (pp. 142–147).

Immunological activities and homogeneity of the materials are investigated by means of one or more different immunodiffusion techniques (e.g., in the cellulose-acetate membrane and in an agarose gel) and by an im-munodisc electrophoresis procedure. The antigens are examined against the

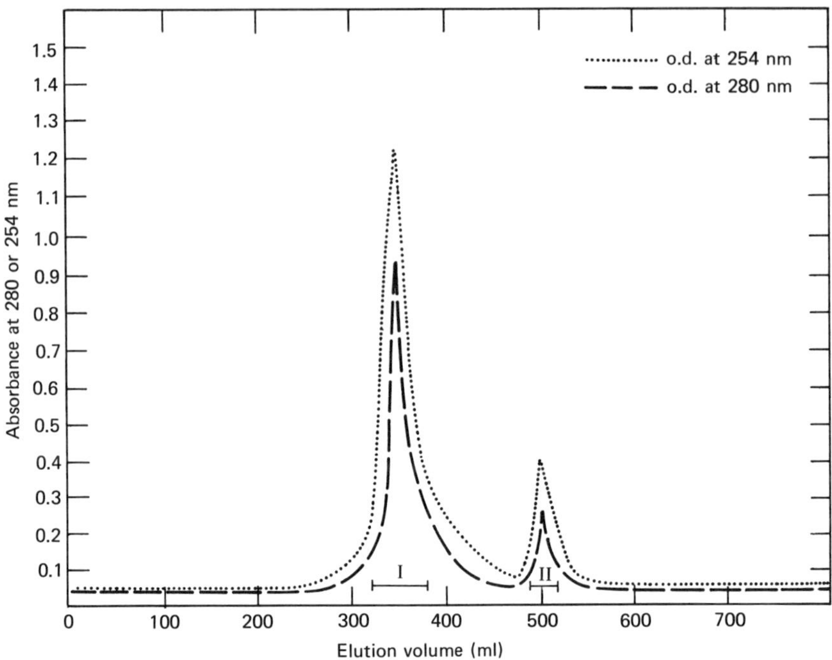

Figure 14. A graph representing the separation of nucleoproteins by the preparative polyacrylamide-gel electrophoresis.

antisera produced against the initial material and the individual purified fractions.

4. Preparation of Lipid Antigens

The most comprehensive methods of lipid fractionation are those of Anderson et al. (1940), Table 15, Williams and Dubos (1959), and Folch et al. (1957) for total lipids, Geiger and Anderson (1939) for "firmly bound" lipids, and Westphal et al. (1952) or Johnson (1955) for lipopolysaccharides. The Rothstein and Hiatt (1956) and Blumer's et al. (1969) techniques for isolating lipid antigens from bacteria are also recommended. An interesting method of extraction and gas chromatography of lipids was described by Abel et al. (1963).

Williams' and Dubos' technique of lipid preparation, used originally for the isolation and fractionation of lipids from mycobacteria, is presented diagrammatically in Table 16. Lipid fractions obtained by this method may be divided into subfractions according to one of the following procedures. First, the fractions, diluted or suspended in water, are treated with ethanol added to 33% volume concentration and precipitated in the presence of

Table 15.   Scheme of the Fractionation of Lipids
(Anderson and Seibert, cf., Seibert, 1950)

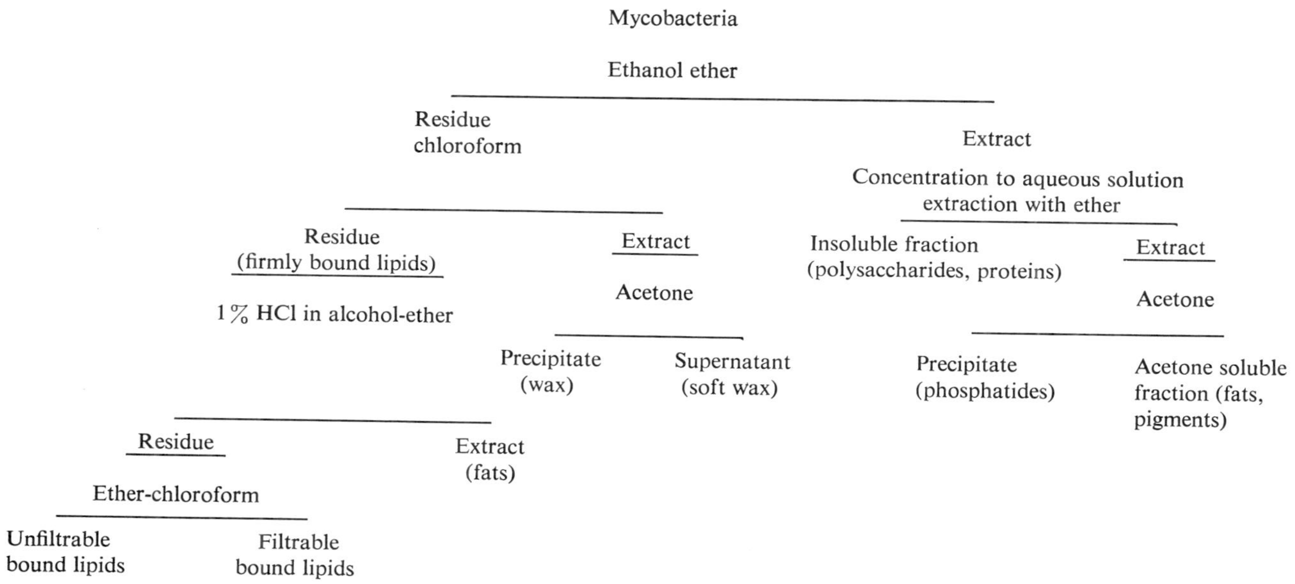

Mycobacteria

Ethanol ether

Residue — chloroform

Extract

Concentration to aqueous solution extraction with ether

Residue (firmly bound lipids)

Extract — Acetone

Insoluble fraction (polysaccharides, proteins)

Extract — Acetone

1 % HCl in alcohol-ether

Precipitate (wax)

Supernatant (soft wax)

Precipitate (phosphatides)

Acetone soluble fraction (fats, pigments)

Residue

Extract (fats)

Ether-chloroform

Unfiltrable bound lipids

Filtrable bound lipids

Table 16. Diagram of the Fractionation of Lipids (Williams and Dubos, 1959)

Bacteria
— Acetone at 40°

Acetone extract: Residue
acetone-soluble   — Methanol at 60°
fats, pigments

                          Methanol extract:
                          "waxes," pigments,
                          phosphatides (?)
                          lipopolysaccharides (?)

                          Concentrated
                          4 × at 50°

Precipitate: Supernatant
hard "wax"   Concentrated
                          20 × at 50°

          Precipitate: Methanol-soluble residue: pigments,
          soft "wax"   oils, salts, soft "wax"

          Petroleum ether
          at 30–60°

Insoluble   Solution:
residue: soft "wax"
hard "wax"

          Petroleum ether
          at 30–60°

Insoluble   Solution:
residue: soft "wax"
hard "wax"   to be dried
                          with acetone

0.5% sodium chloride, at 4° during 17 hours. The precipitate is resuspended in water and reprecipitated in the same manner a second time, then washed, resuspended in water, and dialyzed. This represents the subfraction 1. The other subfraction is recovered from the supernatant after the evaporation of ethanol and concentration.

The second method of subfractionation of lipid fractions depends on precipitation with a methanolic solution of cupric acetate. The copper is then removed from the separated precipitate and supernatant by bubbling hydrogen sulfide through the methanol solutions of all subfractions.

Crude phospholipids can be purified or fractionated according to the Akashi and Saito (1960) method. In this method, the phospholipids are boiled with 30 ml of ethanol, then cooled at 0°, giving a cold ethanol soluble and an insoluble fraction. The ethanol is now distilled off from the soluble fraction; and this fraction is dissolved in a small amount of ether and poured into a ten times greater volume of ice-cold acetone to precipitate an acetone-insoluble fraction in the supernatant.

According to Blumer et al. (1969), the lipids are extracted from bacteria with a 1:1 mixture of methanol and benzene for 5 minutes. The homogenate is centrifuged and the supernatant fluid is decanted and dried at 15° on a rotary evaporator.

The Isolation of Firmly Bound Lipids by the Geiger and Anderson Method. The firmly bound lipids can be isolated with an acidified alcohol-ether mixture. The extraction of firmly bound lipids is preceded by the removal of a portion of the polysaccharides from the bacterial cells. For this purpose, the bacteria are suspended in a diluted ethyl alcohol added in the proportion of 300 ml of 25% alcohol to 100 g of bacteria. The mixture is then filtered, and the supernatant fluid is treated with alkaline lead acetate and ammonia to sediment a polysaccharide.

The residue of bacterial cells may be extracted in a Soxhlet apparatus, heated in water bath at 50°, with a mixture consisting of 1 liter of alcohol, 1.5 liter of ether, and 45 ml of concentrated hydrochloric acid. On completion of the extraction, the residual particulate material is centrifuged and washed with a mixture of alcohol and ether until the washings become neutral on litmus. The resultant residue is extracted with alcohol-ether, and with a 1:1 mixture of ether and chloroform. The extracts are filtered through Chamberland candles and concentrated to a dry mass under reduced atmospheric pressure. This material is then dissolved in a small volume of ether and poured into two to five volumes of cold alcohol. The resultant precipitate must be separated from the supernatant by filtration and washed on the filter with ethyl alcohol. The supernatant should be concentrated and dried in vacuo, yielding a lipid fraction. The precipitate is dissolved in ether and treated with acetone. A slight flocculate occurs that should be collected by centrifugation. It represents the firmly bound lipid fraction.

Cholesterol Extraction. The cholesterol can be extracted into petroleum ether according to the following technique (Abell et al., 1952). The lipoprotein or lipid source is first saponified with a freshly prepared alcoholic solution of potassium hydroxide (1-ml sample and 10-ml KOH solution). The mixture is heated in an oven at 40° for 55 minutes and then cooled at room temperature.

Cholesterol is extracted with petroleum ether (10 ml), added to the lipid mixture. Add 5 ml of distilled water, seal the tubes, shake them vigorously, and centrifuge the material at 1000 rpm for 5 minutes. Collect the petroleum ether layer and allow the petroleum ether to evaporate in a vacuum oven under a stream of nitrogen, or by standing overnight at room temperature.

The Lipopolysaccharide Preparation. The methods of the lipopolysaccharide preparation, devised by Westphal et al. (1952), Johnson (1955), and Jenkin and Rowley (1959) and Adams et al. (1969) are very useful, and may be selected according to the aim of the actual resource. Adam's et al. technique is presented in Table 17.

Westphal's Method of the Lipopolysaccharide Preparation. Bacteria (10 g of dry weight) are suspended in 160 ml of distilled water and mixed with 265 ml of 75% phenol, prepared by adding 65 ml of water to 200 g of liquified phenol (Table 18). The mixture is left at 3 to 5° or 65 to 68° for 30 minutes with occasional shaking, then centrifuged at 3000 to 4000 rpm. The upper aqueous phase should be collected. The remaining material can be washed with water, centrifuged, and the upper layer combined with the first supernatant. This fluid is now dialyzed for 2 to 3 days against tap water and 1 day against distilled water, then concentrated to a 40- to 50-ml volume. Lipopolysaccharide is precipitated from the dialyzate with six volumes of ethyl alcohol or acetone mixed with a small volume of saturated alcoholic solution of sodium acetate. The sediment is collected by centrifugation, washed with alcohol and acetone, and dried in vacuo. An alternative to the alcohol precipitation is centrifugation of the dialyzate at 150,000 × g for 2 hours (Bain and Knox, 1961). The product obtained is more easily water soluble than that precipitated with alcohol. If the dialyzate contains nucleic acids apart from the polysaccharides, ethanol should be added in two steps: first, one volume of ethanol to precipitate nucleic acids, and then the centrifugation and concentration of the supernatant six volumes of ethanol to precipitate the polysaccharides. The polysaccharides may be purified by reprecipitation.

The lipopolysaccharide may also be purified by acetylation (Adams et al., 1969, Table 17). For this purpose, the lipopolysaccharide-containing material is mixed with acetic anhydride (3.0–4.0 g/100 ml) and shaken for 1 hour at room temperature. The mixture is then placed in an ice bath. A few drops of perchloric acid are added, and the mixture is stirred for 2 to 3 hours and left at 0° overnight. The solvents are then removed by evaporation, and the acetylated material is extracted with a chloroform: methanol (50:50) mixture, which removes the acetylated lipopolysaccharide.

Johnson's Method of the Lipopolysaccharide Preparation. Dried bacteria are suspended in anhydrous diethylene glycol (ten times their weight) by mechanical agitation, held at 35° for 24 hours, and collected by centrifugation. This procedure should be repeated twice. The combined extracts are dialyzed at 3 to 5° against distilled water, concentrated by electroultrafiltration, and electrodialyzed.

The dialyzate is then suspended in cold distilled water, treated with cold 95% alcohol(four volumes), and left at 0 to 3° for 1 hour. After centrifugation in a refrigerated centrifuge, the sediment is suspended in cold

Table 17. Preparation and Purification of Lipopolysaccharide
by Adams' et al. (1969) Method

Bacteria

Washed (freeze dried)

Extraction
in 75% phenol,
68° for 30 minutes

Phenol layer	Aqueous layer
(discarded)	
	Dialyze, freeze dry
	Solids
	Stir in water, centrifuge at 44,000 × *g* for 15 minutes

Insolubles	Solubles
Acetylation	(mostly RNA)

Chloroform insolubles	Chloroform solubles
	Deacetylation
	Lipopolysaccharide
	Chloroform extraction

Chloroform solubles	Chloroform insolubles

**Table 18.   Diagram of the Fractionation of Bacteria
by Westphal's et al. (1952) Method**

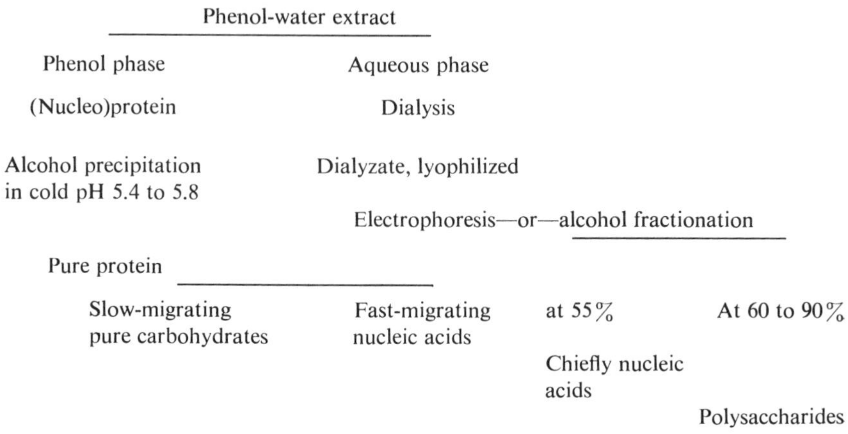

Phenol-water extract

Phenol phase	Aqueous phase
(Nucleo)protein	Dialysis
Alcohol precipitation in cold pH 5.4 to 5.8	Dialyzate, lyophilized

Electrophoresis—or—alcohol fractionation

Pure protein

Slow-migrating pure carbohydrates	Fast-migrating nucleic acids	at 55%	At 60 to 90%
		Chiefly nucleic acids	
			Polysaccharides

distilled water, dialyzed against distilled water at 0 to 3°, and centrifuged at 3000 × *g* in a refrigerated centrifuge for 4 hours. The supernatant is collected. The sediment should be washed three times with cold distilled water, and washings combined with the supernatant, recentrifuged, and lyophilized.

Preparation of Carotenoid Pigments. According to the Starr and Stephens (1964) method, bacterial cells are first extracted for a few minutes with absolute methanol (50 ml/g of moist cells) in a steaming water bath. This mixture is then cooled and centrifuged to remove the cells. The methanolic extract is collected and mixed with an equal volume of petroleum ether and enough distilled water to give a methanol concentration of 90%. This mixture is gently shaken in a separatory funnel and left to separate a petroleum ether epiphase and methanol hypophase. The upper phase should be evaporated to dryness in an evaporator and saponified with 3% methanolic KOH for 3 hours at 40°. An equal volume of petroleum ether and enough distilled water are then added to give 90% methanol concentration. Two phases are to be separated by means of a separatory funnel. The petroleum-ether epiphase containing "hydrocarbons" is removed, washed, dehydrated with sodium sulfate, and dried in vacuo. Individual carotenoid hydrocarbons (i.e., carotens) in the residue can be separated by the column chromatography.

The KOH-methanol hypophase is transferred into diethyl ether by the addition of that solvent and then distilled water. The ether layer is then washed free of the methanol-KOH with water, freed of water with a saturated solution of sodium chloride and anhydrous sodium sulfate, and dried in vacuo. The deesterified carotenoid alcohols can be separated by adsorption chromatography on columns of magnesia-Celite.

The original methanolic cell extract containing carotenoid alcohols and salts of acids is then mixed with methanolic KOH to a final KOH concentration of 3%. This solution is heated at 40° for 5 minutes; two volumes of diethyl ether and enough distilled water are added to separate two layers in a separatory funnel. The ether layer, which contains carotenoid alcohols, should be washed, dehydrated, and evaporated to dryness.

Salts of carotenoid acids can be recovered from the aqueous phase by the addition of dilute hydrochloric acid followed by extraction with diethyl ether.

Another method of extraction and a technique of the quantitative determination of bacterial pigments were described by Mathews and Sistrom (1995), and an alumina-column chromatography of microbial pigments was reported by Ebina et al. (1962).

The Lipoprotein Preparation. The lipoproteins occur as soluble or insoluble complexes. The solubility is due to the presence of the protein component. Lipoproteins may be separated efficiently by ultracentrifugal floatation. The lipoprotein preparations may be centrifuged either at the original density or at an increased density conferred by the addition of concentrated salt solutions, such as 153.0 g of sodium chloride or 354.0 of potassium bromide per liter. According to Havel et al. (1955), the lipoproteins are centrifuged at 105,000 × g for 24 hours at 12 to 15° in the 40 or 40.3 rotor of a Spinco ultracentrifuge, Model L or L2. The lipoproteins possessing a density lower than the solvent density are concentrated in a top layer. The layer can be separated and collected by placing the tube in a tube-slicing device. The lipoprotein preparation may be washed by centrifugation in salt solution of the same density as used for the original centrifugation.

Separation and purification of the lipoproteins is best conducted by the gel filtration on columns composed of 4 and 6% agarose gel (Margolis, 1967), using the eluting fluid consisting of 0.5 M NaCl containing 0.1 M potassium phosphate buffer, pH 7.0, and 0.1 g/l of the sodium salt of EDTA. Toluene (1 drop/l) is added to prevent bacterial growth.

The molecular weight of lipoproteins can be determined from the relationship:

$$MW = \frac{4\pi NR^3}{(3\bar{V})(1.46)}$$

where N = Avogadro's number, $\bar{V}$ = partial specific volume of the lipoprotein, R = Stokes radius of the lipoprotein, and the factor 1.46 is a correction for hydration of the macromolecule.

5. Preparation of Polysaccharide Antigens

Polysaccharide fractions from bacterial cells or cell walls can be obtained by extraction with a variety of chemicals, such as antiformin (Salton, 1952), alkali (Casper, 1937; Kwapinski, 1965), formamide (Fuller, 1938), diluted acetic acid (Kwapinski, 1956, 1960), trichloracetic acid (Smith et al., 1962), sulfosalicylic acid (Kwapinski and Snyder, 1961), phenol (Alexander et al., 1950), urea (Stacey et al., 1951), ethylene glycol or diethylenel glycol (Morgan and Partridge, 1941), pyridine (Akiya, 1953), or with the chelating agents, for example, ethylenediamine tetracetic acid and hot sodium chloride solution (Jann et al., 1968).

Fuller's Formamide Method of Polysaccharide Preparation. In this method as modified by Ullmann and Cameron (1969), the lyophilized cells are extracted in formamide (1 g of dry cell walls and 40 ml of formamide) in an oil bath at 150° for 20 minutes. If purified cell walls are used as the initial material, they are extracted directly in formamide as above. The solubilized cells are dialyzed overnight at 4° against buffered saline (pH 7.4) to remove formamide, and then are digested with pronase (1.0 mg/ml) at 37° for 4 hours to remove protein. The material is dialyzed at 4° against distilled water. The extract is centrifuged, and the supernatant is poured into 2.5 volumes of 95% ethyl alcohol containing 1% hydrochloric acid. The resultant sediment is removed, and the supernatant is mixed with an equal volume of acetone (Zittle and Harris, 1942). The sediment is then collected and extracted with distilled water. Five volumes of acetone containing 1% hydrochloric acid are added to the aqueous extract to precipitate the crude polysaccharide fraction which should be dried with alcohol and ether.

This fraction can be purified in the following way. The crude preparation of polysaccharide is dissolved in distilled water and neutralized with 1 *N* hydrochloric acid. Any flocculent material should be removed. The clear liquid is treated with five volumes of acetone acidified with hydrochloric acid, and the resultant precipitate is collected and dried off.

This dried precipitate is dissolved in 4% acetic acid and treated with Lloyd's reagent, added gradually up to the concentration of 0.02 g of Lloyd's reagent per 1 ml of the super solution. The sediment formed is removed by centrifugation, and the supernatant is dialyzed against distilled water for 16 hours. The dialyzate, flocculated with five volumes of acetone acidified with concentrated hydrochloric acid (5 to 6 drops/100 ml), contains the purified somatic polysaccharide, which should be dried over phosphorus pentoxide or lyophilized.

Extraction of Polysaccharides with Urea (Stacey et al., 1951). A mixture of equal weights of moist bacteria and urea is stirred at 37° for 12 hours. After more urea is added, the incubation is prolonged by a further 8 hours.

The liquid is then diluted with about one-fourth volume of distilled water and centrifuged at a high speed repeatedly. The supernatant fluid should be adjusted to pH 6 with diluted acetic acid, recentrifuged, and filtered through a Seitz pad. The filtrate is treated with three volumes of ethyl alcohol. The precipitate can be fractionated into soluble and insoluble portions by extraction with 2% sodium acetate four times.

Kwapinski's Technique of the Preparation of Polysaccharide Antigens. This technique is diagrammatically presented in Table 19. Crude polysaccharide fractions extracted at each stage are purified in the following manner. The fraction is first suspended in 10% acetic acid and boiled for 10 minutes, then filtered. The filtrate is treated with an equal volume of chloroform, shaken in a separatory funnel for 15 minutes, and allowed to separate layers. The upper layer is collected, dialyzed, and lyophilized, yielding a purified polysaccharide fraction.

Another method of isolating polysaccharide fractions from bacteria (Kwapinski and Snyder, 1961) is often helpful in obtaining serologically

Table 19. Diagram of Chemical Extraction of Polysaccharide Antigens
(Kwapinski, 1965)

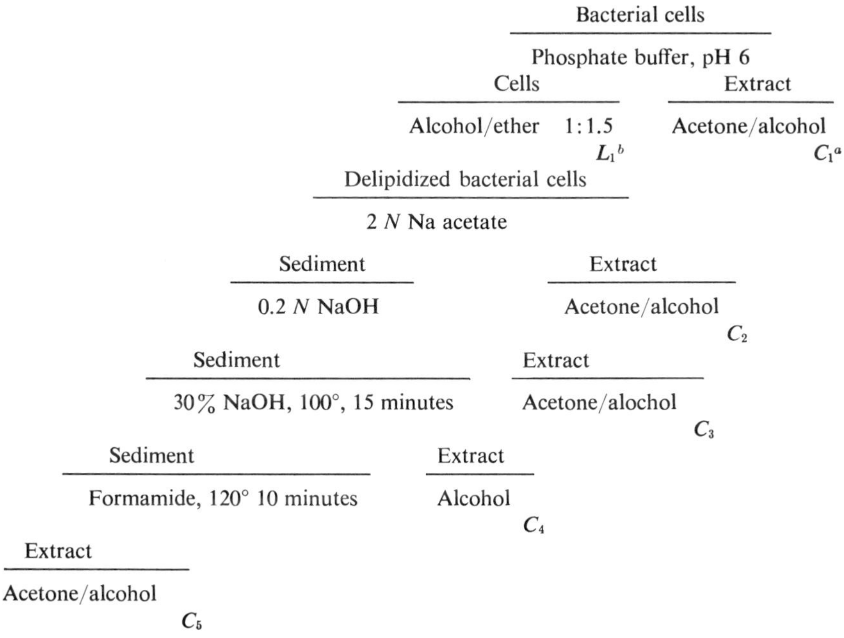

Bacterial cells
____
Phosphate buffer, pH 6
Cells   Extract
_______________   ___________________
Alcohol/ether 1:1.5   Acetone/alcohol
$L_1{}^b$ $C_1{}^a$
Delipidized bacterial cells
____
2 N Na acetate
Sediment   Extract
_______________   ___________________
0.2 N NaOH   Acetone/alcohol
C_2
Sediment   Extract
___________________   ___________________
30% NaOH, 100°, 15 minutes   Acetone/alochol
C_3
Sediment   Extract
___________________   ___________
Formamide, 120° 10 minutes   Alcohol
C_4
Extract
____
Acetone/alcohol
C_5

[a] C = polysaccharide fraction.
[b] L = lipid or lipopolysaccharide fraction.

specific polysaccharides. In this technique, disintegrated or whole cells are suspended in a 1:3 mixture of 7.5% sulfosalicylic acid ether, and extracted at 2° for 12 to 24 hours on an electric shaker. The mixture is then layered in a separatory funnel. The bottom layer is removed, centrifuged at 25,000 × g to remove any fine particles, dialyzed for 3 days against distilled water, and lyophilized. Incidentally, a lipid fraction can be recovered from the upper layer and a protein fraction from the interphase.

The Pyridine Isolation of Polysaccharides. In the Akiya method (1953), bacterial cells dried with acetone and delipidized with ether and alcohol are extracted repeatedly with ten parts (*v/v*) of 50% pyridine at 37° for 24 hours, each time. Pyridine extracts are pooled, passed through a bacterial filter, heated in a steam bath at 50° to remove pyridine water, and dialyzed for 2 days. The dialyzate is cooled at 0°, treated with one-half volume of acetone, and the precipitate is removed by centrifugation. The polysaccharide is sedimented from the supernatant by adding acetone to obtain one molar concentration and is then dissolved in water. An equal amount of acetone should be added to the aqueous solution at 0°, and any precipitate is removed by centrifugation. The purified polysaccharide is now precipitated from the supernatant with a larger amount of acetone. This precipitate should be collected by centrifugation, dissolved in water, electrodialyzed and lyophilized.

The TCA Method of the Polysaccharide Extraction. In this technique by Smith et al. (1962), bacterial cells are extracted with ice-cold 10% trichloracetic acid. After centrifugation, the supernatant is shaken with diethyl ether to extract and remove trichloracetic acid. The hypophase is then collected and adjusted to pH 7.0 with ammonium hydrochloride. Polysaccharides are precipitated from this liquid by adding ten volumes of 95% ethyl alcohol.

Cellulose Extraction. Cellulose may be extracted in 10% HCl. The extract is evaporated on a boiling water bath, dissolved in 3% HCl, and saturated with H_2S. The precipitate thus formed is discarded by centrifugation. The supernatant is dissolved in 1 *N* sodium hydroxide solution and precipitated with ethyl alcohol, yielding purified cellulose.

6. *Preparation of Protein and Nucleoprotein Antigens*

Most proteins and nucleoproteins of microorganisms can be extracted at ph 8.5 to 11 but sometimes at lower pH values, for example, 2 to 2.5, with various buffer solution, such as distilled water adjusted to pH 7.6, 0.1 *M* borate buffer containing 0.85% sodium chloride, 0.02 *N* sodium carbonate, 0.05 1 *N* sodium hydroxide, 10% urea, or 70 to 90% phenol. Details of various immunochemical techniques for protein or nucleoprotein preparation may be found in the papers published by Lancefield and Perlmann (1952), Heidelberger and Menzel (1934), Chambers and Flosdorf (1936),

Stamp and Hendry (1937), Moralez-Otero and Gonzalez (1938), Wong and T'Ung (1939), Sevag et al. (1938), Mudd et al. (1938, 1939), Smadel et al. (1942), Smolens and Mudd (1943), Chargaff and Seidel (1949), Kwapinski (1960, 1965), and Onoue et al. (1961). Kwapinski's fractionation methods, one dealing with the protein or nucleoprotein fractions isolated separately from cell walls or cytoplasm, the other with the total cell material, are represented diagrammatically in Tables 12 and 14, respectively.

Isolation of Bacterial Nucleoproteins (Chargaff and Seidel, 1949). Nucleoproteins are extracted from mechanically disintegrated bacteria with 0.1 *M*, pH 8.5, borate buffer for 2 days, at 2°. The extract is freed from particulate matter by centrifugation at 4000 rpm for 30 minutes, followed by filtration. The filtrate is then dialyzed against distilled water for 48 hours, concentrated by evaporation to one third of the original volume, and dialyzed again for 72 hours. This fluid, containing mostly nucleoproteins and a quantity of glycogen, should be preserved with 0.01 ethylene mercurithiosulfate. Glycogen can be removed from the extract by centrifugation at 31,000 rpm. The supernatant is dialyzed once more and evaporated in vacuo, giving a partially purified nucleoprotein fraction. The yield of this fraction is usually equivalent to 2 to 4% of the original material.

The nucleoprotein fraction can be further purified by electrophoresis or by chemical fractionation. In the latter procedure the crude nucleoprotein dissolved in borate buffer at pH 8.4 is treated with diluted acetic acid until a slight precipitation occurs, usually at pH 4.3. The sediment is cooled for 3 hours, centrifuged, and washed with an ice-cold 0.05 *M*, pH 4.3, citrate buffer, then dissolved in the pH 8.4 borate buffer, dialyzed for several days, and lyophilized. The powdery fraction obtained can be further purified with ammonium sulfate. In this procedure the fraction is dissolved in distilled water and treated with an equal volume of a saturated solution of ammonium sulfate. The sediment formed contains a protein fraction which should be centrifuged, washed with a one-half saturated ammonium sulfate, dissolved in a pH 8.2 phosphate buffer, dialyzed, and lyophilized. The pure nucleoprotein fraction may be recovered from the supernatant, which is dialyzed for several days to remove the electrolytes, and then lyophilized. Lyophilization sometimes renders the nucleoprotein fractions insoluble, and to prevent this they should be suspended in a 0.1 *M* glycine saline buffer containing 0.5% gelatin (de Brujin, 1960).

Preparation of Purified Protein Antigens (Moralez-Otero and Gonzalez, 1938). The bacteria, ground with sand, are extracted with 0.02 *N* sodium carbonate overnight in a refrigerator and filtered through a Berkefeld candle. The filtrate is concentrated to one-twentieth volume by ultrafiltration, and after the addition of 0.5% phenol as preservative is refiltered. The

Table 20.   Preparation of Nucleoprotein Fractions (Kwapinski, 1965)

Bacterial cells
(disintegrated)
____

Ether-alcohol 1.5:1.0

Delipidized bacteria _______ 0.05 N NaOH

Extract _______ 1:2, Benzene + 1 N alcoholic NaOH

Residue _______ 0.2 N NaOH

Extract _______ 10% TCA

Benzene phase _______ L_1

Alcohol-aqueous phase _______ 10% TCA to the precipitation point

Residue _______ 0.5 N NaOH

Extract _______ 10% TCA

Precipitate _______ 2 N Na acetate

Residue _______ 85% phenol

Extract _______ 10% TCA

Precipitate _______ 2 N Na acetate

Sediment _______ 0.1 N NaOH

Precipitate _______ $N_1{}^b$

Extract
————
Acetone
+ 1% HCl

Precipitate
Precipitate
Sediment
Sediment
————
2 N Na acetate
0.2 N NaOH
10% TCA

Precipitate
————
1 N NaOH
centrifugation

Sediment
————
0.2 N NaOH

Extract
————
10% TCA

Precipitate
————
N_2

Extract
————
Dialysis

Extract
————
10% TCA

Precipitate
————

N_4
N_3

Dialyzate
————
10% TCA

Precipitate
————

N_5

[a] L = lipid fraction.
[b] N = nucleoprotein fraction.

protein is precipitated with 50% trichloracetic acid, centrifuged, and washed with 10% TCA until the washings are colorless. The acid is removed by washing with anhydrous ether.

Separation and Identification of Proteins by Electric Current (Protein Mapping). Different proteins present in a mixture may be separated by the isoelectrofusing Svensson et al. (1962), Vesterberg et al. (1967), gel electrophoresis (Raymond, 1964), or, most efficiently, by a two-dimensional technique (Wrigley, 1970). By the two-dimensional electrofocusing-electrophoresis technique, more proteins are separated and characterized more selectively than by any other technique; and the results are well reproducible.

The Density Gradient Isoelectrofocusing. The electrofocusing method utilizes differences in electric charges, isoelectric points, solubility and velocity at a pH range of proteins and other polymers. This method permits effective and reproducible separation of different proteins, while other polymers freed from the proteins can be further and more easily purified.

The electrofocusing method of Vesterberg et al. (1967) or Svensson et al. (1962) is employed. The ampholine electrofusing equipment used in this laboratory consists of a jacketed, water cooled at 10° micro- or macrocolumn, a linear gradient former, peristaltic pump used to empty the column, a fraction collector, a double beam continuous monitor and an automatic recorder. One percent (v/v) ampholyte gradient for the isoelectrofusing is made depending on a pH range, estimated in pretrials as the most suitable for distinct separation of individual proteins. The pH of the focused fractions are measured to determine their isoelectric points, with a pH meter reading directly to 0.001 of a pH unit.

A current of 850 V and 15 to 20 mA is applied for 36 to 48 hours at 2 to 4%, the descending 2 to 5 ml fractions are collected by a fraction collector, and the electrofocusing process is terminated when the current through the column has reached a constant value, about 2 to 3 mA. The pH value of each fraction is measured at the temperature of the column to determine the isoelectric points of the focused components.

The chemical composition of materials collected in individual tubes are determined by the double beam continuous monitor in terms of the absorbance at the 210-, 254-, and 280-nm wave lengths. Identification of other polymers which can not be detected at these wave lengths, is done by a color reaction, specific for saccharides and phosphatides.

Preparative Polyacrylamide Electrophoresis. The equipment for the electrophoresis consists of an electrophoresis column, a linear gradient former, a peristaltic pump, fraction collector, a double beam continuous monitor, and an automatic recorder (Fig. 15).

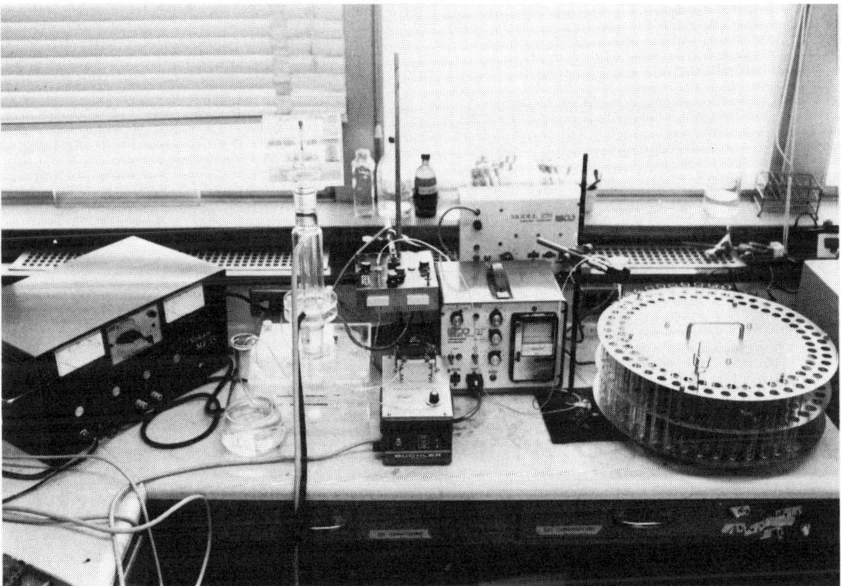

Figure 15. The preparative polyacrylamide-gel electrophoresis equipment (left to right: a jacketed column, peristaltic pump, monitor, and automatic recorder).

In the method described by Raymond (1964), discontinuous gel and buffer systems of polyacrylamide gel electrophoresis are used. Packing and running gels consist of 7% cyanogum-41 in 0.3 M Tris-HCl, pH 8.9. The spacer gel is 4% cyanogum-41 in 0.3 *M* Tris-HCl, pH 6.7; the electrode buffer is 0.005 *M* Tris, 0.04 *M* glycine, pH 8.3; 0.1% TMED (*N, N, N'* , *N'*-tetramethylene-diamine) and 0.1% ammonium persulfate. The system is equilibrated by a 1 hour prerun at 200 V. The electrophoresis is conducted at room temperature, at 400 V for 2 hours. The descending fractions are collected by an automated fraction collector at 6 to 8° and monitored by the double beam continuous monitor at 254 nm and recorded automatically. The eluted materials are plotted against the absorbency values (Fig. 16).

The Two-Dimensional Electrofocusing-Starch Gel Electrophoresis Technique (Wrigley, 1970). In this method, a mixture of proteins is applied to the top (acid end) of a polyacrylamide gel (3 × 60 mm) containing 2 *M* urea and carrier ampholytes in the pH ranges 5 to 7 and 7 to 9 for gel electrofocusing. After the completion of electrofocusing, the unfixed gel is inserted into a 3-mm white slot across one end of a starch gel for electrophoresis (Graham, 1963) for the second dimension run. The starch gel electrophoresis is carried out in aluminum lactate at pH 3.1.

The difference of migration on a starch gel varies inversely with the size and directly with charge at the pH of electrophoresis.

The Lancefield and Perlmann Technique for Preparing Antigens. The bacteria are suspended in a saline solution adjusted to pH 2 to 2.5 with 1 *N* hydrochloric acid and left at 95° in a water bath for 10 minutes, then cooled and adjusted to pH 7.5 with 1 *N* sodium hydroxide. The extract is separated from the debris by centrifugation. The sediment is then washed with saline at pH 7.5, and extracted again with a saline solution. The protein antigen is precipitated from the combined supernatant by adding 6 *N* hydrochloric acid to obtain pH 2.0.

The precipitate should then be dissolved in a small volume of phosphate buffer, pH 8, and treated with ribonuclease, added to a final concentration of 0.001 mg/ml. During a 5-hour digestion period the extract is dialyzed in cellophane tubing at 37° against *M*/10 phosphate buffer, pH 8; chloroform should be added as preservative. The dialysis against phosphate buffer continues for several days at 3°. The dialyzate is then fractionated with ammonium sulfate, and the most serologically active fraction is collected, dialyzed at 3°, and lyophilized (Fig. 12). This method was originally used for preparing protein antigens from the streptococci.

The Smolens and Mudd Technique for the Protein Antigen Preparation. The bacteria are first extracted for 17 to 20 hours with diulte hydrochloric acid, pH 1.8, at 50 to 56°. The supernatant is treated with 1 *N* NaOH, and the precipitate is removed by centrifugation. The precipitate can be washed with distilled water, pH 7.0, and the washings combined with the supernatant to produce a crude extract.

The extract should be mixed with an equal volume of saturated ammonium sulfate solution at 2 to 4°. The resultant precipitate is collected, washed with a half-saturated ammonium sulfate solution, dissolved in water and dialyzed for 48 hours against distilled. The dialyzate should be clarified by centrifugation and treated with a half volume of saturated picric acid solution. The resulting precipitate is dissolved in water and dialyzed against distilled water until the yellow color disappears. The dialyzate is clarified by centrifugation and lyophilized.

Methanol can be substituted for picric acid (Onoue et al. 1961). Methyl alcohol is added slowly, at 0 to 5°, to a final concentration of 13 to 25%, or, as required, to precipitate protein fractions. Precipitates are collected by centrifugation at 10,000 rpm, dialyzed against cold distilled water, and lyophilized.

Preparation of Flagellin. Flagellin may be produced by Kobayashi's et al. (1959) technique or by slight modification of this method (Ada et al.,

1964). According to the latter procedure, the flagella, prepared as described on pp. 37–39), are first treated with 1 N HCl, added at one-twentieth volume of the 0.5% flagella suspension. The solution is left at room temperature for half an hour, and then centrifuged at 80,000 $\times$ g for 1 hour, at 4°. The supernatant is collected, neutralized with 1 N NaOH and passed through a sterilized pad, or chromatographed on a column of hydroxylapatite. The soluble protein may be polymerized either by salting-out procedures, such as cycles of freezing and thawing, or by addition of strong salt solutions. A convenient procedure for the protein polymerization is the addition of 2 volumes of cold, saturated ammonium sulfate to the filtrate. The precipitating filtrate is left at 4° for 12 to 16 hours and centrifuged at 20,000 $\times$ g for 15 minutes. The precipitate containing flagellin-protein is then dissolved in a small volume of distilled water and dialyzed against water.

Preparation of Toxic Proteins (Jenkin and Rowley, 1959). The bacteria suspended in a 2.5-M urea solution, which solubilizes proteins, are disintegrated in an ultrasonic disintegrator. The urea extract is fractionated with ammonium sulfate, added successively to give 1.9 M, 2.8 and 3.8 M solution, each step separated by centrifugation at 1200 $\times$ g and collection of supernatants. The second and third deposits are combined, dissolved in 0.0066 M phosphate buffer, pH 7.3, and reprecipitated with ammonium sulfate, at 2 to 8 M. The precipitate should be dissolved in 0.0066 M phosphate buffer and centrifuged at 20,000 $\times$ g. The supernatant is recentrifuged at 78,000 $\times$ g, yielding a deposit which represents a purified toxic protein.

Mucopeptide Preparation. Intracellular mucopeptides may be obtained from the liquid portion of disrupted cells from which noncombined carbohydrates have been removed, for example, by Fuller's (1938) method. The residue is centrifuged, washed with $M/15$, pH 7.2 phosphate buffered saline, and digested with lysozyme at 37° for 18 hours. The mixture is then centrifuged, and the supernatant contains crude mucopeptide (Krause and McCarty, 1961).

Mucopolysaccharides may be precipitated from solution with cetylpyridinium chloride added to the final concentration of 0.2%. The precipitate is settled in 12 to 18 hours at 4° and washed with ethanol saturated with potassium acetate (Di Ferrante, 1967).

7. *Preparation of Nucleic Acids*

Nucleic acids are usually bound to the proteins or polypeptides but can be released rather easily by extraction in diluted trichloracetic acid, acetic acid, or perchloric acid. The presence of nucleic acids can be detected spectrophotometrically; they exhibit absorption in the 254 to 260-nm region.

Of many techniques designed for nucleic acid preparation, the Mach and Vassali (1965), Oishi and Sueoka (1965), and Adesnik and Levinthal's (1969) methods are recommended for RNA, whereas Marmur's (1961) and Rudin and Albertsson's (1967) methods are recommended for DNA preparation. However, other techniques reported below prove to be useful for obtaining nucleic acids from particular sources.

RNA Extraction and Purification. The most appropriate methods for extraction of cellular and bacterial ribonucleic acid have been published by Mach and Vassali (1965), Oishi and Sueoka (1965), and Adesnik and Levinthal (1969). The Mach and Vassalli method permits the isolation of all the RNA in undegraded and uncontaminated form. If a source of nucleic acid contains an appreciable amount of ribonuclease, the enzymatic hydrolysis during all steps of extraction and purification should be inhibited by bentonite (1 mg/ml) or by polyvinyl sulfate (3 to $4 \times 10^{-4}\%$). The organs or bacteria to be used for extraction of nucleic acid must be kept frozen, and all steps of the following procedure must be performed at 0 to 4°. Frozen materials, serving as a source of ribonucleic acid, are first homogenized in a mixture of equal volumes of fresh phenol and a 0.1 M Tris or acetate buffer, pH 5, containing 0.5% sodium dodecyl sulfate and 0.5% 1,5-naphthalene disulfamate; use 6 ml of phenol and 6 ml of buffer per gram of the initial material. The homogenate is then heated at 65° for 6 minutes and quickly cooled in an acetone-dry ice bath. Centrifuge the mixture at 2000 $\times$ g and collect the aqueous phase. Add an equivalent amount of fresh buffer and phenol to the remaining interphase, shake it at 20° for 10 minutes, centrifuge the mixture, and collect the aqueous phase. Pool the aqueous phases and repeat the extraction twice more, at 20° for 10 minutes, each time with half the volume of phenol. Transfer the collected aqueous phase to 0.1 M sodium chloride, and add $2\frac{1}{2}$ volumes of ethyl alcohol, cooled at −30°. Leave the mixture at 0° for 3 hours; centrifuge the precipitate of RNA at 10,000 $\times$ g for 50 minutes and dissolve it in water. Reprecipitate the RNA with one volume of 4 M potassium acetate and one volume of chilled ethanol. Leave the mixture for 2 hours at −30° and centrifuge it. Dissolve the RNA pellet in distilled water and homogenize it. Reprecipitate the RNA to purify the preparation. The purified RNA preparation must not give a reaction with the diphenylamine reagent.

Successive, fractional extraction of different fractions of ribonucleic acid may be attained according to Georgiev's et al. (1963) method. The extractions are performed at increasing temperatures, ranging from 20 to 65°.

RNA Preparation by Oishi and Sueoka's (1965) Method. Bacterial cells obtained from the early stationary phase are washed in distilled water and resuspended in 0.01 M Tris (pH 7.4) solution containing 0.0005 M $MgCl_2$. A DNase (10 μg/ml) and lysozyme (1 mg/ml) preparation is added, the suspension is subjected to eight cycles of freezing and thawing, after which sodium dodecyl sulfate is added to a final concentration of 2%. The lysed bacteria are then extracted with an equal volume of water-saturated phenol, while shaken for 30 minutes at room temperature. The mixture is centrifuged, and the aqueous phase is collected. Upon the addition of 2.5 volumes of cold ethyl alcohol to the aqueous phase, the RNA is precipitated. The precipitate is collected by centrifugation and dissolved in 1.5 ml of the Tris $MgCl_2$ buffer, followed by ethanol precipitation, applied twice.

Purification of RNA preparations can be obtained by filtration of the crude material through a methylated albumin-Kieselguhr column (Oishi and Sueoka, 1965).

RNA Preparation by Adesnik and Levinthal's Method. The RNA is extracted from protoplasts obtained by the technique of Flessel et al. (1967). In order to prepare protoplasts, the bacterial cells are exposed to lysozyme at 0° at a concentration of 400 μg/ml for 5 minutes. After the bacterial cells have been converted to protoplasts, the protoplasts are collected by centrifugation and lysed by the addition of a sodium dodecyl sulfate buffer consisting of 1.5% sodium dodecyl sulfate, 0.1 M NaCl, 0.01 M $MgCO_2$, and 0.01 M Tris-HCl, pH 7.4. The protoplast lysate is extracted twice at room temperature with a mixture of phenol, *m*-cresol, 8-hydroxy-quinoline (Kirby, 1956). The aqueous layer is collected from the reactant mixture and mixed with 1/10 volume of 3 M sodium acetate, pH 5.5. The nucleic acid is precipitated from this aqueous liquid with three volumes of absolute ethanol on standing overnight at −20°. The precipitate is dissolved in 1 ml of 0.3 M sodium acetate, pH 5.5 containing 0.25% sodium dodecyl sulfate, and precipitated again with ethanol on standing for 3 hours at −20°. The final precipitate is washed with 67% ethanol and dried in vacuo for 15 minutes.

A technique for nucleic acid fractionation using a weak ion exchanger "Ecteola-cellulose" was published by Murase (1961). Crude material for this fractionation is obtained by extracting delipidized bacteria with 1 N sodium chloride, chloroform, and deoxycholate, at pH 7.0, followed by precipitation with ethanol.

Extraction of Infectious RNA from Viruses. The technique, as described by Hinuma and Hummeler (1961), is applied as follows: 10 ml of a virus suspension is mixed with 2 ml of 0.02% Versene, and the mixture is extracted twice with tap water saturated phenol at 40° for 2 minutes. The phenol is extracted by five successive additions of ether, which is removed by bubbling nitrogen.

Another method of obtaining infectious RNA was published by Gierer and Schramm (1956).

Deoxypentose Nucleic Acid Preparation by Marmur's (1961) Method. Bacteria harvested during the logarithmic phase of growth are lyzed by sodium lauryl sulfate at a final concentration of 16% at 60° in 10 minutes, then cooled to room temperature. If the bacteria are insensitive to this detergent, they can be lyzed with lysozyme at 37° in 30 to 60 minutes. This is followed by extraction with sodium lauryl sulfate at 60° for 10 minutes. The extracts should be treated with ribonuclease to remove RNA, according to Saito and Miura's (1963) method.

DNA Isolation Method by Rudin and Albertsson's (1976) Method. This newer method for the isolation of deoxyribonucleic acid from microorganisms consists of a multistep liquid-liquid extraction with an aqueous polymer two-phase system, and selective extraction of nucleic acids by changing the ionic composition of the system.

The following reagents are used:

1. Duponol ME, recrystallized twice from hot ethanol and washed with ether, used as a 25% solution in 45% ethanol.
2. Chloroform.
3. Isoamyl alcohol
4. Lysozyme, grade I.
5. Dextran 500.
6. Polyethyleneglycol (Carbonex 6000).
7. 40% stock solution in water, 0.1 M Li$_2$HPO$_4$.

The phase system consists of calculated amounts of the stock polymer solutions, mixed with distilled water and buffer solutions to obtain a system of the desired composition.

Procedure. Bacteria harvested in the late logarithmic phase are centrifuged and resuspended in 0.15 M NaCl solution containing 0.015 M sodium citrate. To obtain a crude lyzate, 29 mg lysozyme are added per 3.5 g of bacteria, suspended in 25 ml of the 0.15 M NaCl, 0.015 M sodium citrate. The suspension is incubated at 37° for 30 minutes, following which 2 ml of Duponol solution are added together with solid sodium chloride added to a final concentration of about 4 M. The lyzate is then shaken with an equal volume of a 24:1 mixture of chloroform and isoamyl alcohol for 20 minutes, and centrifuged at 6000-7000 $\times$ g for 10 minutes. The upper layer, containing the nucleic acids is collected and recentrifuged at 40,000 $\times$ g for 20 minutes.

The next parts of the procedure are conducted at 4° as follows: To the lysate (20 g) are added: 6 g dextran, 12 g polyethyleneglycol, 2 g buffer and 4.7 g solid NaCl. The phase separation is accomplished by brief centrifugation. The upper phase is collected and substituted with an equal volume of a fresh upper phase consisting of a mixture of 17 g of polyethyleneglycol 6000 and 183 % *g* of 4 M sodium chloride. This part of the procedure is repeated four times in order to remove the bulk of proteins and low molecular weight RNA.

To collect DNA from the upper phase, to the upper phase (10 ml) are added: 3.5 ml of 40% polyethyleneglycol, 4 ml of 0.1 *M* Li_2HPO_4 and distilled water to 20 ml. In the phase system thus formed, the DNA is formed mainly in the upper phase, and the yield is close to 100%. Polyethyleneglycol can be removed by extraction with chloroform, and the DNA is dialyzed against a buffer. Alternatively, polyethyleneglycol may be removed with 40% $(NH_4)_2SO_4$. The DNA in this case is found in the lower phase. Other methods for the DNA purification are: the column chromatography on methylated albumin-coated Kieselguhr or hydroxylapatite, or a preparative ultracentrifugation in a CsCl gradient.

The DNA preparation is purified in the following manner: a 5 *M* solution of sodium perchlorate is then added to the lyzed suspension to a final concentration of 1 *M,* and this mixture is shaken with an equal volume of a 24:1 (*v/v*) chloroform-isoamyl alcohol mixture for 30 minutes. The resultant emulsion is separated into three layers by centrifugation at 5000 to 10,000 rpm for 5 minutes. The upper, aqueous phase, containing nucleic acids, is collected. Nucleic acids are precipitated by gently layering two volumes of ethyl alcohol and are dispersed in a small volume of dilute saline-citrate.*

The concentrations of sodium chloride and citrate are then increased to 0.15 and 0.015 *M,* respectively, by adding enough concentrated saline-citrate solution. The prepared fluid is shaken again with an equal volume of chloroformisoamyl alcohol for 15 minutes, centrifuged, and the supernatant is withdrawn. The procedure of deproteinization should be repeated until very little protein is seen on the interface.

The final supernatant is precipitated with ethyl alcohol and dispersed in dilute saline-citrate solution. The pentose nucleic acid is removed from this fluid by digestion at 37° for 30 minutes with ribonuclease added to a final concentration of 50 μg/ml. The resultant liquid is again deproteinized as described above. The supernatant should be precipitated with ethyl alcohol and the drained nucleic acid dissolved in dilute saline-citrate. The deoxypentose nucleic acid is precipitated twice with 0.54 volume of isopropyl alcohol added dropwise in the presence of saline EDTA, which inhibits the DNase activity. (Saline EDTA contains 0.15 *N* NaCl and 0.1 *M* ethylenediaminetetra-acetate at pH 8.) The final precipitate is washed in increasing portions of ethyl alcohol.

* Dilute saline-citrate contains 0.015 *M* sodium chloride and 0.0015 *M* trisodium citrate, pH 7.0 ± 0.2. The concentrated saline-citrate solution consists of 1.5 *M* sodium chloride and 0.15 *M* trisodium citrate.

Teichoic acids, which are phosphate polymers containing either glycerol or ribitol residues joined through phosphodiester linkages, can be isolated from cell walls of certain bacteria by the method of Armstrong et al. (1958).

8. Preparation of Semisynthetic Antigens

The structure of semisynthetic antigens consists of a protein, artificially coupled to an ion or a chemical compound of low or medium molecular weight, which confers a serological specificity on this complex. The following radicals were coupled to the proteins: aniline, *p*-aminobenzoic acid, *p*-aminobenzene, sulfonic acid, *p*-aminophenyl arsonic acid, *p*-toluidine, *p*-nitro-aniline, 4-aminoantipyrine, *p*-aminoantipyrine, phenolfthalein, aminophenol, glucosides, colitose (3-deoxy-l-fucose), and aliphatic acids. Most of radicals were conjugated to proteins in vitro (Fell and Rodney, 1943; Pauling, 1947; Ogata et al., 1952). Some compounds, for example, phenolfthalein, cholesterol, and lecithin, were conjugated *in vivo* with serum or tissue proteins by injecting or feeding the colloidal radicals to animals (Rosenthal, 1938). The methods of Ogata et al. (1952) and Fell and Rodney (1943) have been chosen as patterns for the preparation of azoprotein antigens, the first one being the method of choice.

The Ogata et al. Technique. The diazo solution is prepared in the following manner: 5 g of arsanilic acid (atoxyl) is dissolved in 60 ml of 1 N hydrochloric acid, cooled in a freezing bath containing ice and salt, and diazotinized by adding a 10% solution of sodium nitrate, using a starch iodide paper as indicator. After 20 minutes, 1 g of urea is added to this mixture, which is then diluted with cold water to 100-ml volume. The diazo compound is coupled with a protein by mixing this solution with a cold 5% solution of purified proteins, at pH 8.0 to 8.5, and leaving the mixture in an ice-box overnight. The azoprotein is then precipitated by cautiously adding dilute hydrochloric acid. The azoprotein preparation may be purified by dissolving this precipitate in a dilute solution of sodium carbonate, followed by centrifugation and reprecipitation with dilute hydrochloric acid. This procedure can be repeated four to seven times until the supernatant becomes colorless. The final fluid must be dialyzed against tap water for 5 days, against distilled water for 2 days, and finally electro-dialyzed.

The arsenic to protein ratio in an azoprotein preparation can be estimated by determining the nitrogen content and arsenic content, the latter by Sandell's (1942) method.

The number of determinant groups per protein molecule can be calculated according to the Boyd and Hooker (1934) formula:

$$\text{As}\ \% = \frac{100R}{Fc}$$

where R is the arsenic-nitrogen ratio; Fc is the conversion factor, for example, the azoprotein to azoprotein ratio, calculated from the following formula:

$$Fc = 6.62(1 - 0.373R) + 3.05R$$

The Fell et al. Technique. This procedure is employed mostly for the diazotization of *p*-aminobenzoyl histamine with subsequent coupling to a protein; but it can be chosen as a general pattern of preparing conjugated antigens. In this technique, 92 g of *p*-aminobenzoylhistamine, dissolved in 1800 ml of water containing 110 ml of concentrated hydrochloric acid, and chilled in ice to 5°, is treated with 10% sodium nitrite added until a very slight excess is shown by starch iodide paper.

This diazonium salt mixture is added at once to 6000-ml volume of despeciated horse serum globulin (containing 29 mg N/ml) diluted 1:3 with distilled water, acidified with hydrochloric acid, and warmed to 30°. Subsequently, about 1 kg of sodium bicarbonate is added rapidly, with vigorous stirring. The mixture is left for 15 minutes, then adjusted to pH 7.4 and treated with sodium sulfate added rapidly to 23% concentration. The resultant precipitate must be centrifuged, and dialyzed overnight against running distilled water.

V. IMMUNOCHEMICAL METHODS FOR SEPARATION AND PURIFICATION OF POLYMERS

Native nonparticulate antigens, obtained by disruption or extraction of cells and tissues consist of different hetero- and homopolymers, which are soluble in water or in organic solvents. The polymers components of a soluble antigen preparation can be separated by a suitable physical or physicochemical procedure.

The polymer constituents of antigen preparations may be separated on the basis of different size, polydispersity, molecular weight and electric charge of the macromolecules. Accordingly, the techniques applied for the separation of antigens may be divided into five categories: (a) filtration, (b) differential gradient centrifugation, (c) electrophoresis, (d) column chromatography, and (e) immunosorption. Combinations of two or more of these methods may also be employed.

1. Separation of Antigen-Polymers by Dialysis and Ultrafiltration

Separation by dialysis consists in differential transport of solutes of different sizes across a porous barrier separating two liquids by the driving force of a concentration gradient. Small solutes, which are able to pass the porous barrier, diffuse freely through the membrane, whereas larger solutes do not pass the barrier. Equilibrium dialysis consists in adjusting electrolytic concentration.

In the ultrafiltration (reverse osmosis), the solutes possessing a certain size and suspended in a solvent are forced through the membrane barrier by considerably higher pressure on one side of the barrier than on the other.

The membrane used for dialysis (Visking casing) are made of viscose or cellulose (cellophane). The pore size of the membranes can be determined by the measurement of actual dialysis rates of solutes of known size under standard conditions. The rate of diffusion of the retentate from a dialysis bag to the outside aqueous solution of a low concentration of salts follows first-order kinetics.

Dialysis is usually carried out by suspending the dialysis bag, containing a retentate, in distilled water or a dilute buffer solution contained in a large container. The dialysis process is expedited by stirring of the diffusate with a magnetic bar rotating the specimens, and by continuous flow exchange of dialyzate fluid. A very convenient and efficient apparatus for multiple-specimen dialysis is Oxford dialyzer (Fig. 16), an apparatus designed by Craig and Konigsberg (1961) in which both the retentate and the diffusate are stirred which shortens the dialysis time considerably. Further improvement of the dialysis technique has been provided by the counter-current dialyzer (Craig and Stewart, 1965).

The concentration dialysis employs a dialyzing medium consisting of a solution of polyvinyl pyrrolidine K-30. The solution is prepared by adding 5 oz of PVP powder to 1000 ml of normal saline, brought to a boil. The medium is stirred and poured to a microdialyzer tank.

Electrodialysis is a rapid procedure for removal of low-molecular weight substances from a solute by a combined action of osmosis and electrophoresis. By this technique, all the electrolytes are removed in a short time whereas complete removal of salts by the dialysis alone requires the application of large volumes of ultrapure water over a long period of time. The electrodialysis is performed in a plastic dialysis unit consisting of three chambers, separated by membranes with a suitable porosity (Fig. 17). A receiving fluid is placed in the outer two chambers, and the material to be dialyzed is placed in the central compartment, which can be static or recirculating. If concentration of the sample in the center chamber is desired, or hypertonic solution of 20% water-soluble polyvinyl pyrrolidine or 100% sucrose is placed in the outer compartments. If demineralization is desired, the outer chambers are filled with distilled water. The sample is pumped into the lower part of the center chamber and exits from the upper part. After appropriate flow rates in the outer chambers have been established,

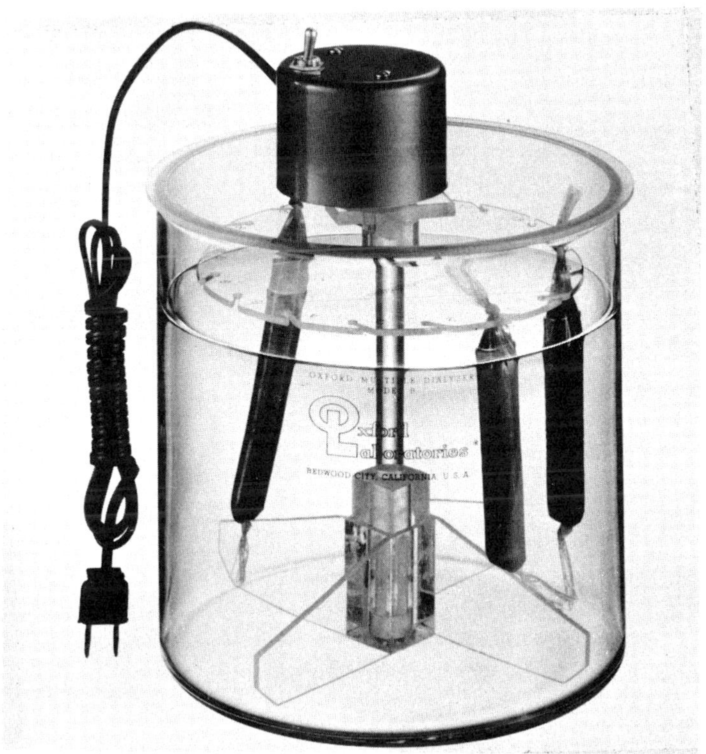

Figure 16. Multiple, electric dialyzer. Specimens placed in a cellophane tubing are attached to a rotating plate and are then rotated by an electric motor through a dialyzing buffer. The bags bump against four vertical baggles, thus agitating both the samples and the buffer for optimum dialyzing efficiency.

the electrodes of the dialysis unit are connected to a d.c. power supply to receive a current of 150 mA. The electrodialysis is usually complete in 3 hours.

Membrane ultrafiltration relies on selective molecular separation of solutes with different molecular dimensions. The membranes (DIAFLO UM1, UM2, and UM3) act as molecular screens that reject solutes at the membrane/solution interface and retain solutes with a larger molecular size and weight (Table 21).

The material to be ultrafiltered, dissolved in water, is passed across a suitably supported membrane, under the pressure of 10 to 100 psi, by means of compressed nitrogen (Fig. 18). Water and solutes below the retention ("cut-off") level pass through the membrane as ultrafiltrate. Retained substances are progressively concentrated upstream of the membrane. The

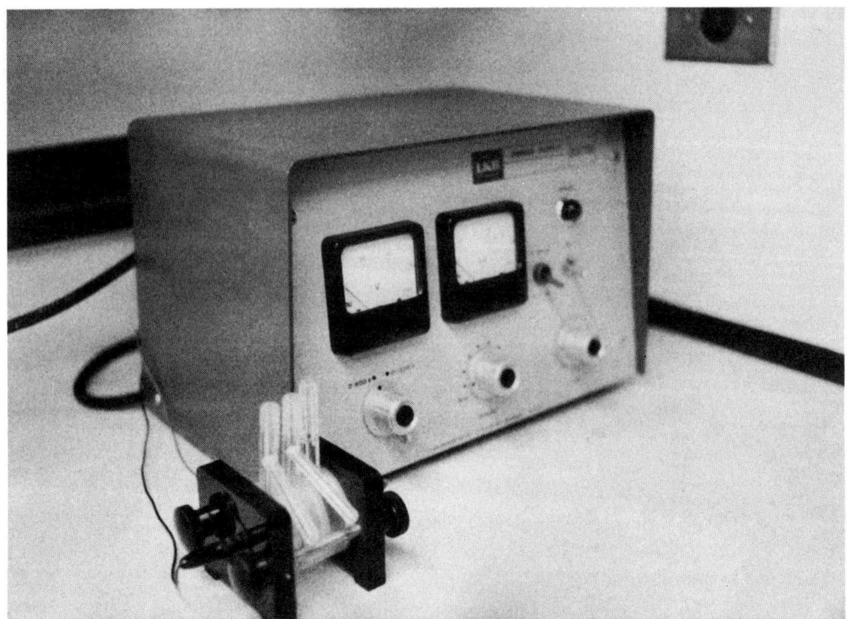

Figure 17. The electrodialyzer, consisting of an electrodialysis cell and a power supply. The material to be dialyzed is placed in the plastic electrodialysis cell which is equipped with appropriate membrane filters. The electrodialysis cell is connected to a water source and the power is supplied to the cell at 150 mA.

ultrafiltration is continued until the original solution reaches the required concentration or until sufficient ultrafiltrate free of unwanted substances has been collected. To reduce further the amount of micromolecular compounds, the retentate may be diluted with water to the original volume and passed again through the selected membrane.

The ultrafiltration can be carried continuously by adding the solvent at the same rate at which the ultrafiltrate is withdrawn.

2. *Separation of Antigen-Polymers by Preparative Gradient Centrifugation*

Centrifugal force is used for distribution of solute and solvent. The particles in solution are obtained under the centrifugal force at terminal velocity which increases with differences in their size, mass, or density relative to the solution and decreases with viscosity of the solution and deviations from spherical shape. The terminal velocity is measured and expressed by sedimentation coefficients which are computed from an observed terminal velocity, divided by the strength of the centrifugal field. The unit of sedimentation is the coefficient S, equal to 10^{-13} second. Values of sedimentation coefficient are frequently converted to standard conditions on infinite dilution in water at $20°$ and denoted at $S^0_{20,w}$ or as S_{20w}.

Table 21.   Retention Characteristics of Diaflo Membranes[a]

MW		Bacteria rickettsiae viruses high MW proteins
		← Apoferritin (480,000 MW)
70,000		
	XM-100	DNA (10 MW) ← Immunoglobulins (160,000 + MW)
60,000		
50,000		
		← Human albumin (67,000 MW)
	XM-50	
		← Hemoglobin (64,000 MW)
40,000		
		← Ovalbumin (45,000 MW)
30,000		
	PM-30	
		← *t*RNA (27,000 MW) ← Myoglobin (17,800 MW)
20,000		
	PM-10	← Polypeptides peptides
10,000		
	UM-10	
1,000	UM-2	← Raffinose (594 MW)
500	UM-05	← Sucrose (342 MW)

[a] Each membrane retains 90% or more of the compounds shown at a higher level. Vertical distances between membranes are roughly proportional to retention.

The centrifugal force, which is a gravitation-like force, acts at a distance on particles in solution and is proportional to the radius and the square of the angular speed. The time needed to sediment or float particles by velocity methods is related almost directly to the volume used and inversely to the square of the speed used. The following are the main centrifugation methods:

1. The moving-boundary method is used to clarify solutions or suspensions. Transport of particles in the solvent may proceed toward the bottom of the tube (sedimentation) or toward the top of the tube (floatation).

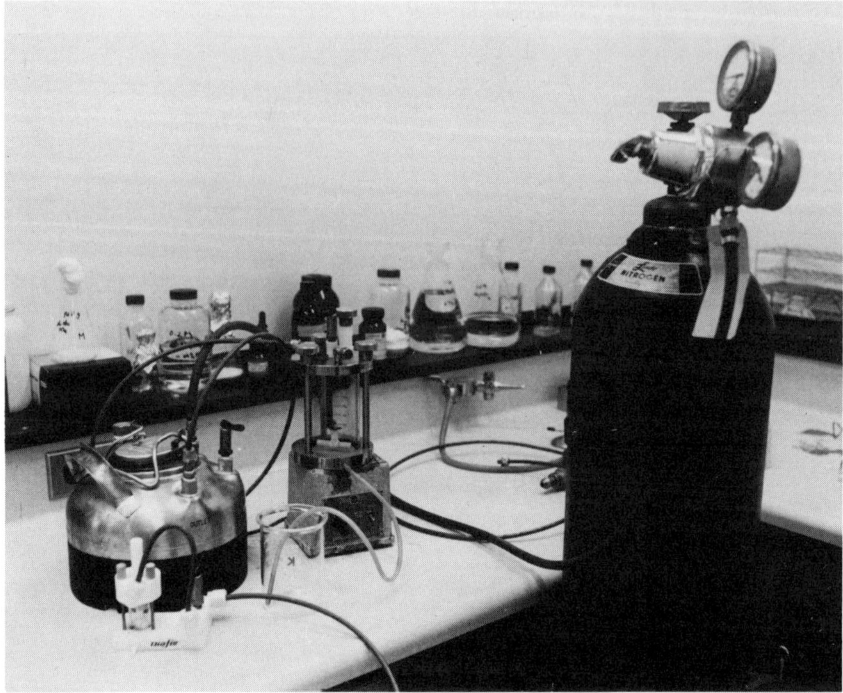

Figure 18.   Ultrafiltration system, consisting of a stirring assembly equipped with an appropriate, high permeability membrane, a liquid reservoir, and a gas supply cylinder.

2. The moving-zone centrifugation depends on the velocity separation of a band or zone of a faster component completely free of slower components in one cycle of centrifugation. This separation is usually obtained by employing a density gradient on which a small sample is layered.

Density gradients can be made by using different concentrations of sucrose, sodium nitrate, potassium bromide, potassium tartrate, cesium chloride, and others. The gradients may be produced by layering three different concentrations of a compound, beginning with the most concentrated and ending with the least concentrated solution or using a gradient forming apparatus (Fig. 19). The end layers should be one half the volume of intervening layer. To produce a continuous gradient of either linear or nonlinear shape, it is recommended to allow the gradient material to diffuse overnight before layering the sample and centrifuging. However, for special techniques in which relatively low centrifugal force is used, such as for separation of and purification of bacteria obtained from an organ or tissues, the undisturbed step gradient is recommended.

The sucrose gradient is prepared as follows (Martin and Ames, 1961). The gradient extending from 5% (*w/v,* 0.146 *M*) to 20% (0.58 *M*) cold sucrose in 0.05 *M* Tris HCl buffer at pH 7.5 is made. Samples of 0.2 ml, containing not more than 2% (*w/v*) protein are layered. A SW-39 swinging bracket rotor and 4.6-ml linear gradient is used.

Accelerate the rotor for 10 seconds and advance the speed dial to 39,000 rpm and centrifuge for 17 hours at 3°. Decelerate without the brake. Fractions are collected by dripping out the bottom or by forced flow out of the top. The fractions are assayed to determine the center of the zone of activity.

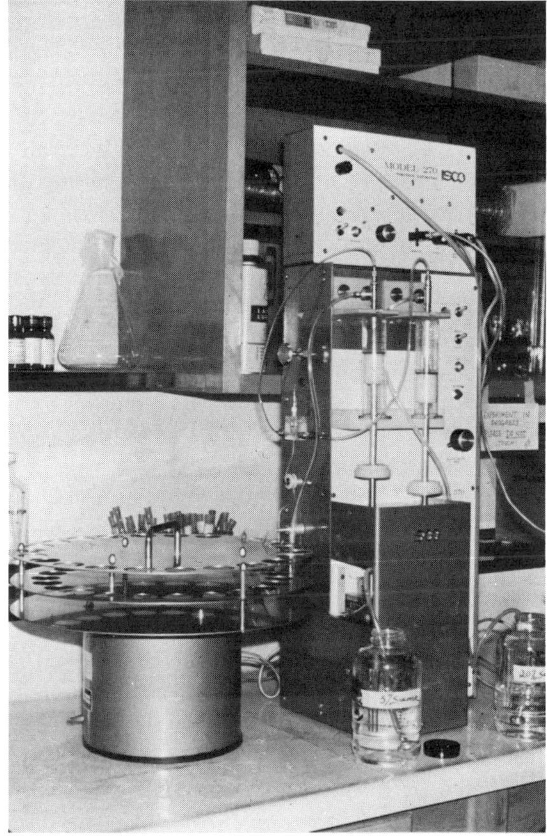

Figure 19. The automatic gradient former (right) and a rotary fraction collector (left).

The average *s*-rate (sedimentation coefficient) is calculated from the movement represented by the distance or volume between the center of the starting zone and the center of activity from the equation:

$$s*t'' = \Delta \overline{ST} \left[\frac{(\text{rpm})_{\text{max}}}{(\text{rmp})} \right]^2$$

The correction of S coefficient to 20% in water by equation shown below must be made by determining the composition (density and viscosity) of the gradient at a midpoint between initial and final zones.

$$S_{20,w} = \left(\frac{1 - \bar{v}p20,w}{1 - \bar{v}p} \right) \left(\frac{\eta}{\eta_{20},w} \right) S*$$

Gradients. Sucrose is the most common material for density gradients. Commercial sucrose contains ribonuclease and absorbes UV light. Most of the ribonuclease can be removed by treatment with decolorizing charcoal, adding 5–10 gm of charcoal per 100 ml of a sucrose solution containing 600–700 mg/ml and boiling gently for 5 to 10 minutes. This suspension is then filtered through a pad of charcoal in a Büchner funnel. Glycerol gradient columns may be used instead of sucrose, generally with similar results. Sucrose and glycerol, however, have a high osmotic pressure if used at effective concentrations, which may cause deterioration of some particulate matter. Gradients with a low osmotic pressure may be obtained by employing polymers such as polyvinyl pyrrolidine, polysucrose (Ficoll), or polyglucose.

Potassium tartrate, potassium citrate, and cesium chloride are also used for preparing instant gradients with generally good results, except that the stability of some particles may be effected by these salts. Concentrations of these salts vary from 3 to 7 or 8 *M*.

Equilibrium Centrifugation in Sucrose Gradients. Step-wise gradients, consisting of sucrose solutions ranging from 15 to 60% (*w/v*) are made in 0.02 *M* Tris HCl buffer (pH 7 to 7.5) and placed in centrifuge tubes to fit the SW 39 rotor of an ultracentrifuge and left at 4° for 12 to 24 hours before use. The material to be purified by sucrose gradient centrifugation is layered on top of the sucrose gradient, and after loading the rotor, the tubes are centrifuged at a desired speed, for example, 26,500 rpm at 4° for 12 to 18 hours. The rotor is deccelerated without breaking and the contents of tubes are removed through a needle which pierces the bottom of the tube. A number of fractions, ranging from 12 to 20, are collected per tube, and the density is estimated by refractometry at room temperature.

Discontinuous Sucrose Gradient Centrifugation. The discontinuous sucrose gradient according to Rowley and Turner's (1964) method is made in lusteroid tubes of the SW 39 Spinco rotor by successive layering of 1 ml amounts of 40, 35, 20, and 10% sucrose made in 1 M NaCl. The gradient is left at 4° for 24 hours and then layered with 1 ml of a material to be separated or purified by the gradient. Centrifuge the gradient for 18 hours at 35,000 rpm. Pierce each tube with a 25-gauge needle and allow the liquid to flow slowly into tubes containing 3 ml of saline. The protein content of each sample, if a proteinaceous material, is used as a sample, and is read at 280 nm in a spectrophotometer.

The Ficoll Density Gradient. The gradient is prepared from a Ficoll (a polysucrose possessing high molecular weight and low viscosity, Pharmacia Inc., New Market, N.J.) dissolved to 50% in distilled water and dialyzed at 2 to 4° for 24 hours. A better method for deionization of Ficoll is by means of a mixed bed resin (AG-501-x8(D), Bio-Rad) at a concentration of 10-g resin/50-g Ficoll (Gorczynski et al., 1970). The deionization is carried out at 4° with constant stirring for 4 hours, and then repeated. The resin is removed by filtration through gauze. The dialyzed or deionized Ficoll is diluted at 2, 4, 6, 8, 10, 14, 16, and 20% in 0.25 M sucrose, 0.01 M MgCl$_2$, and 0.03 M Tris buffer (pH 8.1). The Ficoll solutions (3 ml) are carefully layered one after another and left at 4° for 48 to 60 hours. The sample (9 ml) is layered on top of the gradient and centrifuged at 57,000 $\times$ g for 30 minutes or as required. The opaque zones are removed with a capillary pipette (Ghosh and Murray, 1969).

A linear Ficoll gradient is obtained using two chambers, one containing low density Ficoll and a mixing chamber filled with an initially high density Ficoll solution. The low density material is pumped into the mixing chamber at half the rate that the dense material is pumped out. The sample is introduced into both chambers at equal concentrations (Gorczynski et al., 1970). Gradients are centrifuged at 3800 $\times$ g in an SW 25 rotor. Fractions (1 ml) are collected by upward displacement using dimethylphthalate (1.14 g/ml) as a displacement medium (Shortman, 1968).

The Cesium Chloride Density Gradient. The cesium chloride gradient is prepared by overlaying 1 ml of cesium chloride solution of density 1.46 with 1 ml of solution of density of 1.36 and further overlayered with 1 ml of solution of density 1.26 placed in a 5-ml Lusteroid centrifuge tube. The gradients are prepared at 2 to 4° and are used immediately after the material sample (1 ml) is placed on top. The tubes, in case of purification of viruses, are centrifuged at 2 to 4° at 35,000 rpm in the SW 29 L rotor of the Spinco Model L ultracentrifuge for 2.5 to 3.5 hours. The centrifuge must be stopped without using the braking mechanism. The virus or virus components are obtained from the opalescent bands. The bands are removed with a hypodermic syringe by piercing a hole through the side of the tube or from the top using a hypodermic needle with the beveled tip removed. Cesium chloride is removed by dialysis against distilled water.

The isopycnic gradient in this procedure is formed during the centrifugation of a dense solution, and particles form bands at their own densities.
Solutions of rubidium, cesium chloride, cesium formate, or cesium sulfate
may be used to form the gradient.

Cesium chloride is added to a particle suspension in a phosphate-buffered
saline to adjust the density to a final density of 1.33. The suspension is
centrifuged in the SW 39 rotor of the Spinco Model L ultracentrifuge at
$110,000 \times g$ for 40 hours at 6°. The centrifuge is allowed to stop without
braking, and the fractions are collected by piercing the base of the centrifuge with a hypodermic needle and collecting drops.

Isodensity Technique. The isodensity, buoyant density, or isopycnic
value of a substance is a characteristic which refers to the density of a solution in which the agent neither sediments or floats when subjected to a centrifugal field. The isodensity method is mainly used for purification of subcellular particles and viruses. If the agent is suspended in a solvent of
approximately the buoyant density, the size of the agent determines the
time needed for the particles to reach their positions. Concentration and
purification of the agent can be reached without pellet formation.

3. Separation of Antigen-Polymers by Electrophoresis

Migration of molecules in the electric field depends on their electrophoretic mobility and the resistance of supporting medium.

Mobility (μ) of particles in an electric field is proportioned to the potential gradient applied, and it may be expressed and measured in the following
terms:

$$\mu = \frac{\text{rate of migration}}{\text{potential gradient}} = \left[\frac{\text{cm/second}}{\text{V/cm}}\right] = \left[\text{cm}^2/(\text{V})(\text{second})\right]$$

Although the mobility is a characteristic property of the particle, it varies
in certain limits depending on the pH, the ionic strength, and the composition of the supporting electrolyte. The mobility of molecules depends on
their individual net electric charge, corrected for ions present in the surface
of shear, its size and shape, and the ionic strength of the liquid medium.
The net charge is influenced not only by the state of ionization of the acidic
and basic groups, as expressed by the pH of a medium, but also by the
binding of buffer ions to the molecules migrating in it. The electrophoretic
mobility is expressed mathematically by the following equation:

$$\mu = \frac{D}{4\pi\gamma} \left[\zeta + 5a^5 \int_\infty^a \frac{\psi(r)}{r^6} \, dr - 2a^3 \int_\infty^a \frac{\psi(r)}{r^4} \, dr\right]$$

where $\psi(r)$ is the potential occurring in the ionic atmosphere; zeta the
potential of the surface of shear, γ the coefficient of viscosity of the sup-

porting medium, a the particle or molecule radius, D the dielectric constant, and μ is the electrophoretic mobility for a molecule or particle.

The zone electrophoresis is used for the separation of the components or fractions present in a mixture, whereas the free-boundary electrophoresis is a method for determination of mobilities of charged particles. In the zone electrophoresis, a mixture of polymers or molecules is separated into discreet zones, after a migration of the particles in an electric field from an initial narrow zone of sample. The supporting, stabilizing medium is provided by filter paper, cellulose-acetate membrane, starch grain, synthetic polymer beads (e.g., Pevikon), or gel media, for example, agar, acrylamide, or starch. The gel-electrophoresis technique is divided into nonsieving techniques, where agar, agarose, or cellulose acetate are used, and techniques producing separation by the molecular sieve effect when acrylamide or starch are employed as supporting media.

The molecular sieving action enhances the resolution of antigenic materials by anticonvection, according to different charges by causing a separation relative to the size of molecules or particles. Although usually the differences in size and charge provide for a good resolution of the molecules, sometimes the differences in charge and size may be mutually canceling; for example, some immunogolbulins may be superimposed on much larger molecules, and proteins varying considerably by size of molecules may move as a single band. This action is further improved by gradient gels and by a two-dimensional gel-electrophoresis. In the gradient gel-electrophoresis, molecules are driven through gradually decreasing pores until they are brought almost to a stop in order of their size (the pore-limit electrophoresis). The electrophoresis may be conducted either in the vertical or in the horizontal position, but the vertical gel-electrophoresis is preferable because of its superior resolving power and the possibility of employing larger samples of material. The two-dimensional gel-electrophoresis techniques employ the horizontal position for both dimension.

In the two-dimensional procedures, the material resolved in one system is transferred into a second system for further separation and purification (Raymond, 1964; Margolis and Kenrick, 1969). The two-dimensional gel-electrophoresis technique has been improved further by the introduction of sigmoid gradients (Wein, 1969). The sigmoid gradients, coupled to a two-dimensional electrophoresis, account for a rapid separation of complex polymer mixtures. Optimal zone separation by the electric current is signified by very narrow fractions occurring at large distances from each other. Diffusion of bands in agar gel is relatively greater than in the polyacrylamide or starch gels, but the application of a high-voltage to the electrophoresis in agar often results in a very sharp resolution of substances. Most proteins can be separated by the polyacrylamide-gel electrophoresis at pH 8.0 to 9.5, whereas many polysaccharides are resolved at a lower pH value ranging from pH 4 to 6.0. Nucleic acids require a pH value varying from 6.5 to 7.5, and phospholipids can be resolved in Kwapinski's and McEwan's buffer, adjusted to a desired pH ranging from 8.9 to 10.0, and consisting of:

Tris	5.16 g
Glycine	3.48 g
Tween-80	20 ml
Distilled water	980 ml

Highly polymerized materials, for example, complexes consisting of protein, polysaccharide and nucleotides are soluble at a very narrow pH range, apparently due to a considerable diversity of the isoelectric regions of different constituents.

The One-Dimensional Polyacrylamide Electrophoresis. The original technique (Ornstein, 1964; Davis, 1964) has been improved by the application of a nonlinear gradient (Minden and Farr, 1969). For the nonlinear gradient polyacrylamide electrophoresis, stock and working solutions are the same as used for the Davis' technique (Tables 22–24), but the gels are prepared at the concentrations of 3.75, 4.75, and 12%. The stock Tris-glycine buffer, pH 8.3, is diluted 1:5, and the ammonium persulfate solution is adjusted to 0.145%. Pyrex tubes (12 cm and 6 mm) are marked from the upper end at 3.5, 4.5, 5.5, 7, and 1 cm, and filled with 12% acrylamide solution to the 7-cm mark, followed by the overlaying of 12% acrylamide solution to the 5.5-cm mark. The 4.75% is then introduced to the 4.5-cm mark and the 3.75% gel to the 3.5-cm mark. The tubes are water-layered, and the gels are exposed to a fluorescent light to polymerize (Fig. 20). The tubes are then inserted onto a buffer compartment of the disk-electrophoresis apparatus (Fig. 21), a 0.2–0.6-ml sample (± 300 μg) in 40% sucrose is layered over the 3.75% gel by displacement of buffer over the top of the gel. Electric current of 5-mA tube is applied for 90 to 120 minutes, or until the bromophenol blue tracking dye has reached the 11-cm mark. The gels are then removed from tubes and stained with an appropriate staining solution (see p. 142) and decolorized, either statically by elution or electrophoretically.

The decolorization by electrophoresis is completed within 15 minutes whereas the decolorization by elution takes a few hours. The transverse gel rod destainer (Fig. 22) consists of a plastic unit holding two carbon electrodes. The gel slabs are placed horizontally in a special Perspex frame, and the cell is sealed by a foam plastic strip. The compartments containing the electrodes are filled with 7 to 10% acetic acid. The apparatus is connected to a power supply which delivers 100 mA for each gel slab, while it is cooled with circulating water.

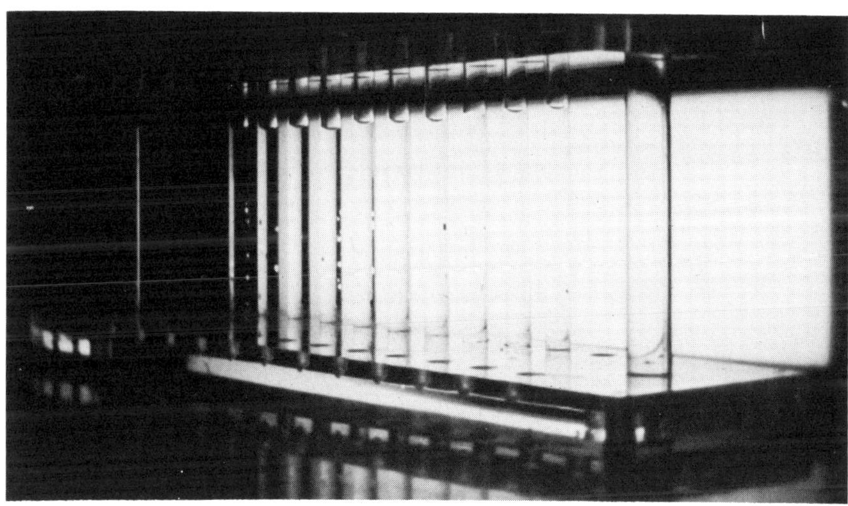

Figure 20. Polymerization rack exposed to a fluorescent light for polymerization of the acrylamide gel.

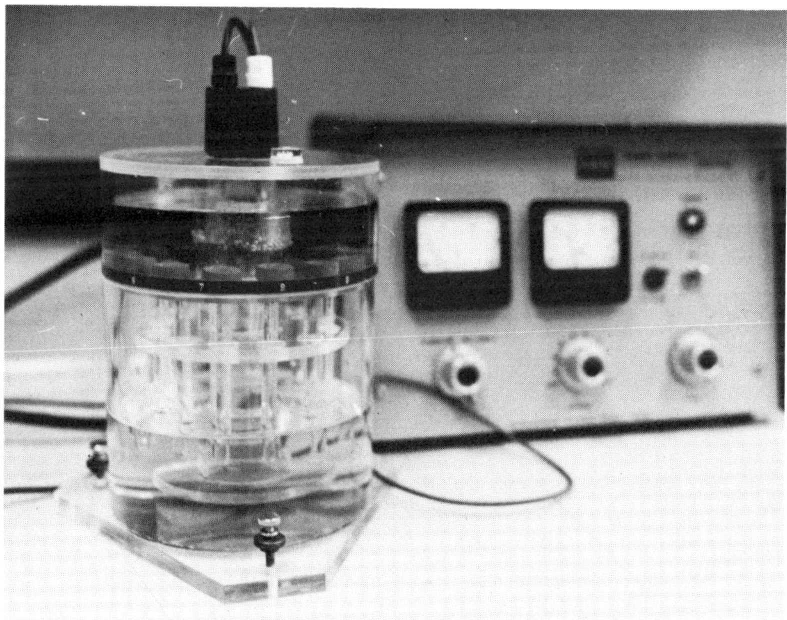

Figure 21. The analytic disk-electrophoresis apparatus with a power supply.

Table 22. Cationic Gel System (Running pH, 2.7)

	Volume Ratios	Components/100 ml			pH (25°)
Lower gel	1	Acrylamide	30	g	
		bisacrylamide	0.8	g	
	2	1 N KOH	12	ml	
	2	acetic acid	53.2	ml	2.9
		temed	0.24	ml	
		Potassium persulfate	120	mg	
	1	riboflavin	2	mg	
Upper gel		Acrylamide	10	gm	
	1	bisacrylamide	0.8	g	
		1 N KOH	24	ml	
	1	acetic acid	1.47	ml	6.7
		temed	0.1	ml	
	2	Potassium persulfate	60	mg	
		riboflavin	1	mg	
		Components/Liter			
Upper buffer		Glycine	28.1	g	
		Acetic acid	3.05	ml	4.0
Lower buffer		Acetic acid	43	ml	
		1 N KOH	120	ml	4.3

These buffers can be used at 1/10 strength.

Micromethod of Polyacrylamide Electrophoresis. The micromethod described by Felgenhauer (1967) allows to separate and detect as little as 1 to 3 μg of single protein, as opposed to several hundred micrograms of protein required for a macroelectrophoresis.

In the micromethod, the lower polyacrylamide gel is composed of 10.5% acrylamide, 0.78% N, N'-methylenebisacrylamide, 0.08 vol % N, N, N', N'-tetramethylethylenediamine, 5.25 mg % $K_3Fe(CN)_6$, 0.5 M Tris HCl (pH 8.75), 14.5% glucose, and 0.07% ammonium persulfate. The gels are degassed at 4° for 3 minutes under aspirator vacuum with occasional shaking.

The upper gel consists of 3% acrylamide, 0.75% N, N'-methylenebisacrylamide, 0.5 mg % riboflavin, 32 mM phosphoric acid, 59 mM Tris (pH), and 10% glucose.

Table 23. Cationic Gel System (Running pH, 4.3)

	Volume Ratios	Components/100 ml			pH (25°)
Lower gel	1	Acrylamide	30	g	
		bisacrylamide	0.8	g	
	1	1 *N* KOH	24	ml	
		acetic acid	8.8	ml	4.3
		temed	0.24	ml	
	2	Potassium persulfate	60	mg	
		riboflavin	2	mg	
Upper gel	1	Acrylamide	10	g	
		bisacrylamide	0.8	g	
	1	1 *N* KOH	48	ml	
		acetic acid	2.87	ml	6.7
		temed	0.1	ml	
	2	Potassium persulfate	60	mg	
		riboflavin	2	mg	

	Components/Liter			pH (25°)
Upper buffer	Acetic acid	8	ml	
	beta alanine	31.2	g	4.5
Lower buffer	Acetic acid	43	ml	
	1 *N* KOH	120	ml	4.3

These buffers can be used at 1/10 strength.

Capillary tubes (10-cm long with 1-mm internal diameter) are filled from the bottom by an aspirator, first with 1 cm of distilled water and then with 6 cm of lower gel, drawn by continuous aspiration. The capillary tube, still attached to the aspirator, is immediately set on a plasticine in the vertical position. The whole procedure is conducted at 4°.

The gels are then polymerized, and the remaining water is expelled by centrifugation at a very low speed for 1 to 2 minutes. The bottom of centrifuge tubes is covered by a cotton plug. The upper gel is inserted into the top of the capillary tube by a 3-cm-long hypodermic needle attached to an injection device. Entrapped air is expelled by gentle centrifugation. A small amount of water is injected into the capillary tube and the air is again removed by centrifugation. The gel is then photopolymerized, and the remaining fluid is removed by centrifugation.

Table 24.   Reagents for Acrylamide Electrophoresis

	Anionic Gel System (Running pH, 9.3)		
	Volume Ratios	Components/100 ml	pH (25°)
Lower gel	1	Acrylamide 30 g bisacrylamide[a] 0.8 g water to volume	
	1	Tris[b] 18.15 1 1 N HCl 24 ml temed 0.24 ml water to volume	9.1
	2	Ammonium persulfate 0.14 g water to volume	
Upper gel	1	Acrylamide 10 g bisacrylamide 0.8 g water to volume	
	1	Tris 2.23 g 1 M H_3PO_4 12.8 ml temed 0.1 ml water to volume	6.7
	1	Riboflavin 2 mg water to volume	
	1	Ammonium persulfate 80 mg water to volume	
	Components/Liter		
Upper buffer		Tris 5.16 g glycine 3.48 g water to volume	8.91
Lower buffer		Tris 14.5 g 1 N HCl 60 ml water to volume	8.07

[a] N,N'-methylenebisacrylamide.
[b] 2-Amino-2-hydroxymethyl)-1,3-propanediol.
[c] N,N,N',N'-tetramethyl ethylenediamine.

The sample (10–30 μg of protein in 5 μl) is supplemented with 1 μl of 50% glucose and 1 μl of a 1:8 diluted saturated solution of bromphenol blue. The sample is introduced by means of a 1-cm needle, and it is spun onto the surface of the gel.

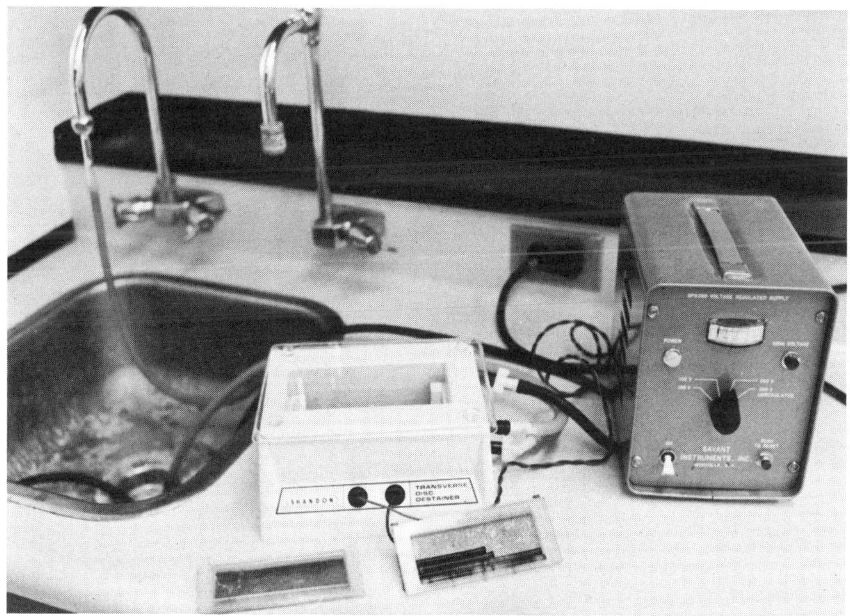

Figure 22.   An electric transverse destainer with the power supply apparatus.

The unfilled part of the capillary tube and the portion containing the plasticine is cut off, and the tube is inserted into perforated plastic caps, which fit into the holes of a disc electrophoresis apparatus. Filled tubes are kept in a water-saturated chamber. The running buffer is a 49.5 mM Tris 0.38 M glycine (pH 8.3) buffer. A constant current of 0.02 to 0.06 mA per tube is applied.

After the electrophoresis, the tubes are centrifuged to remove the remaining fluid and sealed by a piston of paraffin. The gel thread is pushed out with a close-fitting stylet into a staining bath, containing 0.5% Amido Black in 5% acetic acid. The gels are stained for 30 minutes, rinsed in water and destained in 2% acetic acid.

The gels may be scanned at 546 nm in a densitometer using a slot of 3 nm × 0.2 mm.

The resolution obtained by the micromethod is comparable to that obtained by a conventional disk-electrophoresis.

The Two-Dimensional Acrylamide Electrophoresis (Margolis and Kenrick, 1969).   Acrylamide slabs are made of 2.7% acrylamide with 5% cross-linkage, 0.5% dimethylaminoproprionitrile, and 0.5% ammonium persulfate, leaving a free 1- to 2-cm space for application of a sample. The bottom of the tube is sealed with a cellulose-acetate membrane. After a polymerization time, the unpolymerized solution on the surface of the gel is washed away. The gels are prerun in a disk-electrophoresis apparatus at 50 V in a selected buffer for 1 hour, after which a 10-μl sample, previously dialyzed against the same buffer, is placed on top of the gel. If more diluted samples are used, it is recommended to add 10% sucrose to the dialysis solution. To trace the progress of electrophoretic migration, one sample is tagged with Coomassie brilliant blue (Fazekes de St. Groth et al., 1963) and all the gel slabs are subjected to an electric field of 70 V for 1 to 2 hours. Since the gel rods are semifluid, they cannot be handled in the usual manner. It is recommended to expel the gels under buffer with the aid of a rubber teat. The gels are gently transferred into wider tubes.

The second dimension of the electrophoresis is conducted in gradient gels prepared in glass cells according to Margolis and Kenrick's (1968) method. The cells have a diameter of 82 $\times$ 82 $\times$ 5 mm and sucrose is omitted. Either linear or concave gradients may be used although the concave gradients are preferable. The concave gradients are prepared by means of a tall, flat, rectangular vessel with an adjustable partition. Upon the completion of this stage, the gels are pipetted onto the surface of the gradient slabs. The slabs are placed into the electrophoresis apparatus, and run for 24 hours in Tris-EDTA borate buffer, pH 9.2, at 6°, using a 70-V current falling from initial 25 to final 10 mA. After the electrophoresis, the gels are stained with 0.3% Amido Black solution for 8 to 16 hours and destained by continuous washing in 7% acetic acid with or without the aid of current.

Double Disk-Electrophoresis by Racusen (1967). This technique depends on a single system allowing the simultaneous separation of oppositely charged proteins. The system consists of two discontinuous buffer systems which provide concentrating and running conditions for anionic and cationic proteins in a single sample.

The apparatus used for the double disk-electrophoresis consists of two separate gel tubes joined by a 3-cm section of clear plastic hose pierced with a small opening through which a sample solution is injected. One gel tube is filled with a weak acid, for example, taurine (pK_2 8.7) and its potassium salt, and the other tube contains a weak base, such as imidazole, pK 7.0, and its chloride. The sample is introduced into the plastic hose where it is polymerized, and it provides the ionic connection between the two gel tubes.

The composition of gels is as follows: (a) Cation running, buffer, pH 8.1: (running pH of 7.5): 1.2 ml of 1 *M* KOH, 0.75 g taurine, 25 μl tetramethylethylenediamine, diluted to 10 ml. (b) Anion running gel buffer, pH 7.7 (running pH of 8.3): 1.2 ml of 1 *N* HCl, 0.5 g imidazole, and 50 μl tetramethylethylenediamine, diluted to 10 ml with distilled water.

Running gels are prepared by mixing 2 volumes of one of these buffers with 2 volumes of a solution of 20 g acrylamide, 0.8 g N, N'-methylenebisacrylamide, 7.5 mg potassium ferricyanide, and distilled water to 100 ml, with 4 volumes of 0.14% ammonium persulfate in distilled water. The mixture is pipetted into the glass tubes to within $\frac{1}{8}$ in. of the top and layered with water. Polymerization occurs in 10 minutes, indicated by the appearance of a refractile zone below the initial layer.

The sample gel contains 200 μl of distilled water containing bromphenol blue or safranin 0 as tracking dye, 150 μl of 1% aqueous tetramethylenediamine, 150 μl of a solution containing 4 mg of riboflavin in 100 ml of water, 150 μl of 40% acrylamide solution, and 10% aqueous N, N'-methylenebisacrylamide and 1.75 ml of a sample dissolved in 0.025 M phosphate solution, pH 7.0. The components of sample gel are mixed quickly and 1 ml of the mixture is injected into the sample chambers. A piece of plastic film is then slid over the drop to seal off air, and the chambers are exposed to bright fluorescent light until the gel has become opalescent.

The units are then placed in a disc-electrophoresis apparatus, filled with the following solutions: negative electrode reservoir, 0.038 M taurine and 0.0038 M KOH; positive electrode container, 0.038 M imidazole and 0.0038 M HCl. An electric current of 100 V is applied for 2 hours.

The Sigmoid Gradient Polyacrylamide Gel Electrophoresis. The principle of Wein's (1969) method is similar to the combined paper electrophoresis and chromatography. Thus a protein mixture is separated electrophoretically on a rectangular gel slab first in one direction and then separated further in a second direction which is perpendicular to the first direction. The sigmoid concentration gradients of polyacrylamide gel are prepared in a special apparatus by filling a rectangular gel compartment in the diagonal direction with an exponentially increasing concentration of acrylamide. The gradients are sigmoid with references to the migration path of the protein samples.

In practice, the sample of a material is layered on top of a photopolymerized gel inside the sample well of the apparatus. Electrophoresis is conducted in the first direction at 4° and 40 mA (approximately 250 V) for 90 to 120 minutes. This is followed by the electrophoresis in the perpendicular direction; the sample well is discarded and the extending photopolymerized gel is removed. The gel slabs are detached after the completion of electrophoresis from the plexi glass plates with a stream of diulted acetic acid, using a syringe. The slabs are stained with Coomassie blue (Meyer and Lamberts, 1965) and destained by washing in a mixture of water, methanol, acetic acid, and glycerol (50/40/7/2.5).

Preparative Column Electrophoresis. Although the best resolution and separation of proteins, nucleic acids, phospholipids, and polysaccharides has been obtained by preparative polyacrylamide gel electrophoresis, the preparation and purification of the material may also be attained by means of Sephadex G-25 gel electrophoresis (Porath, 1968) or by preparative electrophoresis in a horizontal gel (Avrameas and Uriel, 1964). The latter method combines a single electrophoretic run to separate components of a mixture with a simultaneous recovery of resolved components by continuous elution. An electrophoresis-elution unit has been designed and produced for this technique.

The electrophoresis-convection method depends on a mild physical fractionation of proteins in solution by a technique utilizing a combination of electrophoretic and convective transport of the components of a sample to achieve separation (Cann et al., 1949). A semicontinuous modification of this technique was described by Timasheff et al. (1953). Separation of a mixture of proteins by this technique is obtained by successive immobilization of the components and transport of the mobile components from the top to the bottom reservoir in a special electrophoresis-convection apparatus.

Starch-Gel Electrophoresis. In the starch-gel electrophoresis, separation of polymers is obtained due to the different electric charge and molecular size of molecules. The resolution power of the starch-gel medium varies with the concentration of starch and the composition of a buffer. The discontinuous system of buffers is by far most suitable for a good separation of components of a mixture. The starch-gel electrophoresis, originally described by Smithies (1959), has been improved by preparing the gel in buffers containing a disassociating agent (Poulik, 1960). A two-dimensional method has been developed by Poulik (1964, 1966). In the latter method, a regular starch-gel is used for the first dimension, and a starch-gel prepared either in urea or in urea and mercapto-ethanol is employed for the second dimension.

The Vertical Starch-Gel Electrophoresis (Smithies, 1959). The starch medium is placed in plastic trays measuring 32 × 12 × 0.6 cm and possessing removable antiplates. The starch-gel is prepared by suspending specially hydrolyzed starch of high quality (manufactured by Connaught Medical Research Laboratories, Toronto) in borate buffer at the concentration specified on every batch of the hydrolyzed starch, but the concentration must be increased by about 10% when Tris-citrate buffer is employed. An alternative buffer consists of 8 *M* urea and 0.35 *M* glycine solution, pH 8.8 (Cohen and Porter, 1964). The suspension of hydrolyzed starch in a buffer must be filtered through gauze, following which filtrate is heated with a constant agitation until the starch becomes viscous and then loses the viscosity gradually and becomes more transparent. At this stage, the gel is degassed under vacuum for a short time, and the clear gel is placed in the tray, the bottom of which has been coated with a thin layer of mineral oil. A cover coated with mineral oil, except the immediate region of the gel-former, is placed in 10 minutes on the warm gel. The cover is secured in position by flat weights, each 13 cm in width. The gel is allowed to stand for 6 hours, after which the cover is removed and the slots are walled off with hot petrolatum jelly. Samples of the material are applied to the slots; the slots are covered with warm petrolatum jelly and the gel surface is covered in Saran wrap. The end plates of the plastic tray are then removed, and the tray is placed upright in the lower electrode vessel. The exposed upper surface of the gel is connected with the buffer in the upper electrode vessel by means of a filter paper wick.

A voltage gradient of 4 to 5 V/cm is applied for 18 to 20 hours at room temperature. After the run, the gel is cooled at 4° for 1 hour and then removed from the tray and placed on the slicing tray. With a dermatome knife, the upper part of the gel is separated from the lower part. One half of the gel is stained with a dye solution for 1 to 2 minutes and then decolorized in the tank of the decolorizing machine and washed for 3 hours. Final decolorization is conducted in a fresh decolorizing solution overnight.

Tris Buffer. Tris 9.2 g, citric acid (monohydrated) 1.005 g and distilled water 1 liter, pH 8.5 to 8.6. This buffer is used for preparing the gel. The tank buffer, used in the electrode vessel, consists of 18.5 g of boric acid and 2.5 g of NaOH dissolved in 1 liter of distilled water.

The Dye Solution. Amido Black 10B and Buffalo Black NBR are the recommended dyes for starch-gel electrophoresis. The dye solution is prepared by dissolving 6 g of Buffalo Black in a mixture of methyl alcohol (405 ml), glacial acetic acid (90 ml), and distilled water (405 ml), and filtered through two layers of gauze. The decolorizing solution is the above mixture containing no dye.

Fjellström's (1963) Modification of Preparative Starch-Gel Electrophoresis. The starch-gel is prepared with Tris-citrate acid buffer containing 0.0005 M sodium EDTA and 20 mg ascorbic acid/100 ml buffer. The starch-gel electrophoresis is performed according to Poulik's (1957) technique employing a discontinuous system of buffers. The serum or globulin preparation is applied in a volume of 0.3 to 0.4 ml to three pieces of Whatman No. 1 filter paper (0.6 × 9 cm), placed on top of each other and put in a slit at one-third of the length from the cathodic end of the gel and at right angles to the direction of current flow. The electrophoresis is carried for 3 to 4 hours and then discontinued. Strips 1 to 2 cm wide are then cut off the edges of the gel parallel to the direction of migration and are divided horizontally in two parts. One part is stained with Amido Black 10B to be used as a guide for cutting the main gel so that each piece of the cut gel mainly contains single electrophoretic fractions. The protein is eluted from starch-gel after the pieces of gel are frozen and thawed. Each thawed piece of the gel is placed into a cylinder which possesses a thin sheet of porous polyethylene plastic on its bottom; in centrifugation the contents of the gel passes through while the starch substance is retained. Centrifugation is conducted at 4° at 30,000 × *g* for 10 minutes. The eluate is collected and may be concentrated under negative pressure through ultrafiltration through a collodion membrane.

The Two-Dimensional Starch-Gel Electrophoresis. According to Poulik's (1964) method, the material is first separated by a vertical starch-gel electrophoresis in the discontinuous system of buffers (first dimension) after which the portion of the gel in which the diluted material was run, is removed, sliced in two, and stained with an Amido Black 10B solution for detection of the zones of separated materials. In the second dimension, the electrophoresis is carried out in specially made plastic trays (200 × 280 × 6 mm). The starch-gel may be of the same nature as for the first dimension, or a urea starch-gel may be employed. The starch-gel is poured into the plastic trays and covered with a glass plate. Slots, 6-mm wide, are then cut out across the gel, 5 cm from the intended anodal end of the gels. Starch blocks containing the separated components in the first dimension cut out from the unsliced center portion of the first dimensioned run are placed into these slots. The gels are covered with Saran wrap to prevent evaporation and left at room temperature for 5 hours. After this period of equilibration and reaction, a second-dimension electrophoretic run is performed in horizontal position. The gel is connected with the electrode buffer by means of filter paper wick and a voltage gradient of 5.0 V/cm is applied for 16 hours. The gels are then cooled at 4° for 1 hour and sliced. One half is stained with an Amido Black 10B solution and decolorized in 1% acetic acid. The other half may be used for immunological analysis.

The High-Voltage Agar-Gel Electrophoresis. The sample to be subjected to the high-voltage electrophoresis (Wieme, 1964) is applied to a narrow slot cut with a piece of Whatman no. 3 MM filter paper in a 1.6-mm-thick agar layer on supporting glass slide. The liquid sample is immediately applied to the slot. The gel is connected with the buffer chambers by means of wet filter-paper wicks. The buffer has the ionicity ranging from 0.03 to 0.06. A recommended buffer is 0.05 *M*, pH 8.4 barbital buffer, used for the separation of proteins. At a lower ionic strength, the conductivity of the medium is increased and the electric field is markedly distorted. At higher values, the cooling of the plate becomes difficult. The agar gel is cooled and sealed with petroleum ether, placed in a central chamber, whereas the buffer is poured into two lateral electrode vessels. The agar-coated glass slides are supported by two large agar blocks of the composition identical to that of the electrophoresis slide.

Before the application of electric current, the petroleum ether is cooled to 12° by continuously pumping air. The agar slide is equilibrated for 1 minute. The current is applied and the tension at the electrodes is increased slowly (about 1 minute) to permit the temperature gradient to establish itself. The constant voltage at the electrodes is then set to a desired value, ranging from 60 to 150 V, for 1 to 2 hours.

After the electrophoresis, the agar slides are removed, washed in saline and stained with an Amido Black B solution, and decolorized (see p. 119).

Preparative Zone Electrophoresis on Powder Blocks. Block electrophoresis is perhaps the simplest preparative electrophoretic method. Its greatest usefullness appears to be in the area of isolation of carbohydrate antigens, complement components and immunoglobulins, and purification of ferritin-globulin conjugates. Two or more samples may be separated simultaneously on one block, and the separated material can be cluted from the area of the block where it is located at the completion of electrophoretic run. The original method (Kunkel and Slater, 1952) has been improved by Müller-Eberhard and Kunkel (1959).

In this method, the optimal supporting medium consists of a synthetic polymer of polyvinyl chloride and polyvinyl acetate (Pevikon), which has a great advantage over potato starch as it does not interfere with carbohydrate determinations. The supporting medium should be washed with distilled water and with several liters of electrophoresis buffer on a sintered glass (coarse) filter before it is used for pouring the block. This procedure removes small particles which might cause a turbid appearance of block eluates. The Pevikon supporting medium consists of 50% Pevikon C-870 and 50% liquid. The block for electrophoresis is prepared by pouring a thick, homogeneous suspension of the washed supporting medium prepared in a buffer into a supporting arrangement. This arrangement consists of a glass plate (50 × 30 cm or 50 × 60 cm) and two lucite bars (50 × 1.5 × 1.5 cm) placed on the glass plate along its 50-cm side. The plate and bars are covered with thin polyethylene sheeting. Excess fluid is removed by means of thick filter paper which should be tightly attached to the other two sides of the glass plate and anchored with suitable weights. When the block has solidified and its surface has been smoothed with a spatula, a sample of a material to be separated is applied. Before the application of the sample a narrow slit is made with a spatula at a site approximately 10 cm away from the cathodal end of the block. Then 10 to 20 ml of a sample is applied to a smaller block although a larger block may receive 20 to 40 ml. The slit is closed with a spatula and the block surface is covered with polyethylene sheeting. The block is transferred to a cold room and its ends are connected with the electrode chamber by means of buffer soaked towels. The electric current is applied with a potential gradient of 3 to 4

V/cm on the block, and the electrophoresis in carried out for a desired time (usually 20 to 25 hours) on a 30-cm plate.

The fractions are recovered at the end of the electrophoretic run after the block has been disconnected. The block is cut into 1.5-cm-wide segments and the solute from the segments is eluted by displacement filtration. The segment may be pressed onto the bottom of a small sintered (coarse) glass funnel and overlayed with a few milliliters of a buffer. The funnel is then inserted into a sucton bottle. A vacuum is applied and the solution is filtered.

The carbohydrate block electrophoresis is carried out in a 0.1 M sodium borate buffer, pH 9. Borate buffer interacts with carbohydrates and causes neutral carbohydrate molecules to acquire an electric charge. Pevikon C-870 or Geon 426 are the most suitable supporting medium. Acid hydrolysates of polysaccharides are placed in the slot of prepared blocks and subjected to electrophoresis in 0.1 or 0.05 M sodium borate, pH 9.0 to 9.2, at 4° for 12 hours with a potential gradient of 8 V/cm (Müller-Eberhard and Kunkel, 1959). A 2-ml sample of a carbohydrate containing solution is applied to a slit 6 to 8 cm in length to obtain the best separation. To visualize the initial band of carbohydrate, a drop of phenolphthalein is added to the sample. In the above experimental conditions, various hexoses can be separated from each other quantitatively.

The Density Gradient Electrofocusing. The electrofocusing method depends on the condensation of ampholytes, for example, proteins, into an isoelectric spectrum of discrete zones, located at points of a pH gradient corresponding to the pI value of the individual ampholytes. The electrofocusing method utilizes differences in electric charges, isoelectric points, solubility and velocity at a pH range of proteins and other polymers. This method permits effective and reproducible separation of different proteins, while other polymers freed from the proteins can be further and more easily purified.

The electrofocusing method of Vesterberg et al. (1967) or Svensson (1962) is employed. The ampholine electrofocusing equipment (Fig. 23) used in this laboratory consists of a jacketed, water cooled at 10° micro- or macrocolumn, a linear gradient former, peristaltic pump used to empty the column, a fraction collector, a double beam continuous monitor, and an automatic recorder. Ampholyte carriers for the electrofocusing are selected depending on a pH range, estimated in pretrials as the most suitable for distinct separation of individual proteins. The pH of the focused fractions are measured to determine their isoelectric points, with a pH meter reading directly to 0.001 of a pH unit.

A current of 850 V and 15 to 20 mA is applied for 36 to 48 hours, and the electrofocusing process is terminated when the current through the

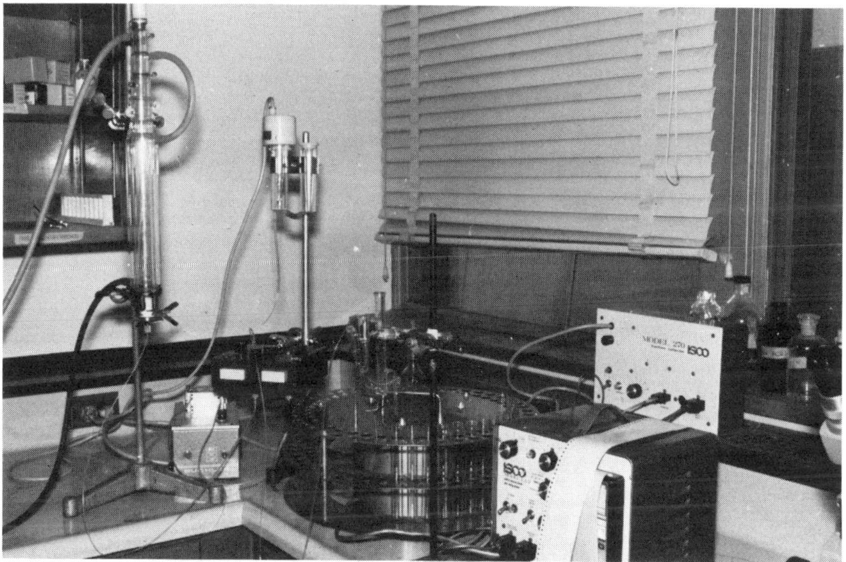

Figure 23. The isoelectric focusing equipment (right to left: an ampholline column, peristaltic pump, monitor, power supply, fraction collector, and automatic recorder).

column has reached a constant value, about 2 to 3 mA. The pH of each fraction is measured to determine the isoelectric points of the focused components. The selected materials are dialyzed or filtered through a Sephadex G-25 (fine) gel to remove the ampholytes.

The chemical composition of materials collected in individual tubes are determined by the double beam continuous monitor in terms of the absorbance at the 254 and 280-nm wave lengths. Identification of other polymers, which can not be detected at these wavelengths, is done by a color reaction, specific for saccharides and phosphatides.

The isoelectric focusing method has been greatly simplified by Luner and Kolin (1970). The latter technique allows to obtain clear-cut condensation marking the isoelectric pH within a few minutes and complete fractionation within about 15 minutes. The pH gradient is generated by utilization of the temperature dependence of pH. The pI of the focused fractions is determined by measuring the local temperature within each of the isoelectric zones by a thermistor.

The apparatus developed for the modified and simplified isoelectric focusing and fractionation in a thermal pH gradient consists of a water jacketed U tube mounted in a Lucite block framework. Electrodes are inserted into one of the two compartments of the U tube. The ends of the U tube are submerged in a buffer solution which fills the compartment harbouring the electrodes. A voltage of about 300 V is maintained, and the current of the order of 9 mA is passed through the apparatus. The 0° and 50° solutions are circulated through the jackets. Since no apparatus based on Luner and Kolin's method is available commercially thus far, it is recommended that interested readers consult the original paper details of this method.

The Continuous Particle Electrophoresis. Polymers possessing sufficiently different electric charges and molecular weights are separated from each other when dissolved in a suitable buffer solution and subjected to a double-dimensional electric field. Constitution of a suitable buffer may be predetermined by the disk electrophoresis pretrials, intended to select a solvent, temperature, and time, which provide optimal resolution of an analyzed material. Many crude materials containing a mixture of nucleic acids, proteins, polysaccharides, and phospholipids yield separate constituents when subjected to an electric field, at 33°, in a buffer of pH 7.4 to 7.6, possessing the following composition:

Tris	5 g
Tartaric acid	4 g
Sodium tartrate	3 g
Octyl phenoxy-polyethoxyethanol (Triton X-100)	2 ml
Distilled water	986 ml

In a CPE apparatus (Fig. 24), a mixture of polymers is subjected for 8 to 24 hours, to an electric current of 400 V and 300 mA at 33° or at a lower temperature, depending on the physical consistency and chemical composition of the polymer source. The gradually separated materials are collected in 92 test tubes, which are screened for the presence of nucleic acids, and proteins, at 254- and 280-nm wave lengths, preferably after the concentration or lyophilization. The liquids are also examined for the presence of saccharides and phospholipids by suitable, qualitative chemical tests or by the following cytochromatoscopic procedure: a few drops of a solution from each tube are transferred onto four chromatography papers, which are subsequently dried at 70° for 2 minutes. The paper sheets are then sprayed with one of the following reagents:

1. The 0.15% ninhydrin solution in acetone, for detection of amino sugars, upon heating at 105° for 3 to 5 minutes.

2. A solution consisting of equal parts of 2.5% oxalic acid and 1% alcoholic solution of alinine, or a color reagent consisting of 1.66 g of 0-phthalic acid and 0.91 ml aniline dissolved in 48 ml of 1-butanol, 48 ml of ethyl ether and 4 ml of water, for detection of saccharides on heating at 105°.

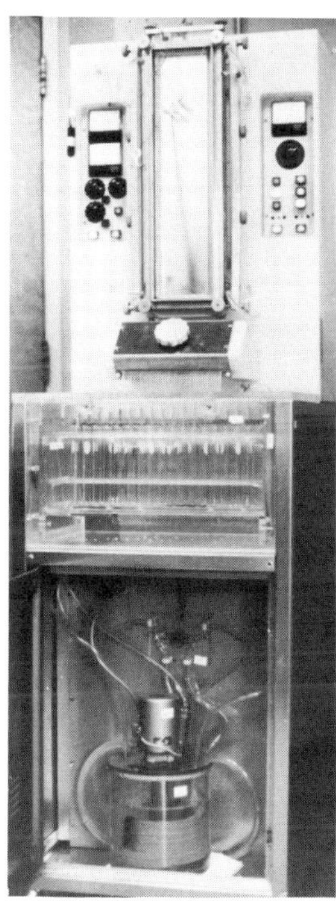

Figure 24. The continuous particle electrophoresis apparatus. The materials are separated in the central chamber by an electric current in two dimensions and the separated fractions are collected in test tubes maintained in the space situated under the table of the apparatus.

3. A solution of acridine orange, for nucleic acids.

4. Rhodamine solution of Dragendorff's reagent, for the detection of lipids.

The last two paper sheets are examined in the UV light. This procedure permits initial determination of the chemical nature of collected polymers, and elimination of tubes possessing no material. The data thus obtained provide a guidance for a selection of physicochemical and quantitative chemical methods for further purification and examination of the polymers.

4. Separation of Antigen-Polymers by Chromatography

Diffusion of molecules in dilute solution is inversely related to the frictional forces it must overcome to move at a steady rate. The frictional force, in turn, depends on the radius and weight of the molecule. Separation of different polymers depending on the difference in molecular weight and polydispersity may be attained by the gradient dilution, precipitation chromatography and most of all, by permeation chromatography. The gradient dilution and precipitation chromatography depend on the partitioning of a polymer between a mobile solution phase and a supported stationary, condensed phase in accordance with the solubility of a given molecular weight. Fractionation by the permeation chromatography method is due to the increasing exclusion of column volume with increasing hydrodynamic volume of polymer chains. It appears that the largest chains have the least column volume accessible to them; and since their flow is retarded least, they are eluted first. An alternative explanation of the mechanism proposes that since large molucules have larger average velocity than small molecules, the large solute particles elute out earlier than the small particles.

The *thin layer chromatography* is often the most rapid and effective technique for separation of polymers (Otocka and Hellman, 1970). The method depends on the resolution of complex mixtures by adsorption. Solutes are deposited at one point on a supported layer of adsorbent and eluted by a solvent which is drawn up the absorbent by capillary action. As the solutes migrate, the distances, measured by their Rf values, increase with eluting power of the solvent and decrease as the strength of their own adsorption on the substrate increases. The thin layer chromatography seems to be an ideal technique for the study of polymer separation by adsorption. One of the most suitable substrates for thin layer chromatography is alumina or silica gel.

Technical details for a thin layer chromatography are as follows: samples of a polymer (10–20 μg) are deposited as spots along a line, 2 cm from one edge of the adsorbent layer. The adsorbent plates are mounted in a sandwich type cell or an Eastman chromogram apparatus. Gradient elutions are conducted in a cylindrical tank with the flexible plate curved along the inner wall. The elution in a gradient is carried for 20 to 60 minutes. At the end of the run, the plates are dried and the samples are visualized. The polymers can be separated by the thin layer chromatography using either a constant solvent possessing a mixed composition or a gradient solution. Fractionation in the thin layer chromatography occurs by both solubility and adsorption mechanisms.

The gradient dilution thin layer chromatography can be employed for the determination of molecular weight distribution of polymers by means of scanning densitometry (Otocka, 1970).

Column-Gel Chromatography (Filtration) Methods. Filtration through columns of aqueous gels made of cross-linked dextrans permit the separation of solutes mainly on the basis of the molecular size differences (Fig. 25). Cross-linked dextrans (commercial name Sephadex) are useful for fractionation of solutes possessing molecular weights ranging from several hundred to several hundred thousand. The principle of separation process on Sepha-

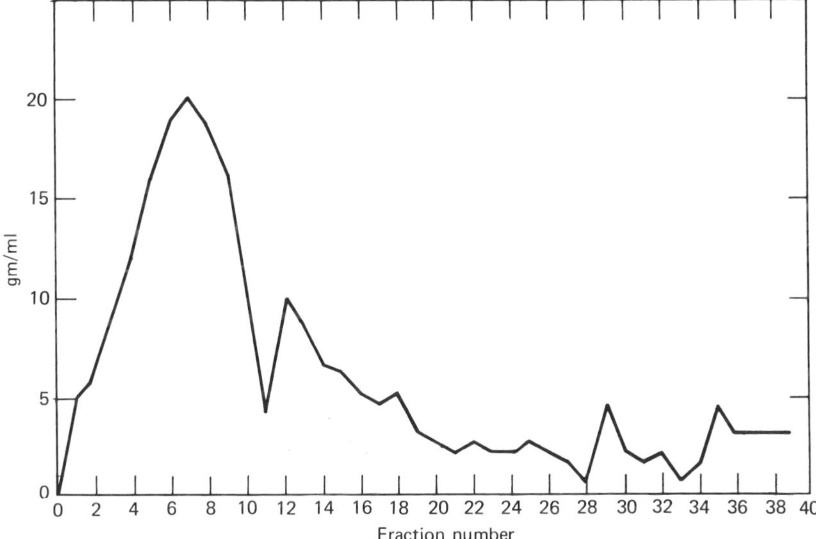

Figure 25. A graph representing the separation of different glycoprotein fractions by column filtration on Sephadex G-200.

dex columns is that large solutes which cannot enter the gel pores emerge first at the void volume (the volume of liquid surrounding the gel in a column). Small solutes which penetrate the gel pores freely are retarded and emerge at a volume $V_0 + V_i$, where V_i is the volume of liquid inside the gel particles. Apart from the property of gel filtration, Sephadex gel absorbs aromatic compounds, which may be advantageous for separation purpose.

Filtration or chromatography on Sephadex columns is relatively independent on the pH value and ionic strength of the eluants. The degree of separation achieved on a Sephadex column depends on the column height to diameter, since a column with a high ratio provides more stages of fractionation. Long columns with better resolution are preferred to short columns. The most commonly used columns have the dimensions of 1×205 cm and 2.5×205 cm for analytical and preparative purposes. A sample containing between 100 and 300 mg of a dry mass may be deposited on such columns. The 1-cm column may be operated by simple gravity flow at a rate of 8 to 12 ml/hour. Higher flow rates broaden the peaks. With the 2.5-cm-diameter column an amount of dry mass as large as 1500 to 2000 mg may be processed, and the flow rate is maintained below 20–40 ml/ hour. The ionic strength of the eluant to be used for Sephadex G-25 and G-50 columns should be equivalent to about 0.1 M NaCl; for G-75 to G-200 columns, the ionic strength of the eluant must be equivalent to about

1 *M* NaCl. The following eluant has been designed for the separation of cytoplasm components on Sephadex G-200 columns (Kwapinski, 1972). The eluant consists of 0.1% Tween 80, 0.15 *M* sodium perchlorate, and 0.15 *M* Tris-hydroxymethylaminomethane (pH 7.0–7.2), or an alternative eluant: 0.2 *M* Tris, 0.7 *M* NaCl, 0.1% Tween 80. The gel is made in a solvent consisting of 0.2 *M* Tris, 0.1% Tween 80 and 0.7 *M* NaCl.

The Sephadex gel to be used for packing a column is prepared according to the specification of Sephadex gels (Table 25). The prepared gel is suspended in a larger volume of a selected buffer in a beaker and after a settling period of 20 minutes, the supernatant containing some fine particles is decanted off.

The column should be packed without trapped air bubbles. For this purpose, it is recommended to fill the column with a buffer to a height of about 25 cm and then add a uniform suspension of the gel. After most of the gel has settled, the excess buffer is taken out from above the gel leaving some 10-cm layer above it. More gel suspension is then added until the required height of column is reached. Before the column is used for an experiment, it should be calibrated with a known mixture of proteins and a low-molecular-weight neutral solid. For the separation of heat-labile mate-

Table 25. Specification for Preparing Sephadex Gel Columns

Type	Water Regain (g/g Dry Gel)	Bed Volume (ml/g Dry Gel)	Fractionation Range	Particle Size (μ)
G-10	1.0 ± 0.1	2–3	Up to 700	40–120
G-15	1.5 ± 0.1	2.5–3.8	Up to 1500	40–120
G-25	2.5 ± 0.2	5	100–5,000	
Superfine				10–40
Fine				20–80
Coarse				100–300
G-50	5.0 ± 0.3	10	500–10,000	
Superfine				10–40
Fine				20–80
Coarse				100–300
G-75	7.5 ± 0.5	12–15	1,000–50,000	40–120
Superfine			3,000–70,000	10–40
G-100	10.0 ± 1.0	15–20	1,000–100,000	40–120
			4,000–150,000	
Superfine				10–40
G-150	15.0 ± 1.5	24–30	1,000–150,000	40–120
Superfine				10–40
G-200	20.0 ± 2.0	30–40	1,000–200,000	40–120
			5,000–800,000	
Superfine				10–40

rials, for example, most of protein antigens, it is recommended to use jacketed, water-cooled columns (Fig. 26).

Chromatography on Polyacrylamide Gels. Polyacrylamide gel columns allow the fractionation of substances largely on the basis of molecular size, acting as molecular sieves. Polyacrylamide gels have been used to desalt and defractionate polysaccharides, nucleic acids, proteins, and peptides (Hjerten and Mosbach, 1962; Lea and Sehon, 1962). The gel grains are prepared from the monomers, acrylamide and $M.N'$-methylenebisacrylamide. The N,N'-methylenebisacrylamide acts as a cross-linking agent. The optimum polyacrylamide gel composition for a particular material to be separated must be determined experimentally, but a general relationship between the amount of acrylamide, (a) N',N'-methylenebisacrylamide, and (b) the volume of buffer (m) is expressed by the equation:

$$T = \left[\frac{a + b}{m} \times 100 \right] \% \qquad (w/v)$$

where T stands for the total concentration of the two monomers.

A general rule is that the higher the molecule weight of the substance to be separated, the lower is the gel concentration required for an adequate separation.

Polyacrylamide gel spheres are prepared by suspension polymerization. Thus an aqueous solution of the monomers is dispersed into spheres in a hydrophobic liquid which contains a stabilizer preventing aggregation of the spheres. A special apparatus, equipped with a motor, is used for preparation of polyacrylamide and agarose spheres (Hjerten, 1967). The column is packed with the polyacrylamide spheres polymerized for 45 to 60 minutes by feeding the column to the height of about 10 cm and then pouring a dilute suspension of the polyacrylamide spheres into the column tube. The flow rate is set at 3 ml/(hour)(cm^2). If the flow rate above is exceeded, it is recommended to repack the column to obtain good separation.

Gel grains of dextran and polyacrylamide can be used for chromatographic molecular sieving of substances with molecular weight below 1 million only. Agarose, a polysaccharide gel, permits fractionation of substances with molecular weights ranging from 50,000 to several millions and of submicroscopic particles.

Agarose spheres are prepared in much the same way as polyacrylamide spheres. A warm agarose solution is dispersed into spheres in an organic liquid by stirring in the presence of a stabilizer and gelation occurs by decrease in temperature. The agarose spheres and gel is prepared in the same apparatus as used for polyacrylamide sphere preparation. Typically, agarose gels with the nominal sphere diameter of 0.05 mm and columns with the

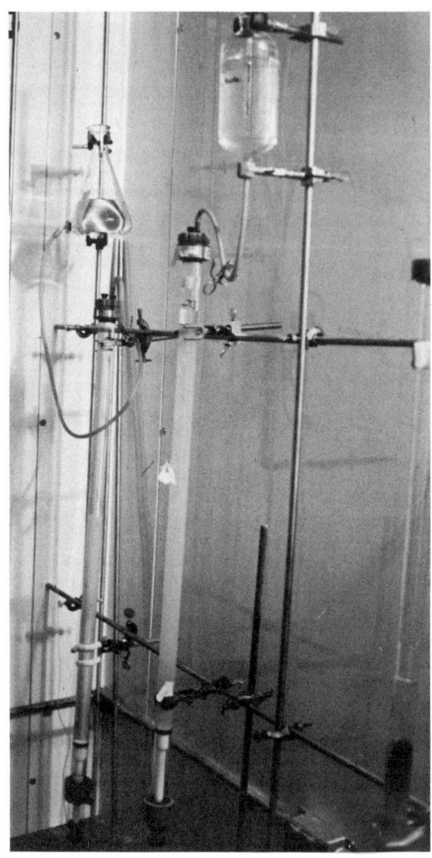

Figure 26. The column gel-filtration apparatus, consisting of a water jacketed column filled with a gel slurry and a refrigerated unit containing an automatic fraction collector.

dimensions of 2.0 × 95 cm are used. Also 0.1 M Tris HCl + 0.2 M NaCl, pH 8.0, is employed, and a 1-ml sample is placed on the column. Chromatography on agarose columns is suitable for purification of high-molecular weight substances, for fractionation of submicroscopic particles and for isolation of proteins from these particles or from whole cells (Hjerten, 1967).

Cellulose Ion Exchange Chromatography. Of a wide variety of cellulose ion exchangers, the most popular and the most recommended exchangers are DEAE (Diethylaminoethyl-), ionic form − $OCH_2CH_2\overset{+}{N}H$ $(C_2H_2)_2$, and CM-cellulose (Carboxymethyl-) gamma, ionic form − $OCH_2CH_2CO_2^-$.

The separation of proteins on cellulose ion exchangers seems to depend chiefly on the electrostatic interactions of the polyelectrolyte protein with the oppositely charged adsorbent. The relative affinity of a protein molecule depends on its charge density. This affinity may be modified either by an alteration of the charge of solute and/or depth of the adsorbent, or by increasing the concentration of buffer salts whose ions also possess affinities for the adsorbent. The choice of a cation or an ion exchanger depends on the charge of the protein at the selected pH. The DEAE cellulose is used for separation of acidic proteins whereas the CM-cellulose is employed for the basic proteins. Chromatography on ion exchange columns is sensitive to temperature changes and therefore the temperature has to be maintained at a precise level within 5°.

Technique. Approximately 15 g of the dry cellulose ion exchangers is used to pack a column of 2.5 × 25 cm. The cellulose is suspended in about 600 ml of 0.5 *M* NaOH + 0.5 M NaCl, and the suspension is stirred until free of trapped air bubbles. After settling for half an hour the cloudy supernatant is decanted, the cellulose is resuspended in a 600 ml of 1 M NaCl, left to settle and decanted again and then filtered by suction on a Büchner funnel through two pieces of filter paper and washed with several hundred milliliters of 1 M NaCl.

According to the Huisman and Dozy (1962) method, modified by Suhrland et al. (1968), the DEAE cellulose column is layered with 0.5 ml (10 to 15 mg) of a material dissolved in initial buffer and is washed with 0.005 *M* sodium phosphate buffer, pH 8.6. The elution is carried out with 100 ml volumes of ten buffers of increasing sodium chloride concentrations and decreasing pH value. A linear gradient of the eluting buffer is delivered to the column from a Technicon Autograd. The flow rate is maintained at 2 ml/minute with a constant infusion pump. The effluent is constantly monitored by an Automatic UV Analyzer at an appropriate wave length. The 10-ml aliquots are collected in a fraction collector, and the optical density of the solution is determined in a spectrophotometer.

Carboxymethyl Cellulose Chromatography. Carboxymethyl cellulose column is prepared by filling a glass column (2 × 25 mμ) with carboxymethyl cellulose suspended in 0.01 *M* acetate buffer, pH 5.5 (Porter, 1958).

5. *Separation of Antigen-Polymers by Immunosorption*

Immunosorbents are preparations containing either an antibody and capable of specific removal by absorption of a respective antigen from mixtures of antigens, or an antigen and capable of a specific antibody from a mixture of different antibodies possessing different immunological specificities. A useful immunosorbent possesses a high capacity for a corresponding or homologous antigen and low solubility. The following immunosorbents are endowed with these properties: cellulose-linked antibody preparations, disulfide-linked antibody preparations, thiolated protein antigens, and antigens adsorbed to Sephadex or Kieselguhr (Stephen et al., 1966). Thiolated protein antigens are used to absorb specific antibodies following which the antigen is removed from acid solutions of the thiolated antigen-antibody complexes with a bifunctional organomercurial compound, for example, 3,6-bis-(acetoxymecurimethyl) dioxan, to yield pure antibody in free solution (Singer et al., 1968). An antibody preparation may be thiolated for the absorption of an antigen, which is then released in a free pure form after the removal of antibodies. A technique designed for this purpose by Stephen's et al. (1966) is applied in the following manner.

Preparation of the Immunosorbent. To a gamma globulin concentrate containing the desired antibody (10 ml), N-acetyl-homocysteine thiolactone (60 mg in 1 ml of water) and carbonate buffer, pH 10.6 (10 ml), are added. The mixture is left at 0° for 30 to 40 minutes, after which the reaction is stopped by the addition of a 0.4 M, pH 7.0, phosphate buffer (40 ml). The mixture is filtered through a Sephadex G-25 column equilibrated with 0.05 M, pH 7.0, phosphate buffer. The thiolated protein emerges at the void volume of the column.

The thiolated protein is lyophilized and cross-linked to form insoluble polymers according to the following method (Benesch and Benesch, 1958).

The lyophilized thiolated antibody protein is diluted with a 0.05 M, pH 7.2, phosphate buffer to form a paste. An excess of the cross-linking solution is added to obtain rubber like product. The aggregated polymer, formed after standing at 0° for 1 hour with occasional stirring, is dispersed in phosphate-buffer saline (30 ml) by homogenization. The mixture is then centrifuged; the sediment is collected and washed in the phosphate-buffer saline and recentrifuged. This process is repeated until the supernatant contains less than 10 μg protein/ml. The product is washed twice with sodium acetate-HCl solution, pH 1.0, and twice with phosphate-buffer saline.

The washed suspension of disulfide-linked protein is added to 4 volumes of Sephadex G-200 suspension, which has been equilibrated with a phosphate-buffer saline. A column of 2.5-cm diameter and of 10-cm height is prepared and washed with phosphate-buffered saline.

The capacity of the immunosorbent preparation for its antigen is determined in a preliminary run on a small sample of the antigen eluted with phosphate-buffered saline. In the main experiment, a mixture of antigens is placed on the column and eluted with a phosphate-buffered saline. The protein profile of the effluent is followed by measuring E 280 and assaying individual fractions for heterologous and homologous antigens. The heterologous antigens and a residuum of uncombined homologous antigens descent from the column according to their respective molecular weight. The fraction may be concentrated with polyethylene glycol or by freeze-drying.

It is recommended to purify the eluates by recycling them on a Recychrom apparatus (LKB Produkter, Stockholm) five times or more before using the material for clinical analysis, as described by Birkbeck and Stephen (1970).

The cross-linking solution consists of 1.82 g potassium ferrocyanide, 4.86 g ammonium chloride, and 7.1 ml aqueous ammonium per 100 ml of distilled water.

Phosphate buffer, pH 7.0, 0.4 M consists of 4.76 g of $Na_2PHO_4 \cdot 12H_2O_4$ per liter and 2.5 g of $NaH_2PO_4 \cdot 2H_2O$ per liter.

Sodium acetate-HCl solution, pH 1.8 comprises 100 ml 0.1 M sodium acetate and 1 ml concentrated hydrochloric acid.

6. *Separation of Components of Immunocomplexes*

Several methods have been proposed for liberation of antigens from an antigen-antibody complex, however, antigens can only seldom be completely separated from an antibody complex without denaturation. Partial dissociation of antibody from complexes may be attained by methods which employ acid or alkali alone or in combination with heat, denaturation agents, or enzymes; but these methods are too drastic to obtain satisfactory yield of nondenaturated antibody. Antibody combined with pneumococcal polysaccharides was successfully released from the complex by means of strong salt solution (Heidelberger and Kabat, 1938), but this method is seldom applicable to other antibodies. Other methods for separation of antigens from serological complexes employ nonaqueous solvents, such as liquid ammonium or sulfur dioxide (Rees and Singer, 1956), ultrasonic waves, treatment with reagents which break hydrogen bonds (thiocyanates, iodides, salicylates, and urea), but with little success.

Aqueous carbon dioxide in the absence of salt is able to detach antibodies from many immune complexes or nearly neutral pH level (Mitz, 1957). The latter method was modified, improved by Tozer et al. (1962), and used successfully for the separation of immunoglobulins from the complexes with antigens.

Chapter Three

PHYSICOCHEMICAL CHARACTERIZATION OF ANTIGEN PREPARATIONS

The active groupings of particulate antigens that are most likely to react with a specific antibody are those situated on the surface of cells, mycelia, appendages, and spores. It is unlikely that antigens contained within the nondisintegrated structures may take any active or specific part in the serological reaction. After the disruption of structural elements, either by artificial means or in natural conditions in the infected host, a number of chemical substances can be released. Substances with molecular weights over 5000 can act as immunogens and display immunological specificities which differ or are similar among a group of compounds, and may immunize the host individually.

The cellular somatic "O" antigen of vegetative cells and spores can be studied only with regard to physical properties, such as thermal destruction point or the susceptibility to denaturating substances. Other particulate antigens, such as cell and mycelial membranes, appendages (flagella and fimbriae), and cytoplasmic membranes, can be characterized as to their physical and chemical properties if prepared in a pure state. It must be borne in mind, however, that most of these particulate antigens represent a network of various chemical complexes and antigenic fractions.

The cell walls and appendages are examined with regard to their thermal destruction point and denaturation by alcohol, phenol, and mineral acids. The serological activities of the particulate antigens are not necessarily completely destroyed by heat; sometimes only the specificity is changed under exposure to moderately high temperatures. The chemical composition of these cellular components is studied by measuring the amounts of nitrogen, carbohydrates, and phosphorus, and by the chromatographic determination of sugars, polyols, and amino acids. Techniques selected for the individual physical and chemical investigations are presented below. Chemical or antigenic constituents, isolated from the microorganisms and purified to a reasonable degree, are examined more precisely by using various selected techniques presented in the following sections. The general principle of measuring the immunological activities of antigen preparations is the determination of the minimum quantity of an antigen giving a serological reaction with a constant amount of anti-serum. The titer of an antigen preparation should, if possible, be expressed in relation to a standard antigen preparation. A most accurate determination of the amount of antigen involved in a serological reaction is attained by chemical estimation of the amount of the antigen preparation occurring in the precipitate.

It should be anticipated that the physical, chemical, and antigenic state of isolated fractions will be altered to a lesser or greater degree during various chemical operations. If, however, a cautious preparation of several samples of a material repeatedly yields very similar fractions, these may be valid cell constituents.

I. DETERMINATION OF PHYSICAL PROPERTIES OF ANTIGENS

The following physical characteristics of isolated immunochemical fractions should be determined: 1) the dry weight, consistency, and color; 2) the solubility in water, dilute alkali (0.1 M sodium hydroxide), 5% acetic acid, in alcohol, ether, and benzene; 3) the physical homogeneity; 4) the sedimentation constant; and 5) the electrophoretic mobility. In respect to lipid fractions, the melting point may be determined by means of the Fisher-Johns apparatus. Once the dry weight of individual fractions has been estimated (after drying to a constant weight at 70° *in vacuo*), the yield of each fraction is calculated in relation to the total dry mass of cells or to the individual cell constituents. It is also advisable to estimate the yield of each fraction in relation to the total dry mass of particular classes of chemical material such as polysaccharides, proteins, or lipids.

1 Dry Weight Determination

The dry weight value is an operational concept, referring to a particular drying condition. The details of the procedure follow.

Prepare a known solution or suspension of the purified material. Dry a sample of the material containing at least 5 mg of starting solid to constant weight over phosphorus pentoxide (P_2O_5) or silica gel in a vacuum oven (Fig. 27) at 70° for 4 to 6 hours, or at 45° for 1 to 2 days if the sample is to be saved. Quicker drying is attained in the Abderhalden drying pistol (Kimble Glass Co., Vineland, N.J.), attached to a high vacuum pump (0.2 mm of mercury) or to a house vacuum. Determine the weight in Cahn's electrobalance or microbalance three times during the period of 3 days. Estimate the content of the dry material per milliliter of the original solution or suspension.

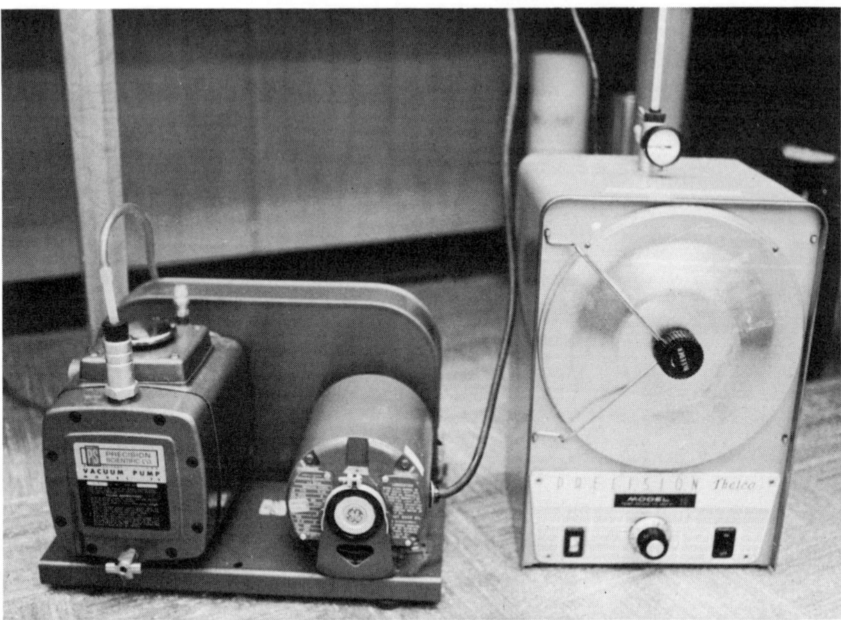

Figure 27. A vacuum oven connected to a vacuum pump.

2. *Ash Value Determination*

Ash value is a correction factor for metals and nonvolatile salts, which may be present in the sample. The ash value is determined after the combustion of a sample at 700° in a combustion glass tubing or a micromuffle (Steyermark, 1961).

3. *Molecular Weight Determination*

The molecular weight and diffusion coefficient of a purified agent may be determined by a sedimentation equilibrium method. The technique depends on a balance between sedimentation and diffusion. Sedimentation constants are determined by the ultracentrifugation method of Svedberg and Pederson (1940). The purified agent is placed in a double-sector cell of an analytical ultracentrifuge and is centrifuged at a speed that gives at equilibrium a concentration at the bottom of the cell about three times that of the top. The precise average molecular weight is computed from the equilibrium photograph. Estimates are made of nonideal heterogen- and association-coefficients (Adams and Filmer, 1966).

Approximate molecular weights may be calculated from the sedimentation coefficients by Archibald's (1947) method.

The molecular weight of mucopolysaccharides may be determined by a combined sedimentation-diffusion method (Constantopoulos et al., 1969).

The diffusion study is carried out in the Rayleigh synthetic boundary cell in a Spinco Model E ultracentrifuge.

II. DETERMINATION OF PURITY, HOMOGENEITY, AND PHYSICOCHEMICAL IDENTITY OF ANTIGEN PREPARATIONS

Effectiveness of the separation and purification procedures is controlled by a homogeneity test, performed with the highly concentrated materials, obtained at each phase of the separation and purification. The homogeneity is tested by a qualitative, polyacrylamide disk electrophoresis, cellulose acetate electrophoresis, a high voltage flat-plate electrophoresis, preparative ultracentrifugation (Schachman and Harrington, 1954), immunodiffusion, or immunoelectrophoresis, or a combination of these methods. The disk electrophoresis together with the cellulose acetate immunodiffusion or immunoelectrophoresis, or a combination of the disk electrophoresis and disk immunoelectrophoresis are used most frequently for the homogeneity estimation in this laboratory.

Of many types of electrophoresis, the acrylamide gel electrophoresis and the cellulose-acetate electrophoresis are most suitable procedures for the determination of heterogeneity, although electrophoresis on filter paper is generally satisfactory. Immunoelectrophoretic separation of the fractions or antigens can be combined with "schlieren" scanning (Pierce, 1962).

Testing for homogeneity or heterogeneity must be conducted over a wide range of pH and ionic strength to determine whether the tested substance in the varies conditions migrates as a single boundary. However, the resolution of electrophoretic pattern into multiple boundaries does not necessarily indicate heterogeneity since multiple boundaries may sometimes occur due to the interactions between a substance (particularly a protein) and the buffer components. On the other hand, a minor component, occurring in a lower concentration and having the electrophoretic mobility approaching that of the major component, may result in nondetectability of the minor component as a separate boundary.

The most suitable and convenient support for the zone electrophoresis is polyacrylamide gel and cellulose acetate membrane, except where large sample volumes are used. Filter paper is employed with large samples as a supporting medium, particularly for high-voltage electrophoresis, for example, peptide mapping or fingerprinting. Zone electrophoresis in agar offers no advantage over electrophoresis in cellulose acetate membranes with small samples except for comparison studies with immunoelectrophoresis, but polyacrylamide gels and hydrolyzed starch gels are often useful because of the special resolution produced by these supporting media due to the dual action of polyacrylamide and starch gels as anticonvection supports and molecular sieves.

1. Polyacrylamide-Gel Electrophoresis

The gel slabs for the polyacrylamide gel electrophoresis are made of the monomeric mix consisting of 2:1:4:1 mixture of the following constituents:

1. Acrylamide monomer (Eastman No. 5521)   30 g
   N,N'-methylamine bisacrylamide (Eastman No. 8383)   1 g
   Distilled water   123 ml
2. 0.28% N,N,N',N'-tetramethylethylenediamine (TEMED) solution
3. 0.14% ammonium persulfate solution in water
4. Glycine   29 g
   Tris   6 g
   Distilled water   980 ml

The electrolyte solution, pH 8.1, is prepared as a stock solution from 29 g glycine, 6 g Tris, 5.5 ml NHCl, and 975 ml water.

The antigen source, of which polymer categories are to be determined by the disk electrophoresis, is dissolved in 2 to 5% urea or sucrose solution at a suitable pH, and 0.2 ml, containing 0.2 to 1.0 mg of dry weight, is placed in the upper gel, followed by 0.05 ml of 0.5% bromphenol blue, overlaid by an electrolyte. A current of 1.25 mA/gel slab is applied for approximately 30 minutes or until a blue or purple tracking ring of an indicator outlining the salt front has descended 45 mm to the mark located 1 cm from the bottom end. A current of 2.5 mA per tube is used thereafter until the blue line has entered within 0.5 cm from the bottom of the tube.

For the separation of proteins by polyacrylamide gel electrophoresis, Gesteland and Staehelin (1967) method as adapted by Hoober and Blobel (1969) is recommended. For this technique 7.5% acrylamide gels are used, the upper and lower gel solutions contain 2.5 and 5 μg of ribo-flavin per milliliter, as catalyst, and are used in the volume of 0.2 and 1.7 ml, respectively. The acrylamide gels are photopolymerized with white fluorescent lamps for 1 hour. After the gel containing tubes have been inserted in the disk electrophoresis apparatus, a constant current of 1 mA/gel is applied for the first 30 minutes, followed by 3 mA/gel for 2 hours, at room temperature.

After the electrophoretic run, remove the tubes from the disk electro-phoresis apparatus and place them in a dish of distilled water. Using a syringe filled with distilled water and equipped with a long, thin needle, remove the gel from the inside of the tube by gently moving the needle around the side of the tube and squirting water in gently, until the gel slips out. Lift the gel in fingers and place it in a staining test tube.

Stain the gel by filling the tube past the top of the gel with a stain. Plug the tube with a rubber plug and leave it for the required time; decant and pour 7% acetic acid.

The gel slabs are destained either in a Transverse Disk Destainer or in a disk electrophoresis apparatus with 7% acetic acid using a 50- to 100-V electric current and 50 to 100 mA per destaining tube. Individual classes of polymers are distinguished by selected staining procedures (Fig. 28). Rs values (the ratio between the distance run by a band to the distance travelled by a dye-tracer) are calculated, and patterns produced by the separated polymer zones may be recorded either manually or by the aid of a Chromoscan (Fig. 29, 30).

The polyacrylamide gel disk electrophoresis is supplemented by a *complementarity examination* (Kwapinski, 1972). In this method, a comparison is made between the electrophoregram patterns, formed by individual and pooled antigen preparations, as follows: polyacrylamide gel slabs set in triplicate are loaded with one of the following materials: (a) 0.1 ml of a material and 0.1 ml of buffer, (b) 0.1 ml of another preparation and 0.1 ml of buffer, or 0.2 ml of a mixture of (a) and (b), preincubated at 37° for 1 hour. The total number and pattern of bands, their Rs values and thickness are determined and photographed or sketched upon the completion of an electrophoretic run, staining, and destaining. Coalescent bands

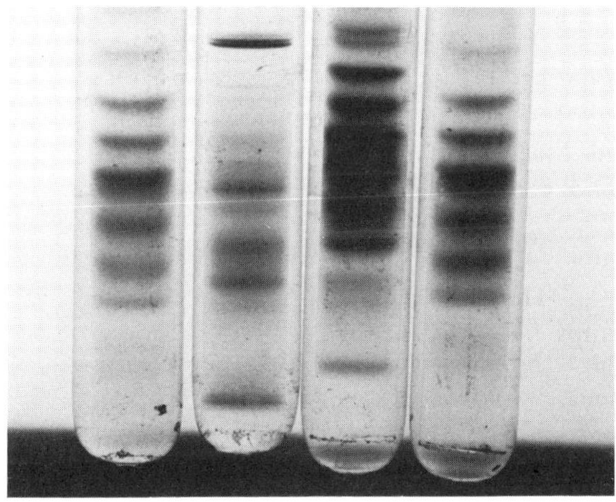

Figure 28. Protein bands separated by the analytical disk electrophoresis and stained with an Amido Black 10B solution and destained in 7% acetic acid.

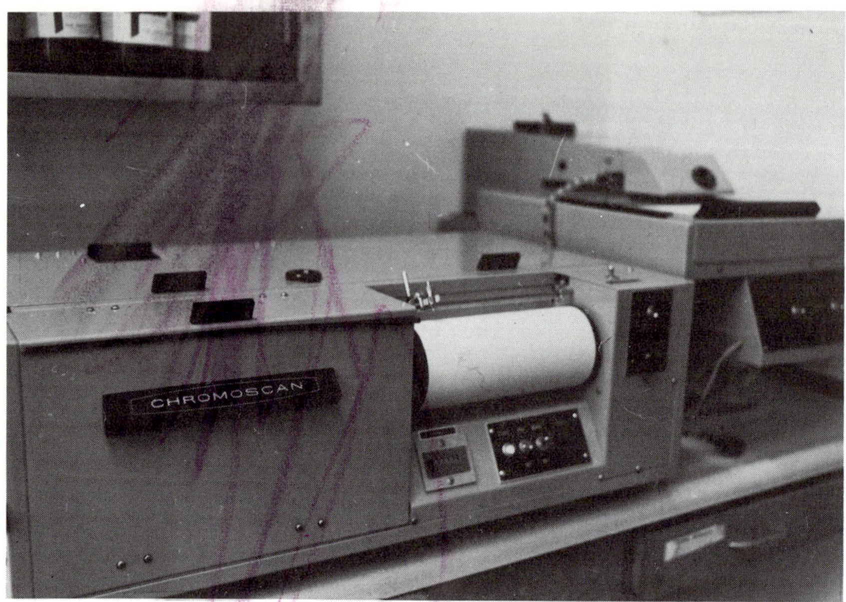

Figure 29.   The Chromoscan with an attachment for scanning and recording of thin-layer chromatograms.

with approximately double thickness are formed in the third tube if physicochemical properties of the polymers in (a) and (b) are identical. The polymers that are physicochemically different form separate bands, located in different zones.

Polyacrylamide Disk Electrophoresis of Nucleotides (Wikman et al., 1969). RNA preparations are first digested with a ribonuclease. For this purpose, an RNA preparation is dissolved in 0.04 *M* Tris-acetic acid, pH 7.2, 0.02 *M* sodium acetate, and 0.02 *M* EDTA and digested with 1 unit of RNAse/10 μl of the solution at 37° for 30 minutes. At the end of the incubation period, sufficient 55% sucrose is added to make a final concentration of 10% sucrose and 50-μl aliquot of the digest is immediately applied to the polyacrylamide gel.

A 4% stock solution of polyacrylamide gel contains 3.875 g polyacrylamide and 0.125 g bisacrylamide/100 ml buffer, which consists of 0.016 *M* sodium acetate, 0.0016 *M* EDTA, and 0.32 M Tris-acetic acid, pH 7.2. A 2.8% polyacrylamide gel contains 2.675 g of acrylamide and 0.125 g of bisacrylamide. To the gel are added 20 μl of *N,N,N',N'*-tetramethylenediamine and 10% ammonium persulfate, 0.66 ml/40 ml of gel solution, and the mixture is allowed to polymerize in glass tubes (0.5 ×

7.5 cm). After the polymerization, the gels are cooled at 4°. A prerun is made at 5 mA/tube for 30 minutes at 24° in a buffer containing 0.04 M Tris-acetic acid, pH 7.2, 0.02 M sodium acetate, 0.002 M EDTA, 0.5% sodium lauryl sulfate, and 0.01% glycerol. After the prerun, a 0.01 to 0.1 mg of the hydrolized RNA sample, dissolved in a buffer containing 5% to 10% sucrose, are layered on the gels. The electrophoresis is conducted at 5 to 6 mA/gel slab and a current of 10 V/cm, until the bromphenol blue marker migrates to the end of the gel.

The polyacrylamide gel electrophoresis of oligonucleotides and nucleic acids is essentially conducted in the identical conditions, although the pH of the buffer is usually increased to 7.8 to 8.0.

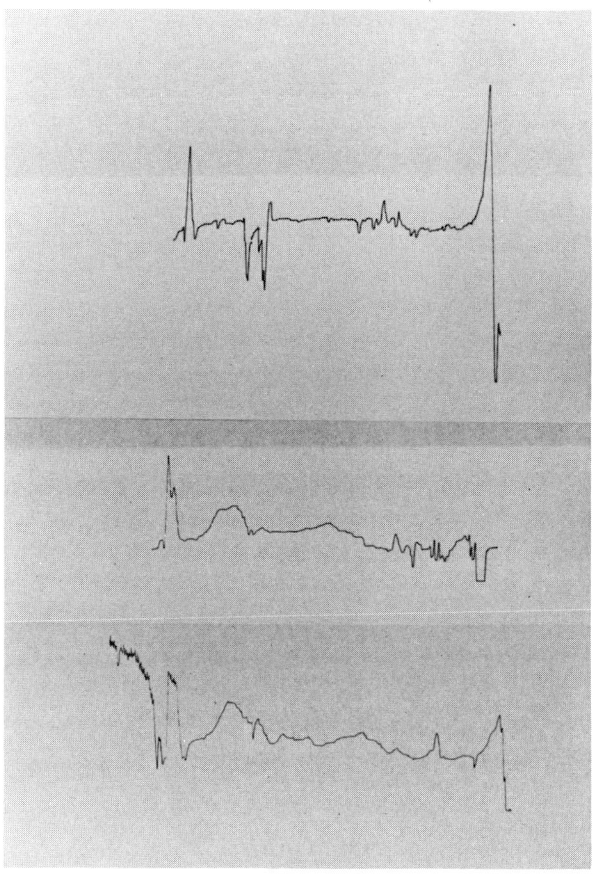

Figure 30. Different patterns of the polymers separated by the analytical disk electrophoresis and recorded by Chromoscan, equipped with an attachment for scanning of gel slabs.

The gels are then examined either unstained in the UV light or upon staining. The staining is obtained by soaking the gels for 1 hour in a 0.2% methylene blue solution made in 0.2 M sodium acetate-acetic acid buffer, pH 4.7. The background is then destained by several washings in 500 ml of distilled water over a period of 8 to 16 hours. The absorbance of polymers separated in the gel is scanned in a Chromoscan.

The Rs values for each of the oligonucleotide bands, relative to the Rs values of the bromphenol blue are determined in the Chromoscan. The unstained gels are scanned in the Chromoscan fitted with a deuterium lamp and an interference filter with a maximum transmission at 280 nm. Gels are held in a parallel sided quartz container and scanned with a live beam about 0.8 by 0.05 mm. The minimum detectable amount of the RNA and related materials is about 0.05 μg. The Rs value of an oligonucleotide band is its fractional mobility to the mobility of the midpoint of the marker peak.

Oligonucleotides can be eluted from the polyacrylamide gel by the elution of sliced gel slabs in 0.05 M, pH 5.0 sodium acetate.

Polyacrylamide Disk Electrophoresis of Mucopolysaccharides. The acrylamide gel is prepared by dissolving Cyanogum-41 and 0.2 g of ammonium persulfate in 1 ml of a 0.1 M phosphate buffer, pH 11.4, containing sodium formate (Hilborn and Anastassiadis, 1969). The pH value is critical for separation of mucopolysaccharides, whereas sodium formate improves the compactness of bands. The gel solution is filtered and supplemented with 1 ml of dimethylaminopropionitrile (1 ml/100). The electrophoresis is carried out on gel slabs or on strips of Whatman No. 3 filter paper, soaked in the gel solution. The electrophoregrams are stained with 0.5% solution of Alcian Blue made in 3% acetic acid, and destained in 3% acetic acid. Reference acetic mucopolysaccharides are hyaluronic acid, heparin, and chondroitin sulfate.

Detection of Polymers in Polyacrylamide Gel. The following dyes can be used for the detection of protein bands, arranged in the order of decreasing sensitivity: nigrosine, naphthol blue-black, Ponceau S, Lissamine green, Coomassie brilliant blue.

Nigrosine Staining	Staining solution:
Nigrosine	0.5 g
1 M acetic acid	450 ml
0.1 M sodium acetate	450 ml
Glycerol	100 ml
	Destaining solution:

2% acetic acid containing 10% glycerol

Stain for 2 minutes; destain for 1 hour. Protein bands retain black color.
Naphthol Blue-Black Staining: Staining Solution

Amido black 10B	5 g
Glycerol	150 ml
Glacial acetic acid	100 ml
Distilled water	95 ml

Destaining solution:

Glacial acetic acid	100 ml
Glycerol	150 ml
Distilled water	750 ml

Stain for 30 minutes and destain for 15 to 30 minutes. Protein bands stain dark blue.

Polysaccharide Detection. Polysaccharides and simple saccharides can best be detected with an α-naphthol or anthrone reagent.

The α-naphthol reagent:

1.	α-naphthol	144 g
	EDTA	38 mg
	Distilled water	100 ml
2.	*p*-phenylendiamine	216 mg
	EDTA	38 mg
	Distilled water	100 ml
3.	3% hydrogen peroxide solution	

Mix (1), (2), and (3) in the ratio 1:1:0.2.

Immerse gel in the reagent for 10 minutes. Wash in running tap water for 10 minutes. Purple color indicates saccharides.

The anthrone reagent:

Purified anthrone	0.2 g
Ethyl alcohol	8 ml
Distilled water	30 ml
Sulfuric acid	50 ml

Stain for 5 minutes, destain in 10% sulfuric acid for 10 minutes. Saccharides stain green to blue.

Mucopolysaccharides stain most readily with 0.1% alcian blue in 5% acetic acid.

Detection of Nucleic Acids. Zones of nucleic acids in gel can be detected either by viewing unstained gel slabs at 260-nm wavelength in a Chromoscan fitted with a deuterium lamp and interference filter or by applying specific staining reagents. The most recommended dyes for nucleic acids are acridine orange and acriflavine. Toluidine blue O staining is often used, but the destaining is a lengthy process. Bands containing DNA alone can be identified by a reaction with a diphenylamine reagent, and RNA may be detected with a phloroglucinol reagent.

Acridine Orange Staining: Acridine Orange Solution

Acridine orange	2 g
Lanthanum acetate	1 g
15% acetic acid	97 ml

Destaining solution:

15% acetic acid

Stain for 4 hours and destain for 30 to 45 minutes. View the bands in UV light.

Acriflavine Staining (Kwapinski, 1972):

Reagents

1. Acriflavine dihydrochloride — 1 g
   Potassium metabisulfite — 2 g
   Hydrochloric acid (concentrated) — 13 ml
   Distilled water — 184 ml
2. Periodic acid — 1.2 g
   1 *M* sodium acetate — 10 ml
   Butyl alcohol — 90 ml
3. Acid alcohol:
   Hydrochloric acid (concentrated) — 1 ml
   70% ethyl alcohol — 90 ml

Procedure

Immerse gel slabs in the solution 2 for 10 minutes; wash briefly in distilled water; transfer to solution 1 for 20 minutes, and wash in solution 3 for 10 minutes.

Examine the gel slabs in ultraviolet light.

The bands of nucleic acid show a green or orange fluorescence.

Immerse gel slabs in the solution 2 for 10 minutes; wash briefly in distilled water; transfer to solution 1 for 20 minutes; wash in acid alcohol for 5 to 10 minutes. Examine in UV light.

The DNA Staining: Diphenylamine Reagent

Diphenylamine	2.0 g
Glacial acetic acid	98 ml
Sulfuric acid (concentrated)	5 ml

Apply the diphenylamine reagent for 1 hour at 37°. Destain in acetic acid for 10 minutes. The DNA containing bands are colored blue.

The RNA Staining: Phloroglucinol Reagent

1.	Phloroglucinol	25 g
	Concentrated HCl, glacial acetic acid, water (1:2:1)	75 ml
2.	Ferric Chloride	0.1 g
	Concentrated HCl, glacial acetic acid (1 + 6)	99.9 ml

Apply reagent 2 for 50 minutes at 40°, the reagent 1 for 4 minutes, and leave the slabs at room temperature for 10 hours. DNA does not interfere with the color.

Phospholipid Detection: Reagent

60% $HClO_4$	10 ml
0.7 N HCl	150 ml
5% ammonium molybdate	40 ml

Expose the gel slabs to the reagent at 40° for 1 hour. Viewing with strong UV light brings out the blue zones of phospholipids and phosphates.

Lipid Detection. Lipid bands in gel can be detected by staining with 0.05% alcoholic solution of Rhodamine B, or with 0.5% Sudan IV or Sudan Black solution, made in 50% warm ethyl alcohol. The Rhodamine B stained bands are detected in the UV light. The Sudan IV or Sudan Black solutions are applied for 30 minutes and the slabs are destained quickly in 50% ethanol and then in 40% ethanol until all background has disappeared. An alternative procedure consists of staining in a saturated Sudan Black solution made in propylene glycol, and destaining in a 50% propylene glycol solution.

Lipids and lipoproteins can be stained with Oil Red "O" solution, made by dissolving 0.5 g of Oil Red "O" in 100 ml of 50% ethyl alcohol. The dye solution should be left at 37° for 24 hours and filtered. The gel slabs are stained for 2 hours and then washed with 50% ethyl alcohol until the excess dye has been removed.

Polysaccharide-protein, lipoprotein, nucleoprotein, liposaccharide, each forming a separate band in the gel, can be detected by a stepwise staining, destaining, and restaining, aimed at a successive detection of each part of a chemical complex.

In the case of the disk electrophoresis of a complex, containing nucleic acids, the gel slabs may first be examined in the UV light to determine the position of nucleic acids and then the same slabs are stained with suitable reagents to reveal other parts of the complex.

Investigation of the Homogeneity of RNA Preparation by the Disk Electrophoresis Technique (Richards et al., 1965). The following solutions are used for the preparation of polyacrylamide gels and as buffers for the electrophoresis:

Reservoir solution:	Diethylbarbiturate acid—0.03 *M*.
	Tris—0.0033 *M*, pH 8.9.
Large pore solution:	Hydrochloric acid—0.05 *M*.
	Tris—0.0503 *M*.
	Cyanogum 41—5 g/dl.
Small pore solution:	Hydrochloric acid—0.05 *M*.
	Tris—0.243 *M*.
	Cyanogum 41—10 g/dl.

The large and small pore solutions must be degassed under vacuum to remove dissolved oxygen which could inhibit the polymerization, add 1 volume of a stock solution of 0.01% riboflavin to 40 volumes of each pore solution. Fill the electrophoresis tubes, closed by small rubber stopper or wrapped in parafilm at one end, with the small pore solution. Carefully layer distilled water over the gel top, 5 mm high. Polymerize the gel by exposing it to a fluorescent light supplied by a 25-W fluorescent lamp, for 20 minutes. Polymerization is signified by the appearance of a slight opalescence in the gel. Pour off the excess liquid and blot the surface of the gel. Pipette 0.5 ml of large pore solution on top of the gel and add a water layer, and polymerize the gels again. Apply the sample of RNA absorbed on a filter paper disk, placing it on top of the large pore gel. A second paper disk soaked in 0.001% bromphenol blue, a dye migrating in the same direction as the RNA may be placed next to it. The remaining length of the tube is filled with a slurry of acid-washed sand in reservoir buffer to prevent back diffusion of the RNA. Remove the stoppers from the tubes and insert the tubes into the disk electrophoresis apparatus. Apply an electric current at 6 mA/tube, using the reservoir buffer. The electrophoresis is continued until the anion front has migrated about $\frac{2}{3}$ of the length of the small pore gel. After the electrophoresis, extract the gel from tubes by careful rimming with a dissecting needle and expelling with gentle water pressure into a beaker of water. Transfer the gel slabs into the fixative stain solution and leave them in the solution for a few hours or overnight.

The fixative stain solution consists of 1% lanthanum acetate, 2% acridine orange, and 15% acetic acid. Destaining is best conducted in an electric destaining apparatus by passing a current of 50 mA/gel until the gel is clear, usually for 20 minutes. The residual unbound dye is removed by soaking the gel slabs in water for 50 minutes. The RNA containing bands are orange-red stained.

2. *The Cellulose Acetate Membrane Electrophoresis*

The electrophoresis on cellulose acetate membranes may be conducted as a macro- or microprocedure and accordingly, 9 to 12 cm × 2 to 3 cm or 7 × 2 cm strips of cellulose acetate membrane (CAM) are used. The electric contact between cellulose acetate strips and the buffer is provided by filter paper wicks 4 to 5 cm in length. The electrophoresis is conducted in a universal electrophoresis apparatus equipped with a power supply, preferably with a constant-current device and capable of delivering up to 25 mA and 400 V.

The application line on cellulose acetate strips are marked with non-diffusible ink or a soft grease pencil. The strips are floated on the surface of a selected buffer and then submerged in the buffer. The buffer-impregnated CAM strips are blotted lightly between sheets of filter paper and then placed on the bridge of an electrophoresis tank and connected to the buffer by means of the wet paper wicks. The sample is applied on the CAM strip as a straight streak by means of a micropipette or preferably a special applicator, leaving a 5 to 6 mm margin on both sides of the applied sample. The place for application of the sample should be determined for each substance in buffer system, but the usual application spot is $\frac{1}{3}$ to $\frac{1}{2}$ of the distance from the cathode end.

CAM Electrophoresis of Proteins. An electric, preferably constant current, is applied, 0.4 to 0.5 mA/cm of wick with the initial potential gradient of 25 V/cm of strip which gradually decreases during the run. The separation of polymer mixtures is usually attained within 2 hours.

On the completion of electrophoretic run, the CAM strip is transferred into a denaturant, for example, 3% sulfosalicylic acid or 5% trichloroacetic acid in case of proteins, for 15 minutes. The staining method depends on the nature of separated material, if known, or as predetermined by suitable qualitative chemical tests designed to detect proteins, carbohydrates, nucleic acids, or lipids. The recommended staining procedures have been described under the section dealing with polyacrylamide gel disk electrophoresis.

Ponceau S dye is particularly convenient for staining proteins but nigrosin is a more sensitive stain. Ponceau S dye is used as 0.2% solution made in 3% trichloroacetic acid. The CAM strip, fixed in 3% sulfosalicylic acid or 5% trichloroacetic acid for 5 minutes, is stained in the Ponceau S solution for 5 minutes. Wash the strips in 5% acetic acid with a few changes until the background is colorless. Blot the CAM and dry it at room temperature.

Nigrosin is applied as 0.002% solution made in 2% acetic acid and the staining of CAM strips is carried out for about 2 hours following which the strips are rinsed in tap water, blotted, and dried at room temperature.

Naphthalene black (naphthol-black) is almost as sensitive as nigrosin for detection of proteins. The dye is used as 0.2% solution made in a 1:9 mixture of glacial acetic acid and methyl alcohol. The CAM strip is stained for 10 to 15 minutes after which the excess stain is removed by immersing the membrane in a 10% methanol solution of acetic acid.

Other dyes, for example, light green or azocarmine B are less appropriate for detection of proteins.

The CAM strips may be cleared and made transparent by immersing the membranes in liquid paraffin, white Moore oil No. 120, cotton seed oil, or in another white oil. The cleared strips can be used for scanning of separated fractions.

Elution of protein bands from the cellulose acetate strips may be obtained by applying 0.1 M NaOH to a Ponceau S stained strip and precipitating the protein with 0.1 ml of 40% acetic acid, if required. The protein bands, or bands containing other materials, may be cut out and completely dissolved leaving the separated fractions in solution. The CAM strips may be dissolved in a 1:10 mixture of ethyl alcohol and methylene chloride or in a mixture of equal volumes of acetone and methylene chloride.

CAM Electrophoresis of Glycoproteins (Arai and Wallace, 1969): Reagents

1. Barbital buffer, 0.075 M, pH 8.6, 2.76 g diethylbarbituric acid and 15.4 g diethylbarbiturate, dissolved in 1 liter of deionized distilled water.
2. 95% ethyl alcohol.
3. 0.8% periodic acid.
4. Schiff reagent: 6 g of basic fuchsin, dissolved in 1200 ml of distilled water at 90°, cool to 50° and filter; add 30 ml of 2 N HCl and 4 g of potassium metabisulfite. Allow to stand at 4° overnight. Add 3 g of powdered activated animal charcoal, mix, and filter. Add 40 ml of 2 N HCl.
5. 0.5% potassium metabisulfite in 0.1 N HCl, freshly made.
6. 0.01 N HCl.
7. 0.1% trichloroacetic acid in absolute methyl alcohol.
8. Clearing solution: 25 ml of clacial acetic acid and 75 ml of absolute methyl alcohol.

Perform the electrophoresis on cellulose-acetate membrane at 250 V for 20 minutes, using the barbital buffer. Remove the membrane and place it in 15% ethyl alcohol for 5 minutes and in 0.8% periodic acid solution for 10 minutes. Wash the membrane in distilled water for 3 minutes, and stain it in the Schiff reagent for 15 minutes, in the potassium metabisulfite-HCl solution for 3 minutes, and in 0.01 N HCl for 5 minutes. Transfer the membrane to absolute alcohol for 2 minutes and to the TCA-methanol solution for 30 seconds. Clear the membrane, spread on a glass slide in the clearing solution for 30 seconds, and dry it at room temperature. Densitometric quantitation is performed at 550 nm.

CAM Electrophoresis of Lipoproteins. The recommended method for lipoprotein and lipid is the staining with 0.05% alcohol solution of Rhodamine B for 5 to 10 minutes, followed by the detection of lipoprotein or lipid bands in the UV light. An alternative method (Kohn, 1961) employs the ozone Schiff technique.

The electrophoresis on CAM is relatively sensitive since as little as 5 μg of a polymer mixture can be successfully separated into the components.

The recommended buffer for protein electrophoresis (Laurell et al., 1956) consists of the following.

Barbitone	1.5 g
Sodium diethylbarbitone	10.8 g
Distilled water to 1000 ml	

The solution above is used for impregnation of the CAM strips. It should be diluted in a proportion of 5 volumes of buffer to 1 volume of distilled water to serve as a buffer for the electrophoresis tank. Thymol may be added as preservative using 5 ml of 5% thymol solution made in isopropyl alcohol per 1 liter of buffer.

The buffer concentration in the tank should be such that at 0.4 mA/cm width of the CAM strip, the initial voltage would be 200 V, falling to 150 V by the end of the run. The lower the buffer concentration, the greater the rate of mobility with increase in the width of the bands.

3. The Paper Zone Electrophoresis

The paper zone electrophoresis is more widely employed in immunochemical studies, because of its relative simplicity. Electrophoretograms are usually prepared on Whatman filter No. 1 or 3, although strips of cellulose acetate membrane filters sometimes are more advantageous (Kohn, 1957). After a 0.05- to 0.01-ml sample is put on the paper soaked in buffer, electrophoresis is carried out either with 310-V electric current applied across the electrodes for 2 hours, or with 120 V for 16 hours at room temperature.

A barbiturate* or borate buffer,† pH 8.6, is used. Electrophoretograms are dried at 105° and sprayed with a selective dye to reveal the presence and position of the fractions.

Carbohydrates can be detected with an acidified aniline phthalate reagent, viewed against an ultraviolet lamp (Consden and Stainier, 1952), or by spraying with a solution of periodic acid, potassium iodine solution, and Schiff's fuchsin reagent (Köiw and Grönwall, 1952).

Sugar Electrophoresis. Sugar molecules, which normally do not possess a sufficient charge to be separated in an electric field, are made charged when complexed to the borate ions. A high-voltage electrophoresis (Mabry et al., 1965; Kwapinski, 1972) permits a more rapid separation of sugars than a low-voltage ionophoresis (Consden and Stanier, 1952). Since the distance travelled within a given time by a molecule is directly proportional to the applied potential, the sugars are separated from each other more efficiently by the application of high potential gradients, ranging from 50 to 120 V/cm. Foster (1952) has applied a potential of 1200 V, and Kwapinski et al. (1971), has applied a voltage of 900 V for his technique of the flat-plate electrophoresis of carbohydrates (Fig. 31).

4. Sugar Ionophoresis

The borate buffer, pH 7.0, 8.0, 8.6, 9.2, and 9.7, used as an electrolyte solution for this technique, consists of 0.2 *M* boric acid and 0.05 *M* sodium chloride and varied volumes of 0.05 *M* borax, except that 0.1 *M* sodium hydroxide is used instead of borax to adjust the solution to pH 9.7. A pH 10.0 borate buffer consists of 7.44 g boric acid per liter of 0.1 *N* NaOH. The suitable pH value of a borate buffer for an individual sugar sample must be predetermined.

The sugars are applied to Whatman No. 1 paper, dipped in the buffer, blotted, and placed in a rectangular glass frame in order to keep the paper stretched horizontally. The ends of the paper should be dipped in the buffer solution. The samples and 1% standard sugar solutions are applied along a starting line 12 cm from the cathode end of the paper. The ionophoresis is run at room temperature at a potential of about 310 V for about 2 hours.

---

* Barbiturate buffer, pH 8.6 and 0.125 ionic concentration, consists of:

Veronal (diethylbarbituric acid)	8.712 g
Sodium hydroxide	1.893 g
Sodium acetate	6.476 g
0.1 *N* hydrochloric acid	60 ml
Distilled water, up to	1 liter

† M/5 borate buffer, pH 8.6, contains:

45 ml of 1.24% aqueous boric acid
55 ml of 1.9% $Na_2B_4O_7 \cdot 10H_2O$ solution

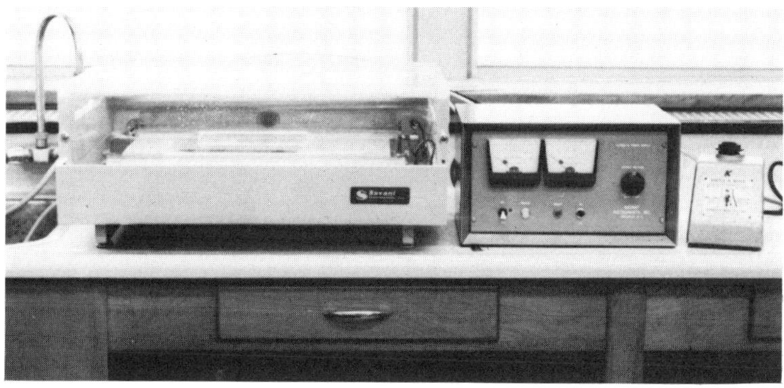

Figure 31. The flat-plate electrophoresis apparatus consisting of a flat-plate chamber connected to tap water for cooling and to a high voltage power supply.

At the end of the ionophoresis, the paper is removed and dried and the sugars are revealed with a suitable reagent, for example, aniline hydrogen phthalate reagent on heating at 100 ot 100° for a few minutes, and then viewed in ultraviolet light. The monose spots show an intense fluorescence. The mobilities [$cm^2/(V)(second)$] are calculated from the distance between the sugar spot and proline or creatinine which have run on the same paper, the effective length of the paper, voltage, and time. If an alkaline buffer is used, it is recommended to add a few drops of glacial acetic to overcome the alkalinity of the buffer. For most monoses, a buffer possessing pH 8.0 to 8.6 is adequate.

Hexosamines and hexuronic acids may be separated in nonborate buffers because of their different electric charges. A sample analyzed for hexosamines and hexosamine-uronic acids is first treated with a 1:1 mixture of 5% sodium nitrite and 33% acetic acid, left for 10 minutes and applied to Whatman No. 1 paper. After the electrophoresis in a pH 10.0 borate buffer, at 20 V/cm for 2 to 3 hours, the paper is dried, sprayed with 1% indole in ethanol containing 5% HCl, and heated at 100° for 1 minute. The anyhdro sugars give orange-yellow color (Williamson and Zamenhof, 1963).

5. *The High Voltage Electrophoresis for Sugars*
Buffers:

1. A 0.1 *M,* pH 9.2 borate buffer, containing 38.1 g of sodium borate per liter.
2. A pH 7.3 buffer prepared by adding 2 *M* NaOH dropwise to 0.5 *M* boric acid (30.9 g of boric acid per liter) until the pH 7.3 is attained.

The sugar sample, consisting of oligosaccharides or hydrolyzates containing monosaccharides, and 0.5% solutions of standard sugars in 10% isopropanol (25 μl) are applied 12 cm from one end of a sheet of Whatman No. 3 MM paper (57 $\times$ 23.5 or 27 $\times$ 47 cm). The paper is then dipped through the buffer until all but 2 cm to either side of the origin has become saturated. The paper is placed on the support rack and the remaining area is sprayed lightly with buffer. The rack is then placed into the electrophoresis tank (Fig. 32) so that the origin rests near the negative (cathode) terminal. The buffer is overlayered by a cooling medium, for example, Varsol. The tank is cooled by circulating an antifreeze through a refrigeration unit and the coils of the chamber. The electrophoresis at pH 9.2 is carried at the operating potential gradient of 24 V/cm length and the current of 5 mA/cm width, at 10 to 15° for $2\frac{1}{2}$ hours. At pH 7.3, the operating potential of 40 V/cm and the current of 1 to 2 mA/cm is applied for 2 hours.

After the completion of the electrophoresis, the paper is removed from the tank and dried at 90° for 30 minutes. The sugars are detected with a diphenylamine-*p*-anisidine reagent, freshly prepared and filtered. This re-

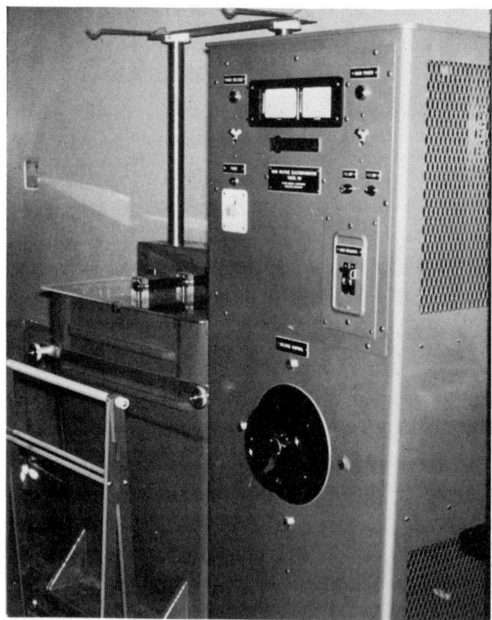

Figure 32. The high voltage electrophoresis apparatus consisting of a large tank in which the paper carrying specimen is immersed and a power supply delivering the voltage up to 10,000 V.

agent consists of equal volumes of 2% diphenylamine in acetone containing 8.8% orthophosphoric acid. The chromatographic paper is dipped through the reagent, and acetone and ethanol are evaporated by drying at room temperature for 20 minutes. The paper is then placed in a vented chromatography oven at 85° with a relative humidity of 50%, for 10 to 15 minutes, or until characteristic colors of individual sugar bands have appeared. The sugars migrate from the cathode to the anode in the following order: galacturonic acid (the fastest), glucose, galactose, mannose, rhamnose, maltose, and sucrose (the slowest sugar).

Individual sugars are identified by mobility and color, as well as by the rate of color development. Mobility rates are determined in relation to the mobility of glucose at pH 9.2 and of ribose at pH 7.3. Colors are as follows: green color of glucose, galactose and mannose, gold color of rhamnose, xylose and fructose, copper color of arabinose and deoxyribose, galacturonic- and glucuronic acid, yellow color of fucose, and yellow-green color of ribose.

An alternative reagent for the detection of sugars is the aniline phthalate reagent, consisting of 1.7% aniline in water-saturated *n*-butanol. The paper dipped in this reagent is heated at 100° to 105° for 10 minutes.

Neither of the above reagents develop some substituted sugars, for example, amino sugars. Amino sugars are detected with an indole reagent which induces a yellow color of amino sugars on a light pink background.

6. *The Lipid Electrophoresis*

Lipids or lipoproteins can be separated by electrophoresis on starch, polyvinyl, or on filter paper, using techniques described by Durrum et al. (1952), Kunkel and Trautman (1956), Reissel et al. (1966) and Kwapinski (1972). The thin layer electrophoresis (Reissel et al., 1966) and Kwapinski's (1972) high-voltage electrophoresis are most efficient in the separation of lipids, phospholipids, and lipoproteins; but Durrum's et al. technique has its application occasionally.

7. *Thin Layer Electrophoresis of Lipoproteins*

The supporting media, spread on 20 × 20 cm glass plates, are a potato starch slurry in a 0.1 *M*, pH 8.6, barbital buffer, containing 0.001 *M* EDTA, Silica Gel, or cellulose.

Glass plates are coated with the potato starch slurry at a thickness of 0.37 mm, following which the plates are dried until the surface becomes dull and nonreflective in appearance. The phospholipid sample is applied about 5 cm from the intended cathodal end of the plate.

The plate is placed in the tank, and wicks of Whatman 3 MM filter paper are placed between the buffer reservoirs and the ends of the starch layer.

Electrophoresis is conducted at 600 V and 18 to 20 mA for 2 hours to allow the material to migrate approximately 10 cm toward the anode. The plates are then removed from the apparatus, dried, and sprayed with 0.4% ninhydrin in acetone solution to develop the protein part of the lipoprotein. The lipid part of the phospholipid is detected with a warm, saturated solution of Oil Red 0 in 60% ethanol. Standard solutions of lipids, such as cholesterol, cholesterol oleate and triolein are applied in the amounts varying from 25 to 100 μg in a volume of 5 μl.

Lipids such as glycerol ether diesterases can be detected with 0.2% ethanol solution of 2′,7′-chlorofluorescein (Wood and Snyder, 1967).

Saponification of lipids can be attained by refluxing the material with a several-fold excess of 1.0 N ethanolic KOH for 1 to 2 hours. The unidentified lipids can be transesterified by refluxing in 2% H_2SO_4 in methanol for 2 hours. The products are then separated by the TLC system on the Silica Gel G coated plates by developing in a chamber containing hexane-diethyl ether (90:10).

Phospholipids can be identified by a tricomplex staining procedure, using 0.005% acid fuchsin in water and 0.2% uranyl nitrate and 0.01 N HCl as spray reagent (Hooghwinkel and Van Niekerk, 1960). The lecithin spots appear stained red against a slight background color.

8. *High Voltage Electrophoresis of Phospholipids and Lipids*

Phospholipids are saponified as follows: 50- to 100-μg samples are suspended in 1 ml of 1 N KOH, made in 80% ethyl alcohol. The ampoules are sealed, and incubated at 140° for 6 hours and then cooled. The saponified material, in aliquots of 5 to 10 μl, is placed on cellulose acetate strips or on Whatman 3 MM paper, impregnated with a 1:10 mixture of paraffin oil and ether, and dried. The electrophoresis is conducted at 6500 V and 360 mA for 5 to 6 hours in the following solvent:

Tris	8 g
Glycine	2 g
Tween-80	50 ml
Distilled water	540 ml (pH 9.0–9.5)
Methyl alcohol	400 ml

placed in a tank, cooled by circulating water.

According to the Durrum et al. (1952) technique, a lipid-containing sample is placed on Whatman 3 MM paper, and the electrophoresis is run in a veronal buffer, pH 8.6, ionic strength 0.05. Lipids are then "developed" by means of a solution of Oil Red O in 60% ethyl alcohol. Spots of lipids are red-colored.

An alternative staining of lipidograms, with a saturated Sudan black B solution, is conducted by placing the electrophoretogram, dried at 80°, in a bath containing this dye solution for 3 hours (Ribeiro et al., 1961). The paper is then washed three times for 15 minutes in 50% ethyl alcohol. Lipids appear as blue-black spots on a pale blue background.

9. The Protein Electrophoresis

Electrophoretic separation and identification of proteins is attained most effectively by a polyacrylamide disk electrophoresis (Kwapinski, 1972), which is preferred to the electrophoresis on cellulose acetate membranes and on filter paper.

10. Polyacrylamide Disk Electrophoresis of Proteins

A protein sample, dialyzed overnight at 4° against 0.01 *M,* pH 6.7, sodium phosphate buffer, is diluted with an equal volume of glycerol, which maintains stable interphase between the applied specimen and upper buffer, and necessitates no sample gel. The sample is applied in a volume ranging from 0.05 to 0.08 ml containing 10 to 50 μg protein nitrogen for best resolution.

The power source is initially set at 20 mA per 12 tubes until all bromphenol blue rings have passed into the concentrating gels, following which the current is increased to 50 mA per 12 tubes. The electrophoresis is continued until the ring of bromphenol blue marker is approximately 30 mm from the origin, which is the concentrating-resolving gel interphase in the resolving gel. The gels are stained with buffalo black, and the free stain is removed by electrophoresis at 50 mA per 12 tubes with 7% aqueous acetic acid (Fig. 28).

The Rs values for each band are determined with bromphenol blue as the reference. Scanning of the bands can be attained in a densitometer, equipped with an integrator attachment or in a Chromoscan (Fig. 29).

According to Durrum's (1951) method, electrophoresis is conducted for 16 hours at 110 V on a Whatman filter paper No. 1 or 3, in a veronal buffer, pH 8.6, or in an acetate buffer. Acetate buffer, pH 4.5, contains 350 ml of $M/1$ acetic acid and 100 ml of M/1 sodium acetate. In the two-dimensional electrophoresis (Markam et al., 1956), paper strips are first run in one of these buffers, then the central part of the electrophoretogram is cut out and put on another strip of filter paper, placed rectangularly to the previous direction, and electropohresis continues for another period of 16 hours. The electrophoretogram is dried at 105° and developed either in a bromophenol blue, naphthalen black, or amido black 10B solution. The first solution can contain either 100 ml of absolute ethyl alcohol, 100 ml of bromophenol blue, and 5.0 g of mercuric chloride, or 500 mg of bromo-phenol blue, 50 ml of glacial acetic acid, and 50 g of mercury chloride per liter of distilled water. The electrophoretogram is immersed in this stain for 30 minutes, then washed in 0.5% acetic acid four times, 10 minutes each time. When the filter paper dries off partially, it should be either exposed to the fumes of ammonia or dipped for 3 minutes in a buffer, pH 6 to 7, to detect the dark blue spots of protein.

The naphthalen black 12B is used as a saturated solution in methyl alcohol mixed with 10% acetic acid. Before staining, the electrophoretogram should be dried at 100°, fixed for a few minutes in 10% alcohol solution of mercuric bichloride, and dried. The filter paper is then immersed in a naphthalen black solution for 10 minutes, washed in a 9:1 mixture of methyl alcohol and acetic acid until the washings show no color, and finally in 60% methanol containing 1.2% of acetic acid and 0.2% of hydrochloric acid. A saturated solution of amido black 10B in a 9:1 mixture of methanol and glacial acetic acid is applied for 10 minutes, followed by washing with the solvent mixture. Electrophoretic mobility of the immunochemical fractions or subfractions can be measured and evaluated by comparison with the standard preparations of albumin, globulins, polysaccharides, or lipids. Amounts of the separated protein fractions can be determined densitometrically with the aid of the Eppendorf photometer, or spectrophotometrically.

In the first procedure, the electrophoresis strips are made transparent and passed through a densitometer. The extinction readings are plotted on a graph, and the resulting curve is measured planimetrically. For the spectrophotometric study, the electrophoresis strips are first colored and cut in strips, each containing a single protein fraction. The dye is then extracted with a solution of sodium hydroxide, and extinctions of the extracts are measured in a spectrophotometer. If a fraction shows the mobility of albumin, the recorded result must be multiplied by a correction factor of 1.4 since the affinity of albumin for dyes is greater than of other proteins.

III. SEPARATION OF COMPONENTS OF HETEROGENEOUS FRACTIONS

If a thorough immunochemical analysis of a complex, natural antigen-source is intended, the subsequent step in research is separation and recovery of individual immunochemical components. This may best be accomplished by one or more of the following methods: isoelectrofocusing, preparative polyacrylamide, gel electrophoresis, gel filtration and differential gradient centrifugation (see pp. 90, 103, 125). Chemical partitioning of the immunochemical constituents, used more frequently before the advent of the techniques above, may sometimes (together with anion-exchange chromatography) be employed as a preliminary or conjoint procedure, under carefully controlled conditions of pH, temperature, and concentration. In these procedures, slight solubility differences are exploited. Heterogeneous polysaccharide materials are dissolved in distilled water or in 5% acetic acid, and are treated with cold absolute ethyl alcohol added in a gradually increased concentration. Whenever the fluid becomes turbid, the mixture is left for several hours in the refrigerator and the precipitated subfraction is separated by centrifugation.

Heterogeneous proteinaceous materials are dissolved in 0.1 N NaOH chilled at 2°. To this solution is added a 5 to 10% TCA in the cold to separate the components at the increased pH levels. Alternatively, a saturated solution of ammonium sulfate or sodium sulfate may be used.

Lipids are dissolved in ether or benzene and are tested with acetone added in gradually increased amounts, and determined qualitatively by the Folch et al. (1957) method. Details of other procedures of subfractionation are given by Geiger and Anderson (1939) and Gubariev and Lubenec (1951).

Chromatographic Separation of Polymers. According to the Peterson and Sober (1956) technique, the ion exchange chromatography is set up on diethylaminoethyl (DEAE) cellulose. Columns, 2.5 by 50 cm, containing 14 g of the ion exchanger, are packed under a hydrostatic head of 15 in. The solution of heterogenous protein fraction is poured on the column and eluted by gradients of pH and ionic strength, at a flow rate of 80 to 100 ml/hour; 10-ml portions are collected with an automatic fraction collector and can be examined spectrophotometrically at the ultraviolet wavelengths of 360 and 280 nm.

The following buffers can be used for the elution of subfractions (Glenchur et al., 1962):

0.005 M phosphate buffer, pH 8.0.
0.003 M phosphate buffer, pH 7.0.
0.05 M NaH$_2$PO$_4$ solution.
0.10 M NaH$_2$PO$_4$ containing 0.20 M NaCl.
0.10 M NaH$_2$PO$_4$ containing 1.0 M NaCl.
0.10 M NAH$_2$PO$_4$ containing 2.0 M NaCl.

IV. CHEMICAL ANALYSIS OF ANTIGENS

The scope of chemical analysis of antigen preparations depends greatly on the yield of fractions and can be either limited to essential tests or extended to a more comprehensive study (Table 26). If the bulk of material is to be reserved for immunological investigations, and if the yield of certain fractions or subfractions obtained from the microorganisms is below 20 mg, only chromatographic analysis and qualitative tests for carbohydrate (the Molisch test) and protein (the Millon test), and nucleic acids (the Korson test) can be carried out.

Chemical analysis of complex structural preparations, such as cell walls or flagella, should consist of the determination of all four major types of macromolecular substances, the lipids, proteins, nucleic acids, and polysaccharides. Chemical analysis of the purified immunochemical constituents is usually planned in accordance with their essential physiochemical characteristics.

1. Chemical Analysis of Lipids

The essential chemical examinations of lipids are the nitrogen and phosphorus determinations and the chromatographic analysis of phosphatides and fatty acids. Fatty acids may be determined quantitatively by titration (Trout et al., 1960), but the most exact technique for the determination of fatty acids is the gas chromatography (Jamieson and Reid, 1965; Wilson et al., 1966; Moss and Lewis, 1967; Plackett et al., 1969). The gas chromatography equipment for automated procedure, used in Kwapinski's research laboratories, is shown in Fig. 33. Separation and identification of fatty acids by a paper- or thin-layer chromatography is much less convenient and less accurate.

Total nitrogen can be estimated by Kjeldahl's (1883) method as modified by Elek and Sobotka (1926), Markham (1942), or Bathurst and Mitchell (1958), or by Rommers and Visser's (1969) spectrophotometric technique. Methods for phosphorus determination by Chen's et al. (1956), Bartlett (1959), or Murkejee and Sri Ram (1964) are recommended. The percentage of phosphorus multiplied by 25 gives an approximate content of phospholipids in the material examined.

Chromatographic analysis of phosphatides can be conducted by Skidmore and Entenman's (1962) or Renkonen and Renkonen's (1959) or Marinetti's et al. (1957) method. The two-dimensional technique of Skidmore and Entenman is recommended. The chromatography of long-chain fatty acids is carried out by the Spiteri (1955) technique, as modified by Kwapinski (1959), or by the thin layer chromatography (Mangold, 1961; Morgan, 1962). The phospholipids are hydrolyzed by heating the material in sealed ampoules with 1.7 N methanolic HCl at 100° for 4 hours. The hydrolyzates are taken to dryness under reduced pressure at 75°. The dry material is then dissolved in a small volume of distilled water for chromatography.

The Two-Dimensional Thin-layer Chromatography of Phospholipids (Skidmore and Entenman, 1962). Glass plates, thoroughly cleaned with a detergent and with a 5% solution of potassium hydroxide in ethanol, are coated with Silica Gel G. Samples dissolved in a 2:1 mixture of chloroform-methanol are applied to the plates. The chromatograms are developed first

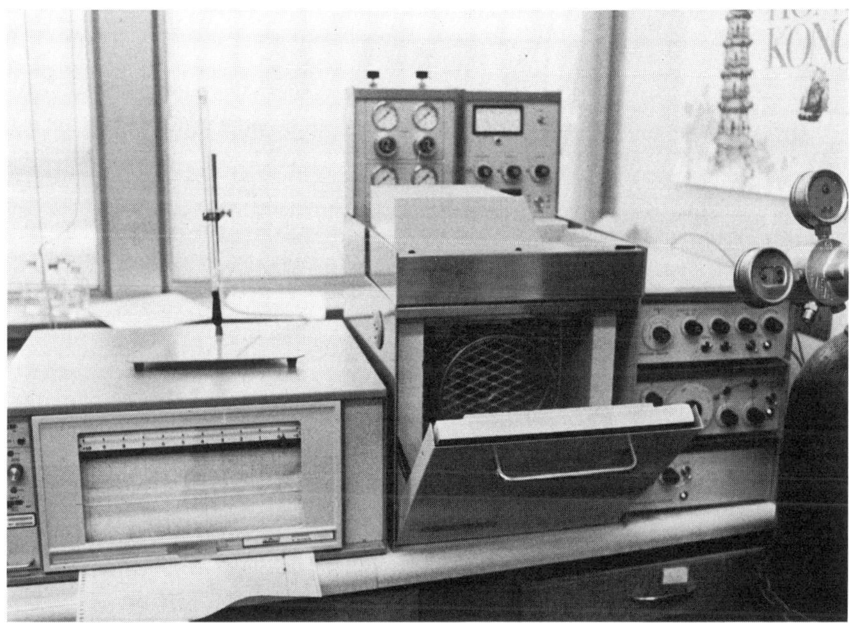

Figure 33.   The gas chromatography equipment, consisting of the basic oven unit, accommodating glass or steel columns, and a complete detector system as well as a linear recorder.

in solvent I (chloroform-methanol-7 N ammonium hydroxide, 60:35:5) until it moved a predetermined distance (usually in 1 hour). The plates are then dried, rotated 90° clockwise, and placed in solvent II (chloroform-methanol-7 N ammonium hydroxide, 35:60:5), for about 1 hour.

After drying the chromatogram, the lipid spots are detected by exposing the plate face down in an iodine atmosphere (in a plastic box containing a few cooling crystals). Dark yellow spots appear, and they should be marked. After the spots have disappeared on air, the plate is sprayed by one of the required reagents, for example:

1. Ninhydrine (0.3 g) in 5 ml lutidine + 95 ml n-butanol saturated with water, to detect amino phosphatides (red-violet spots at room temperature).

2. Molybdate reagent (4% ammonium molybdate, 25 ml, 1 N HCl, 10 ml, 60% perchloric acid, 5 ml) to detect phosphatides (blue spots appearing at room temperature).

3. Ferric-chloride-sulfosalicylic acid reagent ($FeCl_3 \cdot 6H_2O$, 0.1 g, sulfosalicylic acid, 7.0 g, water, 25 ml, diluted to 100 ml with 95% ethanol) to detect phosphate groups (white fluorescent spots appearing on a purple background in the UV).

Table 26. Schedule for Chemical Analysis of Antigen Preparation

Type of Material	Essential Tests	Milli-grams Required	Additional Tests	Milli-grams Required
Proteins	Nitrogen content	10	Amino and imino acid content	20
	Phosphorus content	10	Gas chromatography of amino	20
	Protein content	10	acids	
	Amino acid TLC	20	Autoanalysis of amino acids	20
	Disk electrophoresis	20	Terminal a-a determination	20
	Peptide mapping	20	Chromatography of saccharides	10
	Carbohydrate content	10	and lipids	
Polysac-charides	Saccharide content	10	Ketose content	10
	Nitrogen content	20	Pentose content	10
	Phosphorus content	20	Glucosamine content	10
	Chromatography	10	Sugar finger-printing	10
	Disk electrophoresis	10	Chromatography of amino and	10
			fatty acids	
Nucleic acids	Phosphorus content	20	Autoanalysis of purines and	20
	Nitrogen content	20	pyrimidines	
	Ribose (deoxyribose) content	5	HV-Nucleotide mapping	10
			Termal denaturation deter-mination	20
	TL chromatography	10		
	Buoyant density determi-nation	10	Molecular weight determi-nation	20
	Nucleotide electrophoresis	10		
Lipids	Nitrogen content	20	Paper chromatography of fatty	10
	Phosphorus content	20	acids and phosphatides	
	Disk electrophoresis	20	Cholesterol, phospholipid, and	50
	Gas chromatography	20	cerebroside content	
			Melting point	100
			Neutralization number	100
			Iodine number	100
			Saponification number	100

4. Ammoniacal silver nitrate reagent for detection of glycerol and inositol. Dry plates are sprayed with a 1:1 mixture of 0.1 N $AgNO_3$ and 7 N ammonium hydroxide and are heated at 110° until dark brown spots appear.

5. Dragendorf's reagent for choline. Dry plates are sprayed with a 4:1: 20 mixture of solution I, II, and water. Solution I contains 1.7 g $Bi(NO_3)_3 \cdot 5H_2O$ diluted to 100 ml with 20% acetic acid. Solution II consists of 40% KI in water. Free choline produces orange spots at room temperature.

6. Hydroxylamine ferric chloride reagent for *esterified fatty acids*. The reagent consists of two solutions.

Solution 1: 10 g hydroxylamine · HCl dissolved in 25 ml water, diluted to 100 ml with ethanol, supplemented with 26 ml of saturated aqueous NaOH, diluted to 200 ml with ethanol, and filtered.

Solution 2: 10 g $FeCl_3 \cdot 6H_2O$ are dissolved in 20 ml 37% HCl and shaken in the solution with 300 ml ether. The plates are first sprayed with solution 1, dried briefly, and then sprayed with solution 2. Purple spots appear on a yellow background.

The most sensitive reagent for the detection of phospholipids consists of a mixture of the following solutions 1 and 2 (Vaskovsky and Kosletsky, 1968).

Solution 1: 16.0 g of ammonium molybdate is dissolved in 120 ml distilled water.

Solution 2: To 80 ml of solution 1 are added 10 ml of concentrated hydrochloric acid and 10 ml of mercury; the liquid is shaken for 30 minutes, and filtered.

Final Reagent: To 40 ml of solution 1 are added 200 ml of concentrated sulfuric acid, and diluted to 1 liter with distilled water.

The chromatogram of phospholipids is sprayed with the final reagent, without heating. The phospholipids produce blue coloration on a white background. Phosphates, fatty acids, and cholesterols give no color.

Cholesterol and cholesteryl esters are detected with Lowry's (1968) reagent, consisting of 50 mg $FeCl_3 \cdot 6H_2O$ in 9 ml of water, 5 ml of glacial acetic acid, and 5 ml of concentrated sulfuric acid. The chromatograms are sprayed with this solution and heated at 100° for 2 to 3 minutes. Characteristic red to violet color is given by cholesterol. The color is unstable and darkens gradually.

Thin-Layer Chromatography of Phospholipids. A good solvent for the separation of phospholipids by the thin-layer chromatography consists of a 65:25:4 mixture of chloroform, methanol and water. The separation is improved by the application of a two-dimensional chromatography (Skidmore and Entenman, 1962). The chromatography is run first in the solvent consisting of chloroform, methanol, and 7 *N* ammonium hydroxide (60:35:5) and then in the second direction, using a system consisting of chloroform, methanol, and 7 *N* ammonium hydroxide (35:60:5).

Total phospholipids are detected by immersing the plate in a closed container with iodine crystals and iodine vapors. Amino nitrogen groups are detected with 0.2 to 0.5% ethanolic solution of ninhydrine. Phosphate is detected with acid molybdate (Vaskovsky and Kosletsky, 1968), glycolipid with an anthrone and diphenylamine reagent and choline with Chargaff's reagent (Waldi, 1965).

To minimize streaking, it is recommended to coat glass plates with a stationary phase of Silica Gel G buffered with borate buffer at pH 8.0. Thirty grams of Silica Gel G are suspended in 60 ml of borate buffer. This suspension is spread on glass plates, which are then dried at room temperature for several hours and activated at 100° for 1 hour. The plates should be stored over a dessicant and be reactivated at 100° for 1 hour before use (Bunn et al., 1969).

Chromatography of Long-Chain Fatty Acids. According to Kwapinski's (1965) procedure, the lipids are first separated by heating a 5 to 10 mg sample, suspended in 2 ml of 1 N alcoholic solution of sodium hydroxide, sealed in an ampoule, at 100° for 12 to 15 hours. An amount of 0.005 to 0.01 ml of the saponified material is then transferred on a sheet of Whatman No. 2, 4 or 1 filter paper, which has been previously impregnated in 10% etheric solution of paraffin oil, and dried. The 0.01 molar alcohol solution of such standard fatty acid preparations as palmitic, C_{16} (hexadecanoic), stearic, C_{18} (octadecanoic), oleic, C_{18} (*cis*-9-octadecanoic), linoleic, C_{18} (octadecadienoic), lauric, C_{12} (dodecanoic), behenic, C_{22} (docosanoic), and others, if required, should be placed 2 cm apart on the same sheet of filter paper for the Rf standardization. Chromatograms are developed for 12 to 24 hours in 85% acetic acid, dried for 2 to 3 hours at 70° or at room temperature, and immersed for 30 minutes in a 0.2% cupric acetate. The papers are then washed for 1 hour with running tap water and left for 2 to 3 minutes in a 0.2% solution of $K_4Fe(CN)_6$. By this treatment, pink spots of saturated and nonsaturated higher fatty acids appear. To differentiate the nonsaturated from other fatty acids, a parallel chromatogram should be immersed for 15 seconds into 1% solution of potassium permanganate, and washed in running tap water for 10 minutes. The nonsaturated high fatty acids occur as brown colored spots. The higher fatty acids must be identified by calculating their Rf values in comparison with the standards.

The method described is often used together with the circular technique of Nowotny et al. (1958).

Circular Chromatography of Long-Chain Fatty Acids (Nowotny et al., 1958). This technique is a modification of the Kaufmann and Nitsch (1954) method. To obtain a good separation of fatty acids, filter-paper disks are first impregnated with a fraction of petroleum oil obtained by repeated distillation at 200 to 210°. Filter-paper disks (20 cm in diameter) soaked in the petroleum fraction should be wiped off between two layers of filter paper and dried at room temperature for 1 hour. Lipid samples (10 to 20 mg) are suspended in 10 ml of 5N HCl and hydrolyzed in the steaming bath for 8 hours. Hydrolyzates are then mixed with 20 ml of ether and shaken to dissolve lipids in ether. This step is to be repeated three times.

Etheric extracts are then collected, dried over sodium sulfate, and finally pervaporated. The solid material is dissolved or suspended in 0.2 ml of benzene, and small amounts of this solution are put on the impregnated filter paper.

Chromatograms are developed for 16 hours in an 85% acetic acid solution which has been saturated with the isolated lipid fraction. Chromatograms are then dried at 80°, immersed for a few minutes into a 0.5% solution of cupric acetate in 0.05 N sodium acetate, rinsed for 1 hour in running tap water, and placed for 30 minutes in a 0.5% potassium-ferrocyanid solution in 0.1 N HCl. Chromatograms should then be washed in running tap water and dried at room temperature.

Long-chain fatty acids appear in the form of pink-red bands. Unsaturated fatty acids can be detected by exposing the chromatogram for 15 minutes to an atmosphere saturated with osmium-tetroxide. The saturation is attained by placing a few O_5O_4 crystals in a closed dark beaker. Bands of unsaturated fatty acids stain greyish-black.

The method described is very sensitive, as it permits detection of as little as 5 μg of fatty acids.

The Thin Layer Chromatography of Fatty Acids. According to Mangold (1961), a lipid sample, dissolved in a minimal amount of chloroform-methyl alcohol (2:1) is applied in bands on 20-cm² glass plates coated with a 0.5-mm-thick layer of Silica Gel G (Merck) or alumina and dried. After the application of lipids, 1.5 to 2 cm from the lower edge, the plates are developed in the ascending manner, with a 90:10 mixture of hexane and diethyl ether, placed in glass containers lined with filter paper saturated with the developing solvent (Mangold, 1961; Wood and Snyder, 1967). After 30 to 40 minutes, when the solvent has moved over 100 mm, the lipid fractions separated are located by spraying the edges of the chromatogram with an aqueous bromothymol blue or with 0.05% ethanolic solution of Rhodamine B and observed in UV light, in the case of the latter reagent).

Chromatography of lower fatty acids can be carried out by the methods of Read and Lederer (1951), Brown and Hall (1950), Hack (1953), Fink and Fink (1949), or Isherwood and Hanes (1935). The following technique, based on the method of Reid and Lederer (1951), has been satisfactorily used by the author. An amount of 10 to 20 mg of a lipid fraction suspended in 2 to 3 ml of 25% solution of ammonium hydroxide is heated for 3 to 4 hours at 90° to transform fatty acids into ammonium salts. The mixture is then centrifuged, the sediment suspended in 1 to 2 ml of distilled water, and 0.01 to 0.05 amounts are placed on a sheet of Whatman No. 1 or No. 2 filter paper which has been previously saturated with fumes of ammonia; 0.1 M solutions of standard lower fatty acids are placed on the same sheet for control purposes. The solvent consists of primary *n*-butyl alcohol saturated with an equal volume of 1.5 *N* ammonia. The chromatogram is developed for 15 to 20 hours in the butanol phase of this solvent whereas the water phase is placed in a Petri dish on the bottom of the jar. The chromatogram is then dried by using a fan, and it is sprayed with a developer composed of a 1:5 mixture of 0.04% aqueous solution of bromocresol red and alcoholic solution of formaldehyde adjusted to pH 5.0. The sheet is left for 2 to 3 minutes in an atmosphere saturated with 3% ammonia. Fatty acids occur as bright yellow spots on a purple background.

Free Fatty Acid Determination (Trout et al., 1960):

Reagents

1. Titration mixture consists of a Nile Blue solution extracted with heptane and diluted 1:10 with absolute methyl alcohol. The extraction is conducted by adding successive volumes of heptane to 0.02% aqueous solution to Nile Blue, and conducting the extraction in a separatory funnel until the heptane is colorless.

2. Extraction mixture: redistilled heptane (100 parts), redistilled isopropyl alcohol (400 parts), 1 *N* sulfuric acid (10 parts).

3. O.018 *N* sulfuric acid.

4. 0.02 *N* sodium hydroxide.

To 2 ml of sample containing fatty acids in a glass-stopper test tube, add, with shaking, 10 ml of the extraction mixture, followed by 6 ml of redistilled heptane and 4 ml of distilled water. Shake the mixture for 2 minutes. Collect the upper layer and shake it with an equal volume of 0.018 *N* sulfuric acid. Centrifuge the content at about 300 × *g* for 5 to 10 minutes. Collect 3 ml of the upper heptane layer and add it to 1 ml of the titration mixture. Titrate free fatty acids with 0.02 *N* sodium hydroxide while the sample is being agitated with a stream of nitrogen.

Standards consisting of 0.5 micromole of recrystallized higher fatty acids per milliter of heptane and blanks are subjected to the same treatment after being washed with the 0.05% sulfuric acid before titration.

Triglyceride Determination (Van Handel, 1961):

Reagents

1. Chloroform, redistilled.

2. 95% ethanol, redistilled.

3. 0.07 *N* (0.4%) alcoholic solution of potassium hydroxide. The stock solution consists of 2 g of potassium hydroxide dissolved in 5 ml of distilled water and diluted to 100 ml with absolute ethyl alcohol. The stock solution should be diluted 1:5 with redistilled 95% ethyl alcohol for the test.

4. 0.2 *N* sulfuric acid.

5. 0.02 *M* (0.5%) sodium metaperiodate.

6. 5% sodium disulfite.

7. Chromotropic acid, prepared as follows: add 30 ml of cold distilled water to 600 ml of concentrated sulfuric acid. Dissolve 2 g of chromotropic acid in 200 ml of distilled water and filter it through Whatman No. 1 filter paper into a brown bottle. Add the sulfuric acid solution to the chromotropic acid solution.

8. Standard triglyceride solution consisting of a purified triglyceride (0.5 to 0.1 mg/ml of redistilled chloroform). This stock solution should be diluted as required with redistilled chloroform, usually to obtain final concentration of triglyceride of 0.03 mg/ml.

9. Silicic acid, 100 to 200 mesh (Clarkson Chemical Co., Williamsport, Pa.).

Extract lipids by adding the lipid source (1 ml) to a chloroform:methyl alcohol (2:1) mixture, 20 volumes. Agitate the mixture for a short while and centrifuge it. Collect the chloroform-methanol layer and evaporate it to dryness under nitrogen or in a vacuum oven at 40°.

Glycerides may be separated from phosphatides by extraction with a solution containing 2 g of silicic acid per 5 ml of chloroform, added to the dried sample. Agitate the mixture and then add 20 ml of chloroform. Filter the content through a shark skin filter paper. Remove chloroform in a vacuum oven or by heating the content of the tube in a boiling water bath.

Saponify the material containing triglyceride by adding 0.5 ml of alcoholic potassium hydroxide solution and heating the mixture at 60 to 70° for 20 minutes. Add 0.5 ml of 0.2 *N* sulfuric acid and heat the tubes for 10 to 12 minutes in a boiling water bath, until the smell of alcohol has disappeared.

Oxydate the triglycerides by adding 0.05 ml of 0.025 *N* periodate solution per tube. Shake the tubes for 10 minutes and add 0.05 ml of 5% bisulfite solution or 0.5 *M* sodium arsenite. Shake the contents and allow to stand for 10 minutes. Add 5 ml of chromotropic acid. Centrifuge until clear and heat the mixture at 100° to 105° for 30 minutes in the absence of light. Read optical density at 570 nm.

The standards contain chloroform solutions of purified triglyceride standard preparations, to be treated in the same manner as the samples. The blank contains chloroform alone.

The Gas Chromatography of Lipids (Jamieson and Reid, 1965). The quantitative determination of fatty acids by the gas-liquid chromatography is preceded by the conversion of fatty acids to the corresponding methyl esters. The methyl esters may be prepared either by a transesterification procedure or by esterification (saponification) procedure.

The transesterification method is as follows: A mixture of a lipid preparation (1 g) and 0.2 M sodium methoxide in methanol (1.6 ml) is heated under reflux for 40 minutes. The mixture is then cooled and acidified with 2 N sulfuric acid, and the resulting mixture is added into an equal volume of cold, saturated sodium chloride solution. The methyl esters thus produced are extracted with 3 × 10 ml portions of light petrol (b.d. 40–60°) and the extracts are washed with small portions of ice-cold water until the washings become neutral. The light petrol extract is dried over anhydrose sodium sulfate for 30 minutes and after filtration the bulk of the light petrol is removed by distillation.

Here is a description of the esterification (saponification) procedure: a mixture of the lipid (1 g) and 7.8% potassium hydroxide in 95% ethanol (5.0 ml) is heated under reflux for 3 hours. The resulting solution is poured into an equal volume of cold water, and the unsaponifiable material is removed by extraction with ether. The aqueous layer, containing potassium salts of the fatty acids is acidified with 2 N sulfuric acid. Free fatty acids are extracted with 3 to 10 ml portions of diethyl ether. The extracts are dried for 30 minutes over anhydrous sodium sulfate and the ether is removed by distillation. The fatty acids are esterified by heating under reflux for 4 hours with 550 ml methanol containing 1% sulfuric acid. The resulting solution is added to an equal volume of distilled water and the methyl esters are extracted with three 10-ml portions of diethyl ether. The ether extracts are washed with an aqueous sodium bicarbonate solution and finally with distilled water. The ether extract may be dried for 30 minutes over anhydrous sodium sulfate and after filtration the ether is removed by distillation.

Gas-Liquid Chromatography Technique. The methyl esters of fatty acids are separated on a gas chromatograph (Perkin Elmer 800) with a dual flame ionization detector or on an Argon Chromatograph with strontium-90 ionization detector. When the first chromatograph is used, stainless steel columns (6 ft × $\frac{1}{8}$ in.) are packed with butanediol succinate on HMDS Chromosorb W (80–100 mesh) (8:92, w/w). The temperature is programmed to the desired temperature, ranging from 180 to 210° at a rate of 3.3°/minute. The flash heater temperature is set at 300° and the flow rate of nitrogen is set at 30 ml/minute. Samples are injected onto the chromatography column by means of a Hamilton microsyringe.

The areas under the peaks found on the graph automatically recorded are obtained by multiplying the peak height by the width of $\frac{1}{2}$ peak height and the percentage areas are determined by the internal normalization technique (Scott and Grant, 1964).

The Plackett's et al. (1969) technique of gas-liquid chromatography employs glass columns (5 ft × $\frac{1}{4}$ in. o.d.) tacked with 15% ethylene glycol

succinate or 2% silicone gum on Diatoport S, or 3% cyanoethyl silicone on
Gas Chrom Q (Applied Science Laboratories, State College, Pa.). Methyl
esters of fatty acids are chromatographed on the ethylene glycol succinate
columns and silicone gum columns are 185° or 203° or on the cyanoethyl
silicone columns at 180°.

The gas chromatography equipment consists of a gas chromatograph
equipped with a flame detector, linear temperature program, automatic at-
tenuator and a 1-mV recorder. Chromatograms are recorded from the columns in the presence and in the absence of normal methyl esters of fatty
acids internal standards. Equivalent chain lengths of the unknown fatty
acids are measured relative to the internal standard according to Miwa's
(1963) method. Quantitative determinations of fatty acids are made by the
estimation of peak areas from the product of height and width at $\frac{1}{2}$ height.
All the values are normalized to 100%.

The Gas Chromatography of Fatty Acids. According to Moss and
Lewis' (1967) technique, the methyl esters of fatty acids are prepared as
follows: fatty acids are first extracted by direct saponification of the fatty
acid source under nitrogen with 15% potassium hydroxide in 50% methanol, for 4 hours at 70°. Nonsaponifiable material is extracted in an 1:1
ether and hexane mixture, and discarded. The aqueous layer is acidified to
pH 2 with concentrated hydrochloric acid, and the fatty acids are extracted with 3 portions of the ether-hexane mixture. The extracts are then
evaporated at room temperature under a gentle stream of nitrogen. The residue is mixed with 2 ml of Boron-Trichloride-Methanol Reagent (Applied
Science Lab., State College, Pa.). The mixture is heated at 80° for 5 minutes, cooled and transferred to a separatory funnel containing 30 ml of the
ether-hexane mixture and 30 ml of distilled water. After shaking the mixture, the ether-hexane layer is collected and evaporated to dryness under a
ready for the injection into columns. For the gas-liquid chromatography, a
Barber-Colman (Model 5000) Gas Chromatograph, equipped with a
hydrogen flame ionization detector and a disk integrator recorder, is employed. The following parameters are pertinent for the procedure: injection
temperature, 220°; texture temperature, 230°. Column temperature is set
initially at 110° for 5 minutes and is then programmed to 195° at 5°/min-
ute. The carrier gas is nitrogen.

U-tube glass columns are used, packed with a polar phase, represented
by 12% ethylene-glycol adipate on Chromosorb P (80-100 mesh) or on
the nonpolar phase composed of 2% SE methyl silicone rubber gum (SE
30) coated on Chromosorb P. Three to 5 μl of the methyl esters may be
analyzed for 60 minutes after the injection of the material to the columns.
Peaks of the fatty-acid methyl esters are identified by comparison of reten-
sion times on the columns with those of highly purified methyl ester stand-

ards (Applied Science Laboratories, National Institute of Health). Peak areas are determined from the disk integrator data. The percentage of each fatty acid is calculated from the ratio of the area of its peak to the total area of all peaks.

The Gas Chromatography of High-Molecular-Weight Fatty Acids. A dual column chromatography apparatus equipped with a flame ionization and strontium-90 detectors is used for the chromatography method described by Wilson et al. (1966). The stationary phase in the column is 40–50 mesh Anachrome-ABS. The liquid phase is 1% SE 30. The carrier gas is nitrogen, flowing at a pressure of 12/psi and at the flow rate of 136 ml/minute. The temperature of the flash heater is set at 175°, and the temperature of the detector is 250°. The fatty acid methyl esters are dissolved or solubilized in hexane and are injected into the columns by Hamilton 1-μl microsyringes.

The quantitative measurement of a large number of fatty acid methyl esters is determined very precisely by the method of relative molar response. The relative molar response of a particular substance is defined as the peak area obtained for 1 mole of an unknown expressed relatively to the peak area of 1 mole of a standard. The relative molar response is plotted against the carbon number. The peak areas for each of the fatty acid methyl esters is converted to relative peak areas. The areas under the curves and the relative molar response are calculated and compared to the theoretical relative molar response of standard fatty acid methyl esters. The actual molar response is the area under the curves in arbitrary units obtained with the integrator.

Chemical characterization of the lipid fractions can be completed by the determination of the iodine, acid, saponification, and acetyl figures, the estimation of percentages of cholesterol (Schoenheimer and Sperry, 1934), phospholipids, cerebrosides (Brand and Sperry, 1941), and free fatty acids, and by the isolation of individual fatty acids on chromatographic columns (Hoffmann et al., 1955), or by fractional crystallization at low temperature (Brown and Kolb, 1955). It may also involve the determination of chemical formula and molecular weight after Gubariev and Pustovalov (1956) or Geiger and Anderson (1939). However, the latter investigations are rather beyond the scope of immunochemical analysis as they require considerable amounts of material.

2. Chemical Analysis of Polysaccharides

The chemical study of polysaccharides should include the determination of total nitrogen content and carbohydrate (by Dubois et al., 1956 or by the thymolsulfuric acid reaction of Shetlar and Master, 1957), and the chromatographic identification of monosaccharides. These assays may be extended by the chemical determination of reducing sugars (Nelson, 1944;

Park and Johnson, 1949), glucose (Marks, 1959), ketoses (Lunt and Sutcliffe, 1953, or Dische and Borenfreund, 1951), heptose [Osborn's (1963) modification of Dische's (1953) method], pentoses (Mejbaum, 1939; Dische and Schwartz, 1937), deoxypentoses (DeDeken-Grenson and DeDeken, 1959; Burton, 1956), methylpentose (Dische and Shettles, 1948; Rondle and Morgan, 1955), hexosamine (Ludowieg and Benman, 1967; Belcher et al., 1954; Tracey, 1952; Johansen et al., 1960), lactose (Malpress and Morrison, 1949), tyvclose and abequose (Westphal et al., 1954), o-acetyl groups (Hestrin, 1949), N-acetylhexosamine (Reissig et al., 1955), total acetyl groups (Ludowieg and Dorfman, 1960), uronic acids [Kuhn's (1958) modification of Dische's (1950) method], 6-deoxyhexoses and hexoses (Heyns and Mueller, 1965), 2-keto-deoxyoctonate (Aminoff, 1961), acetylneuraminic acid or sialic acid (Warren, 1959), polyols (Frahn and Mills, 1959), and sucrose (Raybin, 1937). Glucose and galactose may be determined with Glucostat and Galactostat reagents (Worthington Biochemical Corp.). More detailed studies of the chemical structure of isolated sugars, according to the methods of Anderson and Crighton (1939), or Gubariev and Lubenec (1951), are beyond the scope of immunochemical analysis of microorganisms. Terminal saccharides in the polysaccharide determinants can be accurately estimated by the technique of Staub et al. (1959).

The nitrogen determination is carried out either by the micro-Kjeldahl method, as modified by Elek and Sobotka (1926), Markham (1942), or Bathurst and Mitchell (1958), or by Rommers and Visser's (1969) spectrophotometric technique.

The sugar contents can be determined either by one or more of the following techniques: Morris' (1948) anthrone method, modified by Trevelyan and Harrison (1950) and by Fairbain (1953); the reducing technique of Johnston (1965); the phenol technique of Dubois et al. (1956) or Borel et al. (1952). The modified Morris method, the Park and Johnson submicro method, and Dubois et al. technique are recommended. The Morris anthrone method is more specific for sugars than the reducing assays, and it does not require hydrolyzation of materials prior to the test. The Park and Johnson submicro technique is a very sensitive assay which allows the detection of as little as 0.5 μg of reducing sugars. The reduction methods are not applicable for fractions other than those containing pure or almost pure carbohydrates. If the yield of a polysaccharide fraction is low or if the bulk of the material is to be reserved for serological studies, the minimum of qualitative tests should include the α-naphthol reaction (Dische, 1955) and the paper chromatography of sugars.

Muramic acid may be separated from hexosamines on charcoal-celite columns (Perkins and Rogers, 1959). Other individual saccharides may be separated and identified by electrophoretic or chromatographic methods, or by a combination of these two methods. Although the electrophoresis is generally a more rapid and efficient method, it has no particular advantage over chromatography in case of saccharides due to the relative electric inertness of the saccharide molecules. Only if complexed with borate ions, saccharides display sufficient electric charges.

The high-voltage electrophoresis of neutral sugars is conducted by Mabry's et al. (1965) method. Amino sugars tend to show trailing on the electrophoresis, which may be eliminated by converting them to neutral sugars by ninhydrin oxidation (Stoffyn and Jeanloz, 1954). Sugars, to be separated by the electrophoresis, are hydrolyzed with 3 N HCl at 103° for 1 hour, dried over phosphorus pentoxide in a vacuum and dissolved in distilled water (Ullmann and Cameron, 1969). Salts are removed with Dowex 50 (H+ form), added to the solution of sugars (or amino acids) until the pH of the mixture has become almost neutral. The mixture is then filtered, and the resins are washed on the filter with distilled water. The filtrate is dried in vacuo over phosphorus pentoxide.

The sugar finger-printing technique (Ingram, 1958) is a combination of paper electrophoresis and chromatography. In this method, acid hydrolyzates or lysozyme-digests containing sugars are applied to Whatman 3 MM paper which has moistened with a volatile buffer consisting of pyridine, glacial acetic acid and distilled water (10:0.4:90). The electrophoresis is conducted at pH 6.4 for 2 hours at 14 V/cm after which the paper is dried and is subjected to ascending chromatography in a solvent consisting of *n*-butanol, glacial acetic acid, and distilled water (3:1:1) overnight. The fingerprints are dried at room temperature and sprayed with a suitable sugar-detecting reagent and left at 35° until colors develop fully.

Acid hydrolysis of a sugar-containing material may be attained by suspending a sample in 12 N HCl and leaving it at 4° for 6 days or at 37° for 1 to 2 days.

Electrophoresis of Glycoproteins (Arai and Wallace, 1969). The electrolyte solution used for electrophoresis on cellulose-acetate membrane is provided by a barbital buffer (0.075 M, pH 8.6), prepared by dissolving 2.786 g diethyl barbituric acid and 15.40 g sodium diethyl barbiturate in 1 liter of deionized distilled water. Electrophoresis is conducted for 20 minutes at 250 V. After the electrophoresis, the membrane is placed in 95% ethyl alcohol for 5 minutes, and then transferred to 0.8% periodic acid for about 10 minutes. The membrane is washed in distilled water for 1 minute and rewashed in another aliquot of distilled water for 2 minutes. The membrane is then stained for 15 minutes in Schiff's solution. The Schiff solution is obtained by dissolving 6 g of basic fuchsin in 1200 ml of distilled water at 90°, filtering and adding 30 ml of 2 N HCl, 4 g of potassium metabisulfate, and 3 g of powdered, activated animal charcoal; the mixture is shaken, filtered, and supplemented with 40 ml of 2 N HCl. The membrane is stained with Schiff's reagent, placed in a 0.5% potassium metabisulfate solution in 0.1 N HCl for 3 minutes and then soaked for 5 minutes in 0.01 N HCl. The membrane is finally washed in absolute alcohol for 2 minutes and placed in a 0.1% trichloracetic acid-methanol solution for 30 seconds.

The chromatographic identification of monosaccharides and related substances can be satisfactorily performed by employing two different types of assays. The first type, which elicits a range of color reactions given by various sugars, is represented by the Partridge (1949), Jermyn and Isherwood (1949), Cummins and Harris (1956), Salton and Marshall (1959), and Kwapinski (1959, 1960) techniques. Glucosamine and inositol, which cannot be detected by these assays, may be revealed by a reducing chromatographic technique, for example, the method of Trevelyan et al. (1950) or Gillissen et al. (1955). Other useful chromatographic methods were published by Bacon and Edelman (1951), Aronoff (1956), and Gordon et al. (1956). The following chromatographic technique has been used by Kwapinski's research group: 5- to 20-mg samples of material suspended in 1 to 2 ml of 1.5 N sulfuric acid are hydrolyzed for 3 to 5 hours at 100°. Ion-exchange resin hydrolyzates prepared by means of Dowex 50 (X_4:H$^+$ form) of 200 to 400 mesh are equally or more suitable. The hydrolyzate is adjusted to approximately pH 4.5, using barium hydroxide or barium carbonate. The resulting sediment is discarded by centrifugation, and 0.01- to 0.1-ml amounts of the hydrolyzate and of 0.1% sugar standards are placed in duplicate on Whatman filter paper No. 2 or No. 4, or preferably on the glass plates coated with MN 300 cellulose blended in a 1:24 mixture of alcohol and water (Kwapinski et al., 1971). Alternatively, the plates are coated with Kieselguhr G (Merck), one part, blended for 1 minute with 0.02 M sodium acetate (three parts) and spread at a thickness of 0.5 mm. The plates are dried at room temperature for 24 hours (Bell and Talukder, 1970). The paper chromatograms are run descending for 12 to 24 hours, whereas the TL chromatograms are developed for 4 hours, in a solvent composed of primary n-butyl alcohol, 98% ethyl alcohol, glacial acetic acid, and distilled water mixed in the ratio of 10:5:2:1, or in a solvent consisting of pyridine, ethyl acetate and distilled water (3:5:5). One chromatogram is immersed for 1 to 2 seconds in a 4% acetone solution of silver nitrate, and dried for approximately 5 minutes at 105°, then dipped for 30 seconds in a 0.5 to 1.0 N alcohol solution of sodium or potassium hydroxide. The excess of silver oxide is finally removed by immersing the

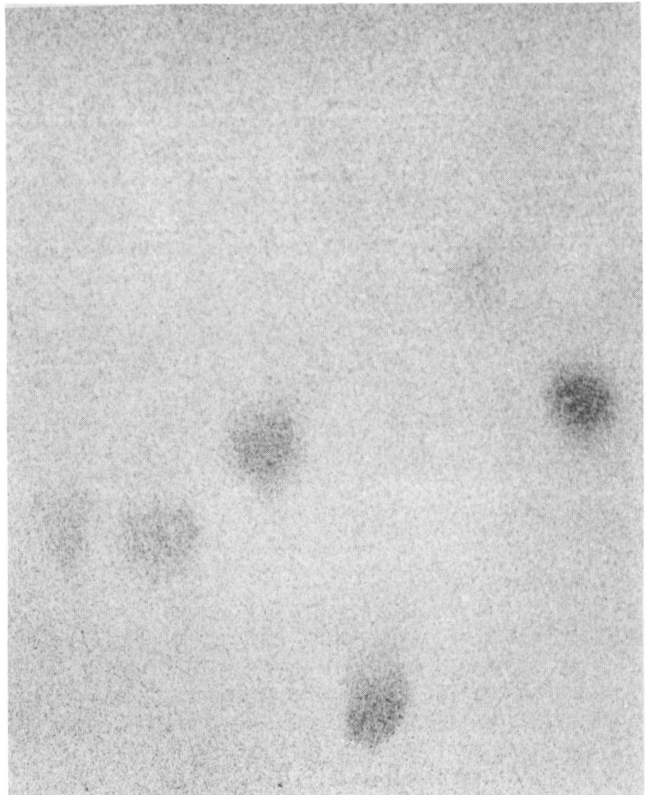

Figure 34.   Saccharides separated by Kwapinski's method of the thin-layer chromatography (left to right: xylose, rhamnose, glucosamine, arabinose, glucose, and galactose).

sheet for 2 to 3 minutes in 6 N ammonia and rinsing it in tap water for 30 minutes. Saccharides are identified by the determination of the Rf or RF_R values as compared with those of the appropriate standards (Fig. 34).

$$Rf_R = \frac{Rf \text{ of examined saccharide}}{Rf \text{ of rhamnose}} \times 100$$

The other chromatogram may be simultaneously developed with an aniline-oxalic acid detector (se below) or run in a second solvent (the two-dimensional chromatography). In the latter case, the paper or the coated glass plates are turned by 90° and run for 2 to 4 hours in Kwapinski and Snyder's (1961) solvent consisting of propylene glycol, acetone, ethyl alcohol, and distilled water (6.5:50:23.5:20), or in a mixture of pyridine, n-butyl alcohol, and distilled water in the proportion of 3:7:2. A satisfactory separation of monosaccharides can also be obtained in the Jermyn and Isherwood (1949) solvent, as modified by Torheim (1963). It consists of ethyl acetate, pyridine, and distilled water (5:2:5). Another useful solvent for TL chromatography of sugars contains ethyl acetate, propan-2-ol and water in the ratio of 8:2:1 (Stahl and Kaltenbach, 1961). The chromatograms are then air dried and sprayed with a solution of equal parts of 2.5% oxalic acid and 1.0% alcoholic solution of aniline. Alternatively, a saturated aqueous solution of aniline oxalate can be used (Torheim, 1963). After drying the chromatograms for 10 to 15 minutes at 100 to 105°, colors and locations of monosaccharide spots are recorded and compared with a map of standards. Color of hexose is brown, of pentoses pink, and of rhamnose yellow. Pentoses can also be distinguished from other monosaccharides with the orcinol-$FeCl_3$ reagent (Rosenberg and Zamenhof, 1961). Other useful saccharide detectors are benzidine-acetate (Aronoff, 1956) and a 4:1 mixture of 1% alcohol solution of cadmium chloride and 1% alcoholic solution of aniline (Kwapinski, 1965), and a reagent consisting of 4-aminobenzoic acid (2 g), 3-carboxy-4-hydroxybenzenesulfonic acid (3 g), and stannous chloride (1 g) in 100 ml of 80% aqueous acetic acid (Bell and Talukder, 1970. The chromatograms (filter paper or plates) sprayed with the reagent are heated at 100° for 15 minutes. Pentose give cerise color; aldohexoses brown-yellow; hexuloses yellow; 6-oleoxyaldohexoses yellow or yellow-pink.

Stable color of sugars is produced by Pridham's (1956) reagent, consisting of 4-methoxyaniline (*p*-anisidine) hydrochloride (1 g) dissolved in MeOH (5 ml) containing sodium dithionite (100 mg) and butan-1-ol (95 ml). The sprayed chromatograms are heated at 130° for 15 minutes. All classes of sugar show brownish color on Kieselguhr-coated plates, but selective colors are found on paper chromatograms.

Preliminary identification of monosaccharides and related substances by these chromatographic techniques may be supplemented by certain additional tests. Glucose can be differentiated from galactose by a glucosidase test (Roth et al., 1965), or by employing the specific oxidases (Glucostat and Galactostat, Worthington Bioch. Co., Freeholt, N.J.). Heptoses are detected after periodate oxidation as formaldehyde (Jones et al., 1963), and ketoheptoses (sialic acid) are detected by Klevstrand and Nordal's (1950) reagent. Hexosamines may be detected with ninhydrin or by the more specific reagents such as acetylacetone-*p*-dimethylaminobenzaldehyde or sulfamate (Payne and Kieber, 1954; Williamson and Zamenhof, 1963). Ninhydrin is only applied if no amino acids are present in the hydrolyzate. The chromatogram is sprayed with 0.15% solution of ninhydrin in acetone, ethyl alcohol, or *n*-butyl alcohol saturated with water and heated at 100°. A purple color of the amino groups is shown. According to Payne and

Kieber's method, the chromatogram is first sprayed with a mixture consisting of 10 ml of 1% acetyloacetone in *n*-butyl alcohol and 0.5 ml of an alcoholic solution of potassium hydroxide (made of 5 ml of 50% KOH and 20 ml of ethyl alcohol), dried for 5 minutes at 105°, sprayed with Ehrlich's reagent, and heated for 5 minutes at 90°. Hexosamines occur as cherry-red colored spots. (Ehrlich's reagent consists of 1 g of *p*-dimethylamino-benzaldehyde, 30 ml of ethyl alcohol, and 30 ml of concentrated hydrochloric acid.) Hexosamines can also be detected with Warren's (1960) thiobarbiturate reagent, but the most sensitive reagent for the identification of hexosamines and hexosamine-uronic acids is the indole reagent (Williamson and Zamenhof, 1963).

A sample examined for the presence of hexosamines and hexosamine-uronic acids is first wetted with a 1:1 mixture of 5% sodium nitrate and 33% acetic acid, left for 10 minutes, dried, and sprayed with a reagent consisting of 1% indole in 95% ethanol containing 5% HCl. The paper is then heated at 100° for 1 minute. The anhydro sugars appear as orange-yellow spots.

To detect 2-amino-2-deoxy sugars, the chromatogram is first wetted with a 1:1 mixture of 5% sodium nitrate solution and 33% acetic acid for 1 to 2 minutes and dried at 100°. The paper is then sprayed with 12% ammonium sulfamate, wetting it completely, and dried at 100°. Finally, the chromatogram is sprayed with 1% ethanolic solution of indole containing 5% HCl and heated at 100° for 1 minute or at 80° for 2 minutes. The 2-amino-2-deoxy sugars produce bright orange-yellow spots on a pale pink ground. Glucosamine may be distinguished from galactosamine by a procedure devised by Stoffyn and Jeanloz (1954) or Hornung (1963). Muramic acid is identified by Strange's (1956) technique, polyhydric alcohols by the method of Bradfield and Flood (1950), or Hackman and Trikojust (1952). Deoxy sugars are detected with the following reagents (Warren, 1960): (a) 0.5 *M* sodium periodate in 0.05 *N* sulfuric acid, (b) ethylene glycol, acetone, concentrated sulfuric acid (50:50:3), and (c) 6% aqueous solution of sodium-2 thiobarbiturate. The chromatogram is sprayed successively with the reagent a and left for 15 minutes, the reagent b for 10 minutes, and reagent c for 5 minutes at 100°. Red spots of deoxy sugars give red fluorescence if viewed in ultraviolet light.

N-acetylamino sugars are detected by Salton's (1959) modification of Partridge's (1948) method. Salton's reagent is less susceptible to heating with alkali, presence of salts and concentration of hydrochloric acid, and it is capable of detecting as little as 1 *μ*g of *N*-acetylglucosamine or *N*-acetyl-galactosamine. The reagent consists of a mixture of 10 ml 2% solution of *p*-dimethyl-amino-benzaldehyde in glacial acetic acid, 30 ml *n*-butanol and 0.4 ml concentrated hydrochloric acid. The ethanol-borate mixture consists of equal volumes of 95% ethanol and 0.05 M sodium borate. The chromatogram of sugars containing N-acetylaminohexoses is first sprayed with the ethanol-borate mixture to moisten the papers fully, steamed for 10 minutes in a steam oven, and sprayed with the p-dimethyl-amino-benzaldehyde reagent. A purple color is indicative of acetylhexoses.

Ketoses (fructose or sorbose) may be detected with a mixture consisting of equal parts of 0.3% alcoholic solution of naphtoresorcin and 2% trichloracetic acid. When the mixture is dried for 5 minutes at 105°, red spots of ketoses appear. Fructose is distinguished from sorbose by comparing the Rf values with the respective standards. Aldopentose may be detected with p-anisidine hydrochloride, aniline phthalate, and phloroglucinol-acetic acid (Hough, 1950).

Hexuronic acids, which show a dark blue color, may be detected with the same reagent by drying at room temperature. More sensitive chromatographic methods for uronic acids were published by Horrocks (1949), Gee and McCready (1957), and Corden (1964). According to Young and Corden's (1964) method, galacturonic acids are identified by an ascending solvent-colorization system provided these compounds are not accompanied by other acids. By this procedure, different uronic acids are satisfactorily separated and localized in a single operation. The solvent-indicator system consists of 50 mg bromophenol blue and 60 mg of sodium formate dissolved in 77% ethanol-88% formic acid (85:15, v/v). The chromatogram (on Whatman No. 4 paper) is developed for about 8 hours, or until the solvent front has risen to about 30 cm from the origin, and the paper is hung in a fume hood to dry, for about 1 to $1\frac{1}{2}$ hours.

The wet chromatograms are initially yellow, but the background turns bright blue within an hour, whereas the spots of galacturonic acids remain yellow. N-acetylneuraminic acid and derivatives can be chromatographically separated and stained according to the procedure by Barry et al. (1963) or by Warren (1960).

The quantitative paper chromatography of saccharides is conducted in the following manner: a chromatogram is first set and developed in a usual manner, then dried. The chromatogram sheet is then divided into longitudinal strips, 4 cm wide, and cut in two. One strip should be sprayed with a saccharide reagent to locate positions of individual saccharides. The parallel strip is cut accordingly to yield pieces containing separate monosaccharides. These should be eluted with 5 ml of distilled water coming from a separatory funnel. Eluates are examined for amount of saccharides by an appropriate chemical test.

Gas Chromatography of Sugars. Sugars to be used for a gas chromatography analysis must be converted into trimethylsilyl derivatives by the following technique (Brooks et al., 1970): the cells serving as source of carbohydrates are suspended in formamide (1 ml), and the mixture is heated in an oil bath at 165° for 20 minutes, and then cooled. To this mixture, an acid ethanol (0.1 N HCl in 90% ethanol) is added (2.5 ml), and the mixture is centrifuged in the cold at 3000 × g for 20 minutes. The supernatant is collected and precipitated with acetone (5 ml). The precipitate formed at 4° is collected by centrifugation and dissolved in a solution containing 1.66 ml of 0.3 M ammonium acetate and 0.23 ml of concentrated HCl. The mixture is sealed in a screw-cap tube and hydrolyzed in a boiling water bath for 3 hours, and cooled and dried in a vacuum rotator at 40°. The sugar preparation is then dissolved in pyridine, and the trimethylsilyl (TMS) derivatives of sugars are prepared according to Farshtchi and Moss' (1969) method.

The Gas-Liquid Chromatography Analysis. The 5 μl of the hexane of solution TMS derivatives is injected into a gas chromatograph, equipped with flame ionization detectors and dual glass columns (0.3-cm i. d. by 7.3 m in length). The columns are packed with Chromosorb W (AW-DMCS, HP) and coated with 3% OV-1. The instrument is temperature programmed immediately after the injection of a sample from 80 to 265° at a linear increase of 5°/minute. The detector temperature is 290°; the injector inlet temperature, 250°; the electrometer attenuation, 10^2; and helium flow, 38 ml/minute. A recorder input signal of 1 mV is used with a chart speed of 30 in./hr. Identification of saccharides is made by comparing the retention time of known sugars with those of unknown compounds. Rhamnose should be identified more precisely on a polar column (0.3-cm i. d. by 4.9-m length) packed with tetracyanoethylated pentaerythritol on Varaport 30 100/120 mesh at 120° with nitrogen as the carrier gas at the rate of 38 ml/minute.

An alternative gas chromatography technique for the analysis of sugars, according to Adams et al. (1969), is applied as follows: the sugar preparations are first hydrolyzed in sealed glass tubes in 1 N sulfuric acid at 100% for 12 hours. The hydrolyzate is neutralized with barium carbonate following which the monoses are reduced with sodium borohydride to their corresponding alditols which are subsequently acetylated (Albershcim et al., 1967). The acetylated alditols are placed on straight glass columns (120 × 0.5-cm i. d.), packed either with 10% w/w neopentyl glycol sebacate polyester on 80–100 mesh Chromosorb W, or with 9.5% ECNSS-M on 100–120 mesh Chromosorb Q (Applied Science Laboratories). The analysis in a Pye Argon Chromatograph fitted with a strontium 90 ionization detector is conducted at 204° with the first column or 190° with the second column. The relative proportions of individual sugars are calculated from the areas under the corresponding peaks.

3. Chemical Analysis of Proteins

Proteins are characterized by the determination of the nitrogen, phosphorus, and by the identification of composing peptides and amino acids.

Chemical investigations may be extended by the titration of amino acids and imino acids (Troll and Cannan, 1953; Housewright and Thorne, 1950) and the determination of carboxyl groups (Ellenbogen and Brand, 1955). The isolation of individual amino acids on the chromatographic columns (Moore and Stein, 1951) and the study of their optical configurations (Galajev, 1955), and the estimation of molecular weights are reserved for more advanced immunochemical investigations. The molecular weight of proteins may be determined in a relatively simple way by gel-filtration on a Sephadex G-200 column at 25° and 40° (Leach and O'Shea, 1965).

Total nitrogen content is usually determined either by Kjeldahl's (1883) method as modified by Elek and Sobotka (1926), Markham (1942), or Bathurst and Mitchell (1958), or by the spectrophotometric technique of Rommers and Visser (1969); α-amino nitrogen can be estimated according to Sobel et al. (1945). Total and protein nitrogen should be determined separately in the nucleoprotein fractions. In these cases, the total nitrogen is first estimated; then the protein is separated by precipitation with phosphotungstic acid or trichloracetic acid, and the remaining nonprotein nitrogen is determined. Protein nitrogen is calculated from the difference between the total and nonprotein nitrogen.

Contents of the protein can be determined by one of the colorimetric techniques, for example, the Folin and Ciocalteu (1927) assay; Weichselbaum's (1946) Biuret method, modified by Ditterbrandt (1948), Robinson and Hogden (1940), or Lowry et al. (1951); the xanthoprotein technique (Machaboeuf et al. 1947), the ninhydrin method (Kunkel and Ward, 1950), and the measurement of ultraviolet absorption spectra. Selection of the most adequate procedure in each case depends greatly on the amino acids occurring in the material studied.

Identification of Peptides by Electrophoresis. To determine the peptides composing a protein molecule, the peptides must first be released by trypsin, chemotrypsin, pepsin, or papain digestion, and then separated and identified. The most efficient technique for peptide separation is a combination of high-voltage electrophoresis and chromatography.

Trypsin Digestion. To yield peptides, most, but not all, native proteins must be denatured prior to the digestion in the following way: the protein is dissolved at 4 to 10% concentration in 6- to 10-M urea, and the solution is diluted to a 2.8-M urea concentration, at which trypsin and chemotrypsin are fully active. A 0.2- to 0.3 M, pH 8.3 to 8.4 ammonium bicarbonate buffer is satisfactory for trypsin and chemotrypsin digestion; the pH can be readjusted during the digestion with ammonium hydroxide, read against a phenol red indicator. Trypsin digestion is conducted by adding twice recrystallized trypsin to the diluted protein at the 2% final concentration and incubating the digestion mixture in a shaker at 25 to 35° for 24 to 48 hours or until no insoluble material is visible. At the end of the digestion, the urea can be removed by absorbing the peptides in a small column of Dowex 50-2X 100 mesh, in the hydrogen form. The peptides are eluted with 4M ammonia. The final mixture of peptides must be free of salts to secure satisfactory separation of peptides. If the urea denaturation is to be omitted, the proteins should be dialyzed against 0.01 M, pH 8.3 to 8.4 ammonium bicarbonate for 8 hours at 4°, and then diluted to 1 to 2% concentration in 0.2 to 0.3 M, pH 8.4 ammonium bicarbonate (Meltzer et al., 1964).

Pepsin Digestion. Pepsin digestion is conducted as follows: pepsin dissolved in 0.1 M sodium acetate, pH 4.5 is added to a globulin preparation dissolved in the same buffer using 1 mg of enzyme to 50 mg protein. The mixture is incubated at 37° for 8 hours after which time the pH is adjusted to 8.0. The digestion products are precipitated three times in 18% sodium sulfate and the final precipitate is dissolved in a small amount of water and dialyzed against 0.15 M Tris-HCl, pH 7.2.

Papain Digestion. The protein to be digested is dissolved in 0.1 M sodium phosphate buffer, pH 7.0, containing 0.1 molar cysteine and 0.002 M ethylenediamine-tetraacetic acid. Papain is added in the ratio 1 mg/100 mg of protein to be digested. The digestion mixture is incubated at 37° for 16 hours and then dialyzed against 0.009 M K_2HPO_4, 0.001 M KH_2PO_4, pH 7.9 buffer. The digest is adjusted to a desired concentration and applied directly to the Whatman No. 3 or 3 MM filter paper, or to a TLC plate in the amount equivalent to 1 to 5 mg of peptide. For the quantitation, the digest may be lyophilized and weighed, and aliquots are dissolved in distilled water to contain 1 mg/0.02 ml.

Separation of peptides can be accomplished by: (a) a combination of paper chromatography and the high-voltage electrophoresis, (b) a combined thin-layer chromatography and the flat plate electrophoresis (Fig. 31), (c) a combined chromatography and flat plate electrophoresis on cellulose sheets.

Separation of Peptides by Combined Paper Chromatography and High-Voltage Paper Electrophoresis. The descending chromatography is set up in a solvent consisting of *n*-butanol-acetic acid-water (4:1:5), separated into two phases. The lower aqueous phase is used as a solvent. Chromatograms are run for 16 to 20 hours or more at room temperature. At the end of the chromatography time, the paper is dried at about 70° in a ventilated chromatographic drying oven. A line is drawn from the origin at the edge of the paper to the direction of chromatography marking the line of partially separated peptides. If the chromatography is combined with electrophoresis, the paper is dried in a stream of cool air.

The electrophoresis is carried out in a pH 3.7 buffer, consisting of pyridine, acetic acid, and water (1:10:289). The chromatogram is wetted with the buffer before being placed in an electrophoresis tank. The electrophoresis at 43° to 44° is run at 2000 to 3000 V and 75 to 150 mA. The filter paper is then removed, dried at 70°, and stained with a reagent suitable for peptides and specific amino acids. The following reagent is recommended: 0.5 g ninhydrin, 100 ml acetone, and 10 ml of a solution consisting of 1 g cadium carbonate, 20 ml acetic acid, and 80 ml distilled water. The paper is dipped in this liquid and incubated at room temperature over concentrated sulfuric acid, in a sealed container. Alternatively, the paper may be sprayed with 0.25% ninhydrin solution in acetone and dried overnight at room temperature.

Individual peptides are identified by matching the colored spots of peptides with a map of known, synthetic peptides or by identification of constituting amino acids in the eluates, obtained by soaking the corresponding area of the filter paper in distilled water and hydrolizing the material in 6 N HCl. Semiquantitative information may be obtained by the scanning of maps in a recording densitometer with a 500-nm interference filter, or in a Chromoscan fitted with the attachment for thin-layer chromatograph scanning. The maps may be photographed with a back-lighting such as provided by an x-ray view box, for records and comparison. A 500-nm interference filter greatly enhances the contrast of the photographs.

The order in the combined HV electrophoresis-chromatography may be reversed. According to Meltzer's et al. (1964) method, the HV electrophoresis of peptides is first run employing one of the following buffers, selected in accordance with the individual physicochemical properties of proteins and peptides: (a) a pH 6.4 buffer consisting of 10% pyridine, 0.4% acetic acid, and 89.6% water; (b) a pH 3.5 buffer consisting of 0.33% pyridine, 3.33% acetic acid, and 96.33% water; and (c) a pH 1.9 buffer consisting of 4.7% formic acid, 7.5% acetic acid, and 89.8% water.

The chromatography follows in a direction differing by 90° performed with the following solvent systems: (a) the upper layer of a mixture of 40% n-butanol, 10% acetic acid, and 50% water; and (b) 35.9% pyridine, 35.9% isoamyl alcohol, and 28.2% water (Wang and Fudenberg, 1969). The most recommended combination of buffer and chromatography solvent comprises the pH 3.5 buffer and the upper layer of the 4:1:5 mixture of butanol, acetic acid, and water.

The electrophoresis of amino acids is carried out in a pH 2.0 acetic acid: formic acid buffer (Smith, 1960), using hydrolyzates of proteins or peptides, made in 5 to 6 *N* HCl, heated at 100° for 12 to 18 hours. The amino acid spots are detected with a ninhydrin-collidine reagent.

Separation of Peptides by Combined TLC and Flat Plate Electrophoresis. The TLC chromatography is conducted for 1 to 2 hours in one of the following solvents which should be chosen according to the essential physicochemical characteristics of peptides: (a) neutral solvents: 96% ethanol-water (70:30), or *n*-propanol-water (70:30); (b) basic solvents: *n*-propanol-34% ammonium hydroxide (70:30), or chloroform-methanol-34% ammonium hydroxide (40:40:20); (c) acidic solvents: 96% ethanol-water-acetic acid (70:20:10), or *n*-propanol-water-acetic acid (70:20:10).

The flat plate electrophoresis is carried out in the second direction at 950 to 1000 V and 30 mA for 1 hour in a solvent consisting of pyridine-acetic-water (1:10:289). The plate is then dried at 100°, and the peptides are detected with a 0.5% ninhydrin in alcohol spray or with a chlorine-*o*-toluidine solution.

According to Ritchard's (1964) method, peptides are first separated on (Eastman) cellulose-sheets by the chromatography in a solvent consisting of 96% ethanol and water (70:30); 5 μl of a solution of methyl red in 60% aqueous ethanol are placed 1 in. from either side of one corner to trace the progress of chromatography. The chromatography is usually completed in 4 to 5 hours following which the electrophoresis is set up in a second direction, utilizing a solvent containing pyridine-glacial acetic acid and water (4:40:2000). The electrophoresis is run for 90 minutes in a flat plate system, at a constant voltage of 940 V, at −1°. The peptides are then detected upon spraying with a 0.5% ninhydrin solution in methanol, and drying at 100° for 1 to 4 minutes.

Arginine and tyrosine can be identified specifically by Acher and Crocker's (1952) method, histidine by Sanger and Tuppy's (1951) method, and proline by Atfield and Morris' (1961) technique.

Separation and Identification of Amino Acids. Amino acids composing the purified protein preparation are most readily separated and identified by the electrophoresis, gas-liquid partition chromatography, the column chromatography, paper chromatography, or by a combination of these methods. A very efficient, rapid, and relatively simple method for separation of most amino acids and dipeptides is the ion exchange paper electrophoresis (Selegny et al., 1970). Very good separation of amino acids is also achieved by the ion exchange resin column filtration (Hamilton, 1966), and particularly by Munier and Thommegay's (1967) combination of the thin-layer chromatography and high-voltage electrophoresis on cellulose-powder or on 3 MM filter paper.

The electrophoretic mobility (u) of an ion in an ion exchange paper/ buffer solution system may be expressed by the following equation which refers to the "limiting distribution coefficient":

$$u = \frac{k_1}{P^0 + k_2}$$

where k_1 and k_2 are characteristic constants which may be determined experimentally and the P^0 is porosity of the ion exchange paper. The Rf and (u) values are interrelated, as shown by the equation:

$$u = \frac{k_1}{(1/\mathrm{Rf}) + k_2}$$

The ion exchange paper electrophoresis may be employed alone or in a combination with chromatography. The charge on the amino acid molecule alters depending upon the pH of a medium employed. In this procedure, an exchange takes place between an amino acid molecule in solution and the counter-ion of the resin particle. The supporting medium consists of resin particles incorporated into a cellulose matrix. The following types of ion exchange papers are recommended: a strongly acid exchange paper SA-2 containing particles of the sulfonic type, Amberlite IR-120, and a weakly acid exchange paper WA-2 with particles of the carboxylic rating IRC-50. Ionization of carboxylic groups of amino acid molecules also undergoes modification by the pH and the ionic strength of a medium.

The electric current of 25 to 28 V/cm is applied for 4 to 6 hours in $M/$ 20 sodium citrate buffer, pH 2.3, using the WA-2 paper. Strongly charged papers produce small spots of amino acids, separated in a short time over relatively short migration distances.

Chromatographic analysis of proteins in terms of the composing amino acids can be performed by Dent's (1948) two-dimensional technique or its modifications, by Toenius and Kalb (1951), Williams and Synge (1951), Cummins and Harris (1956), Kwapinski and Snyder (1961), or Kwapinski (1964). It is convenient to set up a "circular chromatography" assay (Rao and Wadhwani, 1956) prior to the regular chromatography to obtain preliminary information of the number and types of amino acids. In the Cummins and Harris technique, chromatograms are prepared on Whatman no. 4 filter paper, and the solvents are a phenol-water (4:1) mixture in an atmosphere of ammonia and NaCN, and 2,6-lutidine:ethanolic-water: diethylamine (55:25:18:2) mixture.

Kwapinski's (1964) two-dimensional chromatographic technique is conducted as follows: 5- to 10-mg samples of a material are hydrolyzed in 5 N hydrochloric acid for 15 to 20 hours in an oven at 105 to 110°, preferably under a reduced pressure. The hydrolyzates are decolorized with active decolorizing charcoal (Norit NK) on a sintered glass disk washing the Norit with water, centrifuged, and either evaporated *in vacuo* or in a boiling water bath. Alternatively, hydrolyzates can be desalted on the ion exchange resin (Dowex 50 × 4, H$^+$ form). Amounts of hydrolyzates ranging from 0.01 to 0.1 ml are placed on a sheet of Whatman no. 2 or no. 1 filter paper. The chromatogram is first run for 16 to 24 hours in a solvent consisting of propylene glycol, acetone, ethyl alcohol, and distilled water (6:5:50:23.5: 20), then dried at 100°, turned by 90°, and developed for another 16 hours in a solving consisting of primary *n*-butanol, ethyl alcohol, acetic acid, and redistilled water (10:5:1:2). An even better separation of amino acids can be obtained by diluting the latter solvent 2:1 with a 20% aqueous phenol. The paper sheet is then dried and sprayed with, or immersed in, a 0.15% solution of ninhydrin (triketo-hydrindene hydrate) made in *n*-butanol saturated with water, in acetone, or ethyl alcohol, and heated for 3 to 5 minutes at 105°. The Rf or Rf$_L$ coefficients are calculated by comparison with standard amino acids run simultaneously. The Rf$_L$ coefficients are calculated according to the formula

$$\text{Rf}_L = \frac{\text{Rf of unknown amino acid}}{\text{Rf of a leucine standard}} \times 100$$

Amino acids can be easily differentiated by applying a polychrome stain technique (Barrollier et al., 1956). Relative molecular proportions of the amino acids can be estimated by the Salton and Marshall (1959) method as follows. Chromatograms are dipped into a 5% ninhydrin solution made in acetone and phosphate buffer, pH 9.5. Colors are eluted with a mixture of acetone and water (3:1 *v/v*) and the extinctions determined spectrophotometrically at a wavelength of 570 nm. Diaminopimelic acid is estimated by reading at 540 nm the optical density of an eluate in 70% alcohol prepared from a spot corresponding to DAP on a chromatogram.

Amino acids can also be located by the ultraviolet irradiation technique of Fowden (1951). The amino-acid spots located on the filter paper may be then eluted by Kornberg and Patey's technique (1957), and amounts of amino acids can be quantitatively determined by the Yenn and Cocking (1955) method.

The Gas Chromatography of Amino Acids. The gas chromatography of amino acids according to McBride and Klingman's (1968) method employs a single flame ionization detector gas chromatograph equipped with a strip-chart recorder, a digital readout integrator, and a printer. (An alternative instrument consists of a gas chromatograph equipped with two single flame ionization detectors and a dual-channel strip-chart recorder.)

The most suitable column packing consists of a Gas Chrom A (60 to 80 mesh) used as a solid support and 1.2% PDEAS as stationary phase, or Chromosorb W coated with 3% OV-1 (Brooks et al., 1970). These materials must be carefully prepared and conditioned for the chromatography. Glass columns (110 $\times$ 0.4 cm i.d.) are packed by slow addition of the coated support and by gentle tapping of column until packing settled. The ends of the columns are packed firmly with glass wool, washed in hot 50% nitric acid, rinsed with water, and dried at 100° for 48 hours. The stationary phase is dissolved in acetone or chloroform and then transferred to the support. The column packing are conditioned for 12 or more hours from 175° to 230° with a nitrogen flow rate set at a given volume between 20 and 38 ml/minute.

Amino acid derivatives for the chromatography are prepared by adding an aqueous solution of the sample to 1.2 N HCl in methanol and leaving the mixture at room temperature for 30 minutes. The excess solvent is then removed under vacuum using a Virtis Centrifugal Bio-Dryer. Approximately 0.1 ml of 1.2 N HCl in butanol is added and the solution is mixed at room temperature and after heating at 100° for 5 minutes to dissolve the sample. The mixture is then immersed in oil at 100° for $2\frac{1}{2}$ hours following which the excess solvent is removed under vacuum. Approximately 50 μl of CH_2Cl_2 and 25 μl of trifluoroacetic anhydride is then added, mixed, and left at room temperature for 2 hours. According to Brooks and Moore's (1969) technique, 9 parts of TFA are used to 1 part of a pyridine reagent. Excess solvent is removed under vacuum. The sample is taken up in a small (e.g., 1 to 2 μl volume) of chloroform and is injected directly into the column.

The column temperature is initially set at 67 to 70° for 7 minutes and the final temperature is 200° or higher. The program rate is set at 2°/minute, and the flame ionization detector base and exit transfer lines at 250°. The inlet temperature is initially 70°. Nitrogen is introduced as a carrier flow at 35/minute and the hydrogen at 45 ml/minute and air at 300 ml/minute. The chart speed is 0.25 in/minute.

According to Adams' et al. (1969) method for gas-liquid partition chromatography of amino acids, a preparation containing amino acids is first refluxed in a mixture of methanol (4.2 ml) and concentrated hydrochloric acid (0.8 ml) for 8 hours. This material is then placed on (2.73 m $\times$ 3 mm) straight glass columns, packed with two different materials: (a) 10% w/w neopenthyl glycol sebacate polyester on 80–100 mesh chromosorb W, or (b) 9.5% ECNSS-N on 100–120 mesh chromosorb Q, and chromatographed at 195° or 187°, respectively. A gas chromatograph equipped with a flame ionization detector is employed for these studies.

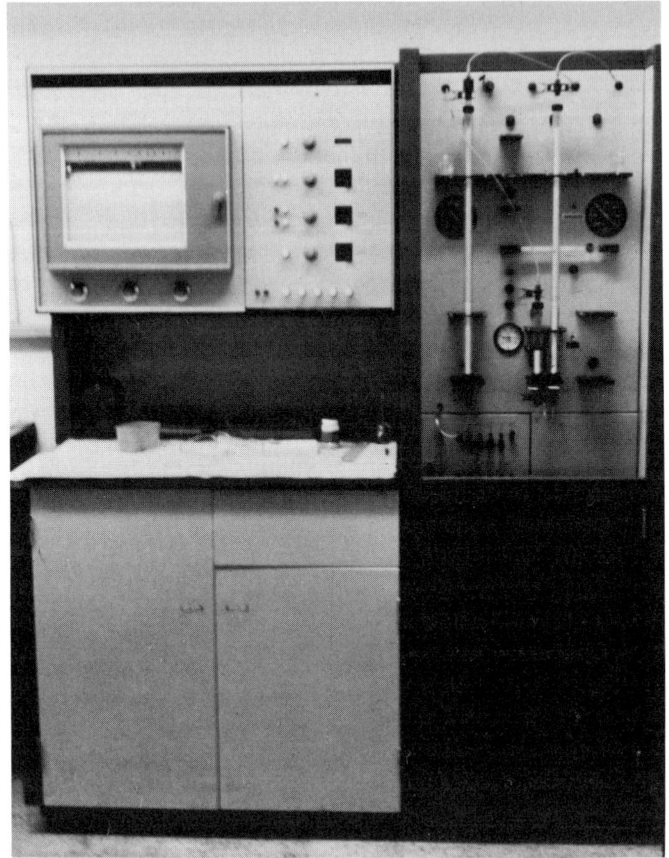

Figure 35. The amino acid analyzer (right to left: columns, a control panel, and an automatic recorder).

Quantitative Determination of Amino Acids. The most accurate method for quantitation of different amino acids is the analysis in a (Spinco Model 120 L) Automatic Amino Acid Analyzer (Fig. 35), employing Crumpton and Wilkinson's (1963) or Dus' et al. (1966) technique. The material used as a source of amino acids must first be hydrolyzed in 6 *N* HCl under reduced pressure, at 110° for 20 hours.

N-Terminal amino acids can be determined by the fluorodinitrobenzene method (Porter, 1957).

4. *Immunochemical Analysis of Nucleic Acids*

Immunochemical analysis of nucleic acids consists in the determination of: (a) the type of nucleic acid, (b) the conformation of molecules, and

(c) susceptibility to enzymatic digestion, and by the isolation, purification, and identification of the antigenic determinant.

The chemical examination of nucleic acids comprises the determination of phosphorus, pentose, and deoxyribose or deoxyribonucleic acids contents, and the electrophoresis and chromatographic analysis of constituents of nucleic acids (nucleosides and purine and pyrimidine bases).

The concentration of a purified nucleic acid preparation in a solution may be determined by measurement of absorbancy at 260-nm wavelengths. If the solution only contains the ribonucleic acid, the concentration of RNA is calculated by applying the conversion factor of 33.16 according to the equation (DeDeken-Grenson and DeDeken, 1959):

$$\frac{\mu g \ RNA}{ml} = \text{O.D. at 260 nm} \times 33.16$$

The conversion factor is based on the basis of 9.0% phosphorus content in the RNA (Magasanik, 1955). The average content of phosphorus in DNA is 9.4%.

If the nucleic acids are present in a combination with phospholipids, the content of nucleic acid may be calculated approximately from the phosphorus data. The percentage of phosphorus in nucleic acid is obtained by subtracting the percentage P in lipid from total phosphorus in a sample. By applying a conversion factor of 9.89 and multiplying it by the figure of phosphorus in nucleic acid, an approximate percentage of nucleic acid may be calculated. The amount of ribonucleic acid in a preparation free of polysaccharides may be approximated from the ribose content by multiplying the ribose data by 2.3 (which is the conversion factor for ribose content in ribonucleic acid).

Phosphorus can be estimated by Fiske and Subbarow's (1926), Chen's (1956), Murkerje and Sri Ram's (1964), or Harvey's (1953) method. Chen's (1956) and Murkerje and Sri Ram's (1964) techniques are most recommended for immunochemical research. If a preparation contained purified RNA, its amount may be calculated from the phosphorus content by multiplying it by the factor of 11.1, considering that the RNA contains 9% phosphorus. The contents of pentoses is determined by Mejbaum's (1939) method, the ribonucleic acid by Webb's (1956) method, and deoxyribonucleic acid according to various modifications of Dische's method, by Webb and Levy (1955) and Burton (1956). An automatic analysis of purines and pyrimidines, simultaneously with the amino acids, if required, may be performed on a modified (Beckman-Spinco) Amino Acid Analyzer according to Bonnelycke's et al. (1969) method.

i. *Immunochemical Characterization of DNA.* The following criteria are used to identify the deoxyribonucleic acid: changes of the extinction coefficient, viscosity, buoyant density, optical rotation, light scattering, and transforming ability of DNA on heating DNA preparations in neutral solutions (Marmur et al., 1963). These changes occur at the temperature level at which the native double-strand structure collapses to form a denaturate molecule.

Determination of the DNA Concentration. Concentration of DNA in a purified DNA preparation can be measured either by the ultraviolet absorption at 260 or 267 nm using a DNA standard such as calf thymus DNA, or by Kissane and Robins' (1958) fluorometric method. The latter method is more sensitive than the ultraviolet absorption technique. The fluorometric method modified by Colli and Oishi (1970) is applied as follows.

A measured amount of dried DNA preparation is placed in a number of tubes to which 20 μl of a 2M-DABA aqueous solution are added (DABA, 3,5-diamino-benzoic acid dihydrochloride. MAK, methylated albumin-Kieselguhr). The tubes are capped, shaken, and incubated at 60° for 30 minutes. Immediately after the incubation, 2 to 8 μl samples are withdrawn from the tubes with a Hamilton microsyringe and transferred to a fluorometer cell containing 2 ml of 0.6 N perchloric acid. Blanks consist of the DABA solution which has been extracted three times with 20 mg of acid washed charcoal (Norit A). The reaction tubes are washed to remove possible contamination with deoxyribose. Fluorescence is determined in the Eppendorf Fluorometer equipped with an Eppendorf filter which passes the exciting light of 405 and 436 nm, placed before the low pressure mercury light source. Emitted fluorescent light is isolated by a combination of a Eppendorf filter (400–3000 nm) and a Kodak Wratten filter No. 8 which blocks light below 460 nm. These filters are placed before the photomultiplier tube. The output of the photomultiplier tube is connected to a Honeywell potentiometric recorder.

DNA measurements by the fluorometric, ultraviolet absorption, indol, and dimethylamine methods agree with each other within an error of ±5% of the measurements performed accurately.

Determination of DNA Base Composition by Thermal Denaturation. Thermal denaturation of DNA may be determined most conveniently with an automatic thermospectrophotometer, according to Stenderup and Bak's (1968) method. The equipment consists of an ultraviolet spectrophotometer, containing a thermostatted cuvette holder (Unicam, SP874). The cuvette holder is heated by circulating water whose temperature may be raised at a constant rate. The temperature is measured in a control cuvette containing the platinum resistance of a Gilford linear thermosensor. The temperature and extinction are recorded on a Mosley x-y, Model 2D-4M autograph. The extinction is recorded in the temperature interval from 60 to 100°.

A standard sample of pure DNA in saline citrate adjusted to give an extinction of about 0.7 is used in parallel with the tested DNA preparation. The blank contains adenine of the same extinction in saline citrate to correct for thermal expansion.

The Tm values are determined as midpoint of the extinction-temperature curves between the extinction at 69° and extinction at maximal hyperchromicity, as designed by Rogul et al. (1965), and an average can be expressed by the equation: $Tm = 69.3 + 0.41$ (G-C). The mean base composition is calculated from Tm by the formula (Marmur and Doty, 1962):

$$\text{mole } \% \text{ GC} = \frac{Tm - 69.3}{0.41}$$

and expressed as % GC. (Tm is the melting temperature of one-dimensional crystallites, characterized at the midpoint of the transition, and is linearly related to the average DNA base composition.)

Molecular Weight Determination of DNA. Molecular weight of purified DNA may be determined by alkaline-sucrose gradient centrifugation, employing 5% to 20% sucrose, 0.9 M NaCl, 0.1 M NaOH, and 0.001 M EDTA. The molecular weight (M) is calculated from the equation (Studier, 1965):

$$S_{20,w}^{o} = 0.0528 \, M^{0.400}$$

The molecular weight of a standard DNA can be determined by sedimentation velocity in the Spinco Model E Analytical Centrifuge.

ii. *Separation and Identification of Nucleosides.* Constituents of nucleic acids can be separated by chromatographic methods, such as filter-paper chromatography (Gerlach et al. 1965), thin-layer chromatography, thin-layer electrophoresis, and gas-liquid chromatography. The latter method is especially sensitive and fast. The procedure described by Jacobsen et al. (1968) permits the analysis of microgram quantities of ribonucleic acid by gas-liquid chromatography of trimethylsilyl derivatives of the ribonucleosides. The thin-layer chromatography, however, sometimes proves to be more convenient due to its simplicity. By the thin-layer chromatography technique designed by Buteau and Simmons (1970), principle nucleoside constituents can be determined quantitatively.

Nucleosides are released from molecules of DNA by the digestion of DNA with DNAse and phosphodiesterase: the DNA preparation is dissolved in 1.0 ml 0.0004 M MgSO$_4$, buffered at pH 5.0 with acetate buffer, 0.02 M. Deoxyribonuclese (1 μg/5 DNA) is added and the mixture is left at 37° for 5 hours. The pH of the digestion mixture is adjusted to 8.0 with 0.1 M Tris (hydroxymethyl) aminomethane buffer, pH 9.6. Phosphodiesterase and alkaline phosphatase are then added (1 μg/5 μg DNA) and the mixture is shaken overnight at room temperature. The digestate is adjusted to pH 7.0 with 0.1 *N* HCl, after which a 24:1 mixture of chloroform and isoamyl alcohol (two volumes) is added. The mixture is agitated for a few minutes and centrifuged at 1250 × *g* for 5 minutes to remove the proteins.

Chromoplates for this procedure are prepared in the following manner: 15 g MN 300 PEI cellulose (Brinkmann Instruments, Westbury, N.Y.) are washed several times with 10% NaCl, distilled water, 0.4 *M* triethylammonium tetraborate, and again with distilled water. The cellulose is then homogenized in 65 ml distilled water and spread on 20 × 20-cm glass chromoplates at 500-μ thickness with a spreader. The plates are allowed to dry overnight, after which the plates are immersed at one end in 0.1 *M* boric acid which migrates upwards to the tops of the plates in order to cleanse the cellulose, and then the plates are dried again.

Chromatography is run in a solvent consisting of 0.02 *M* ammonium acetate, pH 4.8 and 95% ethyl alcohol (1:1). The solvent migrates to within 1 to 2 cm of the top of the plate, following which the plate is air dried. The plates are turned by 90° for the second dimension of the chromatography in 0.1 *M* boric acid which is terminated when the liquid has migrated half-way. The nucleosides are located under ultraviolet light. Quantitation of the separated nucleosides is conducted after the elution of areas containing nucleosides with 0.1 *N* HCl, followed by filtration through Whatman's No. 1 filter paper. The absorbance is measured at the wavelength of maximal adsorption at pH 2 for each compound (255, 258, 267, and 280 nm for deoxyguanosine, deoxyadenosine, thymidine, and deoxycytidine, respectively), as compared with relative absorbance of known concentrations of each type of the deoxyribonucleosides.

The average Rf values for deoxyguanosine, deoxyadenosine, thymidine, and deoxycytidine were found to be, respectively, 0.62, 0.75, 0.86, and 0.76.

Another good method for the thin-layer chromatography of nucleosides is the procedure described by Hedgcoth and Jacobson (1968). The solvent systems used for this technique are: (a) isopropyl alcohol/water, conc. HCl (65/18.4/16.6), and (b) *tert*-butyl alcohol/methy/ethyl ketone/water/concentrated ammonium hydroxide (40/30/20/10). The chromatograms are dried at room temperature and examined in short-wave uv light in a Chromato-vue viewing chamber, except for dihydrouridine, which is detected by Fink's et al. (1956) reagent.

The Base Ratio Analysis (Wyatt, 1951). The DNA preparation is first hydrolyzed in a very small volume (0.02 ml) of 70% (concentrated) perchloric acid at 100° for 1 hour. The hydrolyzate is then cooled at room temperature and neutralized with 4 *N* potassium hydroxide. Centrifuge the mixture and collect the supernatant. Deposit the material on Whatman's No. 1 filter paper and partition it by descending chromatography for 18 hours in a 170:41:39 mixture of isopropanol, hydrochloric acid, and water. Dry the chromatogram in air and scan it with an ultraviolet light. For quantitative estimation of bases, elute the fluorescent spots with 0.1 N hydrochloric acid overnight at room temperature. Determine each base quantitatively by measuring absorption in a spectrophotometer using the following constants: adenine, MAX = 260, EM = 13,000; thymine, X = 262, EM = 7950; guanine, X = 250, EM = 11,000; cytosine, X = 275, EM = 10,500.

Determination of the Conformation of DNA. The DNA preparation is first denatured by the following procedure (Chen et al., 1956): dissolve native DNA in 0.01 M Tris-HCl, pH 7.4, 0.14 M NaCl; incubate the solution at varying temperatures for 10 minutes, and dilute it into a chilled buffer consisting of 0.01 M Tris-HCl, pH 7.4, 0.14 M NaCl, 1.5×10^{-4} M MgCl$_2$, and 0.1% bovine serum albumin. Determine serological activity of the DNA by the microcomplement fixation test (Levine et al., 1960) or by another suitable serological test.

Determination of the Renaturation. The extent of renaturation of DNA may be determined by estimation of the loss of serological activity caused by base pairing (Levine et al., 1966). The renaturation is measured in the following manner: the DNA preparation is suspended in 0.15 M NaCl and is terminally denatured by heating at 100° for 10 minutes. Make serial dilutions of the termally denatured DNA in a preheated salt solution. At varying times of incubation at a desired temperature, aliquots are removed and rapidly diluted into a cold Tris-HCl buffer. The serological activity of these solutions of DNA is determined by complement fixation tests. The temperature of 50° is found to be the optimum incubation temperature for most of the testing of DNA preparations.

The thermal denaturation temperature (Tm of the DNA) and the mole percentage (GC) are determined by employing the equation derived by Marmur and Doty (1962):

$$\text{mole } \% \text{ GC} = \frac{T\text{m} - 69.3}{0.41}$$

The thermal denaturation temperature is measured with a DU monochrometer equipped with a Gilfort Model 2000 multiple sample absorbance recorder.

Determination of DNA Base Composition by the High-Voltage Analysis (Schildkraut and Maio, 1969). The DNA preparation (0.08 ml) is first digested with pancreatic deoxyribonuclease (50 μg/ml), in 0.005 M Tris, pH 7.0, containing 0.005 M MgCl$_2$ for 30 minutes at 37°. The suspension is then heated at 100° for 5 minutes, adjusted to 0.02 M, pH 8.8, with NaOH and glycine buffer, and digested with 0.01 unit of a snake venom phosphodiesterase a 37° for 30 minutes. The solution is applied to Whatman No. 3 paper and subjected to a high voltage electrophoresis in a sodium citrate buffer, pH 3.5, at 6000 V for 2 hours. Bases are detected in the UV light.

ii. *Immunochemical Characterization of RNA.* A complete characterization of ribonucleic acid preparation depends on the determination of the size, nucleotide composition, kinetics of synthesis (using radioactive labelling), and template activity (the ability to stimulate cell-free protein synthesis).

Determination of the Size of Nucleic Acid. Approximate determination of the size of ribonucleic-acid molecules may be accomplished by the sucrose-gradient centrifugation using a gradient from 5 to 20% sucrose. Incorporation of 0.5% of sodium dodecyl sulfate in the gradient is helpful for fractionation of bacterial RNA (Gilbert, 1963). Each fraction obtained from the gradient is assayed for absorption at 260 nm. The RNA can also be fractionated on methylated albumin columns and on Sephadex columns.

Determination of the Polynucleotide Linkage. A chemical method for the estimation of polynucleotide chain linkage (Midgley, 1965) depends on the reaction of RNA with sodium periodate which results in the oxidation of only the terminal ribose molecule with unsubstituted hydroxyl groups. Oxidized ribose reacts with radioactive isonicotinic acid hydrazide in a 1:1 stoichiometric relation with RNA chains. The radio active RNA-isonicotinic acid hydrazone is then precipitated and counted. An alternative method (Lane, 1965), depends on the finding that on alkaline hydrolysis of RNA, ribonucleoside, and ribonucleoside-diphosphate are released from each chain. The nucleosides or the nucleoside-diphosphate is then identified and measured.

Analysis of Nucleotide Composition. Different ribonucleotides may be separated by the high-voltage electrophoresis, low-voltage paper electrophoresis, ion exchange chromatography, and column chromatography on methylated albumin Kieselguhr, or by a method of reverse phase chromatography relying on the ion exchange and differential solubility (Kelmers et al., 1965). Other methods for nucleotide and nucleic acid separation are the partition chromatography on Sephadex G-25 (Tanaka et al., 1962), chromatography on DEAE columns with gradient elution at elevated temperatures (Baguley et al., 1965), and the counter-current distribution technique (Apgar et al., 1962). The high-voltage electrophoresis and the counter-current distribution techniques are most recommended. An alternative method is the cation exchange chromatography (Katz and Comb, 1963). In the latter method, small columns (0.9 × 5.0 cm) of Dowex 50-H+ are used. The columns are prewashed with 3 N HCl, with water until neutral, and finally washed with 0.05 N HCl. The elution is conducted with distilled water which first releases GMP alone and then CMP and AMP together. The absorbance, due to each of these two nucleotides, is calculated from the extinction absorption values of the mixture at 257 and 279 nm in 0.05 N HCl from the equations:

$$x = \frac{2.32\ (A_{257}) - A_{279}}{2.08}$$

$$y = A_{279} - 0.238x$$

where x is the absorbency at 257 nm due to AMP alone, y is the absorbency at 279 nm due to CMP alone, and A is the absorbance of the mixture.

High-Voltage Electrophoresis of Ribonucleotides (Monjardino, 1969). RNA preparations are hydrolized at 37° for 18 hours in 0.3 N KOH using 1 mg of RNA/ml. The pH of the hydrolyzate is adjusted to 7.0 with perchloric acid, and the occurring precipitate of potassium perchlorate is spun down. A clear supernatant is concentrated in a rotory evaporator before being applied to the coated plates. Glass plates are coated with a cellulose (MN 300) suspension to the thickness of 500 nm, and dried in an oven at 100°.

The sample is applied to the plate at 6 cm from one end as a band 1.0 to 1.5-cm wide. The plate is then immersed in a jar containing a 0.02 M, pH 3.5, buffer up to 2 or 3 cm below the spotted band. The origin is on the side of the negative electrode. The 3 MM Whatman wicks are connected with the plates and the other end is dipped in the buffer. The voltage of 650 V is applied, giving a voltage gradient of approximately 50 V/cm and the current is about 3 to 5 mA. The electrophoresis is carried out at 4° for 90 minutes. The plates are then dried under an infrared lamp, and the bands are located and penciled round under UV light (245 nm).

The base composition can be detected by scraping off the bands and eluting overnight in 0.1 N HCl. The eluants are examined at the appropriate wave length (CMP 279 nm, AMP 257 nm, GMP 257 nm, UMP 260 nm). Conversion of the μg values is made by applying millimolar extinction coefficients, determined from commercial preparations of the corresponding 5′-nucleotide, dissolved in 0.1 N HCl.

High-Voltage Mapping of Nucleotides (Sanger et al., 1965). Digestion of nucleic acids may be performed in a capillary tube; 10–50 μg of nucleic acid, dissolved in 10 to 50 μl of 0.02 M Tris buffer, pH 7.4, containing

0.002 M EDTA, and 20 μg of a nuclease or deoxyribonuclease preparations are incubated for 30 minutes at 37°.

The digest is then deposited on a 4 × 60 cm cellulose acetate strip, wetted by floating on the buffer, about 10 cm from the cathode end. A colored marker (a 2% orange G solution) is placed on each side of the digest. The ionophoresis is run at 3000 V until the yellow marker has reached the anode buffer (about 2 hours) or a little longer.

Mononucleotides may be released from oligonucleotides by the hydrolysis in 0.2 N NaOH at 37° for 16 hours in drawn-out melting point tubes, or by digestion with pancreatic ribonuclease using 0.2 mg pancreatic nuclease per milliliter of 0.001 M EDTA − 0.01 M Tris buffer (pH 7.4) containing 5 to 10 μl of nucleotide sample. The mixture is drawn into the capillary tube, sealed at the drawn-out end, and incubated at 37° for 30 minutes. The samples are then treated with 0.1 N HCl to breakdown cyclic phosphates, in the following manner: 0.5 N HCl is put on a polythene strip. The tip of the capillary tube is broken and the digest is squeezed out, mixed with 0.5 N HCl and sucked back into the capillary which is then resealed and incubated at 37° for 1 hour. The digest is subjected to ionophoresis at pH 3.5, 3000 V. The nucleotides are identified by their position in comparison to the position of standard nucleotides, or the nucleotide areas are eluted with water and subjected to alkaline hydrolysis for further analysis. The digest is applied to Whatman No. 52 paper or onto the cellulose pulver coated glass plate for ionophoresis at pH 3.5 and 60 V/cm for 1 to $1\frac{1}{2}$ hours.

The following buffer systems can be applied for ionophoresis: pH 3.5, 0.5% pyridine-5% acetic acid (v/v), pH 1.9, 2.5% formic acid-8.7% acetic acid (v/v), pH 6.5, 10% pyridine-0.3% acetic acid (v/v), and pH 3.5, 5% acetic acid adjusted with ammonia to pH 3.5; 1% acetic acid adjusted with ammonia to pH 4.1; 0.5% acetic acid adjusted with ammonia to pH 4.4; 0.25% acetic acid adjusted with ammonia to pH 4.9; and 1.7 ethyl morpholine adjusted with acetic acid to pH 7.9.

Nucleotides are detected by the absorbency in UV light.

Determination of terminal residues of nucleotides can be accomplished by Sanger's et al. (1965) method, utilizing specific action of phosphomono-esterase and phosphodiesterase.

The sequence of larger oligonucleotides may be estimated by partial digestion with venom or spleen phosphodiesterase. The overall percentage composition of a molecule of nucleic acid is calculated from the individual sequence and frequency, and these data should coincide with those obtained by total alkaline hydrolysis.

Template Activity Measurement. Certain types of RNA, for example, messenger RNA, have the ability to act as a template in protein synthesis and to stimulate the incorporation of amino acids into hot TCA-insoluble material in cell-free extracts. A method for the template activity measurement has been described by Nirenberg and Mathei (1961).

V. INVESTIGATION OF BIOLOGICAL PROPERTIES OF ANTIGENS

The biological properties of antigens can be fully determined by investigating their serological activity and specificity, specific immunogenic strength, stimulation of nonspecific immunity, allergic (anaphylactic) and pyrogenic properties, toxicity, and influence on phagocytosis and on the bacteriophage-bacterium interaction between bacteriophages and the sensitive bacterial cells. Useful data may also be obtained from a stimulographic assay.

The following serological tests are recommended for an investigation of immunological activities and specificity of antigen preparations:

1. Cross-agglutination absorption and immunofluorescence tests involving intact or disintegrated cells, separated cell membranes, or other anatomical structures. This assay reveals reactions depending on the antigens situated on the surface or in the superficial layers of intact cells or their anatomical constituents.

2. Complement fixation test to determine the antigen activity versus a constant amount of antiserum.

3. Indirect hemagglutination or immune hemolytic test to estimate the affinity of homologous and heterologous antiserum to the soluble antigens absorbed onto the erythrocytes.

4. The diffusion precipitation technique to test the homogeneity of an antigen preparation and immunological relationships among various antigens.

Adequate immunological techniques for these investigations are described in subsequent chapters.

1. Determination of the Immunogenic Potency of Antigens

The purpose of these studies is to estimate the class of prepared antigen (complete antigen, hapten, or haptid) and to evaluate the immunizing ability of the isolated antigen preparations by testing the protective power of induced antibodies against an infection with virulent or toxic microorganisms. A number of different tests are used for these investigations.

To determine the antigenicity of DNA molecules, for example, the following immunological assays have been applied: the precipitation, complement fixation, passive cutaneous anaphylaxis, and immunofluorescence technique (Deicher et al., 1959).

The immunogenic power of antigens is estimated by injecting animals with each antigen preparation found active in the preceding serological test. Rabbits are immunized intravenously, whereas guinea pigs are mostly injected intraperitoneally. Usually four to five injections are given over a 2-week period. In some cases, a better immune response is obtained by 3 to 5 daily injections of gradually increased doses of an antigen. Serum samples, obtained from these animals in 7 to 10 days after the last injection, are examined for the presence of antibodies. If the serum reacts with the homologous antigen used for immunization, this antigen is classified as a complete antigen. If the result is negative, the antigen may be regarded either as hapten or haptid, depending on whether it reacted in a direct or an indirect serological test or in a blocking test with the antiserum, produced against the whole bacteria. Antisera prepared for these investigations can also be used for systematic studies on the antigenic structure and immunological relationships of microorganisms and in studies on the passive immunity.

The protective value of the antibodies produced can be investigated by three types of experiments. First, experimental animals showing a high antibody titer are exposed to a lethal or infective dose of corresponding microorganisms. Second, a larger group of guinea pigs, mice, or hamsters is injected subcutaneously or intramuscularly with a dose of 1 to 3 mg of antigen preparation, two to three times, and a week later challenged with the live microorganisms. Third, antiserum samples withdrawn from the immunized animals can be injected into another group of normal animals to be challenged with the infectious microorganisms. Injections of the antiserum should be repeated on the successive 2 or 3 days. After a period of observation, the survival index is calculated according to the formula:

$$\frac{\text{number of survived animals}}{\text{total number of animals}} \times 100$$

All surviving animals are sacrificed and carefully autopsied. Complementary histological examinations and sometimes culture tests, to determine whether the injected microorganisms have been eliminated from the activity or passively immunized host, may be made. The data are collected and analyzed statistically (Hill, 1956; Boyd, 1956; Sokal and Michener, 1958). The mortality of 50% animals (LD_{50}) can be estimated by plotting the recorded data against the dosage of an antigen preparation on a logarithmic probability paper (Boyd, 1956). The best fitting line is drawn, and the dosage corresponding to the intersection of this line with the 50% ordinate is recorded.

The immunity measurement, according to Sulitzeanu's (1955) technique, is carried out in the following way. A group of mice receives an intraperitoneal injection of killed microorganisms. After an appropriate time, these animals are challenged with a standard dose of live bacteria. Subsequently spleen counts of the immunized and control animals are made by a culture technique. The degree of immunity is determined from the equation:

$$\text{protection index} = \frac{\text{mean spleen count of control group}}{\text{mean spleen count of immunized group}}$$

An index of 5 or higher is regarded as indicative of a significant protective effect.

The immunogenicity of an antigen preparation or a vaccine, which confers active protection against microorganisms affecting the respiratory tract, may be studied affectively by Ribi's et al. (1968) method. Groups of mice are infected intratracheally with a dose of mycobacteria sufficient for the entry of 40 to 50 bacilli into the lungs. Alternatively, a challenge, large dose of tubercle bacilli may be administered intravenously. At 4 weeks after the challenge, the mice are sacrificed, and the lungs are inspected for the presence of macroscopically visible tubercles. Lesions found in the lungs and spleen are enumerated. The lungs are weighed, homogenized, and suspended in saline. Aliquots of the suspension are planted on a culture medium. The results are expressed as the number of viable mycobacteria per 100 mg of lung tissue. The immune response in case of mycobacteria is manifested by a significant reduction in the proportion of lungs containing grossly visible tubercles and by the reduced amount of challenge tubercle bacilli found in the lungs of immunized mice as compared to the unvaccinated control. An additional criterion is the number of mycobacteria in spleens.

The Nonspecific Immunity Stimulation Test. This test suggested by Rowley (1956) is set up in the following manner. Groups of mice are injected intravenously with 10 to 50 μg of a fraction dissolved in 0.1 ml of saline. The control mice receive 0.2 ml of saline only. After 48 hours, the mice are challenged intraperitoneally with a virulent strain of another microorganism suspended in saline or in a 1.75% (w/v) solution of hog gastric mucin which increases the virulence of some bacteria. The number of deaths is recorded and compared with the number of deaths in the control group.

2. Determination of the Toxicity of Antigens

Toxicity of antigen preparations can be determined *in vitro* by the demonstration of morphological effects on organ explants (Heilman, 1968), by comparing the number of Trypan blue-positive macrophages which have been exposed to a toxin to the macrophages maintained in a solution containing no toxic materials. (The number of the toxin-exposed macrophages should increase, Kessel et al., 1966.) Other methods for the determination of toxicity are the inhibition of the growth of fibroblasts maintained in a tissue culture (Bergman and Nilsson, 1963), and the study of tissue-damage and lethal effect of the preparation for mice or other animals (Woods et al., 1961). The most commendable method for toxicity determination is the study of effects of the toxins on tissue cultures (Bergman and Weibull, 1969). Ancillary symptoms of toxic reaction are leukopenic, glycemic, and thermal reactions. The ancillary reactions are studied on groups of rabbits injected intravenously with a dose of 2 to 10 mg of individual antigen preparations. The minimum dose causing one or several of the toxic reactions should be determined in each case.

Semiquantitative Determination of Toxicity. The medium for toxicity determination (Bergman and Weibull, 1969) consists of a suspension of HeLa cells and fibroblasts obtained from human fetuses, suspended at a final concentration of 100,000 to 200,000 cells/ml in the Parker 199 medium supplemented with 2% calf serum. The toxic preparation is dissolved in a 0.85% sodium chloride solution; 0.2 ml of the toxic solution and 0.5 ml of cell suspension are placed on ringed glass slides, and the cells are allowed to attach to the slides for 4 hours at 37°. The rings are then taken out; the slides are placed in cuvettes containing 14 ml of the tissue culture medium and left for 18 hours, after which the cells are fixed in Carnoy's fluid and stained with haematoxylin according to Weigert's method. The cells are examined as described by Bergman (1963).

Primary skin toxicity is studied by injecting in a horizontal row a series of dilutions of an antigen preparation into the closely clipped skin of four or five rabbits. The toxin of *Serratia marcescens,* which has primary toxicity, is injected for comparative purposes. Sites of the skin injections are examined for the presence of lesion at 12, 24, and 48 hours. Diameters of the lesions are measured with a planimeter.

The leukopenic reaction is indicated by a significant decrease of the leukocyte number in blood samples withdrawn in 1 to 6 and 24 hours after the antigen injections.

Hyperglycemia occurring 6 to 24 hours after the injection of an antigen preparation is another evidence of toxicity.

Thermal reaction, caused by the pyrogenic action of an antigen preparation injected intravenously, is determined by measuring temperatures of a group of rabbits before and after the injection, at 1, 2, 4, and 8 hours or at 30-minute intervals (Beson, 1947). The material tested should be dissolved in serile, nonpyrogenic isotonic saline. The use of tri-R electronic thermometers can be advantage. (Normal body temperatures of rabbits vary be-

tween 39.0 and 39.6°.) The temperature figures read after the injection of
a pyrogen may be plotted against the time in days, and the area beneath
the curve is measured with a Keuffel compensating planimeter. The vernier
reading of the planimeter is taken as an "index of fever" (Bennett, 1948).
The temperature curve can be drawn more accurately if temperatures are
taken with thermometers fixed under the skin of experimental animals
(Westphal et al., 1952) or by using a Foxboro Rabbit Scanner and Fever
Recorder. Apart from temperature changes, the alterations in total leukocyte counts and differential leukocyte and thrombocyte counts are made at
intervals. The pyrogenicity can be semiquantitatively evaluated in terms of
the minimum pyrogenic dose, which is the smallest amount, in micrograms,
of a dried material per kilogram of rabbit weight that elicits a febrile reaction. Pure pyrogens can be obtained by trypsin-digestion at pH 8.5 of bacteria, autoclaved at 121° for 20 minutes and layered with toluene. The
digest is then centrifuged; the supernatant should be collected, dialyzed, and
lyophilized (Nesset et al., 1950).

Lesions can vary from a pink coloration and slight induration to a
reddish coloration of the periphery with a discolored and necrotic center
and an intense induration. The dermotoxic activity of an antigen preparation can be determined quantitatively by the estimation of the skin lesion
dose (SLD_{50}) according to Larson et al., (1960). The lesions due to intradermal injections of varying amounts of an antigen preparation may be
scored 72 hours after the injection according to Miles' et al. (1957) technique. In this method, the major and minor axes of a lesion are measured,
and the square root of product of the major axis multiplied by the minor
axis is calculated. A number of different dilutions of an antigen preparation
can be injected into a single rabbit, but five to seven rabbits should be used
for reproducibility. The lesions observed may be studied histologically after
they have been excised surgically and fixed in 10% formalin or Bouin's
fixative. The exercised and formalized materials are embedded in paraffin,
sectioned, and stained with hemotoxylin and eosin or hemotoxylin and
chromotrope 2 R.

Primary skin reactivity to an injected antigen preparation is often a reliable indicator of its local toxicity or the issue-damaging power. The minimal reacting dose (MRD) or minimal necrotizing dose (MUD) can be
used as a measure of the tissue-damaging power of an antigen. The test is
conducted by injecting intradermally into rabbits 0.1-ml volumes of progressive dilutions of the test material in saline, buffered at pH 7.4. The
highest dilution, or the equivalent in dry mass, causing withn 2 to 3 days a
visible reaction in the skin (red coloration, papula, or focus of necrosis)
denotes 1 MRD or 1 MND.

Cytometric Assay of the Toxicity.   The toxic effect of antigen preparations on cells can be measured by the Carpenter et al. (1962) tissue-culture technique. Suspensions of spleen cells are prepared by 10-minute trypsinization of minced guinea pig spleen in a 0.2% trypsin solution prepared in phosphate-buffered saline. The cells are washed with warm Hanks' balanced salt solution (HBSS)* and resuspended in a tissue-culture medium at a concentration of 5×10^6 cells/ml. The medium consists of 40% fresh guinea pig serum, 59% Hanks' BSS, and 1% antibiotic solution containing penicillin, dihydrosterptomycin, and neomycin in the concentration of 125 μg, 125 μg, and 1.25 units/ml, respectively.

Various amounts of the antigen preparations can be added to the tissue cultures and incubated at 37° for a time period.

The cytotoxic effect of an antigen preparation is estimated by the cell survival index (CSI), determined by dividing the mean cell count of the test culture by the mean cell count of the control culture tubes as represented by the equation:

$$\text{CSI} = \frac{\text{average cell count of test culture}}{\text{average cell count of control culture}}$$

The Intestinal Toxicity Test.   According to Jensen's technique (1959), segments of an ileum removed immediately from a chloroform-killed guinea pig are placed in oxygenated Ringer solution bath. Controls receive 1 ml of a histamine solution. The toxic effect is noted as contractions in the ileum segments which are recorded on a kymograph.

The lethal toxic effect of an antigen preparation is tested on groups of ten white mice or guinea pigs. Individual mice should weigh about 20 g and guinea pigs about 300 g. Various amounts of the material, ranging from 0.1 to 3 mg/gram weight of mouse, and between 1 to 10 mg/gram weight of guinea pig, are injected intraperitoneally or intravenously. The medium lethal dose (LD_{50}) corresponds to the amount of antigen preparation which causes death of 50% of the animals in 24 to 96 hours. It can also be calculated by a graphic probit method (Weiss, 1948). Standard errors and 95% confidence limits are estimated by the method of Irwin and Chessman (1935). The minimal lethal dose (MLD) is at present used less

---

* HBSS (Hanks' balanced salt solution) consists of 1 volume of stock solution A, 1 volume of stock solution B, and 18 volumes of glass-bidistilled water. Immediately before use, 2.5 ml of sterile 1.4% $NaHCO_3$ solution is added per 100 ml Hanks' solution.

Stock solution A.   NaCl, 100 g; KCl, 8 g; $MgSO_4 \cdot 7H_2O$, 4 g; bidistilled water, 800 ml; $CaCl_2$, 2 g; bidistilled water up to 1000 ml; chloroform, 2 ml.

Stock solution B. $Na_2HPO_4 \cdot 12H_2O$, 3.04 g; KH_2PO_4, 1.2 g; glucose, 20 g; bidistilled water, 800 ml; 0.4% phenol red solution, 100 ml; bidistilled water up to 1000 ml; chloroform, 2 ml.

frequently for the estimation of the antigen toxicity; it has been employed mostly for the evaluation of toxins. The MLD is determined in the following manner (Lepow and Pillemer, 1952). Serial dilutions of a preparation are made in $M/15$ phosphate buffer of pH 7.0 and injected subcutaneously into 250-g guinea pigs. Mice or rats can be used instead of guinea pigs. The smallest amount of test material, in milligrams, causing the death of animals in a arbitrarily chosen time, expresses the MLD.

3. Testing of the Antigen Influence on the Bacteriophage-Bacterium Interaction

The test depends on the inhibition of lytic action of bacteriophages by the absorbed specific antigens or components of bacteria. According to the Burnet and Freeman (1937) technique, serial dilutions of an antigen preparation are incubated with a standard dilution of phage for 4 hours at 45°; 0.02 ml of these mixtures are then spread on an agar plate, previously inoculated with a young broth culture of bacteria, and incubated at 37° overnight. The number of plaques is counted, and the end point is estimated by the corresponding concentration of antigen preparation which reduced the number of plaques from the standard dilution of phage to 20%.

The technique devised by Kwapinski (1965) consists of two procedures:

1. A suspension of bacteriophages is mixed with a solution of immunochemical fraction and incubated for 30 to 90 minutes at 37°, then sedimented in an ultracentrifuge, and washed with a 0.1 M phosphate buffer, pH 7.0.

2. Lytic action on the sensitive bacteria of the pretreated and control bacteriophages is tested. Effective lytic dilutions (titers) of the pretreated and control bacteriophages are determined. On the solid media, numbers of "plaques" produced by similar concentrations of both lots are estimated, and the inhibition of lysis is expressed by the percentage (LI %), according to the following equation:

$$\text{LI } \% = 100 - \left(\frac{f}{c} \times 100 \right)$$

where f and c are numbers of plaques formed by the pretreated and nontreated bacteriophages, respectively. Bacteriophage analysis is very sensitive and provides interesting data on the antigenic relationships among the microorganisms.

4. Stimulographic Analysis of Antigen Preparations

Stimulographic analysis (Kwapinski and Merkel, 1960) depends on a selective stimulation by certain polymerized substances extracted from microorganisms of the growth of other indicator microorganisms.

In this technique, agar plates made of 1.5% saline or buffered purified agar are flooded with a suspension of an indicator bacterium or yeast and dried at 37°. Sterile filter-paper disks, 5 mm in diameter, made of Whatman paper No. 2, saturated in 0.5% solutions of the fractions for examination, are then placed on the plates. They are incubated at 37 or 25° for 1 to 2 days, and inspected through a stereomicroscope. Stimulation of growth is denoted by the formation of a ring or halo consisting of colonies of the indicator microorganisms around a disk containing a stimulatory substance.

A high degree of species-specificity of the stimulatory bacterial fractions has been discovered by this technique. This method can provide valuable supplementary data on biological characteristics of antigen preparations.

VI. SELECTED QUANTITATIVE CHEMICAL TESTS

1. Nitrogen Determination

The nitrogen determination depends essentially on the measurement of ammonia obtained by the reduction of nitrogen present in an organic matter on acid digestion. The ammonia is then either titrated directly with acid against an indicator, or it is first reacted with hypochloride to produce chloramine which in turn reacts with phenol to form indophenol, quantitated spectrophotometrically (Rommers and Visser, 1969). An older colorimetric method, which employs Nessler's reagent, has been published by Koch and McMeekin (1924).

The original Kjeldahl's method for the determination of nitrogen as ammonia has been modified by Elek and Sobotka (1926), Markham (1942), and Bathurst and Mitchell (1958). The procedure has been automated by Marten and Catanzaro (1966) and modified by Berthelot (1969). All the methods are equally sensitive, and the choice of a technique for nitrogen determination depends mainly on the availability of the appropriate equipment. Rommers and Visser's method is generally very convenient.

From the nitrogen quotient, obtained by one of the techniques, the equivalent protein may be calculated approximately by multiplying the nitrogen quotient by the factor 6.25 to convert the figures into protein-milligrams.

Nitrogen Determination by Elek and Sobotka (1926):

Reagents
    1. Digestion mixture:
            0.38 g Cu SO$_4$ · 5H$_2$O.
            0.13 g K$_2$SO$_4$.
            0.30 g selenium.
            100 ml concentrated sulfuric acid.
    2. 50% (or saturated) solution of sodium hydroxide.

3. 2% boric acid.

4. The Tashiro indicator, consisting of 1 part of the Tashiro's stock solution, 1 part of 96% ethyl alcohol, and 2 parts of distilled water, mixed before use. Stock solution is a 4:1 mixture of 0.1% (twice recrystallized) methyl red in 95% ethyl alcohol and 0.1% methylene blue in water.

5. $N/70$ HCl, prepared exactly by weighing in air the constant boiling HCl, collected between 0.75 volume and residual.

6. Nitrogen standard, in the form of ammonium sulfate, obtainable as certified primary standard (Fisher No. A-938). To obtain a standard stock solution containing 60 μg N/ml, weigh 140.83 mg of the ammonium sulfate, and dissolve with distilled water to 500 ml.

Procedure. Place 10-mg samples in 2 ml of the digestion mixture in Kjeldahl flasks or suitable Pyrex-glass test tubes and boil the contents (on an electric rack, Fig. 36), until 15 minutes after clarification of the resultant liquid. Transfer the fluid quantitatively into the distillation bulb of Markham's (1942) apparatus (Fig. 37), add 6 ml of 50% NaOH, rinse with distilled water, and add one boiling stone. Distill ammonia into 5 ml of 2% boric acid diluted with 5 ml of distilled water and containing 2 to 3 drops of Tashiro's indicator. Titrate with $1/70$ N HCl from a monostat or Scholander burette until the distillate turns pink.

Calculate the contents of nitrogen in milligrams according to the formula:

$$N = \text{ml } N/70 \text{ HCl} \times 0.2$$

The experimental error is about $\pm$ 0.01 mg of nitrogen.

Spectrophotometric Nitrogen Determination. The Rommers and Visser (1969) method is applied for nitrogen determination in samples containing 0.05 to 20μg of nitrogen.

Reagents

1. 5% aqueous solution of boric acid.
2. 8% aqueous solution of phenol (stable for several months).
3. 3 M sodium hydroxide solution.
4. 5% aqueous solution of chloramine-T ($CH_3 \cdot C_6H_4 \cdot SO_2 \cdot NClNa \cdot 3H_2O$, stable for several months).
5. Nitrogen standard, consisting of 3.819 g of ammonium chloride, dried at 110°, and dissolved in distilled water to give 1 liter of a solution. This standard nitrogen solution contains 1 mg/ml^{-1} of nitrogen.
6. All solutions are prepared from analytical grade reagents.

Procedure. The nitrogen containing sample is first digested as described in Elek and Sobotka's method (see above) to reduce nitrogen to ammonia. Transfer the sample quantitatively to a 50-ml graduated flask. Add 5.0 ml

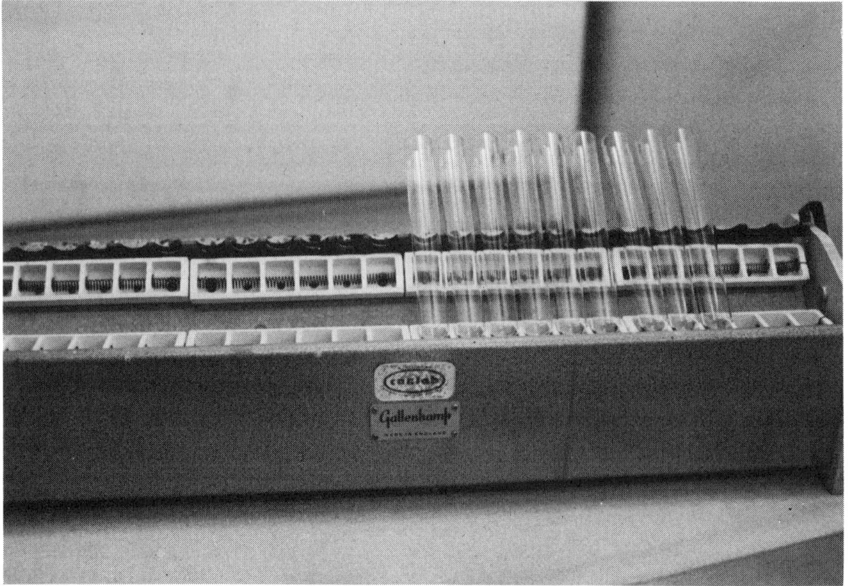

Figure 36. An electric Kjeldahl's rack.

of boric acid solution and dilute the whole to about 25 ml with distilled water. Cool the flask at 3°. Add, with swirling, 4.0 ml of chloramine-T solution. After 20 seconds exactly, add rapidly, with thorough mixing, 10 ml of phenol solution and heat the flask in a water bath at 60° for 16 minutes exactly. Remove the flask from the water bath and add 5.0 ml of the sodium hydroxide solution. Cool the flask at room temperature under running tap water and add distilled water to the 50-ml mark and mix. Measure the absorbance at 625 nm in a spectrophotometer, using a reagent blank as a reference solution (Fig. 38).

The reagent blank consists of 5.0 ml of boric acid solution, supplemented with distilled water to about 25 ml and then processed as described above.

A calibration graph is prepared from readings made on the standard ammonium chloride solution containing known and varying amounts of nitrogen, diluted to about 25 ml with distilled water and then processed in the same manner as the test sample and the blank.

The indophenol formed during the reaction described above may be extracted with isobutyl alcohol (Namiki et al., 1964). In this procedure, the processed sample is poured quantitatively into a separating funnel. Add 18 g of sodium chloride and shake the solution until most of the salt has dissolved. Add 10 ml of isobutyl alcohol and shake the mixture for 1 minute. Pipette off the excess solution. Filter the isobutyl alcohol layer through a fast running filter paper into an absorptiometric cell. Measure the absorbance at 625 nm with a reagent black as reference solution. The reagent blank should be extracted with 10 ml of isobutyl alcohol for 1 minute. The extraction procedure sometimes gives lower figures than the unextracted samples.

In the automatic analyzing system designed by Ferrari (1960), continuous supply of the digestion mixtures to the digestor is provided by the multiple proportioning pumps. The digestion is carried out in a continuous digestion module. Combined streams of a sample and digestion solution are fed into the digestion vessel. In the adjacent and combined parts of the autoanalyzer, the digestion solution receives alkaline treatment which leads to the liberation of ammonia from the ammonium sulfate derived from the sample. The solution is then sent through a mixing coil to a solution of alkaline phenol, followed by the introduction of 5 to 6% sodium hypochloride solution. This procedure yields an intensely blue-colored product, which is either indophenol or a closely related substance. The product is measured at 625 nm wavelength.

Automated Nitrogen Determination. The digestion of a sample and quantitative determination of ammonia are conducted by a Technicon Analyzer (Technicon Instr., Co., Chertsey, Surrey) and the results are calculated by an IBM computer or by an electronic desk calculator.

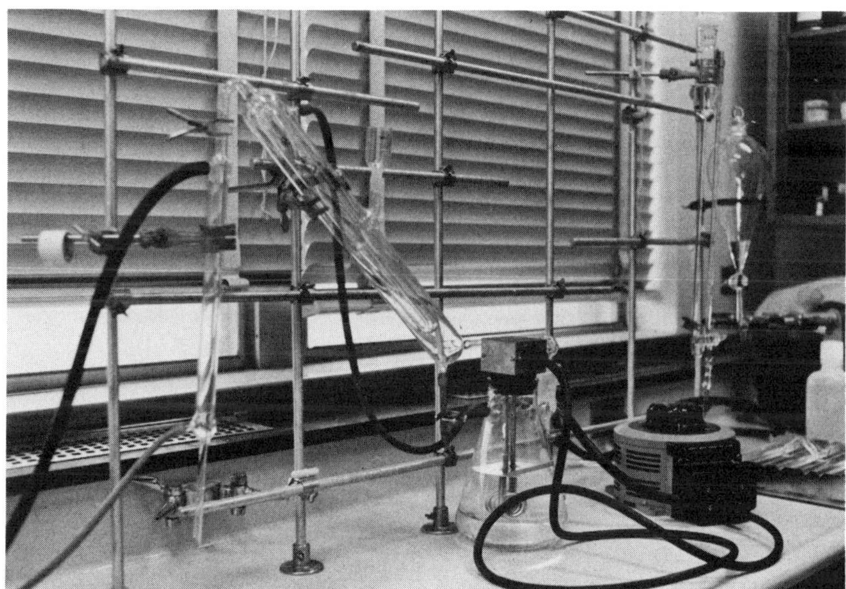

Figure 37. Markham's distillation apparatus for nitrogen determination.

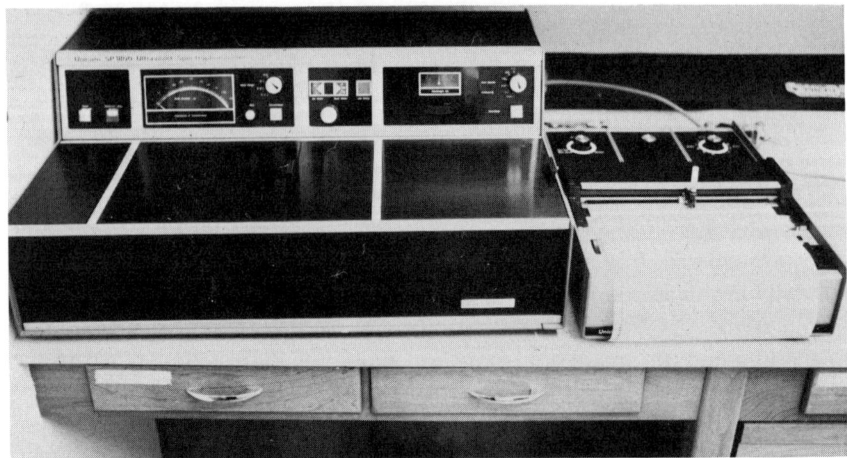

Figure 38.   Automatic spectrophotometer equipped with an automatic recorder.

The basic apparatus for automatic determination of nitrogen has been described by Marten and Catanzaro (1966) and a modified assembly for automatic digestion and color development is shown in Fig. 39. In the automatic digestor, a fluid stream may be heated to the temperature determined by the boiling point of the digestion mixture. The stream of digesting fluids is retained for 5 minutes in the revolving helix, and the digested sample(s) are automatically respirated and sampled into the color development where an extinction (E) value proportional to nitrogen in the original sample is obtained and determined.

The calculation of results by computer depends on a comparison of the extinction values from test and standard solutions. Punch cards are punched with code numbers for standard solutions and samples on one card, corresponding weights for nitrogen for standard and test samples on a second card, and corresponding peak extinction values from the chart recorder on a third card. A suitable computer program corrects for any base-line drift in every run.

The intensity of color developed are effected by certain heavy metals and other cations; an error thus produced in the determination of nitrogen must be considered when a completely unknown sample is analyzed.

Since the accuracy of the automatic digestion unit is not always satisfactory, Berthelot (1969) recommends the digestion of a sample of organic material by the procedure shown below and the use of the automated system only for determining ammonia in aqueous solutions using the indophenol-blue reaction (Rommers and Visser, 1969). Figures obtained for

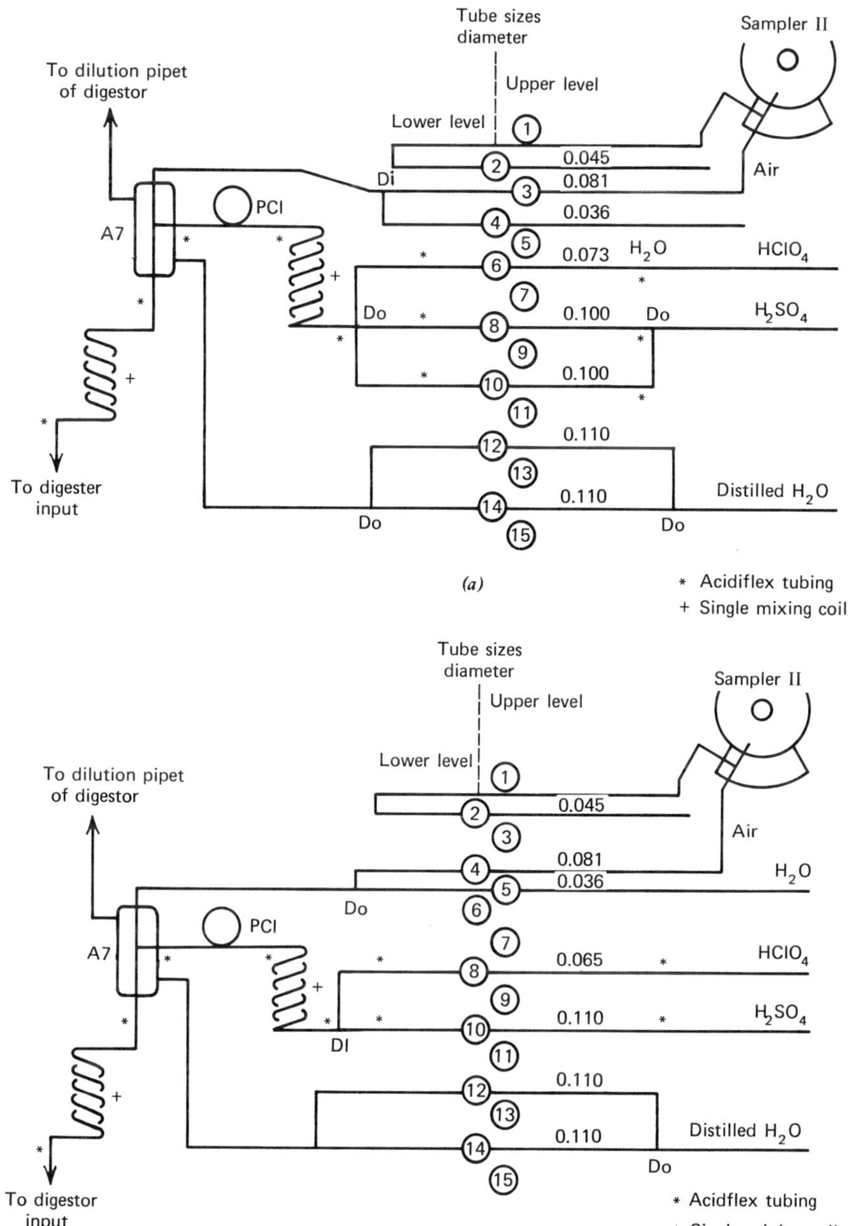

Figure 39. A flow diagram of a Nitrogen AutoAnalyzer (Davidson et al., 1970).

nitrogen determination in acid digests by the automated and the standard distillation procedures are in close agreement.

Reagents

Digestion mixture. a 90% solution of sulfuric acid containing 2% of perchloric acid (72%) and 0.02% *w/v* of selenium dioxide.

Mercury catalyst. 7% *w/v* solution of mercury sulfate in 10% *v/v* sulfuric acid.

Sodium hydroxide. 35% *w/v,* containing 4% *w/v* of EDTA disodium salt.

Alkaline sodium phenate. 486 g of phenol dissolved in water added to 1 liter of 40% *w/v* sodium hydroxide and made up to a total volume of 2 liters.

Sodium hypochlorite solution. 5% *w/v* aqueous solution of sodium hypochlorite is prepared by dilution of the 15 or 10% solution of sodium hypochlorite available commercially.

Procedure: A sample containing between 5 and 50 mg of nitrogen is placed in a 500-ml Pyrex Kjeldahl flask graduated at 550 ml. Three Kjeltabs M (Thomson and Capper, Liverpool), each containing 5 g of potassium sulfate and 0.25 g of mercury oxide, and 25 ml of concentrated sulfuric acid (sp. gr. 1.84), are then added. The mixture is heated carefully until white fumes appear and then it is boiled briskly for 2 hours.

Nitrogen Determination by Nessler's Reagent (Koch and McMeekin, 1924). Nitrogen is first converted to ammonium sulfate on digestion of a sample with sulfuric acid, as in the Elek and Sobotka's (1926) method; but the ammonia is detected and determined quantitatively by the reaction with Nessler's reagent, as a colored compound. The details of the technique follow.

Reagents

1. Concentrated sulfuric acid, analytical reagent grade, specified low in nitrogen.

2. 30% hydrogen peroxide.

3. Nessler's reagent, consisting of mercuric iodide and potassium iodide dissolved in a sodium hydroxide solution (the reagent is available commercially).

4. Ammonium sulfate nitrogen standard (Fisher's certified primary standard, No. A-938).

Procedure. Add 0.5 ml of reagent 1 to 1 to 2 ml volume of a sample, containing 20 to 300 μg of nitrogen, and digest the material under heat for 1 hour. Cool the mixture, add one drop of reagent 2 and digest for 20 minutes. Cool the tubes, add distilled water to the 35-ml mark, and add 15 ml of Nessler's reagent. Read the samples atfer 30 minutes, at 440-nm wavelenth.

Subtract the reading of the reagent blank from the reading of the standard and the unknown. Divide the corrected absorbency of the unknown by the corrected absorbency of the standard, and multiply the quotient by the nitrogen of the standard in milligrams.

2. *Phosphorus Determination*

The methods described below are generally equally sensitive and convenient, although according to our experience, Chen's et al. (1956) and Murkerje and SriRam's (1964) methods proved to be most suitable for the determination of phosphorus in different preparations of microbial antigen.

Phosphorus Determination by Chen's et al. (1956) Method:
Reagents

1. 6 N sulfuric acid, 1 volume, distilled water, 2 volumes, 2.5% ammonium molybdate, 1 volume, 10% ascorbic acid, to be prepared freshly each day. The 6 N sulfuric acid is prepared by diluting 18 ml of concentrated sulfuric acid to 108 ml with water.
2. Perchloric acid 72%.
3. Hydrogen peroxide 30%.
4. Trichloracetic acid 10%.

Procedure. A sample containing up to 8 gamma of phosphorus is placed into a graduated centrifuge tube and adjusted to the volume of 4 ml with distilled water. The reagent blank consists of 4 ml of distilled water. A phosphorus standard is tested in parallel. Pipette 4 ml of reagent 1 to each tube, cap with parafilm, mix, and place rack with all tubes in 37° for $1\frac{1}{2}$ to 2 hours. Cool the mixtures for a few minutes and read absorbance at 820 nm against the blank.

It is assumed that the content of P in deoxyribonucleic acid is 9.4% (Gulland et al., 1947).

Inorganic Phosphorus. Inorganic phosphorus is determined on the supernatant fluid obtained by the precipitation or proteins and nucleic acids with trichloracetic acid. The procedure is as follows: add 0.5 ml of a sample to 2 ml of 10% trichloracetic acid. Mix well, centrifuge, and collect the supernatant fluid. Use 0.5 ml of the liquid for the determination of phosphorus.

Organic phosphate is calculated by subtracting the value for inorganic phosphorus from the total phosphate.

Lipid Phosphorus. Extract the sample with alcohol-ether (3:1). Add 0.5 ml of the sample to 9.5 ml of alcohol-ether and place in a hot water bath at 80° until boiling occurs. Remove the tubes, cool them, and readjust to 10 ml with alcohol-ether. Ash 5 ml of filtrate or supernatant liquid or evaporate and ash the alcohol-ether extract (in case of lipid phosphorus) in the following manner. Add 4 drops of concentrated sulfuric acid and 2.0 ml of concentrated nitric acid to the sample if a protein containing material is used. Heat over a boiling bath until white fumes or sulfur dioxide appear. Add 2 drops of 72% perchloric acid to each tube and heat until the liquid becomes clear. After cooling, add distilled water, and adjust the volume to 25 ml in a volumetric flask. Take aliquots and determine absorbency at 820 nm.

The sensitivity of Chen's method is further enhanced by the following modification (Ames and Dubin, 1960). To a 0.3-ml sample of a hydrolyzate are added 0.7 ml of the following ascorbic acid-molybdate mixture: 10% ascorbic acid (1 part), 0.42% ammonium molybdate · H_2O (6 parts) in 1 N sulfuric acid.

*Total Phosphorus Determination (Murkerje and Sri-Ram, 1964):
Reagents*

1. 30% hydrogen peroxide.
2. 1.5 N H_2SO_4.
3. Acid molybdate reagent.

Procedure. Add 0.5 ml of 1.5 N H_2SO_4 and one drop of 30% hydrogen peroxide to 0.02 ml sample. Heat the reactants in a 120° air or oil bath until the water has evaporated and the residue turns dark. Add a second drop of hydrogen peroxide and continue to heat until the solution clears up and then turns dark. Repeat this process until the residue remains colorless. Add 1 ml of distilled water and cool to room temperature. Add 0.5 ml of the acid molybdate reagent; mix and add 0.5 ml of the reducing agent. Mix the reactants and allow to stand for 30 minutes. Read the color at 820 nm.

The blank contains 0.5 ml of 1.5 N sulfuric acid. Standards contain different amounts of phosphorus standard in 0.02 ml. The following calculation can be made:

$$\frac{\text{absorbance of unknown}}{\text{absorbance of standard}} \times 10 = \text{mg of total} \; \frac{P}{100} \; \text{ml}$$

$$\left(\text{mg total} \; \frac{P}{100} \; \text{ml} \right) - \left(\text{mg inorganic} \; \frac{P}{100} \; \text{ml} \right) = \text{mg organic}$$

$$\frac{P}{100} \; \text{ml mg organic} \; \frac{P}{100} \; \text{ml} \times 25 = \text{mg} \; \frac{\text{phospholipid}}{100} \; \text{ml}$$

The factor for conversion of inorganic phosphorus to phospholipid is derived from the composition of lecithin.

The P conversion factor for DNA is 9.4.

Total Phosphorus Estimation by Fiske and Subbarow's (1926) Method: Reagents

1. 10 N sulfuric acid (450 ml of concentrated sulfuric acid added to 1300 ml of distilled water).

2. Molybdate I: 2.5% ammonium molybdate in 5 N H_2SO_4 (25 g of ammonium molybdate dissolved in 200 ml of water + 500 ml of 5 M sulfuric acid).

3. Molybdate II: 2.5% ammonium molybdate in 3 N sulfuric acid, prepared as reagent 2 but with only 300 ml of 10 N sulfuric acid.

4. Molybdate III: 2.5% aqueous solution of ammonium molybdate.

5. 10% trichloracetic acid.

6. Standard phosphate (5 ml = 0.4 mg of phosphorus). Dissolve 0.350 g of pure monopotassium phosphate in water. Add 10 N sulfuric acid up to 1 liter in a volumetric flask.

7. 15% sodium bisulfite.

8. 20% sodium sulfite.

9. 0.25% 1, 2, 4-aminonaphtholsulfonic acid; dissolve 0.5 g of the substance in 195 ml of 15% sodium bisulfite, add 5 ml of 20% sodium sulfite.

Procedure. Boil a sample suspended in 2.5 ml of 10 N sulfuric acid until fumes appear, add 1 to 2 drops of concentrated nitric acid, and boil until no color remains. Transfer the contents of the flask quantitatively into a 50-ml volumetric flask with 35 ml of distilled water. Add 5 ml of molybdate III and 2 ml of the reagent 9. Dilute to the mark with water and read in a spectrophotometer at 820 nm.

With samples containing very small amounts of phosphorus use 0.5 ml of molybdate III and 0.2 ml of reagent 9, make up to 5-ml volume with 2 N sulfuric acid and heat in boiling water for 20 minutes.

Automated Method for Phosphate Estimation (Bide, 1969). The Auto-Analyzer system for the phosphate determination consists of a sampler, two proportioning pumps, a constant-temperature bath, digestor, and N-method colorimeter-recorder with a range expender (Fig. 40). The original paper of Bide (1969) must be consulted for the details of the procedure. The inorganic phosphate may be assayed by the automated Technicon N-4b method (Ferrari, 1960).

3. Protein Determination

Protein Determination by UV Absorbency Determination (Waddell, 1956). Absorption maximum for proteins is at about 280-nm wavelength; but a greater sensitivity, accuracy, and specificity of protein determination is attained by the use of absorption at 215 and 225 nm. Protein concentrations are derived from the differences between the absorbances at 215 and

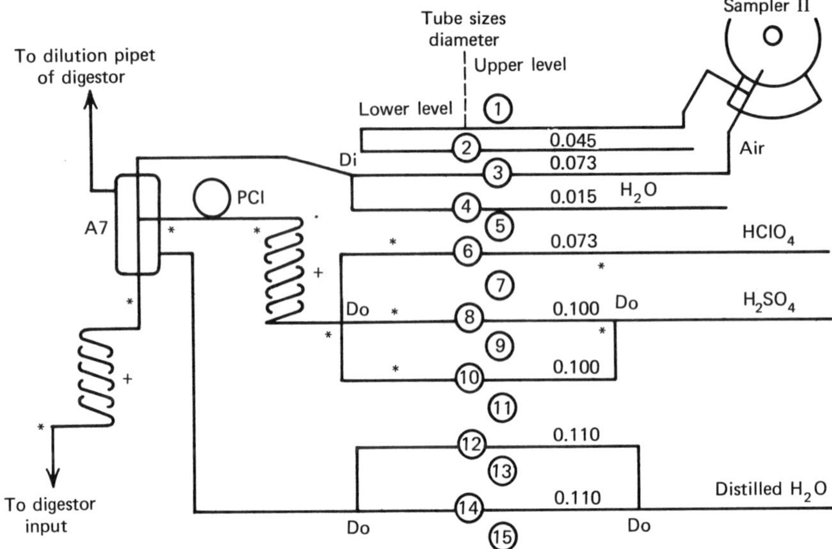

Figure 40. A flow diagram of a Phosphorus AutoAnalyzer (Bide, 1969).

225 nm. The absorption maximum exhibited by proteins in the region of 280 nm is due to the presence of aromatic amino acids, and the intensity of absorption depends on the proportions of these amino acids in the protein molecule. Proteins, however, differ considerably with regard to the absorptions in the spectral region, and nucleic acids and nucleotides interfere. An intense absorption at the spectral range between 200 and 250 nm depends mainly on the peptide bonds, but proteins differ among themselves in their absorption in this spectral region. The use of the difference between the absorbance at 225 and at 215 nm rather than the absorbance at a single wavelength minimize the error from nonprotein constituents of a material. The absorbance of a protein solution is measured at 215 and at 225 nm using diluent as the blank. If the absorbance at 215 nm exceeds 1.5, the protein solution is further diluted. The absorbance at 225 nm is subtracted from that of 215 nm. The difference is multiplied by 155 giving the protein concentration in the diluted solution expressed in milligrams per milliliter.

If proteins occur together with the nucleic acids, the absorption can be measured at 280 and 260 nm, and the concentration of proteins or nucleic acids is determined either from a monogram (Warburg and Christian, 1942), or by applying a conversion factor (Table 27). Ultraviolet absorbancy is the most rapid and simplest of all assays but it is most prone to errors due to the contamination with nonprotein material.

Colorimetric Protein Determination (Inchiosa, 1964): Reagent

$KNaC_4H_4O_6 \cdot 4H_2O$	12 g
1 N NaOH	200 ml
Potassium iodide (KI)	5 g
Distilled water	1000 ml

Procedure. Add 5 ml of the reagent to 5 ml of a protein material. Allow to stand for 30 minutes to solubilize proteins. Measure turbidity (in the Klett colorimeter against water as the blank using No. 54 filter or using a spectrophotometer). Add 0.15 ml of 5% $CuSO_4 \cdot 5H_2O$/5 ml of sample. Leave the tubes at room temperature for 30 minutes. Read the absorbance as before. The blank consists of equal parts of water and reagent, and a standard is prepared from a crystalline bovine albumin.

Protein nitrogen of an unknown sample is calculated from the colorimeter readings, according to the following equation, which refers to an analysis of final sample volume in the colorimeter tube of 5.0 ml:

$$\text{protein N} =$$

$$\left[\left(\text{unknown final reading} \right) - \left(\text{turbidity} \times \frac{5.00}{5.15} \right) - \text{reagent blank} \right]$$

$$\times \frac{\text{N of standard}}{\text{standard final reading-reagent blank}}$$

The factor 5.00/5.15 in the formula corrects the initial turbidity reading for the amount of dilution of the sample by addition of 0.15 ml of $CuSO_4$ solution.

Biuret assay is less sensitive than Folin-Cicocalteu and ninhydrin, but it is precise.

Colorimetric Determination of Protein by Lowry's et al. (1951) Method: Reagents

1. 2% Na_2CO_3 in 0.1 N NaOH.
2. 0.5% $CuSO_4 \cdot 5H_2O$ in 1% sodium tartrate. Mix 1 ml of the reagent 1 with 50 ml of reagent 2 just before use.
3. Folin reagent, prepared according to Folin and Ciocalteu (1927). This reagent is also available commercially.

Procedure. Add 1 ml of mixed reagent 1 plus 2 to 0.2 ml of test material containing 1 to 5 μg of nitrogen, leave for 10 minutes at room temperature, add 0.1 ml of Folin reagent, previously titrated to phenolphthalein and diluted to an acidity of 1 N. Mix vigorously and read the solution, after 30 minutes, in a spectrophotometer at 750 nm.

Table 27. Conversion factors for Protein Estimation by Ultraviolet Absorption

Ratio 280/260	% Nucleic Acid	B_{280}	Factor for 1.0 cm Cell at 280 (Factor $\times$ O.D.$_{280}$ = mg/cc)
1.75	0	2.08	1.10
1.60	0.25	2.14	1.07
1.50	0.50	2.19	1.05
1.40	0.75	2.25	1.02
1.30	1.00	2.31	0.99
1.25	1.25	2.36	0.97
1.20	1.50	2.42	0.95
1.15	2.00	2.53	0.91
1.10	2.50	2.65	0.87
1.05	3.00	2.76	0.83
1.00	3.50	2.87	0.80
0.96	3.75	2.93	0.78
0.92	4.25	3.05	0.75
0.88	5.00	3.22	0.71
0.86	5.25	3.27	0.70
0.84	5.50	3.33	0.69
0.82	6.00	3.44	0.67
0.80	6.50	3.56	0.64
0.78	7.25	3.73	0.61
0.76	8.00	3.90	0.59
0.74	8.75	4.07	0.56
0.72	9.50	4.24	0.54
0.70	10.75	4.52	0.51
0.68	12.0	4.80	0.48
0.66	13.5	5.14	0.45
0.65	14.5	5.37	0.43
0.64	15.25	5.54	0.41
0.62	17.5	6.05	0.38
0.60	20.0	6.62	0.35
0.49	100	24.8 (n.a.)	

Biuret Test (Ditterbrandt, 1948). Biuret reagent is prepared as follows. Dissolve 9.0 g of sodium potassium tartrate in 400 ml of 0.2 N NaOH; add 3.00 g of $CuSO_4 \cdot H_2O$ of potassium iodide, make up to 1 liter with a CO_2-free 0.2 N NaOH.

Procedure. Add 1.5 ml of Biuret reagent to a 1.0-ml sample (20 to 400 μg of protein nitrogen), standards and blanks, incubate at 37° for 30 minutes, read at 550 nm in a spectrophotometer.

Ninhydrin Method (Kunkel and Ward, 1950).

1. Ninhydrin reagent: 0.4 g of ninhydrin in 12.5 ml of ethylene glycol monomethyl ether and 40 ml of $SnCl_2 \cdot 2H_2O$ dissolved in 25 ml of citrate buffer. Cirtate buffer, 0.2 M, pH 5.0, contains 2.101 g of citric acid monohydrate and 20 ml of $N/1$ MaOH made up to 100 ml.

2. Diluent consisting of equal volumes of *n*-propanol and distilled water.

Procedure. Add 0.5 ml of ninhydrin reagent to 0.1-ml sample (1 to 20 μg of nitrogen) and blanks, heat in boiling water for 20 minutes. Add 2.0 ml of the diluent, mix. Clarify by centrifugation if necessary. Read at 570 nm wavelengths.

4. Saccharide Determination

Determination of total sugars by Dische's (1955) Method. The test depends on the spectrophotometric determination of ultraviolet-absorbing chromogens (furfuraldehyde, crotonaldehyde), which evolve on a reaction of carbohydrates with α-naphthol in strong sulfuric acid.

Reagents

1. Sulfuric acid, 89 volume %.
2. 2% alcoholic solution of α-naphthol, freshly prepared.

Procedure. Add 4.5 ml of 89% sulfuric acid to 0.5 ml of the test material solution (5 to 25 mg of sugar). Set up a water blank and standard sugar control simultaneously. Heat the tubes in boiling water for 3 minutes, cool, add 0.2 ml of reagent 2, and shake.

A red color develops in the presence of hexoses, pentoses, and methylpentoses. The reaction can be evaluated qualitatively, or quantitatively by a reading made after 6 hours, in a spectrophotometer at a suitable wavelength. Absorption maxima are: hexose at 570 nm, pentose at 550 nm, and heptose at 560 nm wavelength.

Determination of Total Sugars and Related Substances (Dubois et al., 1956): Reagents

1. 80% phenol by weight, prepared by adding 20 g of glass distilled water to 80 g of redistilled phenol.
2. Sulfuric acid (concentrated).

Procedure. Samples (5 to 25 mg) containing sugars must be hydrolyzed with 2 N HCl (5 ml) at 100° for 3 hours, filtered and dried at 45°. The residue is deionized by passage through a small column of Dowex X_4, CH_3COO^- form, 100–200 mesh and then through a Dowex X_4H^+ form, column (Lopes and Inniss, 1970). A similar and normally satisfactory technique calls for the evaporation of HCl, after the hydrolysis, over a boiling water bath, and dissolving the pellet quantitatively in distilled water.

A 2 ml of a solution (containing between 10 and 70 gamma of sugar) or a water blank is mixed with 0.05 ml of 80% phenol and 5 ml of concentrated sulfuric acid. Alternatively, 1 or 2 ml of a sugar solution, 1 ml of 5% phenol in water, and 5 ml of concentrated sulfuric acid are employed. The tubes are allowed to stand for 10 minutes at room temperature and for 10 to 20 minutes at 25 to 30°. Absorbance is determined by measuring the characteristic yellow-orange color at 490 nm for hexoses and at 480 nm for pentoses and uronic acids. The amount of sugar is estimated by reference to a standard curve prepared for an individual saccharide type or group occurring in the examined sample. All solutions should be prepared in triplicate to minimize errors, resulting from accidental contamination with cellulose or lint. The absorbance is a dimensionless ration equal to:

$$\log_{10} \frac{T \text{ solvent}}{T \text{ solution}}$$

where T is the transmittance.

The absorbance maximum for pentoses, methyl pentoses, and uronic acids is at 480 nm, for hexoses and methyl hexoses 485 to 490 nm. Some methylated pentoses and their methyl glycosides show selective absorption between 415 and 420 nm.

Anthrone Reaction for Total Hexoses. This reaction, originally devised by Dreywood (1946), and modified by Trevelyan and Harrison (1952) and Fairbairn (1953), is carried out as follows.

The reagent consists of 0.1% solution of purified anthrone in 72% sulfuric acid. The 72% sulfuric acid is prepared by diluting 760 ml concentrated sulfuric acid, sp. gr. 1.84, with distilled water, made up to 1000 ml. Anthrone is purified by Gilman and Blatt's (1941) technique.

Pipette 10 ml of anthrone reagent to a number of tubes kept in a water bath at 10 to 15°. Layer a 5-ml sample (50 to 250 μg of carbohydrate) above the reagent. Set up, simultaneously, blanks and glucose or dextran standards. Shake each mixture vigorously, heat at 100° for 12 minutes, cool, and read the blue color at 625 nm wavelength.

Submicromethod for Determination of Reducing Substances. The assay (Park and Johnson, 1949) depends on the formation of Prussian blue (ferric ferrocyanide) from ferricyanide in the presence of reducing saccharides.

Reagents

Solution I, 0.05% potassium ferricyanide.

Solution II, containing 5.3 g of sodium carbonate and 0.65 g of KCN per liter.

Solution III, containing 1.5 g of ferric ammonium sulfate, 1 mg of Duponol "ME dry" in 1 liter 0.05 N H_2SO_4.

Procedure (Slightly Modified by Carsten, cf. Kabat, 1961). To 1-ml sample add 0.25 ml of solution I and 1.0 ml of solution II and heat in boiling water bath for 15 minutes. Cool rapidly and add 2.5 ml of solution III. Make up to 5-ml volume in one 5-ml Pyrex volumetric flask, mix, and read after 15 minutes at 690 nm in a spectrophotometer. A standard solution of glucose or other reducing sugar is set in parallel. The test is very sensitive, the range of the method being 1 to 9 μg of glucose in a 1 to 3 ml sample.

Heptose Determination. According to Osborn's (1963) modification of Dische's (1953) method, heptoses are determined as follows.

To two samples (0.5 ml) containing heptose, add slowly 2.25 ml of dilute sulfuric acid. Shake in the cold for 3 minutes. Transfer the tubes to 20° water bath for 3 minutes, and to a boiling water bath for exactly 10 minutes. Cool and add 0.05 ml of 3% cysteine-HCl to one sample, the other sample serving as blank. After exactly 2 hours, read absorbances at 505 and 545 nm. Correct for nonspecific absorbance in the blank, which has not received cysteine solution.

Reagents

1. Dilute sulfuric acid: 6 volumes of concentrated sulfuric acid and 1 volume of distilled water.

2. 3% aqueous cysteine-HCl solution.

Hexosamine Determination. Hydrolyzates for the hexosamine determination are prepared according to the following procedure (Boas, 1953). The sample (5–10 mg) is suspended in 3 N HCl (2 ml), sealed in an evacuated ampule and heated at 100° for 9 to 10 hours. The hydrolyzate is evaporated to dryness, dissolved in distilled water (1 ml), adjusted to pH 1.0 with 1 N HCl, and filtered through a small column of Dowex 50W, X_4, H^+ form, 100–200 mesh. The column is first washed with distilled water, and the hexosamine is eluted with 0.5 N HCl (Lopes and Inniss, 1970).

Hexosamine Determination by Elson and Morgan's (1933) Method, as modified by Belcher et al. (1954):

Reagents

1. Acetyloacetone solution: 0.2 ml of acetyloacetone dissolved in 10 ml of $N/2$ Na_2CO_3 immediately before use.

2. Aldehyde-free absolute ethyl alcohol.

3. Ehrlich's reagent, containing 0.8 g of *p*-dimethylaminobenzaldhyde, 30 ml of absolute alcohol, and 30 ml of concentrated hydrochloric acid. This solution can be stored in a refrigerator for up to a week.

Procedure. Hydrolize solutions of samples with 2 to 4 N HCl for 2 hours, centrifuge, evaporate supernatants to dryness in a vacuum desiccator over phosphorus pentoxide and NaOH pellets.

Add 1.0-ml amounts of acetyloacetone solution from a 1.0-ml analytical pipette to the hydrolized samples, as well as to blanks and the standard solutions containing 10 to 100 μg of glucosamine hydrochloride, stopper the flasks, and place them in boiling water for 30 minutes. Cool flasks to room temperature, add 3 ml of absolute alcohol, mix vigorously, leave in a water bath at 37° for 30 minutes, cool, and read in a spectrophotometer at 540 nm.

N-Acetyl Hexosamine Determination. According to the principle of this test (Reissig et al., 1955), *N*-acetyl hexosamines react with *p*-dimethylamidobenzaldehyde in a sodium carbonate solution on heating, producing a chromogen, the intensity of which intensity is determined at 544- or 585-nm wavelength.

Reagents

1. Potassium tetraborate solution: 24.7 g of boric acid and 9 g of potassium hydroxide are dissolved in 500 ml of distilled water adjusted to pH 9.1 with a potassium hydroxide solution and made up to 1 liter (pH 8.9 when diluted sixfold).

2. p-dimethylamidobenzaldehyde solution: 10 g dissolved in 100 ml of glacial acetic acid, containing 12.5% (v/v) 10 *N* HCl. Dilute the reagent with 9 volumes of glacial acetic acid before use.

Procedure. Add 0.05 ml of the potassium tetraborate solution to 0.25-ml volume of the sample, standards containing between 1 and 10 μg of *N*-acetylglucosamine and blanks containing distilled water. Heat the solutions for exactly 3 minutes in a boiling water bath and cool them in tap water. Add 1.5 ml of the *p*-dimethylamidobenzaldehyde solution, mix the contents and place the tubes in a water bath at 37° for 20 minutes. Cool the solution in tap water and read immediately in the spectrophotometer at 544 or 585 nm wavelength.

$$N\text{-acethylhexosamine} \times 1.238 = \text{hexosamine}$$

Glucosamine may be differentiated from other hexosamines by Lüdowieg and Bennaman's (1967) technique.

Pentose Estimation (Mejbaum, 1939). Hydrolyze the polysaccharide preparation in 1 *N* HCl in a boiling water bath for 5 hours; centrifuge the hydrolyzate and neutralize it with 1 *N* NaOH.

Reagents

1. 5% orcinol solution in 96% ethyl alcohol.
2. 0.02% $FeCl_3$ solution in concentrated hydrochloric acid.

Procedure. Add 0.5 ml of orcinol solution and 5 ml of $FeCl_3$ solution to 1-ml samples of neutralized hydrolyzate of a polysaccharide. Heat in boiling water for 20 minutes; cool. Measure the intensity of green color in a colorimeter at 670 nm.

Pentose Determination by Cysteine-Sulfuric Acid Method (Dische, 1949). Add 4 ml of concentrated sulfuric acid to 1 ml of the test material (10 to 50 μg of pentose); shake the mixture for 1 hour at room temperature. Add 0.1 ml of 3% aqueous cysteine-HCl solution and mix. After 10 to 30 minutes measure the color extinction in a spectrophotometer. Pentoses are determined by the differences between D_{390} and D_{424}. Pentoses can be determined by this procedure even in the presence of hexoses and methylpentoses.

Methylpentose Determination (Dische and Shettles, 1948). The method relies on the observation that methylpentose has no absorption at 430 nm whereas hexoses, pentoses, and uronic acids have symmetrical absorption curves such that their absorption at 430 and 396 nm is the same. Therefore, subtraction of the first value from the last value corrects for all absorption except that due to methyl pentose.

Reagents

1. Sulfuric acid: Concentrated sulfuric acid (6 parts) and distilled water (1 volume).
2. 3% aqueous solution of cysteine hydrochloride.

Procedure. Add 4.5 ml of cold sulfuric acid solution to 1 ml of an ice-cold sample solution (containing 3 to 10 μg of methyl pentose) with constant shaking in an ice bath. Transfer the tubes to a boiling water bath for 3 minutes, and then transfer them into a room temperature bath. Add 0.1 ml of cysteine hydrochloride solution, mix the liquids, and leave them at room temperature for 2 hours. Measure the absorption at 396 and 430 nm. The difference between these two estimates is proportional to methyl pentose content of the solutions.

In some instances, heating of the samples in a boiling water bath for 10 minutes rather than 3 minutes is advantageous.

Rhamnose and fucose produce equal color intensities.

A modification of Dische and Shettles' method has been published by Gibbons (1955).

5. Uronic Acid Determination

The test depends on a reaction between uronic acids and carbazole to form colored furan derivatives.

Reagents

1. 0.1% carbazole solution in 95% ethyl alcohol; carbazole (Eastman-Kodak) must be recrystallized twice from benzene.

2. Acid-buffer mixture, made of 19.5 volume of concentrated sulfuric acid and 0.5 volume of 1 *M,* pH 9. sodium tetraborate.

Procedure.   To 0.7 ml volume of a sample add 6.0 ml of the reagent 2. Heat the mixture in a boiling water bath for 15 minutes. Cool the mixture in tap water. Add 0.2 ml of 0.1% carbazole solution. Heat the mixture in a boiling water bath for 10 minutes. Cool the liquid and measure the color at 530 nm against a blank containing 0.7 ml distilled water and processed as the test sample.

6.   *N-acetylneuraminic Acid Determination*
i.   *Warren's (1959) Method*
Reagents

1. Sodium meta periodate 0.2 *M,* in 9 *M* phosphoric acid.
2. Sodium arsenite, 10%, in a solution of 0.5 *M* sodium sulfate and 0.1 *N* H_2SO_4.
3. Thiobarbituric acid, 0.5%, in 0.5 *M* sodium sulfate solution.
4. Cyclohexanone.

Procedure.   The 0.2 ml of a sample containing up to 0.05 μ mole of N-acetylneuraminic acid is added to 0.1 ml of the periodate solution, shaken, and left at room temperature for 20 minutes; 1.0 ml of the sodium arsenite solution is then added and shaken until a yellow-brown color disappears; 3.0 ml of the thiobarbituric acid solution is finally added, shaken, capped with a glass bead, and left in a boiling water bath for 15 minutes, then removed, and placed in cold water for 15 minutes.

A 1.0 ml sample of this solution should be transferred into a tube containing 1.0 ml of cyclohexanone. Alternatively, the entire 4.3 ml volume of the aqueous solution may be extracted with an equal volume of cyclohexanone.

Shake twice, centrifuge 3 minutes, collect the upper (red) cyclohexanone phase. Optical density is to be determined at 549 nm.

The molecular extinction coefficient is 57,000. The amount of N-acetylneuraminic acid present in a given sample can be estimated from the equation:

$$\frac{V \times \text{O.D. } 549}{57} = \frac{4.3 \times \text{O.D. } 549}{57} = 0.075 \times \text{O.D. } 549$$

where *V* is the final volume of the test solution.

Another useful method of the sialic acid determination was published by Barry et al. (1962).

ii. *N-acetylneuraminic Acid Determination by Aminoff's (1961) Method*
Reagents

1. 25 mM-periodic acid in 0.125 N H_2SO_4 (pH 1.2).
2. 2% sodium arsenite in 0.5 N HCl.
3. 0.1 M 2-thiobarbituric acid in distilled water, adjusted to pH 9.0 with 0.1 M NaOH (to be kept in a dark bottle at 4°).
4. Acid butanol: Butan-1-ol containing 5% of 12 N HCl.

Procedure. To a sample (0.5 ml) add 0.25 ml of the periodate reagent and heat it at 37° for 30 minutes. Reduce the excess of periodate with 0.2 ml of the reagent 2. Add 2 ml of reagent 3 after 1 to 2 minutes. Heat the solution in a boiling water bath for 7.5 minutes. Cool the colored solution in ice-water. Add 5 ml of acid butanol and shake. The separation of two phases is expedited by a short rapid centrifugation. Collect the butanol-layer. Measure the intensity of the color at 549 mn. The color extinction is directly proportional to the concentration of N-acetylneuraminic acid, read from a standard curve. N-acetylglucosamine, glucosamine, ribose do not give a color under the test's conditions. Deoxyribose reacts and gives intense color at 532 nm.

7. *2-Keto-3-deoxyoctonate Determination.* The sample to test for the presence of 2-keto-3-deoxyoctonate must be hydrolyzed with 0.2 N H_2SO_4 at 100° for 15 minutes and then tested with Aminoff's reagent.

8. *Acetyl-Group Determination*
Reagents

1. 0.35 M Hydroxylamine HCl.
2. 1.5 M Sodium hydroxide.
3. Alkaline hydroxylamine: 0.35 M hydroxylamine HCl (1 part), 1.5 M NaOH (1 part).
4. 0.75 M perchloric acid.
5. Ferric-perchloric acid solution: a mixture of 1.9 g of $FeCl_3 \cdot 6H_2O$ in 5 ml of concentrated HCl, and 5 ml of 70% perchloric acid is evaporated to dryness and diluted to 100 ml with distilled water.
6. The reagent for acetylation, prepared by absorbing dry HCl into refrigerated absolute ethanol. A 2-M solution is then prepared by titration of the above solution with standard alkali.

Procedure. A sample (containing 1.0 to 10 micromoles of acetyl) is first evaporated to dryness in a vacuum dessicator over anhydrous $CaCl_2$ by use of an oil pump. Add 0.5 ml of 2 N HCl-methanol solution to the dry sample. Cool the mixture for a few seconds with a mixture of solid CO_2methanol and seal the ampoule containing the material with an oxygen torch. Heat the tube at 100° for 4 hours.

The deacetylation tube is then opened and placed in a chamber of a glass-distillation apparatus and evacuated to 30 mm Hg, at 35 to 45°, for 20 to 40 minutes.

After the distillation, methyl acetate is determined in the collected distillate in the following manner: add 1.0 ml of distilled water and 2.0 ml of alkaline hydroxylamine solution. Shake the tube: leave it at room temperature for 10 minutes. Add 2.0 ml of 0.75 M perchloric acid and 1.0 ml of ferric perchloric acid solution. Read the color in 5 to 10 minutes at 520 nm. The quantity of methyl acetate is estimated by comparison with ethyl acetate standards.

9. *Deoxyribonucleic-Acid Determination*

Deoxyribonucleic Acid Determination by Burton's (1956) Modification of Dische's (1930) Method: Reagent. The 1.5 g diphenylamine in dissolved in 100 ml of glacial acetic acid, mixed with 1.5 ml of concentrated sulfuric acid; and 0.5 ml of an aqueous solution of acetylaldehyde (16 mg/ml) on the day the reagent is to be used.

Procedure. Dissolve the material being examined in 0.5 M perchloric acid. (An extract in 5% TCA may also be used; perchloric acid should be added to the extract, to 0.5% concentration.)

Add 2 ml of diphenylamine reagent to 1 ml of a solution of the test material. Heat at 30° for 16 to 20 hours. Read the blue color at 600 nm.

Interference by salts and reagents is minimized by precipitation of nucleic acid with cadium as follows: 1 to 10 ml volume of a solution containing 20 to 200 μg of nucleic acid per milliliter is added to sufficient volume of a 1 M $CdCl_2$ to attain 0.2 to 1 M final concentration of cadium. The liquid is adjusted to pH between 4 and 9. The mixtures are allowed to stand for 5 to 10 minutes at 40° and then centrifuged. The supernatant is discarded, and the precipitate is washed twice with 3 ml of 0.1 M $CdCl_2$. The precipitate can be used for RNA and DNA determination directly or after hydrolysis in 0.1 N HCl at 90° for 20 minutes.

DNA Determination by DeDeken-Grenson and DeDeken's (1959) Method. A deoxyribonucleic acid preparation is dissolved in 5% perchloric acid and heated for 20 minutes at 37°. The hydrolyzate is diluted with 5% perchloric acid to a suitable concentration for spectrophotometry and measured at 267 nm. A conversion factor of 32.94, estimated on the basis of 9.22% phosphorus content in DNA (Chargaff, 1955) is used for the following calculation:

$$\text{O.D. at 267 nm} \times 32.94 = \mu\text{g deoxyribonucleic acid per milliliter}$$

DNA Determination by Dische (1944), as Modified by Stumpf (1947):
Reagents

1. 5% aqueous solution of cysteine hydrochloride.
2. 70% sulfuric acid.

Procedure. To 0.1 to 0.5 ml of the RNA solution add 0.05 ml of 5% cysteine hydrochloride solution and 5.0 ml of 70% sulfuric acid. Leave the mixture for 10 to 15 minutes at room temperature. Read the developing pink color at 490 nm in a spectrophotometer.

10. Ribonucleic-Acid Determination

RNA Determination by Hatcher and Goldstein's (1969) Method:
Reagent

1. 2 g of orcinol (5-methylresorcinol), recrystallized from benzene is dissolved in 35 ml of ethanol and diluted to 50 ml with *n*-butanol.
2. 0.5 g of ferric chloride, dissolved in 100 ml of concentrated hydrochloric acid.

Procedure. 1.0 ml of the orcinol reagent 1, mixed with 3.0 ml of the ferric chloride reagent 2 is added to 1.0 ml of a dialyzed hydrolyzate of nucleic acid. After heating at 90° in a water bath for 30 minutes, the solutions are cooled to room temperature, diluted as necessary, and the absorbance is measured against an appropriate reagent blank at 660 nm.

11. Cholesterol Determination
Reagents

1. Absolute alcohol, redistilled.
2. Petroleum ether, redistilled.
3. Acetic acid.
4. Sulfuric acid.
5. Acetic anhydride, free from HCl.
6. 33% potassium hydroxide.
7. Alcoholic KOH solution, prepared by adding 6 ml of 33% KOH to 94 ml of absolute alcohol.
8. Cholesterol standard: 0.4 mg/ml in absolute alcohol.
9. Modified Liebermann-Burchard reagent: 20 volumes of acetic anhydride, chilled below 10°, 1 volume of concentrated sulfuric acid, kept in cold, 10 volumes of glacial acetic acid added and the mixture is warmed to room temperature (to be used within 1 hour).

Procedure. To 5 ml sample add 5 ml of alcoholic KOH and heat the mixture at 37 to 40° for 55 minutes. Cool at room temperature, add 10 ml of petroleum ether, mix; add 5 ml of distilled water, shake vigorously for

1 minute. Centrifuge at slow speed for 5 minutes, until the emulsion breaks to form two layers.

Transfer an aliquot of the petroleum ether layer to a small dry bottle. Evaporate petroleum ether in a water bath at 60° by blowing air stream into the tube. Cool to room temperature. Add 6 ml of the modified Liebermann-Burchard reagent. Cork the bottles and leave them in a 25° water bath for 30 to 35 minutes. Read the optical density at 620 nm.

The optical density equivalent to 1 mg of cholesterol is calculated from the reading of the standards as follows:

$$\frac{\text{optical density of standard}}{\text{mg cholesterol in standard}} = S$$

and applying the following equation:

$$\frac{\text{mg cholesterol}}{100 \text{ ml}} = \frac{\text{O.D. of unknown}}{S} \times \frac{10}{\text{volume petroleum ether aliquot}}$$
$$\times \frac{100}{\text{volume sample}}$$

The blank consists of 6 ml of color reagent.

Standard solutions of cholesterol contain dilutions of the original amount of 0.4 mg/ml cholesterol, which are mixed with 0.3 ml of 33% potassium hydroxide solution, incubated at 37 to 40° for 55 minutes, and then extracted with petroleum ether and further processed as the test sample.

12. Procedures for Hydrolysis and Concentration of Antigen Preparations

i. *Method for Obtaining Acid Hydrolyzates.* Suspend 5 to 50 mg of a material in 0.5 to 1 ml of distilled water and add an equal volume of reagent grade concentrated HCl to obtain final 6 N HCl solution, in a 5-ml ampoule. Place the ampoule in a dry ice-alcohol bath until the liquid solidifies. Attach the ampoule to a high-vacuum pump and evacuate it to 50 μ Hg of pressure or less. After a full evacuation of that ampoule, lift it from the dry ice-alcohol bath and seal off the ampoule at the narrow neck with a pin-point oxygen gas flame. Place the ampoule at 110° for 24 to 48 hours, preferably in a mechanical forced draft recirculating oven.

Any precipitate visible after the hydrolysis must be removed by centrifugation. Remove the HCl evaporating the liquid to dryness, over NaOH pellets in a vacuum dessicator, while the ampoule has been placed inclined at about 15° from the horizontal. Evaporation of a larger volume of liquid can be attained in a rotary evaporator.

ii. *Basic Hydrolysis of Peptides, Polypeptides, and Proteins.* Basic hydrolysis is conducted by heating the material with 76 mg of $Ba(OH)_2 \cdot$

H₂O in 0.5 ml of water at 112° for 22 hours in evacuated sealed tubes. The barium is then precipitated with carbon dioxide, and the precipitate is washed with a small volume of water (Gold and Blackman, 1970).

iii. *Enzymatic Digestion of Peptides.* The digestion is carried out in 0.1 *M* *N*-ethylmorpholine-acetic acid buffer at 30°. The pH values for different enzymes are as follows: pH 8.0 for alpha chymotrypsin and pronase, pH 7.5 for carboxypeptidase and aminopeptidase. Concentration of the enzyme and times of digestion have to be worked out for individual experiment.

Tryptic digestion is accomplished satisfactorily by the following procedure (Smyth, 1967): diphenylcarbonyl chloride treated trypsin, dissolved in 2 *M* urea, is added to a protein solution in the proportion of 0.09 mg/ml of trypsin per 5 mg/ml of protein. The digestion is carried out at 28° for 2 hours while the pH is maintained at 8 by periodic addition of dilute ammonia (Gold and Blackman, 1970).

iv. *Concentration of Antigen Preparations.* Dissolved antigen preparations may be concentrated by: freeze-drying (lyophilization), pervaporation, ultrafiltration, evaporation with a nitrogen stream, or by the exposure to hydroscopic materials, for example, Carbowax, pyrollidone, and Sephadex G-200. Selection of a suitable method depends on the heat stability, molecular size, and general chemical nature of the antigen. Heat-sensitive materials should be concentrated by the lyophilization, ultrafiltration, electrodialysis, or by the exposure to dry Sephadex G-200, in the cold. Some of these methods, and particularly the freeze drying occasionally causes insolubility of a lyophilized material. Sephadex G-200 often proves to be a satisfactory simple agent for the concentration of various materials. The antigen solution is placed in dialysis tubing and immersed in dry Sephadex G-200 granules. This method often proves to be superior to the freeze drying and concentration-dialysis against polyvinyl pyrrolidone or polyethylene glycol since the recovery of antigenic material is much higher than by the other methods (Birkbeck and Stephen, 1970).

Concentration of Proteins. Drying of proteins from the frozen state *in vacuo* sometimes causes a denaturation of complexes of proteins with lipids on freezing and drying. If the material has not been properly dialyzed, the lyophilization causes considerable increase in salt concentration.

An alternative method for concentrating protein solution is the removal of water by dialysis of the protein solution against concentrated solutions of dextran or polyethylene glycol, or by absorption of the water by shaking the protein solution with dispersed, cross-linked dextran (Sephadex). Removal of the water with Sephadex sometimes causes considerable loss of trace proteins by absorption on the gel particles.

A more efficient method for concentration of proteins is Curtain's (1964) method utilizing rods of dried hydrophilic gel to remove the water under a constant ionic strength maintained. The rods are prepared by polymerizing an aqueous solution containing 15.2 g/100 ml acrylamide and 0.8 g/100 ml *N, N*-methylenebisacrylamide. The polymerization is initiated by adding 0.4 g of ammonium persulfate and 0.2 ml of dimethylaminopropionitrile to each 100 ml of the monomer solution. The rods are then produced in the silicone-coated glass tubes. The coating is accomplished by dipping glass tubes in undiluted Dri-film chlorosilane for 30 seconds. The gel rods are removed from the tubes by pushing with a close fitting glass rod and are washed with distilled water for 48 to 72 hours with changes of water every 6 hours. The gel slabs are cut into convenient lengths and dried to 20% of their original diameter with a cool air at 4°. The rods may be kept indefinitely in a dessicator over phosphorus pentoxide. For concentration of protein solutions, the dry rod is dipped in the solution held in a test tube. A tenfold concentration may be obtained by this technique within a few hours.

13. *Statistical Analysis and Interpretation of Data*

Data obtained by the immunochemical tests must be properly recorded, organized, analyzed, and interpreted before logical conclusions can be drawn. Numerical data, collected from the measurements and counts, are first organized and presented in the form of tables and graphs. Relevant information is extracted from the organized measurements and figures by a statistical analysis of data.

A statistical analysis of immunochemical data depends on determination of the mean, the median, the range, and the standard deviation as well as the association coefficients. The association coefficients are frequently utilized for a statistical interpretation of data, since the similarity coefficients may be compared and statistically evaluated.

Larger volumes of immunological data are processed with the aid of a computer, applying arithmetic methods to classify the antigens and their sources on the basis of overall similarity to one another. Reactions of antigens with an antiserum are encoded on the corresponding intersections by the numeral symbol 2, whereas the lack of interaction is expressed by the numerical symbol 1. Provisions are also made for an occasional lack and undecided information, recorded as no answer. The numerical data are then fed into a computer together with a suitable program, such as Warburton's (1967) VA 310 program. The encoded immunological characters are compared and the shared and nonshared attributes of pairs of processed antigen preparations are counted. The overall similarity or affinity between each antigen-pair is determined, and the numerical ratio of similar characters to the total characters is compared and expressed numerically in the form of a similarity index (similarity score and similarity percentage). Affinities between different antigens are often evident in the data provided by the computer. Alternatively, the similarity coefficients produced by the computer are arranged, somewhat arbitrarily, in a decreasing order starting with the pairs of antigens which showed the highest similarity coefficient and ending with the lowest value. From the affinity table thus produced, groups of closely related antigens (strains) are depicted by maximizing the similarities of antigens enclosed in a group and minimizing possible intercluster similarities (Lessel and Holt, 1970).

The most sophisticated analysis of the affinities depends on a mathematical extraction of variables from the data, that is, printing of selected portions of the data (Seal, 1964; Quadling, 1967). The derived variables or dimensions are then arranged in order of relative importance, or may be plotted in a two- or three-dimensional diagram.

Relationships between the processed antigen preparations can be represented by a simple, two-dimensional table, in case of a relatively small amount of characters. A great volume of the computed data ought to be summarized, and presented graphically as a shaded similarity gradient or matrix. Presentation of the summarized affinities in the form of a bar diagram or a dendogram is less appropriate.

14. Buffers

Borate Buffered Saline, pH 7.3

NaCl	8.5	g
Boric acid	1.94	g
Sodium borate (borax)	1.9	g
Distilled water to	1	liter

Phosphate Buffered Saline (PBS)

Solution A: $NaH_2PO_4 \cdot H_2O$, 27.6 g/liter.
Solution B: $Na_2HPO_4 \cdot 12H_2O$, 71.63 g/liter and 8.5 g of NaCl per liter.

0.01 M Phosphate in Saline, pH 7.0

16.5 ml of solution A.
33.5 ml of solution B.
8.5 g of NaCl.
Distilled water to 1 liter.

0.02 M phosphate in saline, pH 7.0. 33 ml of solution A, 67 ml of solution B, 8.5 g of NaCl, and distilled water to 1 liter.

0.05 M phosphate in saline, pH 7.1.   70 ml of solution A, 180 ml of solution B, 5.7 g of NaCl, and distilled water to 1 liter.

Tris-HCl Buffer (pH 7.2–9.0, 0.015 M)

Solution A: Tris 24.23 g/liter.
Solution B: 1.0 N HCl.

To 250 ml of solution A add n ml of solution B per liter, and dilute to 1 liter.

	Solution B	
	pH	(ml/liter)
	7.2	44.2
	7.4	41.4
	7.6	38.4
	7.8	32.5
	8.0	26.8
	8.2	21.9
	8.4	16.5
	8.6	12.2
	8.8	8.1
	9.0	5.0

pH	A (ml/liter)	B (ml/liter)	C (ml/liter)	A (ml/liter)	B (ml/liter)	C (ml/liter)
8.6	409	100	0	403	100	100
8.8				509	200	0
8.9				321	200	0

Barbital Sodium-Sodium Acetate-HCl, pH 2.6–9.4 Buffer

Solution A: barbital sodium 29.43 g/liter, sodium acetate (trihydrate) 19.43 g/liter.
Solution B: 1.0 N HCl.
Solution C: 8.5% NaCl.

To 200 ml of solution A and 80 ml of solution C, add n ml of solution B, and dilute to 1 liter.

Solution B	
pH	(ml/liter)
2.62	64
3.62	56
4.66	40
5.32	32
6.12	28
6.5	27
6.99	24
7.25	22
7.42	20
7.66	16
7.90	12
8.18	8
8.55	4
8.68	3

Tris-Boric Acid-EDTA, pH 8.5 Buffer

Tris, 109 g, 0.5 M boric acid (30.9 g), and 0.02 *M* EDTA (5.76 g), dissolved in distilled water to 1 liter. Dilute with 19 volumes of distilled water and adjust the liquid to pH 8.5.

Tris-HCl buffer 0.1 *M* Tris, 0.2 *N* HCl, 0.2 *M* NaCl, pH 8.0 buffer.

Dissolve 12.11 g/liter Tris and 11.69 g/liter NaCl in two-thirds of buffer volume using deionized distilled water and add 1.0 N HCl to pH 8.0.

EDTA-NaOH Buffer, 0.15 M, pH 7.4. Dissolve 55.84 g of EDTA disodium in 1 liter of distilled water and add 1 *M* NaOH to pH 7.4.

Barbital-Barbital Sodium-NaCl, pH 7.4–9.0 Buffer

Solution A: barbital, 4.605 g/liter.
Solution B: barbital sodium, 103.09 g/liter.
Solution C: sodium chloride, 29.2 g/liter.

pH	A (ml/liter)	B (ml/liter)	C (ml/liter)	A (ml/liter)	B (ml/liter)	C (ml/liter)
7.4	648	10	90	639	10	190
7.6	409	10	90	403	10	190
7.8	645	25	75	636	25	175
8.0	814	50	50	401	25	175
8.2	514	50	50	506	50	150
8.4	648	100	0	639	100	100

Veronal-Acetate Buffers, pH 5.6–8.38. The buffers may be prepared from three stock solutions A, B, and C possessing the following compositions: (A) sodium acetate anhydrous 6.276 g; sodium 5,5-diethylbarbiturate 15.770 g; $MgCl_2$ 0.5 ml of 1.0 M; $CaCl_2$ 0.5 ml of 0.3 M; distilled water to 11; (B) HCl 38.30 ml of 1.0 N; $MgCl_2$ 0.125 ml of 1.0 M; $CaCl_2$ 0.125 ml of 0.3 M; distilled water to 250 ml; (C) NaCl 9.01 g; $MgCl_2$ 0.5 ml of 1.0 M; $CaCl_2$ 0.5 ml of 0.3 M; distilled water to 11. To prepare a buffer with the desired pH value and the ionic strength of 0.15 M, the three stock solutions are mixed in the proportions shown below.

Composition of Veronal-Acetate Buffers (Ibe and Wardlaw, 1964)

pH	HCl (Solution B) (ml)	Veronal-Acetate (Solution A) (ml)	NaCl (Solution C) (ml)	Calculated Ionic Strength
5.60	5.15	10	84.85	0.148
6.13	4.92	10	85.08	0.148
6.70	4.65	10	85.35	0.148
7.08	4.20	10	85.80	0.149
7.65	3.00	10	87.00	0.151
8.38	0.20	10	89.80	0.155

Michaelis' Acetate-Veronal Buffer: Basic Mixture

Sodium acetate	19.428 g
Sodium veronal	29.428 g
Sodium chloride	34.0 g
Distilled water to	1000 ml

Add 5.0 ml of the mixture above to 7.0 ml of N-HCl, 13.0 ml distilled water, and 0.25 ml of 1 M $CaCl_2$. Adjust the buffer to pH 6.1.

Veronal-Acetate Buffers Stock Solutions

Solution A:	Distilled water	500 ml
	Sodium acetate, trihydrate	9.714 g
	Sodium diethylbarbiturate (Veronal)	14.714 g

First boil the water (to expel dissolved CO_2); then allow to cool before adding and shaking in the solids.

Solution B: Sodium chloride 8.5% aqueous (prepared with CO_2-free distilled water).

Solution C: $N/10$ HCl.

pH	$N/10$ HCl (ml)	Reagent A (ml)	Reagent B (ml)	Distilled Water (CO_2 Free) (ml)
2.62	16.0	5	2	2.0
3.20	15.0	5	2	3.0
3.62	14.0	5	2	4.0
3.88	13.0	5	2	5.0
4.13	12.0	5	2	6.0
4.33	11.0	5	2	7.0
4.66	10.0	5	2	8.0
4.93	9.0	5	2	9.0
5.32	8.0	5	2	10.0
6.12	7.0	5	2	11.0
6.75	6.5	5	2	11.5
6.99	6.0	5	2	12.0
7.25	5.5	5	2	12.5
7.42	5.0	5	2	13.0
7.66	4.0	5	2	14.0
7.90	3.0	5	2	15.0
8.18	2.0	5	2	16.0
8.55	1.0	5	2	17.0
8.68	0.75	5	2	17.25
8.30	0.5	5	2	17.5
8.16	0.25	5	2	17.75

The Barbiturate-Acetate Buffer, 0.125 M, pH 8.6. This consists of:

Diethylbarbituric acid	8.712 g
Sodium acetate	6.476 g
Sodium hydroxide	1.893 g
0.1 N HCl	60 ml
Distilled water to	1 liter

Sodium Citrate (0.05 M) Buffers, pH 2.2–5.28

pH	2.2	3.28	4.25	5.28
Sodium citrate (gm)	19.6	19.6	19.6	34.4
HCl (concentrated) (ml)	16.5	12.3	8.4	6.5
Distilled water to ml	1000	1000	1000	1000

Acetate Buffer, 0.1 M, pH 3.6–5.6 (Walpole, 1914)

Solution A: 0.2 M acetic acid (11.55-ml glacial acetic acid/liter).
Solution B: 0.2 M sodium acetate (sodium acetate · $3H_2O$, 27.2 g/liter).

pH	Solution B (ml/liter)	pH	Solution B (ml/liter)
8.1	24.5	9.1	118.0
8.2	30.0	9.2	132.0
8.3	36.0	9.3	146.5
8.4	43.0	9.4	160.5
8.5	50.5	9.5	173.0
8.6	50.9	9.6	184.5
8.7	68.5	9.7	194.5
8.8	79.0	9.8	203.0
8.9	90.5	9.9	211.0
9.0	104.0	10.0	218.5

Boric Acid-NaOH-KCl Buffer

Solution A: boric acid, 12.4 g/liter and KCl, 14.91 g/liter.
Solution B: 0.2 M NaOH.

To 250 ml of solution A add *n* ml of solution B.

pH	Solution A (ml/liter)	Solution B (ml/liter)	pH	Solution A (ml/liter)	Solution B (ml/liter)
3.6	463.0	37.0	4.8	200.0	300.0
3.8	440.0	60.0	5.0	148.0	352.0
4.0	410.0	90.0	5.2	105.0	395.0
4.2	368.0	132.0	5.4	88.0	412.0
4.4	305.0	195.0	5.6	48.0	452.0
4.6	255.0	245.0			

Borate buffer, pH 8.6, contains:

45 ml of 1.25% aqueous boric acid.
55 ml of 1.9% $Na_2B_4O_7 \cdot 10H_2O$ solution.

Borate-NaOH buffer, pH 8.6 for immunoclectrophoresis electrode-vessels:

Boric acid 18.38.
$N/1$ NaoH — 60 ml.
Distilled water up to 1000 ml.

Glycine-HCl buffer, pH 2.0–3.4
Solution A: glycine, 150.14 g/liter.
Solution B: 1 M HCl.

Solution A (ml/liter)	Solution B (ml/liter)	pH	Solution A (ml/liter)	Solution B (ml/liter)
59.0	100	2.0	—	—
71.5	100	2.2	25.0	44.0
89.2	100	2.4	25.0	32.4
116.0	100	2.6	25.0	24.2
157.0	100	2.8	25.0	16.8
222.0	100	3.0	25.0	11.4
324.0	100	3.2	25.0	8.2
486.0	100	3.4	25.0	6.4
		3.6	25.0	5.0

Phosphate Buffers, pH 5.3–8.0: Stock Solutions

Solution A: *M/10 Disodium hydrogen phosphate:*
Disodium hydrogen phosphate, anhydrous (Na_2HPO_4) 10% aqueous, 141.98 ml.
Distilled water, 859.02 ml.

Solution B: *M/10 Sodium dihydrogen phosphate:*
Sodium dihydrogen phosphate ($NaH_2PO_4 \cdot H_2O$) 10% aqueous, 138.05 ml.
Distilled water, 861.95 ml.

pH	Solution A (ml)	Solution B (ml)	pH	Solution A (ml)	Solution B (ml)
5.3	2.6	97.4	6.7	43.3	56.7
5.4	3.2	96.8	6.8	49.1	50.9
5.5	4.0	96.0	6.9	55.1	44.9
5.6	5.1	94.9	7.0	61.1	38.9
5.7	6.4	93.6	7.1	66.6	33.4
5.8	8.0	92.0	7.2	72.0	28.0
5.9	9.9	90.1	7.3	76.8	23.2
6.0	12.3	87.7	7.4	80.8	19.2
6.1	15.1	84.9	7.5	84.1	15.9
6.2	18.6	81.4	7.6	87.0	13.0
6.3	22.5	77.5	7.7	89.4	10.6
6.4	26.7	73.3	7.8	91.5	8.5
6.5	31.7	68.3	7.9	93.2	6.8
6.6	37.5	62.5	8.0	94.7	5.3

KH_2PO_4-NaOH Buffer, pH 5.8–7.9

    Solution A: 0.2 M KH_2PO_4 (KH_2PO_4, 27.21 g/liter).

    Solution B: 0.2M NaOH.

To 250 ml of solution A, add n ml of soluiton B, and dilute to 1 liter.

pH	Solution B (ml/liter)	pH	Solution B (ml/liter)
5.9	23	7.0	145.5
6.0	28	7.1	160.5
6.1	34	7.2	173.5
6.2	40.5	7.3	185
6.3	48.5	7.4	195.5
6.4	58	7.5	204.5
6.5	69.5	7.6	212
6.6	82	7.7	217.5
6.7	96.5	7.8	222.5
6.8	112	7.9	226.5
6.9	129.5		

Phosphate Buffer, 0.056 M, pH 7.   The stock solution is prepared by combining the following two solutions:

4.76 g $Na_2HPO_4 \cdot 12H_2O$/liter   and   2.5 g $NH_2PO_4 \cdot 2H_2O$/liter.

Modified Brock's stock solution contains the following salts in 1000 ml of distilled water: 170 g of NaCl, 2.7i g of KH_2PO_4, 11.3 g of Na_2HPO_4 (or 28.5 g of $Na_2HPO_4 \cdot 10H_2O$). The stock solution must be diluted 1:20 with distilled water prior to use.

Formate Buffer, pH 3.023.   The 136 ml of formic acid (90%) and 51.2 g of sodium hydroxide are dissolved in distilled water and made up to a final volume of 16 liters.

M/5 Maleate Buffer Solutions: Stock Solutions

    Solution A: Maleic acid   46.4 g
                      Sodium hydroxide $N/1$ 400 ml
                      Distilled water sufficient to make volume up to 1 liter.

    Solution B: Sodium hydroxide $N/1$.

pH	Solution A (ml)	Solution B (ml)	Distilled Water (ml)
4.6	50	0.5	49.5
4.8	50	1.0	49
5.0	50	1.8	48.2
5.2	50	2.8	47.2
5.4	50	4.0	46
5.6	50	5.8	44.2
5.8	50	7.6	42.4
6.0	50	10.0	40
6.2	50	12.5	37.5
6.4	50	14.5	35.5

Citrate Buffer, pH 3.0–6.2 (Lillie, 1948): *Stock Solutions*

Solution A: 0.1 M solution of citric acid (21.01 g in 1000 ml).

Solution B: 0.1 M solution of sodium citrate (20.41 g $C_6H_5O_7Na_3 \cdot 2H_2O$ in 1000 ml); the use of the salt with $5\frac{1}{2}$ H_2O is not recommended.

Thus x ml of solution A $+$ y ml of solution B are diluted to a total of 100 ml.

x	y	pH
46.5	3.5	3.0
43.7	6.3	3.2
40.0	10.0	3.4
37.0	13.0	3.6
35.0	15.0	3.8
33.0	17.0	4.0
31.5	18.5	4.2
28.0	22.0	4.4
25.5	24.5	4.6
23.0	27.0	4.8
20.5	29.5	5.0
18.0	32.0	5.2
16.0	34.0	5.4
13.7	36.3	5.6
11.8	38.2	5.8
9.5	41.5	6.0
7.2	42.8	6.2

Citrate-phosphate buffer, pH 2.6–7.0 (McIlvaine, 1921): *Stock Solutions.*

Solution A: 0.1 M solution of citric acid (19.21 g in 1000 ml).
Solution B: 0.2 M solution of dibasic sodium phosphate (53.65 g of $Na_2\text{-}HPO_4 \cdot 7H_2O$ or 71.7 g of $Na_2HPO_4 \cdot 12H_2O$ in 100 ml).

Thus x ml of solution A + 6 ml of solution B are diluted to a total of 100 ml.

x	y	pH
44.6	5.4	2.6
42.2	7.8	2.8
39.8	10.2	3.0
37.7	12.3	3.2
35.9	14.1	3.4
33.9	16.1	3.6
32.3	17.7	3.8
30.7	19.3	4.0
29.4	20.6	4.2
27.8	22.2	4.4
26.7	23.3	4.6
25.2	24.8	4.8
24.3	25.7	5.0
23.3	26.7	5.2
22.2	27.8	5.4
21.0	29.0	5.6
19.7	30.3	5.8
17.9	32.1	6.0
16.9	33.1	6.2
15.4	34.6	6.4
13.6	36.4	6.6
9.1	40.9	6.8
6.5	43.6	7.0

Glycine-NaOH Buffer, pH 8.6–10.6 (Sørensen, 1909): *Stock Solutions*

Solution A: 0.2 M solution of glycine (15.01 g in 1000 ml).
Solution B: 0.2 M NaOH.

Thus 50 ml of solution A + x ml of solution B are diluted to a total of 200 ml.

x	pH	x	pH
4.0	8.6	22.4	9.6
6.0	8.8	27.2	9.8
8.8	9.0	32.0	10.0
12.0	9.2	38.6	10.4
16.8	9.4	45.5	10.6

Glycine-HCl Buffer, pH 2.2–3.6: Stock Solutions

Solution A: 0.2 *M* solution of glycine (15.01 g in 1000 ml).

Solution B: 0.2 *M* HCl.

Thus 50 ml of solution A + *x* ml of solution B are diluted to a total of 200 ml.

x	pH	*x*	pH
5.0	3.6	16.8	2.8
6.4	3.4	24.2	2.6
8.2	3.2	32.4	2.4
11.4	3.0	44.0	2.2

Carbonate-Bicarbonate Buffer, pH 9.2–10.7 (Delory and King, 1945):
Stock Solutions

Solution A: 0.2 *M* solution of anhydrous sodium carbonate (21.2 g in 1000 ml).

Solution B: 0.2 *M* solution of sodium bicarbonate (16.8 g in 1000 ml).

Thus *x* ml of solution A + *y* ml of solution B are diluted to a total of 200.

x	*y*	pH
4.0	46.0	9.2
7.5	42.5	9.3
9.5	40.5	9.4
13.0	37.0	9.5
16.0	34.0	9.6
19.5	30.5	9.7
22.0	28.0	9.8
25.0	25.0	9.9
27.5	22.5	10.0
30.0	20.0	10.1
33.0	17.0	10.2
35.5	14.5	10.3
38.5	11.5	10.4
40.5	9.5	10.5
42.5	7.5	10.6
45.0	5.0	10.7

Tris (hydroxymethyl)aminomethane-maleate (Tris-maleate) Buffer, pH 5.2–8.6 (Gomori, 1955): *Stock Solutions*

Solution A: 0.2 M solution of Tris acid maleate (24.2 g of tris (acid or 19.5 g maleic (hydroxymethyl)aminomethane + 23.2 g of maleic anhydride in 1000 ml).

Solution B: 0.2 M NaOH.

Thus 50 ml of solution A + x ml of solution B are diluted to a total of 200 ml.

x	pH	x	pH
7.0	5.2	48.0	7.0
10.8	5.4	51.0	7.2
15.5	5.6	54.0	7.4
20.5	5.8	58.0	7.6
26.0	6.0	63.5	7.8
31.5	6.2	69.0	8.0
37.0	6.4	75.0	8.2
42.5	6.6	81.0	8.4
45.0	6.8	86.5	8.6

Gey's Solution

Solution A consists of: 70.0 g NaCl
3.7 g KCl
3.01 g $Na_2HPO_4 \cdot 12H_2O$
0.237 g KH_2PO_4
10.0 g glucose
0.1 g phenol red
Distilled water to 1 liter

Solution B contains: 0.42 g $MgCl_2 \cdot 6H_2O$
0.14 g $McSO_4 \cdot 7H_2O$
0.35 g $CaCl_2$
Distilled water to 100 ml

Solution C is a 2.25% solution of $NaHCO_3$.

Dilute solution A (10 ml) in 80 ml distilled water. Autoclave each solution at 10 psi. To the diluted solution A add 5 ml solution B and 5 ml solution C and adjust final liquid to pH 7.8 (orange color) with CO_2.

Preservation of Buffers. Buffer solutions which are not used immediately must be preserved with Merthiolate and pentachlorophenol (or *n*-caprylic acid) to prevent deterioration by bacteria and molds.

Antibacterial Reagent

| Merthiolate | 1 g |
| Distilled water | 199 ml |

Add 1.0 ml of this solution per 1000 ml buffer to make a 1:200,000 final dilution of Merthiolate (Thiomersal). Alternatively, use 0.1% aqueous sodium azide solution.

Antimold Reagent

| Pentachlorophenol | 100 mg |
| 95% ethyl alcohol | 10 ml |

Add 0.1 ml of this solution per 1000 ml buffer. Alternatively, use 0.1 ml octanoic (*n*-caprylic) acid per liter to make a final 1:10,000 dilution.

Chapter Four

ANTIBODIES

I. IMMUNOCHEMICAL DEFINITION OF ANTIBODIES

Antibodies represent a specific group of animal proteins, the immunoglobulins, which are distinct from other immunoglobulins by the capability of complexing with antigenic determinants of complementary combining sites on antibody molecules.

The combining site or complementary area constitutes a relatively small portion of the antibody molecule, equivalent to 0.4 to 0.1% of the surface of an immunoglobulin molecule, with the approximate dimensions of 34 $\times$ 12 $\times$ 7 Å (Campbell and Bulman, 1952; Kabat, 1960). The combining site appears to have a shape of cavity formed by the immunoglobulin molecule with its van der Waals contour group (Karush, 1956). The complementary region or active sites occur in the number from 2 to 5 and are distributed asymmetrically on an immunoglobulin molecule. Antitoxic groups, for example, are positioned relatively closely together on one side of the antitoxin molecule. Immunochemical activity of an antibody molecule may thus be exhibited by less than the total active site. Due to the presence of more than one active site on an immunoglobulin molecule, a single antibody molecule may link several molecules of a multivalent antigen. A limited enzymatic degradation of the immunoglobulin molecule does not diminish its combining activity.

The immunological specificity of antibodies refers to their avidity, that is, their ability to only combine with the substances bearing a unique physicochemical feature, the corresponding antigenic determinant. The specificity has been defined by Landsteiner (1945) as "a disproportional action of a number of similar agents on a variety of related substrates." The specificity of antibodies provides a powerful tool for the detection, identification, and differentiation of antigens. The antibody specificity and avidity is determined by the amino acid sequence in the variable segment of the H chain and to a lesser extent in the L chain which determines the secondary and tertiary folding of the chains. But essentially the specificity depends on the stereochemical architecture of the combining site of antibody molecule which is basically a function of the spatial orientation of its electrons and the binding force of energy. The antibody combining region is exclusively associated with the heavy chain of immunoglobulins whereas the light chain serves to prevent the aggregation or denaturation of the heavy chain and thus contributes to the immunological activity. The combining constants of various antibody molecules are different in respect to the antigen determinants and depend on the source and origin of particular antibodies. The physical and serological properties of some antibodies differ from the nonantibody protein substances by so little that they are almost identical with the normal immunoglobulins. Free amino groups seem to be essential for the reactivity of antibody molecules.

At least five distinct classes of immunogloblins endowed with an antibody activity have been identified by the antigenic analysis, and designated as IgG, IgM, IgA, IgD, and IgE immunoglobulins (Table 28). The immunochemical structure of the IgG molecule is shown in Fig. 41 (Fougereau and Edelman, 1965). Each class of immunoglobulins has been subdivided into a number of individual subclasses. For example, four IgG subclasses are known.

The immunoglobulins are distributed in the body in approximately equal proportion in blood plasma and in the extravascular fluid. About $\frac{1}{4}$ of the circulating immunoglobulins is replaced daily. A healthy adult synthesizes from 2 to 5 g of immunoglobulin daily, but the synthesis may be increased as much as 7 times in response to an infection. Immunoglobulins are produced by plasma cells and their precursors and by lymphocytes. Immunoglobulins, especially the low molecular weight plasma immunoglobulins ($3s\gamma_1\alpha$-globulin), are excreted to urine (Poortmans and Jeanloz, 1967).

The molecule of the IgG antibody-immunoglobulin observed in the election microscope appeared as a markedly nonspherical structure, which consists of three cylinders. This structure seems to possess two hemispherical sites (Valentine and Green, 1967, Fig. 42). This structure has also been inferred from the studies on rotational motions of antibody molecules (Yguerabide et al., 1970). At the junction of the F_{ab} segments of antibody globulin there is a flexible joint which may be biologically significant in facilitating the formation of antibody-antigen complexes.

Molecules of the γM immunoglobulin revealed on electromicroscopy possess a spider-like structure with five legs varying in length and often joining a central ring. The central part of the structure, measuring about 150×170 Å is usually clearly visible but sometimes very flexible leglike structures have been observed with a total span of about 350 Å. Human and rabbit α macroglobulin occurs as a more rigid symmetric structure measuring 100×200 Å and resembling the letter Ж (Svehag et al., 1967).

The IgG immunoglobulin is present in equal amounts in plasma and extravascular fluid and has the longest half-life of 20 to 28 days. It comprises

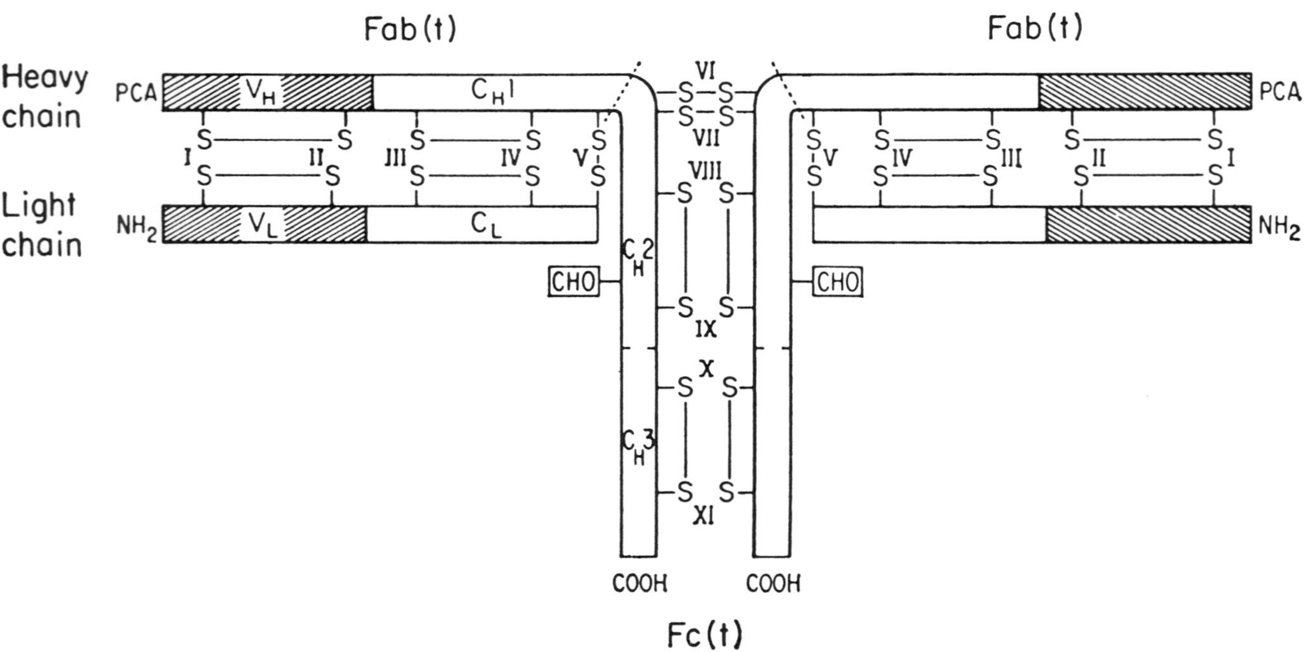
Fab(t)
Heavy chain
Light chain
PCA
NH2
V_H
V_L
C_H1
C_L
CHO
Fc(t)
C_H2
C_H3
COOH
I
II
III
IV
V
VI
VII
VIII
IX
X
XI

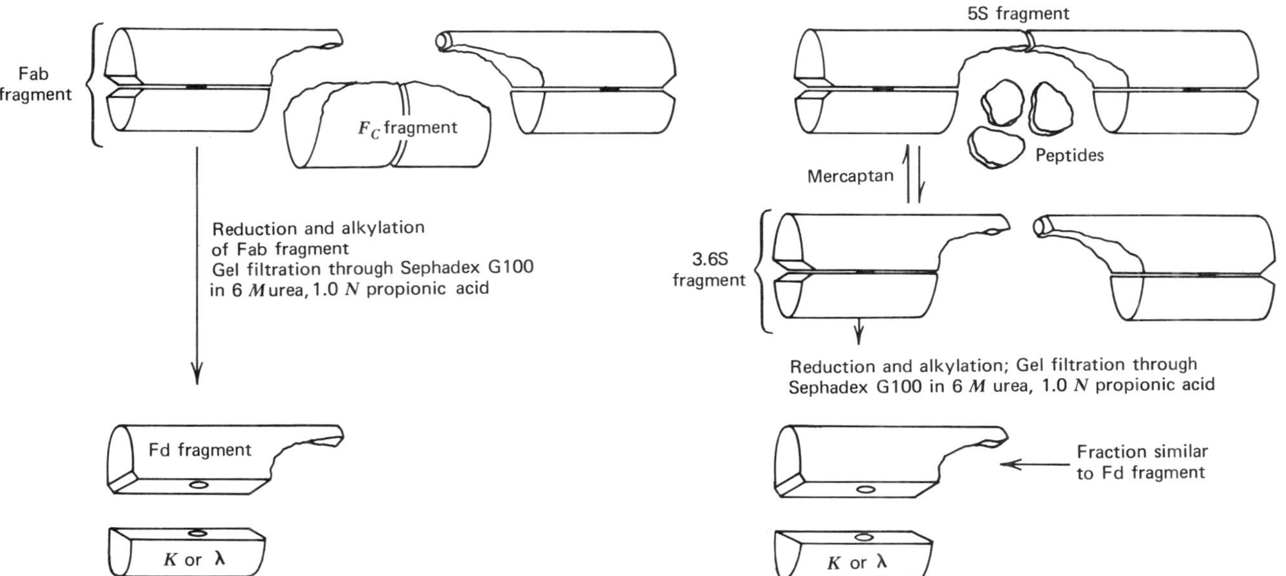

Figure 41. Structural models of the IgG molecule (Edelman, 1970, Fougereau and Edelman, 1965.)

Table 28.   Physicochemical and Biological Properties of Immunoglobulins and Other Proteins of Human Plasma

Protein	Electro-phoretic Mobility	Molecular Weight	Sedimentation Constants $S_{20°,w}$	Percentage Carbohydrate	Concentration (mg/100 ml Plasma)	Biological Function and Characteristics
Prealbumin	α_0	61,000	4.2	0.5	10–40	Binding of thyroxin.
Albumin	α_0	69,000	4.6	0.08	3500–5500	Osmotic functions, metabolic protein (amino acid) pool, plasma transport of anions, cations, dyes, pigments, drugs, and so on.
α_1-Lipoprotein	α_1	200,000	5.0	1.5	290–770	Transport of fats, lipids, hormones, and fat-soluble vitamins.
α_1-Acid glycoprotein	α_1	44,100	3.1	41.4	55–140	Electrophoretic heterogeneity due to genetically determined polymorphism.
α_1-Antitrypsin	α_1	45,000	3.4	12.4	200–400	Proteinase, inhibits trypsin and chymotrypsin.
α_1-Glycoprotein	α_1	50,000	3.8	13.3	15–30	Functions unknown.
Transcortin	α_1		3.0	14.1	~7	Binding and transport of cortisol.
4.6S-Postalbumin	α_1		4.6	10.0	~20	Functions unknown.
Tryptophan-poor α_1-glycoprotein	α_1	60,000	3.3	13.8	5–12	Functions unknown.
$\alpha_1 x$-Glycoprotein	α_1		3.9	22.7	40–60	Functions unknown.
Thyroxin-binding globulin	α_1	40,000–50,000	3.3		1–2	Binding of thyroxin (together with prealbumin).
Inter-α-trypsin-inhibitor	$\alpha_1 \cdot \alpha_2$		6.4	9.1	40–70	Trypsin and proteinase inhibitor.
Gc-globulin (Gc 1-1) (Gc 2-1) (Gc 2-2)	$\alpha_1 \cdot \alpha_2$	50,800	3.7	4.2	30–55	Genetically determined Gc-groups (Gc 1-1, 2-1, 2-2); immunologically identical but with different electrophoretic mobility. Biologic functions unknown.

Protein		Molecular weight				Comments
Haptoglobin	α_2	85,000	4.4	19.3	50–220	Binding of free hemoglobin in plasma, regulation of renal threshold for hemoglobin; Hb-Hp-complex possesses peroxidase activity; 3 major hereditary phenotypes: Hp 1-1, Hp 2-1, and Hp 2-2, controlled by two allelic autosomal genes (Hp 1 and Hp 2).
(Hp 1-1)			4.3; 6.5			
(Hp 2-1)			7.5			
(Hp 2-2)						
Ceruloplasmin	α_2	160,000	7.1	8.0	20–45	Cooper-binding glycoprotein with oxidase activity. Binds more than 90% of serum copper.
Cholinesterase	α_2	$\sim$300,000	$\sim$12		0.8–1.1	Involved in the degradation of acetylcholine; inhibition by organic phosphorous compounds. Exists in at least 5 phenotypes.
α_2-Lipoprotein(s)	α_2	5–20,000,000	$S_f > 12$	1.7	150–230	Transport of lipids and triglycerides. Continuous spectrum of densities and molecular sizes of α_2-lipoproteins.
α_2-Macroglobulin	α_2	820,000	19.6	8.4	150–350	Plasmin and trypsin inhibitor.
					175–420	
α_2-HS-glycoprotein	α_2	49,000	3.3	13.4	40–85	Designations HS derived from names Heremans and Schmid. Solvents used in isolation procedures (Z = Zinc sulfate, Ba = Barium acetate). Biological functions unknown.
Zn-α_2-glycoprotein	α_2	41,000	3.2	18.2	2–15	High content of tyrosine and tryptophan. The Zn refers to Zinc acetate used in the purification procedure. Biological functions unknown.

(Continued)

Table 28 (*Continued*)

Protein	Electro-phoretic Mobility	Molecular Weight	Sedimentation Constants $S_{20°,w}$	Percentage Carbohydrate	Concentration (mg/100 ml Plasma)	Biological Function and Characteristics
α_2-Neuramino-glyco-protein	α_2		3.7	42.6	15–25	Trace protein with high neuraminic acid (17%) and total carbohydrate content. Functions unknown.
Erythropoietin	α_2	30,000				Erythropoietic function; also produced by some tumors (Polycythemia)
β-lipoprotein	β_1	3,200,000	$S_f = 3$–12	1.8	290–950	Transport of glycerides, cholesterol, phospholipids, hormones, and lipid-soluble vitamins. Shares antigenic properties with α_2-lipoprotein(s). Ag and Lp phenotypes. Continuous spectrum of S_f 3–12 lipoproteins which differ in lipid contents, molecular weight, and density.
Transferrin	β_1	90,000	5.5	5.8	200–400	Binding of plasma iron, normally 30% saturated; serum iron transport participating in regulation and control of iron absorption and protection from iron intoxication. Genetically determined polymorphism, variants demonstrable by starchgel electrophoresis.
Hemopexin	β_1	80,000	4.8	22.6	70–130	Heme-binding glycoprotein, binds 1 mole heme, but no hemoglobin. Salmon red color of the heme-

						hemopexin complex distinct from the brown color of methemalbumin.
Fibrinogen	β_1	341,000	7.6	2.5	(200–450) (mean–300)	Essential factor of blood coagulation system. Converted to fibrin by clotting enzyme thrombin.
Plasminogen	β_1	143,000	4.3		20–40	Conversion into plasmin (fibrinolysin). Lysis of blood clots by this protease.
β_2-glycoprotein I	β_2	40,000	2.9	18.8	15–30	Unknown.
β_2-glycoprotein II	β_2		3.7	5.7	12–30	Unknown.
Immunoglobulin G (IgG) or γG-globulin Mol. formula: $\gamma_2 k_2$ or $\gamma_2\lambda_2$		150,000	6.5–7.2	2.9	800–1600	Antibodies against bacteria, viruses, and toxins; Rh antibodies, antinuclear Factors; carriers of Gm-antigenic determinants. γG globulin subclasses (γG1–γG4).
Immunoglobulin A (IgA) or γA-globulin Mol. formula: $(\alpha_2 k_2)^n$ or $(\alpha_2\lambda_2)^n$		1. Serum γA-globulins 180,000 + polymers 2. Secretory γA-globulins 390,000	7; 9,11,13 15,17 $\sim$11.4	7.5	90–420	Antibodies to a variety of antigens. Predominant immunoglobulins in many body fluids.
Immunoglobulin M (IgM) or γM-globulin Mol. formula: $(\mu_2 k_2)^5$ or $(\mu_2\lambda_2)^5$		950,000	18–20	11.8	♂60–250 ♀70–280	Natural antibodies, such as ABO isoagglutinins; antibodies to gram-negative microorganisms; autoantibodies, such as rheumatoid factors; miscellaneous antibodies, including heterophile antibody, and reagins.

(Continued)

Table 28 (*Continued*)

Protein	Electro-phoretic Mobility	Molecular Weight	Sedimentation Constants $S_{20°,w}$	Percentage Carbohydrate	Concentration (mg/100 ml Plasma)	Biological Function and Characteristics
Immunoglobulin D (IgD) or γD-Globulin (γD) Mol. formula: ($\delta_2 k_2$) or ($\delta_2 \lambda_2$)		155,000	6.2 to 6.8	11	0, 3–40	Unknown.
Immunoglobulin E (IgE) or γE-Globulin (γE) Mol. formula: ($\epsilon_2 k_2$) or ($\epsilon_2 \lambda_2$)		196,000	7.9		0.01–0.14	Reaginic activity, Praussnitz-Küstner activity.
Free light chains	$\gamma \cdot \alpha_1$	22,500 45,000	2.2 3.4	Traces		Occurrence in trace amounts in normal human serum and urine. Carry inv-antigenic determinants; common to all immunoglobulins; 2 types (K and L).
$C'1$			18		2–3	When activated it initiates complement fixation reactions. Heat labile. $C'1$ complex dissociates into $C'q$; $C'r$ and $C's$.
$C'1q$	γ_2		11.1			
$C'1r$	β		7			
$C'1s$	α_2		4			
$C'2$	β_1		6		1	Heat labile.
$C'3$	β_1		9.5	3.03	80–140	Inactivated by Zymosan. β_1C-globulin is present only in fresh serum. On aging, $C'3$ is split into two faster moving fractions, the inactive β_1A and α_2D. β_1G is a hemolytically inactive reaction product with sedimentation values similar to that of β_1C.
β_1A	β_1	75,000				
α_2D	α_2					

C′4	β_1	10.0	20–40	Inactivated by hydrazine, C′1 esterase, and antigen-antibody complexes.
C′5	β_1	8.7	3–5	Relatively heat stable.
C′6	β_2	5–6	1	Heat stable.
C′7	β_2	6–7		Heat stable.
C′8	γ_1	8		Relatively heat stable.
C′9	$\alpha_2 \cdot \alpha_1$	4		

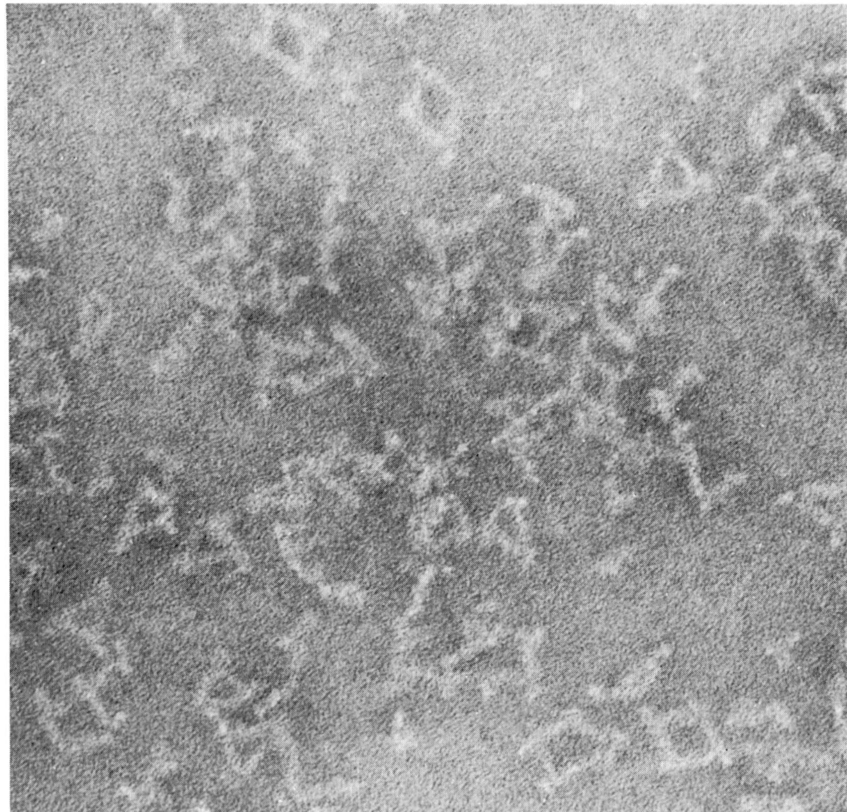

Figure 42.   The physical structure of the IgG molecule, observed in electron microscope (Valentine and Green, 1967).

85 to 90% of the immunoglobulins in adult serum. A great majority (80%) of antibacterial, antivirus-, and antitoxin antibodies present in the serum belong to IgG immunoglobulin class. Normal human plasma contains between 800 and 1600 mg of IgG per 100 ml. The IgG molecule has an approximate molecular weight of 150,000 to 160,000 and a sedimentation constant of 7S. The molecule of the IgM immunoglobulin is much heavier, as it possesses a molecular weight of 950,000 and a sedimentation constant of 19S. The 19S gamma globulins dissociate to 7S units on treatment with reducing agents in the absence of urea. It is estimated that approximately six 7S subunits comprise a mole of 19S protein. The 19S antibodies are formed mainly in the early stages of primary immunization and are followed by antibodies of the 7S variety (Fig. 43). Secondary immunization

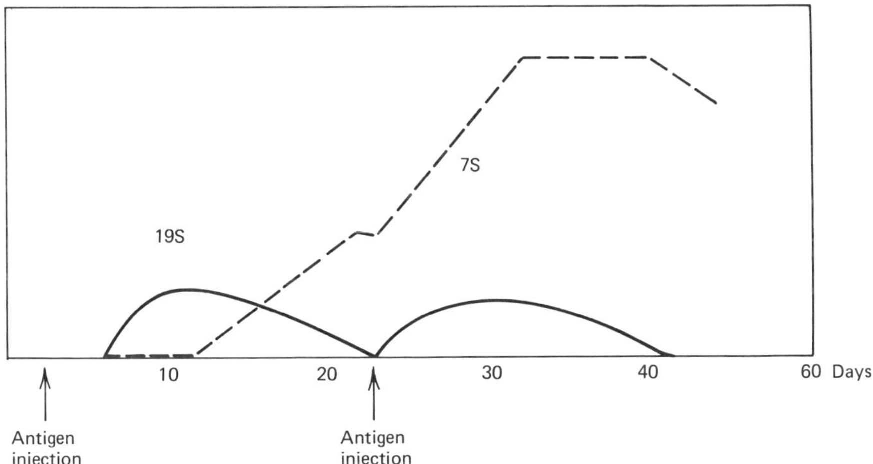

Figure 43. A diagram of the primary and secondary antibody response to an antigen.

elicits mainly 7S antibodies. Approximately 10% of the total antibody protein in serum is of the IgM type. The most common IgM immunoglobulins are cold agglutinins, antibodies specific for lipopolysaccharide antigens of Gram-negative bacteria, bacteriolytic reagins, and heteroantibodies. A normal serum of a human adult contains 60 to 170 mg of the IgM immunoglobulin per 100 ml. The IgM immunoglobulin occurs mainly in the intravascular compartments. It has a half-life of 5 days and it is the chief class of immunoglobulins synthesized in the neonatal period. In the immunization, IgM is the first immunoglobulin to appear in the circulation.

The IgA immunoglobulin represents 10% of the gamma globulins in human serum; it occurs in the average, relative concentration of 150 to 250 mg/100 ml of serum and has a half-life of 4-6 days. Globulin molecules constituting the IgA immunoglobulin display different sedimentation constants and molecular weights, ranging from 180,000 to 390,000 or more, but approximately 90% of the IgA molecules have a sedimentation constant of 7S and molecular weight of 180,000. The heavier molecules of the IgA class are more common than the lighter molecules in parotid saliva, tears, colostrum, and in the nasal, bronchial, and intestinal secretions (coproantibodies). The predominant immunoglobulin molecules in external secretions are chiefly the 11S IgA molecules.

The IgD immunoglobulin, which has approximate molecular weight of 160,000 and the 7S sedimentation constant, represents roughly 3 mg % of normal serum proteins. The IgE immunoglobulin occurs in very small concentrations in serum and possesses an approximate molecular weight of 160,000 and a sedimentation constant of 8S; it represents most of the T-K antibody (reagins).

Molecular weights of the immunoglobulins may be determined by Archibald's (1947) technique utilizing the approach to equilibrium procedure.

Antibodies are destroyed by heat. Heat destruction is minimal at pH 7.0 but it increases at lower or higher pH. High concentration of salts, glycerol, or sugar delay the thermal destruction of antibodies. There are certain differences in the heat resistance of various antibodies; for example, flagellar antibodies are often more thermostable than the corresponding somatic antibodies, which may be indicative of different physicochemical structures. Ultraviolet rays render antibody nonprecipitable (Hanan, 1952). Electrons in a dose of 2 million rep. at 2° inactivate immune antibody almost completely, but isoagglutinins are more resistant. Formaldehyde addition or acidification of serum renders many antibodies nonprecipitable, possibly owing to the formation of complexes between the various serum proteins.

The valence of antibodies is approximately 2, as suggested by results obtained with ultracentrifugation, electrophoresis, and equilibrium-dialysis measurements (Eisen and Karush, 1949; Marrack et al., 1951; Singer and Campbell, 1952; Plescia et al., 1952; Becker, 1953; Karush, 1956; Weigle and Maurer, 1957).

II. THE SYNTHESIS OF ANTIBODIES

The capacity of certain animals to respond to a specific antigen has developed during the evolution of vertebrates and is transmitted as a unigenic Mendelian dominant trait. The mechanism of the antibody synthesis has not been elucidated, and the lack of facts can hardly be filled by the various hypotheses (the instruction-, the selection-, and germ-line theories). The instruction theories are based on the principle of participation of antigen as a template which directs antibody synthesis. In the selection theories, it is postulated that antigen selectively stimulates those particular cells in a population which are fortuitously capable of producing antibodies specific for the antigen. The germ line theory assumes that the genome of the antibody-producing cell possesses all the necessary information to code for all antibody specificities. According to the latter theory, inducible cells are pluripotential and may be induced to turn on the appropriate codons in order to synthesize specific antibodies.

According to the concept of acquired cellular immunity, the immunity results from activities of cells rather than humoral antibodies. Acquired cellular immunity depends on both nonspecific and specific factors. Delayed sensitivities depend on a specific recognition mechanism which involves specific antigen-antibody interaction.

According to Kwapinski's (1972) quantum-theory of immunogenesis, the immunogenicity is viewed as a transfer of an energy quantum from an inductor molecule to a nascent globulin molecule, endowed with a greater and more flexible potential conformational configuration than the configuration of mature molecules. The fundamental phenomenon in the immunogenic reaction can be the hybridization of outer orbitals of interacting atomic loci of the two interacting molecules, accompanied by an exchange and rearrangement of energy in space. The transient complex is subsequently annealated, and the immunoglobulin molecules, possessing the quantum of (specific) energy, held by stereochemically specific conformations, obtained during the reaction with the inductor molecule, are replicated by the mediation of s- and m-RNAs. The inductor-specific configuration and conformation of the immunoglobulin molecule is maintained for a relatively short time until its potential of energy is modified. Immunochemical properties of molecules and immunochemical phenomena can best be studied, determined, and described in terms of stereochemistry and quantum chemistry. By these criteria, the induction and formation of specific sites on immunoglobulin molecules, and the interactions between the stereochemically and energetically compatible molecular areas of "antigen" and "antibody" are explained as specific interactions between electrons of outer orbitals, leading to the formation of aggregates.

Antibody is specific for the antigens that have induced its formation. Antibody formation consists of two phases, an induction phase and a production phase. Specific information for the anamnestic response is stored in lymphoid cells. The capacity of animals to form antibodies against certain antigens is genetically determined. Avidity of a specific antibody is increased by prolonged stimulation with an antigen.

Studies on the antibody synthesis in vitro (by spleen cells from pre-immunized animals) have shown that antibody production is associated with a considerable increase in the rate of synthesis of RNA and DNA and of cell proliferation. The antibody is formed due to an active metabolism in the competent cell and the antibody is synthesized *de novo* and secreted. Antibody synthesis is mediated by short-lived messenger RNA. During the antibody synthesis, light peptide chains are formed rapidly on small polyribosomes and they migrate to large polyribosomes which slowly form H chains. The H chains unite to form complete antibody molecules. Secretion of the antibody is an energy-dependent process. The simultaneous antibody response to two antigens depends on two distinct populations of cells.

The antibody is released chiefly by selective secretion of the secretory product from the antibody-synthesizing cells. The antibody can be secreted as early as 20 minutes after synthesis. Some antibody-synthesizing cells dialyze, thus releasing an additional amount of antibody.

The antibody response is usually very potent, relative to the amount of antigen. Thus 1 mg of an antigen can elicit the formation of as much as 100,000 mg of antibody immunoglobulins (Cohn and Pappenheiner, 1949).

The chemical composition of antibodies formed in various animals may differ. Thus the amino acid composition of rabbit antibodies is different from that of equine and human immune globulins.

Antibody globulins of some animals, for example, of the horse, seem to be heterogeneous in chemical constitution, since a variety of N- terminal groups was found in preparations of horse immune globulins (McFadden and Smith, 1955).

The antibody secreting cells are large blasts. The antibody first appears within the perinuclear space between the two membranes of nuclear envelope. The blasts then diminishes in size whereas endoplasmic reticulum containing antibody proliferates until it finally occupies all of the cytoplasm. Antibodies are also produced by lymphoplasmacytes which arise from small lymphocytes and by another type of cell, which has not been fully identified. The antibody-producing cells are highly specialized to the production of antibodies for an individual antigen, as proved by experiments of Coons (1958) and Nossal and Lederberg (1958). It is assumed that these cells have unique sequences of nucleotides in segments of the chromosomal deoxyribonucleic acid, which are genes for the globulin synthesis. It is probable that each maturing cell of the reticuloendothelial system spontaneously produces small amounts of antibody corresponding to its own genotype. Ready antibody molecules pass into the blood stream, circulate with the blood, and may be absorbed by some cells or tissues to form sessile antibodies.

Antibodies can also be synthesized along the intestinal tract or in the mucous membrane of the vagina, being excreted directly into the human bowel or into the lumen of the vagina (Koshland, 1953). As revealed by animal experiments, fecal antibodies appear in the feces soon after the primary injection of antigen, and reach the highest concentration on the fifth day, whereas the highest titer of serum antibody is noted on the ninth day (Burrows et al., 1947). Similar data were found for antibodies from vaginal mucus (Straus, 1961). Antibodies have also been found in the *humor vitreus* (Bozsoky, 1960) and in pleural exudates. Bacterial agglutinins, isohemagglutinins, and diphtherial antitoxin have been found in saliva and parotid fluid (Kraus and Konno, 1963). The classes of IgA, IgG, and IgM immunoglobulins were detected in saliva by Tomasi et al. (1965); but the antibacterial activity depends on the IgA immunoglobulin (Brandtzaeg et al. 1968). Bactericidal antibodies to *Salmonella typhosa* and *Shigella dysenteriae* were found in human parotid fluid as natural antibodies (Evans and Mergenhagen, 1965).

The rate and yield of antibody production depend, at least under experimental conditions, on such factors as the purity or complexity of the antigen preparation, the molecular weight and size of the antigen and its serological potency, the affinity of plasma cells and lymphocytes to the antigen, the immune readiness of the antibody producing system, and the dose of antigen and technique of immunization.

Most antigens, and especially purified antigens, diffuse from the site of injection quickly, so that excision of the antigen depot atfer a few hours or even after a few minutes does not prevent its spread in the host, or the subsequent production of antibodies (Roberts, 1931; Westwater, 1940). Traces of antibodies may be detected in the blood 8 to 10 hours after the injection of an antigen, but they are at a definite level in several days. Certain purified antigens leave the host through the urinary system so quickly that the stimulation of antibody-producing cells is ineffective. The first introduction of an antigen into the host, either under natural or artificial conditions, may promote an early and rather slow antibody formation (the primary response). After reaching a peak level, the antibodies decline gradually and in a few months cannot be detected. A subsequent introduction of the antigen causes a more rapid and more abundant antibody formation (secondary or anamnestic response), and the level of antibodies in this case declines rapidly.

Antibody formation is suppressed by irradiation "from within," for example, by the action of ^{131}I labeled particles such as viruses (Webber, 1964). The primary antibody response is radiosensitive. Sublethal x-ray irradiation of an animal, applied in a month, a few days, or even a few hours prior to the antigen injection, causes a decrease of the antibody production but has no such effect when the antibody has already appeared in the serum (Benjamin and Sluka, 1908; Craddock and Lawrence, 1948). Focal x-irradiation of the site injected with an antigen may even enhance the antibody production (Graham et al., 1956). An animal x-irradiated before the application of an antigen may recover its capacity to produce antibody through the injection of isologous bone marrow (Makinodan et al., 1955). Cortisone acetate delays or inhibits the local and general antibody formation (Hayes, 1953). Sodium salicylate and structurally related compounds, in a concentration equal to 80 mg/ml or more, inhibit antigen-antibody reactions in vitro (Friend, 1953).

The reason for a more vigorous antibody response to certain antigens than to others is obscure. Some investigations seem to suggest that antigens with higher molecular weights are able to induce a more rapid production of antibodies than antigens of lower molecular weights. For example, precipitins to bovine γ-globulin (its molecular weight being 180,000) were detected in rabbits in 7 to 15 days, whereas antibodies against bovine serum albumin (molecular weight of 69,000) appeared in 15 to 29 days (Janeway, 1953; Dixon et al., 1954). Similarly, precipitins to human γ-globulin in immunized chickens were detected earlier than those for bovine serum albumin (Abramoff and Wolfe, 1956).

Intact cells injected into animals stimulate the formation of antibodies to each structural element (Vennes and Gerhardt, 1959) and probably to all antigenic components. However, isolated antigens more readily induce antibody formation and a more vigorous immunological response than those incorporated in the cell structure. Isolated antigens can more easily provoke the antibody production whereas those present in intact cells, and especially in their deeper layers, can hardly be as effective. The immunization of rabbits with isolated fractions of streptococci produces a more effective antibody response than the injection of intact bacteria (Kwapinski, 1965). Immunization with purified antigens should be regarded as more efficient than, and preferable to, immunization with crude preparations or crude extracts of microorganisms.

The amount of antibody in the serum generally increases following each consecutive injecton of an antigen. However, sometimes a relative decrease of the antibody titer can be noticed at the fourth or fifth injection. The specificity of an antiserum, which primarily depends on the physiological state of the animal producing the antibody, usually decreases in the course of a prolonged immunization. The specificity of an antiserum is a function of the time of immunization and of the amount of antigen injected. With a prolonged immunization course, minor immunogenic substances accompanying a major antigenic component have a better chance to exert their immunizing effect. However, even under identical experimental conditions, specificities of the antisera may vary from animal to animal. The temperature of the host also seems to influence the immune response; for example, a higher immunity against tetanus toxoid was obtained when immunized mice were kept at 35° than at 25 or 6° (Ipsen, 1952).

Simultaneous injection of a number of individual antigens usually induces a qualitatively and quantitatively satisfactory antibody response to each of the antigens introduced (Huntoon and Craig, 1921; Corrigan, 1925; Heidelberger et al., 1948; Harris et al., 1954). Injection of a mixture of antigens may sometimes be more effective in stimulating antibody formation than immunization with individual antigens. For example, individual mammalian and avian antigens introduced in a mixture of 14:35 gave a greater yield of precipitins than was obtained by separate injections (Hektoen and Boor, 1931). Sometimes, however, the production of antibodies to some antigen mixtures may be lessened, probably as a result of the antigen competition phenomenon (Michaelis, 1904; Boyd and Bernard, 1937). For example, Abramoff and Wolfe (1956) noticed that the yield of antibodies to each of two different antigens mixed and injected simultaneously into chicken or rabbits was lower than after separate injections. A reduction of the antibody response to a previously used antigen was especially marked. It may be assumed that the more active antigens, which are quickly absorbed by cells of the reticuloendothelial system, can saturate reactive sites of antibody-producing cells so that few sites remain free and able to absorb molecules of other, less active antigens. According to Abramoff and Wolfe (1956), antigens with a high molecular weight may be more effective in binding reactive sites of antibodies than those of low molecular weight.

Antibody populations, formed against two or more (related) antigens may differ qualitatively. Thus upon the injection (in chicken) of two related antigens, spaced by 45 days, two qualitatively different antibody populations were produced. Antibodies specific for the second antigen proved to be of primary-response quality whereas the antibodies which cross-related with the first antigen were of secondary-response quality (Gilden and Tokuda, 1963).

Host factors influencing antibody production include the physical condition and immunological state of the host animal, the affinity to antigens of individual animal species, and efficiency in producing antibodies. For example, the New Zealand and Dutch strains of rabbits are more efficient in the production of (precipitating) antibodies than other strains of rabbits. The age of animals, the diet and other environmental conditions, such as *in vivo* temperature, and the route through which antigens enter the host play an important part in the yield of antibodies.

Some species of animals are better producers of antibodies to certain antigens than other species. Rabbits are usually capable of producing a great variety of antibodies. However, they do not form antibodies to certain purified antigens, for example, to capsular polysaccharides of pneumococci or to the carbohydrate Vi antigen, which induce antibody responses in man. Rabbits sometimes respond poorly to *Nocardia* antigens, whereas guinea pigs injected intraperitoneally with the same antigens produce high titers of antibodies (Kwapinski, 1965).

Some polysaccharide substances, for example, zymosan, which do not ordinarily promote antibody formation in rabbits, may provoke an antibody response when injected in an emulsion of adjuvants.

Antigens do not induce antibody formation in animals in a state of immunological tolerance. Immunologically unresponsive periods occur in the fetal or immediate newborn period or after the x-irradiation of the whole body (Billingham et al., 1956). The antibody production may be retarded or stopped altogether at extremely low body temperature, at least in some species of animals. For example, frogs kept at 22 to 27° are able to produce hemolysins but they do not form any antibody at temperatures between 8 to 10° (Allen and McDaniel, 1937).

III. CLASSIFICATIONS OF ANTIBODIES

Antibodies may be conventionally classified according to their origin, to their host specificity, or to the characteristics of immunological reactions in which they are involved. Most of known antibodies are free, circulating immunoglobulins, but some immunologically specific immunoglobulins occur as "cell-associated antibodies," playing an important part in the phenomena of cell-mediated immunity. "Cytophilic antibodies" are immunologically specific antibodies which after being discharged from antibody-synthesizing cells become adsorbed to other cells through "cytophilic bonds" of the Fc segment of IgG immunoglobulin molecule.

Two types of antibody, the natural and the immune, are differentiated depending on whether the antibody occurred without any obvious external stimulus or followed either an infection by microorganisms or experimental introduction of the antigen. The term "natural antibodies" is customarily applied to isohemagglutinins, which are hereditary, and to "normal" bacterial antibodies, which sometimes occur in low concentrations in human and animal sera. These "normal" bacterial antibodies, however, seem to differ only quantitatively from immune bacterial antibodies. The diagnostic insignificance of the former and the significance of the latter type of immune bodies should not obscure their identical immunological origin. Thus it is suggested that the term "natural antibodies" or "hereditary antibodies" should be limited to immune bodies which, like the isohemagglutinins, are specific "biochemical organs" (Hirszfeld et al., 1924), appearing in the serum at certain times in the life of the individual, and they are inherited. Stimulation of the formation of these antibodies by certain antigens of beans which are serologically similar to, or identical with, the blood group substances, has not yet been proved sufficiently.

Natural or hereditary antibodies against foreign red blood cells appear within a few months after the birth, attain a peak concentration by the age of 10 years and slowly decrease in the following years. Human serum contains natural antibodies against the erythrocytes of some other human beings, and against rabbit, guinea pig, sheep, ox, horse, and pigeon erythrocytes. Natural antibodies of the rabbit react with the erythrocytes of human beings, guinea pigs, sheep, and horses. The reactivity of normal antibodies with certain red blood cells should be considered in selecting appropriate systems for hemagglutination tests.

Immune antibodies are produced by the host in response to an apparent or inapparent infection by microorganisms, or following the experimental introduction of antigens. The rate of antibody response and especially the actual concentration and persistence of antibodies depend greatly upon the individual characteristics of antigens and hosts, and on the environmental or experimental conditions cited above. An acute invasion of a host with a large number of virulent microorganisms through an appropriate site of entry may cause a greater stimulation of the antibody-producing system than the intake of microorganisms with food, which is followed by the disintegration of many antigens by enzymes of the alimentary system.

The frequent occurrence of low-titer antibodies against *Enterobacteriaceae* in pigs probably results from the intake by these animals of a considerable number of various intestinal bacteria with the food contaminated by excreta. The presence of such antibodies in rabbits, guinea pigs, and horses probably arises from similar causes. The occurrence of antibodies against *Diplococcus pneumoniae, Streptococcus pyogenes,* or *Staphylococcus aureus* in apparently healthy human beings may result from frequent and repeated "carrier state." Any disturbance of the delicate biological balance between a microorganism and host, established in the "carrier state," can stimulate the antibody-producing system.

Antibodies are divided into three different groups, according to their host-specificity: (a) autoantibodies, produced against host's own antigens; (b) isoantibodies, formed by an individual in response to antigens of another individual of the same species; and (c) heteroantibodies, directed against antigens of another species.

Classification of Antibodies Based on the Characteristics of Immunological Reactions. The affinity of antibodies for homologous and related antigens varies within certain limits; hence three types of antibodies have been distinguished (Haurowitz, 1942): low grade, imperfect, and special. Low-grade antibodies are so imperfectly adapted to determinant groups of the antigen that only loose, reversible bonding is formed, and no precipitate is produced directly. Imperfect antibodies are only precipitated by the homologous antigen. Special antibodies are reactive with, and precipitated by, the homologous and heterologous antigens containing adequate determinant factors, which correspond to the active site of the antibody.

Cold agglutinins are usually IgM molecules with type K light chains. The K-chains possess either aspartic acid or glutamic acid as the N-terminal amino acids (Cohen and Cooper, 1968). Peptide chains of cold agglutinins may be prepared by Chaplin's et al. (1965) method.

Most immunological tests are carried out *in vitro,* but some, for example, the mouse protection test, are conducted *in vivo.* Reactions *in vitro* of antibodies with a homologous antigen may bring about observable changes in the physical properties of reactive mixtures used in the conventional serological tests. Thus complete or bivalent and incomplete or univalent antibodies are distinguished. Each group is further divided into subgroups according to the types of serological reaction they undergo. Complete antibodies occur as precipitins, agglutinins, hemagglutinins, hemolysins, bacteriolysins, complement fixing antibodies, bacteriotropins, or ablastins. They can be detected by direct serological tests, for example, the precipitation, agglutination, hemagglutination, complement fixation, immunohemolysis, or bacteriotropin test. Incomplete antibodies are classified as agglutinoids, cryptagglutinoids, and aggloids. They may be detected by indirect tests, for example, the antiglobulin, albumin, or saline blocking test, or by special physical tests involving the measurement of a change in the viscosity or in the optical rotation. Immunological tests used for the diagnosis of some infections are shown in Table 29.

Table 29. Tests Used for Immunological Diagnosis of Infections

Infecting Microorganism	Immunological Reactions	Allergens Used in Intradermal Tests
Actinobacillus mallei	CF, A	Mallein, a culture filtrate.
Actinobacillus pseudomallei	CF, A	
Adenovirus	CF, N	
Bacillus anthracis	P	
Blastomyces	CF, PH	
Bordetella pertussis	CF, A, MP, OP	
Brucella	A, F, CF, G, OP	*Brucella* polysaccharide, culture filtrate, heat killed bacteria.
Chlamydia	CF, N	
Coccidioidomyces	CF	
Corynebacterium diphtheriae	ID	
Coxiella burnetii	A, CF	
Coxsackie virus	N, CF	
Dengue virus	N, LF	
Diplococcus pneumoniae	C	
Haemophilus ducreyi		Killed culture.
Haemophilus influenzae	C	
Herpesvirus	N, CF	
Histoplasma capsulatum		Histoplasmin, a culture filtrate.
Leptospira	A, AA, AL	
Listeria	CF	
Lymphogranuloma vener. chlamydia	CF, N	Inactivated virus culture.
Measles virus	CF, N, HI	

(*Continued*)

Table 29 (*Continued*)

Infecting Microorganism	Immunological Reactions	Allergens Used in Intradermal Tests
Mononucleosis inf. agent	Paul-Bunnel test	
Mumps virus	CF, N, HI	
Mycobacterium leprae	H, CF	Lepromin (boiled lepromatous tissue).
Mycobacterium tuberculosis	PH, CF, H	PPD, tuberculin.
Mycoplasma	MGA	
Myxoviruses	CF, HI	
Neisseria gonorrhoeae	CF, FA, F	
Neisseria meningitidis	A	
PAP *virus*	MGA, CH	
Pasteurella pestis	P, PH	
Pasteurella tularensis	A, PH, OP	Killed bacteria.
Polio virus	N, CF, F, OP	
Poxvirus variolae	N, CF, HI, F	
Ricksettsia prowazeki	A, CF, PH, OP	
Rickettsia rickettsii	CF, A	
Rift Valley fever virus	NT	
Rubella virus	N	
Salmonella	A, PH	
Shigella	A	
Toxoplasma	CF, N	
Treponema pallidum	CF, F, I, IA, AT, PT, FA	
Trypanosoma	CF	
Vibrio comma	A	
Yellow Fever virus	N, CF	

A	= agglutination test	HI	= hemagglutination-inhibition test
AA	= agglutinin-absorption test	IA	= immune adherence test
AL	= agglutination-lysis test	I	= immobilizing test
CA	= cold agglutination test	ID	= immunodiffusion test
CF	= complement fixation test	N	= neutralization test
C	= capsular test	PH	= passive hemagglutination test
F	= flocculation test	P	= precipitation test
CH	= cold hemagglutinin test	OP	= opsono-phagocytic test
G	= γ-globulin test	MGA	= *Streptococcus* MG agglutination
H	= hemolytic test	MP	= mouse protection test
HeI	= hemolysin-inhibition test	FA	= fluorescent antibody test

IV. METHODS OF ANTISERUM PREPARATION

Sera used in serological tests are obtained from human beings or animals suffering from infectious diseases or are artificially produced by injections of antigenic materials into animals. For the purpose of immunization, soluble antigen preparations are sterilized by filtration. Insoluble antigens can be sterilized with 0.2% formalin or 0.3 to 0.5% phenol. Antigens treated with the disinfectants for 12t o 18 hours are then centrifuged and washed with sterile saline. All antigen preparations may be preserved with 0.01% merthiolate.

Important factors in the artificial immunization are the selection of reactive animals, the route of injection, the dose of the antigen preparation, and the number and schedule of injections.

Antisera are produced mostly in small laboratory animals, such as rabbits, guinea pigs, or chickens. Horses, sheep, goats, and cattle are used for the commercial production of large quantities of antitoxins and antibacterial sera. Monkeys and human beings are only occasionally selected for special experimental immunization. Rats, mice, and hamsters are seldom used since they yield little serum.

Normal and immune sera occasionally contain, at low titers, some antibodies which probably arose from a natural uptake of certain antigens. Therefore, animals to be used for artificial immunization should ideally be bred under conditions lessening the chance of acquiring common microorganisms from the environment. Before an immunization is started, serum samples of the laboratory animals must be tested for the presence of "natural" antibodies versus antigens to be injected and against some common microorganisms, such as enteric bacteria, staphylococci, and streptococci. These antibodies must not be present in serum samples from animals to be used for immunization.

Antigens are injected into animals intravenously, intraperitoneally, or subcutaneously and less frequently through the intracutaneous or intramuscular route. Materials like fungal mycelia, which cannot be adequately homogenized for intravenous injections, should be extracted with a 2:1 mixture of ether and alcohol. The delipidized material can be easily homogenized and injected intravenously whereas the extracted lipids are dried off, suspended in saline, and injected intramuscularly or subcutaneously.

Materials introduced into the peritoneal cavity enter the blood stream rather rapidly, but they diffuse slowly from subcutaneous or intracutaneous depot. The speed of antigen diffusion from a depot depends considerably on the degree of its purification. Purified protein or polysaccharide antigens, for example, enter the blood stream more rapidly than more complex or crude antigen preparations. Rapid diffusion of an antigen into the blood stream, followed by a quick excretion through the urinary system, may not sufficiently stimulate the antibody-producing cells. A prolonged deposition of antigens in the subcutaneous tissue is often beneficial for the antibody-production. The outward flow of antigens from a subcutaneous depot can be retarded by adjuvants.

Doses of an antigen preparation vary according to the nature of the antigen. Immunization with highly toxic materials should begin with very small amounts and gradually increase. For example, 0.1 ml of 1:10 dilution of a culture filtrate of *Clostridium tetani* is the starting dose for a rabbit. Nontoxic antigens can be injected in larger amounts. For example, doses starting with 0.2 mg and increasing gradually by 0.2 mg up to 2.0 mg are adequate for most nontoxic antigen preparations. Immunization with several or more smaller or gradually increased doses injected a few days apart is for many antigens more effective than the inoculation of a single large dose. However, some antigen preparations (e.g., those of the *Actinomycetales* or corynebacteria) cause a satisfactory antibody response when injected, in gradually increasing doses, in each of five consecutive days. In other cases a schedule of two to three periods consisting of three daily injections followed by a 1- to 2- weeks rest gives the best result.

Suspensions of bacteria used for immunization contain usually 10^8 to 10^9 cells/ml. Suitable techniques for the determination of quantity of bacteria are (a) the progressive-dilution culture method, (b) the spectrophotometric density determination by comparison with a standard suspension of bacteria, and (c) the relative count procedure. In the last technique (Wright, 1902), a bacterial suspension is mixed with an equal volume of fresh, citrated human blood. A drop of the mixture is spread in a thick layer on a microscope slide and colored with Wright's stain. The number of bacteria seen among 200 erythrocytes is estimated. Assuming that normal blood contains about 5,000,000 red blood cells per centimeter, the number of bacteria per milliliter is calculated from this simple formula:

$$\text{number of bacteria per milliliter} = (\text{number of bacteria counted}) \times 2500$$

Injections of an antigen, given either at daily or weekly intervals, should be continued only until a maximum or satisfactory titer of circulating antibodies is reached. Additional injections beyond a peak level of antibodies have no effect. The amount of circulating antibody is a function of the amount being produced and the amount being destroyed (Koshland et al., 1950). The number of minor antibodies is usually greater after a long-term immunization than after a short series of injections. The titer of antibodies decreases slowly when the immunization is stopped, but it can remain on a level not lower than 70% of the maximum titer for several weeks or months. An additional injection in this period of the same antigen or a serologically unrelated protein can bring about a rapid increase of antibodies (the anamnestic reaction). However, boosters carrying heterologous proteins can diminish or alter the specificity of the antisera and elicit a fatal anaphylactic reaction.

Antibodies against many particulate antigens, such as Gram-negative bacteria or erythrocytes, appear in the blood of immunized animals in a short time ranging from 2 to 5 days after a single intravenous injection. The immunization time is somewhat longer, ranging from 2 to 3 weeks in the case of soluble antigens, such as toxins or polysaccharide fractions, and may be as long as 2 to 3 months with some bacteria of the order *Actinomycetales*. Subsequent injections of the same antigen are followed by a more pronounced secondary response, with a more rapid and higher rise of the titer than the first introduction of the antigen; and the antibody persists for a longer time.

The following immunization schedule (Kwapinski, 1969) has proved, in numerous experiments, to invariably yield satisfactory antibodies.

An antigen preparation containing approximately 1% solids is injected at 3 to 5 day intervals by the following routes and in the following sequence.

> 0.3 ml subcutaneously
> 0.4 ml intramuscularly
> 0.4 ml into a food pad
> 0.4 into another food pad
> 0.4 ml intravenously
> 0.5 ml subcutaneously

The serum is collected 7 days after the last injection if it proves reactive with its antigen. Otherwise, the injections are repeated, increasing the dose twofold.

Barth's et al. (1965) schedule for the production of hyperimmune serum involves four daily interperitoneal injections of an antigen or a vaccine at 2-week intervals. The animals (mice) are bled by cardiac puncture 1 week after the last injection.

The antibody content of a serum should be tested periodically. For this purpose, 1 to 2 ml of blood are withdrawn each time, allowed to clot, and the serum is separated by centrifugation. Final bleeding is performed in 5 to 7 days after the last injection which yielded the maximum antibody titer. The bleeding of guinea pigs from ear vein is greatly facilitated by a sucking glass bell or an illuminated apparatus devised by Entel and Weinhold (1957), or Markham and Kent (1951). A method of bleeding mice from the ophthalmic venous plexus was published by Riley (1960). The serum is then separated from the clotted blood and centrifuged until clear. Feed should be withheld from animals for 24 hours before bleeding to avoid an accumulation of lipids in the serum in high concentration. Alternatively, the excess of lipids can be removed by storing the serum at $0°$ for 3 to 5 days and centrifuging at 2000 to 5000 $\times$ g. The lipid is brought to the surface, and clear serum can be withdrawn with a Pasteur pipette. Another method of serum clarification is by filtration through a precooled Seitz pad with an average pore diameter of 5 μ. The serum can be stored at $-30°$ for many months or even for years. Sera that are not likely to be used in a few weeks or months should be desiccated in vacuo from the frozen state in a lyophilizer. They can also be preserved for some months if mixed with disinfectants such as 0.08% Merthiolate, 0.1% phenol, 0.1% tricresol, 0.5% chloroform, or 0.1% sodium azide. Formalin is not recommended as a preservative of antisera. It has been found that formalin, added in the proportion of 1 ml of 0.2% formalin solution per 9 ml of serum, may cause a slight reduction of activity of immunoglobulins.

V. IMMUNE TOLERANCE

An usual immunological reaction in adult animals to repeated small doses of an antigen is that after an initial antibody production, starting 1 to 2 weeks after the first injection, the rate of antibody synthesis is gradually reduced until very little or no specific antibody is produced. A similar phenomenom of progressive reduction of antibody synthesis occurs after an intermittent circulation of soluble complexes in rabbits (Andres et al., 1963).

Immunotolerance (a tolerance state) in an animal to specific antigen may be produced by:

1. Antigen overloading, caused by the administration of large doses of a foreign antigen into adult animals leading to the immunological paralysis (Dixon and Maurer, 1955).

2. Repeated injection of an antigen into neonatal animals, causing a specific immune tolerance apparently due to the continuous circulation of soluble immunological complexes.

3. Injections of antigen-antibody complexes, resulting in a continuous circulation of the complex acid in a subsequent loss of ability to synthesize the specific antibodies (Boyns and Hardwicke, 1968). Antibody infusion at or immediately after the injection of antigen can suppress subsequent antibody formation Möller and Wigzell, 1965).

The immune tolerance may be broken or terminated by the injection of a closely related antigen into the tolerant animals.

VI. ADJUVANTS

The formation of antibodies can be enhanced by boosting some antigens with adjuvants. In these cases, potent antibodies are produced after a lesser number of injections of antigen-adjuvant mixtures than of an antigen alone, and titers of antibodies increase at least fivefold and persist in the host for a longer time. The disadvantage of the use of adjuvants can be the production of antibodies against minor antigenic contaminants and against antigenic constituents of the adjuvants.

The synergistic effect is exhibited by a variety of nonantigenic or antigenic substances such as alum hydroxide, kaolin, charcoal, lanolin, tapioca, solid paraffin, paraffin oil, a light mineral oil, Bayol F, Arlacel A, phosphorylated hespiridin, magnesium salts, calcium salts, staphylococcal toxoid, and autoclaved mycobacteria (Saenz, 1912; Ramon et al., 1935, 1938; Freund, 1936; Salk and Laurent, 1952; Jensen and Francis, 1953).

The enhanced formation of antibodies may be attributed to a local inflammation caused by adjuvants, or to the retarded absorption of antigens deposited in subcutaneous depots. Killed mycobacteria, used in complete Freund's adjuvants, provoke the formation of local granulomas at the site of injection; these granulomas consist of epithelioid cells which are thought to produce antibody. A marked hyperplasia of the regional lymph nodes of the spleen can follow an injection of adjuvants (Fishel et al., 1952). It is also possible that droplets of antigen-adjuvant mixtures drain to the regional lymph node and stimulate antibody-forming cells, or they are deposited by blood circulation in the antibody-forming organs, the spleen and bone marrow.

Complete antigen-adjuvant preparations consist of an antigen incorporated into the aqueous phase of water-in-oil emulsion, the oily phase containing killed mycobacteria. *Mycobacterium tuberculosis,* often used in the adjuvant emulsions, can be replaced by saprophytic mycobacteria, for example, *Mycobacterium phlei, Mycobacterium butyricum,* or *Nocardia asteroides* (Lipton and Freund, 1950), as well as by a "wax fraction" isolated from *Mycobacterium tuberculosis* according to Anderson's method (1929, 1939). According to the technique of Freund et al. (1940), modified by Fishel et al. (1952), adjuvants are prepared in the following manner. About 60 to 70 mg of killed dried tubercle bacilli (the strain $H_{37}Rv$) are mixed with 50 ml of paraffin oil and ground in a mortar. A mixture composed of 500 mg of an antigen dissolved in 25 ml of saline and 25 ml of aquaphor (an oil emulsifier) is added to this adjuvant emulsion, under constant stirring.

Another adjuvant (Uhr et al., 1957) consists of 8.5 parts Bayol F, 1.5 parts Arlacel A, and 2 mg/ml of lyophilized *Mycobacterium butyricum* per an equal volume of the antigen suspension. The immunizing agent can be precipitated with alumina before the antigen-adjuvant emulsion is prepared. Thus a suspension of bacteria or a culture filtrate in a volume of 100 ml is mixed with 4.66 ml of 10% $AlCl_3$, and this fluid is adjusted to pH 7 by adding 20% sodium hydroxide. The final liquid is diluted 1:1 with a saline solution.

The antigen-adjuvant mixtures are usually injected intramuscularly in a volume of 0.5 ml thrice at weekly intervals, in different sites of the animals body, or into each of the four footpads (toepads). Another schedule for the immunization of antigen-adjuvant emulsions (containing 10 mg of protein per milliliter is as follows: two intramuscular injections of 0.5 ml of the antigen-adjuvant mixture, two intramuscular injections of 0.25 ml, and two intraperitoneal injections of 0.25 ml of the emulsion, spaced by 7-day periods. The serum is tested for the presence of antibodies 2 to 4 weeks after the last injection.

In view of the new findings that 10% saline suspensions of carbonyl iron (carbonyl iron-starch) or kaolin injected with antigens enhanced greatly antitbody response (Levine and Sowinski, 1970), comparable to that produced by oily emulsions of mycobacteria, the use of the latter type of adjuvants is not recommended.

VII. THE ANTIBODY PRODUCTION IN VITRO

Antibodies can be produced *in vitro* by isolated fragments of tissues and by single plasma cells or lymphocytes in adequate environmental conditions. Hemolysins, hemagglutinins, bacteriolysins, bacterial agglutinins, and antitoxin have been detected in cultures of lymph nodes or spleen maintained in a homologous blood plasma. The antibody-synthesizing capability may be tested *in vitro* essentially on organs obtained from preimmunized animals.

The effect of an antigen on DNA synthesis by splenic cells in vitro may be determined by Dutton and Eady's (1964) procedure.

Antibody Production by Organs and Tissues in Vitro. According to the procedure described by Stavitsky (1954), spleen and lymphoid glands removed aseptically from animals are placed in Fischer's (1948) medium containing 20% sterile, normal rabbit serum with 100 units of penicillin and 50 μg of streptomycin per milliliter. Fragments of these organs are blotted, weighed, and placed in sterile, 13 × 100 ml tubes containing 1 ml of Fischer's medium, and plugged with sterile rubber stoppers. Tissue fragments of nonimmunized animals are at this stage exposed to an antigen preparation added to the culture medium. Tubes are rotated for 21 to 24 hours at 37° in a roller tube apparatus, at the rate of one revolution every 3 minutes. Tissue fragments are then removed, washed with saline, and homogenized in 1 ml of saline. The tissue culture medium and saline washings are combined, centrifuged at 1000 × g for 30 minutes, left at 56° for 30 minutes, and the supernatant is tested against a homologous antigen by an adequate immunological test.

Various antibodies, such as *corynebact. diphtheriae*-antitoxin, *Brucella* and *Salmonella* agglutinins, hemagglutinins, and hemolysins, were obtained by this or a similar technique (Stavitsky, 1955; Steiner and Anker, 1956; Grabar and Corvazier, 1960).

Antibody Production by Single Cell. Antibody production by single cells may be tested by the following techniques:

1. The localized immunolysis test in gel (Jerne and Nordin, 1963; Ingraham and Bussard, 1964).
2. Specific erythrocyte aggregation test (Zaalberg, 1964).
3. Fluorescein-labelled antigen in sections of tissue (Coons et al., 1958).
4. A microdroplet assay in which a microdrop containing a single cell is assayed for antibacteriophage antibody (Attardi et al., 1959).
5. Immunoadherence (Mäkelä and Nossal, 1961).
6. Specific inhibition of bacterial movement in the microdrop by flagella antibody (Nossal, 1962).
7. Autoradiographic technique (Pick and Feldman, 1967).
8. Antigen-bentonite adherence test (Baker et al., 1966).

The localized immunohemolysis assay depends on the detection of the immune hemolysin, secreted by antigen-producing cells, by revealing complement-dependent hemolytic plaques, formed around the cells on reaction with erythrocytes. A method analogous to the plaque hemolysis technique is the localized bacteriolysis technique (Schwartz and Braun, 1965). The localized hemolysis technique has been modified for use with polysaccharide antigens absorbed onto erythrocytes and with soluble polyamino acid antigens (Landy et al., 1964; Walsh et al., 1967). Techniques for the determination of direct interactions between the relevant antigen and the antibody-producing cells, as opposed to the complement-dependent immune lysis, are the autoradiographic plaque technique (Pick and Feldman, 1967) and the antigen-bentonite adherence technique (Baker et al., 1966). An immunocytoadherence technique (Mäkelä and Nossal, 1961) relies on the principle of bacterial immunocytoadherence onto antibody-forming cells. The bacteria adherent to the antibody forming cells cultured in a solid cultured medium give rise to bacterial colonies which can be enumerated under low power magnification.

The Specific Erythrocyte Aggregation Assay. According to Zaalberg's (1964) method, the potential antibody-forming cells are derived from spleens obtained from mice immunized with sheep red cells by intraperitoneal injection of 10^9 cells twice a week for 3 consecutive weeks. Six days after the last injection, the spleen is removed and a homogeneous suspension of cells is prepared. The washed spleen cells are suspended in a test tube at 10^7 cells/ml of a tissue culture medium containing 1% washed sheep erythrocytes. The test tubes are incubated at 37° in a roller tube apparatus for 2 hours. The cells are then pipetted into a haemocytometer and counted under a microscope. It is observed that nucleated, antibody-producing spleen cells are surrounded by agglutinated sheep erythrocytes and the number of agglutinated erythrocytes clustered around a cell appears to reflect the amount of antibody produced by that cell.

This method is suitable for the determination of the number of antibody-forming cells in a lymphoid tissue after different routes of immunization as well as for the differentiation of antibodies produced after immunization with two different antigens, such as sheep and fowl erythrocytes. The use of the erythrocytes possessing different morphology makes it possible to decide whether the cell cluster around a single lymphoid cell consists of a mixture of the two red cell types or a single type. The two different types of cells can be coated with various antigens.

Potassium cyanide at 0.01 M added to the culture medium containing immunized lymphoid cells stops cellular antibody formation.

VIII. PREPARATION OF TISSUE ANTIBODIES

Antibodies can be extracted from tissues with distilled water adjusted to pH 7.6 or with a cold saline. Tissues are at first disintegrated by the procedure of three alternative rapid freezing at 80° and thawing at 37°. The fragmentated tissue is then suspended in cold saline, homogenized in a chilled Ten Broeck homogenizer, and centrifuged at 5° for 30 minutes. The supernatant represents a crude source of the tissue antibody.

IX. PREPARATION OF COPROANTIBODIES

The coproantibody or fecal antibody seems to be separate from the serum antibody. Coproantibodies are produced in local sites along the intestinal tract.

Coproantibodies were found in enteric cholera in guinea pigs and in the dysentery caused by *Shigella flexneri* or *Shigella sonnei*. Coproantibodies seem to reach the highest titer and start to decline before serum antibody levels began to rise (Burrows et al., 1947; Koshland et al., 1950; Barksdale and Ghoda, 1951).

Coproantibodies can be isolated from fecal samples by means of the procedures reported by Koshland et al. (1950) and Barksdale and Ghoda (1951). Excreta are collected in a collecting funnel equipped with a brass screen, attached to the metabolism cage (Burrows et al., 1947) and homogenized in a Waring blender for 30 seconds. This material treated with 0.5% formalin can then be extracted with physiological saline, and centrifuged at 5% for 30 minutes at 3000 × g. The supernatant is collected, centrifuged again at 4000 × g, and stored in the cold. Prior to use in a complement fixation test, it is inactivated at 50° for 30 minutes, adjusted to pH

7.0 with 0.1 N HCl, and recentrifuged at 4000 $\times$ g for 20 minutes. To minimize its anticomplementary activity, the fecal preparation should be diluted in the ratio 1:5 with a 1:80 solution of a normal serum.

X. PREPARATION AND PURIFICATION OF SERUM IMMUNOGLOBULINS

Antibodies are found predominantly in the blood plasma. Minor amounts of antibodies can be detected in the cerebrospinal fluid, exudates, feces, and various tissues. Serum proteins constitute 6 to 7% of dry weight of the blood serum. Globulins account for approximately 1.4 to 3.5 g or an average 39% of the total protein of normal serum (14% α-globulin, 14% β-globulin, and 11% γ-globulin); albumin represents 3.6 to 5.5 g or an average 57% and fibrinogen 5% of the total serum protein. Blood plasma can be fractionated to more than 30 identifiable substances, ranging from serum albumins to various enzymes (Table 28), by means of gel chromatography and electrophoresis immunosorption and chemical fractionation.

Separation of Antibody-Containing Serum Proteins by Precipitation. Separation of proteins containing antibody immunoglobulins can be attained by dilution of the serum with water at low temperature, or by the precipitation with neutral salts, such as ammonium or sodium sulfate, with ethyl alcohol, or by a partition chromatography or electrophoresis. According to Kendall's (1937) procedure, 50 ml of saturated ammonium sulfate are added to 100 ml of undiluted human serum to precipitate euglobulins. After the centrifugation, the euglobulin is purified by dissolving it in 50 ml of distilled water and adding 25 ml of a saturated ammonium sulfate solution slowly with stirring. Various globulin fractions, the euglobulin, pseudoglobulin 1, and pseudoglobulin 2, may be precipitated at successive concentrations of 13.5, 17.4, and 21.5 to 26% of sodium sulfate, while the albumin remains in solution (Kibrick and Bronstein, 1948). Globulins containing antibody can be precipitated at 16% concentration of sodium sulfate or at final 50% saturation of ammonium sulfate. Each globulin fraction or total globulins are dialyzed for 3 to 5 days in the cold against distilled water, to remove the salt completely, then concentrated or lyophilized. The fraction containing most antibody activity is determined by a serological test with the homologous antigen. Most antibodies are confined to the pseudoglobulin fraction, and less frequently to the euglobulin fraction.

Precipitation by dialysis is conducted by suspending a bag containing serum in distilled water. When most electrolytes leave the dialyzate, a precipitate containing the euglobulin fraction is formed whereas pseudoglobulins and the albumin remain in solution. Precipitated euglobulins are soluble in dilute electrolyte solutions, for example, in physiological saline.

Alcohol precipitation of antibody-containing plasma fractions (Felton, 1931; Cohn et al., 1946; Deutsch, 1952) depends on a gradual increase of the ethyl alcohol concentration in the plasma under controlled pH. According to Felton's procedure the antiserum is poured slowly into 20 volumes of cold distilled water with continuous stirring, and left at 2 to 4° overnight. If the flocculate does not settle readily, 1 ml of 1 M phosphate buffer, pH 6.8, is added per liter of water used. The precipitate should be centrifuged off in the cold, then resuspended in a small volume of cold distilled water, and dissolved by addition of a 10% solution of sodium chloride. This solution is diluted approximately five times, and held at 37° for 2 hours upon the addition of ethyl mercury-thiosalicylate as preservative. The fluid is finally clarified by centrifugation and filtration through a 0.45μ-porosity membrane filter.

Cohn's technique No. 6 is presented diagrammatically (Table 30). The temperature is at all stages maintained between -2.5 and $-5°$ to prevent denaturation of the proteins. Five major fractions are separaed from human plasma, and they can be further subfractionated by an additional alcohol precipitation. A modification of this method (Steffanini, 1954) is presented in Table 31. Most antibodies are found in the subfractions II $-$ 1,2,3 and III $-$ 1 (Enders, 1944, and others). Chromatographic isolation of the antibody-containing serum globulins is carried out by Porter's method (1955).

The most accurate separation of individual serum proteins is obtained by electrophoresis. Separation in an electric field of antibody-carrying serum proteins is conventionally conducted in the electrophoresis-convection apparatus (Cann et al., 1949) or by starch electrophoresis (Kunkel and Slater, 1952; Poulik, 1959, 1964).

On electrophoresis, in the ascending boundaries, the first to ascend is albumin, followed by alpha 1 and alpha 2 globulins, beta globulin, fibrinogen, and γ globulin coming last. In the descending boundaries, albumin is

Table 30.   Fractionation of Plasma Proteins by Cohn's et al. (1946) Method

pH	Alcohol Concentra- tion (%)	Fraction	Composition of the Fraction				
			Fibrinogen (%)	Albumin (%)	α Globulin (%)	β Globulin (%)	γ Globulin (%)
7.2	8	I	61	7	8	15	9
6.8	25	II + III	5	4	6	48	37
5.2	18[a]	IV-1	0	—	89	10	1
5.8	40	IV-4	0	16	46	38	0
4.8	40	V	0	95	4	1	0

[a] By diluting the supernatant with water.

Table 31.   Modified Ethanol Fractionation of Plasma Proteins[a]
(Stefanini, 1954)

Plasma			
pH 5.8; $r/2$ 0.04, Ethanol 19%, 5 P.V.			
Filtrate Fraction IV-V-VI		Precipitate Fraction I-II-III	
pH 5.8, 0.02 M Zn(Ac)$_2$ 5 P.V., Ethanol 19%		pH 5.4, 0.60 M Glycine, 2 P.V., Ethanol 15%	
Filtrate Fraction VI	Precipitate Fraction IV-V	Precipitate Fraction I-III	Filtrate Fraction II
Traces of IV-V	*Albumins*	β_1-Lipoproteins	*γ-Globulins*
α_1-Glycoprotein	β_1-Metal combining protein	β_1-Lipid poor euglobulins	
α_1-*Protein*	α_2-Glycoproteins	Ceruloplasmin	
β_1-*Protein*	α_2-Mucoproteins	*Isoagglutinins*	
Urea	α_1-Lipoproteins	Profibrinolysin	
Glucose	Iodoproteins	*Cold-insoluble globulin*	
Small peptides	Choline esterase	Fibrinogen	
	Alkaline phosphatase	Prothrombin	

[a] The fractionation is carried out at $-5°$.

followed by delta globulin, alpha 1 and alpha 2 globulin, followed by beta globulin, fibrinogen, and γ globulins (Figs. 44 and 45).

Cohn's ethanol fractionation method has been modified by Steffanini (1954) as shown in Table 31. Antibody-containing fractions can also be satisfactorily separated by paper electrophoresis and eluted with saline from fragments of the electrophoretogram (Witmer, 1952; Kwapinski and Madalinski, 1955). Purity of the immunoglobulin preparations is determined by the immunoelectrophoresis using antisera produced against the individual classes of immunoglobulins.

Anti-IgG serum is produced by immunization of rabbits and goats with IgG mixed in incomplete Freund's adjuvant.

Anti-Fc antiserum is obtained by absorbing an antirabbit IgG serum with rabbit-Fab produced by digestion of the IgG serum with pepsin.

Antiimmunoglobulin reagent is obtained most efficiently by the following immunization schedule (Triftshauser et al., 1970): goats of mixed breeds weighing between 40 and 125 lb and 1 to 4 years of age, thoroughly examined, tuberculin tested and deparasitized, are injected (after an initial sample of blood has been withdrawn) with 1 mg/ml of an antigen in saline mixed with an equal volume of complete Freund's adjuvant. Injections are made intradermally into four legs.

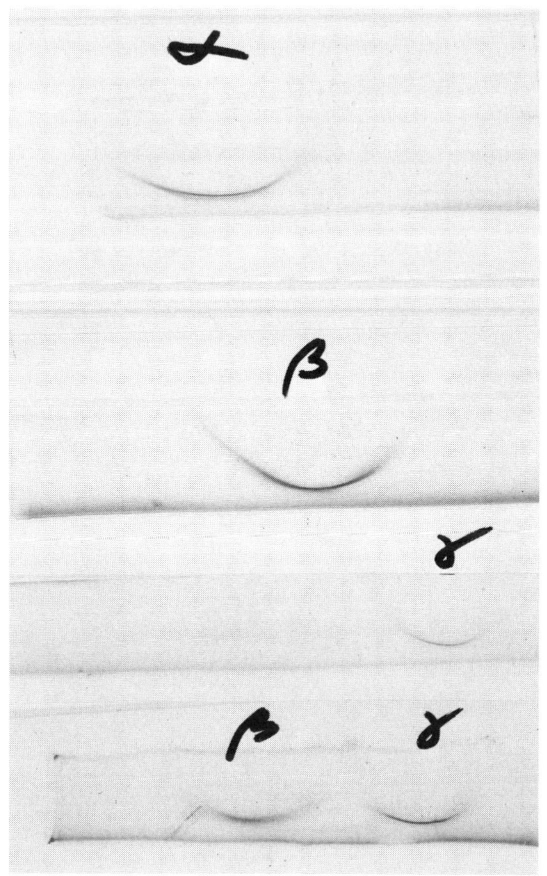

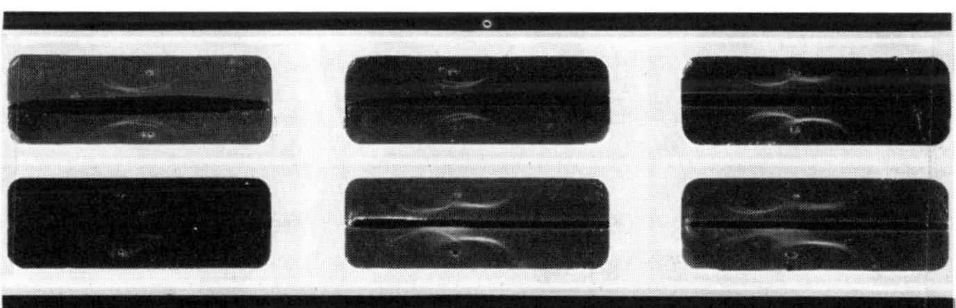

Figure 44. Relative position of purified, immunologically different electrophoretic globulins of the mouse serum (Kwapinski, 1968).

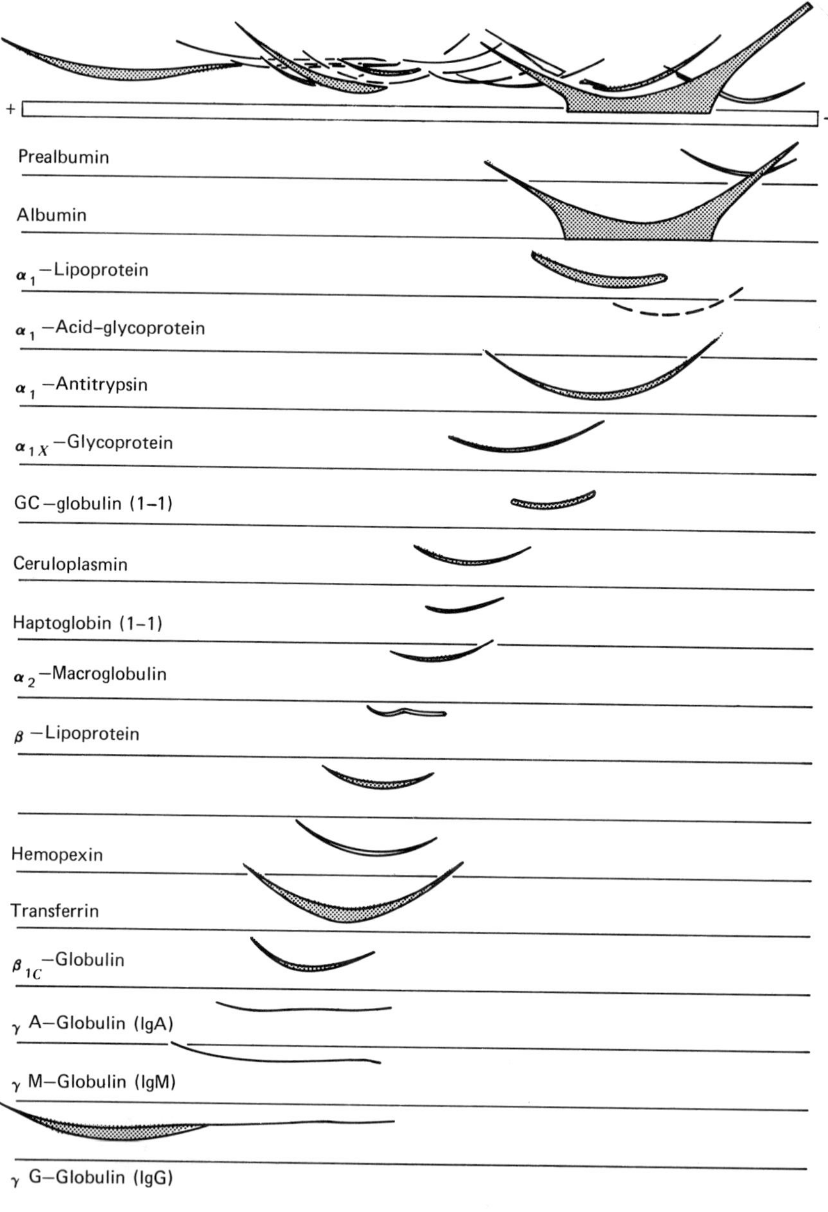

Figure 45. Position of immunoglobulins and other proteins in the immunoelectrophoregram of human serum.

Purification of Antibodies.   Antibodies can be purified either by the removal of intert proteins or absorbed antigens, or by the absorption of the specific immunoglobulins on immunoadsorbents. Inert protein may often be precipitated with zinc chloride (Murdick and Cohen, 1935) by adding $N/10$ zinc chloride to the solution of a crude globulin preparation maintained at pH 7.6, in the proportion of 1 ml of the zinc chloride solution per 100 mg of the globulin nitrogen. The mixture is left for 1 hour at room temperature, then centrifuged. The precipitate is suspended in 0.8% sodium chloride solution, dissolved with $N/10$ HCl, and reprecipitated with $N/10$ NaOH. The precipitate should be removed, and the supernatant containing the purified antibody globulin is analyzed and precipitated isoelectrically as described by Felton (1928).

Syphilitic reagins can be separated from the cardiolipin or similar antigen preparations by ether extraction. According to Davis et al. (1945), the floccules containing cardiolipidreagin complexes are first centrifuged in the cold and washed three times with a cold 0.9% saline. The final sediment is suspended in 1 to 2 ml of 15% sodium chloride and mixed with 10 ml of cold ether, then shaken until most of the solid sodium is dissolved. The ether is then removed by suction, and the remaining fluid is centrifuged in the cold for 15 minutes. The clear supernatant is now dialyzed overnight in a refrigerator against a phosphate buffered saline at pH 7.4. Any precipitate that is found during dialysis is removed by centrifugation. Purified antibody remains in the solution.

Antibodies can be isolated from globulin preparations by a specific absorption on antigens or by a nonspecific absorption on inert particles such as kaolin, followed by elution at an appropriate pH.

Antigen preparations used for specific absorption of the antibody are in the form of intact cells, soluble antigen preparations, or are coupled to the diazonium salts, or absorbed onto an ion exchange resin.

A simple absorption of antibodies with particulate antigens is conducted by adding 1 ml of washed, packed microorganisms to 9 ml of antiserum diluted 1:2 to 1:5 to isolated serum globulin diluted 1:10 to 1:20. The mixture is left for 1 hour at 37° and agitated for 2 hours at 2° on an electrical shaker, then centrifuged for 5 to 10 minutes at 12,000 rpm. Precipitates are washed twice with saline. The antibody can be removed from the antigen-antibody complex by elution at a very high or very low pH range with veronal or another alkaline buffer at pH 10 to 13, with 0.1 M sodium hydroxide, a cold 10% barium chloride, or 10 to 15% sodium chloride at 37° (Heidelberger and Kendall, 1936; Kabat and Mayer, 1948; Liu and Wu, 1938; Kleinschmidt and Boyer, 1952; Kwapinski, 1965).

Antitoxins, particularly the diphtheria antitoxin, can be separated from its antigen by exposing toxin-antitoxin precipitates to 0.1 N glycine-HCl buffer at pH 2.5 to 3.0 at 26° for 18 hours (Turner and Boyer, 1952) or by heating to 50° in dilute acetic acid (Ramon, 1923). The polysaccharide antibody can be purified by extracting the specific precipitate with 15% sodium chloride followed by dialysis (Heidelberger and Kendall, 1936). Another method of purifying the antihapten antibody was published by Karush and Marks (1957).

Total antibody absorbed in a concentrated serum is greater than in a diluted serum; but the relative amount of absorbed antibody is less from the concentrated than from a diluted serum (Eisenberg and Volk, 1902). Antibodies are less susceptible to denaturation than protein antigens.

Antibody Preparation and Purification by Immunosorbents. Specific antibody-immunoglobulins may be absorbed on physical complexes consisting of an antigen adsorbed to inert particles, and then eluted. The following substances are known to adsorb proteins: charcoal, kaolin, Pyrex glass, cholesterol, collodion, polystyrene latex, polyacrylamide, bismuth, gallate, alizarine, ferric and ammonium oxides, resin, and cellulose treated with chitosan.

However, the amount of proteins adsorbed onto these sorbents is relatively small. More efficient are sorbents consisting of antigens linked to an insoluble support or to chemical bonds, e.g., the diazo bond or amide bond.

The *antibody purification* by diazotized compounds were designed by Sternberger and Pressman (1950) and Weetall (1967). The first technique employs soluble antigens and is based on a modification of the antigen so that it can still precipitate specific antibodies but can now be removed from solution under conditions in which the dissociation of antigen-antibody complex takes place. The other method utilizes bacteria, polymerized by tetrazotized benzidine.

According to Sternberger and Pressman's technique, a protein antigen is coupled with either the diazotized *p*-aminobenzenearsonic acid or diazotized *o*-aminobenzoic acid. The coupled antigen is added in an optimum amount to antiserum and is left at 37° for 2 hours and at 5° for 44 hours. The precipitate is then centrifuged in the cold, washed twice with chilled saline, and once with chilled distilled water. The washed precipitate is dissolved in 20 ml of saturated calcium hydroxide solution and left for 5 minutes. The antigen is removed with calcium aluminate. Thus 1.5 to 2 ml of a freshly prepared suspension of calcium aluminate is added to the dissolved precipitate, at pH 12, shaken for a few seconds, and centrifuged for 10 minutes at RCF1600. Sediment containing the antigen is removed and the colored supernatant containing the antibody globulin is rapidly adjusted to pH 7.2 to 7.5 with 0.1 *N* HCl, under constant stirring. Any colored precipitate formed is collected by centrifugation. The clear supernatant contains the first fraction of purified antibody. Other antibody fractions can be recovered from the collected sediment by dissolving repeatedly in 20 ml of saturated calcium hydroxide solution and precipitating with 1.5 ml of the calcium aluminate suspension. The suspension of calcium aluminate is prepared by adding saturated calcium hydroxide solution to 0.8 ml of 2.0 M aluminate chloride solution until pH 12.0 is reached. The calcium aluminate precipitates under vigorous stirring. This suspension should be concentrated to about 4 or 5 ml by centrifugation.

Weetall's Method for the Purification of Antibodies. The bacteria are first washed three times in 0.1 M NaOH and 0.1 N HCl, resuspended in distilled water, and polymerized by the addition of tetrazotized benzidine in the proportion of $\frac{1}{10}$ of the weight of (acetone-dried) bacteria. The tetrazotized benzidine is prepared by the Campbell et al. (1970) method. Sodium nitrate is added to the mixture in the amount of 2 moles/1 mole of benzidine, maintaining the pH at 9.2. The reaction is continued overnight at 4°. The polymerized cells are washed on a Büchner funnel with 0.1 N NaOH, 0.1 N HCl, and acetone, successively. The immunosorbents can be stored at $-20°$.

The immunoadsorbent columns (1.5 × 5.0 cm and 2.5 × 50 cm) are prepared with a mixture consisting of the acetonedried polymerized bacteria and 5 times their weight of nonionic cellulose. The immunoadsorbent columns are washed with 0.1 M HCl, 0.1 M phosphate in 1% saline solution, pH 7.0, and 1% sodium chloride solution, successively, until little or no adsorption is detectable in the effluent at 280 nm.

In order to isolate and purify specific antibodies, the antiserum is layered over the immunoadsorbent bed which is then washed with 1% sodium chloride solution until no ultraviolet-adsorbing material is detectable in the column effluent. The antibodies are eluted at 4° with 0.05 M phosphate made in 1% saline, pH 2.3.

The collected eluate is concentrated with powdered sucrose and dialyzed against 0.01 M NaHCO$_3$ in 1% saline, pH 8.2. The purity of antibody is determined indirectly by applying the following equation:

$$\frac{(P_s - P_n)}{P_s} \times 100 = \text{percentage of purity}$$

where P_s refers to the total quantity of protein eluted at pH 2.3 when a specific antiserum was filtered; P_n represents the total protein eluted from the same column through which an equal volume of nonspecific rabbit serum had passed.

Immunospecific isolation of antibodies from a serum by the adsorption on a water-insoluble complex of poly-D-alanyl-rabbit serum albumin-cellulose (Robbins et al., 1967), is carried out as follows: the immunosorbent (1 g) is suspended in an antiserum (40–70 ml) and stirred overnight at 4°. The mixture is then centrifuged and the supernatant is removed. The cellulose conjugate is washed with PBS with centrifugation. This washing is repeated until the absorbency at 280 nm of the washing fluid is negligible. The adsorbed antibody may be dissociated from the immunoadsorbent by means of a specific hapten or antigen dissolved in PBS, followed by the elution with 0.1 *M* acidic acid.

A technique for absorption of serum antibodies on the antigen-resin particles, followed by the elution of antibodies at an altered pH was published by Isliker (1953) and Campbell et al. (1961).

Absorption of Antibodies on Inert Particles. Antibody immunoglobulins may be adsorbed to kaolin, or on diethylaminoethyl-(DEAE) cellulose.

Purification of Antibodies by Absorption on Kaolin (Klobusitzky, 1938). The antiserum diluted with three volumes of distilled water is mixed with kaolin and a sufficient amount of 1 *N* nitrous acid to adjust the pH to 3.8. The ratio of diluted antiserum, in milliliters, to kaolin, in grams, should correspond to 100:25. The mixture is agitated for 6 hours at room temperature, then centrifuged. The sediment must be collected and resuspended in 2% aqueous solution of glycol at the original volume of diluted serum. The fluid is adjusted to pH 9.4 with 1 *N* sodium hydroxide. The mixture is now agitated for 6 hours at 38° and centrifuged. The kaolin sediment should be removed, the supernatant fluid adjusted to pH 7.4, and the antiserum concentrated by means of ultrafiltration through a membrane, made of 10% collodium in glacial acetic acid.

Isolation of Immunoglobulins by Zone Electrophoresis. The electrophoretic method is perhaps the most efficient procedure for immunoglobulin preparation, but the yield of antibodies thus obtained is relatively low. Here is the recommended Murgita and Vas' (1970) method. The supporting medium consists of equal amounts of polyvinyl chloride particles (Geon 427, Goodrich Chemical Company) and polyvinyl chloride, polyvinyl acetate copolymer (Pevikon C-870, Mercer Chemical Corporation, New York) is prepared as a thick slurry with barbital buffer, 0.025 *M,* pH 8.5 and poured into plastic trays. The water-jacketed trays are placed into the electrode vessels, each filled with 4 liters of barbital buffer. The electrodes are cooled with ice-cooled water circulating through the water-jackets. Two blocks are connected in parallel to a power supply and the electrophoresis is carried out at a constant potential of 600 V and a current of 70 mA (35 mA/block).

Further purification of the immunoglobulins is conducted by density-gradient electrofocusing at a constant voltage of 600 V and approximately 15-mA current. The electrofocusing process is terminated when the current to the column reaches a constant value of 2 to 3 mA. The column is emptied with a peristaltic pump and the effluent is continuously monitored by a Uviscan unit. The pH of each fraction is measured to determine the iso-electric points of the focused components.

XI. PREPARATION OF INDIVIDUAL CLASSES OF IMMUNOGLOBULINS

The human IgG may be obtained from normal human sera. Human IgE, IgA, and IgM are obtained from patients suffering from myelomas. The IgA, IgM, and IgG immunoglobulins are purified on anion-exchange and gel filtration columns. The ion exchange chromatography is conducted by Sober and Peterson's (1956) method. Serum samples, dialyzed against the starting buffer, are eluted from the column by a series of phosphate buffers: the starting buffer, 0.01 M, pH 7.9 and 7.4, and buffers of decreasing pH (7.2, 6.2, 6.0, 4.8) and increasing molar concentrations (0.05, 0.10, 0.15 and 0.30) or phosphate. Some samples are pooled and further purified by filtration through Sephadex G-200 equilibrated in 0.15 M NaCl (Trifts-hauser et al., 1970).

The IgG occurs in a relatively crude form in the Cohn fraction II prep-aration: it may be purified by diethylaminocellulose chromatography (Strauss et al., 1964).

The IgA can be isolated from human parotic secretion by Tomasi's et al. (1965) method, or from human collostrum by Cebra and Robbins' (1966) technique.

The F(ab')$_2$ or the pepsin split IgG is prepared by Harboe's (1965) method. The pepsin digestion is carried at 37° at pH 4.0 for 24 hours using the enzyme globulin ratio of 2:100 (w/w).

Concentration of immunoglobulin preparations is determined by single radial immunodiffusion (Brandtzaeg et al., 1968). Concentrations of F(ab')$_2$ preparations are calculated from the optical density recorded at 280 nm (Tray, 1966).

Monospecific rabbit antisera to the heavy chains of IgG, IgA, and IgM are prepared by Brandtzaeg's et al. (1968) method.

The IgG may be obtained from the serum of man and various primates by successive precipitations in 18 and 14% sodium sulfate followed by a block electrophoresis in a barbital buffer, pH 8.6, 0.1 mμ and by the gel filtration on a Sephadex G-200 column using 0.02 M Tris and 0.15 M NaCl, pH 8.0 (Wang and Fudenberg, 1969), see Fig. 46.

Normal serum γ_2-globulin may be obtained as column fraction II, puri-fied by filtration through a Sephadex G-166 column equilibrated with pH 8.0, 0.15 M phosphate buffered saline (Tan and Epstein, 1965).

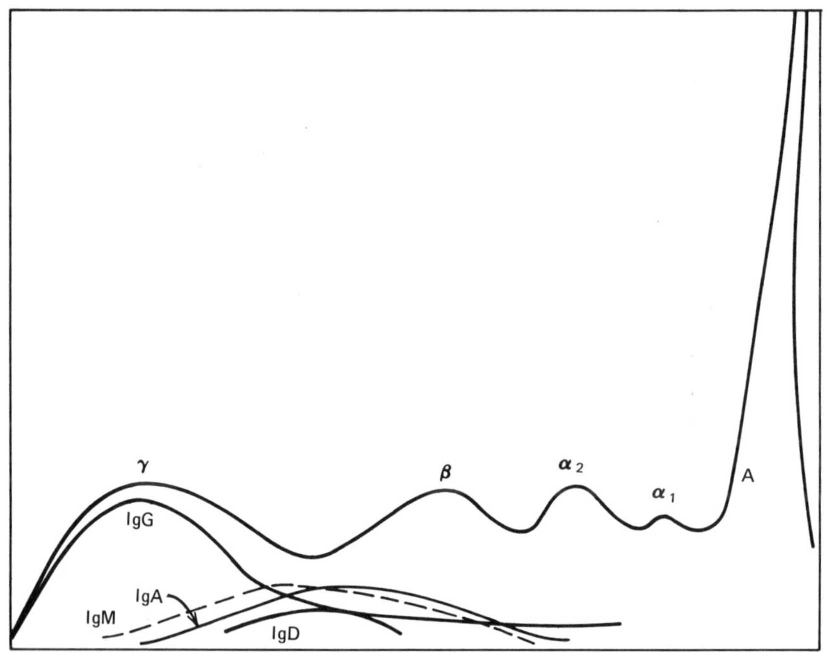

Figure 46. Occurrence of immunoglobulins in relation to the electrophoretically separated serum globulins and albumin.

The Sephadex G-166 is a mixture two parts of G-200 to one part Sephadex G-100 by weight. This mixture has a faster flow rate and permits better protein separation than does G-200 alone.

The $\gamma_1 M$ protein may be obtained from the sera of patients having macro-globulinemia from peak I. The $\gamma_1 A$ protein is obtained from peak I of a serum of a patient with multiple myeloma, and two globulins from peak II.

The IgG Immunoglobulin Preparation and Purification. Very efficient and convenient methods for the preparation of IgG immunoglobulins depend on the anion-exchange choromatography of whole serum on the diethylaminoethyl cellulose (Sober and Peterson, 1958; Strauss et al., 1963; Aalund et al., 1965; Reif, 1969). Reif's method is especially recommended for the preparation of IgG immunoglobulin with a specified purity. This procedure utilizes a single batch absorption of serum with DEAE-cellulose.

Preparaton of DEAE-Cellulose. The precycled anion-exchange cellulose DE52 is suspended in 0.01 M, pH 8.0 phosphate buffer in the ratio of 1:5.5. The mixture is stirred and adjusted to pH 8.0 with 1 N HCl. The cellulose is left to settle for 30 minutes, the supernatant is decanted to remove fines, and the cellulose is resuspended in a slightly larger volume of the phosphate buffer. The cycle of settling of cellulose, decantation, and resuspension is repeated three times.

The equilibrated cellulose can be preserved by adding 0.3 ml toluene in 10 ml chloroform to the buffer above the cellulose. Before use, the supernatant containing preservative is decanted, and the cellulose is washed with 0.01 M, pH 8.0 phosphate buffer in a Büchner funnel containing two layers of Whatman No. 1 filter paper. The cellulose is then sucked dry for 30 seconds to leave a cake of wet cellulose on the paper.

Separation of IgG Immunoglobulin from Serum. The serum diluted with 3 volumes of distilled water is added to the wet cellulose at the ratio of 1 ml of undiluted serum to 1.5 g (dry weight) 5–8 g (wet weight) of DEAE-cellulose. The smaller the quantity of DEAE-cellulose, the more impurities occur in the final product. The serum-cellulose mixture is equilibrated by stirring it thoroughly every 10 minutes for 1 hour at 30°. The equilibrated mixture is poured into a Büchner funnel, sucked dry for a few seconds, and washed rapidly three times with a small volume of 0.01 M, pH 8.0 phosphate buffer. The combined effluent contains the purified γG globulin preparation, which can be concentrated by pressure dialysis, or less sufficiently by a combined dialysis against 0.003 M, pH 8.0 phosphate buffer and lyophilization.

The cellulose can be reused after regeneration. For regeneration, the used cellulose is washed on a Büchner funnel with 2 N NaCl, sucked dry, and washed with 5 volumes of 2 N NaCl containing 0.03% Tween 80, to remove lipids. The cellulose is then resuspended in 5 volumes of the same saline solution, refiltered, washed on the filter with 12 volumes of distilled water, and resuspended in 5 volumes of 0.01 M, pH 8.0 phosphate buffer. Subsequently, the cellulose is treated with 0.1 N NaOH, added in the ratio of 012 ml/g of wet weight of cellulose. The suspension is stirred during 10 minutes, and then the cellulose is allowed to settle, and the supernatant is decanted. Finally, the cellulose is washed twice with 5 volumes of 0.01 M, pH 8.0 phosphate buffer.

Separation of the 19S and 7S Immunoglobulins. The safest procedure for the preparation and separation of the 19S and 7S immunoglobulins is the filtration through a Sephadex gel. The 19S macroglobulin 7S gamma-globulin preparation can be obtained by filtration of a serum through a Sephadex G-200 column (2.5 × 90 cm), overlayed with 10 ml of serum and eluted at the rate of 4–9 ml/hour with 0.2 M NaCl − 0.1 M Tris buffer, pH 8.0. The 3-ml fractions are collected, and protein concentration is measured at 280 nm. The first peak corresponds to 19S macroglobulin and the second peak corresponds to 7S gamma-globulin (Fig. 47). The peaks are collected and concentrated by vacuum dialysis (Borel et al., 1968).

The γM Immunoglobulin Preparation.   The most suitable source for γM immunoglobulin is human serum from Walderström's macroglobulinemia. Initial steps in the technique are the precipitation of euglobulin fraction on dissolving the serum in tenfold volume of distilled water, and dialysis in the cold. The precipitate is dissolved in 0.1 *M* Tris-HCl − 0.15 *M* NaCl, pH 8.0 or 0.15 *M* NaCl; the precipitation is repeated 3 to 6 times to free the preparation from any γG-globulin.

The γM preparation can be freed from other immunoglobulins most efficiently by gel filtration on Sephadex G-200 using 0.1 *M* Tris-HCl − 0.15 *M* NaCl, pH 8.0, with 5% sucrose added to the sample to aid penetration of the Sephadex. The purity of the γM immunoglobulin preparation is determined by analytical ultracentrifugation, immunodiffusion, immunoelectrophoresis, or starch gel electrophoresis (Putnam et al., 1967).

Preparation of Heavy Chains of Immunoglobulins.   The heavy chains are prepared from purified IgG's preparations dissolved in 0.55 *M* Tris buffer, pH 8.2, at a concentration of 20 mg/ml. Nitrogen is flushed through this solution for 5 minutes and 2-mercaptoethanol is added to the final concentration of 0.1 *M*. The mixture is maintained under nitrogen for 1 hour at room temperature and then placed in an ice bath. Crystalline iodoacetamide is then added to a final concentration of 0.11 *M*. The solution left in the ice bath for one hour is dialyzed against 0.15 *M* NaCl in a cold room overnight. The liquid is centrifuged; the supernatant is collected and dialyzed against 1 *M* acetic overnight in a cold room and filtered through a

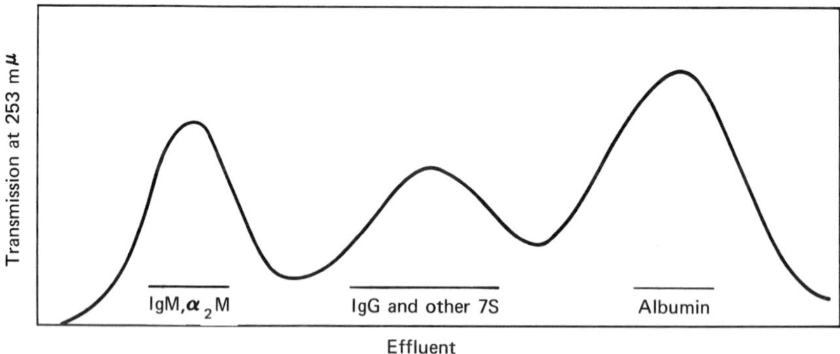

Figure 47.   Separation of human plasma proteins and recovery of immunoglobulins by Sephadex G-200 filtration.

Sephadex G-100 column (in 1 *M* acetic acid) to separate the heavy chains from the light chains (Fleischman et al., 1962).

Separation of the L and H chains is often more efficient on the Sephadex G-166 columns (Tan and Epstein, 1965).

Separation of 7S and 19S Antibody Immunoglobulins on differential gradient. Separation of the 7S and 19S antibodies by sucrose gradient (Bishop, 1966) is accomplished as follows: a 10 to 40% (*w/v*) sucrose gradient in isotonic saline is prepared. When the gradient has been formed, 0.5 ml of cold, 1:2 diluted serum is layered on the top. The serum boundary is blurred by gentle stirring with the pipette tip. Using the swinging-bracket rotor (SW-39), the gradient mixture is centrifuged at 35,000 rpm for 18 hours at 10°. The 19S serum component occurs close to the bottom of the tube whereas the 7S component is present in the upper half. Serial fractions are obtained from the bottom of the tube by drip-out.

XII. ISOLATION OF INDIVIDUAL ANTIGEN-ANTIBODY COMPLEXES

Separation of immune complexes from other materials can be accomplished by a CO_2-treatment and ultracentrifugation procedure (Tozer et al., 1962, Table 32), the pepsin digestion of proteinaceous antigens, or by the separation of antigen from immunoglobulin on a gel column, sectioning the gel column, and eluting the components.

Methods for *antitoxin purification* by the digestion of toxin-antitoxin floccules with pepsin or trypsin were published by Pope and Healey (1939), Petermann and Pappenheimer (1941), and Northrop (1942).

According to Northrop's (1942) technique, the floccules resulting from a toxin-antitoxin reaction are treated with 0.025% solution of pepsin at pH 3.0, in the absence of electrolytes, at 23 to 25°, for 2 to 6 hours, then centrifuged. The inactive protein component is removed by adjusting the supernatant to pH 4. The resulting precipitate is removed, and the supernatant is collected. It should contain free antitoxin which can be concentrated, purified further by ammonium sulfate precipitation, and then dialyzed and lyophilized.

According to Smith's et al. (1962) procedure, the antigen-antibody complexes are first separated as parallel planes in the gel using a specially designed diffusion cell. The gel is then frozen and cut into sections with a freezing microtome. Sections containing individual antigen-antibody complexes are suspended in a phosphate-buffered saline, pH 7.3, and left at room temperature overnight. The precipitate is then removed by centrifugation.

The buffered saline (pH 7.3) contains in 1 liter of water: 4.2 g of NaCl, 8.096 g of Na_2HPO_4, and 2.438 g of KH_2PO_4.

Table 32. Separation of Antibody from Immunological Complexes
(Tozer et al., 1962)

Antigen-antibody

Wash in water.
Dissolve in
aqueous CO_2

Aqueous CO_2 solution

Ultracentrifuge in
SW 39 rotor at
150,000 $\times$ *g* for
330 minutes at 23°

Supernatant		Deposit	
Remove CO_2 *in vacuo*. Add 0.9% NaCl, hold overnight at 2°. Centrifuge at 1100 $\times$ *g* for 15 minutes.		Redissolve in aqueous CO_2. Ultracentrifuge at 150,000 $\times$ *g* for 720 minutes.	
Supernatant	Sediment (discarded)		
Concentrate ($\times$3) by pressure dialysis in 0.9% NaCl; centrifuge at 1100 $\times$ *g* for 20 minutes.		Supernatant Treatment	Sediment (discarded)
Supernatant	Sediment (discarded)	Supernatant	Sediment (discarded)

Antibody

XIII. DETERMINATION OF THE AFFINITY OF ANTIBODY FOR ANTIGEN

The most accurate method for estimation of the affinity of antibody immunoglobulins to an antigen is the equilibrium-constant determination method. By this technique, both the free and bound antibody can be determined quantitatively. The procedure (Kronvall et al., 1970) is as follows.

Purified antibody globulins are first labeled with ^{125}I; 50 to 500 μg of the ^{125}I-labeled immunoglobulin is added to a measured amount of a particulate antigen (example: 1×10^9 to 1×1^{10} bacteria per 2-ml final volume). The mixture is incubated for 30 minutes at room temperature or at 37°, and centrifuged at 10,000 rpm to collect the particle pellet. The radioactivity count in this material is measured in an automatic gamma-counting system (e.g., a Nuclear-Chicago Automatic Gamma Counting System, Model 1075). On the assumption that each molecule of the immunoglobulin reacts with one antigen site, a Scatchard (1949) plot estimating the number of antigen residues maximally available is applicable. In this manner, all the data necessary for calculation of the equilibrium constant according to the following formula are supplied:

$$K = \frac{(MGpa)}{(MG)(pa)}$$

where (MGpa) is the molecular concentration of immunoglobulin bound to antigen, and (MG)(pa) are the molecular concentration of free immunoglobulin and free antigen residues, respectively.

XIV. COMMON PROCEDURES OF SEROLOGICAL TECHNIQUES

Technical procedures applied to many serological assays are the antiserum concentration, the dilution technique, the serum inactivation, and antiserum absorption, and determination of the strength of an antiserum.

1. Antiserum Concentration

Antiserum may be concentrated gently by partial lyophilization, ultrafiltration, water-absorption, or pervaporation. Concentration by the ultrafiltration is conducted at 4° with an ultrafiltration cell, Model 50 and diafloultrafiltration membranes, type UM-20E (Amicon).

2. The Dilution Technique

There are three types of dilution techniques: the twofold dilution procedure, the fractional dilution procedure, and the photometric dilution procedure, with the accuracy rising in that order.

The diluent most commonly used is buffered saline, that is, a 85% solution of sodium chloride buffered at pH 7.0 to 7.2 with 0.01 M phosphate. Lower concentrations of sodium chloride, such as 0.2 to 0.3%, are recommended for tests with cells which tend to clump spontaneously. Certain ions and salts, KF, KCL, KBr, KI, and KCNS, must be avoided because of their inhibitory influence on the formation of specific precipitates. Amino acids and acetylated amino acids in relatively high concentrations (about 0.75 M), inhibit serological reactions (Kleinschmidt and Boyer, 1952).

A simple, routine dilution procedure depends on making serial twofold dilutions of a serum or antigen, such as 1:10, 1:20, 1:40, 1:80, 1:160, and so on. For this purpose, constant volume, for example, 0.2 or 0.5 ml of diluent, is first placed in a row of tubes. An equal volume of a serum or antigen solution is then added to the first tube, mixed, and transferred from one tube to the next, ending with the last, from which the excess amount of fluid is discarded.

The process of dilution and dispensing of the reagents is greatly expedited and is made more accurate by means of a semiautomatic electric dilutor (Aminco, Fig. 48).

The relatively large experimental error inherent in this procedure makes a close reproduction of the titration end point difficult (Curnen and Horsfall, 1947). The precision of the routine dilution procedure is increased by applying two series of twofold dilutions, in which one series represents the geometric mean of adjacent dilutions in the other row (Von Magnus, 1951).

The fractional dilution (Horsfall and Tamm, 1953) is set up in three rows of standard, 13 × 100-mm tubes with 10 or more tubes in each row. Each tube, except the first in each row, receives 1.9 ml of buffered saline. The first tube in all rows obtains 0.91, 1.58, and 1.89 ml of diluent and 3.50, 2.70, and 1.90 ml of the original 1:10 dilution of the serum or an

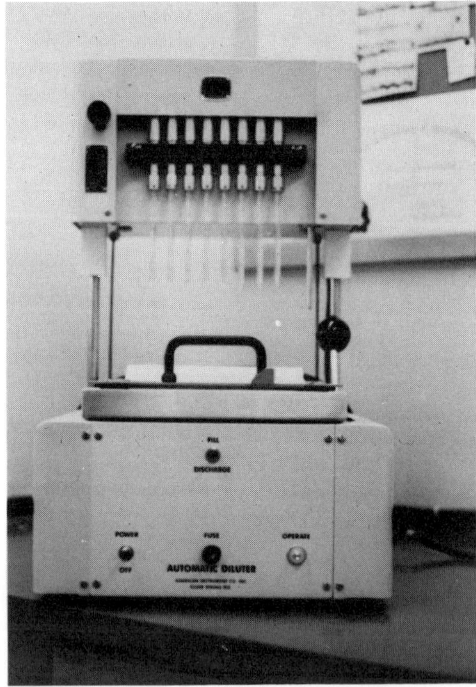

Figure 48.   Semiautomatic electric dilutor.

antigen. The initial dilutions in the tube 1 in rows A, B, and C are thus $10^{-1.1}$, $10^{-1.2}$, and $10^{-1.3}$, respectively. Beginning with this tube in each row a series of twofold dilutions is then made by transferring a 1.9-ml volume to the next tube. Finally, 0.5 ml of each dilution is placed in three rows of tubes.

The fractional dilution can be arranged in the harmonic, linear, and centred series (Ingram, 1962). In the harmonic series, concentrations take values of the reciprocals of successive whole numbers, $1, \frac{1}{2}, \frac{1}{3}, \frac{1}{4}, \frac{1}{5}$. In practical work, dilutions are made by putting out increasing volumes of a diluent into a row of tubes and adding a constant unit volume of the recipient to each one.

Photometric dilution procedures were described by Miller and Stanley (1941) and Hirst and Pickles (1942).

Dilutions and, consequently, titers of antibodies or antigens can be expressed more adequately by logarithms to the base $2(\log_2)$ as suggested by Vennes et al. (1957). In a twofold dilution series 1:2, 1:4, 1:8, 1:16, 1:32, . . . , $1:2''$, the corresponding $\log_2$ values follow directly as 1, 2, 3, 4, 8, . . . , n. If the initial dilution is other than 1:2, the $\log_2$ should be added to the subsequent 2^n dilution series; for example, in a dilution series of 1:10, 1:20, 1:40, 1:80, . . . , $1:10x^{2n}$ the resulting $\log_2$ values are 3.32, 4.32, 5.32, . . . , $3.32 + n$. In the case of fractional dilution procedures, titers are expressed as common logarithms. A table of logarithms to the base 2 has been published by Finney et al. (1955).

The end point or titer of antibody reactivity by any dilution technique arbitrarily determines the concentration of antibodies in relation to their hypothetical concentration in the nondiluted serum. A titer informs of the lowest concentration of serum antibody which gives an observable reaction. The relative potency of a serum may be determined by comparison with the titer of a standard serum having a known concentration of antibody, estimated perferably by chemical measurement of antibody nitrogen. If titers of the standard and the test serum are y and x, respectively, the relative potency (P) of a serum being examined is calculated thus:

$$P = \frac{x}{y}$$

3. The Serum Inactivation Procedure

The heating of a serum at temperatures not exceeding 63° inactivates the complement, so that it becomes temporarily nonhemolytic. The complement in human sera is sufficiently inactivated in 30 minutes at 56°. It is recommended that animal sera should be heated at 60° for 30 minutes or at 62° for 3 minutes to eliminate the complement and certain nonspecific factors which are sometimes present in animal sera (Roberts, 1945).

4. *The Serum Absorption Technique*

A greater amount of a substance is absorbed by unit surface if its amount increases. The absorption is, however, not in the direct proportion to the amount, but to some root value of it.

Absorption of sera is most widely used for the removal of heterophile or heterologous antibodies. Antisera can be absorbed with particulate or soluble antigens, and the antigen-antibody complexes are then removed by centrifugation. The effect of absorption with particles is proved by a blocking reaction. To avoid overabsorption, the procedure must be completed as quickly as possible, preferably within 6 hours.

In the absorption technique by Kopeloff and Kopeloff (1949), a serum inactivated if applicable, and diluted 1:10, is mixed with an equal volume of an antigen suspension, incubated for 1 hour at 37.5°, centrifuged, and absorbed with the antigen two more times. The final centrifugation for 30 minutes is conducted at 40,000 × g. The absorption of certain antibodies by heterologous antigens is sometimes more effective if carried out at two different temperatures, first by incubation at 37° for 1 to 2 hours, with constant shaking, then at 2° for 2 to 3 hours, followed by centrifugation at about 30,000 × g.

Techniques for the absorption of antisera with viruses were published by Bedson et al. (1949) and Fodor and Adams (1955). In the procedure described by Bedson et al., the virus preparation is added to the antiserum and left for 1 hour at room temperature and overnight at 4° with occasional shaking, then passed through a Seitz filter, and centrifuged at 20,000 × g for 30 minutes. Clear supernatant containing the absorbed serum is withdrawn by the aid of a fine Pasteur pipette. Additional centrifugation at 40,000 × g is sometimes required to remove completely antigen-antibody complexes.

5. *Decomplementation of the Serum*

Decomplementation of the serum may be attained by absorption with sensitized stromata. According to Klein's technique (1960), approximately 20 × 10⁹ sensitized stromata are required per 1 ml of a guinea pig serum, and this mixture is incubated for 30 minutes at 37°. The absorption is repeated twice. All C′1 and C′4 components are removed in a short time, while the removal of C′2 and C′3 proceeds at a slower rate. Stromata can also be prepared according to the Winn et al. (1953) method (see p. 286).

6. *Determination of the Strength of Antiserum*

Potency (*P*) or strength of antisera is usually expressed as the antiserum titer (*T*), which refers to the end-point of an immunological test, and is inversely proportional to the serum potency, as indicated by the equation (Reif et al., 1963):

$$P = \frac{100}{T}$$

The comparison of results of serological reactions carried out with homologous and heterologous antisera or antigens can be evaluated by computing ratios of titers according to the formula (Burnet and Lush, 1940):

$$\frac{\text{heterologous titer}}{\text{homologous titer}} \times 100$$

7. *Automation of Immunological Procedures*

A fully automated procedure for turbidity determination, in numerous samples, designed by Hucke and Roche (1959-1960), may be adapted for immunological work, in which the examination of turbidity in large series is required. According to the fully automated technique, all samples enter the laboratory through the receiving station where a weight-dilution master card containing the necessary sample information is produced. The information is punched on a key punch card. The samples reach the reading station where light transmissions are recorded and turbidity readings are automatically determined and recorded on another card. The weight-dilution card and turbidity reading card are sent to the IBM 650 electronic computer, which produces an output card on which all the original sample information and the computed potency of the sample has been recorded.

The weight-dilution master contains information about sample weight, dilution, and estimated potency. The sample, in the meantime, progresses through the laboratory in a group called a test. Each test consists of a standard, the samples to be examined and reagent blanks arranged into racks of test tubes. The test mixtures are incubated and proceed to the reading station where a punch card containing transmission readings is produced for every row of tubes, of a standard or a sample. The identification of a sample is in the form of a six-digit code.

After the code is entered on the keyboards, the spectrophotometric readings are made, which is done by pouring the contents of the test tube into the cuvette and pressing the read-out button on the keyboard. Pressing the read-out button activates the digital voltmeter, control consol, and key punches. The digital voltmeter converts the voltage output of a spectronic 20 to a digital pulse acceptable for punching by the control consol. The consol controls the punching of the date, keyboard information, position number and transmission reading on the IBM card. The cards produced at the reading station and the weight-dilution master cards are fed through an IBM 650 electronic computer. The computer may carry as many as 2000 program steps on each sample and 600 sample potencies may be computed in just 6 minutes. The automated method is free of errors common to manual operation.

XV. THE IMMUNOLOGICAL REACTION

Specific attraction between the antigen and antibody depends on intermolecular forces and radicals with opposite fields of force, or on short-range forces, such as those of van der Waals, and Coulomb's attraction, and upon sufficiently large areas of the complementary configuration (Marrack, 1938; Pauling, 1945).

Reaction between an antigen and antibody at the surface of molecules results in the formation of an antigen-antibody complex which probably consists of a network of alternate antigen and antibody molecules. Alterations in the conformation or in molecular flexibility related to the antigen-antibody reactions may be detected by fluorescence polarization measurement. Fluorescence polarization is particularly suited for following the changes in the rotary motion of molecules which accompany reactions between molecules.

Antigen-antibody equilibria and kinetics are measurable by the fluorescence polarization, and results on macromolecular equilibria may be interpreted according to the equation:

$$\text{ligand} + \text{receptor} \rightleftarrows \text{complex}.$$

Biomolecular reactions between antigen and antibody molecules are very rapid at least in most cases, since they occur with a rate constant approaching 1×10^7 M^{-1} second and yet they only require activation energy of 4 to 12 cal/mole. In most antigen-antibody reactions, as many as six linked organic residues of an antigen molecule participate in the reaction with certain active antibody sites, but in some cases, the haptenic groups are relatively small. The active site of an antibody surface is able to accommodate a range of sizes of antigenic determinant groups.

These reactions depend on weak forces, such as Coulombic forces, between charge groups which vary inversely as the square of the distance between the groups, polar forces including hydrogen bonds occurring between nonionic groups and varying inversely as the sixth power of the distance between groups, and van der Waals forces of very short range, that are basically attractive and compressive and vary inversely as the seventh power of interatomic distances. Firm binding between the antigen-antibody molecules necessitates several points of force constant and several weak bonds.

It is possible that haptenic groups are not homogeneous entities but surface constituents capable of taking on a wide spectrum of structures depending on the environment (structural heterogeneity). Some haptenic groups protrude outwards from the surface while others lie imbedded in a protein surface.

Antigen and antibody molecules appear to unite in a reversible bimolecular association (Ab + Ag $\rightleftarrows$ AbAg), as concluded from the fluorescence polarization studies of antigen-antibody interactions and from an empirical rate law, applied to wide initial concentrations of antigen and antibody (Dandliker and Levison, 1967).

A hapten is bound to an antibody globulin according to the low of mass action and may be represented by the equation:

$$K = \frac{[Hb]}{(n[Ab] - [Hg])[Hf]}$$

where AB is antibody-bound hapten, Hf free hapten, n antibody valent, (AB) total antibody concentration, and $n(Ab) - (Hg)$ concentration of antibody unoccupied by hapten.

Reactions of antibody with haptens may be studied by equilibrium dialysis.

Relative concentration of the three components, Ab, Ag, and Ab Ag, in a reaction mixture, in any system at an equilibrium is represented by the value of the equilibrium constant, K. The end point of a serological reaction thus observed is determined by the amount of antibody or antigen (depending on whether antibody or antigen is being determined) and it does not take into account the amount of free antibody or antigen, respectively, present in a reaction mixture.

Antibody molecules interacting with antigen molecules become distorted by the physical stresses involved in the reaction. Following this distortion, antigen determinants, which would be hidden within the antibody molecule, may become exposed. The distorted immunoglobulin antibody molecules may give rise to anti-antibodies.

The amount of antibody combined with a molecule of antigen is relative to the molecular weight of antigens(Brunius, 1936). Simple serological reactions, according to the most accepted assumption, occur in two stages. The first stage, in which a specific combination between those two principal components of the immune system takes place rapidly, is followed by a secondary, slower reaction of aggregation which takes 1 to 3 minutes. The latter stage is considered nonspecific by a majority of investigators. The antibody globulin seems to possess a small amount of attached lipid which enhances the intensity and the visible shape of certain serological reactions, especially of the precipitation, probably by providing nuclei, around which a specific precipitation is initiated (Heidelberger, 1939).

Antisera extracted with ether yield smaller amounts of precipitates, but their precipitating power is restored by small amounts of extracted lipids (Horsfall and Goodner, 1936).

The second, visible phase of serological reaction is usually accelerated as the temperature rises from 0 to 20° or 40° due to the increased Brownian movement which may cause more frequent collisions between the reacting molecules or particles. The optimum temperature for different serological systems varies from 1 to 55°, according to the species of micro-organisms, the type of antigen, and the class of serological reaction. At temperatures over 55°, dissociation or a partial denaturation often occurs. Certain agglutinins and hemagglutinins combine with specific antigens at low temperatures but dissociate reversally at 37°. Mechanical agitation accelerates the visible stage of antigen-antibody reactions, probably because of the increased frequency of collisions between reacting molecules or particles.

The role of electrolytes in the serological reaction is probably the reduction of negative charges on particles to a critical value of about 15 mV, which results in their aggregation. However, electrolytes in 0.01 to 0.1 N concentrations decrease the cohesiveness of such particles or increase their attraction for water, thus reducing the tendency to aggregation. The action of electrolytes on various immune systems varies considerably. For example, the precipitation of antigens with mammalian antisera is best observed in 0.8 to 1.0% salt concentrations, but it decreases in 2 N or higher concentrations, whereas chicken, pheasant, and owl antisera precipitate with homologous protein antigens in 8% and poorly in 0.5% sodium chloride solution (Goodman et al., 1951).

The optimum hydrogen ion concentration for most immunological tests is between pH 6.5 and 8.5, but some reactions may occur within a wide range of pH between 4.5 and 9.5. The failure of antigen and antibody to form precipitates at pH levels above 10 and in low salt concentrations is attributed to electrostatic repulsion between antigen and antibody complexes. Antigen-antibody complexes can dissolve or dissociate at high salt concentrations and also in the antigen or antibody excess. Immune reactions, especially the precipitation, can be reversibly inhibited by certain small molecular compounds, for example, salicylate, hydrobenzoates, and some amino acids (Friend, 1953).

It is still not clear whether different antibodies participate in various types of serological reactions, as believed by Gottlieb et al. (1953) and others, or whether different types of serological reactions can be exhibited by the same antibody according to experimental conditions. Any rigid attitude to these biological phenomena must be avoided, since a close observation reveals that characteristics of immune sera vary. For example, certain antisera produced by injections of disintegrated microorganisms react with the homologous antigens in the agglutination, tube precipitation, diffusion precipitation, complement fixation, and hemagglutination test, depending on physicochemical characteristics of the antigen, the species of animals immunized, and varying schedules of the immunization and immunological test. In contrast, other antisera obtained by the same technique react only in the complement fixation test. Antisera from individual rabbits immunized with the same antigen and by an identical schedule often differ in their antibody titers (Grabar and Williams, 1953; Grabar, 1958; Kwapinski, 1965). This variation in the immune response is probably genetically determined.

Reactions in vitro between soluble antigen macromolecules and corresponding antibodies result in the formation of a precipitate. Antibody molecules reacting with an antigen present on the surface of a particulate antigen, such as bacterium or mammalian cell, cause clustering of the particulate antigens, and the formation of clumps or agglutinates. Antibodies reacting with the antigens present on structures responsible for mobility, for example, flagella, immobilize them by binding a number of these structures. Toxic or infectious agents reacting with their specific antibodies may become nontoxic or noninfectious as the result of interactions with the antibodies.

Five principal and ten individual types of immunological reactions can be differentiated according to the physicochemical characteristics of the antigens and substrates involved. Principal types of immunological reactions are agglutination, precipitation, immunolysis, neutralization, and opsonization. Individual immunological reactions are hemagglutination, flocculation, precipitation, immunodiffusion, complement fixation, immune hemolysis, and bactericidal, augmentation, opsonin, and bacteriotropin tests. According to Talmage (1959), precipitation and the toxin neutralization involve antigen molecules with a valence of 6, antibody molecules with a valence of 2, and an optimal ratio of antigen and antibody. Agglutination involves a suspension of 10^8 particles/ml, each particle containing 6×10^5 sites. Comparison of sensitivities of some immunological tests is presented in Table 33.

The intensity of an immunological reaction is ordinarily greater at higher concentrations of the antigen or the antibody, or both reactants, with the exception of the region of "prozone." The serological reaction in the prozone is nonobservable or it diminishes at greater concentrations (low dilutions) of antiserum, but it is noticed clearly at higher serum dilutions. Prozones occur most commonly in old antisera or in some fresh sera heated at 56° for 1 hour or more. The prozone is most readily observed in the quantitative agglutination or precipitation test and also in the complement-fixation reaction. The prozone can be eliminated by centrifugation at $2000 \times g$ for 15 minutes before reading the test.

Table 33.   Sensitivity of Immunological Tests

Immunological Test	Minimum of Antibody N (μg) Detectable or Needed	Author
Precipitation		
Interfacial test	0.2–0.5	Finger and Kabat (1958)
Tube precipitation	0.1	Stats and Bullowa (1942)
Immunodiffusion	0.1–0.3	Kwapinski (1965)
Radioimmunoelectrophoresis	0.003	Staub and Raynaud (1965)
Flocculation	0.02–0.1	Kwapinski (1965)
Agglutination		
Qualitative	0.05	Heidelberger and Kabat (1934)
Quantitative	0.02–0.1	
Hemagglutination, passive	0.001	Wright and Feinberg (1952)
Immune adherence-hemagglutination	0.0005–0.02	Tachibana and Klein (1970)
Hemagglutination-inhibition	0.001	Wright and Feinberg (1952)
Coombs reaction	0.01	Staub and Raynaud (1965)
Indirect hemolysis	0.001	Kwapinski (1965)
Bactericidal test	0.001	Muschel and Treffers (1956)
Complement fixation	0.05	Wallace et al. (1950)
Toxin-neutralization	0.012	Koshland and Engleberger (1957)
Fluorescent antibody test	1.0	Kwapinski (1965)
Immune chromatography test	0.2	Miguel et al. (1960)
Anaphylaxis		
Passive, general	3.0	Ovary and Biozzi (1954)
Passive, local	0.003	
Schultz-Dale reaction	0.008–32	Staub and Raynaud (1965)

XVI. RELATIVE IMMUNOLOGICAL SPECIFICITY

Cross-reaction refers to the immunological reactivity of two or more antigens with the same serum or to the reactivity of two or more sera with one antigen. Cross-reactivity is regarded as indicative of immunological relationships between the coreacting systems, based on similar or identical structural groupings within their molecules. The reactivity of an antibody with a number of antigens of different origin and chemical composition is conditioned by the existence of a special and common determinant group, to which the active site of the antibody corresponds. Antigens which possess a common determinant group, apart from a number of other individual and different determinant groups, can be differentiated from each other by a cross-absorption procedure. The cross-reaction assay may reveal the following immunological phenomena:

1. If an antiserum contains antibodies against an antigenic determinant which is possessed by two different antigen preparations, it reacts with

both, but often to a variable extent. An immune reaction is stronger with an antigen containing a greater than with that having a smaller amount of an individual determinant grouping.

2. If the homologous antigen possesses two determinant groups, one of which is common with another antigen preparation under test, the same amount of the latter preparation absorbs less antibody than the homologous antigen. Immunological reactions given by heterologous but related antigen preparations are weaker in comparison with the homologous system, and a serum absorbed by the heterologous antigen is still able to react with its homologous antigen. These differences depend on a variable quantity of an antigenic determinant in the homologous and heterologous antigen preparation. Cross-reactions amongst various groups of microorganisms are frequent as illustrated in Table 34. Certain antigens or haptens may be found in biologically distant groups of plants and animals. An example is the serological reactivity of antipneumococcal sera with dextrans, dextrins, hemicelluloses, and glycogens, isolated from various higher plants and animals.

Degree of the immunological cross-reaction (C) is determined by the percentage of antibody (A) which reacts with a related antigen (y), relative to its reaction with the homologous antigen (a) (Kabat, 1961), as represented by the equation:

$$C = \frac{PAy}{PAa} \times 100 - \frac{TAa}{TAy} \times 100$$

In case of two different antisera (A and B), cross-reacting with each other's homologous antigen (a and b), the percentage (D) of dual cross-reacting antibody is defined as the reciprocal of the homologous specificity index, multiplied by 100 (Reif et al., 1965):

$$D = \frac{PAb}{PAa} \times \frac{PBa}{PBb} \times 100 = \frac{TAa}{TAb} \times \frac{TBb}{TBa} \times 100$$

Relative immunological *specificity* may be determined by the "specificity ratio," which is defined as the ratio of potencies of either a single antiserum reacting with two antigens, or a single antigen reacting with two antisera. The specificity ratio is calculated from the specificity index (S), which in case of testing relative specificities of antisera A and B for the same two antigens X and Y is represented by the equation:

$$S = \frac{PAx}{PAy} \times \frac{PBy}{PBx} - \frac{TAy}{TAx} \times \frac{TBx}{TBy}$$

where P is potency and T is titer (Reif et al., 1965).

Table 34. Phyloantigenic Relationships of Microorganisms (Kwapinski, 1972)

In case of an antiserum reacting only with its homologous antigen but not with other related antigen, the relative specificity of the antiserum exceeds the specificity ratio $PAa/P_{\min}$, where PAa is the potency of antiserum A against its homologous antigen a, and $P_{\min}$ is the minimum potency detectable with the antigens used. The percentage of cross-reacting antibody in this antiserum is less than $P_{\min}/PAa \times 100$ (Reif et al., 1965).

No antiserum must be regarded as "absolutely specific" until it has been examined against all existing antigens.

Chapter Five

THE AGGLUTINATION TEST

I. PRINCIPLES OF THE AGGLUTINATION ASSAY

The agglutination consists of clumping of cells and other particulate matters, covered by a specific antibody called agglutinin, in the presence of certain ions. The immunological reaction takes place on the surface of insoluble particles, and the antigens involved in the agglutination are those situated on the surface of cells. According to Bordet's theory, the agglutination of cells by an antibody consists of two phases, one of which is a specific combination of agglutinins with the homologous antigen, and the other is a specific aggregation of sensitized particulate antigen in the presence of electrolytes. Bacterial cells sensitized with a homologous antibody react as hydrophobic colloids. When the surface potential of these bacteria is reduced below 13 mV by the action of electrolytes, the clumping takes place. Marrack's theory (1934) postulates that the antigen-antibody reaction is totally due to specific forces, and both phases of agglutination are mediated by a chemical attraction between the antigen and antibody sites. Molecules or particles of the antigen and antibody probably combine alternately to build a three-dimensional lattice or a mosaic.

Agglutination and precipitation are reversible reactions, occurring essentially under equilibrium conditions. These reactions may be represented by the equation:

$$\frac{Ag + Ab \rightleftarrows (AgAb)}{\text{large aggregates}} + \frac{Ag \rightleftarrows Ag2Ab}{\text{excess soluble}}$$

If a large excess of antigen is present, antigen-antibody complexes are soluble and the size of the complexes decreases with increasing antigen concentration.

The agglutination test is technically simple. It should, however, be standardized for reproducible results. An estimated concentration of bacterial suspension, a buffered diluent, that temperature and the time of incubation must be maintained in accordance with standard conditions. Reference sera should be included in each series of the test. It is recommended that international standard antisera* be used if available, and that results of the agglutinin determination be expressed by the antibody units, to assure comparable results. A unitage system suggested by Stabbleforth (1954) requires standard antisera with known titers, or local standards made by comparison with the international standards. Agglutinin units may be calculated by applying the following modified formula:

$$X = \frac{Y \times E}{S}$$

where X = the calculated antibody units per milliliter
     Y = the number of antibody units in an ampoule of a antiserum
     S = the titer of standard serum reconstituted as indicated by the supplying institute and tested against a certain suspension of cells
     E = the titer of examined serum tested against the same antigen suspension.

Certain sera fail to agglutinate particulate antigens at lower dilutions, although clumping occurs at greater dilutions ("the prozone phenomenon"). In another zonal phenomenon, a marked agglutination is observed at the lower dilutions, no clumping in a midzone, and a range with pronounced agglutination at top dilutions. The prozone sera can be produced by heating or by air slowly bubbling through the agglutinating sera, which suggests that the alteration of proteins plays a part in the prozone reaction. The "prozone phenomenon" can also be caused by substances preventing collision of bacterial cells and by an increased viscosity or the accumulation of an excessive quantity of colloidal material in the serum (Mudd and Mudd, 1927; Jones and Orcutt, 1934).

The test sera should be clear and translucent. Most antisera need not be inactivated, since the agglutination titer of some sera, for example, the antistreptococcal sera, may be slightly reduced owing to the heating at temperatures between 56 and 62°. If, however, a serum exhibits a non-specific agglutination, it should be heated at 56° for 15 to 30 minutes to abolish zone inhibitions (Renoux, 1954; Hunter and Colbert, 1956).

The diluent employed in the agglutination test is either a 0.85 or 0.3% sodium chloride solution, or, preferably, a buffered saline solution, and the pH of these fluids must not be lower than 6.0.

---

* International standards of anti-typhoid sera are produced by Lister Institute of Preventive Medicine, London, England, and international standards of anti-*Brucella abortus* sera are supplied by Statens Seruminstitut, Copenhagen, Denmark, and by the Ministry of Agriculture and Fisheries, Veterinary Laboratory, Weybridge, England.

The agglutination test can be carried out either in (0.5 × 8 cm) test tubes, in capillary tubes, or on glass slides. Special techniques are provided to study the agglutination reaction in the agar gel or on filter paper.

Cells of bacteria, microfungi, rickettsiae, and of higher plants and animals can be used as particulate antigens for the agglutination test. They may be colored with methylene blue or Harris' stain as modified by Luoto (1953)) to provide a better contrast in the test tube, and preserved with sodium ethyl-mercurithiosalicylate (Merthiolate, Thimerosal) added to the 0.01% final concentration. The cells are usually suspended in 0.85% solution of sodium chloride, but a pH 7.0 buffered saline is preferable. However, to prepare suspensions of certain microbial cells, which are liable to the autoagglutination (e.g., the streptococci, corynebacteria, mycobacteria), a 0.3% solution of sodium chloride is used. The cells showing the auto-agglutinability despite this procedure can be extracted either with $N/2$ NaOH or with alcohol-ether for 30 to 60 minutes, washed with saline, and resuspended in a 0.3% sodium chloride solution. It must be considered, however, that by such a treatment the cells may be voided of certain antigens. Homogenous suspensions of mycelia in a 1% dextrose or in a normal saline solution are prepared by grinding in the mycelia a Duall tissue grinder (Kontes Glass, Co., Vineland, N.J.), operated at 900 rpm (Guidry and Trellers, 1962), or by the homogenization in high-speed electric homogenizer, a Mickle electromagnetic disintegrator or a sonic oscillator.

Living cells or cells killed by a prolonged heating at 56 to 60° or by chemical disinfectants like formaldehyde, phenol, or Merthiolate, can be used in the agglutination test, depending on the physicochemical nature of particular antigens to participate in a serological reaction. Cells must sometimes be pretreated with adequate substances to uncover a cellular antigen situated in a deeper layer of cells; for example, the K antigen of streptococci is made accessible for antibodies by treating these microorganisms with a hyaluronidase preparation. For more information concerning cellular antigens, see pp. 35–42.

The concentration of cells for the agglutination test depends largely on the species of microorganisms, but it usually varies between 500,000 and 1,000,000 cells/ml. The number of cells in a suspension can be estimated either by counting them directly in a Petroff-Hauser chamber at 400 to 600× magnification or by the indirect Wright's (1902) method as well as by a culture assay or by a turbidimetric technique. Determination of cell concentration by a culture assay employs serial dilutions of a stock cell suspension in 1-ml volumes, which are inoculated to a suitable solid culture medium. After a period of incubation, colonies are counted and the concentration of original suspension is determined on the assumption that each colony developed from a single cell. The figure calculated must be multiplied by the dilution factor to obtain the number of cells per milliliter.

The measurement of bacterial density by the determination of transmitted or scattered light is based upon Beer's law, which correlates the density of a bacterial suspension to a linear calibration constructed for each bacterial species or strain, within a range in which a linear relationship applies to the logarithms of transmittance π and bacterial density. If two types of metameter of transmittance (T) are applied, the optical density thus expressed shows a linear relationship to bacterial density or cell concentration over the whole range of transmittance values, except of the extreme ends. The bacterial suspensions are correlated to standard curve prepared previously by a linear calibration for the bacterial strain (Lamanna and Mallette, 1954). A modification of this procedure by Kurokawa et al. (1962) can be used for the transformation of logarithms of transmittance (T) to give a metameter of T showing a linear relationship to the bacterial density through the whole range of T values. In this method, sampling and dilution are eliminated and cell concentrations are expressed by the relative optical densities.

The standardization of bacterial suspensions according to a barium sulfate standard (McFarland, 1907) consists in adjusting the opacity of a bacterial suspension to that of a standard tube containing an amount of barium sulfate suspension. Ten standard barium sulfate suspensions are prepared in uniform tubes, according to the following pattern: 1% solution of chemically pure barium chloride is added to 10 tubes in amounts increasing from 0.1 ml in the first tube to 1.0 ml in the last. The total volume of the fluid in each tube is then made up to 10 ml with a 1% solution of chemically pure sulfuric acid and the tubes are sealed. Densities of the suspension in individual standard tubes correspond approximately to the amount of bacteria per milliliter (Table 35).

Table 35. Preparation of McFarland's Density Standard

Tube	1% BaCl$_2$ (ml)	1% H$_2$SO$_4$ (ml)	Bacteria per milliliter (Number $\times$ 10^6
1	0.1	9.9	300
2	0.2	9.8	600
3	0.3	9.7	900
4	0.4	9.6	1200
5	0.5	9.5	1500
6	0.6	9.4	1800
7	0.7	9.3	2100
8	0.8	9.2	2400
9	0.9	9.1	2700
10	1.0	9.0	3000

A bacterial suspension can be adjusted to the desired density, relative to a tube number in the McFarland scale by diluting 1 ml of bacterial suspension with a measured amount of sterile saline until the densities match. The number of bacteria per milliliter is then calculated by multiplying the dilution factor by the number of cells corresponding to the matched standard tube.

The optimal cell concentration for the agglutination test depends not only on the absolute number of cells but also on certain particularities of species of microorganisms. Thus the optimal cell concentration in each case should be determined in a preliminary agglutination test with one or several reference sera, if available. This assay is carried out in the following manner (Lennette et al., 1952; Kendrick, 1933). Serial dilutions of the antigen are made in 2-ml volumes, and 0.2-ml aliquots of each dilution are delivered into seven to nine rows. Serial antiserum dilutions are made in 2-ml volumes, and 0.2-ml aliquots of each dilution are distributed in the rectangular direction to the rows containing antigen dilutions. A control series should be included, to consist of various antigen dilutions and a diluted known negative serum, to check for a nonspecific agglutination. The mixtures are incubated at 48° for 3 hours and left at 4° overnight. The incubation temperature and time may vary according to conditions selected for the test proper. The unit of antigen to be used in the test proper is represented by the highest dilution of an antigen suspension which gives a strong agglutination in the presence of the highest dilution of antiserum or of a positive reference serum.

II. TECHNIQUES FOR AGGLUTINATION TEST

1. The Test-Tube Agglutination Test

Serial twofold dilutions of serum, ranging from 1:5 to 1:640 or more, are made in a volume of 0.1, 0.25, or 0.5 ml by means of a calibrated capillary pipette. The same or a larger volume of the antigen suspension is added to each tube. Two control tubes are inserted, one containing an equal volume of saline and the antigen suspension, and the other a volume of the original serum dilution and an equal volume of saline. Besides, two control rows for the whole series of the test are included to contain a reference positive or negative serum diluted identically with the main row and the antigen suspension.

The test mixtures are shaken vigorously and incubated for a time period. The incubation temperature and time vary, depending on particular techniques, around 20, 37, 48, 50, 52, and 56°, and between 2 and 12 hours. The clumping of agglutinated cells can be expedited by rocking or centrifugation than a steady incubation of test mixtures even for a longer time period. In the first case, the test tubes are rocked for 2 hours at room temperature on a rocker operated by a small motor. If the latter technique is applied, the test mixtures are centrifuged for 10 minutes at 500 × g, shaken to dislodge the agglutinated particles from the bottom of tubes and read either with the naked eye or through a magnifying glass, while tubes are held against a black screen and a constant light source. By these procedures, the agglutinin titer is expressed as the reciprocal of the highest dilution of the serum showing clumps distinctly visible in the main row, whereas all the controls, except the row containing a positive reference serum, should show no agglutinates. Commonly, the degree of agglutination is expressed in terms of 1+ to 4+ reaction, as shown in Table 36. The agglutinating power of serum may be expressed more accurately by the unitage or logarithm system, as described on p. 285.

Table 36.   Interpretation of Tube Agglutination Test

Agglutination Observed	Degree of Agglutination
Large agglutinates in a clear fluid	4+
Medium-sized clumps in a slightly turbid fluid	3+
Small clumps in a turbid liquid	2+
Very small clumps and fluid	1+
No clumps, turbid liquid	0

2. *The Capillary-Tube Agglutination Test*

This assay was first devised by Hudson and Mudd (1935) and Luoto (1953) and improved by Luoto and Mason (1955), Luoto (1956), and Cozad and Larsh (1960). According to Luoto's technique, the test is set up in capillary tubes about 9 cm long, with an inside bore diameter of 0.4 mm. Approximately one third of the tube is filled, by means of capillary action, with a colored antigen suspension, and two thirds with a non-diluted or serially diluted serum. The tubes are inverted and placed in a vertical position in a clay or wax block. In a screen test, the reactant mixtures are incubated either at 37° for 2 hours or at room temperature for 4 hours. In case of a quantitative serum titration, the incubation is prolonged to 5 hours at 37° or to 24 hours at room temperature. The tubes are examined in a light passing directly from above the tubes. In the case of a positive result, blue-black colored floccules or rings are macroscopically visible in the lower or central part of tubes. The highest serum dilution, showing either floccules or a ring, is taken as end point. The same test may be conducted not only with the serum but also with a milk or whey sample.

The capillary-tube test is especially useful when small amounts of antigens are available. It is as sensitive as complement fixation test and gives reproducible results.

End points of the agglutination can be determined more precisely by optical measurement of the sedimentation rate of agglutinated cells.

3. The Slide Agglutination Test

This test is set out either on cover glass by adopting the "hanging drop" technique or on microscope slides, in Petri plates, or on pieces of stiff paper. Small paraffin circles, about 5 mm in radius, are placed on the slides to prevent spreading of the liquid.

According to the technique of Castañeda and Silva (1942), as slightly modified by Kauffmann (1950), a loopful of antiserum at a given dilution is mixed with a loopful of an antigen suspension, for example, of rickettsiae, on a cover glass rimmed with petroleum jelly. A hollow-ground slide is placed over the glass, and the preparation is inverted. A series of serum dilutions may be made by transferring a drop of one serum dilution to the neighboring microdrop of saline on a cover glass or a glass slide (Castañeda, 1945) by means of a wire loop, of 4 to 5 mm outside diameter, or with a fine capillary pipette. A microdrop of a colored antigen, which has been standardized in the presence of a known homologous antiserum, is then added to each serum dilution and to two controls containing saline or a homologous antiserum. The "hanging-drop" preparations are incubated for 15 to 30 minutes, rotated on a phonograph plate at 15 rpm, and examined by means of a low-power microscope objective for the presence of agglutinates. Preparations made on microslides are incubated in a large Petri plate containing a piece of wet cotton wool to prevent drying.

The "drop test" described by Powell and Jamieson (1942), which has been originally suggested by Castañeda et al. (1940), is set up either on microslides, or on pieces of hard surface cardboard, or a stiff paper. A single small drop of citrated blood or serum is mixed with one drop of a suspension of colored antigen which is made in a sodium citrate solution and containing over 10^8 bacterial cells/ml. After a short time of incubation, results of the test are read by observing granulation or clumping of blue colored cells, which is indicative of a positive serological reaction.

The results of the slide agglutination and "drop test" is commonly expressed in terms of 1+ and 4+ degrees (Table 37).

A selective agglutination test published by Castañeda (1942) may sometimes be useful for a rough typing of sera or antigens. Antigens used in this test are stained in different colors and standardized to give a comparable slide agglutination. Equal amounts of suspensions of both antigens are mixed on a slide with a drop of an appropriate antiserum dilution. A

Table 37. Expression of Results of Slide
Agglutination Test

Amount of Agglutination (%)	Degree of Agglutination
100 (complete)	4+
75	3+
50	2+
25	1+
Trace	±
No agglutination	−

ring is formed in a short time at the edge of the mixture, showing the color of a homologous antigen, for which a preference is exhibited by the antiserum.

4. The Microagglutination Test

The Takatsy (1955.) and Sever's (1962) "microtiter system" has been applied for a microagglutination test by Galton et al. (1965). The equipment or this micro-technique consists of disposable plastic plates (3.25 × 5 in.) containing 96 U wells, each holding 0.125-ml volume of liquid, spiral steel diluting loops calibrating to deliver 0.025 ml, loop delivery tester of special blotter material, and plastic pipette droppers calibrated to deliver 0.025 ml.

The microagglutination test is set up by diluting hyperimmune sera or unknown sera in a twofold series in a final colume of 0.25 ml using the calibrated loops and a buffered saline as diluent. The antigen suspension is adjusted to a density of 25 to 30 nephelometer units in a Coleman No. 7 nephelometer. The 0.025 ml of the antigen suspension is delivered by a means of the pipette dropper into each dilution of serum making a final volume of 0.05 ml. The plastic trays are rotated for a short time and then covered with a porous tape to prevent evaporation during the following incubation for 3 hours at 30°.

The test is read by observing agglutinates by placing the plates on a microscope stage and the observing through dark-filled condenser and a 10× objective. A zoom dissecting microscope equipped with 20 wide field occulars and a 2× supplemental lens and allowing a magnification ranging from 40 to 120×, is most satisfactory for the observation of agglutinates. A black glass stage is placed on the microscope stage and the lamp of the microscope is so adjusted that the light strikes the top surface of the plate at an approximate 45° angle. The degrees of agglutination are recorded as 1+ when 25% of the bacteria have clumped, 2+ with about 50% clumped cells, 3+ with approximately 75 clumped and 4+ with 75 to 100% agglutination. The end point is taken from the highest dilution of the serum showing a 2+ reaction.

5. *The Electron-Microscopy Aggregation Test*

The principle of this immunological test is the detection, by an electron microscope, of antigen-antibody aggregates. The test may be set up indirectly, that is, by the pre-incubation of antigen-antibody mixture and then applying it to a grid, or directly, allowing the antigen-antibody reaction to occur on the grid.

In the *indirect technique* (Höglund, 1967), a particulate antigen preparation and an antiserum are first incubated at 37° for 1 hour and then a drop of the suspension is placed on a grid and observed under an electron microscope. An immunological reaction between antigen and antibody is indicated by the presence of aggregates of particles, as observed under the $20,000$ to $60,000\times$ magnification.

In the *direct technique* (Yanagida and Ahmad-Zadeh, 1970), the antibody is applied to an antigen based on a collodion coated grid and revealing the reaction by the detection of a dense layer zone around the antigen-antibody complex at $20,000$ to $60,000\times$ magnification. Details for this test are presented below. One microdrop of particle or cell suspension (about 5 to 10^{11} particles/ml) is placed on a grid, which after 30 seconds is washed off with a drop of distilled water. The grid is flooded with the antigen preparation side down on an antiserum solution, either unabsorbed or absorbed, in a small plastic tube with a stopper. The grid is incubated in the antiserum at 37° for 1 to 4 hours after which it is washed with three drops of distilled water and stained negatively by a drop of 2% sodium phosphotungstate at pH 7.0 for 30 seconds. Excess water or phosphotungstate is removed with filter paper. The grid is mounted into an electron microscope, and the specimens are investigated at 80 kV. Photomicrographs are taken at the magnification ranging from 20,000 to 60,000 times.

The particulate antigen or particles, which have reacted with the antiserum, appear as structures surrounded by haloes or a dense layer of material, 1 to 300 Å wide.

6. *The Slide-Centrifuge Agglutination Test*

The slide-centrifuge agglutination test (Kwapinski, 1972) depends on bringing agglutinogens and agglutinins into contact by the gravity force, and on rapid concentration of the complexes on a cellulose-acetate membrane. The test is conducted by the aid of a cytocentrifuge (Shandon Co.) in the following manner:

1. Arrange constituents of each plastic chamber in the cytocentrifuge in the following order: a glass slide, a cellulose-acetate strip (Serometrics), and a punched, water-absorbing filter-paper strip (Fig. 49).

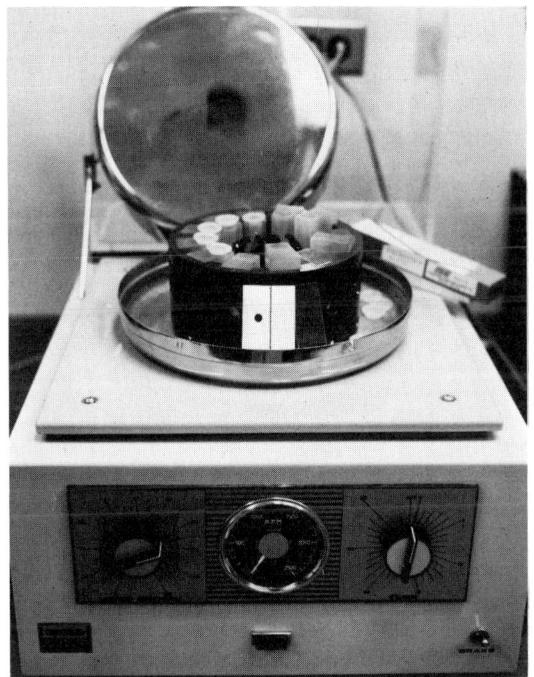

Figure 49. The cytocentrifuge adopted for immunological tests.

2. Incubate a mixture consisting of 0.1 ml of antiserum or an immuno-globulin preparation and 0.1 ml of antigen solution for 1 to 2 minutes at a desired temperature.

3. Transfer the mixture to a plastic compartment of the cytocentrifuge and spin the mixture at 1000 rpm for 5 minutes.

4. Wash off the noncombined material of the reaction mixture from the acetate strip in two changes of 1 *M* NaCl for 2 minutes.

5. Stain the cellulose strip in 0.001% Ponceau S stain solution or in 1:10,000 nigrosin solution, or in 1:100 Giemsa stain solution for 15 minutes.

6. Wash the membrane in 7% acetic acid for 2 minutes in case of Ponceau S stain and in distilled water for 1 minute.

7. View the cellulose strip against a fluorescent light through a 10× magnifying glass.

Antigen-antibody complexes occur in the form of a red-stain clump of amorphous material on a pale-pink background (Fig. 50). Controls consisting of a heterologous, nonrelated antigen and the antibody or consisting of the antigen mixed with a normal serum produce no clumps.

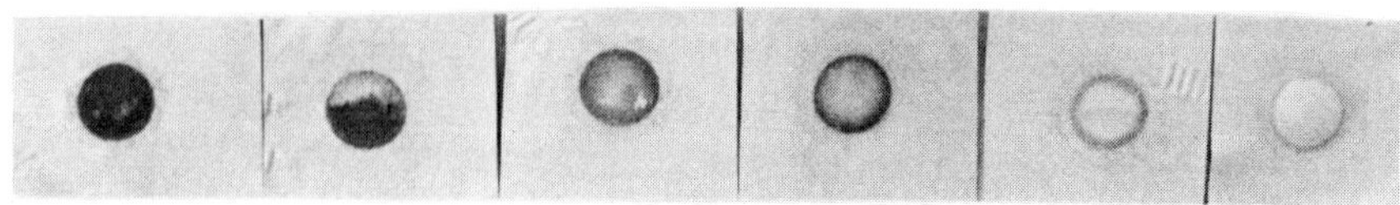

Figure 50. Clumps of bacteria agglutinated by an antiserum, deposited on cellulose-acetate membrane at antiserum dilutions 1:10 to 1:160.

7. *The Agglutinin-Absorption Test*

This procedure is based on the absorption of antiserum with a heterologous strain and testing the absorbed serum against the homologous bacterium. If both strains have common antigens, the absorbed serum will fail to agglutinate homologous bacteria. An antiserum containing a number of different specific antibodies or reactive groupings (*a, b, c*), treated with corresponding antigens, *A, B, C,* loses one, two, or all antibodies according to the use of one, two, or all antigen preparations. Any biological preparation bearing one or more of these antigens or determinants is able to absorb and, consequently, to neutralize a corresponding number of antibodies, while others remain noncombined. For example, an antigen possessing the determinants *B, C,* and *D* removes antibodies b and c from the abc serum, leaving the *a* antibody free; a biological preparation bearing determinants *A, D,* and *E* removes antibodies *a* and *c* while the *b* antibody remains uncombined. The antiserum abc absorbed with either of these antigen preparations is still able to react with the homologous antigen *ABC,* owing to the remaining antibody *a,* in the first case, or *b* in case of the absorption with the antigen complex *A, C, E.* By means of a cross-absorption technique, antigenic relationships amongst various microorganisms may be studied, either in the agglutination or another serological test.

Absorption of antibodies from antiserum or globulin preparation is accomplished according to Kwapinski's (1969) technique in the following manner: equal volumes of the particulate antigen used in a concentration varying from 2.0 to 5.0 $\times$ 10^{10} particles or cells/per milliliter and antibody source are mixed and incubated at 37° for 2 hours and at 4° for 6 hours on an electric shaker. The mixtures are then centrifuged at 23,500 $\times$ *g* for 10 minutes; the supernatant is carefully collected and recentrifuged for 5 minutes at the same speed. Another portion of the particulate antigen may be added to the supernatant, if required, and the procedure is thus repeated. The final supernatant is concentrated to $\frac{1}{2}$ volume with polyacrylamide gel pellet or by partial lyophilization. The efficiency of absorption ought to be controlled by conducting a serological test with the supernatant and the sorbent. No reaction should occur if the absorption has been complete.

According to the technique of Spicer and Rachstein (1931) the ratio between the mass of bacterial cells and the serum volume to be absorbed should be calculated by applying a coefficient equal to 2.7. Multiplying the mass, in milligrams, of packed bacterial cells by 2.7 gives the amount of 1:10 diluted serum which should be mixed with the bacteria to assure a satisfactory absorption. The mixture is incubated in a water bath at 45° for 2 hours with occasional shaking, then centrifuged at 4000 × g for 30 minutes. Clear serum is serially diluted in 0.2 or 0.3 ml volumes and mixed with an equal volume of the suspension of nonhomologous bacteria. Three controls are set simultaneously, containing (a) dilutions of a serum absorbed with the homologous strain of bacteria, and a suspension of nonhomologous bacterial cells, (b) the nonabsorbed serum with a homologous antigen, and (c) equal volumes of the antigen and saline.

8. *The Mixed Agglutination Test*

The mixed agglutination test (Coombs et al., 1956, 1961) depends on the observation that an antibody combined with its specific antigen on a cell may have a free combining site capable of reacting with another molecule of its specific antigen. The free combining sites participating in the mixed agglutination are revealed by antigens attached to a red-cell indicator. Thus two types of cells participate in the mixed agglutination reaction: the cells under study, and indicator cells usually are erythrocytes.

The test is set up in 50 × 100 mm siliconed tubes by placing two drops of serum diluitons and two drops of a tissue cell suspension. The mixtures are incubated at room temperature on a slowly revolving machine. The tissue cells are then centrifuged at 200 × *g* for 5 minutes in a refrigerated centrifuge and washed twice in a cold diluent, then resuspended in one drop of the normal rabbit serum diluent (NRS) diluent. The NRS consists of one part of a heat-inactivated normal rabbit serum and 199 parts of saline buffered at pH 7.2. This suspension is mixed with one drop of the red-cell indicator suspension (e.g., a 0.5% ox red blood cells), and the mixture is centrifuged at 200 × *g* for 2 minutes to bring the cells into contact. The deposited cells are then lifted gently with a siliconed capillary tube and placed on a siliconed slide, covered with a siliconed cover slip, sealed with paraffin wax, and examined microscopically.

The procedure for mixed agglutination test designed by Milgrom and Kano (1965), is as follows: monolayer cell cultures are exposed to an antiserum used in varying dilutions and incubated at room temperature for 3 hours. The cultures are then washed, and an indicator system consisting of sheep erythrocytes sensitized with human antiserum to sheep erythrocytes is added, following by a rabbit antiserum to human gamma globulin. Adherence of the indicator erythrocytes to the monolayer cell culture is interpreted as a positive result of the reaction.

This test was used to detect A and B antigens in primary cell cultures of human fetal organs and to detect the blood group B antigen in cell cultures of rhesus monkey kidney (Kano, 1966).

The mixed agglutination tests have also been applied to the identification of the species of origin of tissue cells, blood groups, and to the demonstration of isoantigens in the culture tissue cells.

9. *The Growth Agglutinaton Test*

In this test, described by Wynne et al. (1953), a specific antiserum is diluted serially from 1:2.5 to 1:640 in 2.0- or 2.5-ml volumes of a culture medium. A control tube contains the medium alone. Each tube then receives one drop or 0.025 ml of an 18- to 24-hour liquid culture of bacteria. After 18 to 24 hours' incubation at 37°, the contents of tubes are examined grossly for the presence of the agglutinated growth. The highest agglutinating serum dilution is determined.

10. *The Agglutination-Lysis Test*

This test is reported in the chapter on immune hemolysis (p. 454).

11. *The Leukocyte-Agglutination Test*

According to the Steinberg and Martin (1944) technique, 0.05 ml of a saline suspension of leukocytes (27,000 cell/ml) is added to 0.5-ml volumes of an inactivated serum, made in a series of dilutions from 1:10 to 1:5,120. The tubes are shaken for 3 minutes, incubated in a water bath at 37° for 1 hour, shaken again, and left overnight in the refrigerator. Contents of tubes are then examined and observed for the presence of clumped cell. A diffuse cloudiness is seen if no agglutination has occurred. Microscopic readings at a medium magnification are also made by examining drops of reaction mixtures on a glass slide. Positive reaction is indicated by the presence of clumped leukocytes, with individual cells unrecognizable in the aggregates.

Patterns of the distribution or aggregation of leukocytes on the bottom of tubes can be more easily observed with the aid of an inverted microscope, as suggested by Beran and Dausset (1963).

12. *The Sensitized-Bacteria Agglutination Test*

This test is based on a principle similar to that of the hemagglutination test, that is, on the reaction between the antibody and an antigen adsorbed on the cell surface. The reaction was first described by Roberts and Jones (1941) and slightly modified by Roberts (1945). The test can be performed in the following manner. Cells of *Serratia marcescens* are washed with a saline, then suspended in distilled water and exposed to the flowing steam for 30 minutes. The killed cells should be resuspended in a saline, buffered at pH 6.5, to a concentration equivalent to 0.5 mg of the microbial nitrogen per milliliter. An amount of this stock suspension is mixed with a solution or a suspension of the antigen in an approximate ratio of 1:5. After the incubation at 37° for 9 to 15 hours, the "sensitized" bacterial cells are centrifuged at 500 × g for 10 to 15 minutes, and washed twice with a saline solution warmed at 37°. The cells are now suspended in 15 to 20 ml of warm saline and centrifuged at 8000 × g for 5 minutes to separate larger clumps. The supernatant is collected and diluted to a concentration corresponding to the optical density of a suspension of 0.2 mg (dry weight) or finely ground Pyrex glass per milliliter, which represents 125,000,000 bacterial cells per milliliter. Merthiolate should be added as preservative.

The test is set up by adding 0.25-ml volumes of sensitized cells to 0.5-ml aliquots of a serially diluted, fresh or inactivated serum. The following controls are included:

1. Two tubes containing 0.5-ml saline and 0.25 ml of sensitized cells.
2. A series of dilutions of a known, positive and negative, serum mixed with the sensitized antigen.

These mixtures are incubated for 2 to 6 hours at 40 to 42°, and examined immediately or when left overnight at 5°. The contents of tubes can be centrifuged for 10 minutes at 500 × g and examined with the aid of a lens against the indirect light from an ordinary 100-W desk lamp placed against a black background. The tubes are gently shaken. Finely granular agglutinates are observed if the test is positive.

This method is more sensitive than the ordinary precipitation or collodion test. Cells of *Serratia marcescens* were used as carriers of the following antigens: tuberculin (Muetter, 1945), poliomyelites virus (Roberts and Jones, 1941, 1942), and distemper virus (Weil et al., 1944), and were tested with immune or convalescent sera. An antigen obtained from the spinal fluid of pigs infected with the hog cholera (swine fever) virus could also be absorbed on the *Serratia marcescens* cells, rendering them agglutinable by the antihog cholera virus hyperimmune sera (Weil, 1942).

13. The Spore Agglutination Test

Equal 0.2-ml volumes of the antispore serum dilutions and a spore suspension are mixed and left at 4° for 30 to 60 minutes and then recentrifuged for 4 minutes. Results are read by gently tapping the tube to shake up the deposit (Tomcsik and Baumann-Grace, 1959).

III. CHEMICAL DETERMINATION OF AGGLUTININS

Common agglutination techniques, in which the potency of sera is evaluated either by titers or units of agglutinins, are only arbitrarily quantitative procedures, and the experimental error can be as high as 50% or more. An exact evaluation of the serological potency of antisera may be attained by the chemical determination of agglutinins, as described by Heidelberger and Kabat (1934). In this method, accurately measured volumes of washed particulate antigens are added to measured volumes of an antiserum. Increase of the nitrogen content of the agglutinated particles, washed with saline, over that of controls containing the saline instead of antiserum is determined chemically. For this assay, bacterial cells are killed by heating at 60° for 45 minutes or with 0.5 to 1% formalin, incubated for 10 to 12 hours, and then washed repeatedly with 0.9% saline until the supernatant no longer gives a Biuret test. The cells are suspended in a volume of saline so that each milliliter of the suspension is an equivalent of 0.15 to 0.25 mg of nitrogen. A volume of 2 to 3 ml of the uniformly mixed bacterial suspension is then added from accurately measured pipettes to several samples of the antiserum or test serum. The volume of serum may vary between 0.5 to 3 ml, depending on its serological potency. Blanks contain either the bacterial suspension and saline instead of serum, or a serum and saline without bacteria. The contents of tubes are thoroughly mixed and incubated at 37° for 2 hours, then left in an ice box overnight. If the bacteria tend to flocculate, the tubes are gently agitated every 15 minutes for the first 2 hours. After standing overnight, the tubes are centrifuged once or twice in the refrigerated centrifuge at 500 × g. Supernatants should be completely decanted and the tubes allowed to drain. The drained tubes are immersed in ice water, and the precipitates are washed twice with 3.0 ml of a cold saline, and centrifuged. The tubes are finally drained again, and the precipitates suspended in water are quantitatively transferred to micro-Kjeldahl flasks to be analyzed for the nitrogen content according to one of the procedures for a micro-Kjeldahl technique.

The blanks and nitrogen standards are tested in a similar manner. The agglutinin nitrogen, expressed in milligrams, is calculated for the volume of a serum used by subtracting the nitrogen figure of the bacterial suspension blank and nitrogen of the serum blank from the nitrogen figure of the test sample. Multiplying the agglutinin nitrogen figure by the coefficient of 6.25 the approximate contents of agglutinin protein, in milligrams, may be calculated for the serum volume used. The agglutinin content of a serum, in milligrams per milliliter, is obtained by dividing the figure of agglutinin contents by the amout of milliliters of the serum employed in the test. This method is especially useful in the quantitative determination of the agglutinin content of a serum versus different variants of the same microorganism. It is not suitable for the determination of the agglutinin quantity of very weak antisera, containing less than 0.02 mg of antibody nitrogen per 5 ml of serum. According to Heidelberger and Kabat (1934) an amount of 0.002 to 2.0 mg of the antibody nitrogen per 1 g of bacterial nitrogen is required to bring about agglutination.

IV. DIAGNOSTIC TECHNIQUES OF AGGLUTINATION TEST

Many agglutination tests, for example, the Widal, Weil-Felix, Wright, and the *Streptococcus* MG test are widely used for immunological diagnosis of salmonelloses, rickettsioses, brucellosis, and atypical pneumonia, respectively. The following techniques have been selected and presented below as most suitable for diagnostic purposes.

1. The Widal Agglutination Test

The Widal test, as designed by Felix and Bensted (1954), is set up in round-bottomed tubes, about 2 in. long and $\frac{1}{2}$ in. in external diameter. Patient's serum is diluted in the geometric progression from 1:25 to 1:1:1,600 in 0.5-ml volumes of a saline solution and mixed with equal volumes of the O- or H-antigen preparation of *Salmonella typhosa*, *Salmonella paratyphi* A, and *Salmonella paratyphi* B. The selection of agglutinogen is sometimes extended to include representative strains of serogroups C, C_2, and D (*S. choleraesuis, S. newport,* and *S. anatum*) or other groups prevalent in the area. A test for the Vi-agglutinins with viable bacteria is set up in parallel. Control tubes receive 0.5-ml volumes of saline and the antigen suspension adjusted to the density of tube 5 or 6 of McFarland's scale. For a more uniform testing, international standard agglutinating horse sera or substandards are recommended. Standard antisera are produced by the Lister Institute for Preventive Medicine, London.

The test mixtures are incubated at 37° for 2 hours and left at 2 to 4° for 20 hours, then allowed to stand at room temperature and observed for the presence of agglutinates after 10 minutes, 1, and 2 hours in case of the *H*-agglutination, or after 2 hours only, in case of the *O*- or Vi-agglutination. Tully and Gaines (1961) recommend incubation of the *H*-agglutination test tubes at 52° for 2 hours, and the *O*-agglutination mixtures at 37° for 18 hours; as diluent, a 0.5% phenolized saline should be used to prevent bacterial contamination. The *O*-agglutination occurs in the form of large granules floating in the clear fluid, and it consists of bacterial cells aggregated by polar attachment, to form a regular, crystal-like structure in two dimensions (Pijper, 1938). Flagellar *H*-agglutination is flocculent, with the cells attached to each other through their thickened and entangled flagella. The Vi-agglutinates are in the form of small, rather granular clumps, which are conditioned by the side-to-side attachment of cells.

The serum dilutions giving definite agglutinations with the *O-, H-,* and Vi-antigens, are recorded; no clumping should be observed in the control tubes. The titer of somatic and flagellar antibodies equal to 1:80 or a higher serum dilution is indicative of an active typhoid infection. Lower titers are often found in the sera of *Salmonella* carriers, in convalescents, and in immunized people.

For a "rapid" agglutination test, by Bass and Watkins, are used very concentrated suspensions of bacteria. The agglutination can be observed in a few minutes.

2. The Microscopic Widal Agglutination Test

A series of blood serum dilutions is prepared as for an ordinary Widal test, and a loopful of each solution is placed on a cover glass. A control cover glass obtains one drop of saline. A loopful of a 12- to 24-hour broth culture of *Salmonella* or a saline suspension of these bacteria is added to each drop. Hollow-ground slides, previously ringed with petrolatum, are placed over each cover glass, turned over, and incubated at 37° for 2 hours. The mixtures are examined for the presence of agglutinates under a medium or high magnification of the microscope. The clumped bacteria are motionless and gathered in tangled masses or balls, whereas nonagglutinated bacteria move freely as separate cells.

3. The Weil-Felix Agglutination Test

The antigen is prepared, by the technique of Zarafonetis (1945), from a 24-hour culture of *Proteus* OX-19, OX-2, or OX-K growing on the peptone agar. Only nonmotile strains should be used for preparing the somatic antigen for this test. Thus the growth of *Proteus* OX-19 must be checked microscopically for the nonmotility, then harvested in a saline solution, to which 0.5% formalin has been added to kill the bacteria. The suspension is left at room temperature for about 24 hours, then centrifuged and washed thrice with saline, and finally resuspended in a buffered saline, pH 7.1, containing 0.5% formalin as a preservative. "Stock" solutions prepared in this manner should be standardized for the optimum dilution to be employed in the test, by titrating the diluted antigen suspension against positive reference sera. The Weil-Felix test is set up by adding 0.5-ml volumes of adequate suspensions of *Proteus* OX-19, OX-2, or OX-K to the progressive serum dilutions, made in 0.5-ml saline. Control tubes receive saline instead of the serum. The tubes are shaken and placed in a water bath at 37° for 4 hours, and left for 18 hours at 4°.

The agglutinin titer is expressed in terms of a final serum dilution in which at least one half of the amount of the antigen added appears in clumps. Agglutination titers of 1:80 or higher are considered significant. In some cases, titers exceeding a serum dilution of 1:50,000 are noted. The Weil-Felix test is widely used as a diagnostic measure in suspected cases of rickettsioses (Table 38). The reactivity of sera from cases of rickettsioses with the specific strains of *Proteus* OX-19, OX-2, and OX-K depends on a serologically specific polysaccharide component occurring in these bacteria and in certain pathogenic species of rickettsiae.

Table 38. Agglutination (+) of Proteus in Rickettsioses

OX-19	OX-2	OX-K	Rickettsiosis
4+	1+	—	Epidemic typhus
4+	1+	—	Murine typhus
4+	1+, 4+	—	Spotted fever group
—	—	—	Rickettsial pox
—	—	4+	Tsutsugamushi disease
—	—	2+	Sennetsu rickettsiosis
—	—	—	Q fever

4. The Wright Agglutination Test

This test, used for detection of the *Brucella* antibody, is set up by mixing 0.5-ml aliquots of various saline dilutions of a serum, ranging from 1:25 to 1:3,200, with 0.05 ml of nondiluted or 0.5 ml of a 1:10 dilution of a standard phenolized suspension of *Brucella abortus*. A control tube contains saline and the antigen alone. The samples are incubated at 37° for 24 to 48 hours. Incubation for 48 hours is recommended as accounting for more uniform titers and a lower incidence of the prozone phenomenon. Agglutinates are detected by the aid of a magnifying glass. Agglutination in a serum dilution equal to, or higher than, 1:100 is regarded as abnormal. For a rapid demonstration of *Brucella* agglutinins, the Huddleson (1943) technique with a concentrated *Brucella* suspension is used.

5. The Streptococcus MG Agglutination Test

The antigen for this test is a suspension of cells of a nonhemolytic streptococcus (*Streptococcus* MG). To prepare this suspension, a 48-hour digest broth culture of the microorganism is first centrifuged; the sediment is washed three times with sterile saline, resuspended in saline, and heated in a water bath at 100° for 30 minutes. The suspension of killed bacteria should be centrifuged, the sediment washed with saline, resuspended up to a standard density, and preserved with 1:10,000 Merthiolate.

The test is arranged as follows. A series of twofold serum dilutions ranging from 1:5 to 1:320 is made in 0.5 ml of saline. A control tube receives 0.5 ml of saline only. Another control row consists of a serial dilution of a rabbit serum immunized with the *Streptococcus MG*.

Each tube then receives 0.5 ml of the *Streptococcus* MG suspension; thus final dilutions in each tube are twice increased. All tubes are incubated overnight in the water bath at 37° and inspected for the presence of agglutinates.

The agglutination titer exceeding 1:20 serum dilution is regarded as significant. An elevated titer of the anti-*Streptococcus* MG agglutinins is found in 30 to 40% of the cases of primary atypical pneumonia.

6. *The Treponema Agglutination Test*

The antigen for this test, devised by Hardy and Nell (1955), is the Nichols strain of *Treponema pallidum* obtained from rabbit testicular syphilomas. Equal 0.1-ml volumes of the antigen suspension and a serum, usually diluted at 1:10 in a saline containing 0.005 methylendiamine tetracetate, adjusted to pH 7.6, are used in the test. For the quantitative assay, a series of twofold serum dilutions is incubated in a water bath at 37° for 18 hours. A large drop of each mixture is then examined by the dark-field microscopy. The presence and size of clumps of treponemas are recorded. The highest serum dilution giving a definite agglutination is taken as its titer. According to the authors, the specificity of this test is equal to that of the treponemal immobilization test.

7. *The Rickettsial Agglutination Test*

Three different procedures of the rickettsial agglutination test, by Hudson (1940), Lennette et al. (1952), and Ormsbee (1964), have been selected for presentation. According to our experience, the sensitivity of all three methods is alike, and these tests are simpler and as reproducible as the complement fixation test with rickettsial antigens. The agglutination test according to Hudson's method is carried out using a purified suspension of the rickettsiae, obtained from lungs of infected white mice or rats by the disruption of infected cells and a differential centrifugation of the released cell contents. For the agglutination assay, equal 0.25-ml volumes of the antigen suspension and serial dilutions of a serum tested are incubated for 4 hours at 40°, and left overnight in the cold. Results are read both after the incubation at 40° and after the tubes have been left in the refrigerator overnight.

The Lennette et al. (1952) Technique of the Rickettsial Test. Prior to the test proper, an optimal unit of the antigen is determined by a "checkerboard" or "box-titration" in the following manner: serial twofold dilutions of a purified saline suspension of rickettsiae are distributed in 0.2-ml aliquots into a number of 13 × 100-mm tubes. Each tube then receives a progressively higher serum dilution in 0.2-ml volume. Control tubes contain a standard negative serum in dilutions identical with those of the test serum, or saline and the antigen suspension. The mixtures are incubated at 48° for 3 hours and left at 4° overnight, then read. The unit of antigen to be employed in the test is 0.25 ml of the highest dilution of a rickettsial suspension giving a strong agglutination in the presence of the highest serum dilution. This dilution of the antigen is used in the test proper.

The test proper is carried out by mixing 0.25-ml aliquots of an appropriate antigen dilution with an equal volume of serial twofold saline dilutions of the serum being examined. After the incubation at 48° for 3 hours and at 4° overnight, the agglutination titer is determined by the highest serum dilution giving a definite agglutination of rickettsiae.

The Ormsbee (1964) Agglutination-Resuspension Test for the Detection of Anti-Coxiella (Q-Fever) Antibodies. This test involves the use of a purified antigen suspension and the centrifugation and resuspension of this antigen after exposure to antiserum. The antigen preparation consists of the coxiellae collected from the yolk sacs of infected embryonated chicken eggs, are inactivated with formaldehyde, and purified by a continuous flow, high salt-ether technique, and adjusted to a concentration of 200 μg/ml of 0.15 M NaCl. The sera are serially diluted in 25% bovine serum in 0.15 M NaCl. Mixtures of 0.25 ml of antigen and 0.25 ml of varying serum dilutions are placed in round-bottomed tubes and incubated in a water bath at 37° for 30 minutes. The tubes are then centrifuged at 2000 × g for 10 minutes. After centrifugation, the tubes are repeatedly flipped with a finger. If the agglutination has occurred, the sediment dislodges from the bottom with some difficulty in the form of visible particles which quickly sink to the bottom of the tube. The suspending medium remains clear. If no agglutination has occurred, the pellet can be easily resuspended to form an opalescent suspension without any visible particles.

V. EVALUATION AND APPLICATIONS OF THE AGGLUTINATION ASSAY

Agglutination test is more sensitive than precipitation test for detecting small amounts of antibody, since relatively few antibody molecules can effectively link together large numbers of particulate antigens to produce easily visible clumps, whereas the precipitin reaction is limited by the amount of antigen-antibody aggregate which can be observed. Small amounts of precipitins, however, may be detected by means of a precipitinogen, adsorbed to large inert particles or cells.

Agglutination tests were successfully applied to the following types of investigations:

1. The identification and classification of microorganisms, for example, *Salmonella, Shigella, Escherichia, Proteus, Klebsiella, Haemophilus,* with standard antisera.

2. Studies on antigenic structure variations of the antigenic potency, and antigenic relationship between microorganisms. Examples: studies of the relationship between *Salmonella typhosa* and other species or types of *Salmonella* (Weiner and Price, 1956), *Escherichia, Haemophilus, Shigella,*

Klebsiella, and *Actinomyces israelii* (Kauffmann, 1948; Weiner and Price, 1956; Kwapinski, 1960).

3. The detection in the sera of vaccinated or infected people and animals, of circulating antibodies, for example, *Haemophilus pertussis* agglutinins (Bordet and Gengou, 1906; Mishulov et al., 1939; Evans and Maitland, 1939; Miller and Silverberg, 1939), *Brucella* agglutinins (Angle et al., 1942; Huddleson, 1943; Castañeda, 1945; Eisle et al., 1947; Griggs and Case, 1948; Murduch et al., 1950; Miles, 1954; Carpenter, 1955), *Salmonella* and *Shigella* agglutinins (Weil and Saphra, 1955), *M. tuberculosis, Streptococcus,* and *Staphylococcus* agglutinins (Meynell, 1954; Kwapinski, 1959), *Treponema* agglutinins (Hardy and Nell, 1955), *Histoplasma* agglutinins (Cozad and Larsh, 1960), *Coxiella burneti* agglutinins (Lennette et al., 1952; Luoto, 1953, 1956; Luoto and Mason, 1955), agglutinins against *Rickettsia prowazeki* and other species of rickettsiae (Castañeda, 1945), agglutinins reacting with *Proteus* OX-19, OX-2 or OX-K (Zarafonetis, 1945), *P. tularensis* agglutinins and others.

The agglutinin-absorption test is used for the study of antigenic structure and relationships of various microorganisms and for the differentiation of species and types of bacteria.

Chapter Six

THE PRECIPITATION TEST

I. PRINCIPLES OF THE PRECIPITATION REACTION

The precipitation test depends on the reaction of a soluble antigen with the corresponding antibody in the presence of ions. The union between the antigen and antibody results in the formation of amorphous, powdery, or flocculent precipitate. The ions aid the reaction apparently by depressing the surface potential below 12 to 15 mV, needed for the aggregation of hydrophobic complexes. Specific precipitates are only very slightly soluble in saline or water, as indicated by the average figures of 1 to 2 μg of nitrogen per milliliter of saline. The antigen particles participating in the precipitation reaction are 0.2 μ or less in diameter, whereas larger particles and cells reacting with the antibodies produce agglutinates which differ optically from the precipitates. Antibodies participating in both the precipitation and agglutination reactions are essentially identical. Two types of precipitins, "R" and "H," are differentiated. The R antibody, which is classically produced in rabbits, forms precipitates in a wide range of antigen-antibody ratio, and these precipitates are insoluble in an excess of the antigen. The H precipitin, which is formed most readily in horses against most protein antigens, produces immune complexes within only a narrow range of the antigen-antibody ratio, and these precipitates are readily soluble in either the antigen or antibody excess (Boyd, 1956; Augustin, 1957).

Initial combination between the precipitinogen and precipitins occurs within a few seconds, but a much longer time is required for a complete precipitation. The rate of the precipitate formation depends on the type of antibody, the proportion of antibody and antigen in a reacting mixture, and is influenced by the temperature, salt concentration, pH value, and protein and lipid constituents of the serum.

The proportion of an antigen preparation to the antiserum, which forms particles of the precipitate most rapidly and most abundantly, is termed the optimal ratio of antiserum. The optimal ratio may be estimated by adding a constant quantity of antiserum to a series of dilutions of the antigen (Dean and Webb, 1926) or by mixing a constant amount of antigen with varying concentrations of antiserum (Ramon, 1922; Martin, 1943). The first procedure is applicable mostly for the flocculation test (see p. 374). If the antigen or antibody is in excess of the optimum amount, it delays the formation of particles of the precipitate; at a certain excess of antigen, the precipitation can be prevented entirely. However, other nonspecific factors, such as those responsible for the Danysz phenomenon, or the presence of active complement can also retard or diminish the precipitation reaction. The precipitation is accelerated by polypeptide polysine (Stahmann and Mathews, 1954) or 0.001% tannic acid in 0.1% ferric chloride solution (Kwapinski, 1965).

The kinetics of the aggregation in the precipitation reaction are studied more precisely by measurement of the turbidity as a function of time. The amount of antibody precipitated from most of the horse antisera, and to a lesser degree from rabbit immune sera, is usually greater at $0°$ than at $37°$, but in other cases the reverse is true. Thus the optimum temperature must be selected for individual serological systems, especially in the quantitative precipitation test.

The 0.1 M concentration of sodium chloride seems to be optimal. An increase of the salt concentration above 0.15 M usually brings about a considerable decrease in the specific precipitate. An exception is the precipitation of fowl antibodies by an antigen which is greater at a higher salt concentration, close to 1.5 M or 8% $NaCl$ (Goodman et al., 1951). The effect of pH changes varying from 6.4 to 7.8 is negligible.

Procedures designed for the precipitation test can be classified within one of three following groups: (a) the interfacial or ring precipitation test; (b) the tube precipitation test; and (c) the gel precipitation test (see Chapter 7). Qualitative precipitation tests consist in the observation of antiserum and/or antigen dilutions at which a turbidity occurs. By the quantitative methods, the amount of precipitate formed or the amount of precipitin-nitrogen combined to antigen is determined. Quantitative estimations are made either by the gravimetric determination of precipitates, chemical determination of certain constituents of precipitates, or measurement of the intensity of the light scattering.

Reagents required for the precipitation test, the antigen preparation, and the serum and saline solution must be perfectly clear, since even slightly turbid reagents obscure the reading of the test. The serum should be used in a high concentration, undiluted or only diluted up to 1:5, since the amount of precipitate rapidly decreases with the dilution of antiserum. The reason for the need of a large amount of precipitins is that the total vast surface area occupied by fine precipitinogen particles must be "coated" by the antibody (Zinsser, 1930). The rate of precipitation usually follows the rise of temperature to 45 to $50°$; however, a more complete precipitation is often obtained at 0 to 4°. The optimum temperature varies with different antigen-antibody systems.

II. THE INTERFACIAL PRECIPITATION TEST

To study the immunological activity of a soluble antigen preparation by the ring precipitation test, a series of twofold dilutions of the antigen are made in saline, and 0.1-ml volumes are placed in a series of microtest tubes of 3-mm inside diameter. An equal volume of antiserum is added to each tube by immersing a micropipette to the bottom of the tube and allowing the serum to run slowly. A control tube receives 0.1 ml of saline and 0.1 ml of the antiserum. The antiserum is usually used undiluted, since it should have a greater density than the antigen. The serum must be translucent, and, if necessary, clarified by centrifugation. The tubes are left at room temperature or at 37° for 1 to 4 hours, and observed at 15-minute intervals with the naked eye or by the aid of an agglutinoscope.

A precipitate zone is formed at the interface where the concentration ratio of antigen:antibody is optimal, owing to the diffusion of the antigen. The end point and titer are represented by the highest antigen dilution, giving a definite ring precipitation. In doubtful cases, the contents of the tubes are mixed by inversion and the incubation is prolonged for 12 to 48 hours at 2 to 4°, at a room temperature, or at a higher temperature, and inspected for the presence of precipitates. Positive results may be obtained with antigens diluted over one million times.

Important adaptations of the interfacial precipitation test are the forensic precipitin test and the thermoprecipitin test.

1. The Forensic Precipitin Test

The forensic precipitin test is used for identification of the species specificity of blood stains. The blood stain submitted for this test must be thoroughly dried or otherwise well preserved. It is then extracted with a small amount of saline solution. The nondiluted and serially diluted extract is overlayered, in equal volumes, on an antihuman serum of a high titer, and incubated for 20 minutes at room temperature. Five controls are inserted, to contain (a) the blood stain extract and a normal rabbit serum; (b) the antihuman serum and a saline solution; (c) an extract of unstained portion of the material investigated; (d) blood samples from several animal species other than those involved in the test; and (e) several different specimens of a known blood homologous to the antihuman serum.

The positive forensic precipitin test may be regarded as reliable only if the controls 1 to 4 were negative and the control 5 was positive. The antihuman serum for the forensic test is prepared in rabbits by immunization with human blood, plasma, or serum. A series of intravenous doses of 1 to 2 ml, containing roughly 1% protein or 3 to 6 ml of intraperitoneal doses, are recommended by Schiff and Boyd (1942) to obtain a potent antihuman serum.

The forensic precipitin test has also been applied to the identification of the animal origin of other tissues and fluids (e.g., semen, bones, milk, and meat) by using extracts from these tissues or fluids and specific immune sera. Meats and fish products are often identified by the "thermoprecipitin" test with "cocto-antisera."

2. The Thermoprecipitin Test

The thermoprecipitin test or, more correctly, "the thermoprecipitinogen test" is a precipitin assay with antigens extracted at 70 to 100°, usually from diseased tissues. This test was originally introduced by Ascoli (1902) for the immunological diagnosis of anthrax, but it has also been adopted for the diagnosis of plague.

Thermoprecipitinogens are crude antigen extracts obtained by heating, at 70 to 100°, the diseased or decomposed tissues of carcasses, ground with sterile sand, and suspended in 3 to 5 volumes of distilled water or saline. These extracts are mostly prepared from the liver, spleen, and lymph nodes of infected animals since these organs contain most thermoprecipitinogen. Crude extracts can be delipidized with 2 volumes of ether. The aqueous phase is then separated, clarified by filtration or centrifugation, and the clear supernatant is used as antigen for the precipitation test with standard antisera, obtained by immunization of rabbits with killed suspensions of *Bacillus anthracis* or *Pasteurella pestis*.

Thermoprecipitinogens are sometimes prepared from meats and fish products to be identified for the purpose of forensic medicine. These extracts are tested with "cocto-antisera" obtained by immunizing rabbits with heated tissue extracts.

The *thermoprecipitinogen test,* by the Larson (1957) technique, is carried out as follows. The antigen preparation is serially diluted and drawn into capillary tubes, followed by a standard antiserum. After a 3-hour incubation period at 37°, the tubes are left overnight at 2 to 4° before the reading. Any degree of the precipitate is regarded as a positive reaction. The precipitation titers may range from 1:8 to 1:512 or more. A similar test is used for the immunological identification and typing of certain bacteria such as the streptococci.

Bacterial thermoprecipitinogens by Lancefield's (1933) method are extracted at 100° with $N/10$ hydrochloric acid at pH 2.0 to 2.4. Supernatants are then either neutralized with alkali or mixed with 95% ethyl alcohol to precipitate an active fraction. The precipitation test is carried out by overlaying 0.2 ml of undiluted standard antisera with equal volumes of an undiluted and diluted 1:10 and 1:100 precipitinogen solution. A control tube receives the precipitinogen preparation and saline solution instead of antiserum. The tubes are incubated in a water bath at 37° for 10 minutes and examined for the presence of a precipitate ring. If no precipitate ring is formed, contents of the tubes should be mixed and reincubated at 37° for 2 hours. If no precipitates are observed, the tubes must be left at 2° for 12 to 14 hours before the final reading.

3. The Phase-Contrast Microprecipitin Test

The test by Eggers and Sabin (1961) is set up on glass plates used for lantern slides, 7.5 × 10 cm, divided into 12 (4 × 3) squares of about 2.5 × 2.5 cm. A 0.02-M phosphate buffer, pH 7.2, containing sodium chloride at a final 0.13 $M,$ is used as diluent. Approximately 0.01-ml amounts of the antigen suspension and a serum dilution are delivered per square, using an even-cut, no. 23 syringe needle, mounted on a 0.25-ml syringe barrel.

Controls containing either the antigen in saline or a positive and negative serum are included. Test mixtures are incubated at 36° for 4 hours and kept in humidified chambers (large Petri dishes with a piece of wet filter paper) to prevent evaporation. After the incubation, each mixture is covered by a cover slip and observed by the phase-contrast microscopy, using a 10 objective and a 7 or 15× eyepiece. A positive reaction is indicated by the presence of small, medium-sized, or large floccules.

The test was originally used for a study of polio-virus antigens.

4. The Ultramicroprecipitation Test

The ultramicroprecipitation test (Hudson and Mudd, 1935) is an interesting modification of the capillary-tube technique described by Richards et al. (1933). In this modification, capillary tubes having 0.5-mm o.d. and 0.35 mm i.d., made from capillary tubings are used. The reaction solutions are drawn into capillary tubes by the aid of a water manipulator which consists of a glass tube shaped like the barrel of a 2-ml³ glass syringe, with the large end closed by a cemented-on metal cap. A screw, 3 mm in diameter, is provided with a large milled head. Capillary tubes are illuminated by the transmitted light during the introduction of fluids and during the measuring of the length of fluid columns. These operations are observed through a stereomicroscope at the 24× magnification.

Capillary tubings are first filled with an antiserum, usually to the length of ten scale divisions, read on the ocular micrometer scale. This corresponds approximately to 0.1 ml of the fluid. The antigen solution is then introduced to the length of forty scale divisions. The proportion of antiserum and antigen solutions may vary; for example, two scale divisions of the antigen and twenty-six scale divisions of the serum are used in the test for syphilis reagins, whereas twenty scale divisions of serum and of the cell suspension are applied for the blood grouping.

Results of the test are read in 1 to 10 minutes. Precipitation and agglutination tests may be carried out by this microtechnique. This test deserves recommendation since it provides a quick reaction which can be observed continuously, and it requires only minute amounts of reactants.

III. THE TUBE PRECIPITATION TEST

A screening test usually precedes the test proper, which is carried out with serial dilutions of either the antigen or the antiserum. The screening test is set up by placing 0.5 to 1.0 ml of undiluted serum in a narrow tube; larger volumes (2 to 5 ml) of a weak serum are needed. The antigen solution, varying from 1:100 to 1:300, is added at first in a small volume, for example, 0.1 ml, to avoid the inhibition of the precipitin reaction by an excess antigen. The mixture is left at room temperature or at a lower or higher temperature, according to individual requirements of the immunological system. If a turbidity or a precipitate occurs in a few minutes (or in a few hours if the antiserum is weak), the tube is centrifuged for 10 to 15 minutes at 500 $\times$ g, and the fluid is inspected for the presence of a precipitate. In case of a negative reaction at this stage, additional amounts of the antigen solution, for example, 0.3, 0.5, 1.0, and 3.0 ml, are placed in time intervals to allow the aggregation to occur.

The amount and the volume of the antigen found to give a strong precipitation with a constant amount of antiserum is then employed in the serum dilution test.

The antigen dilution or the serum dilution precipitation tests are used for assaying the potency of antigen or antiserum preparations.

The Antigen Dilution Technique. A series of twofold or tenfold dilutions of an antigen preparation, ranging from 1:25 to 1:1,600,000 or from 1:10 to $1:10^7$, respectively, are made with a saline or a buffer solution in 0.2-ml volumes. Each tube then receives 0.2 ml of the antiserum either undiluted or diluted at its optimum concentration, which should be previously determined by titration with a constant concentration of the antigen.

Two control tubes are set, containing (a) 0.2 ml of the lowest dilution and 0.2 ml of "normal" serum, and (b) 0.2 ml of antiserum and 0.2 ml of saline. All tubes are shaken on an electric shaker for 10 minutes and placed for 2 hours at 37°, then left at 2 to 4° for 1 to 7 days.

Precipitates with strong antisera may be noticed within 2 hours, but weak sera can give positive results as late as on the seventeenth day. The last tube showing a definite sediment denotes the end point, and the precipitinogen titer is expressed by the final antigen dilution in that tube.

The amount of antigen in the precipitate can be estimated if a colored or radioactive antigen is used, or if the antigen contains a particular chemical component, for example, hexosamine or methylpentose, which does not occur in the antiserum. In each case, the precipitate is dissolved either in $M/2$ NaOH or in concentrated hydrochloric acid. The amount of a colored antigen is estimated spectrophotometrically. If the antigen is radioactive, a portion of the dissolved precipitate is assayed in a Geiger counter. The particular chemical component of the antigen may be determined colorimetrically by a suitable method (see pp. 209–221). The figures obtained from these tests should be subtracted from controls containing amounts of the antigen, originally added to the antiserum.

The Serum-Dilution Technique. Twofold progressive dilutions of the antiserum, ranging from 1:2 to 1:2048, are made in 0.2 ml of saline or a buffer solution. Equal volumes of the antigen at an optimum concentration are added to each tube. Optimum concentration of the antigen is determined by a preliminary antigen-dilution titration. One control tube receives 0.2 ml of a normal serum, diluted to 1:2, and 0.2 ml of the antigen solution; another control tube contains 0.2 ml of a normal serum diluted to 1:2 and 0.2 ml of saline or a buffer solution. The tubes are agitated for 10 minutes on an electric shaker, then left for 2 hours at 37° and overnight at 0 to 4°. Contents of the tubes should be inspected for precipitates after 2 hours at 37° and after the reaction mixtures are left overnight in a refrigerator. The last tube showing a definite sediment is taken as end point, and the precipitin titer is expressed in terms of a final antiserum dilution in this tube.

It is advisable to estimate the optimum proportion of an antigen and antibody prior to standard diagnostic precipitation tests, by using Culbertson's (1932) or Martin's (1943) method. To determine the optimum antigen-antibody proportion by the Culbertson method, 0.1-ml volumes of undiluted antiserum are added to equal volumes of serial antigen dilutions. The mixtures are incubated for 2 hours at 37° and left overnight in the refrigerator, then centrifuged in the cold. Supernatant fluids are halved and tested for the presence of either the antigen or antiserum by adding equal amounts of a high-titer antiserum or a diluted antigen. Dilutions in which neither the antigen nor the antibody is demonstrated are regarded as being in the optimum neutral zone.

In Martin's assay, a series of twofold antiserum dilutions, ranging from 1:25 to 1:12,800, are mixed with each of decreasing antigen dilutions. The smallest amount of antigen yielding a precipitate is selected for the precipitation test proper.

Quantitative evaluation of the precipitation test is attained with a greater precision by certain quantitative physical and chemical methods presented below.

IV. THE SLIDE-CENTRIFUGE PRECIPITATION TEST

The test (Kwapinski, 1972) depends on accelerating the contact between the precipitinogens and precipitin by gravity force and concentrating the complexes on a small area of a cellulose-acetate membrane. The test is set up as foqllows:

1. Arrange constituents of each plastic chamber in the cytocentrifuge in the following order: a glass slide, a cellulose-acetate strip (Serometrics), and a punched, water-absorbing filter-paper strip (Fig. 49).

2. Incubate a mixture consisting of 0.1 ml of antiserum or a globulin preparation and 0.1 ml of antigen solution for 1 to 2 minutes.

3. Transfer the mixture to a plastic compartment of the cytocentrifuge and spin the mixture at 1000 rpm for 5 minutes.

4. Wash off the noncombined material of the reaction mixture from the acetate strip in two changes of 1 M NaCl for 2 minutes.

5. Stain the cellulose strip in 0.001% Ponceau S stain solution for 15 seconds.

6. Wash the membrane in 7% acetic acid for 2 minutes and in distilled water for 1 minute.

7. View the cellulose strip against a fluorescent light through a $10\times$ magnifying glass.

Antigen-antibody complexes occur in the form of a red-stain clump of amorphous material on a pale-pink background. Controls consisting of a heterologous, nonrelated antigen and the antibody or consisting of the antigen mixed with a normal serum produce no clumps.

V. THE PHAGE-PRECIPITATION TEST

This test, according to the Jerne and Avegno technique (1956), is conducted by mixing equal volumes of serial serum dilutions and phage particles suspended in saline at a concentration equal to 10^{11}, particles per milliliter. The mixtures are incubated at 37° for 2 hours, left in a refrigerator overnight, and then examined for the presence of precipitates.

VI. THE CRP-PRECIPITATION TEST

The CRP-precipitation test reveals the reaction between an abnormal protein antigen of the host and serum antibody prepared by immunization of experimental animals with a purified CRP-antigen preparation. The abnormal, C-reactive protein is capable of reacting with the somatic polysaccharide of *Diplococcus pneumoniae,* and it occurs in the acute phase of various inflammatory diseases including rheumatic fever. The CRP-antiserum is produced by repeated injections of CRP isolated from an exudate or a serum containing this abnormal protein (McCarty, 1947; Kwapinski et al., 1958).

The test, after the Anderson and McCarty (1950) method, is set up in standard capillary tubes (9-mm long and 0.8-mm diameter), or in narrow precipitation tubes of 1-mm diameter. The anti-CRP serum is introduced into the tube and followed by an equal amount of the serum under test. The tube should be placed horizontally to mix its contents, then the fluid is raised to about 10 mm over the base, placed in a plasticine block, and left at 37° for 2 hours or at room temperature for 12 hours. The intensity of the reaction is evaluated by measuring the height of the precipitate settling in the lower portion of tube or by taking the time in which the precipitate occurred and expressing the results in symbols ranging from + to ++++. The observation and measurement of the precipitate are easier if the anti-CRP serum has been stained by methylene blue. A white precipitate is then easily observed on a blue or greenish-blue background.

More accurate results can be obtained when the test is performed with various dilutions of the patient serum. In this case, serum dilutions ranging from 1:2 to 1:128 are made in 0.2-ml volumes of saline, and 0.2 ml of each dilution is pipetted over an anti-CRP serum diluted according to its potency and distributed in 0.2-ml volumes in seven narrow tubes. A control tube contains 0.2 ml of the anti-CRP serum and 0.2 ml of saline. The samples are incubated at 37° or at room temperature, and the development of a precipitate ring is watched during 30 minutes. The tubes may then be left at 2° overnight and results read again. Titer of the CRP test is estimated according to the highest serum dilution at which the precipitate was observed.

VII. QUANTITATIVE PRECIPITATION TESTS

Products of the precipitation reaction may be measured by procedures that reveal their physical or chemical properties. Quantitative evaluation of precipitation tests according to the physical properties of the products may be accomplished either by a gravimetric technique, or, preferably, by determination of the turbidity and optical density, using a turbidimeter, nephelometer, photon reflectometer, or an ultraviolet-light spectrophotometer. The concentration of antigens may be expressed in terms of the dry weight, in milligrams per milliliter of a solvent, or in terms of nitrogen content in the case of antigens containing protein or another nitrogenous material.

The principle for the turbidimetric quantitation of precipitates is as follows: formation of complexes by soluble antibody and antigen molecules causes opalescence or turbidity in the liquid. The rate and extent of turbidity development are usually functions of the relative concentrations of antigen and antibody. Interactions between the precipitinogens and precipitins may thus be measured by determination of the turbidity (Gitlin and Edelhoch, 1951). Precipitates or precipitating antibodies may also be determined quantitatively by means of a spectrophotometer with which the rate of turbidity development, relative to the antibody concentration is measured.

The potency of a precipitin-containing antiserum may be measured directly by the determination of the maximum quantity of antibody nitrogen, found in an immune precipitate, formed in the equivalence zone of the precipitin curve.

1. The Gravimetric and Turbidimetric Methods

The gravimetric determination of the precipitative potency of antisera in terms of the actual antibody content can be carried out by the methods of Heidelberger and Kendall (1929), Culbertson (1932), or Alexander et al. (1945). These methods, however, are accompanied by a considerable error resulting from different combining ratios of the antigen and antibody.

The Turbidimetric Method. Mixtures containing equal volumes of either a serially diluted antigen preparation and a constant amount of antiserum, or a serially diluted antiserum and a constant concentration of the antigen, preserved with Merthiolate at a final dilution of 1:10,000, are prepared for the turbidimetric test. They may be incubated at 25° for a period of time as short as 5 to 10 minutes or as long as 12 to 24 hours, depending on the reactivity and concentration of individual components of the immunological system. Adequate controls containing either antigen or antiserum alone are included. Precipitates resulting from the reaction should be deposited by centrifugation, washed in saline, and resuspended in 2 to 3 ml of saline. Turbidities of these suspensions are then measured by means of either a nephelometer or a photon reflectometer or, less precisely, in a turbidimeter. Turbidity data are plotted on a graph against varying antigen or antiserum dilutions. Turbidity units are arbitrarily estimated in terms of the turbidity given by suspensions of a water-insoluble substance, such as barium sulfate, used in scaled concentrations.

Relative turbidities, estimated by a comparison with turbidity standards by the aid of a nephelometer, may be converted into absolute turbidity units (Scheiffarth et al., 1958) according to the equation:

$$\frac{\text{relative turbidity of reaction mixtures}}{\text{relative turbidity of standards}} = \frac{\text{absolute turbidity of reaction mixtures}}{\text{absolute turbidity of standards}}$$

A similar nephelometric technique was reported by Hoigné et al. (1955).

Another sensitive apparatus for quantitative determination of the turbidity given by reacting mixtures is the photon reflectometer (Libby, 1938). In this apparatus, an opalescence or turbidity shown by suspended particles causes a deflection of the galvanometer which is greater if the turbidity increases. Galvanometric readings are plotted against contents of the antigen preparation, or against antiserum dilutions on a graph.

The potency of an antigen preparation is expressed in milligrams, whereas the antiserum activity is expressed by actual units (U), which are calculated from the following formula:

$$U = \frac{G}{K \times 1/N} = K_2$$

where G = the galvanometer reading

K = the ratio of units to the galvanometric reading

$1/N$ = a new antiserum dilution

K_2 = the ratio of units to milligrams of antigen per milliliter.

An automatic assay of the turbidity was devised by Hucke and Rocke (1960) for large series of tests. It apparently improves the precision of turbidimetric determinations.

2. Quantitative Spectrophotometric Determination of Precipitins

The technique designed by Gitlin (1949) and by Vincent et al. (1970) are recommended. Gitlin's (1949) technique employs a known volume of antiserum, from which the antibody is precipitated with a measured amount of antigen in the region of a slight antibody excess. The precipitate is washed with cold buffered saline, dissolved in 3 ml of 0.1 M NaOH or 0.25 M acetic acid, diluted to the volume of 10 ml and read at 277 nm in the Beckman quartz spectrophotometer.

Simultaneously, the absorption due to a known quantity of the antigen is estimated and subtracted from the absorption of the entire precipitate. This leaves the absorption due to the antibody.

Results may be calculated by substituting in the following equation for AB (antibody in the precipitate, in milligrams):

$$Ab = \frac{Dsp - Dx}{E^{1\%}_{1/cm(aby)}} \times V \times \frac{1000}{100}$$

where Dsp and Dx are optical densities of the specific precipitate or of the antigen in the precipitate, respectively; V is the volume in milliliters of 0.1 N NaOH used to dissolve the precipitate; $E^{1\%}_{1/cm(aby)}$ is the extinction coefficient equal 16.2 of rabbit globulin dissolved in 0.1 N NaOH; it is applicable if a rabbit antiserum has been used in the test. These data allow calculation of the value of 1 mg of antibody.

Vincent's et al. (1970) method is applied as follows: Various dilutions of an antigen and antibody preparation are rapidly mixed at equal volumes (0.2 ml) and transferred to cuvettes with a 1-mm path length. The turbidity developing at 27° is recorded at 350 nm on a spectrophotometer at 15 second intervals. The reference cuvette holds a mixture of buffered saline and antiserum in equal volume and is used to correct for absorbance by serum components such as haemoglobin.

A precipitin curve is obtained by plotting turbidity, expressed in optical density values measured at 350 nm against time (in seconds). The rate of turbidity in the equivalent zone, when higher concentrations of antibody are used, seems to follow the first-order kinetics reaction. In the sensitivity range of a spectrophotometer, the linearity is observed except where macroscopic flocculation occurs in the cuvette. Measurement of the rate of turbidity development can thus be employed to determine the antibody concentration of serum provided high concentrations of reactants are used.

3. Chemical Determination of Precipitins

The chemical determination of precipitins, originally described by Grabar and Oudin (1943), was improved by Heidelberger and MacPherson (1943) and by Heidelberger and Anderson (1944). According to the latter technique, the antiserum or preferably purified serum globulins (see p. 268) are measured accurately in the volume of 0.5 to 4.0 ml with calibrated Ostwald pipettes and added to an antigen in a slight excess. The amount of the antigen to be used can be previously determined by Martin's procedure (1943). The antigen-antibody mixture is carefully mixed by a rotary motion, and the tube is closed with a rubber cup. After the tube is left for $\frac{1}{4}$ to 1 hour at room temperature, or at 37°, and for 2 to 8 days at 2 to 4°, contents of the tubes are centrifuged. The precipitate is washed twice in the cold with a buffered saline. The nitrogen in the material is determined by one of the methods cited on p. 200. The nitrogen of the antigen is subtracted from total nitrogen to calculate the antibody nitrogen. Quantitative determination of the entire precipitin curve is performed by the Beiser and Kabat technique (1952). Various volumes of the antigen are made up to 1.0 ml with 0.85% saline and mixed with 1 ml of the antiserum (all components chilled in ice water). They should be incubated for 1 hour at 37°, and left at 2 to 4° with an occasional shaking for a period of 2 to 8 days, depending on the strength of the serum. For some serological systems, the optimum incubation temperature may be 41 or 45°. Suitable antigen and antibody controls are included in the test. When a chicken antiserum is tested, the concentration of sodium chloride should be increased to 8% to secure the precipitation (Goodman et al., 1951). The precipitates are separated in a refrigerated centrifuge, washed twice with a cold saline, dissolved with a few drops of 0.5 N/NaOH and made up to 2.5 ml with distilled water; 2-ml samples are withdrawn for colorimetric measurements.

The protein content in each precipitate is estimated by the colorimetric determination of tyrosine according to the Folin-Ciocalteu technique, modified by Heidelberger and MacPherson (1943), by Lowry's et al.(1951) Biuret method, or by Moore and Stein's (1948) ninhydrin method, as modified by Kunkel and Ward (1950). Bovine serum γ-globulin is used as a reference standard. Amount of the antibody present in the precipitate is calculated on the assumption that the entire antigen has been precipitated at the equivalence point. Optical density due to the antigen protein is subtracted from the optical density of the whole precipitate. This gives the optical density due to the antibody. Optical density is plotted versus micrograms of nitrogen in the sample as determined by the micro-Kjeldahl technique. The extinction (E) is determined (McDuffie and Kabat, 1956) as the slope of the best straight line fitted through the points:

$$ E = \frac{\text{o.d.}}{\mu\text{g } N \text{ in sample}} $$

The precipitate protein can be alternatively estimated by the nitrogen determination. In this case, precipitates dissolved in $M/2$ NaOH are transferred quantitatively to 10-ml micro-Kjeldahl flasks and analyzed by Kjeldahl's method (1883), as modified by Markham (1942) or Elek and Sobotka (1926). The nitrogen of the antigen is subtracted from the total nitrogen to calculate the antibody nitrogen.

Similar techniques of the quantitative precipitation test were published by Landy and Webster (1952), Kleinschmidt and Boyer (1952), Bowen and Wyman (1953), Osler and Knipp (1957), and Dandliker and Levison (1967).

According to Dandliker and Levison, the antibody is measured at varying antigen and constant antibody concentration. The antigen-antibody mixtures (1.25 ml) are maintained at 37° for 1 hour and left at 4° overnight. Precipitates thus formed are centrifuged, washed with 0.15 M NaCl, and dissolved in 2 ml of 0.2 M NaOH. The optical density of this solution is immediately read at 280-nm wavelengths and the amount of antibody in the precipitate is calculated by assuming that all of the antigen was precipitated at equivalence. The E_{280} results are interpreted by using the separate extinction coefficients (in NaOH) for the antigen and antibody.

According to Osler and Knipp, the amount of protein in the immune precipitate is determined by the ninhydrin technique of Moore and Stein (1948), as modified by Kunkel and Ward (1950). Proteins are first converted into their constituent amino acids by hydrolysis. For this purpose, washed precipitates should be suspended in 0.5 ml of 6.0 N HCl and heated at 110° for 48 hours. The hydrolyzates are then cooled and treated with exactly 2.0 ml of a freshly prepared ninhydrin reagent and 0.5 ml of 6 N NaOH. The tubes are placed for 20 minutes in a boiling water bath. The samples are then diluted with the proposed diluent to a volume varying from 25.0 to 250.0 ml depending on the intensity of the color developed, and filtered. Readings are made in a spectrophotometer at a wave length of 570 nm with a light path of 1.0 cm.

The ninhydrin (triketohydrindene hydrate) reagent consists of a ninhydrin solution diluted 3:1 with an acetate buffer. Ninhydrin solution contains 1.0 g of ninhydrin in 75 ml of methyl cellosolve. Acetate buffer consists of 1360 g of NaOHc $\cdot$ 3H$_2$O, dissolved in 1 liter of warm distilled water, and 500 ml of glacial acetic acid, adjusted to pH 5.5. The reagent may be activated with KCN, by adding 0.5 ml of a $N/100$ aqueous solution of potassium cyanide per 2.0 ml of the ninhydrin reagent prior to use. The propanol diluent consists of equal parts of n-propyl alcohol and distilled water.

The *supernatant test* (Kendall, 1937) is a quantitative precipitation assay adapted to study the homogeneity of antigen preparations. In this test an antiserum is used which contains antibodies to many or all antigens occurring in the original material, from which the antigen tested has been prepared. This serum is added to the supernatants obtained by centrifugation of contents of tubes showing a precipitate of antigen-antibody complexes. If no precipitation now occurs, this is indicative of the absence of even small amounts of antigens other than the ones homologous to either serum.

4. *Ultramicromethod for the Quantitative Precipitin Analysis*

The technique of Glick et al. (1958) allows the use of very small volumes of serum and antigen. In this assay, 10 μl amounts of an antiserum, measured with Lang-Levy pipettes, are mixed with equal volumes of progressing antigen dilutions, in tubes 27-mm long and 4-mm i.d. The test is carried out in triplicate. Blanks contain 0.9% sodium chloride substituted for the antigen. The tubes are held at 37° for 1 hour and left at 2° for 7 days. Each day during this time period the tubes should be gently tapped. They are then centrifuged at 2° for 1 hour at 3800 $\times$ g in a microcentrifuge. The precipitates are washed twice with 0.9% sodium chloride, dried in a vacuum desiccator and dissolved in 20 ml of 1 N NaOH.

For the protein-nitrogen measurement, 50 ml of the bromsulfophthalein reagent is added to each precipitate solution. (The reagent consists of 1 ml of 5% bromsulfophthalein, 100 ml of 1 N hydrochloric acid, 50 ml of 1 M citric acid, and distilled water added to a volume of 250 ml.) The tubes are then centrifuged for 5 minutes at 3800 $\times$ g; 60 ml of the supernatant are withdrawn, transferred to 1 ml of $N/1$ NaOH, and mixed. The absorbance is measured at 580 nm. The protein-nitrogen is calculated by reference to a calibration curve for dye binding. These are prepared with known quantities of protein nitrogen of the serum albumin and the same volumes of reagents.

The contents of a polysaccharide hapten or an antigen in the precipitate can be estimated by a photometric method based either on the reaction of α-naphthol with carbohydrates (Mikulaszek, 1955) or on the determination of fructose (Allen and Kabat, 1957).

VIII. EVALUATION AND APPLICATION OF THE PRECIPITATION TEST

The precipitation test is a sensitive serological technique by which as little as 0.1 μg of certain antigens or haptens, especially the polysaccharides, can be detected. However, the test does not seem to be sufficiently sensitive for the detection of antibodies. The degree of accuracy of quantitative precipitin methods is equal to that of many standard chemical analyses. Only soluble antigens or haptens can be detected by specific precipitation. Major applications of the precipitation test are the following.

1. Identification and typing of microorganisms.
2. Investigations of the serological potency of antigen preparations and on immunological relationships between various antigen preparations. *Examples:* The type-specific substance of *Diplococcus pneumoniae* was found by the precipitation test reactive in dilutions up to 1:8,000,000 with the homologous antiserum (Brown, 1939); the type-specific polysaccharide of *Neisseria meningitis* reacted in a similar dilution with homologous horse antisera (Sherp and Rake, 1935); a species-specific polysaccharide hapten from *Leptospira biflexa* and tissue antigens were found highly active by Witebsky et al. (1955). An interesting application of the precipitin test is the serological estimation of relationships among animal species (Bordet, 1899; Nuttall, 1904).
3. The detection and identification of soluble antigens in host tissues and fluids. For example, a specific precipitable substance (the capsular polysaccharide of *Diplococcus pneumoniae*) has been repeatedly detected in the urine of patients with pneumococcal pneumonia (Dochez and Avery, 1917; Quigley, 1918; Viktorow and Masel, 1934; de Gara et al., 1939). In this test, the urine concentrated by evaporation and alcohol-precipitation has been used often as antigen. Other examples are the *Bacillus anthracis* and *Pasteurella pestis* thermoprecipitinogens detected in carcasses (Ascoli, 1902; Larsen et al., 1957), the serological identification of human blood

stains by the forensic precipitin test, and the identification of meat and fish products with "cocto-antisera."

4. Determination of the antiserum activity, as a control of the efficiency of an animal immunization procedure.

5. The detection of specific precipitins in patients' sera, for example, detection of antibodies precipitating the poliomyelitis virus (Schultz et al., 1931; Kolmer and Rule, 1935), the precipitin reaction with toxoid of *Corynebacterium diphtheriae* (Kuhns and Dukstein, 1957).

Chapter Seven

THE IMMUNODIFFUSION TEST

I. PRINCIPLES OF THE IMMUNODIFFUSION REACTION

The immunodiffusion precipitation test is a method of immunologic analysis of complex biological materials by optically revealing complexes of antigens and antibodies, formed in gel or on the cellulose-acetate membrane. The visible complexes are formed after the diffusion of antigen and antibody molecules toward each other and concentration in an area of optimal proportion. The diffusion of antigen and antibody through semisolid media consists in the migration from a zone of high concentration to areas of lower or no concentration. Individual antigens have a different chemical structure, specific weight, and electric charge, and, consequently, various diffusion coefficients. Constituents of a complex material therefore separate in the gel and may react with the corresponding antibodies in different sites of the gel medium, forming precipitate bands. An immunoprecipitate formed in gel allows immunologically unrelated molecules to pass through the zone of the immunoprecipitate, but antigens and antibodies immunologically similar to those which have formed the particular precipitate cannot penetrate the barrier. The function of an immunoprecipitate as a selective barrier makes it possible to discriminate between, and compare different antigens and antibodies.

The principle of antigen analysis by observing its diffusion in a gel containing homologous antibody was first suggested by Bechhold (1905), who tested the goat serum antigen in a gelatin gel containing homologous antiserum. Similar techniques were adopted by Nicolle (1920) for the study of a ring precipitation given by diphtherial antitoxin diffusing into gelatin gel containing a culture filtrate of *Corynebacterium diphtheriae* and by Hanks (1935) for estimation of the antibody concentration in the immune serum. Gelatin has been replaced by agar as a gel medium for the precipitation test by Reiner and Kopp (1927), who observed precipitation lines when a pig serum diffused through an agar gel containing a homologous rabbit antiserum. The use of nutrient media for the toxin-antitoxin reaction was first suggested by Petrie and Steabben (1943). More sophisticated media have been introduced to the immunodiffusion technique more recently, such as agarose, pectin, alginate, polyacrylamide, and cellulose-acetate membranes, but purified agar is still used frequently for this technique.

The numerous techniques of the immunodiffusion test may be classified in one of the two following categories: the single immunodiffusion (Oudin, 1946), or the double immunodiffusion method. The latter technique may be carried out as a one-dimensional procedure (Oakley and Fulthorpe, 1953), or a two-dimensional procedure (Elek, 1948; Ouchterlony, 1948).

The single immunodiffusion (the band diffusion) test depends on the diffusion of a concentrated soluble antigen preparation through a column of an antiserum containing agar, placed in small-bore tubes. With the preceding diffusion of the antigen, a continuum of decreasing antigen concentration develops. Ring-form precipitates are produced by active immune systems at the equivalence zone of both components, and they move in bands down the tube as concentrations of antigens diffusing into the gel increase.

In the double-diffusion technique, both the antigens and antibodies migrate through a gel. Observable lines of the precipitation appear in the sites of optimal concentrations of two components of an active immune system. The test can be set up in tubes as "a single-dimension immunodiffusion technique" (Oakley and Fulthorpe, 1953; Gispen, 1955; Augustin and Hayward, 1955; Preer, 1956; Glenn, 1956; Parlett and Youmans, 1959), or a semisolid precipitation technique (Munoz and Becker, 1950; Pope et al., 1951, Bowen, 1952), or as a double-dimension technique on plates. In the single-dimension immunodiffusion technique, the antiserum mixed with melted agar or gelatin is placed in a narrow tube. When it solidifies, a layer of plain gel is poured on top. If the antigens react with the serum antibodies, precipitation bands are formed in the gel at specific locations which depend on the diffusion coefficients and relative concentrations of antigens and antibodies. The semisolid precipitation technique differs mostly by a lower agar concentration provided for the test. In the double-dimension technique, antigens and antibody diffuse toward each other through the gel in an agar plate. A special modification of the immunodiffusion is the immunoelectrophoresis, which combines the electrophoretic separation of components of antisera or antigen preparations with their detection by a two-dimensional immunodiffusion procedure.

II. THE SINGLE IMMUNODIFFUSION TEST

The test devised by Oudin (1946) was modified and improved by several investigators, for example, by Becker and Munoz (1949), Surgalla et al. (1952), Jensen and Francis (1953), Jennings (1953), and Glenn (1956).

The test in Jennings' modification is conducted as follows. An antiserum is mixed with an equal volume of 0.5% melted clarified agar, prepared in a saline buffered at pH 6.4 to 7.5 containing 0.001% Merthiolate as a preservative, and cooled to 45°. About 0.5 ml of this serum agar is introduced to tubes, 9-cm long with a 3-mm bore, which have been internally coated with 0.1 or 1.0% agar, then dried to ensure the adherence of the agar column to the glass. The filling of tubes may be done with Wintrobe's capillary pipettes or with a Cartesian diver looder. When the serum agar solidifies, it is superimposed by 0.5 ml of an antigen solution. The tubes are sealed with plasticene or paraffin and incubated in a water bath at 45°.

Precipitate bands can be observed either on removing the tubes from the water bath or by illuminating the tubes beneath the water bath with a beam of light entering water through a slit in black paper from below and behind a holder of tubes. The weight and movement of precipitation bands may be measured and recorded by the aid of an adjusted, travelling microscope (Neff and Becker, 1957).

A migrating zone of specific precipitate is formed if an antigenic component reacts with the corresponding antibody. Each pair of antigen antibody forms a separate precipitation zone in the agar column, and the number of antigen-antibody systems in the agar column. Secondary or "false" precipitates are known to occur sometimes when a very strong antigen is tested against a weak or moderately strong antiserum, or if the temperature varies sharply during the development of the precipitation lines (Wilson, 1958; Crowle, 1960). The migration of precipitate zones away from the agar meniscus occurs at a rate constant in relation to the square root of time (t), provided the antigen concentration is sufficiently high in comparison with the antibody in agar gel. It may be expressed by the equation $h = k \sqrt{t}$, where h is the distance travelled by the leading edge of the band, t is the time elapsed since the antiserum has been overlayered by an antigen, and k is a constant which varies with the antibody concentration in the gel layer and the antigen concentration in liquid layer. It may also be influenced by some contaminants of the antigen layer.

Considering the concentrations of antigens and relationships between the distance (x) moved by the leading edge of the band and the square root of time (t), the migration rate of a precipitate zone is expressed by the following formula:

$$\frac{\delta c}{\delta t} = D \frac{\delta^2 c}{\delta x^2}$$

where D is the diffusion coefficient and c is the concentration of a substance. Quantitative relations between the antigen and antibody in the diffusion medium are expressed by the equation (Becker and Neff, 1959):

$$\frac{Ag}{AbR^1} = \frac{z(1 + \mathrm{erf}z)e^{z2}}{y(1^1 + \mathrm{erf}y)e^{y2}}$$

where $y = k/2\sqrt{D_2}$ and $z = k/2\sqrt{D_1}$. Ag and Ab represent the concentrations of antigen and antibody, respectively; R^1 is the ratio of antigen to antibody at the beading edge of the precipitation band; erf is the normal probability integral; and D_1 and D_2 are the diffusion coefficients of antigen and antibody, respectively.

The rate of diffusion in gel rises parallelly to the increase of temperature and concentration of reactants; it decreases when the viscosity of a semisolid medium decreases. Certain nonspecific substances, for example, glucose and polyvinyl pyrrolidone, increase the rate of the diffusion.

The intensity of the gel precipitation is largely affected by the quantity of an antibody available for reaction, and to a lesser extent by the antigen and salt concentration, as well as by nonantibody serum constituents and the length of incubation time (Oudin, 1952; Wilson and Pringle, 1954; Glenn, 1958).

Intensity of the precipitation in gel is greatly enhanced by cadmium and nickel (Crowle, 1960) and by an increase of sodium chloride. Sometimes a ten times increase of electrolytes is necessary to provide optimal conditions for the immunodiffusion precipitation (Goodman et al., 1951; Goodman, 1958). Glycine, in 0.1 to 0.5 *M* concentration, is also known to intensity the precipitation in agar gel.

It may be noted that normal rabbit serum, and especially the serum albumin, has a combining affinity for certain antigens, for example, for antigens of *Pasteurella pestis* (Ransom et al., 1955). Thus the diffusion of these antigens in the rabbit antiserum may be retarded. It is advisable in such cases to replace the antiserum by isolated globulins.

III. THE ONE-DIMENSIONAL IMMUNODIFFUSION TEST

In this test (Oakley and Fulthorpe, 1953), antigen and antibody diffuse toward each other in a layer of agar. Small tubes, for example, Lamberth's tubes, 5 to 10 cm long, with 0.8-cm i.d., are filled consecutively with two layers of an agar gel. The bottom layer contains 0.5 ml of a mixture consisting of equal parts of 0.5 to 2% melted purified agar, cooled to 60°, and an antiserum. The central layer, containing 2 ml of melted, plain 0.5 to 2% agar is poured when the bottom layer has solidified. A few drops or 0.2 ml of an antigen or hapten preparation, in approximately 0.1% solution, is placed on top when the agar gel is set. The tubes are sealed with fitting glass tops or with rubber stoppers, and incubated for several days at 37°

or at room temperature. The antiserum and antigen preparation diffuse into the central column of the agar gel. Where fronts of the antigen and the corresponding antibody meet in appropriate concentrations, an immune complex is formed which precipitates as a transverse disk in the central agar column. Separate precipitation lines are produced on various levels in the agar column, depending on the diffusion rates and relative concentrations of the antigen and the antibody constituting a serologic system. The precipitation lines appear in a shorter time, for example, in a few hours, if the concentrations of antigen and antibody are high, and the effective incubation time is longer if the concentrations are lower. Unnecessary prolongation of the incubation time, however, may cause "splitting" of a precipitation line, imitating two lines ordinarily resulting from two different serological systems. Lower concentrations of certain antigens tested against a constant antiserum solution cause fainter lines which are situated higher in the central column than in the case of a higher antigen concentration.

Determination and differentiation of various antigens reacting with one antiserum is conducted in a similar manner, by placing a mixture of equal parts of two antigens on the top of an agar column, each in double concentration. Duplication of one or more precipitation zones indicates that the two antigens differ in some respect. The immunologically related antigens produce an intensification of the precipitation zone, owing to additive action of a mixture or two similar antigens.

Positions of the antiserum and the antigen in the single column test can be reversed (Parlett and Youmans, 1959). In this case, the antigen is mixed 2:1 with a purified melted agar prepared in 0.01 M phosphate buffer, pH 7.5, and introduced into narrow, agar-coated tubes to a depth of 2.5 to 3 cm. A second, 0.5-cm deep layer of 1% purified agar, is placed over the first antigen layer. When this solidifies, an undiluted antiserum is placed on top.

Preer's (1956) Modification of the One-Dimension Immunodiffusion Test

Pyrex tubes, of 2-mm i.d. are coated with 0.1% agar, evacuated and cut into 5-cm lengths, and one end is flame-sealed. An undiluted antiserum is then deposited into the tube to a height of 5 mm, and this is carefully overlayered to a similar height with 0.3 to 0.6% Ionagar, made in 0.9% sodium chloride and containing 0.5 M glycine and 0.01% Merthiolate, or in 0.02 M sodium phosphate adjusted to pH 7.0. When the agar solidifies 0.01 to 0.02 ml of an antigen solution is placed on top. The tube is sealed with Picene cement or modelling clay, and incubated at 17 to 25° in the horizontal position.

Precipitation bands are formed in the middle layer of agar in a few hours or days, sometimes as late as 3 weeks, depending on the antibody concentration in the antiserum. Positions of precipitation bands can be determined by measuring, with a magnifier containing a scale, the length of the column of agar and the distance from the antigen-agar interface to the center of the band.

Dilution of the antigen causes a movement of the precipitation band toward the antigen-agar interface, while the dilution of antiserum is followed by the occurrence of the precipitation band nearer to the antiserum agar interface. If the concentration of either component of an immune system is too high, the precipitation occurs in the antigen or antiserum layer.

IV. THE SEMISOLID IMMUNODIFFUSION TEST

Two techniques, published by Munoz and Becker (1950) and Bowen (1952), are described here in some detail. The procedure by Munoz and Becker employs a mixture, in equal proportions, of a diluted antiserum and 0.6% melted agar, which is introduced into the lower one half or two thirds of a glass tube, 6 to 8 cm in length and of 3 mm internal diameter. The tubes are previously coated with 1% agar and dried either at 50° for 12 hours or in vacuo for 1 to 2 hours. An antigen solution is placed on top of the solidified antiserum agar. The tubes are capped with meltable plastic and incubated at 37°.

The gel precipitation can be evaluated quantitatively by measuring the distance of the leading edge of a precipitate ring from the agar meniscus and from a fixed reference point on the tube, by using calipers. The descent of the precipitate ring, in millimeters, is plotted against the square root of time, in minutes, and the slope of the resultant line is determined graphically (Rubinstein, 1954). Error of the measurement does not exceed 0.2 mm.

In Bowen's technique (1952), 0.3 ml of 1.6% melted agar and 0.7 ml of an antiserum warmed to 40° are mixed and placed in a flocculation tube. The antiserum agar is allowed to harden, then overlayered with 2 ml of 0.8% purified agar; when this solidifies, 1.0 ml of an antigen solution is poured on top. All dilutions of agar and antigens are made in 0.02 *M* phosphate, pH 7, buffered saline.

A useful modification of the Oudin test, devised to study reactions of several antigen peraparations with one antiserum, has been described by Surgalla et al. (1952). A simple device used in this technique is called "the antigen comparator cell," and it consists of a small Plexiglass box divided into two parts, the lower, larger, quadrangular compartment and the upper part partitioned into four narrow, cylindrical compartments. Inner walls of all compartments are precoated with 1% purified agar and dried. The lower part of the cell is filled with a mixture of antiserum and agar, so that it extends by about 1 to 2 mm into the four narrow upper partitions. The narrow compartments are filled with different antigen solutions and sealed with paraffin. Precipitate lines are formed at the lower edges of small compartments and down in the larger cell partition.

More accurate evaluation of results of the immunodiffusion test may be attained by the aid of an adjunct called "the serum agar measuring aid" or an improved apparatus called "serum agar measuring integrator" (Glenn, 1956; Glenn and Garner, 1957). Either device is attached to a Libby photon reflectometer, the latter one being also combined with a Spinco Analytrol. The light scattering or transmission through the zone of precipitation in agar is then determined. The serum agar measuring integrator allows the scanning and plotting of an agar column in 5 to 20 seconds, accurately and automatically.

V. THE TWO-DIMENSIONAL IMMUNODIFFUSION TEST

Two original methods of this test, devised independently by Elek (1948) and Ouchterlony (1948), have been modified by various investigators (e.g., Halbert, 1955; Chen and Meyer, 1955; Kaminski, 1955; Parlett and Youmans, 1956; Mansi, 1957; Kwapinski, 1959; Mata and Weller, 1962) to meet particular requirements with regard to the amount and number of antisera and antigen preparations. The Elek test is employed for testing the toxigenicity and virulence of microorganisms, and for the detection of soluble antigens produced by the microorganism in a suitable culture. The Ouchterlony technique is used predominantly for immunochemical analysis of antigenic relationships amongst microorganisms.

1. Elek's Immunodiffusion Technique

The test is based on the precipitation reaction in the agar gel between a toxin diffusing from colonies of toxigenic microorganisms and the homologous antitoxin diffusing from the rectangular direction. The test can be performed in one of the following ways, depending on the type of microorganisms and the physicochemical properties of the secreted soluble antigens.

i. *Elek's (1949) Method.* A filter paper strip, saturated with a sterile antiserum and dried is embedded in the melted medium poured in a Petri plate, and the microorganisms to be tested are streaked with a loop at right angles. The plates are incubated at 37° for 24 to 48 hours or longer, if required, and inspected in the oblique illumination by the aid of a hand lens. (The oblique illumination can be obtained by mounting two pieces of photographic paper between half-plate glass, leaving a strip of about 1 cm in the center.) The precipitation lines occur at an angle of 45° from the line of the growth of microorganisms.

The nutrient medium for the study of the virulence of *Corynebacterium* strains is made by dissolving 20 g of proteose peptone, 3.0 g of maltose, and 0.7 ml of lactic acid in 500.0 ml of distilled water. A 1.5-ml volume of 40% sodium hydroxide is added to this solution, which must be heated to the boiling point, filtered through a filter paper, and adjusted to pH 7.8 by adding a normal solution of hydrochloric acid. At the same time, 500 ml of 3% agar is prepared in 1% sodium chloride and melted. The reaction is then adjusted to pH 7.8, and the liquid is filtered through a paper pulp in a Büchner funnel, and added to the first solution. The prepared medium must be distributed in 10-ml quantities and autoclaved.

The agar plates are poured just before setting the test, by mixing 10 ml of the melted and cooled medium with 2 ml of normal horse serum. The filter paper strips are saturated with a solution of commercial, refined diphtherial antitoxin globulin, diluted to a concentration of 1000 units/ml with a sterile 0.5% solution of phenol made in normal saline.

ii. *Chen and Meyer's (1955) Immunodiffusion Technique.* Sterile filter paper strips, 0.7 to 1.0 mm wide, are soaked in 0.2 to 0.4 mm of the antiserum, and embedded below the surface of an agar medium before it has hardened. The agar plate is then dried at 37° for 1 hour and inoculated with a liquid culture of bacteria. Inoculated plates are placed in an airtight Petri plate container and incubated at 37° for 1 to 3 weeks. Positive test is marked by circular precipitation lines encircling the colony producing the corresponding diffusible antigens. Small glass cups containing the serum and embedded in the agar may be substituted for the paper strip. The test can be employed for both the testing of the toxigeneity and the study on the antigenic relationship of microorganisms.

iii. *The Agar-Cell Culture Immunodiffusion Test.* This technique, which is based essentially on the principle of Elek's test, has been devised (Mata and Weller, 1962) for studies on diffusible virus antigens in the agar gel. It depends on the propagation of virus antigens in the susceptible cells mounted in nutrient agar, and the demonstration of specific diffusible viral components or products by the reaction with a diffusing specific antiserum. Nutrient agar used in this test consists of one volume of Eagle's basal medium containing 5% inactivated horse serum, 0.042% sodium bicarbonate, phenol red and antibiotic (100 units of penicillin and 100 μg of streptomycin per milliliter), pH 7.2 to 7.4, mixed with an equal volume of 2% melted Noble agar.

Nutrient agar is disposed in Petri plates to form a 1.25- to 1.5-mm-thick layer, and holes are cut in the solidified agar. The "cell culture well" is seeded with approximately 500,000 mammal cells, and the plates are incubated for 2 days at 35.5° under 2 to 3% CO_2 in a humidified chamber. The cells are then inoculated with a virus and reincubated.

Subsequently, a 0.025- to 0.3-ml amount of an antiserum is placed in the circumferential well, and each culture cell well receives a drop of Eagle's medium to promote the diffusion of viral antigens. The plates are reincubated for a few days, and precipitation lines are observed with an oblique illumination.

2. Ouchterlony's Immunodiffusion Techinque

The gel medium is made of a purified agar, for example, Nobel agar (Difco), "Ionagar" no. 2, or New Zealand (Oxoid) agar. Impurities occurring in other sorts of agar can be removed in one of the following ways. A 5% solution of agar is melted and centrifuged while hot, or precipitated when hot with 0.5% calcium chloride (Björklund, 1952), or left in a conical cylinder. Alternatively, melted agar may be filtered through Whatman no. 2 filter paper in a Büchner funnel to remove insoluble material. When it solidifies, the lower portion containing the particulate matter is cut off and discarded.

The upper portion of the agar column is cut into small cubes, 2 × 2 cm, and washed with distilled water for 2 days. The final concentration of the agar is then calculated by dry weight determination, and 1 to 2% agar is prepared by the dilution with buffered saline. It is advisable in some cases to add 10% horse serum to the agar, which eliminates nonspecific precipitation lines sometimes observed around serum basins. Alternatively, the nonmelted agar can be washed three times with acetone and three times with distilled water, centrifuged each time, then dried or clarified with bentonite and hyflosupercel (Feinberg, 1956).

To prepare a medium for the test, 0.6 to 2% agar is made in 0.8 to 0.85% saline buffered at pH 7 to 7.5,* containing 0.005 to 0.01% Merthiolate; 0.1% azide or 0.1% mecuric chloride can be used as alternate preservative. Orange G or methyl orange can be added at 0.002 to 0.006% concentration, which provides a better contrasting background, especially useful for the photography of test plates. Two concentrations of agar are recommended, 2.0 and 1.5%. The more concentrated agar is poured into a sterile Petri plate in a thin layer, just to cover the bottom of the dish. (Alternatively, the dish bottom can be coated with silicone.) When this solidifies, sterile metal matrices or special Plexiglass or Perspex templates, rectangular or spherical in shape, are placed on the smooth surface, and another 3.5-mm-high layer of 0.5% agar is poured. Patterns can also be cut in the solid agar with cork borers, and the agar plugs are removed by aspiration. The matrices or molds are removed from the completely solidified agar and the so-fashioned basins are filled with 1:100 to 1:200 solu-

---

* A phosphate-saline buffer, pH 7.2 contains 4.0 g of sodium chloride, 0.7 g of Na_2HPO_4, 0.6 ml of $N/1$ HCl, and distilled water to 500 ml.

tions of antigens or with sera diluted 1:4 or 1:5. The plates are left for several days, up to 2 weeks, either at 20 or 37°, protected from rapid drying by placing them under a large glass or plastic cover. The basins are refilled with antigens and antisera each day in 3 to 4 days. On the fifth day a few drops of saline solution are placed in each basin, and the plates are left in the refrigerator for another 6 to 9 days, if necessary. Reading of precipitation lines is facilitated by illuminating the plates obliquely in the reflected short-wave light supplied by a mercuric lamp.

Agar plates can be replaced by a 4- and 5-mm agar layer placed on larger glass plates, such as photographic glass plates. This permits a simultaneous analysis of many preparations (Kaminski, 1955). For this purpose, rectangular parallel basins, 2 to 4 cm long and 0.5 cm wide, are cut in the agar layer, 0.5 to 1.5 cm from each other. A large reservoir is cut in the center; it is perpendicular to all other smaller basins. The large basin is filled with a 1:4 mixture of antiserum and melted agar, whereas the smaller reservoirs receive various antigens, diluted in the melted agar. This procedure prevents an excessive dispersion of reagents in the agar. If a large number of antigens and antisera are studied, round reservoirs are arranged in a "chess-board" pattern. The diffusion precipitation test should be set up in duplicate to assert the reliability of results.

Precipitate lines are formed in the areas between the antigens and corresponding antibodies, where both components are in equivalent proportions, usually in 1 to 3 days, but occasionally as late as 2 to 3 weeks.

Faint precipitation lines can be intensified by setting the test in an agar gel containing a small, 0.1 to 0.3 M concentration of glycine (Halbert et al., 1955), or stained with 0.1% Thiazine red made in 1% acetic acid. The images can be enlarged by the aid of the Holophot photomicrographic apparatus under the oblique illumination, using a 8.5-fold magnification.

Any precipitate band resulting from the combination between an antiserum and the homologous antigen is usually narrow, long, dense, and sharply defined, whereas that caused by a cross-reacting but a nonhomologous antigen is broader, shorter, and fainter. If a long trough pattern is used for antiserum, the clarity of the precipitation bands at the ends of the row usually deteriorates due to the absorption of fluid contents into the gel, which causes a net flow away from the center of well pattern. This deterioration can be alleviated by increasing the osmatic pressure of the buffer in the trough, either by applying a salt concentration of at least 6% or by incorporating 15 to 20% glycerol in the agar. The reactivity of a cross-reacting antigen remains sometimes undetected, if the relative concentration of the antibody is too low or too high. The minimum antigen concentration required for the precipitate formation is inversely proportioned to the immunological affinity between an antigen and the antibody

(Wilson and Pringle, 1954). If the initial concentration of an antigen and an antibody is in their equivalence ratio, the precipitation bands formed do not migrate. If one of the constituents of a serological system is in excess, the precipitation band moves away from the more concentrated solution. Thus the precipitate band is shifted further from the source of a concentrated antigen than in the case of a more diluted solution of the same antigen tested against a constant antiserum concentration. Similarly, of two different antiserum solutions, tested against a constant homologous antigen concentration, the precipitate line formed by the more concentrated serum is situated at a greater distance from the antibody source than the higher diluted antiserum.

Concentrations of the antigen and antibody follow the integral equation suggested by Stefan in the form given by Svedberg (1928):

$$Cx_1 = C_1 \left(1 - \frac{2}{\sqrt{\pi}} \cdot \int_0^{y_1} \cdot e^{-y_2/dy_1} \right)$$

where $y_1 = \dfrac{X_1}{2\sqrt{D_1 t}}$

Cx_1 = the antigen concentration at any point (X_1) in the agar gel
C_1 = the initial concentration of the antigen
X_1 = the distance from the interface to the point of the antigen concentration (Cx_1)
D_1 = the diffusion coefficient of the antigen
t = time.

The reaction between antigen and antibody is not considered in this equation. If the antigen and antibody have approximately an equal molecular weight, the precipitation line formed is straight. The line curves slightly forward or away from the antibody reservoir, depending on whether the molecular weight of the antibody is greater or smaller than that of the antigen (Korngold and van Leeuwen, 1957).

It is postulated that each homologous system of antigen and antibody forms a separate precipitate line in the agar gel. However, two or more antigen preparations or fractions obtained from the same microorganism may react with one particular antiserum if they possess either a common antigenic component, or if the antibody has various active groups corresponding to all antigens tested.

If two antigens examined by the diffusion precipitation test possess the same determinant group exclusively, the precipitin lines resulting from the reaction with an antibody fuse in the space above and beneath the antiserum basin. This is called "the reaction of identity." If a preparation of antigens, for example, a crude extract of bacteria or a culture filtrate, contains more than one antigen, each being capable of reacting with the tested antiserum (e.g., a serum obtained by the immunization with whole bacteria), several precipitation lines are formed in the agar gel, under each other (Fig. 52).

If the homologous antigen possess two determinant groupings, one of which is in common with another heterologous antigen preparation tested simultaneously, a coalescent precipitation line is formed. This results from the reaction of this common determinant grouping, or common component with the antiserum. A single spur is produced in the space between a homologous antigen and antiserum. One spur on either side of the antiserum basin, apart from a coalescent precipitation line, is produced by two different, heterologous antigen preparations, if each of them possesses two determinants, for example, AB and AC, of which one is common to both preparations.

If two antigen preparations do not possess any common determinant, being serologically nonrelated, but the antiserum contains antibodies with active groups to both, crossing precipitate lines occur. This is termed "the reaction of nonidentity." However, when a weak antiserum is used, the

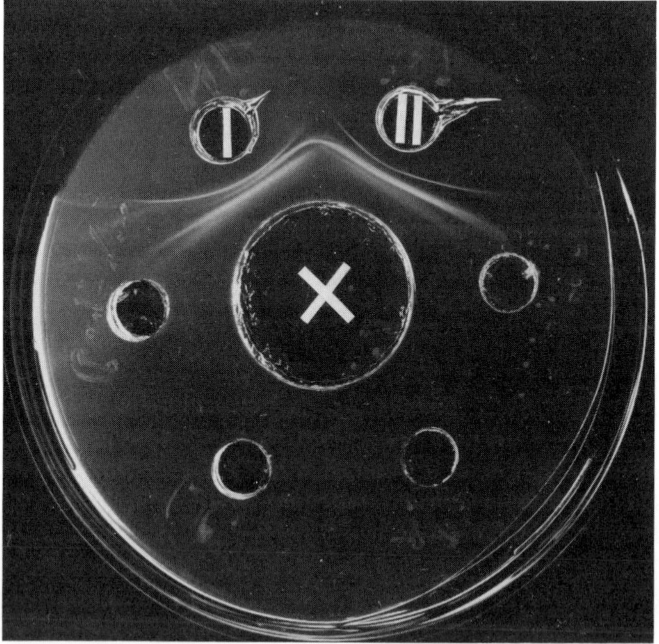

Figure 52. Patterns of precipitation bands formed in agarose gel by two antigens (I and II) reacting with one antiserum (placed in the middle, large trough).

precipitate lines due to unrelated antigens may produce intersections and terminate so that the tip of one line just touches the other instead of crossing, thus simulating a reaction of identity. In these doubtful cases, the test must be repeated by changing the relative concentrations of antigen preparations.

i. *The Paper-Disk Immunodiffusion Test.* The test (Kwapinski, 1965) is set up on plates made of an acetone-purified and water-washed agar of 1.5% concentration in 0.85% sodium chloride, preserved by Merthiolate added to a final concentration of 1:20,000. Sterile strips of no. 1 Whatman filter paper, 2-mm wide and 5-cm long, are saturated with 1:5 dilution of antiserum, dried at 45°, and then placed across the center of the agar plate. Filter paper disks of 5- to 10-mm diameter are saturated in an antigen solution, dried at 45°, and placed on the agar plate, about 2 to 3 mm above and below the quadrangular strip. The plates are left in a wet chamber and incubated at room temperature for several days. Positive reaction is indicated by bands occurring in spaces between the antigens and the antiserum, usually in 1 to 3 days. This test is sensitive, easily reproducible, and especially useful for series with a large number of sera and antigens.

ii. *The Cellulose-Acetate Immunodiffusion Technique (Kwapinski et al., 1970).* The equipment for the test consists of a suitable plastic template, selected from 20 different templates designed by Kwapinski for macro- and microprocedures and for special purposes of the immunological analysis (Figs. 53–56). The template rests on a plastic plate (Immunocell, National Instrument Labs., Rockville, Md.), equipped with a rubber base, on which a cellulose acetate membrane is placed. The membrane is previously floated and soaked in a 0.01 *M, p*H 7.2, phosphate buffer. After the plastic chamber has been reassembled, 0.08–0.16 ml of the antigen solutions are placed in wells, and 0.3 ml of antiserum, or preferably a serum globulin preparation is poured in the well (or in a trough, depending on the type of template used.) If microtemplates are employed, the amounts of antigen and antiserum are reduced to 0.03 and 0.1, respectively. The plates are incubated at 37° in a moist chamber for $1\frac{1}{2}$ to 3 days, and then the membranes are removed, washed in 1 *M* NaCl solution, and stained with 0.2% Ponceau S stain in 3% acetic acid, and then decolorized with 6 to 7% acetic acid. The membranes are examined for the presence of red-colored precipitation bands (Figs. 57–59) in a transmitted light viewer, equipped with a 10× magnifying glass.

The membranes may be cleared in liquid paraffin, decalin, Cotton Seed oil, or in Whitemore oil No. 120 or in a 1:10 mixture of glacial acetic acid and ethyl alcohol. In the latter case, the membranes must immediately be placed on a glass plate since they shrink. Caution must be applied at the clearing of membranes since faint precipitation bands sometimes are not

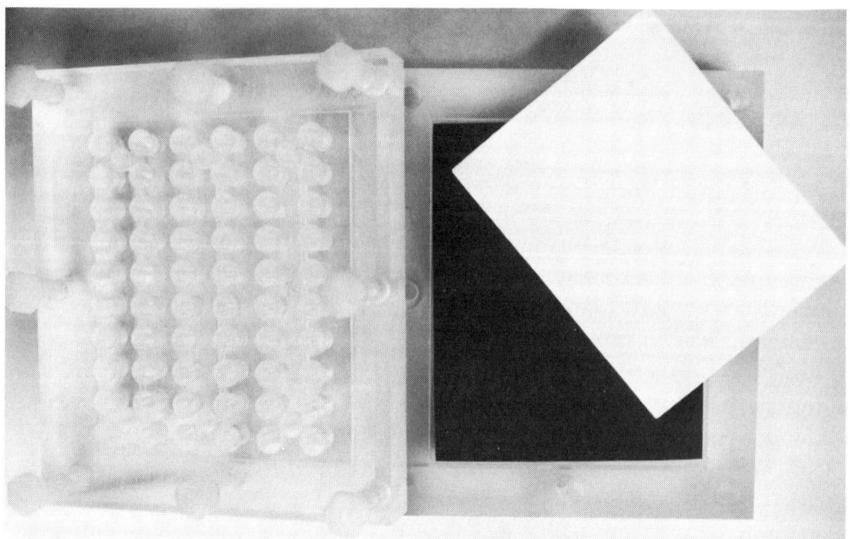

Figure 53. A plastic template and a base equipped with a rubber base and a cellulose-acetate membrane.

visible after the clearing of membrane. It is recommended first to examine noncleared membrane, and utilize cleared membrane mainly for photography. However, if antiserum globulins are used instead of full serum, almost all noncombined protein is eluted on washing with 1 M NaCl, and the background remains colorless so that it does not obscure the visibility of precipitation lines.

In case of nonprecipitating antigen-antibody complexes, the areas occupied by nonprecipitating complexes are detected by flooding the cellulose-acetate membrane after the immunodiffusion with an antiglobulin serum prepared against the globulin of the animal species which provides the first antiserum, followed by the removal of excess protein with 1 M NaCl.

VI. MICROMETHODS OF IMMUNODIFFUSION

Microtechniques of the double immunodiffusion test were devised by Wadsworth (1957), Crowle (1958), Mansi (1957), Grasset et al. (1958), Hennisch (1960), Kwapinski (1965), and Johnson (1967). These techniques permit the use of amounts of reactants as small as 0.025 ml.

i. *Hennisch's Micromethod of Immunodiffusion.* Microscopic slides are uniformly covered with 2 ml of 1.5% prepared agar in Sorensen disodium phosphate, citric acid buffer, pH 7.0, containing 1:10,000 Merthiolate. Seven basins, of 6-mm diameter, at equal distance from one another, are made by means of a metal template. (Basins of 3-mm diameter and 1% agar are employed in the Wadsworth technique.)

The center basin may be filled with an antiserum, and outer basins with antigens. The diffusion period varies from 24 to 36 hours at room temperature or at 37°. The slides, washed in distilled water and dried with blotting paper, may be stained in an Amido Black 10B solution containing 1.0 g of the dye in 1 liter of a 9:1 methanol-glacial acetic acid solution. After 5-minute staining, the slides are washed in a 9:1 methanol-acetic acid solution, then with distilled water and air dried.

Alternative dyes are Thiazine Red R, Crocein Scarlet MOO, Azocarmin G, and Coomassie Blue, each dissolved at 0.1% concentration in 1% acetic acid. Agar slides should be stained in these dye solutions for 10 minutes, then washed for 20 minutes in 1% acetic acid and for 10 minutes in 1% acetic acid containing 1% glycerol.

ii. *Kwapinski's Semimicrotechnique of Immunodiffusion.* This is designed for testing a larger number, for example, 14 to 18, different antigen preparations versus one serum. In this method, macroscopic slides are placed in an adequate plastic frame and first coated with a very thin layer of 1.1% Noble or "Ionagar" in a 0.25 *M,* pH 7.4, barbiturate-HCl buffer. (This buffer consists of 58.1 ml 0.1 *M* sodium diethylbarbiturate and 41.9 ml 0.1 *N* HCl, diluted 1:4 in distilled water.) When the agar hardens, a second, 2- to 3-mm-thick layer of 1.0% agar is poured. A 1-mm-wide

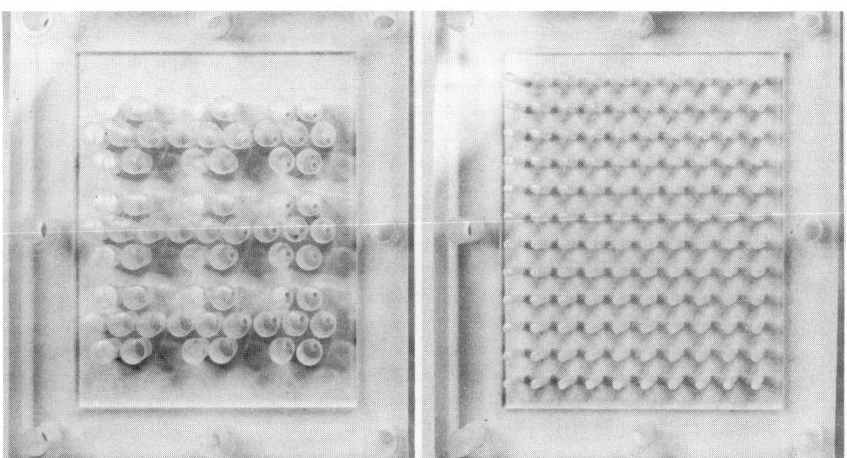

Figure 54. Plastic templates for (left) examination of a single antigen (or antiserum) against six different sera (or antigens), use in different solutions; (right) multiple antigens against multiple sera or their dilutions.

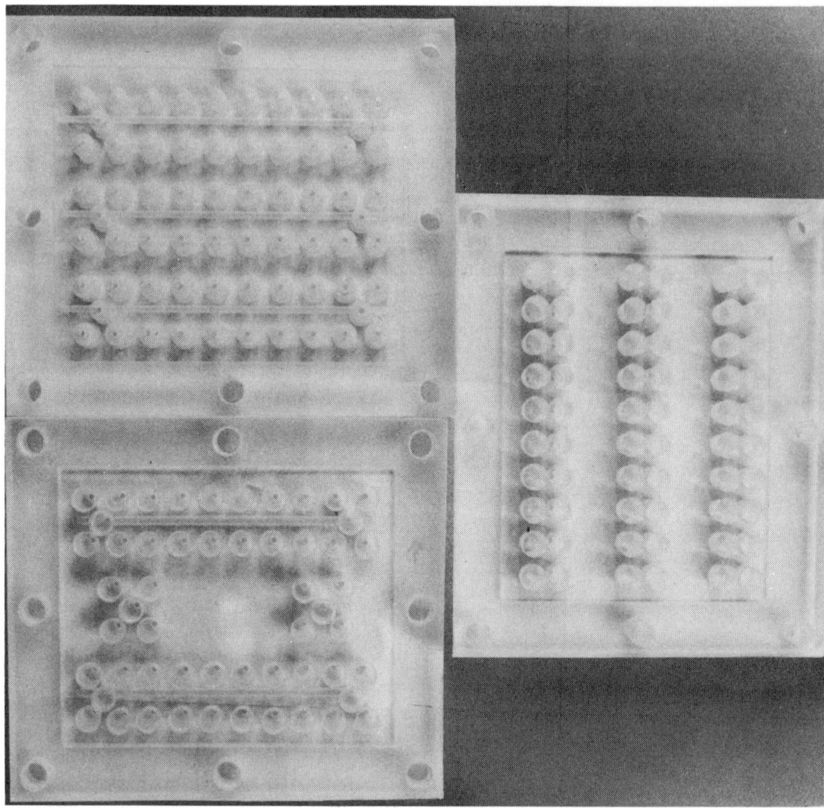

Figure 55. Plastic templates designed for testing of multiple antigens (placed in wells) against an antiserum (in the trough), or of different antiserum dilutions against a single antigen preparation.

trough and 7 to 8 wells (2 mm in diameter), 1 cm apart and 0.5 cm from the central 1.5-mm-wide trough, are then cut on both sides. Wells are cut by means of an adequately prepared capillary pipette. The wells and the central trough are refilled daily for 2 to 3 days, and the agar frames are left overnight at 37, 19, and 3°, respectively. Curved precipitation bands are formed in the space between a well and the trough. Precipitation bands formed by related immune complexes join in the middle between adjacent wells. Precipitation arcs of the nonrelated systems cross at the adjacent ends.

iii. *Johnson's (1967) Microimmunodiffusion Method.* This technique facilitates the detection of faint precipitation bands by employing ultrathin glass plates to support the agar gel and templates. Class plates $\frac{1}{32}$-in. thick, such as those used for binding photographic slides, are very convenient.

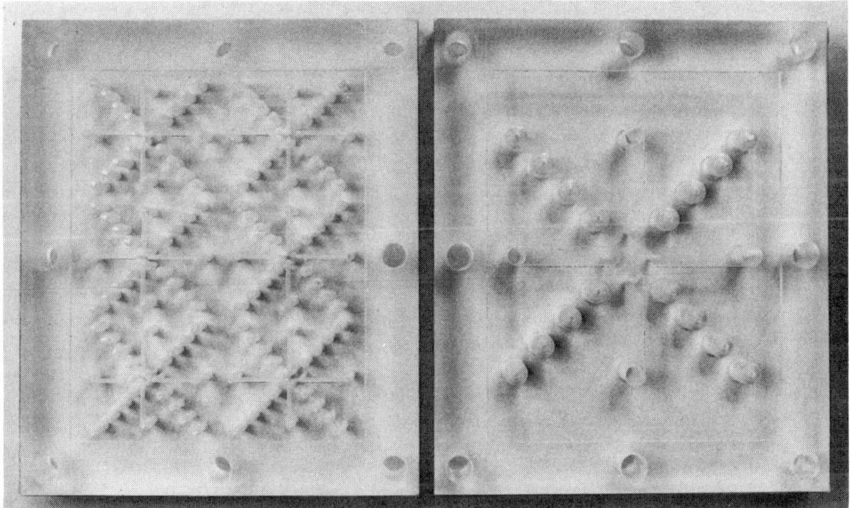

Figure 56. Templates used for the determination of optimal antigen-antibody preparations and for Kwapinski's quantitative immunodiffusion techniques (p. 356).

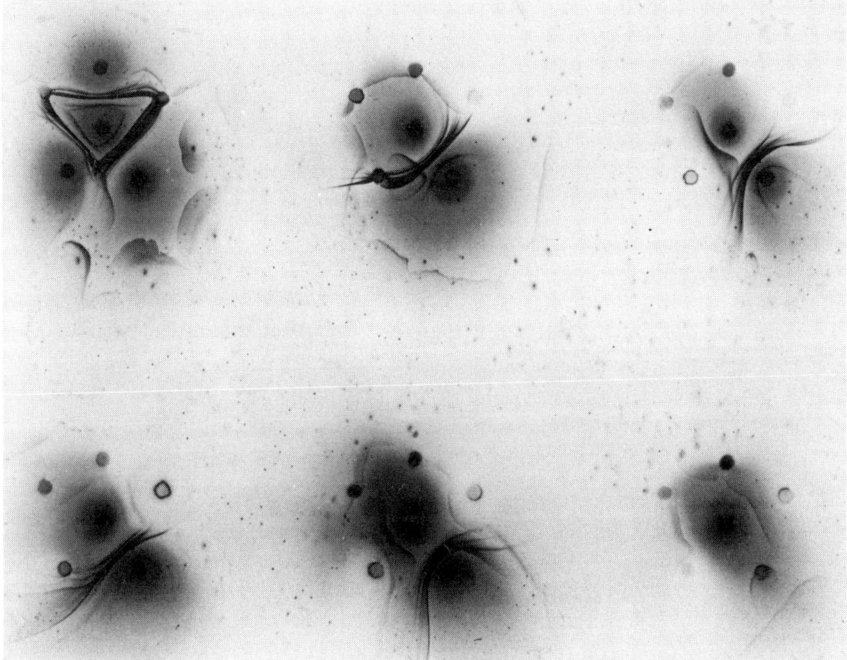

Figure 57. Precipitation bands formed on the cellulose-acetate membrane by the corresponding antigen-antibody systems.

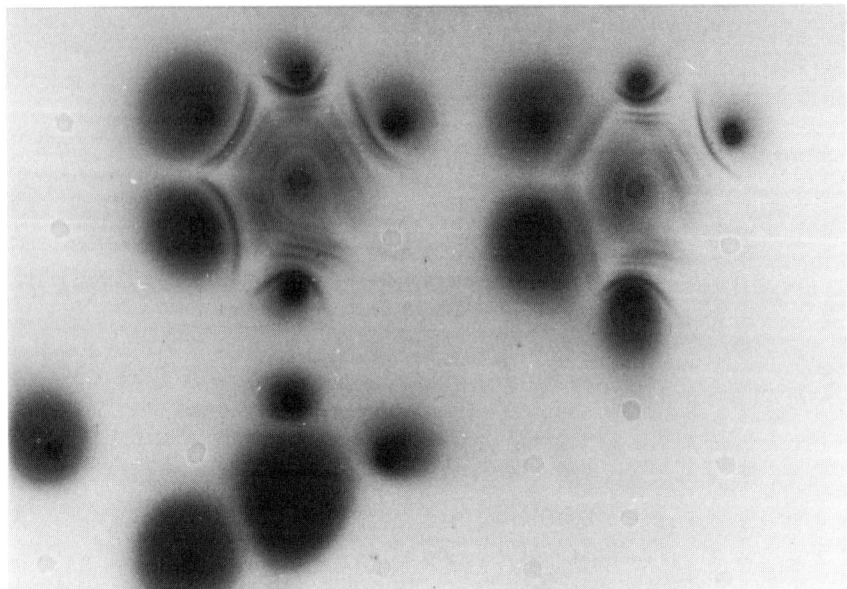

Figure 58. Precipitation bands formed on the cellulose-acetate membranes in the microimmunodiffusion procedure.

Templates are made from $\frac{1}{8}$-in.-thick Plexiglass. Approximately 2 ml of 1% purified agar in barbital buffer, pH 7.4, melted and cooled at 60° are pipetted onto the glass plate. The template is coated on the underside with Desicote (Beckman Instruments Inc., Fullerton, Calif.), and its wells are covered on top with a sticking tape. The templates are warmed and gently lowered onto the agar spurting at one side. When the agar has solidified, the slide is placed in a Petri plate containing moistened filter paper. After 15 minutes, the tape is carefully removed and the reactants are added to the corresponding wells. The slides are then incubated at room temperature for 2 to 3 days. The template thereafter is removed, and the unreactive material present in the agar is leached for 24 hours with several changes of the barbital buffer. The buffer is washed out with distilled water, and the agar is air-dried at room temperature. The plate is then stained with Amido Black 10 solution for 50 minutes, and differentiated in 2% acetic acid until no more stain is removed, rinsed in distilled water and allowed to dry. The slide is then mounted with another clean slide and can be bound in 2 × 2 in. aluminum slide binder. The slides are ready for projection, printing, and photographing.

iv. *Betts and Sewall's (1965) Immunodiffusion Technique for Identification of Blood Stains.* According to Beth and Sewall's method, a saline extract of blood stain is placed in a lateral well cut in 1% Nobel agar (in a 0.05 *M*, pH 8.6 barbital acetate buffer) and tested again on antihuman serum diffusing from a central well. Controls of an extract from the same nonblood stained cloth and antisera versus other animal sera are included. After 18 to 24 hours incubation at room temperature, the agar is exposed to 1% acetic acid to remove unbound proteins and rinsed gently with distilled water. The agarose dried at 50° for 2 hours and stained with 0.5% Amido Black solution and rinsed with a solution consisting of 225-ml methyl alcohol, 50-ml glacial acetic acid, 225-ml distilled water. Blue precipitation bands appear. The test is sensitive and reproducible. It is superior to other methods in which precipitate in tubes is often faint and no records can be made, because the precipitate is a transitory phenomenon.

VII. THE DIFFERENTIAL IMMUNODIFFUSION TECHNIQUE

The diffusion precipitation test usually provides sufficiently clear results for the study of the antigenic structure of microorganisms or their sero-

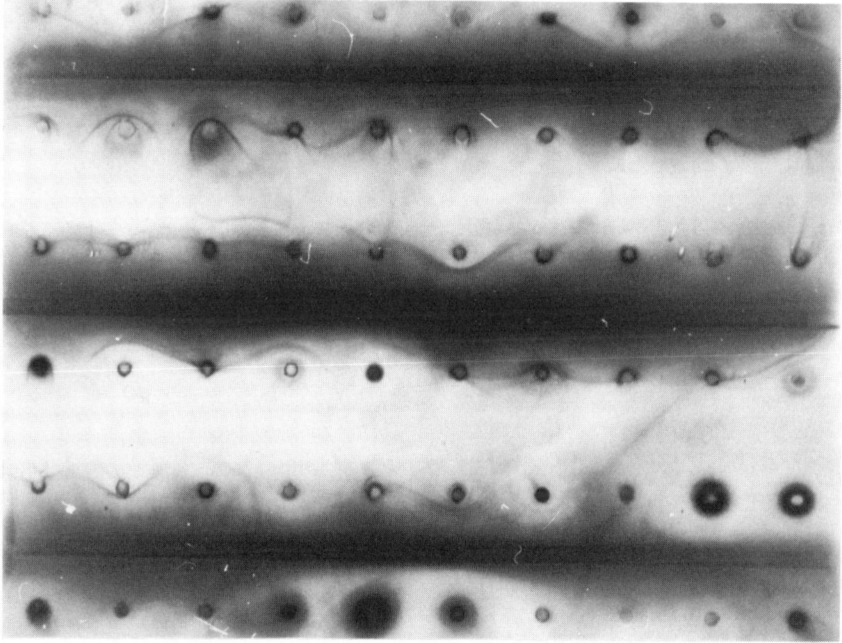

Figure 59. Precipitation bands formed by antigen and antibody reactive in a micro-immunodiffusion test.

logical relationships. However, the interpretation and evaluation of patterns of precipitation lines are sometimes controversial, especially with regard to certain seemingly related immune systems. In such cases, additional immunological studies are recommended, with the aid of absorption procedures devised by Oudin (1946), Oakley and Fulthorpe (1953), Björklund (1952), Feinberg (1957), Schmidt et al. (1965), and Kwapinski (1972), or by using one of the "mutual dilution techniques" described by Gispen (1955), Augustin and Hayward (1955), and Preer (1956). The principle of the immunodiffusion absorption technique is that the absorbents incorporated in agar gel act as barriers to the migration of homologous antigens or antibodies. Heterologous antigens and antibodies are unaffected by the absorbent migrating through the gel and react with the appropriate reagent in the adjacent or opposite well. The details of selected techniques for differential immunodiffusion follow.

1. The Absorption Test

This is carried out by incubating mixtures of small, for example, 0.5-ml amounts of an antigen and an antiserum at 37° for 1 hour and at 8° for 18 to 48 hours. The supernatant obtained after the centrifugation at 850 $\times$ g in a refrigerated centrifuge is assayed in the agar gel for changes in the pattern of the diffusion precipitation. In the procedure devised by Björklund, an antigen preparation or an antiserum is allowed to diffuse into the agar gel prior to the test proper. For this purpose, all basins in the agar plate are filled, for three consecutive days, with one component of the tested serological system (an antigen or a serum). The basins are then filled with the other component of the serological system. Alternatively, the antiserum (or antigen) can be added to the melted agar to replace approximately 25% of saline. The precipitation lines, which would depend on the component introduced into the agar or on related antigens, do not occur, whereas the serological reactions due to other components of the same system are not influenced by that pretreatment.

2. The Intragel Absorption Technique.

According to Feinberg's (1957) technique, as adopted by Schmidt et al. (1965), the sorbent (antigen or antibody) is incorporated into the agar gel, placed in a plate or a slide. Wells are cut and filled with antigens and antisera. If the gel contains an antigen homologous to the antibody present in a given well, the diffusing antibody is immediately precipitated around the well and does not migrate through the gel to react with another antigen placed in an adjacent or opposite well, and possessing determinate groups for the antibody. Similarly, if antiserum has been incorporated in the gel, the homologous antigen is precipitated around the antigen well and does not diffuse outward to meet another, corresponding antibody.

If an antiserum is used as absorbent, it should be inactivated at 60° for 20 minutes and employed in a 10% final concentration in the agar (one part of inactivated antiserum is added to 9 parts of 1% agar, melted, and cooled to 60°). Antigens used as absorbent should be relatively concentrated and diluted 1:5 in a melted agar.

This procedure may be employed as an antigen-antibody absorption technique to investigate immunological relationships or to unmask separate antigen-antibody systems which otherwise might appear as a single precipitation band.

3. *Kwapinski's (1972) Immunodiffusion-Absorption Method*

The test is set up on cellulose-acetate membranes by means of the specially designed, plastic templates (Fig. 60). Antiserum or an antibody-immunoglobulin preparation is placed in the outside, bent-arm trough, whereas the central trough is filled with antigen A and the wells receive the antigen B. On incubation and diffusion of the reactants, the serum first migrates through the zone of antigen B with which the antibody possessing complementary active sites complexes; but the noncomplementary antibody possess the antigen barrier and it may complex with the antigen A and its diffusion's area. Thus if the antigen preparations A and B are immunologically identical and both are complementary to the antibodies, precipitation bands are formed in both diffusion areas. If the antigens are partly related to each other, the precipitation bands are seen at the wells of antigen B and at the trough of antigen A in the areas projected by the free spaces between the wells of antigen B.

4. *Kwapinski's Double-Trough Template Method*

A nonabsorbed antiserum is placed in one trough, whereas an antiserum absorbed with a known antigen is placed in the other, parallel trough. The antigen is deposited in a central, shorter trough. The plate is incubated at 37° for 2 days. The cellulose-acetate membrane is then washed in 1 M NaCl, stained with 0.001% Ponceau S stain, destained in 7% acetic acid, and examined in transmitted light. The lack of a precipitin band on the side of absorbed-antiserum trough indicates immunological identity between the antigen in central trough and the sorbent antigen.

5. *The Mutual Dilution Technique (Preer, 1956)*

In this method, the following seven mutual ratios of diluted antigens A and B, tested against one antiserum are employed:

1. Antigen A diluted 1:100, 1:200, or 1:500.
2. Antigen B diluted 1:100, 1:200, or 1:500, the most adequate dilution of each antigen is that allowing a clear separation of nonhomologous bands.

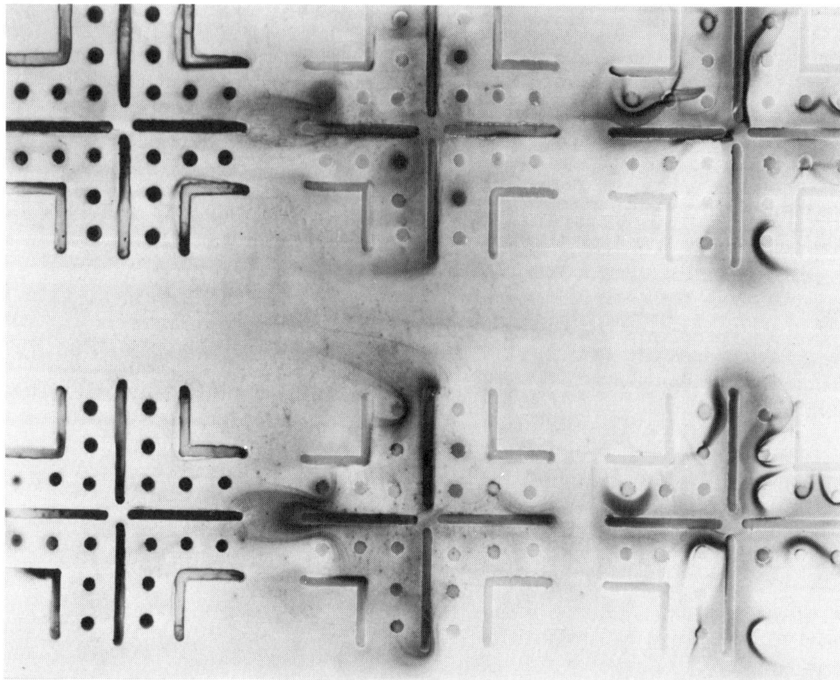

Figure 60. Precipitation bands formed on the cellulose-acetate membrane by anti-bodies complementary to the antigens, examined according to Kwapinski's immuno-diffusion-absorption method (p. 353).

3. The $\frac{7}{8}$ antigen A mixed with $\frac{1}{8}$ antigen B.
4. The $\frac{3}{4}$ antigen A and $\frac{1}{4}$ antigen B.
5. The $\frac{1}{2}$ antigen A and $\frac{1}{2}$ antigen B.
6. The $\frac{1}{4}$ antigen A and $\frac{3}{4}$ antigen B.
7. The $\frac{1}{8}$ antigen A and $\frac{7}{8}$ antigen B.

The controls contain various dilutions, 7:8, 3:4, 1:3, 1:4, and 1:8, made from the initial solutions of each antigen, separately.

The precipitation bands due to identical serologic systems merge, and only single bands are formed in the gel following the reaction of a mixture of two antigen preparations with the antiserum tested. In contrast, two different antigen preparations produce the same pattern of two or more precipitation lines when each of them is tested against an antiserum, whether alone or mixed with the other.

A similar technique and mode of interpretation are employed for the examination of two or more antisera tested against one antigen.

VIII. QUANTITATIVE IMMUNODIFFUSION TECHNIQUES

Semiquantitative methods were described by Wright (1959) and Sewell (1964) for comparison of potencies of different antisera. Quantitative procedures were designed by Feinberg (1957), Fahey and McKelvey (1965), and Kwapinski (1972). The quantitative immunodiffusion technique of Fahey and McKelvey was adapted for immunoglobulin determination by Suhrland et al. (1968).

1. Semiquantitative Immunodiffusion Technique

Immunological potencies of different antisera may be compared by the following technique (Sewell, 1964). A series of antigen dilutions is prepared, and each solution is dispensed into the wells of a plastic tray, followed by a drop of each antiserum added to a drop of each antigen dilution. The immunodiffusion test is set up in an elongated pattern of wells arranged in interlocking hexagons, so that the wells in the upper and bottom row parallel each other but the wells in the center row fall in the space between the wells of the other two rows. The mixtures of antigen and antibody preparations are dispensed into both outer wells. The middle row of wells receives the indicator system, the antiserum and antigen being placed into alternate wells. The characteristics of antigen and antibody preparations used for the test must be studied prior to the test, so that a standard concentration of this reagent can be selected to obtain precipitation bands from between the wells holding the two reagents and so that the line is clear and straight. The plate holding the mixtures and the controls are then placed in an incubator or left at room temperature in a wet chamber. The results are read by the determination of different antigen concentrations with which the antisera thus compared are in equivalence, as shown by the mixture which does not deflect the line formed between the standard reagents. This end point of the test may be clearly defined and it is independent of time and temperature. If, however, the difference in the antigen concentration between successive mixtures is relatively small, the equivalent zone usually extends over several mixtures; in this case, the last mixture containing an excess of one of the reagents is taken as the end point. Different antigen preparations may also be compared in a similar manner using a standard series of dilutions of an antiserum in the mixtures.

A similar test has been proposed earlier by Wright (1959). In Wright's test, equal volumes of antiserum and antigen preparations are mixed, and the excessive antibody or antigen is detected upon the reaction with standard reagents in the immunodiffusion test. The excess reagent is detected by the observation of residual weak line formed between the standard reagents and the mixtures close to the equivalence concentration.

2. Kwapinski's Quantitative Immunodiffusion Technique

In this method, antiserum are placed in the cross-central troughs (Fig. 61) and a single antigen solution is pipetted into each well. The effective antigen dilution (D_e) reactive with antiserum is estimated by, and is proportional to, the distance between a precipitation band thus formed and the well center (in mm):

$$D_e = \frac{A}{r}$$

where A is the original antigen concentration.

3. Quantitative Immunodiffusion Technique of Fahey and McKelvey (1965)

In this technique, adapted by Suhrland et al. (1968), lantern slides ($3 \frac{1}{4} \times 4$ in.) are coated with 12 ml of 1% agar containing 0.8 ml of an antiserum. The agar gel is prepared in the form of 1% solution of Noble

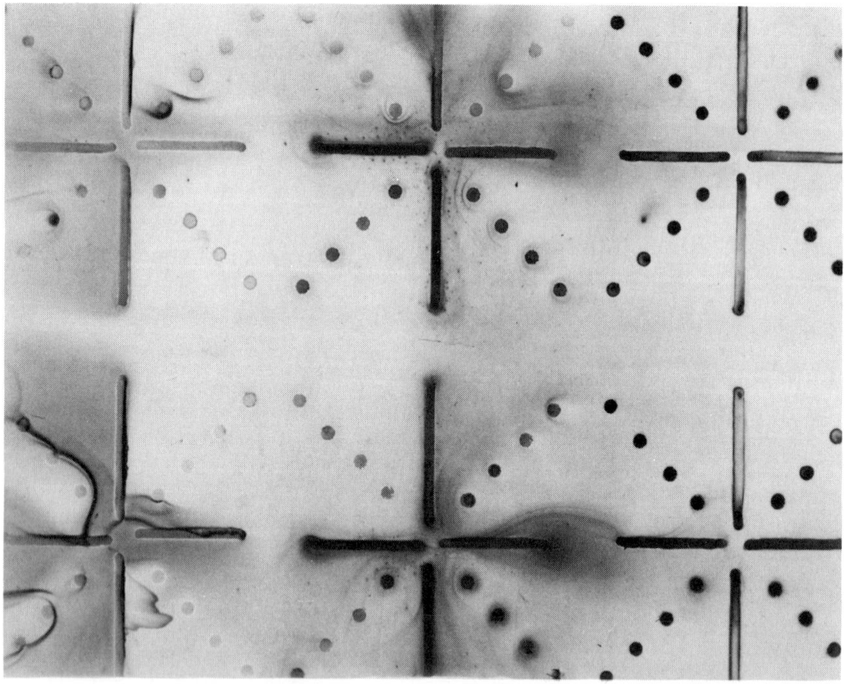

Figure 61. Immunodiffusion-precipitation bands detected by Kwapinski's quantitative immunodiffusion technique (p. 356).

agar in a buffer containing 1.12 g sodium barbital, 2.92 g glycerin, and 0.13 sodium azide dissolved in 130 ml of distilled water. Antigen wells, 4.0 mm in diameter, are cut at 1.2-cm intervals in the solidified agar layer. The antigen wells are filled with 10 μl of different antigen solutions. The slides are incubated in a humid atmosphere at room temperature for 24 hours, and then inspected for the presence of precipitation lines or circles, or photographed. The precipitin ring diameters are measured with a magnified scale, in millimeters, and are plotted on a logarithmic scale against the amount of an antigen or compound in milligrams per milliliters placed in individual antigen wells. Having drawn a standard curve for particular compound and the diameter of precipitate rings determined, the corresponding concentrations of a test compound may thus be determined.

IX. SEPARATION OF ANTIGEN-ANTIBODY COMPLEXES FROM IMMUNODIFFUSION GEL

Antigen-antibody complexes formed over a large crosssection of area in the diffusion agar, kept in a specially designed cell, can be separated as parallel planes by freezing the gel and then cutting sections with a freezing microtome (Smith et al., 1962).

The diffusion cell is made of perspex plate; it consists of central gel space separated from narrow spaces holding the serological agent by a stainless-steel gauze. The gel consists of gelatin or agar, dissolved in warm phosphate buffer saline, pH 7.3 (containing 4.25 g NaCl, 8.096 g of Na_2HPO_4, and 2,438 g of KH_2PO_4 per liter of distilled water), and sodiumazide (0.1%). The gel is poured into the central space and left until solid. The antigen preparation is introduced in the narrow space at one end, and the antibody solution is introduced into the space at the opposite end of the gel chamber. Diffusion or reactants occurs throughout the full length of the gel. The chamber is left at room temperature for 2 to 3 days during which time precipitation bands are formed.

To remove or collect individual antigen-antibody precipitates, the diffusion cell is surrounded with solid carbon dioxide and left for 3 to 4 hours until the gel is completely frozen. The cell is then dismantled and the frozen block of gel is cut on a freezing microtome; 120 mμ sections are cut from the block and collected individually, by a hair brush, in 0.9% NaCl (0.1 ml). The gel is then allowed to thaw, after which it is diluted with phosphate-buffered saline and left at room temperature overnight. The precipitate is collected by the centrifugation at 1200 $\times$ g for $\frac{1}{2}$ hour and washed six times with phosphate-buffered saline.

X. THE IMMUNOCHROMATOGRAPHY ASSAY

The immunochromatography is a combination of chromatography and immunodiffusion, designed for separation and characterization of immunologically active compounds in a gel medium. The separation and characterization by immunochromatography relies on absorptive properties and molecular size. Here is a description of a procedure for immunochromatography (Carnagie and Pacheco, 1964).

Microscope slides are precoated with 0.1% agar and then covered with 2 ml of molten agar and left to solidify. A longitudinal half is removed and a 1.4-mm × 0.2-cm trough is cut in the remaining half of agar, 5 mm from the center of the slide. On the vacant half of the slide, dextran gel columns of reproducible dimensions are prepared. For this purpose, a glass spacer (3.5-mm wide × 0.6-mm thick) is laid next to the cut surface of the agar and a 5-mm wide × 0.6-mm-thick trough is formed between this spacer, and a similar thickness of glass laminated to a second slide. A settled dextran gel is pipetted into a trough and the bed is leveled with a razor blade. The spacer is then removed and the second slide is slid away. The slide with the microcolumn is then placed on a special holder. The wicks are attached, and the columns are equilibrated with 0.1 ml of the following buffer: 0.05 *M,* pH 5.8 phosphate buffer for a DEAE column, or 0.1 M, pH 8.0 phosphate buffer containing 0.5 M sodium chloride for the G-100 Sephadex column. Elution from a DEAE column is attained with 0.1 *M,* pH 5.8 phosphate buffer, containing 0.5 *M* sodium chloride, whereas a 2% agar gel with 1% sodium azide in veronal-HCl buffer (pH 7.2, 0.2 *M*) was used for differ from G-100 column.

After the equilibration of microcolumns, a 2.5-mμ sample of a material to be separated is applied below the feeder wick and is fractionated with an elution buffer. When all the buffer has drained from the reservoir, the wicks are removed, and a drop of hot agar of the same pH and ionic strength as the bed of agar is run along the edge of the bed, placing the dextran gel into contact with the agar. The trough is filled with an antiserum and the slide is left in a humid chamber for 30 to 40 hours. The agar is then washed with buffer and precipitate bands are stained with a solution of Amido Black 10B. Precipitation bands occur in the form of horizontal, slightly curved bands.

The immunochromatography may be set alternatively by embedding a G-200 or G-100 Sephadex agar in a 5-mm trough cut in the center of the agar gel.

The usefulness of the immunochromatography consists in the rapidity of determination of chromatographic properties of immunologically active compounds, used in minute amounts as a preliminary to fractionation on a large scale by conventional methods. The method is particularly useful for characterization of immunologically active polypeptides and similar compounds.

XI. THE IMMUNORHEOPHORESIS (VAN OSS AND BRONSON, 1969)

The immunorheophoresis by Van Oss and Bronson relies on a hydrodynamic transport of molecules and is independent of the isoelectric points of antigen and antibody or of the pH of a medium. It is a procedure designed to bring a greater amount of antigen and antibody diffusing in a medium into an area of precipitation. This hydrodynamic transport of antigen and antibody molecules is attained by continuous evaporation of water from a gel or cellulose medium exactly above the area of the precipitation. Carriers for the immunorheophoresis are gel media, filter paper, or acetate-cellulose membrane. A three-fold increase in efficiency of the immunodiffusion and immunoelectrophoresis has been obtained by this method.

The immunorheophoresis procedure can be applied for uni- and bidimensional immunodiffusion and immunoelectrophoresis.

1. Unidimensional Immunorheophoresis

A supporting tray for the immunodiffusion is filled with 0.05% purified agar, made in aqueous solution of 0.05 M NaCl containing 1% glycerol, to form a 1.5-mm-thick agar layer. Wells of 5-mm diameter are punched 4 mm apart in the solidified agar, and a 2.5-cm-wide band of agar is removed at both edges. This space is filled with 0.05 M NaCl solution containing 1% glycerol; the wells receive an antigen and antibody solution. The plastic tray is now placed in a tank so that it rests on two prongs above the water level which fills the bottom of the tank to a height of 2 cm to assure sufficient humidity. The tank is covered with a plastic plate which has an open slit of 9-mm width in the middle. The slit falls halfway between the antigen and antibody wells. Following an overnight incubation precipitation bands are stained with the Ponceau S stain after the plates have been frozen in an alcohol-dry ice mixture and freeze-dried. The stained plates may be scanned with Analytrol-Densitometer equipped with a microzone scanning attachment or in a Chromoscan.

2. Bidimensional Immunorheophoresis

In this test, first a 1.5-mm-thick agar layer is formed and then a central, 5-mm-wide well and 3 to 6 similar wells around the central area are cut. An outer, 1-cm-wide ring of agar is cut out and removed, and this space is filled with 0.05 M NaCl containing 1% glycerol. The inner well serving as a liquid reservoir is also filled with this solution. The remaining wells receive either an antigen or antibody solution. The Petri dish is covered with a plastic cover which has a hole of 16-mm diameter and above the center of this hole a 9-mm-diameter disk is attached, with two crossed threads. Results of the bidimensional immunorheophoresis tests are inspected after an overnight incubation.

XII. THE IMMUNOELECTROPHORESIS

The immunoelectrophoresis is a combination of electrophoresis and immunodiffusion, carried out in an agar, agarose or starch gel, or on cellulose-acetate membranes. In principle, components of a mixture are separated by an electric current in a gel or cellulose medium and then are allowed to react with an antibody in the same medium. The immunoelectrophoresis is applied as an analytical technique for the study of soluble polymers in mixtures. The electrophoretic transport is facilitated by a buffer possessing a pH value intermediate between the pH of antibody and pH of antigen. The resolution of heterogenous antigenic components can be improved by (a) a longer electrophoretic separation, (b) performing the electrophoresis in a molecular sieving medium, such as starch gel, (c) transferring a gel medium containing separated components to another agar film and allowing the antigen components to react with an antiserum diffusing into the agar, (d) a two-dimensional electrophoresis in which the antigen components separated by an initial electrophoresis are subjected to a second electrophoresis in a direction perpendicular to the first axis, and allowing them to migrate into an antibody containing gel (the antigen-antibody crossed electrophoresis), and (e) the immunofixation electrophoresis. In the last two procedures, the diffusion is considerably minimized during the antigen-antibody reaction, and the resolution thus obtained is superior to the other methods.

The zone electrophoresis in gelified media was described by Gordon et al. (1958), but it was employed for immunodiffusion studies by Grabar and Williams (1953) and modified by replacement of the agar with starch gel (Poulik, 1956), agarose, polyacrylamide, and a cellulose-acetate. Technical alterations and adaptations of the immunoelectrophoresis technique were made by Scheidegger (1955), Skvařila et al. (1958), Grabar (1960), Libich (1959), Cawley et al. (1965), Merrill et al. 1967), and Schild and Pereira (1969). In the immunoelectrophoresis, components of an antigen preparation are first resolved in the electric field on a plate of gel or cellulose-acetate membrane. Antibodies are then applied and allowed to diffuse freely in a linear front from canals cut from the agar or from a template filled with antiserum parallel to the axis of the electrophoretic migration. The antigen preparation diffuses radially into the gel from another discreet zone at right angles to the axis of the electrophoretic migration.

Alternatively, an antigen preparation is first partitioned in the electric field, and the antibody is allowed to diffuse freely at right angles to the electrophoretic axis. Each antigen component separated from a complex preparation may form an arc-shaped precipitation band on its way of diffusion if it meets the corresponding antibody.

1. The Gel Immunoelectrophoresis Techniques

i. *The Immunoelectrophoresis Technique by Grabar and Williams (1953).* An ordinary paper-electrophoresis apparatus or a very convenient immunoelectrophoretic equipment produced by LKB-Produkter, Stockholm, can be used for the immunoelectrophoresis. Two plastic buffer containers on the tank are equipped with platinum wire electrodes and filled with a veronal buffer. This buffer contains 770 ml of $N/10$ soduim barbiturate and 230 ml of $N/10$ hydrochloric acid; it has pH 8.2 and the ionic strength of 0.05.

The gel medium consists of 1 to 1.5% washed agar in pH 8.2 buffer solution. A layer of this agar, 4-mm thick, is poured onto rectangular plates of photographic glass measuring 13×18 cm or on glass slides maintained in a plastic frame. Two strips of filter paper are inserted in the gel layer, one at either end of the plate to provide a contact with the buffer reservoirs. Two lateral canals, 4-cm apart, are molded in the gel layer with glass rods and filled with antiserum when the agar solidifies. Another well, large enough to contain up to 0.2 ml of the antigen solution, is impressed with a mold or cut with a punch. The antigen solution is mixed with melted buffered agar and introduced to this well.

Direct electric current of 100 V and 35 to 45 mA, with a voltage gradient of 3.5 to 5 V/cm of gel layer, is applied for 4 hours. The plates are then removed from the electrophoresis apparatus and left in a wet chamber, at room temperature, for 2 to 5 days, during which time the diffusion proceeds. The wet chamber consists of a glass or plastic box, the base of which is covered with a moist filter paper.

The electrophoretic distribution of protein in the agar layer can be roughly estimated after the electric current is discontinued by a "printing off" procedure. In this procedure, a strip of filter paper is placed along the axis of electrophoretic migration and gently pressed to the gel surface. The paper strip is taken off after a while and can be developed by a suitable color indicator.

Bands of specific precipitates in gel are usually observed during the second day of diffusion. They may be sketched or photographed by using a high-contrast photographic paper and transmitted light. Prior to the photography, the plates must be washed in saline for several days and dried at

37°. They may also be preserved for some time if covered by another glass plate and sealed with a modeling clay.

The speed of the diffusion and formation of precipitates depend on the amounts of antibodies in the immune serum, the size and shape of antigen molecules, and on relative quantities of antigen and antibody.

The motility of resolved components can be determined by placing the patterns of precipitate lines on a mobility scale provided by moving boundary electrophoresis or by the elution technique (Goreczky, 1959). In this technique, the serum is placed on strips of Whatman filter paper 4-cm broad, and the electrophoresis is carried out. The strips are then halved longitudinally. One half is stained after fixation with Amido Black 10B. The other half is cut into pieces 0.5-cm broad; they are placed on a layer of 0.5% blood agar 1.5- to 2.0-mm thick, containing the antigen. These are eluted with Mayer's buffer (see p. 477) containing complement by applying a total 20 to 40 volume of buffer divided into 5 to 10 portions. After the elution, the plates are incubated at 37° for 16 to 18 hours, and results are read by comparison with the control strip.

ii. *Grabar's (1960) Modified Immunoelectrophoresis Technique.* In this simplified procedure, the antigen preparation is first resolved by the electric current, and subsequently an immune serum is allowed to diffuse toward the antigen. A solution of the antigen preparation is placed in a hole molded in the center of agar gel and exposed to an electric field. When the electrophoresis is over, grooves are cut in the gel parallel to the axis of the electrophoretic migration, 5 to 8 cm from the outermost edge of the central hole. They are then filled with the immune sera, and the plates are left for 3 to 5 days in a "wet chamber" at 28°.

Antibodies diffuse at right angles to the axis of the electrophoretic migration while the antigen diffuses outward from the points to which they have been transported by electric current. Specific precipitates can be colored with stains easily fixed by proteins, for example, Azocarmin, Bromophenol-blue, Bromocresol green, Indigo carmin, and Amido Black. The gel precipitate bands are stained, according to the technique of Skvařila et al. (1958), in the following manner. Agar plates are first dried between several layers of filter paper. To stain the protein precipitates, the plates are placed for 3 hours in a 0.05% Azocarmin G solution made in an acetate buffer, pH 3.7. The plates are washed twice in an acetate buffer for 15 minutes, and dried. The other protein dyes are used in 0.1% dilutions made in a solution containing 450 ml of $M/1$ acetic acid, 450 ml of $M/10$ sodium acetate, and 10% glycerol. The agar plates are stained for 4 hours, then washed twice for 1 hour with a solution consisting of 2 parts glacial acetic acid, 15 parts glycerol, and 100 parts distilled water.

Specific precipitates formed by lipo-proteins or lipids can be selectively colored with lipid dyes, Sudan black or Oil Red O. A dye solution for staining lipoprotein precipitates is prepared as follows: 0.025 g of Sudan black is dissolved in 27 ml of 96% ethyl alcohol by boiling for 10 minutes. A volume of 25 ml of distilled water is added, and this is made up to 1 liter with 50% alcohol. The gel plates are exposed to this stain for 24 hours, then washed twice for 30 minutes in 50% ethyl alcohol and dried.

Agar plates can be preserved as permanent records of experiments in the following manner (Uriel and Grabar, 1956). Plates containing precipitate bands are first flooded with 0.9% saline and washed several times in 3 days with saline, and finally with water. The agar films are then placed face downwards on a silicone-coated glass, covered with several sheets of moist filter paper, and dried at 37° to a thin film. The dry films are pried off the silicone coated glass.

iii. *Libich's Immunoelectrophoresis Technique (1959).* A rectangular agar plate is cut into two triangular cells, one of which should be filled with a 1.5% agar-antigen solution, the other with an agar-antibody solution. When the electric current, of the 70-mA intensity, is induced into the plate, both the antigen and the antibody migrate into the reaction area between the cells, in the opposite direction to each other, in the form of a triangle. When the antigen combines with an antibody, a precipitation line is formed; but the excess antigen transgresses the primary line of the equivalence point and migrates towards the anode, while the antibody diffuses towards the cathode.

This method makes possible the determination of antigenic components in a crude toxin or of their antibodies.

iv. *The Direct Immunoelectrophoresis Method.* This method differs from other techniques of the immunoelectrophoresis in that after electrophoresis the surface of agar is flooded with an antiserum instead of placing it in a trough to diffuse. Specific precipitates are formed in a few minutes, but it is advisable to develop the electrophoretograms for 2 to 6 hours overnight. The slides are then washed with saline and stained with thiazine red. By this technique the size, shape, position, and homogeneity of an entire antigen spot in the agar can be visualized. Physicochemical heterogeneity of immunologically related antigenic substances can in some cases be demonstrated better than by a standard immunoelectrophoresis (Wilson, 1962).

v. *Microimmunoelectrophoresis.* Useful micromethods of immunoelectrophoresis were described by Scheidegger (1955), Wadsworth (1957), Skvařila et al. (1958), Tanner and Gregory (1961), Crowle and Lueker (1962), Cawley et al. (1965), Merrill et al. (1967), and Schild and Pereira (1969). Here are details of these techniques.

A 1.0 to 2.0% melted agar prepared in a veronal buffer, pH 8.2, ionic strength 0.05, is placed on small glass or plexiglass slides, such as microscopic slides or larger quadrangular slides measuring 5 × 5, 8 × 8, or 1.5 × 7.5 cm. Microscope slides should be precoated with 0.5% agar for a better adherence of the agar layer proper. Alternatively, slides can be immersed in a water-repellent agent, for example, "Siliclad" (manufactured by Clay-Adams, Inc., New York). Approximately five to seven slides are connected with buffer reservoirs by strips of filter paper inserted into the still liquid agar layer. Spherical basins 2 to 3 mm in diameter or, alternatively, spherical basins and rectangular canals, the latter measuring 2 × 40 mm are cut in the solidified agar layer. Amounts of antigens as small as 0.01 ml are placed in the central basins.

Antigenic components are separated in the Scheidegger micro apparatus under an electric potential of 5 to 6 V/cm in 30 to 60 minutes.

Lateral basins or canals are now filled with an antiserum, and the plates are left in a wet chamber for 24 to 48 hours, at room temperature. After drying, the slides may be stained with Azocarmin G. The excess protein is washed off by soaking the slides for 2 days in a Tris buffer, pH 8.6, consisting of 0.76 M Tris and 0.05 M citric acid.

The starch gel immunoelectrophoresis (Poulik, 1956, 1959) performed by either a single- or double-dimensional technique may often increase the protein resolution and the concentration of components; however, it is technically more complicated and offers no more advantage than the agar-gel methods.

In Cawley's et al. (1965) method, the agar gel is supported by 16-cm strips of photographic film leader. The strips are held in position with a masking tape and are covered with 4 ml of 0.6% molten agar, made in a 0.05 M, pH 8.6, veronal buffer, preserved with 0.1% sodium azide.

vi. *Merrill's et al. (1967) Microimmunoelectrophoresis Method.* The test is set up on glass microscope slides precoated with 1% solution of a purified agar and dried. The precoated slides are then overlaid with a melted, 1% agar made in veronal buffer, pH 8.6, 0.05 M to which an antiserum has been added in the volume of 0.1 to 0.3/3.0 ml of the liquified agar. The slides supporting the agar-antibody solution are left in a moist chamber for 1 to 2 hours. Seven circular wells are punched in a line along the short axis of the slide and the agar is removed from the wells by gentle suction. Antigen solutions are placed in the wells in the volume of 4 μl and the slides are subjected to an electric current at 150 V for 30 to 90 minutes at room temperature. An electrochamber contains a veronal buffer, pH 8.6, 0.1 M. The microscope slides are connected to the electrochambers with filter paper with sufficient thickness to draw 10 mA per slide.

After the electrophoresis, the slides are washed in saline for 24 hours and in distilled water for 1 hour and then dried and stained with Thiazine Red or another suitable dye. The precipitates resulting from a reaction between antigens separated electrophoretically and the serum incorporated in the agar appear in the form of cones attached to the antigen wells, having different length. The length of each precipitate area is plotted against the antigen concentration on an arthimetric scale, and a standard curve is constructed from which unknown concentrations can be determined by the length of their precipitate.

The antigen wells and antiserum troughs are cut along a pattern guided by a cutting guide set placed above the surface of the agar. The wells are filled with an antigen solution and the agar-coated strips are placed in an electrophoretic tank. An electric current of 200 V is applied for 30 to 45 minutes. The strips are then removed from the tank and placed in a moist chamber. The antiserum is placed in the troughs; the chamber is covered with a lid, sealed off with a masking tape, and kept at room temperature for 24 hours.

Excess protein, antigen, or antibody which have not combined with each other and buffer salts are removed by soaking immunoelectrophoretograms in an isotonic saline for 24 to 72 hours. The strips are then soaked in water for several hours to remove saline, dried in an oven or on a histological hood, and stained either with the Amido Black 10B solution for 5 minutes or in Thiazine Red for 20 to 30 minutes. The excess stain is removed in 2% acetic acid. To speed up the removal of unfixed protein and buffer salts, the surface of agar strips may be covered with filter paper and dried in an oven.

The stained strips may be photographed on a dark field illumination of wet strips. The precipitin bands can be intensified by soaking the immuno-electrophotograms in a 1% solution of tannic acid for 24 hours.

Staining solutions: (a) Amido Black 10B, 10 g dissolved in 100 ml of glacial acetic acid and diluted to 1000 ml with distilled water; and (b) Thiazine Red, 0.1 g dissolved in 100 ml of 1% acetic acid.

2. *The Cellulose-Acetate Membrane Immunoelectrophoresis*

The immunoelectrophoresis according to Schild and Perreira's (1969) method, is performed as follows: the antigen is first separated electrophoretically on a cellulose-acetate strip in a suitable buffer. After the electrophoresis, sections of the strip measuring 0.5×7 cm are then cut longitudinally from the central portion of the strip and placed immediately on the surface of glass slides covered with a thin 0.05-cm layer of purified agar. Narrow strips of filter paper moistened with an antiserum are placed on the agar surface on each side of the cellulose-acetate section so that their edges run in parallel to and 0.2 cm from the edges of the cellulose-acetate strip. The slides are kept in a moist chamber for 16 to 18 hours to develop precipitin bands. Upon the completion of incubation time, the cellulose-acetate strips are removed from the agar surface, the slides are washed, and the precipitin lines are stained. To refer the position of precipitation bands to that of the position of an antigen component separated by electrophoresis, the remaining section of the cellulose-acetate strip which has not been exposed to the antiserum is stained with an appropriate dye, for example, Procion brilliant blue (Laver, 1964).

According to Grunbaum's et al. (1963) technique, the antigen preparation is applied on a moist cellulose-acetate strip parallel to the run, by means of a capillary, and is subjected to an electric current of 100 V for 5 to 6 hours. A buffer selected according to the isoelectric point and solubility of the antigen, is employed although a 0.05 *M,* pH 8.6 veronal buffer is often used. After the electrophoresis, the antiserum, or globulin preparation is streaked parallel to the direction of migration, and the cellulose-acetate strip is left in a moist chamber at 37° for 12 to 16 hours. Precipitin arcs develop in the membrane during this time. Immunological identification of individual antigens, forming a precipitation band, is accomplished in two ways: (a) by the comparison of the position of a precipitation band to the location occupied by an antigen, revealed on a stained parallel strip or on a parallel portion of a single strip, not exposed to the antiserum; and (b) by absorbing the antiserum with an individual antigen and applying the absorbed serum to an antigen preparation electrophoresized in parallel with the main strip; consequently, the precipitin line corresponding with this antigen will not be formed.

3. Differential Immunoelectrophoresis Technique   Compositions of two antigen preparations may be compared to each other by means of a differential immunoelectrophoresis, performed on agar-coated slides (Nerenberg, 1962) or in a gel slab (see Disk Immunoelectrophoresis). The first type of the differential immunoelectrophoresis can be performed by one of the following procedures.

i. *The Double-Well Procedure.*   A parallel trough is cut near each long edge of the agar layer, placed on a glass slide, and two wells are cut between and at the beginning of the troughs. The wells are filled with two different antigen preparations and are exposed to an electrical current (see p. 361). After the electrophoresis, both troughs are filled with one antiserum. During the incubation time, precipitation bands formed in the area between the troughs coalesce if the two antigen preparations possess immunologically identical components.

ii. *The Narrow Trough Procedure.*   An antigen preparation is placed in the well and subjected to the electrophoresis. An antiserum is then poured into the narrow trough, positioned near to the antigen source. An antigen mixture is placed in the more distant wide trough on the other side of the antigen source. On diffusion, the antibodies first advance to the electrophoresized antigen; but if they have not combined with the antigen, they pass into the area of antigens diffusing from the wide trough and there they may react with them to form precipitation bands.

iii. *The Interrupted Trough Procedure.*   A horizontal trough is cut in the agar placed on a glass slide, between two antigen wells, along the plane of the slide, except the area where precipitation bands are expected to cross over. There the trough is interrupted. After the electrophoresis of antigens and exposure to the antiserum, a precipitation band, formed by one antigen-antibody complex crosses over the end of the trough and fuses with any arc of immunological identity of the other antigen-antibody complex.

4. *The Disk Immunoelectrophoresis*

The disk immunoelectrophoresis technique depends on the reaction in gel of immunologically active polymers, separated by disk electrophoresis, with the antibodies diffusing at a right angle to the gel slab. Two methods, the macro- and microprocedures (Finkelstein et al., 1966; Felgenhauer, 1968) have been designed.

i. *The Macromethod of Disk Immunoelectrophoresis.*   According to the procedures employed in Kwapinski's research laboratories the polyacrylamide gel slabs recovered from the disk electrophoresis are first washed with 1 M NaCl for 6 hours, and then embedded in 1% melted Noble agar or agarose, poured in a Petri plate and cooled to 55°. (The agar or agarose is made in a Tris buffer, adjusted to the pH suitable for solubility of the original material and preserved with 1:25,000 Merthiolate.) A simultaneously prepared, Amido Black stained gel slab is embedded at a distance of 10 mm from the unstained gel slab. After the agar has solidified, a 2-mm trough is cut in the agar, in parallel to the long axis of the polyacrylamide gel slab; 0.1 to 0.2 ml of an antiserum is placed in the trough, and the test plate is incubated at 37° for 16 to 24 hours. A compound diffusing from a zone in the polyacrylamide gel and reacting with the antibody diffusing from one trough produces an arc directly over the zone whose middle point corresponds to the original position of the band in the parallel, stained slab (Fig. 62).

ii. *The Microdisk Immunoelectrophoresis.*   This technique is a combination of the micropolyacrylamide gel electrophoresis and immunodiffusion

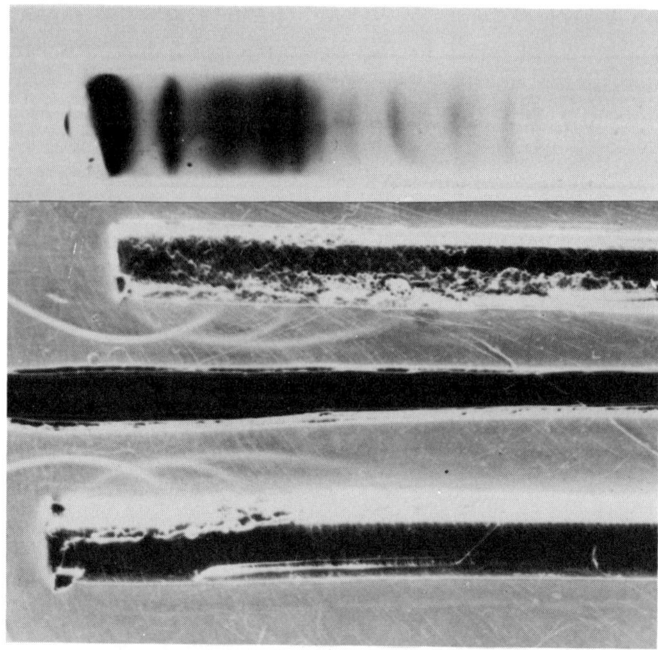

Figure 62.   Immunodiffusion-precipitation patterns arising from reactions between the antibodies diffusing from central troughs and the antigen placed in wells at different distances from the trough.

(Felgenhauer, 1968). Components of an antigen preparation are first separated by Felgenhauer's (1967) technique (see p. 112), except that 6% acrylamide is used for lower gel, which is filled into the capillary from the bottom. Water is overlayered from the top by the injection device. After the electrophoresis, gels are cut at the height of the bromophenol blue tracing band, to be used as the reference point for calculation of Rf values. Gel threads not used immediately should be frozen.

The gel threads, removed from the capillary tube, are placed into small vessels containing 50 to 70 μl of antiserum and incubated at 4° for 17 hours with vigorous shaking. The gel is then washed in saline containing 0.01% Merthiolate for 4 days at room temperature and stained in Amido Black solution, followed by destaining in 2% acetic acid. The optimum antigen-antibody ratio is found by trial and error. An antigen excess may cause doubling of bands. The antiserum may be used many times. Faint precipitation bands and nonvisible reaction products may be detected by the indirect technique, as follows: the gels, recovered from the bath with an antiserum, are washed in a buffered saline and then immersed in an antiimmunoglobulin G serum, directed against the animal species which was the donor of the first antiserum. Precipitation bands appear in these circumstances due to the reaction of the ant-IgG with the antiserum originally combined with the antigens separated by the polyacrylamide microelectrophoresis.

The microimmunodiscelectrophoresis is a very sensitive method, which allows the detection of as little as 0.003 μg of a single protein.

An alternative procedure is the imbedding of the polyacrylamide gel threads into an agar containing a trough filled with antiserum. This technique, however, necessitates the application of 3 times greater amount of proteins than the above described procedure.

5. *The Rheoimmunoelectrophoresis*

In this technique (van Oss and Bronson, 1969), microscope slides coated with melted agar and held in plastic frames are employed as supporting and diffusion medium. An antigen or antibody source is placed in the holes punched in the agar and subjected to an electric current. After the electrophoresis, the second reagent of the immunologic test is placed in a lateral trough cut in the agar, and the tray holding microscope slides is positioned in a plastic container so that both longitudinal sides touch a 0.05 M NaCl solution or a buffer. The chamber is then covered with glass plates except for a gap, parallel to the antiserum trough and open to the air between the antigen wells except for a long, narrow sliver that just sits above the antiserum trough, protecting it from direct evaporation.

6. *The Immunofixation Electrophoresis*

The immunofixation electrophoresis technique (Alper and Johnson, 1969) is conducted as follows: the initial electrophoresis in an agarose, agar, or starch gel is carried out conventionally. After the completion of electrophoresis, an undiluted antiserum is layered over the gel surface, and the gel is placed in a perfectly horizontal position in a moist chamber and left at room temperature for 1 hour. The gel is then covered by a sheet of Whatman no. 1 filter paper moistened with water and 3 sheets of dry Whatman no. 3 filter paper, and on top of this a glass plate weighted with 2 to 3 kg is placed and left for 10 minutes. The plate and filter papers are then carefully removed; the agar plates are washed in normal saline for 6 hours and then in running tap water for 20 minutes, dried in air and stained in 1% Amido Black dissolved in 5% acetic acid, and decolorized in several changes of aqueous 45% methanol containing 10% acetic acid.

The optimal concentration of antigen in the solution to be objected to the immunofixation electrophoresis and reacted with antibody ought to be predetermined. In case of a too high concentration of antigen relative to the antibody concentration, a central clear zone may appear within the specific antigen band and the details may be blurred. An antigen concentration ranging from 5 to 50 mg/100 ml is usually satisfactory.

The bands formed by the separate antigen components reacted with an antibody occur in the form of horizontal, well-defined, short lines. The advantage of utilization of the immunofixation procedure is that nondiffuse precipitation bands occur in a medium. The distance migrated by antibody molecules is extremely short; it is less than 1 mm in agarose and 0.3 to 0.5 mm in the starch gel; thus the diffusion of separated antigen components is essentially restricted to that occurring during electrophoresis. Complexes of antigen and antibody precipitating in an agar gel are trapped and only noncombined material is washed away.

Although the immunofixation electrophoresis is relatively sensitive, its disadvantage is that it requires relatively large quantity, ranging from 0.05 to 0.2 ml of a potent antiserum per sample.

7. The Electrosyneresis

This technique (Abelev and Zvetlov, 1967) is a combination of the electrophoretic and immunoprecipitation analysis, performed simultaneously. The antigen and antibody samples are placed in the gel separately but at such sites that one reactant overruns the other during the electrophoresis. Where this has occurred, an immunoprecipitation is induced, and a stationary band with an immunospecific barrier effect is produced.

XIII. EVALUATION AND APPLICATION OF IMMUNODIFFUSION TEST

The immunodiffusion technique is a rapid and sensitive method for the detection of antigens and antibodies and for the measurement of antigens and immunoglobulins occurring in relatively low concentrations, for example, in dilute biological fluids. The reproducibility of measurement is satisfactory although at low concentrations less reproducibility is observed. The immunodiffusion technique is little affected by the presence of extraneous materials in the reagents, and therefore it allows the determination of a single major system in the presence of minor contaminating systems.

Sensitivity of the immunodiffusion test is high. As little as 2 to 5 μg of the antibody is detectable (Finger and Kabat, 1958); 5 Lf of purified txoids give a definite gel precipitation reaction with 1000 units of antitoxin (Bowen, 1952); the egg albumen has been detected by gel precipitation in a concentration as low as 0.0001% (Preer, 1956). The cellulose acetate provides the most sensitive and convenient medium for practically all immunological systems. However, not all the antigens can be studied by this test. For example, some highly purified haptens of microorganisms, which are able to react with corresponding antisera in the complement fixation test, fail to produce visible precipitation bands in the gel with the homologous antisera. The quantity of the serum antibody to combine with purified antigenic components is sometimes insufficient, though it is adequate to react in other immunologic tests. The nonprecipitating antibodies occurring in some sera or directed against certain antigens can also be responsible for the failure of diffusion tests.

The sensitivity of both the single and the double immunodiffusion techniques is usually comparable, but the latter produces somewhat clearer results, more ready for interpretation. The two-dimension plate test is technically simpler than the other diffusion procedures, for which the adjustment of concentration of the antigen and antibody is sometimes necessary. It permits the direct comparison of various antigens and antisera and the identification of antigens. However, weak antigens sometimes produce precipitates with their antibodies more readily in agar columns than in agar plates.

The Elek test is a reliable method for the determination of toxigenicity. There is an absolute agreement between the results of *in vivo* and *in vitro* tests for the virulence of *Corynebacterium diphtheriae*. The immunodiffusion techniques are the most helpful methods for testing the homo- or heterogeneity of antigen or antiserum preparations.

"False" immunodiffusion reactions can result from the ability of some antigens, for example, lysozyme, fibrinogen, and chicken ovalbumine, alone to produce precipitation lines in agar. A substance occurring in the agar and some inorganic salts are able to precipitate serum constituents at pH values less than 6, and maximally at pH 5 (Wieme, 1959; Kwapinski, 1965). A serum rich in lipids can cause "false," thick precipitation bands. The precipitation may not occur at pH values exceeding 8.2, due to dissolution of precipitates, and in excess of antigen or antibody. The excess antigen or antibody can accumulate in the center column or in the center arch before a sufficient concentration of the other component is reached, thus inhibiting initial precipitation (Parlett, 1961).

The immunoelectrophoresis is often most advantageous in the detailed separation and detection of components occurring in various antigenic preparations and fractions, of microorganism, and of animal and plant tissues, cells, and fluids. Since the immunoelectrophoretic analysis often helps to better separation of antigenic complexes, it is suitable for precise studies on the antigenic structure of microorganisms and macroorganisms. By means of the immunoelectrophoresis and disk-immunoelectrophoresis, even very similar antigens may be separated, and the category of immunoglobulins reactive with an antigen may be determined. It must be noted that the time of electrophoresis and the concentration of antibody in the agar and in the cellulose acetate affects the length of precipitate bands, the test conditions and amounts of antibody must be preexamined and standardized.

The most common application of the immunodiffusion test is in qualitative studies on antigens occurring in the microorganisms and culture filtrates, as well as in cells, tissues, and intracellular fluids of higher organisms. Relative concentrations of individual antigens in complex materials and mixtures may be determined by photometric measurement of the turbidity given in gel by immune systems.

The immunodiffusion has successfully been adapted for testing of the homogeneity and degree of purification of various antigen preparations, and to the detection of antibodies in different hyperimmune and patients' sera. Here are some examples of the application of the immunodiffusion test:

1. Studies of the antigenic potency, structure, grouping of, or immunological relationships between strains of *Mycobacterium* (Lind, 1960, 1961; Sourek and Sir, 1959; Parlett and Youmans, 1959), *Nocardia* and *Actinomyces* and other genera of *Actinomycetales* (Kwapinski, 1965, 1969, 1970–1972), *Vibrio comma* (Misra and Shrivastova, 1961), *Leptospira* (Rothstein and Hiatt, 1956), *Listeria* (Metzger and Smith, 1962), *Coccidioides immitis* (Pappagianis et al., 1961), *Staphylococcus* (Jensen, 1961), *Streptococcus* (Lancaster and Sherris, 1960); Cayeux, 1962), *Pseudomonas aeruginosa* (Homma and Suzuki, 1964), *Pasteurella tularensis* (Carlisle et al., 1962), *Bacterionema matruchotii* (Sibal et al., 1962) outer-cell soluble antigens of corynebacteria (Relyveld et al., 1962), clostridia (Jennings, 1956; Ellner and Green, 1963), and of El Tor virbios (Watanabe and Felsenfeld, 1963), influenza viruses (Jensen and Francis, 1953), poxviruses (Gipsen, 1955; Mata, 1963), adenoviruses and *herpes simplex* virus (Mata, 1963), foot-and-mouth disease virus (Brown and Crick, 1957), poliomyelitis virus (Le Bouvier, 1957; Grasset et al., 1958; Beale and Mason, 1962), *Coxsackie* virus (Schmidt and Lennette, 1962), *Myxomatosis* virus (Chapple et al., 1963), tobacco mosaic virus (Kleczkowski, 1961).

2. Determination of the toxigenicity of microorganisms, for example, *Corynebacterium* of *Clostridium botulinum* (Gendon, 1958).

3. The control of purification of antigens, for example, of staphylococcal enterotoxin (Surgalla et al., 1952), the toxoid of *Corynebacterium diphtheriae* or *Clostridium histolyticum* (Largier, 1957; Ispolatovskaja et al., 1953), and O and Vi antigen preparations of *Salmonella* (Webster et al., 1955; Landy et al., 1955; Baker and Whiteside, 1960).

4. Detection of antibodies in human sera, for example, detection of diphtherial antitoxin, streptococcal antibodies (Halbert et al., 1955), and

mycobacterial antibodies (Lind, 1960; Parlett and Youmans, 1959), and antibody against *Brucella* (Glenchur et al., 1962), *Blastomyces dermatidis* (Abernathy and Heiner, 1961), *Nocardia brasiliensis* (Bojalil and Zamora, 1963), against human blood group A (Kuhns and Dukstein, 1957), the C-reactive protein (Libretti et al., 1957; Kwapinski et al., 1958), and other characteristic proteins in rheumatic sera (Epstein et al., 1951), and DNA antibodies in sera from lupus erythematosus (Deicher et al., 1959).

5. The localization of antibodies in serum and plasma fractions (Goreczky, 1959).

Chapter Eight

THE FLOCCULATION TEST

I. PRINCIPLES OF THE FLOCCULATION REACTION

The phenomenon of flocculation was described by Ramon (1922) and Ramon and Descombey (1926). The flocculation test is a variety of the precipitation in which the reaction between a soluble antigen and a flocculating antibody is manifested in the form of clumps instead of amorphous precipitate. Flocculation occurs over a relatively narrow range of antigen concentrations, whereas the precipitation reaction shows an equivalence zone with a range of increasing or decreasing precipitates on either side. The rate of the formation of flocculates depends on the proportion of antigen to antibody. The speed of the flocculation varies also with changes in temperature and the dilution of test mixtures; even the relation between the level of the bath water and that of reacting mixtures may influence the rate of flocculation (Bunney and Kiamil, 1931).

Flocculating antibodies occur predominantly in the horse antisera produced by the immunization with some toxins or albumins, for example, in antisera reactive with toxins of *Corynebacterium diphtheriae, Clostridium tetani,* or *Clostridium botulinum,* the erythrogenic toxin, human and rabbit serum albumins, chicken albumin, conalbumin, and hemocyanin. Human sera from cases of chronic thyroiditis also contain flocculating antibodies. Larger virus particles combining with the serum antibodies can also produce flocculates or clumps. A special type of flocculating immunologic substances are reagins that are able to react with certain lipid emulsions. Antigens for the flocculation test are crystalline, purified or crude toxins and toxoids, alkaline aqueous extracts, and alcohol-soluble antigens isolated from bacteria or from animal tissues and absorbed onto various inert particles, for example, on collodion, cholesterol crystals, resin, mastix, bentonite, protamine, or metacryl. Lecithin added to such immunologic systems increases the size of antigen particles.

The flocculation test may be carried out qualitatively or quantitatively by a macroscopic technique in tubes, or by a microscopic technique on glass slides. The "fine" or final flocculation test should be preceded by the determination of optimal proportions of the antigen and antibody according to the Dean and Webb technique (1926). In this assay, equal volumes, for example, 0.2 ml of an antiserum diluted 1:10 and of serial twofold antigen dilutions ranging from 1:50 to 1:6200 are incubated at the temperature required. The tube showing a flocculation in the shortest time represents the end point. Based on the result of this preliminary titration a "final" test is conducted with antigen dilutions closely spaced about the preliminary end point.

II. THE ANTITOXIN FLOCCULATION TEST

The macroflocculation test was originally devised by Ramon (1922) to study the reaction between toxins and antitoxins and to evaluate either antitoxins, toxins, or toxoids. It was subsequently adapted to other immune systems, for example, to study reactions between larger viruses and virus antibodies, or between reagins and tissue or bacterial extracts.

In the test based on Ramon's method, amounts of an antitoxin serum increasing from 0.07 up to 0.15 ml by 0.01-ml increments are added to a constant 1-ml amount of a standard toxin, then incubated in a water bath at 44 to 46° and observed frequently. The tube, in which the flocculates have first been noticed, and the flocculation time are recorded. The tube, in which flocculates occur at the earliest, contains the toxin almost completely neutralized by the antitoxin. This can be confirmed by an animal inoculation.

A toxin preparation to be used as an antigen in the test must be standardized previously in the presence of a standard antitoxin serum, which is supplied by Statens Serum Institute, Copenhagen, Denmark. This serum should contain 300 to 1000 antitoxic units per milliliter and show well-defined flocculation in 20 to 30 minutes with several different standard homologous toxins. The standardization of the toxin may be carried out by the determination of its activity in a flocculation test. One Lf dose is the amount of a toxin flocculating most rapidly with one unit of a standard antitoxin. It is calculated as indicated in the equation (Wadsworth, 1939):

$$\text{Lf milliliter toxin} = \frac{\text{antitoxin units per milliliter} \times \text{milliliters of antitoxin serum}}{\text{milliliters of toxin}}$$

The evaluation of a serum being examined by a flocculation test is carried out as follows. Varying amounts of serum are made up to 1.0 ml with saline and mixed with 10-ml amounts of a standard toxin, in tubes 13 × 16 mm in uniform diameter. The tubes are stoppered and mixed with a single, quick up-and-down motion, and incubated in a water bath at 40°.

Readings are made at time intervals in an artificial light against a dark background.

The mixture, in which the flocculation occurs initially, is taken for the estimation of the Lf unit content. If the flocculation occurs simultaneously in two tubes, an approximate estimation can be made. If it is observed in more than two or in the first or last tube, the test must be repeated. The unit content is calculated from the following formula:

$$\text{number of units} = \frac{\text{Lf value} \times \text{milliliters of standard toxin}}{\text{milliliters of undiluted serum}}$$

III. THE TOXIN FLOCCULATION TEST

The test, by Pillemer et al. (1950), is carried out as follows. A standard antitoxin flocculating serum is diluted with $M/15$ phosphate buffer at pH 7.4 to contain 50 Lf/ml; 0.5-ml amounts of this solution are distributed in a series of test tubes. Varying amounts of the toxoid in increments of 20% are added to the consecutive tubes, and the total volume of each is brought up to 2 ml with the buffer. The contents of tubes are mixed and these are incubated at 50° and inspected for flocculation in a transmitted light against a black background. The first tube showing flocculation is recorded, and the flocculation time is symbolized by Kf.

The toxoid should now be so diluted that the indicator tube contains approximately 0.5 ml of the toxoid. The test is repeated as described above, but the toxoid is now added to each tube in increments of 4% by placing the quantity of the toxoid found previously in the "incubator tube" in the middle tube in this series. The Lf content of the toxoid is more accurately determined by this procedure, although the "experimental error" is about 4%.

The contents of Lf per milligram of the protein nitrogen are determined after the dialysis of a 5-ml sample of a purified toxoid, containing between 500 and 200 Lf/ml against 0.15 M sodium chloride at 2°. The dialyzate is then analyzed for the Lf and total nitrogen contents.

IV. THE VIRUS FLOCCULATION TEST

The direct flocculation test with viruses of a larger size, for example, pox viruses, is carried out by mixing in narrow tubes, 0.5-ml volumes of a suspension of virus particles with an equal volume of progressing serum dilutions. The results are read after 2- to 4-hour incubation in a water bath at 37°.

V. THE QUANTITATIVE FLOCCULATION TEST

The flocculation reaction can be more precisely evaluated by a chemical determination of flocculates. In the test, devised for the toxin-antitoxin flocculation reaction by Turner and Boyer (1952), a precise amount of a purified or crystalline toxoid is placed in 1-ml centrifuge tubes and followed by a correct amount of a diluted antitoxic serum.

The mixtures are incubated for 3 hours in a water bath at 45°. The flocculation time for each tube is recorded, and the tubes are left overnight at 2 to 4° and centrifuged. The sediments should be washed twice with chilled 0.15 *M* sodium chloride solution, adjusted to pH 7.0, and dissolved in 1 ml of 0.02% sodium hydroxide. The protein percentage is estimated by using Lowry's et al. (1951) technique.

VI. REAGIN FLOCCULATION TESTS

Some inert, nonantigenic particles, such as cholesterol or oil globules, collodion, latex, resin, mastix, or bentonite particles, are able to absorb antigenic materials, either lipid or protein in nature, which render them reactive with the specific or characteristic antibody-like substances, the reagins. The aggregates resulting from these reactions are easily detectable, and these tests are often more sensitive than an ordinary flocculation, agglutination, or precipitation test. Even nonsensitized particles may be clumped by certain sera which possess high amounts of rheumatoid reagins (Wallis, 1956; Kwapinski et al. 1956).

The group of reagin flocculation tests can be divided into the following types of reaction:

1. The cholesterol flocculation test.
2. The collodion flocculation test.
3. The latex flocculation (fixation) test.
4. The bismuth tannate flocculation test.
5. The resin-particles flocculation test.
6. The virus-protamine flocculation test.
7. The acryl flocculation test.
8. The bentonite flocculation test.
9. The kaolin flocculation test.
10. The barium sulfate flocculation test.
11. The oil-droplets aggregation test.

Here are details of recommended techniques of reagin flocculation tests.

1. *The Cholesterol Flocculation Test*

Antigen preparations for this test, devised predominantly for the detection of syphilis reagins, consist either of crude alcoholic tissue extracts or of purified lipid substances, emulsified with cholesterol and lecithin. The purified reagin-antigen, cardiolipin, is a complex phosphatidic acid containing linoleic and oleic acid, a polyester of glycerophosphoric acid, and glycerol. The sodium salt of cardiolipin has a molecular weight of 2195 (Pangborn, 1941). Other antigen preparations for this test were made according to techniques published by Sachs and Georgi (1918), Kopeloff and Kopeloff (1949), Kline (1930), Klein et al. (1948), or Hunter and Colbert (1956). The optimum amounts of ingredients in the antigen emulsion should be determined by testing the antigens emulsified with the other constituents at different ratios, against reference sera, and comparing the flocculation titers with those revealed by other immunological tests.

The antigen preparation by Sachs and Georgi, as modified by Kopeloff and Kopeloff, is made from an alcoholic extract of beef heart. The extract should be evaporated to dryness over a steam bath and redissolved at 1% concentration in 95% ethyl alcohol. The emulsion is prepared by slowly adding 1 ml of saline solution to 1 ml of the extract, followed after 20 seconds by 4 ml of saline.

The antigen preparation devised by Kline consists of the cardiolipin coated by lecithin and cholesterol. The optimal ratio between the cardiolipin and lecithin seems to correspond to 1:8 or 1:10, that is, 1 mg of cardiolipin and 8 to 10 mg of lecithin per milliliter of ethyl alcohol. The following solutions are used to produce a satisfactory antigen for the reagin-flocculation test:

> 0.2% alcohol solution of cardiolipin.
> 1.0% alcohol solution of lecithin.
> 1.0% alcohol solution of cholesterol.
> 0.85% solution of sodium chloride.

One volume of the cardiolipin solution is mixed with 1.6 volumes of the lecithin solution, and a volume of 0.13 ml of this mixture is added to a fluid containing 0.43 ml of double distilled water and 0.5 ml of the cholesterol solution, followed by 1.22 ml of saline.

The antigen emulsion by the Hunter and Colbert method is prepared in the following manner: 1 ml of 1% cholesterol solution is added dropwise to a 0.85-ml volume of distilled water, at pH 6.0, while the tube is rotated for 20 seconds; 0.1 ml of this mixture is transferred to 0.25 ml of 1% lecithin solution in an absolute alcohol, and shaken vigorously for 15 seconds. The antigen extract should be added to this mixture in an optimum amount or in volumes varying from 0.05 to 3.0 ml and shaken vigorously for 1 minute, followed by 2.5 ml of Eagle's buffered saline. The antigen emulsion is shaken for 30 seconds and may be used undiluted, or diluted 1:4, immediately or within 24 hours, if stored at 2 to 4°. The syphilitic reagins are antibody-like substances which occur in the serum and in the spinal fluid apparently in response to the infection by *Treponema pallidum* and have a selective affinity to tissue lipids.

Various techniques and modification of the reagin flocculation test in the serum or spinal fluid were published by Kahn (1928, 1945), Sachs and Georgi (1918), Kopeloff and Kopeloff (1949), Harris (1946, 1947), Mazzini (1951), and Hunter and Colbert (1956).

The Kahn Flocculation Test. The cardiolipin antigen used in this test consists of 0.1% cardiolipin, 1% purified lecithin, and 0.025% cholesterol in absolute alcohol. The mutual ratio of these constituents can be slightly changed from one lot to another, to render the reagents suitable antigen preparations. Standard antigen preparations, which are commercially available, should be suspended in a volume of saline according to the titer indicated on the bottle. Kahn's test may be conducted qualitatively, quantitatively in a micro- or macrotechnique.

The qualitative macrotest is set up in nine tubes arranged in three parallel rows, to be used for a tested, a standard positive, and a standard negative serum. The antigen suspension, in 0.05-, 0.025-, and 0.0125-ml volume, is distributed in the horizontal direction by using a Kahn antigen pipette; 0.15 ml of each preheated serum is added in the parallel direction. The mixtures are shaken by hand for 10 seconds, left at room temperature for 3 to 7 minutes, and agitated on a shaking machine for 3 minutes. A 1.2% sodium chloride solution is then added in 0.2-, 1.0-, and 1.0-ml volumes to the tubes, respectively, and the results are read immediately. The intensity of the flocculation is expressed arbitrarily in pluses (1+ to 4+); the readings from all three tubes in a row are added and averaged. Reading of doubtful reactions is facilitated by centrifuging the tubes for 10 minutes at $800 \times$ g and resuspending the sediment. The centrifugation enhances the clumping of particles, thus leaving the medium clearer.

The *quantitative Kahn test* is conducted with progressing dilutions of the serum, in 0.15-ml volume, and a constant amount, for example, 0.01 ml, of the antigen suspension. The tubes are shaken for 10 seconds, left for 3 to 7 minutes, and agitated on a mechanical shaker for 3 minutes; 0.5 ml of saline is then added to all tubes, which should be shaken for a few seconds and read. The highest serum dilutions, giving 4+, 3+, or 2+ reactions, are recorded. The quantitative flocculation titer is computed by applying the formula $S = 4D$, where S is the potency of a serum in terms of Kahn units and D is the highest dilution at which a definite flocculation is observed.

The *presumptive Kahn test* is sometimes used prior to the quantitative test. In this procedure, 0.15 ml of a heated serum being tested is added to 0.025 ml of Kahn's antigen. Controls for the whole series of tests include a positive serum, a negative serum, and a saline control of the antigen. The tubes are shaken for 10 seconds, left for 3 minutes, and agitated in Kahn's shaker for 3 minutes; 0.5 ml of saline is then added to all tubes, which are shaken by hand for a few seconds and read.

The Mazzini Flocculation Test. The antigen preparation used in this test usually consists of 0.025% cardiolipin and 0.2% lecithin which gives the 1:8 ratio, and of 0.75 to 0.9% cholesterol dissolved in ethyl alcohol. The antigen adsorbed onto cholesterol must be tested with varying amounts of lecithin in several "reference" positive and negative sera to determine the optimum concentration of lecithin, which largely influences the sensitivity of the test. The maximum sensitivity of the test is secured by an emulsion containing the largest amount of lecithin which has produced clear-cut negative reactions with sera from normal people, the strongest positive reactions with serum samples from syphilis, and the least number of positive reactions with sera from diseases other than syphilis. The antigen preparation is standardized in the following two steps: (a) examination of the dispersibility of the emulsion and (b) determination of the antigen titer.

The *dispersibility* of the antigen emulsion is tested by using a 0.75% solution of cardiolipin, 2.0% alcohol solution of lecithin, 1% alcohol solution of cholesterol, and 40 serum samples of the individuals free from syphilis. Cardiolipin and lecithin are mixed in four or five different ratios, for example, 1:6, 1:8, 1:10, 1:12, 1:14, and 1 ml of each mixture is added to 9 ml of the cholesterol solution. The antigen emulsions are prepared by placing 0.4 ml of each antigen mixture into 0.4-ml volumes of buffered saline, and adding another 2.6 ml of buffered saline solution. The bottles are constantly rotated during this procedure.

Small, 0.03-ml amounts of each serum are now placed in five separate chambers on a glass slide and mixed with 0.01 ml of various antigen emulsions. The slide is rotated for 4 minutes at 160 to 180 rpm by a mechanical shaker or by hand. One drop, or approximately 0.05 ml of 0.9% sodium chloride solution, is then added to each chamber, and the glass slide is rotated for an additional 4 minutes. Results of the test are observed under a low-power microscope objective.

The *antigen-titer determination* is carried out by the same procedure as described above, but a number of strongly or weakly positive sera and false-positive reacting sera are substituted for the negative sera. The cardiolipin:lecithin ratio showing the strongest reactions with the weakly positive sera and the less marked positive reactions with false-positive sera is recorded as optimum.

This "standard" antigen preparation is stored in small, 2- to 4-ml volumes, to be used for the standardization of other lots of reagents.

The Qualitative Mazzini Test.   A 0.03-ml volume of the serum being examined is mixed with 0.01 ml of the cardiolipin emulsion on a glass slide. The slide is rotated for 4 minutes; approximately 0.05 ml of 0.9% sodium solution is then added, and the slide is rotated for another 4 minutes. Results of the test are read under the low-power microscope objective and evaluated as follows:

> No clumping of antigen particles: a negative result.
> Very small but definite clumps: 1+.
> Small clumps: 2+
> Medium-sized clumps: 3+.
> Large clumps: 4+.

The Quantitative Mazzini Test.   This assay differs from the qualitative technique only by the use of serially diluted sera within the range of 1:2 to 1:64 or more if necessary.

Results of the test are reported in terms of dilution units at the point of a 3+ or 4+ positive reaction. For example, if a 2+ reaction has been obtained with the serum diluted 1:16, the result is read in terms of 32 dilution units. The specificity of Mazzini's test is high, ranging from 95.3 to 99.3%, and the sensitivity varies from 64.1 to 86.9%.

The VDRL Microflocculation Test.   The antigen used in this test (Harris, 1946) consists of an alcoholic solution containing 0.03% cardiolipin, 0.9% cholesterol, and 0.21% lecithin. The antigen emulsion is prepared by adding in drops 0.5 ml of the antigen to 0.4 ml of buffered saline while rotating the bottle continuously. Another 4.1-ml volume of buffered saline is then added. The antigen should be tested preliminarily for its ability to give typically positive and negative results with known positive and negative sera, respectively.

Buffered saline consists of 0.093 g of Na_2HPO_4, $12H_2O$, 0.170 g of KH_2PO_4, 10.0 g of sodium chloride, and 1000 ml of distilled water preserved with 0.5 ml of formaldehyde. The antigen may also be stabilized with benzoic acid. For this purpose, 0.1 ml of 1.0% benzoid acid solution in ethyl alcohol should be added per 10 ml of the VDRL antigen emulsion and shaken gently for 10 seconds. The stabilized antigen must be stored at 6 to 10°.

The *qualitative* VDRL test can be carried out either on glass slides or in tubes. In the microtechnique, one drop (1/60 ml) of the antigen emulsion is added to 0.05-ml volume of heated serum, placed on a paraffin-ringed glass slide, and rotated for 4 minutes. The slide is then examined microscopically at 100 magnification. The presence of uniform, either large or small, clumps is indicative of a positive test. Zonal reactions that occur in the excess of a reactive serum component are recognizable by irregular clumping. In the case of a zonal reaction, the serum should be diluted 1:5 and 12:5 and retested.

The *quantitative* VDRL *flocculation test* can be carried out on slides, as described above, but with progressing serum dilutions, or in tubes. In tubes, 0.5-ml volumes of the diluted antigen are added to equal volumes of each serum (or spinal fluid) dilution. The tubes are agitated on a Kahn shaker for 5 minutes, then centrifuged at 500–700 $\times$ g, and re-shaken for exactly 1 minute. The titer of the test is estimated as the reciprocal of a serum dilution in the end point tube showing definitely visible aggregates in a clear or very slightly turbid liquid.

The Kopeloff Technique.   The tested serum is serially diluted in 1-ml volumes. Each serum dilution and a control tube containing 1 ml of saline receive 0.5 ml of the antigen emulsion, and the mixtures are incubated overnight in a water bath at 37.5°. After a preliminary reading, the contents of tubes are centrifuged at 500 $\times$ g for 10 minutes, flipped, and examined again for the presence of floccules.

The highest dilution of the serum in which the floccules have been observed denotes the end point, and the titer is expressed in terms of the final serum dilution in that tube.

The Hunter and Colbert Technique (1956).   A series of twofold serum dilutions made in 0.5-ml volumes of saline is mixed with an equal volume of an antigen emulsion diluted 1:4 in 1% sodium chloride solution. The mixtures are shaken on a Kahn shaker for 5 minutes and centrifuged for 10 minutes at 1000 $\times$ g. The tubes are then shaken again for exactly 1 minute and read immediately in front of a lamp with a black background. A positive reaction is manifested by the presence of clumps in a clear or slightly opalescent fluid.

Results of the reagin flocculation test can be evaluated in terms of reagin units, which corresponds to the serum dilution giving a 2+ flocculation. If the end point tube shows a stronger (3+ or 4+) reaction, an additional titration between the dilutions of these two tubes must be set up, to find the last dilution, at which a 2+ reaction is observed.

The Hunter and Colbert Microflocculation Test.   The test is set up in paraffin or permanent ring glass slides. The undiluted or serially diluted serum is pipetted in 0.05-ml volumes into the rings, followed by one drop of the antigen emulsion delivered by a syringe equipped with a standard needle. Control slides receive either 0.05 ml of saline and one drop of the antigen or 0.05 ml of an initial dilution of the serum or 0.05 ml of non-diluted serum and one drop of saline. In addition, controls of a positive and a negative serum are set up in a similar manner.

The slides are rotated for 4 minutes on a mechanical rotator at a speed of 180 rpm and read immediately at the 100 magnification. Large or medium-sized clumps are observed in the case of a positive reaction. The highest effective serum dilution is taken as end point for calculation of the flocculation titer.

The Rapid Qualitative Reagin Test. This test, a modification by Portnoy et al. (1957) of Harris's slide test, is set up with unheated plasma or serum. Three drops of an examined plasma or 0.05 ml of unheated serum are mixed with one drop of the VDRL antigen in a ring of a paraffin-ringed glass slide. The slide should be rotated for 4 minutes, and examined for the presence of clumps under a 100 magnification of the microscope. Large or medium clumps are indicative of a positive reaction.

The Brucella Flocculation Test. The antigen used for the test (Hunter and Colbert, 1956) is prepared by extracting a 48-hour culture of *Brucella abortus* with 0.25% phenol solution made in 0.85% saline. The extract is then centrifuged and dialyzed in a cellophane bag against running tap water to remove phenol. The dialyzate is made isotonic by adding sodium chloride, and is preserved with 1:10,000 Merthiolate.

The antigen emulsion is prepared by first suspending 1 ml of 1% ethanol solution of cholesterol in 0.85 ml of distilled water, then adding 0.1 to 0.25 ml of 1% alcohol solution of lecithin and 0.05 to 3.0 ml of the *Brucella* extract. The mixture is shaken vigorously for 1 minute, then diluted with 2.5 ml of Eagle buffered saline. The antigen emulsion must be used within 24 hours. The optimal ratio of lecithin to the *Brucella* extract should be determined by titrating positive sera with various mixtures of the extract and with 1% lecithin.

The *microscopic slide test* is set up by pipetting 1 drop of the antigen emulsion to 0.05 ml of serum dilutions placed in paraffin or permanent ring glass slides. A positive and negative serum and saline controls are inserted. The slides are rotated for 4 minutes and read immediately at a 100 × magnification. The occurrence of clumps and their sizes are recorded.

The Macroscopic Tube Flocculation Test. The antigen emulsion, as prepared for the slide test, should be diluted 1:4 with 1% sodium chloride solution and used after 5 minutes. The test is set up by adding 0.5 ml of the diluted antigen emulsion to 0.5 ml of saline dilutions of a serum, ranging from 1:10 to 1:640. The mixtures are agitated on a Kahn shaker for 5 minutes, then centrifuged at 1000 × g for 10 minutes, and agitated on the shaker for exactly 1 minute.

Tubes are examined for the presence of clumps by holding them in front of a reading lamp with a black background. The presence of floccules in a clear supernatant fluid is indicative of a positive test. No clumps and cloudy supernatant are observed if the reaction is negative.

2. The Collodion Flocculation (Agglutination) Test

Collodion-particle techniques for the antibody detection were described by Loeb (1922), and Jones (1927), and modified by Cannon and Marshall (1940), Weir (1941), and Cavelti (1948). The test involves the following procedures:

1. Preparation of collodion particles.
2. Determination of the optimum ratio between the antigen to be absorbed and a collodion suspension.
3. "Sensitization" of collodion particles for the test proper.
4. The test proper.

Methods of preparing stable aqueous suspensions of collodion particles were described by Loeb (1922), Cannon and Marshall (1940), Cavelti (1948), Havens and Lloyd (1949), and Arjona et al. (1954). According to the technique of Cannon and Marshall, a volume of 100 ml of collodion USP (Merck) is poured into approximately 2 liters of distilled water and stirred with a glass rod. The collodion mass separating from the solution is collected after decantation, washed thrice in distilled water, and dried at 40°. A 5% acetone suspension of this material is made by stirring at 40°, and kept in stock. This stock suspension must be treated, prior to use, with a 3:1 mixture of water and acetone (approximately 30 ml of water-acetone mixture is added to 75 ml of the stock solution) while heated at 40° and stirred vigorously. As a result, a heavy gelatinous portion separates from the solution, leaving a clear or slightly cloudy supernatant, which is decanted to a filter flask containing about 300 ml of cold distilled water. The flask is attached to a water-aspirator pump for 2 to 5 hours, until the odor of acetone becomes faint. The suspension is then decanted through a thin cotton filter to remove larger particles of collodion. The filtrate should be centrifuged for 5 minutes at $1000 \times g$, and the sediment resuspended in water, washed to remove acetone completely and centrifuged for 1 minute at 500 to $700 \times g$. The supernatant is used as the stock suspension of particles for the test. Cavelti's method of preparation of collodion particles is diagrammatically presented in Table 40.

The preparation of collodion particles by Arjona et al. (1954) employs crystal violet for staining the collodion particles and making them more easily visible. According to this method, 0.5 g of collodion is mixed with an acetone solution of crystal violet, shaken for 5 to 10 minutes, then transferred to 50 ml of distilled water, shaken for several minutes, and poured into 300 ml of 0.9% sodium chloride solution. This suspension should be shaken for 20 minutes, and left in the refrigerator for 24 hours. During this time, the collodion particles precipitate. The sediment should be washed three times with distilled water and diluted in saline to a final

Table 40. The Schedule of the Collodion Particles Preparation
(Cavelti, 1948)

10% collodium
+ 3 parts of acetone and 1 part of distilled water

Precipitate

+ Acetone
Colloidal solution of collodion particles

+ 3 parts of acetone and 1 part of water
40°, centrifugation at 200 × g

Precipitate

Supernatant

+ Acetone,
evaporation

Filtered through gauze
into cold water

—Combined—

Dry collodion particles

Filtration through gauze, centrifuged
5 minutes at 1000 × g

Precipitate

Supernatant,
centrifuged 1 hour
at 1000 × g

+ Distilled water

Precipitate

Combined + water

Centrifuged

Sediment

Washed in water,
centrifuged 3 minutes
at 1000 × g

Sediment

Supernatant

+ Water
centrifuged

Combined

Supernatant

Diluted 1:20, optical density
adjusted to McFarland's scale no. 2

concentration of 2000 million particles/ml, which corresponds to 6 to 7 turbidimetric degrees of the McFarland scale.

The optimal collodion concentration for use with an antigen is determined in the presence of a reference serum, if available, in the way suggested by Eisler (1941). In this technique, aliquots of 5.0, 3.0, 2.0, 1.0, 0.75, 0.5, and 0.25 ml of the stock collodion suspension are first sedimented by centrifugation. Each sediment is mixed with 1 ml of the antigen solution and 0.1-ml aliquots from each tube are added to equal volumes of serial dilutions of the reference serum. Control tubes receive saline solution instead of serum. The mixtures are incubated for 1 hour at 56°, then 0.5 ml of cold saline is added to each tube to facilitate reading, and the tubes are left in a cold room before reading.

The ratio between the antigen and the collodion suspension, at which the highest flocculation titer has been observed, is employed for the sensitization of collodion particles to be used in the test proper. The sensitization is conducted by mixing collodion particles with an optimum amount of the antigen and incubating this mixture for 15 minutes at room temperature. The sensitized collodion particles are then washed with saline and resuspended at the original volume. Alternatively, the antigen solution and the suspension of collodion particles can be added separately in the optimum ratio to a series of dilutions of the test serum. The test may be set up either in small tubes or on glass slides. The diluent is a 0.85 to 1.1% solution of sodium chloride.

The *test by Cannon and Marshall* is carried out by mixing 1-ml volumes of progressing dilutions of the examined serum with 1-ml aliquots of a suspension of sensitized collodion particles, their turbidity corresponding to tube 5 of the McFarland scale. Reference positive and negative sera and a tube containing 1 ml of saline and 1 ml of sensitized particles should be inserted as controls.

The tubes are shaken, left at room temperature for 10 minutes, then centrifuged for 4 minutes at 300 × g, and shaken again before being examined in front of a black screen for the presence of agglutinates. The highest dilution of a serum showing definite clumps of collodion particles in a clear supernatant fluid is taken as titer.

3. The Latex Flocculation (Fixation) Test

Particles of polyvinyl to toluene latex of $0.77\text{-}\mu$ diameter or polystyrene latex particles measuring between 0.81 to $1.17\text{-}\mu$ (produced by the Dow Chemical Company of the United States) are used in the test. The suspension of latex particles for the assay is prepared in the following manner (Rheins et al., 1957): an amount of 2 ml of the latex preparation is suspended in 20 ml of distilled water, agitated, and filtered through a Whatman no. 40 filter paper. The filtrate is then diluted with saline buffered at pH 8.2 so that 0.1 ml of this suspension mixed with 10 ml of borate buffer gives 70% light transmission in a spectrophotometer at 650-nm wavelength. Borate buffer consists of 50 ml of 0.1 M H_3BO_3, 5.9 ml of 0.1 M NaOH, and distilled water added to 100-ml volume. The suspension of latex particles is sensitized with an antigen, for example, a γ-globulin preparation, by mixing 0.1 ml of the latex suspension with 9.5 ml of buffered saline and 0.5 ml of 0.5% antigen solution. This mixture is kept at 37° for 30 to 60 minutes and used for the latext test.

Another technique for sensitization (Christian et al., 1958) employs 2 ml of the latex suspension mixed with a solution of nucleoprotein antigen in a saline glycine-NaOH buffer, pH 8.2. This mixture is centrifuged at 1500 rpm for 30 minutes. Packed latex particles are washed with buffer and resuspended in 200 ml of buffered saline.

The latex flocculation test (Plotz and Singer, 1956; Singer and Plotz, 1958) is conducted by mixing equal 1-ml volumes of progressing serum dilutions in a borate or 0.1 M glycine buffer with a sensitized latex suspension diluted 1:100. Control tubes receive saline instead of serum. The tubes are incubated at 56° for 2 hours, then centrifuged at 1500 $\times$ g for 3 minutes, and gently tapped. The degree of flocculation and the highest effective serum dilution are recorded. The test may also be conducted with smaller (0.1 ml) amounts of reactants.

In the latex flocculation test by Whang and Neter (1962) equal amounts of antigen dilutions and a 1:50 suspension of latex particles are incubated in a water bath at 37° for 30 minutes, in boiling water for 30 minutes, or in the autoclave at 121° for 15 minutes. The sensitized latex suspension (0.5 ml) is then mixed with antiserum in serial dilutions (0.5 ml). The mixtures are incubated in a water bath at 37° for 90 minutes, then centrifuged at 300 $\times$ g for 3 minutes, and shaken gently before reading.

The test, modified by Valkenburg (1963), differs from the Singer and Plotz's (1956) method by the following details: the 0.81-μ latex particles are stabilized with bovine serum albumin added to a final 0.2% concentration, and the latext is used at 1% concentration. A glycine buffer is employed as diluent, and the reaction mixtures are incubated at room temperature for 24 hours before centrifugation.

A glycine-saline buffer, pH 8.2, is used for the latex flocculation technique of Watson (1965). Serum dilutions are made in a volume of 0.2 ml of the buffer in the wells of a plastic tray, which then receive 0.05 ml of an antigen-coated latex reagent. The plates are rotated and covered with a transparent plastic sheet to prevent evaporation. The wells are observed during the following 15 minutes while the trays are gently tilted over a view box. Flocculation is marked by the aggregation of particles clearly visible.

The latex flocculation test of Bercks (1967), as slightly modified by Salih et al. (1968), is set up in the following conditions: the latex preparation, containing 1.5% (w/v) solids or approximately 1.5×10^{10} particles/ml (0.81-μ diameter), is diluted 1:14 with 0.9% NaCl and added to an equal volume of an antiserum globulin solution, and incubated at room temperature for 30 minutes. The coated latex suspension is then centrifuged at 5000 × g for 30 minutes; the sediment is washed in saline and resuspended in half a volume of 0.2 M Tris-HCl buffer, pH 7.2, containing 0.02% polyvinyl pyrrolidone. Two drops of the antibody-sensitized latex particles are then added to one drop of different, twofold dilutions of an antigen made in the same buffer, on a glass plate painted black on the reverse side. The mixture is gently rocked for 10 minutes and observed for the presence of floccules. Controls consist of (a) the sensitized latex mixed with buffer, (b) nonsensitized latex suspension with the antigen, and (c) the sensitized latex particles with a heterologous antigen. A positive reaction is signified by the presence of loose aggregates within 3 to 5 minutes whereas the lack of flocculation was indicated by a milky suspension.

A maximum sensitivity of the test is obtained in optimum concentration of antiserum globulins used for sensitization of latex particles, which has to be determined prior to the main test.

The Florman and Scoma (1960) Technique for Latex Flocculation. Latex particles to be used for this assay are sensitized by mixing 0.5-ml volume of a bacterial suspension with 0.2-ml volume of a latex suspension and with 4.3 ml of a glycine-saline buffer, pH 8.2. After standing 70 minutes at room temperature, 0.5 ml of the antigen-latex mixture is added to tubes containing a volume of a serially diluted serum. Control tubes receive a nonspecific serum and the antigen-latex mixture. All tubes are agitated, incubated at 56° for 1 ½ hours, centrifuged at 1000 × g for 3 minutes, and read.

A positive reaction is indicated by a clear supernatant, and a negative reaction by a turbid supernatant.

Optimal conditions for the virus absorption on latex particles were found by Aubert et al. to be 1 hour at 37°, and for the latex-flocculation test 2 hours at 56°, followed by centrifugation of test tubes.

Saline flocculation or saline precipitation can sometimes be observed in the serum with a high concentration of the rheumatoid factor (rheumatoid reagins). This phenomenon, which bears a similarity to the flocculation of nonsensitized collodion particles, is induced by a 4:1 dilution of the sedum in 0.85% sodium chloride and incubated at 37° for 2 hours and at 2° overnight (Wallis, 1956; Kwapinski et al., 1956).

4. The Bismuth-Tannate Flocculation Test

In the test designed by Pick and Nelken (1963), particles of bismuth tannate containing 40% bismuth monoxide, insoluble in water, are used as antigen carriers. A suspension of bismuth tannate particles for the flocculation test is obtained by mixing 2 g of bismuth tannate to 10 ml of 0.85% sodium chloride solution and homogenizing the suspension in an homogenizer. Since the suspension of bismuth tannate particles consists of varying sized particles, the suspension is left undisturbed for 30 seconds to allow the larger particles to settle. The suspension is then decanted into another test tube and centrifuged for 3 minutes at 500 × g. The stock suspension prepared from the sediment may be kept in a refrigerator for many weeks. The 0.3 ml of the sediment are added to 9.7 ml of saline for use in the bismuth tannate flocculation test.

Adsorption of an antigen onto the bismuth tannate particles is attained by mixing equal volumes of the bismuth tannate suspension and an antigen solution made in saline and agitating the suspension at room temperature for 30 minutes. The coated bismuth tannate particles are then washed three times in saline to remove the unadsorbed antigen. The antigen-coated bismuth tannate particles are finally resuspended in saline.

A flocculation test is set up by preparing a series of antiserum dilutions in volumes of 0.2 ml using a 1.5% saline solution of normal rabbit serum as deluant. Each tube containing a serum dilution then receives 1 drop of the antigen-coated bismuth tannate particles. Control tubes contain no antiserum or a normal serum instead of antiserum. The tubes are shaken vigorously for 3 minutes and left in a refrigerator for 2 hours. After 2 hours, the tubes are shaken again and left at room temperature for at least 4 hours before the readings are made. Another reading is performed after overnight incubation.

A flocculation of the antigen-coated bismuth tannate particles, caused by antibodies, is signified by an irregular, thick denticular ring or a coarse brownish disk present on the tube bottom. If no flocculation occurs, a regular ring with or without a central point, or a brownish, uniform coating of the whole bottom of tube is observed.

The bismuth tannate flocculation-inhibition test can be carried out by adding the inhibiting antigen to the antiserum 30 minutes before the addition of the antigen-coated particles and comparing the patterns of sedimentation to that of the tubes containing the antiserum which has not been exposed to the inhibiting antigen. Bismuth tannate particles are able to only absorb protein antigens whereas nonprotein antigens are not adsorbable to the particles.

Bismuth tannate may be prepared by allowing an aqueous solution of $Bi(NO_3)_3.5H_2O$ slightly acidified by nitric acid, to react with an alkaline solution of tannic acid. A yellowish precipitate, which occurs in this condition, is washed five times with a large amount of saline and then dried. The powder should be carefully grounded.

5. The Resin-Particles Flocculation Test

Ion exchange resin particles, as carriers of antigens, were introduced by Evans and Haines (1954). The test arranged by Segre (1957) for the detection of viral antigens is conducted in the following manner: a basic anion exchanger, Amberlite IRA-400 Cor IR-4B, should be finely ground and suspended in distilled water. The suspension is allowed to settle for 30 minutes. The sediment is then discarded, and the supernatant fluid is centrifuged at 300 × g for 5 minutes. The sediment should now be collected and washed once in 1.0 N NaOH, and four to five times in distilled water. Finally, packed resin particles are resuspended in the diluent (0.1 *M* tris-(hydroxymethyl-aminomethane) to give 5% light transmittance at 450-nm wavelength. Resin particles thus prepared are coated with an antibody contained in the isolated γ-globulin by adding 1 mg of the γ-globulin preparation, diluted in 1 ml of diluent, to 1 ml of the resin particle suspension. The mixture is shaken during the 10-minute period of incubation at room temperature, then centrifuged at 200 × g for 2 minutes. The packed antibody-coated resin particles are resuspended in 2 volumes of the diluent.

A series of twofold virus dilutions are now made in the diluent containing 2% normal calf serum, used to stabilize the resin particle suspension and to prevent a spontaneous agglutination of these particles. One drop of each virus dilution is mixed on a glass plate with one drop of the sensitized resin particle suspension. After thorough mixing, the plate is rotated for a few minutes and read. Clumping of resin particles is easily observed in the case of a positive reaction.

6. *The Virus-Protamine Flocculation Test*

The test, described by Roberts (1949), and used for studying antipoliomyclitis virus antibodies, depends on the flocculation of viruses absorbed on protamine particles in a specific antivirus serum. The optimal amount of protamine for absorption of virus particles must be determined prior to the test proper. For this purpose, varying quantities of a protamine sulfate solution are added to a constant amount of a partially purified virus suspension, and incubated first at room temperature, then at 43°.

These suspensions of virus-absorbed protamine are transferred to equal volumes of serial twofold dilutions of an inactivated antiserum and incubated at 43° for 3 hours. The amount of protamine which gives the most pronounced flocculation at the relatively high serum dilution is employed as carrier of antigen for the flocculation test proper.

The test is set up by mixing equal volumes of the protamine absorbed antigen and varying dilutions of examined sera. The mixtures are incubated at 43° for 3 hours. The highest serum dilution showing definite floccules is taken as end point and the flocculation titer.

7. *The Acryl Flocculation Test*

Acryl (polymethyl metacryl) plast particles, with the size of 0.5 μ used in the test (Winblad, 1960), are first homogenized in distilled water by shaking them with glass beads. They are then left at room temperature for

20 minutes to sediment larger particles. The supernatant is withdrawn and mixed 10.18 with a borate buffer; 0.5-ml volumes of acryl particles are added to equal amounts of a serum or serum fraction, followed by 1.2 ml of 5% solution of the sensitizing antigen. The tubes are shaken and incubated at 56° for 18 hours, then read. If floccules or a sediment are observed, the reaction is regarded as positive. A uniform suspension is indicative of a negative result.

(The borate buffer used in the test consists of 0.85% sodium chloride, 5.0 ml of 0.1 M boric acid, 5.9 ml of 0.1 M sodium hydroxide, and distilled water added up to 100 ml.)

8. *The Bentonite-Flocculation Test*

This test depends on an immunologic reaction between molecules of an antigen adsorbed onto bentonite particles and a specific antibody. A stock bentonite suspension for absorption of antigens is made as described by Bloch and Bunim (1959): 0.5 g of Wyoming bentonite (B.C. μ or no. 200 standard Volclay) is suspended in 100 ml of distilled water. The suspension is homogenized in a Waring blender for 1 minute, and this procedure is repeated after 5 minutes for another minute. The bentonite suspension is transferred to a 500-ml glass-stoppered graduate which is filled to volume with distilled water, shaken vigorously, and allowed to settle for 1 hour. The supernatant fluid is removed and centrifuged in 100-ml tubes at 300 × g for 15 minutes. The supernatant collected is again centrifuged at 300 × g for 15 minutes. Following this centrifugation, the supernatant fluid is discarded. The sediment is resuspended in 100 ml of distilled water, and homogenized in a Waring blender for 1 minute. This stock bentonite suspension is stable for 6 months.

The bentonite particles are sensitized in the following manner: 100 ml of the stock bentonite suspension are centrifuged at 1000 × g for 5 minutes; the supernatant is discarded, and the sediment is resuspended in 1 ml of distilled water. This sediment is mixed with 2 ml of a solution of an antigen preparation which should usually contain 2- to 5-mg dry mass in that volume. The mixture is agitated in an electric shaker at 37° for 30 minutes to allow absorption. Distilled water to the amount of 15.0 ml is added, and this suspension is carefully mixed, followed by centrifugation at 1000 × g for 5 minutes. The sediment is washed twice with distilled water and resuspended in 5.0 ml of distilled water, to which 1 ml of 0.1% methylene blue is added. After being shaken for 5 minutes, the volume is brought to 10 ml with distilled water. This stained suspension is centrifuged, and the sediment is washed in distilled water, centrifuged again, and finally resuspended in 4 ml of 0.05 M phosphate buffer, pH 7.3, containing 0.1 of 1% polysorbate 80 (Tween 80) to stabilize the suspension (although no stabilization is required for most of antigen preparations). This suspension is the sensitized bentonite antigen for the immunologic test.

The bentonite-flocculation test is set out on glass slides with twelve small rings or indisposable concavity slides (Bozicevich et al., 1958; Bloch and Bunim, 1959; Kwapinski, 1962; Wallace et al., 1966, 1970).

According to Kwapinski's procedure, the inactivated serum under test is serially diluted from 1:5 to 1:640 in saline buffered at pH 7.4. From each dilution a 0.1-ml volume is placed in a corresponding ring on a slide, and one drop of a bentonite suspension "sensitized" with an antigen preparation is added. Control rings receive 0.1 ml of the buffered saline and a drop of the "sensitized" bentonite suspension, or 0.1 ml of the serum diluted 1:5 and one drop of the nonsensitized bentonite suspension. One row of dilutions of a "positive" reference serum, if available, and one row of a "negative" reference serum are also set out as controls for each series of tests. The slide is now rotated on a rotating machine at 100 to 120 rpm for 20 minutes. Results are immediately read under a high dry microscope magnification and expressed in symbols + up to + + + + or − as follows:

> + + + + when all the "sensitized" particles are clumped in floccules floating in a clear fluid.
>
> + + + when approximately three-fourths of the "sensitized" particles are clumped.
>
> + + when half of the particles are clumped and half still remain in a colloidal suspension.
>
> + when only one-fourth of the bentonite particles are clumped.
>
> − a colloidal, turbid suspension with no floccules visible.

The result of the bentonite flocculation test is regarded as positive when a 2+ + or stronger clumping of the "sensitized" bentonite particles is observed in a serum dilution of 1:32 or higher and all the controls are negative except the "positive" reference serum.

According to Wallace's et al. method, 0.1 ml or 2 drops of a serum dilution are placed in the concavities on disposable concavity slides followed by an equal volume of sensitized bentonite suspension. The slides are shaken for 20 minutes (100 rotations/minute) on an Eberbach rotator and read immediately at a magnification 60 times. The antibody titer is read according to the final dilution of serum which caused clumping of all the sensitized bentonite particles. The bentonite flocculation test has been used for detection of tuberculosis antibodies and gonococcal antibodies (Wallace et al., 1966, 1970).

9. The Kaolin-Flocculation Test

The kaolin powder for this test must have a proper absorbent power following heating to redness. (An adequate kaolin powder is available in the Meiji Chemical Company Ltd., Tokyo, Japan.) The kaolin powder should be washed with 5% hydrochloric acid for 24 to 24 hours under constant agitation, then rinsed with deionized water to remove the acid, and dried at 120°. The dry kaolin is then heated to redness for exactly 2 hours in an electric forge, at 800°, cooled, and pulverized mechanically in a porcelain mortar, for 2 $\frac{1}{2}$ hours. At the end of pulverization, an adequate amount of deionized water is added to the mortar to obtain a thick suspension of kaolin, then washed in deionized water, and centrifuged. A standard kaolin suspension is prepared to contain exactly 1.0 mg of kaolin per milliliter of deionized water. This suspension, distributed into glass ampules and sealed, should be heated at 100° for 15 minutes in the Koch apparatus, in two consecutive days. This standard kaolin suspension is usable for at least 1 year.

The sensitization of kaolin with an antigen is carried out as follows (Takahashi, 1962): one part of the antigen solution diluted with 19 parts of a buffered saline, pH 6.6 to 6.8, is mixed with one-half of the standard kaolin suspension. The mixture is incubated at 37° for 30 minutes, with occasional shaking.

The kaolin flocculation test is set up by adding 0.1 ml of the sensitized kaolin suspension to tubes containing varying serum dilutions in 0.5-ml volume, and to a control tube containing 0.5 ml of buffered saline alone. The mixtures are incubated at 37° for 30 minutes, with occasional shaking, then centrifuged at 300 to 500 × g for 5 minutes.

Readings are made by gently shaking the tubes against a sheet of black pasteboard under the fluorescent lamp light. The highest serum dilution showing flocculates is taken as end point and titer.

Diluent used in the test is a TME buffered saline prepared by adding 1 part of TME buffer to 9 parts of 0.85% sodium chloride solution. The TME buffer contains 12.1 g of tris-(hydroxymethyl)-aminomethane, 11.6 g of anhydrous maleic acid, 5.63 g of EDTA (disodium ethylene-diamine-tetraacetate), 0.05 g of Tween 80, and 3.75 g of sodium hydroxide per 1000 ml of deionized water. This solution is adjusted to pH 6.6 to 6.8 with 1 N NaOH. Tween 80 is used to prevent spontaneous flocculation.

10. The Barium Sulfate Flocculation Test

According to Gilboa-Garber and Nelken (1963), the test is set up in the following way: an antigen solution is added to an equal volume of 3% barium sulfate suspension in saline, and the mixture is shaken at room temperature for 2 minutes. The sensitized barium sulfate particles are washed three times in saline and resuspended in a saline containing 10% normal rabbit serum to the original 3% concentration.

To perform the test, serial dilutions of an antiserum are made in 0.2-ml volumes to which 0.05 ml of the sensitized barium sulfate suspension is added subsequently. The serum dilutions are made in a saline containing 10% normal rabbit serum, although the optimal rabbit serum concentration may vary from 5 to 10% as predetermined for each immune system so as to obtain complete negative controls. The control tubes contain the diluent and antigen-coated barium sulfate suspension. The tubes are shaken vigorously, left at room temperature; the pattern of sedimentation is observed at 30 to 60 minutes with a mirror placed underneath the tubes at an angle of 45°.

Flocculation is signified by a sedimentation in the form of denticular curved lines of the deposit whereas a negative result is indicated by a sedimentation in a form of a regular ring.

11. The Oil-Droplets Aggregation Test

This test, devised by Boroff (1938) and Boroff and Tripp (1947), is carried out as follows. The antigen is prepared by emulsifying 5 ml of 0.01% solution of an antigen in 0.1-ml volume of olive oil by the aid of a magnetoconstriction oscillator to a milky, stable suspension. The test may be set up either in tubes or on microslides.

In the first case, equal volumes of progressing dilutions of a serum and an antigen emulsion are placed in a row of tubes, and the mixtures are incubated overnight at 56°. If the test is positive, the agglutinated oil globules accumulate in a creamy layer on the surface of the liquid; the reaction is evaluated by the degree of clearness of the underlying liquid. The fluid remains turbid if no agglutination has occurred.

The slide agglutination test is carried out by mixing one drop of the antigen emulsion and one drop of serum on a microslide. If the result is positive, the oil globules aggregate in large clumps that are visible to the unaided eye. Alternatively, this test may be set out in the following manner. A cover slip is attached to a microslide by means of paraffn placed on two opposite edges of the slip. One drop of the antigen emulsion and one drop of a serum are put rectangularly from opposite directions, under the cover slip, so that they meet in the middle. The cover slip is then sealed and examined with the dark-field microscope for the presence of aggregates of oil drops.

VII. EVALUATION AND APPLICATION OF FLOCCULATION TESTS

The toxin-antitoxin flocculation test is a very sensitive method for the determination of the potency of antitoxins, toxins, and toxoids. The

Brucella-flocculation test has not been employed as widely for the titration of *Brucella* antibodies and for the immunologic diagnosis of brucellosis as the Wright agglutination test. However, in our experience, this flocculation test is more sensitive than the conventional agglutination technique.

Cholesterol-flocculation tests are commonly used for the serological diagnosis of syphilis and, less widely, for the diagnosis of brucellosis and trichinosis. In the latter two cases, phenol extracts of *Brucella abortus* or alkaline extracts of trichinae larvae are used to coat cholesterol crystals. Lecithin is added to enhance the sensitivity of the test (Hunter and Colbert, 1956). The sensitivity of the VDRL test is usually found greater in comparison with other flocculation tests or with Kolmer's complement fixation test. Collodion and latex particles and, to a lesser extent, bentonite particles and oil globules enhance the intensity and sensitivity of certain serological reactions, which show only a very weak precepitation, by converting them into an agglutination reaction. By the absorption of antigens or antibodies on larger, inert particles not only the antibody titers of weak sera increase but also incomplete antibodies can be detected, for which the precipitin test proves to be not sensitive enough.

The collodion flocculation test has been employed to studies of reactions between tuberculin and tuberculous antibodies (Weir, 1941), between antigens of *Diplococcus pneumoniae, Neisseria meningitidis,* or *Neisseria gonorrhoeae* and antibacterial sera (Eisler, 1941), between the viruses of influenza, yellow fever or poliomyelitis and immune sera (Goodner, 1941), between the egg protein or crystalline insulin and their antibodies (Cannon and Marshall, 1941), between tissue antigens and antibodies, to include autoantibodies. The test has also been adapted to the investigation of certain serologically active substances occurring in the viral hepatitis (Havens and Eichman, 1950) and rheumatoid arthritis (Reiholec and Wagner, 1955; Kwapinski and Snyder, 1962). The kaolin flocculation test has been successfully introduced to the immunodiagnosis of tuberculosis. (Takahashi, 1962).

The flocculation tests utilizing sensitized inert particles are more rapid and often more sensitive methods than "passive" haemagglutination tests. The vehicle particles do not require any pretreatment for proteinaceous antigens and the incubation period is very short. The barium sulfate particles, for example, coated with an antigen, are stable and may be preserved for at least 14 days. The sedimentation patterns in the positive and negative tube can be observed for a number of days without a change. Finally, no absorption of antiserum or normal rabbit serum is needed since the barium sulfate particles are antigenically inert.

Latex and bentonite tests and, to a lesser extent, acryl and mastix assays have been used primarily to detect rheumatoid heteroreagins (Kwapinski and Snyder, 1961). Applications of the latex flocculation test have been greatly extended in the sixties to fields such as: the detection of antibodies in leptospiroses and viral infections, and detection of antithyroid antibodies and antinuclear factors. The latex test has also been employed for the examination of antigenic relationships between bacteria (Florman and Scoma, 1960; Aubert et al., 1962; Vosta, 1963). The latex test has been found to be a 25 to 100 times more sensitive test than a tube precipitation test for the identification of isometric viruses (Abu Salih et al., 1968), but about 10 times less sensitive than the passive hemagglutination. The latex-inhibition test (see p. 541) is used for immunological detection of pregnancy. The resin flocculation test has been employed to detect viral antigens.

The oil-droplets agglutination test has been used for the study of serological activity of some soluble antigens, for example, proteins of streptococci (Boroff and Tripp, 1947). Nonspecific reactions which are very seldom observed in these tests are due mostly to an inadequate sort of inert particles used, for example, those larger than $4\ \mu$ in diameter, to a faulty preparation of antigen carriers, or to a long storage of stock solutions.

Chapter Nine

HEMAGGLUTINATION TESTS

Hemagglutination depends on the clumping of erythrocytes either under direct action of hemagglutinins produced by some microorganisms and higher plants, or under indirect influence of specific serum hemagglutinins. Plant hemagglutinins, formed by some species of bacteria, microfungi, viruses, and higher plants, either remain inside or are secreted outside the cells. Most hemagglutinins are predominantly glycopeptides and are able to absorb onto red blood cells bringing them into close contact and aggregation. These substances function as complete antigens, capable of inducing the formation of specific antibodies in animals. Homologous antibodies brought in contact with the corresponding hemagglutinins prevent the agglutination of erythrocytes due to the neutralization of hemagglutinins. Microbial hemagglutinis occur in culture filtrates and supernatants of casein digest broth cultures, in the phosphatide, polysaccharide, and nucleoprotein fractions isolated from certain bacteria and microfungi, and in elementary bodies of some viruses (Table 41).

The serum hemagglutinins are specific antibody globulins that can be induced by the immunization with crude or purified plant hemagglutinins or by an infection with the hemagglutinin-producing microorganisms. Since the specific hemagglutinins can occur not only in the serum but also in other body fluids a general name of "animal hemagglutinins" is proposed for these substances. Animal hemagglutinins may combine either (a) with specific antigens which either occur normally in the cell walls or erythrocytes (isoagglutinogens, isohemagglutinogens) or can be uncovered by certain enzymes or (b) with the antigens absorbed by erythrocytes under artificial conditions. The latter group of sensitizing antigens is appropriately called hemosensitins. The large group of hemagglutination reactions may be classified thus:

1. Direct or active, microbial hemagglutinin tests: the bacterial hemagglutination and the virus hemagglutination.
2. Indirect hemagglutination tests: the hemosensitin hemagglutination, the enhanced hemagglutination, and the conglutination.

Table 41. Hemosensitins of Microorganisms Adsorbable onto
Plain Erythrocytes

Species of Microorganisms	Hemosinsitin Found in	Author
Streptococcus pyogenes	Polysaccharide	Keogh et al., 1948; Kwapinski, 1958
Diplococcus pneumoniae	Polysaccharide	Keogh et al., 1948; Hayes, 1951; Bier, 1951
Neisseria meningitidis	Polysaccharide	Keogh et al., 1958; Jyssum,
Neisseria gonorrhoeae	Polysaccharide	1956; Thomas and Mennic, 1950
Corynebacterium diphtheriae	Polysaccharide	Hayes, 1951; Chen, 1952
Actinobacillus mallei; *Actinobacillus whitemori*	Crude extract	Boyden, 1950; Boyden, 1950
Francisella tularensis	Lipopolysaccharide Polysaccharide	Alexander et al., 1950; Wright and Feinberg, 1952; Charkes, 1959
Pasteurella pestis	Polysaccharide	Amies, 1957; Chen, 1952; Neel et al., 1950; Payne et al., 1956
Pasteurella multocida	Capsular antigen	Chen, 1952; Neel et al., 1950
Brucella abortus	Crude extract	Carrere and Roux, 1952
Haemophilus influenzae	Polysaccharide	Keogh et al., 1957, 1958; Fisher,
Haemophilus pertussis	Crude	1950
Treponema reiteri	Polysaccharide	Pillot, 1969
Veillonella	Lipopolysaccharide	Mergenhagen and Varah, 1963
Erysipelothrix	Polysaccharide	Truszczynski, 1957
Listeria monocytogenes	Polysaccharide	Potel and Degen, 1962
Chromobacterium	Lipopolysaccharide	Davies et al., 1958
Mycobacterium tuberculosis	Saline extract of 90% phenol extracted mycobacteria and polysaccharide fraction of cells and tuberculin	Davies et al., 1958; Middlebrook and Dubos, 1948; Sorkin and Boyden, 1955; Kwapinski, 1959
Klebsiella aerogenes	Polysaccharide	MacPherson et al., 1953;
Klebsiella cloacae	Polysaccharide	MacPherson et al., 1953
Salmonella typhosa	Lipopolysaccharide, Polysaccharide	Keogh et al., 1958; Spaun, 1952; Corvazier, 1952; Landy and Lamb, 1953
Salmonella typhi-murium; *Salmonella derby* *Salmonella pullorum*	Polysaccharide	Keogh et al., 1948
Shigella dysenteriae	Polysaccharide	Neter and Gorzynski, cf. Slopek, 1969
Shigella flexneri		Chun and Park, 1956
Shigella sonnei	Crude, polysaccharide	Hayes and Stanley, 1950; Hayes, 1951
Rickettsiae	Crude extract	Chang, 1953
Candida albicans	Polysaccharide	Vogel and Collins, 1955
Entamoeba histolytica	Crude extract	Kessel et al., 1961

3. Hemagglutination of nonsensitized erythrocytes: the cold hemagglutination, the heterophile hemagglutination, immune hemagglutination, the T-hemagglutination, the bacteriogenic hemagglutination, and the isohemagglutination.

I. THE DIRECT MICROBIAL HEMAGGLUTININ TESTS

The direct or active microbial hemagglutination is caused by the adsorption of certain viscous substances of microbial origin onto the erythrocytes, which results in the conglomeration and sedimentation of red blood cells. Fimbriae or heat labile antigens of fimbriae, which occur in some species of bacteria (e.g., *Escherichia coli, Shigella flexneri*), have been found responsible for hemagglutinating activities of intact bacteria. Only fimbriate strains were able to clump red blood cells (Duguid et al., 1955; Duguid and Gillies, 1957). The hemagglutinating viruses presumably adsorb onto the mucoprotein of the erythrocyte surface. Virus receptors can be destroyed by mucinases produced by many bacteria, particularly by *Vibrio comma*. The virus-caused hemagglutination may be inhibited by specific antibodies, the antihemagglutinins.

Most microbial hemagglutinins are capable of agglutinating erythrocytes of the man, rabbit, guinea pig, mouse, and fowl although the agglutinability of red blood cells of individual animal species by certain microbial hemagglutinins may vary occasionally. For example, *Haemophilus aegypticus* clumps human erythrocytes, but those of monkey, rabbit, and rat are not affected; *Poxvirus variolae* agglutinates only chicken red blood cells (Marennikova and Akatova, 1958). Erythrocytes of the cat are agglutinated by influenza B virus, but not by viruses influenzae A or C, or by the swine influenza virus, mumps, or Newcastle disease viruses (Tamm, 1954). Red blood cells which are ordinarily not liable to the agglutination by virus particles can become agglutinable after the trypsinization. A close correlation may sometimes be revealed between the hemagglutinin content of a strain, and its virulence or antigenic potency. For example, virulent strains of *Haemophilus bronchisepticus* are rich in hemagglutinin, whereas avirulent, nonhemolytic variants do not contain hemagglutinins at all (Keogh et al., 1947). Hemagglutinins occur more frequently and at higher concentrations in the freshly isolated than in subcultured strains. Substances agglutinating red blood cells were also detected in the *Basidiomycetes* (Ford, 1911; Bernheimer and Farkas, 1953), seed-bearing plants (Renkonen, 1948; Boyd, 1950), and in acetone-etheric extracts of certain animal organs infected with viruses.

1. The Bacterial Hemagglutinin Test

Thiele's Technique. This technique provides twofold dilutions of an extract, filtrate, or saline suspension of bacterial cells made in 0.9-ml volumes of 0.9% sodium chloride solution. A control tube contains saline alone. All tubes receive 0.1-ml volumes of a 5% suspension of chicken or human red blood cells and are left at 37° for 1 ½ hours. The end point of the reaction is then determined by the last tube showing complete hemagglutination, whereas the control tube must show no clumping of erythrocytes. Titers of crude preparations of bacterial hemagglutinins usually range between 1:8 and 1:32.

Kwapinski's Technique. An extract or a preparation of bacterial or fungal hemagglutinins is first diluted serially from 1:5 to 1:320 in 0.2-ml volume of the saline buffered at pH 7.0. The volume of liquid in each tube is then made up to 0.4 ml by adding 0.2 ml of buffered saline. An 0.2-ml amount of 1 to 2% suspension of washed, human, rabbit, or chicken erythrocytes is added to all tubes, including two control tubes which contain 0.4 ml of the buffered saline alone. The tubes are shaken and incubated at 37° for 2 to 3 hours, and then left at 6 to 10° for 12 to 16 hours. The hemagglutinin titer is expressed in terms of the highest dilution of the preparation examined, which produces a macroscopically detectable agglutination whereas no agglutination should be observed in the control tubes. The corresponding amount of hemagglutinin in the end-point tube is regarded as one hemagglutinating unit. A similar test was published by Dolby (1958).

A *micromodification* of the test, by Bernheimer and Farkas (1953), employs 0.01-ml quantities of a tested extract, diluted serially in 0.9% sodium chloride, and 0.4 ml of a 3% suspension of human erythrocytes.

A similar test, devised originally for fimbrial hemagglutinins (Gillies and Duguid, 1958), is set up in depressions on a white porcelain tile. One drop of 3% guinea pig erythrocytes is placed in the depressions followed by one drop of a broth culture of fimbriate bacteria taken at various stages of the growth. The tile is rocked to and fro at room temperature for 5 minutes or more and inspected for the presence of clumps.

2. The Microfungal Hemagglutinin Test

Dilutions of filtrates of microfungi growing in a Sabouraud or Kwapinski's semisynthetic medium (p. 12) are made in 0.3 ml of saline buffered at pH 7.2; 0.2 ml of 3% chicken red blood cells suspension is added to each tube, including a control tube containing 0.3 ml of the phosphate buffered saline. The tubes are left at room temperature for 5 hours and at 2° overnight, then read. The highest dilution of the filtrate showing a definite hemagglutination is taken as end point.

3. The Virus Hemagglutinin Test

The virus agglutination of erythrocytes is caused in most cases by the attachment of virus particles to the surface of red blood cells; but some viruses (the viruses of variola, vaccinia, ectromelia, meningo-pneumonitis, and hepatitis contagiosa canis) produce a soluble substance which is separate from the virus particles and elicits the hemagglutinating activity. Virus hemagglutinins behave like enzymes which can destroy the mucoprotein present on the erythrocyte surface.

The following viruses are adsorbable to the erythrocytes causing clumping of the cells: viruses of influenza, parainfluenza, mumps, Newcastle disease, smallpox, vaccinia, measles, St. Louis encephalitis, Western equine encephalitis, Japanese B encephalitis, Venezuelan equine encephalitis, West Nile fever, as well as adenoviruses, Dengue virus, respiratory syncytial virus, and some enteroviruses.

Two reactants participate in the virus hemagglutination test, a virus suspension and a 0.25 to 1.0% erythrocyte suspension. Chicken red blood cells are used most commonly; however, erythrocytes of man, group O, guinea pig, cat, or other mammals may sometimes prove to be more advantageous. Chicken blood is obtained either by cardiac puncture or from the wing vein and mixed immediately with a 5% solution of sodium citrate, in the proportion of 10:1. A 10% stock suspension in saline is prepared by volume from the red blood cells sedimented by centrifugation at 300 × g for exactly 10 minutes. This stock suspension can be kept at 4° and used within a week. Some viruses, for example, Newcastle disease virus, appear to be adsorbed by erythroctyes more completely at 4° than at higher temperatures (Florman, 1947), giving at 40° more distinct and clear-cut results. Thus it is advisable to carry out a virus hemagglutination test at various temperature levels and to choose optimal conditions for a particular virus. Techniques of virus hemagglutination test, by Salk (1944) and Horsfall and Tamm (1953), the test on hollowed plastic trays by Fazekas de St. Groth and Graham (1954), and the spectrophotometric determination of virus hemagglutinins by Hirst and Pickels (1942) are recommended.

The Virus Hemagglutination Test, by Salk. A 0.25% suspension of chicken red blood cells is made from a stock 10% erythrocyte suspension by mixing 2 to 5 ml of this suspension with 100 ml of saline solution; 0.5-ml amounts of the erythrocyte suspension are then added to 0.5-ml volumes of serially diluted virus preparation. Control tubes receive 0.5 ml of the saline solution and 0.5 ml of 0.25% erythrocyte suspension.

The mixtures are shaken and left at room temperature for 2 hours. Patterns of sedimented erythrocytes are examined by observing them through a perforated rack, either directly or at the reflection from a mirror fixed at a proper angle under a small glass-top table. A uniform salmon-pink film covering the entire bottom indicates a strong hemagglutination. If the agglutination is weaker, irregular clumps of cells surrounded by a halo of finely aggregated or nonagglutinated erythrocytes are seen. A small central, compact, sharply demarcated red disk with smooth edges is visible if no hemagglutination occurs. When tubes are tilted horizintally the cells run smoothly down the bottom and do not stick to the margins, as in the case of hemagglutination. The highest dilution of the virus, at which a complete hemagglutination occurred, is taken as end point, and the corresponding amount of the virus is arbitrarily considered as one agglutinating unit.

The Virus Hemagglutination Test, by Horsfall and Tamm. Serial twofold dilutions of a virus suspension are made in 0.4- to 0.5-ml volumes of buffered saline (0.85% NaCl solution, buffered at pH 7.2 with 0.01 or 0.02 M phosphate). Equal volumes of 1 or 0.5% suspension of chicken red blood cells are added to each tube. The mixtures are shaken and left either at 24° or at 40 to 50° for 1 to 3 hours. Readings are made by observing patterns of the red blood cells on the bottom of the tubes, and the end point is taken as the highest dilution showing definite hemagglutination.

The Virus Hemagglutination Test, by Fazekas de St. Groth and Graham. This is set up in hollowed plastic trays, by adding 0.075 ml of a 10% fowl red blood cells to 0.25-ml volumes of serial twofold dilutions of the test material. The mixtures are agitated and results read after 20 minutes' incubation at 18 to 24°.

4. The Spectrophotometric Determination of Hemagglutinins

The virus hemagglutination, and in fact any hemagglutination or agglutination, may be evaluated more accurately by photoelectric measurement of the density of immune systems. This procedure depends on the constant rate of the cells settling. Normal nonagglutinated cells left in test tubes for a short time form the following three layers: (1) a top clear layer devoid of cells, (b) a middle layer of sedimenting cells of uniform density, and (c) a bottom layer of settled cells. The concentration of agglutinated cells and the corresponding density of the middle layer is lower than that of the control, nonagglutinated cells.

The test devised by Hirst and Pickels (1942), as modified by Levine et al. (1953), is carried out as follows. Washed chicken erythrocytes, suspended in 0.9% saline prepared in 0.01 M phosphate buffer at a desired pH to give the concentration of 5.8×10^7 red blood cells per milliliter, are distributed in 6.0-ml volume into a series of 100×13-mm Pyrex tubes. Serial, progressive dilutions of the virus preparation in a volume of 0.5 or 1 ml are added to each tube. The mixtures are held at room temperature for an adequate time, for example, 65 or 75 minutes. The optical densities are determined every 10 minutes by means of a Beckman model B spectrophotometer, at 490 nm. The height of the light beam should be adjusted so as to intercept the liquid column at a certain level below the meniscus, according to the position of the middle layer of the settling cell column. The end point is taken as the quantity of viruses which caused a 50% decrease in the optical density under selected conditions. From the data obtained, the number of hemagglutinating particles is calculated by plotting optical densities against time in minutes. The absolute number of hemagglutinating particles in the suspension is calculated from a dilution which exhibits a linear settling curve. A similar test was described by Drescher et al. (1962).

5. The Platelet Aggregation Test

The test is based on the observation that human blood platelets are able to interact with virus particles which cause aggregation of the platelets. This aggregating action of virus particles, for example, Newcastle disease virus, is inhibited by specific virus antibodies. Platelets are also aggregated by complexes consisting of soluble, or small-size viral antigens and their antibodies.

The platelet aggregation test according to Penttinen and Myllylä (1968) as modified by Palosuo et al. (1970) is conducted as follows: test sera, inactivated at 56° for 30 minutes, are serially diluted in a buffered saline solution and added to different antigen solutions, in equal 0.025-ml volume. Each tube serum receives 0.05 ml of a platelet suspension. The test mixtures are shaken and left at 28° overnight after which the sedimentation pattern of platelet is observed.

Since approximately 15% of individual lots of platelets are not satisfactorily aggregated by soluble immune complexes; thus pools of three individual lots of platelets are to be used.

The direct, active platelet aggregation test is used for detection of agglutinins produced by certain virus particles as a preliminary stage for a platelet aggregation-inhibition test, performed in much the same manner as the hemagglutinin-inhibition test. The platelet aggregation by antigen-antibody complexes is used for measuring antibodies against small size viral antigen. The latter test is very useful in the study on monovalent, antihapten antibodies. The hapten is coupled to a bovine serum albumin (Penttinen et al., 1969). The platelet aggregation test has been found to be 16 times more sensitive than the complement fixation test, applied for determination of antibodies and 100 times more sensitive when antigens are measured.

The platelet aggregation tests were successfully used for detection and measurement of antibodies in cases of herpes simplex, rubella, arbovirus B, and cytomepolovirus infections. The results obtained by this test and by complement fixation test coincide in 98%.

6. *The Cytohemadsorption Test*

A modification of the active virus hemagglutination test, described by Vogel and Shelokov (1957), is based on the adsorption of erythrocytes by monkey kidney cells in the tissue culture infected with influenza virus. The guinea pig or fowl erythrocytes adsorbed by infected cells form characteristic aggregates over the surface of a cell monolayer.

The Mixed Hemadsorption Test (Espmark, 1965, c.f. Melnick, 1969). The test is set up on moderately degenerated tissue culture monolayers infected or presumably infected with viruses. The monolayers are first washed with maintenance medium, following which serial dilutions of an antivirus serum are added. The tubes are incubated for 1 hour at room temperature, drained, and gently washed with the maintenance medium. Each tube holding the monolayer then receives 0.5 ml of sheep red blood cells treated first with the rabbit antisheep red cell serum and then with antigamma globulin serum prepared in a different species. Following a brief incubation, the monolayers are observed at 200 × magnification. The immunological reaction is demonstrated by the presence of erythrocytes aggregated in the areas occupied by virus particles. The last antiserum dilutions showing the hemadsorption is considered as end point, and the titer is expressed in the serum dilution.

The hemadsorption test has been employed to detect and identify viral antigens in monolayer cultures infected with measles, distemper, vaccinia, herpes, and respiratory syncytial viruses. It has also been sued successfully to measure herpes simplex antibodies. The test is more sensitive than the complement fixation and neutralization test, since it gives 100- to 1000-fold higher titers than complement fixation and neutralization tests.

II. THE INDIRECT HEMAGGLUTINATION TESTS

Indirect, passive, or conditioned hemagglutination depend on the clumping of erythrocytes, coated by certain microbial substances, called "hemosensitins," and linked together by a homologous serum which reacts with the hemosensitins. Components of red cells bringing about the adsorption of these antigens are predominantly of lipid nature, as indicated by the following experiments: antigens treated with an alcohol-ether extract of red blood cells lose the sensitizing power, and bacterial antigens exposed to cholesterol and lecithin inhibit the hemagglutination (Boyden, 1950; Neter et al., 1953).

Other morphotic blood elements, leukocytes, and platelets, are also able to adsorb certain bacterial antigens and be agglutinated by antisera (DiNardo, 1958).

Hemosensitins are either polysaccharides or proteins in the chemical character. Polysaccharide antibodies are easily adsorbable to the surface of erythrocytes. Lipopolysaccharides of microorganisms which do not adsorb, or adsorb only slightly, onto red blood cells are often rendered adsorbable after heating at 100° for one hour or under the treatment with 0.25 N NaOH at 37° (Staub, 1954; Landy et al., 1955). Six to 1000 $\mu g/ml$ of lipopolysaccharide are required to coat 2.5% suspension of erythrocytes, as compared with only one tenth of heated preparations (Neter et al., 1956).

Antigens other than polysaccharides or lipopolysaccharides, for example, purified proteins, can be adsorbed only onto altered surface of erythrocytes. This can be attained by exposing red blood cells to substances which are able to agglutinate the erythrocytes at a high concentration and to render them capable of adsorbing various proteins if used at a low concentration. The following substances are known to render erythrocytes susceptible to the agglutination by homologous antisera: diazo compounds, for example, diazotized arsanilic acid, bis-diazotized benzidine, or tetrazotized benzidine (Pressman et al., 1942); periodate; tannic acid (Reiner and Fischer, 1929; Boyden, 1951); pepsin; trypsin; and inulin (Boyden, 1951). Newcastle disease virus exhibits a similar action.

Mechanisms of the adsorption of antigens onto treated or modified red cells are presumably different, since diverse immunochemical components are adsorbed from a solution of a crude antigen preparation or a mixture of various antigens (Boyden, 1953). Usually, several antigens can be adsorbed simultaneously or consecutively onto red blood cells without any apparent blocking of the adsorbity of one antigen by another. This observation is helpful in studies on the antigenic structure of microorganisms. The chemical nature of hemosensitins has not yet been precisely determined. Hemosensitins detected in some microorganisms are listed in Tables 41 and 42.

The Technique of the Indirect (Passive) Hemagglutination Test. Components of the test are a hemosensitin preparation, red blood cells, and test serum. Pleural, peritoneal, or cerebrospinal fluids or secretions of mucous membranes are less frequently examined than the blood serum.

Red blood cells of various species of animals can be used for the test, such as sheep, rabbit, cattle, chicken, duck, and human group ORh- erythrocytes. Chicken red blood cells are used in preference since they clump in a relatively shorter time than erythrocytes of other animals. However, certain antigens can more strongly adsorb onto a particular type of red blood cells, for example, rabbit erythrocytes, thus giving relatively higher titers of antisera (Gernez-Rieux, 1952). Fresh red blood cells collected in 3.5% sodium citrate solution or formolized and stored in frozen

Table 42.   Hemosensitins Adsorbable onto Tanned or Trypsinized Erythrocytes

Hemosensitin Preparation	Author
Streptococcus pyogenes, protein	Boyden, 1951; Kwapinski, 1958
Pasteurella pestis, protein toxin	Landy and Trapani, 1954; Chen and Meyer, 1966
Clostridium tetani, toxoid	Stavitsky, 1954; Sonak et al., 1968.
Clostridium perfringens, α-lecithinase	Stavitsky, 1954
Escherichia coli, filtrates	Neter et al., 1952
Leptospira	Chang and McCoomb, 1954; Rothstein and Hiatt, 1956
Treponema reiteri, protein extract	Lamedica and Robert, 1957
Corynebacterium diphtheriae, toxin, toxoid	Boyden, 1951; Fisher, 1952
Mycobacterium tuberculosis, protein	Boyden, 1951; Meynell, 1954; Cole and Farrell, 1955; Kwapinski, 1959
M. tuberculosis, cytoplasm	Kwapinski, 1964
M. tuberculosis, culture filtrate and tuberculin	Middlebrook and Dubos, 1958; Boyden, 1951; Kwapinski and Pietraszkiewiczowa, 1953; Brodhage and Frey, 1955
PPD	Boyden, 1951; Boyden and Sorkin, 1955; Kwapinski, 1959
Mycoplasma pneumoniae, "crude" antigen	Organick and Resnick, 1966
Bovine Serum Albumin	Wolberg et al., 1969
Human albumin	cf. Boyden, 1953
Antitoxin of *Cl. oedematicus*	Cook, 1965
Guinea pig and horse serum globulins	Boyden, 1953
Hormones	
Pollen extracts	cf. Boyden, 1953

state are equally suitable. The use of formolized cells is advantageous since they are stabilized and consequently the work involved in the titration is greatly reduced.

Formalinization of Erythrocytes by Czismas' (1960) Method, Modified by Daniel's et al. (1963).   One volume of packed red blood cells washed in pH 7.2 buffered saline is mixed with 8 volumes of cold 3% formaldehyde, diluted in pH 7.2 buffered saline. This mixture is poured into a Lusteroid centrifuge tube, tightly corked, and placed at 4° on a rocking dialysis apparatus. After 24 hours 2 volumes of cold, undiluted (approximately 40%) formaldehyde is added to this suspension, and agitation is continued in the cold for another 24 hours. The red blood cells are then centrifuged, collected, and washed ten times in 8 to 10 volumes of saline, and finally resuspended in 6 to 8 volumes of saline. (The pH 7.2 buffered saline solution consists of 286 ml of 0.15 M Na$_2$HPO$_4$, 90 ml of 0.15 M KH$_2$PO$_4$, and 376 ml of 0.15 M NaCl.) Merthiolate should be added to a final concentration of 1:10,000 if this suspension is to be stored for a prolonged time (at −20°).

Erythrocytes are rendered suitable for the adsorption of proteins by the treatment with tannic acid, trypsin, pepsin, a fungal proteinase, ficin, or macrodex (Boyden, 1951; Neter and Gorzynski, 1959). The treatment with tannic acid is carried out in the following manner: 2 ml of a 2.5% suspension of washed, fresh, or formolized sheep erythrocytes made in a saline solution buffered at pH 7 to 7.2 are mixed with 2 ml of a freshly prepared 1:10,000 to 1:40,000 solution of tannic acid in saline. The mixture is held either at 37° or at room temperature for 10 minutes. The cells are then centrifuged, washed twice in a buffered saline, and resuspended in 1 ml of saline to produce an approximately 5% suspension. Tanned cells should be stored at 2 to 4° and used within 24 hours. (The buffered saline, pH 7.0 to 7.2, consists of 23.9 ml of 0.15 M KH_2PO_4, 76 ml of 0.15 M Na_2HPO_4, and 100 ml of 0.85% NaCl.)

Trypsinization of erythrocytes is conducted in the following way (Stulberg et al., 1956). Human ORh-negative or rabbit red blood cells, washed in buffered saline, pH 7.2, are exposed to a 250 μg/ml trypsin solution and incubated for 10 to 30 minutes at 37°. The trypsinized cells are then washed three times with buffered saline.

The treatment of red blood cells with papain follows this pattern. One ml of washed packed red cells is mixed with 2 ml of 0.01% solution of papain in saline buffered at pH 7.3; 1 ml of 0.2% L-cysteine chloride is added as an activator of this enzyme. The mixture is left at 37° for 30 minutes, then centrifuged, and washed twice with an isotonic saline. A similar technique of papainization employs a 20% saline suspension of erythrocytes mixed in equal parts with a papain solution which may consist of 1 volume of 0.25% aqueous papin, 1 volume of 36% disodium phosphate, and 2 volumes of 0.2% L-cysteine hydrochloride. The mixture of cells and papin solution is incubated at 37° for 15 minutes.

The Sensitization of Erythrocytes. An optimal amount of a crude antigen preparation to be used for the sensitization of erythrocytes often corresponds to about 0.01 mg of dry weight in 1 ml of saline per 1 ml of 2% suspension of red blood cells, which is equivalent to 0.5 mg of antigen per 1 ml of packed red cells. However, as little as 0.05 or even 0.005 mg of a purified and active preparation can be sufficient to sensitize the same amount of erythrocytes. The optimal sensitizing amount of an antigen preparation should be determined by titration. For this purpose, several dilutions of the antigen are made in a buffered saline to contain 0.1, 0.2, 0.5, 1.0, and 5.0 mg of the preparation per ml, and are mixed with 1 ml of 2% suspension of normal or pretreated erythrocytes. After the incubation at 37° for 1 hour, the cells are sedimented, resuspended, and added to a series of antiserum dilutions made in 1% normal rabbit serum. The ratio of antigen to antiserum which brings about the highest titer of antiserum is selected for the test proper.

According to Kwapinski's (1959) technique for sensitization of erythrocytes, an amount of 0.5 ml of packed sheep or chicken red blood cells is suspended in 5 ml of an antigen solution and incubated in a water bath at 37° for 1 hour or at room temperature for 2 hours, agitated slowly on an electric shaker. The red cells are then centrifuged, washed twice with buffered saline, and resuspended in a buffered saline at 0.2, 0.25, or 0.5% final concentration. Instead of packed red blood cells, a 5 or 20% suspension is often employed for the sensitization.

The adsorption of antigens onto erythrocytes seems to be partially reversible at 37° so that the hemosensitins can migrate from sensitized to nonsensitized cells (Boyden, 1951). The sensitized cells should be used on the day of their preparation. However, if normal erythrocytes have been coated by an antigen, they can be used in 24 or even 36 hours, usually without any noticeable error. The formalin treated and antigen-coated red cells may be frozen at −70° and stored at −40°.

The sensitization of modified, tanned, trypsinized, or papainized red blood cells can be carried out in a similar manner. The incubation time may be shortened to 1 to 5 minutes, since the absorption of protein antigens onto the modified erythrocytes is a rapid process. If the sensitization of red blood cells proves to be unsatisfactory at 37°, it is advisable to reincubate the mixture of the antigen and erythrocytes at 4° for 12 hours. The following technique described by Stulberg et al. (1956) is recommended as a sensitization procedure for modified red blood cells: 1 ml of packed trypsinized cells is suspended in 10 ml of an antigen solution and incubated at 37° for 1 minute. The sensitized cells are centrifuged at 300 × g for 3 minutes, washed once with buffered saline, and resuspended at 0.5% final concentration. The technique of sensitization of diazotized red blood cells differs, slightly, from the procedure applied to the erythrocytes modified by other substances.

Numerous procedures for the passive hemagglutination test have been designed, but the following methods are recommended: the techniques of Boyden (1953), and Kwapinski and Pietraszkiewiczowa (1953), which are conducted with tanned or normal red blood cells, the Stulberg (1956) method with the enzyme-pretreated erythrocytes, the technique of Stavitsky and Arquilla (1955) with the diazotized red cells, and a slide hemagglutination test by Thalhimer and Rowe (1951).

1. Boyden's Technique of the Hemagglutination Test

Two series of twofold dilutions of inactivated, erythrocyte-absorbed antiserum are prepared in 0.1- to 0.5-ml volumes of a normal rabbit serum, diluted 1:100 with saline. Red blood cells are suspended at 1.25% concentration in a 1:250 diluted rabbit serum. The suspension of sensitized tanned red blood cells is added in equal volume to the first row of tubes, whereas a 1.25% suspension of nonsensitized erythrocytes is added to the other row. Four additional control tubes are set, two of them containing equal volumes of sensitized erythrocytes and buffered saline, and the other two tubes receiving nonsensitized red cells and a buffered saline. It is also advisable to insert two separate rows of tubes containing varying dilutions of a known positive and a negative sera, if available, with the sensitized red cells.

The mixtures are incubated at 37° for 2 hours, and left either at room temperature for 2 to 4 hours or at 4° overnight. The tubes should be examined after 4, 2, and 4 hours, and possibly after another 12 hours, to observe the amount of the most evident difference in the pattern of settled cells in the main and control rows.

A marked difference is sometimes observed within 2 hours, whereas after 12 hours there is a compact button of sedimented erythrocytes in all tubes. The hemagglutination is usually detected by observing the pattern of settling erythrocytes on the bottom of tubes directly or after the centrifugation at 200 × g for 1 minute. The agglutinated red cells form a rather broad disk with ragged edge, whereas nonagglutinated erythrocytes appear in the form of a round button with an even edge. If the hemagglutination is doubtful, the deposits must be resuspended by gently striking the glass. The agglutinated red blood cells resuspend in a form of granules floating in the transparent fluid, whereas the nonagglutinated cells resuspend slowly forming a homogenous, intransparent suspension. The titer of hemagglutinins is expressed in terms of the final dilution of antiserum in the last tube in which a complete or nearly complete agglutination is observed.

A similar test was adapted by Scott et al. (1957) for passive virus hemagglutination reaction. The absorption by viruses, for example, by herpes simplex virus, onto tanned cells is attained by incubating at room temperature for 10 minutes, a 4:1:1 mixture of a pH 6.4 buffered saline, concentrated virus, and 50% tanned red blood cells. The cells are then washed in a 1:100 diluted normal rabbit serum and resuspended in one volume of this diluent. The test is conducted by adding 0.05 ml of these cells to a series of progressive antiserum dilutions in 0.5-ml volumes of the rabbit serum diluent.

Control tubes receive (a) the serum diluent and the virus-absorbed erythrocytes, (b) a normal, noninfected, concentrated allantoic fluid, (c) the virus suspension and untreated erythrocytes, and (d) the suspension of untreated sheep erythrocytes in the serum diluent.

Recordings are made after an incubation at room temperature for 3 hours and at 5° for 16 hours.

A positive agglutination pattern consists of a uniform thin layer of red cells on the bottom of tubes. Negative pattern consists of a round button of sedimented erythrocytes. The agglutination titer is determined according to the highest serum dilution giving a definite "positive pattern."

2. *Kwapinski's Technique for the Hemagglutination Test*

The inactivated serum being tested is diluted in 0.4-ml volumes of a buffered saline from 1:4 to 1:512, in duplicate. One row receives 0.4 ml of a 0.2% sensitized red cells suspension, and the other row obtains 0.4 ml of a 0.2% suspension of nonsensitized, human O Rh-negative erythrocytes or chicken red blood cells. If sheep erythrocytes are employed, the serum must be absorbed with packed sheep red blood cells prior to the test. Two additional control tubes contain 0.4 ml of a phosphate-buffered saline, pH 7.2, and 0.4 ml of the suspension of sensitized erythrocytes. The mixtures are incubated in a water bath at 37° for 1 $\frac{1}{2}$ to 2 hours and left at 2° overnight. The results are read in the usual manner.

The assay with body fluids other than serum, for example, pleural or peritoneal exudates, cerebrospinal fluid, vaginal mucus, and humor vitreous, is carried out according to the similar pattern. Nonspecific reactions at low titers given by some of these materials, especially by mucous membranes secretions, may be removed by freezing and thawing the samples before testing as recommended by Te Punga (1958). The test can also be set up on plastic hollowed trays instead of tubes.

3. *The Middlebrook and Dubos Hemagglutination Test*

The Middlebrook and Dubos technique devised originally for the study on tuberculous antibodies is applied as follows: sheep red blood cells are sensitized with a tuberculin by mixing 1 volume of 2.5% cell suspension with 0.2 volume of old tuberculin diluted with 2 volumes of saline, and incubating this mixture at 37° for 2 hours. The erythrocytes are then washed and resuspended to a 1.25% concentration. The examined sera should be inactivated, diluted 1:5, and absorbed with packed sheep erythrocytes to remove natural agglutinins for sheep red blood cells. The sera are then serially diluted in duplicate, in a volume of 0.25 ml. A 1.25% suspension of sensitized cells is added in the volume of 0.05 ml to each tube of one row, whereas the other row of tubes receives 0.05 ml of 1.5% nonsensitized erythrocytes. A positive serum with a known hemagglutinin titer is inserted in each series of tests. After a 4-hour incubation at room temperature, the mixtures are left at 4° overnight. Readings are made by observing the pattern of red cells rising from the bottom of the gently shaken tube. The nonagglutinated erythrocytes disperse evenly in the fluid, where as the agglutinated cells form large, firmly adhering clumps.

4. Microtechniques of the Hemagglutination Assay

i. *The Slide Hemagglutination Test, by Thalhimer and Rowe (1951).* The test is carried out on glass slides by mixing one drop of a 15% suspension of human O Rh-negative erythrocytes sensitized with an antigen and one or two drops of an inactivated serum being investigated. A drop of nonsensitized erythrocytes mixed with one or two drops of the same serum is provided as a control.

ii. *The Microtiter Hemagglutination Technique (Ransom et al., 1968).* Concentration of the erythrocytes, used as antigen carriers, is adjusted to 10^8 cells/ml with a Colter electronic counter (Drecher et al., 1962). The test is set up in the U-plates which are incubated at 37° for 1 hour and results are read by a settling pattern. The titer read according to the highest dilution of serum showing definite agglutination of cells is expressed as $1 + \log 2$ of the reciprocal of the dilution.

Passive hemolysis test has been carried out by adding complement to the hemagglutination test tubes after the test has been completed and read. After the addition of complement, the mixtures are incubated for 1 hour, the U-plates are centrifuged in a special centrifuge carrier for microtiter plates, and the degree of hemolysis is evaluated in each well on a scale of 0 to 4+.

5. The Electrophoresis-Hemagglutination Test

In this assay by Berg et al. (1955), the test serum is first partitioned by means of a paper electrophoresis. The sensitized erythrocytes are placed on the edge of a still wet electrophoretogram. Serum fractions containing no antibody diffuse through sensitized erythrocytes into the middle of the electrophoretogram. In contrast, the serum fractions containing antibodies cannot diffuse, owing to the absorption onto erythrocytes and to the hemagglutination.

A similar assay for enhanced hemagglutination was published earlier by Kwapinski and Madalinski (1955, see p. 417).

6. The Hemagglutination Test of Enzyme-Pretreated Erythrocytes

The test with trypsinized or papainized red blood cells, which are subsequently sensitized with an antigen, can be carried out by a standard hemagglutination technique. However, the following simple procedure, devised by Stulberg et al. (1956), is recommended for this purpose. To a series of twofold dilutions in 0.5-ml volumes of a tested serum, warmed to 37°, and kept in a water bath at 37°, an equal volume of a 0.5% suspension of trypsinized and sensitized red cells is added. (The sera and red cells suspension are warmed at 37° to deviate the effect of cold agglutinins.) Control tubes contain serum dilutions and nonsensitized, trypsinized erythrocytes or 0.5 ml of saline and 0.5 ml of the sensitized erythrocyte suspension. All tubes are centrifuged after 1 to 2 minutes; the sediments are gently agitated and examined microscopically for the presence of hemagglutinated cells. The end point is indicated by a tube in which the sediment contains at least 50% of agglutinated red cells. In this technique, the non-specific hemagglutination in the control tubes is observed less frequently than in the usual procedure.

Further techniques for the hemagglutination test with the enzyme-modified cells were described by Morton and Pickles (1947), Wright et al. (1955), and Neter and Gorzynski (1959).

7. *The Hemagglutination Test of Diazotized Erythrocytes*

A conjugated antigen for this test, by the technique of Stavitsky and Arquilla (1956), is prepared in the following way: an aliquot of a 0.25 to 0.50 ml (5.5 mg/ml) of bisdiazotized benzidine, made according to the Kabat and Mayer (1948) method, is mixed with 0.25 to 1.0 ml of an antigen solution is isotonic (0.11 M, pH 7.4) phosphate buffer containing 1 to 3 mg of dry substance and 0.05 ml of washed packed sheep red blood cells in 1.6 ml of saline.

The mixture is diluted with 7 ml of 0.11 M phosphate buffer, pH 7.3, and left at room temperature for 10 minutes, then centrifuged at 1700 rpm for 5 minutes. The cells are resuspended in 3.5 ml of 1% saline solution of inactivated normal rabbit serum which has been absorbed with an equal volume of sheep red blood cells. Finally, the cells are recentrifuged and resuspended in 2.5 ml of 1% normal rabbit serum. The following antigen preparations were found adsorbable onto the diazotized red cells: the diphtheria toxoid, bovine serum albumin, egg albumen, bovine γ-globulin, ragweed pollen extract, and insulin.

The test is carried out by mixing equal 0.05-ml volumes of serial dilutions of a serum being examined, diluted in 1% normal rabbit serum and a suspension of diazotized and antigen conjugated red cells. The mixtures are incubated at room temperature for 3 hours. Readings are made immediately and in 12 hours by observing patterns of the cells on the bottom of tubes. The hemagglutination test with diazotized cells gives results of the same order of sensitivity as the technique with tanned erythrocytes.

8. *The Hapten-Conjugate Hemagglutination Test*

In this test, a simple hapten is first combined to the erythrocytes or protein molecules, and this complex is then reacted with the antibodies which are presumed to possess reactive groups for the hapten. The reaction between a hapten and the corresponding antibodies is signified by clumping of the erythrocytes.

The following simple haptens are readily coupled to proteins and erythrocytes: 2,4-dinitrophenyl groups, picryl chloride groups, and 1,3-difluoro-4,6-dinitrobenzene (DFDNB).

The most convenient method for covalent conjugation of erythrocytes with dinitrophenyl groups is presented in Table 43. Coupling with other haptens may be achieved in a similar fashion.

Reagents for this technique are as follows:

1. Ethylenediaminetetraacetate buffer, pH 8.4. EDTA disodium salt dihydrate (17 g) dissolved in distilled water, adjusted to pH 8.4 with 2 *N* NaOH and made up to 1 liter with water.

2. EDTA buffer, pH 7.5: 17 g of EDTA disodium salt dihydrate, dissolved in 0.85% NaCl solution, adjusted to pH 7.5 with 2 *N* NaOH and made up to 1 liter with 0.85% NaCl solution. The osmolarity is adjusted to 300 millimoles/liter by the addition of glucose.

Table 43. Coupling of Erythrocytes to Dinitrophenyl Groups
(Bullock and Kantor, 1965)

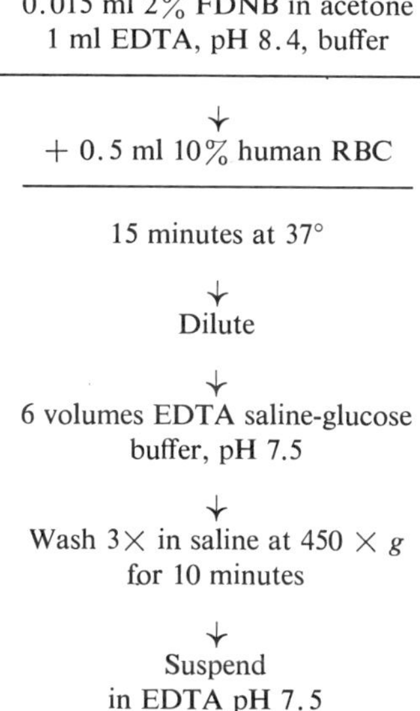

9. *The Dinitrophenyl-Erythrocyte Hemagglutination Test*

The dinitrophenyl-protein conjugates are prepared by Bullock and Kantor's (1965) modification of Eisen's et al. (1953) method as follows: appropriate dilutions of a hapten (2,4-dinitrophenyl-, or picryl chloride-group) preparation, dissolved in dioxane calculated not to exceed 5% of the total volume of protein solution, are slowly added in drops to a protein solution, whose pH is maintained between 8.5 and 9.0 by addition of 5%

sodium carbonate. The mixture is stirred for 4 hours, after which the unreacted hapten is separated by Sephadex G-25 gel filtration.

Protein concentration in the hapten-protein conjugate is determined in terms of nitrogen. The number of hapten groups per mole of protein is estimated by spectrophotometric analysis using a molar extinction coefficient of 17,400 for DNP groups at 360-nm wavelengths, or a coefficient of 15,400 for picryl chloride groups at 347 nm.

To perform the dinitrophenyl-erythrocyte hemagglutination test, according to Bullock and Kantor (1965), twofold dilutions of an erythrocyte-absorbed antiserum are made in 0.25 ml of an EDTA buffer, pH 7.5 (see p. 413) in Dispose trays. To each antiserum dilution, and to a control normal serum, 0.25 ml of hapten-coupled erythrocytes (p. 412) are added. The trays are agitated gently and left overnight at 4°.

The patterns of settled cells in wells are then recorded. The highest antiserum dilution showing strong agglutination of erythrocytes (the cells spread uniformly in the well) is taken as the hemagglutinin titer.

The hapten-conjugate hemagglutination is a relatively sensitive method for detection of antihapten antibodies.

10. *The DFDNB-Erythrocyte Hemagglutination Test*

In this test (Ling, 1961), protein antigens are attached to difluorodinitrobenzene (DFDNB) altered erythrocytes. For this purpose, the group O Rh-negative cells are washed four times in saline and resuspended in saline to a 10% concentration; 1 ml of this suspension is added to 2 ml of EDTA buffer, pH 8.4, containing 0.3 ml of 2% acetone solution of 1,3-difluoro-4,6-dinitrobenzene. After the 30-minute incubation in a 37° water bath, the red cells are centrifuged, withdrawn, resuspended in 2 ml of buffer, pH 8.4, and added to 0.5 ml (10 mg) of a protein antigen. After another 60-minute incubation at 37°, the cells are centrifuged lightly, washed three times with EDTA buffer, pH 7.5, and resuspended in 40 ml of this buffer. Test sera must be absorbed with washed DFDNB-treated cells by incubating, at 4° for 1 hour, mixtures consisting of 0.1 ml of serum, 0.4 ml of the EDTA buffer, pH 7.5, and 0.1 ml of washed DFDNB-pretreated cells.

After the centrifugation, the absorbed sera are serially diluted in 0.25-ml volumes of a pH 7.5 buffer in plastic agglutination trays, and mixed with 0.25 ml of the hapten-conjugated erythrocytes. Controls contain (a) 0.25 ml of the hapten-conjugated erythrocytes and 0.25 ml buffer, and (b) a diluted normal serum and the suspension of DFDNB-treated erythrocytes. The trays are agitated and left at 4°. The end point of hemagglutination is determined by the "settled pattern" method. The EDTA-buffer consists of 1.7% aqueous solution of ethylene-diamine-tetra-acetic acid disodium salt dihydrate adjusted to pH 8.4 with 2 *N* sodium hydroxide.

11. Evaluation and Application of the Passive Hemagglutination Test

The passive hemagglutination test is very sensitive, reliable, and more specific than the agglutination of bacterial cells. As little as 0.001 μg of some antigens can be detected by this immunologic method (Wright and Feinberg, 1952). The hemagglutinin titers are usually 5 to 50 times higher than those of bacterial agglutinins (Neter et al., 1956). Even very scanty precipitating or nonprecipitating antibodies may be detected by a hemagglutination techinque.

A limitation of hemagglutination test is the use of erythrocytes as carriers of antigens. Red blood cells are liable to variations from one batch to another, and this may cause a significant experimental error. Apart from erythrocytes, also hepatic and renal cells, certain bacteria and some inert particles are able to absorb some antigens and become specifically agglutinable by antibodies which are homologous to the absorbed antigens. Cells of *Serratia marcescens* and inert particles, for example, collodion, polystyrene latex, kaolin, or bentonite particles can serve as antigen carriers (see p. 384–394).

The passive hemagglutination test has been successfully applied to the following.

1. The detection of specific antibodies (hemagglutinins) in human sera, as well as in the cerebrospinal fluid, pleural exudates, humor vitreous, and mucus samples. Specific hemagglutinins have been found in infections by *Pasteurella tularensis, Pasteurella pestis, Mycobacterium tuberculosis, Vibrio fetus, Salmonella, Blastomyces dermatidis,* and *Rickettsia prowazeki* (Middlebrook and Dubos, 1948; Gernez-Rieux, 1951, 1952; Takeda et al., 1952; Kwapinski and Pietraszkiewiczowa, 1953; Martin, 1953; Chang et al., 1954; Payne et al., 1956; Te Punga, 1958; Charles, 1959; Kwapinski, 1959).

2. The immunologic tracing of typhoid carriers (Landy and Lamb, 1953; Staack and Spaun, 1953).

3. The testing of diagnostic and therapeutic antisera (Keogh et al., 1947).

4. The determination of antigens and identification of microorganisms, the antigenic analysis, and serological typing of strains and species of bacteria (Gernez-Rieux and Tacquet, 1950; Fisher, 1951; Fenner, 1952; Sieburth, 1957; Kwapinski, 1958; Vosti and Rantz, 1965).

III. ENHANCED HEMAGGLUTINATION TESTS

This class of immunological tests depends on the enhancement by heteroreagins of the agglutination of red blood cells partly sensitized by a homologous antibody. The hemagglutination enhancing factor (the heteroreagin or rheumatoid factor), which occurs most characteristically in the rheumatoid arthritis sera, has a mucoprotein character of the immunoglobulin and an ability to adsorb onto the erythrocytes coated by homologous antibodies and reacts with altered small-molecule 2gG forming reversible large complexes.

The sensitized antigen used in the enhanced hemagglutination test consists of red blood cells, partially sensitized either by a homologous whole antiserum or by isolated serum globulins (Rose et al., 1948; Heller et al., 1949; Svartz and Schlossmann, 1949; Hobson and Gorrill, 1952; Kwapinski et al., 1955; Gibson and Ling, 1956; Ziff, 1954; Svartz and Schlossmann, 1954; Heller et al., 1955; Rheins et al., 1957; Whillans and Fischman, 1958).

1. The Rose et al. (1948) Hemagglutination Test

The most often used antigen for this assay is sheep red blood cells sensitized with half a minimal hemagglutinating unit of an antisheep erythrocyte serum (ASES). The minimal hemagglutinating dose of serum is determined by the following procedures: 0.5-ml volumes of the ASES in progressive dilutions are mixed with 0.5 ml of a 2% sheep erythrocyte suspension and made up with saline to a total volume of 2 ml, incubated at 37° for 1 hour, and held at 2 to 4° overnight. The dilution of antiserum in the last tube which shows a definite hemagglutination denotes its titer. Red blood cells are sensitized for the test proper by adding a volume of 1% suspension of erythrocytes to an equal volume of the ASES solution diluted to contain half a hemagglutinating unit and incubating this mixture at room temperature for 45 to 60 minutes.

The hemagglutination test is set up in the following manner: the inactivated serum under test is serially diluted, in duplicate from 1:10 to 1:2560 in 0.5-ml volume of saline solution. Each tube of the first row receives 0.5 ml of a 1% suspension of sensitized red blood cells, and the tubes of the other row obtain 0.5 ml of a 1% suspension of the nonsensitized cells. Control tubes, set up for the whole series of tests, contain serial dilutions of a reference "positive" and "negative" serum with the sensitized erythrocytes; two other tubes receive saline and sensitized cells. All test tubes are held at 37° for 1 hour and at 2 to 4° overnight, then inverted twice, left for a few minutes, and read. The highest final dilutions of sera showing clumps of agglutinated cells are recorded in all rows of tubes. The results are expressed in terms of geometric differences between serum titers with the sensitized and nonsensitized red blood cells, according to the following formula:

$$\text{DAT} = \frac{\text{the serum titer with nonsensitized cells}}{\text{the serum titer with sensitized cells}}$$

Differential agglutination titer higher than 16 is regarded as significant. High titers of the enhanced hemagglutination are characteristically found in rheumatoid arthritis (see Kwapinski and Snyder, 1962).

Heterophile hemagglutinins which are responsible for the agglutination of nonsensitized erythrocytes can be removed from the test serum by absorption on washed sheep red blood cells, prior to the test proper (Heller et al., 1949). The hemagglutination titer in this assay is calculated from the difference between the hemagglutination titers of test mixtures containing sensitized and those with nonsensitized cells.

2. The Heller et al. (1949) Hemagglutination Test

This assay employs a sheep serum diluent which has the ability to promote the agglutinating capacity of rheumatoid sera. This diluent should step up by 128- to 256-fold the hemagglutinating titer of a positive reference serum but must not increase the basic agglutinating titer of an antisheep erythrocyte serum by more than one fifth, or set up the titer of "negative" sera.

The hemagglutination test is carried out as follows: two series of progressive, twofold dilutions of the erythrocyte absorbed serum are prepared, one in 0.5-ml volumes of a 2% saline solution of inactivated normal sheep serum, and the other in an isotonic saline solution. Control tubes contain positive and negative reference sera and the diluents alone. Equal volumes of a 0.5% suspension sheep red blood cells, sensitized by 1/20 basic agglutinating dose of an antierythrocyte serum, are added to each tube and these are left at 2° overnight. The test is considered positive if the hemagglutination titer of test serum is at least fourfold greater in the serum-diluent than in saline.

3. The Screening Enhanced Hemagglutination Test

The assay by Meijers and Westendorp-Boerma (1958) is carried out on glass slides divided into three parts by paraffin strokes. One drop of the examined serum diluted 1:8 is mixed on the slide with one drop of sensitized cells. (Sensitized cells are prepared by mixing equal parts of 1% suspension of human group O erythrocytes and one fourth minimum agglutinating dose of amboceptor.) After 5 minutes of tilting, the slide is examined for the presence of agglutinates.

4. The Enhanced Hemagglutination Test with Globulin Fractions

The assay, published by Kwapinski and Madalinski (1955), is conducted as follows. The serum (0.02-ml volume) is first absorbed with normal sheep erythrocytes, inactivated at 62° for 3 minutes, and partitioned on a strip of Whatman no. 1 filter paper, by applying the electrophoresis (0.16 mA, 6.5 V/mm) for 16 hours, using a veronal buffer, pH

8.6, with 0.05 ionic strength. Individual globulin fractions are then cut out of the filter paper, guided by a parallel electrophoretogram stained with a solution of Azocarmin B. The corresponding pieces of unstained electrophoretogram are then immersed into 0.5 ml of 0.85% sodium chloride solution and agitated at 37° for 2 hours. Eluates thus obtained are used for the hemagglutination test.

To set up the test, 1 to 2 drops of the undiluted and diluted eluate are mixed on a glass slide with 1 to 2 drops of a 1% sheep erythrocyte suspension, sensitized with a one third minimal hemagglutinating unit of a rabbit antisheep erythrocyte serum. Controls receive the eluate mixed with nonsensitized cells, or saline with sensitized cells. The slides are rotated for 2 minutes, then examined grossly and by the aid of a lens. Clumped cells floating in a clear fluid denote a positive reaction.

5.   *The Ziff et al. (1954) Euglobulin-Hemagglutination Test*

The serum euglobulin fraction, composed chiefly of γ- and β-globulins, is isolated from the specimen under test in the following manner: a serum sample, inactivated and adsorbed with the sheep erythrocytes, is diluted 1:1 in distilled water and dialyzed against distilled water for 48 hours. The precipitated euglobulin is centrifuged, washed in water, and dissolved to the original volume in 0.85% sodium chloride, buffered at pH 8.0.

The euglobulin solution is now diluted serially from 1:4 to 1:512 or higher, in 0.5-ml volumes of saline, and mixed with 0.5 ml of a 1% sheep erythrocyte suspension sensitized by a half hemagglutinating dose of an antierythrocyte serum. After the incubation in a water bath at 37° for 1 hour, the tubes are left at 2 to 4° overnight, and read for the presence of agglutinates. A titer equal to 64 or higher is considered positive.

In a similar test by Svartz and Schlossmann (1954), the kryoglobulin fraction is obtained by diluting inactivated and erythrocyte absorbed serum in the proportion of 1:14 in ice-cooled distilled water. After the sample is left at 2 to 4° for 48 hours, the precipitated kryoglobulin is collected by centrifugation at 2 to 4° for 90 minutes. The hemagglutination test is set up with a 1% suspension of sheep erythrocytes sensitized by two hemolytic units of an antierythrocyte serum.

6.   *The Heller et al. (1955) Immunoglobulin Test*

The test, often termed the FII test, is carried out with erythrocytes sensitized by the second fraction (FII) of human globulin prepared according to the Cohn et al. (1944) method. The optimal dose of the fraction II needed to sensitize red blood cells is determined by testing the erythrocyte sensitized by various doses of the fraction II against a "positive" reference serum, containing rheumatoid heteroreagins.

This assay is conducted as follows. First, the sheep erythrocytes suspended in a buffered saline, pH 8.0, at 33 $\frac{1}{3}$% concentration are tanned in a 1:40,000 saline solution of tannic acid, at 37° for 10 minutes. The cells are then washed twice with saline and resuspended to 33 $\frac{1}{3}$% concentration. A few lots of this suspension are mixed in the 1:2 proportion with various solutions of the human globulin fraction II, incubated at 37° for 30 minutes, then centrifuged, washed with saline, and suspended at 0.25% concentration.

Suspensions of erythrocytes sensitized with various amounts of the globulin fraction II are mixed in equal 0.5-ml volumes with progressive dilutions of a "positive" reference serum and incubated at 2 to 4° overnight. The "negative" reference serum receives 0.25% suspension of nonsensitized, tanned cells, and this must not show the hemagglutination. The smallest amount of fraction II, which brought about the highest hemagglutination titer, is considered optimal. It varies usually between 100 to 150 mg % of a lyophilized preparation of the human globulin fraction II.

The FII test is set up as follows: a serum sample absorbed with sheep red blood cells and inactivated is serially diluted from 1:14 to 1:5600 in 0.5-ml volumes of buffered saline, in duplicate. The first row of tubes receives 0.5 ml of a 0.25% suspension of the FII sensitized sheep erythrocytes, whereas the other row contains nonsensitized, tanned cells. Each series of tests should be accompanied by three additional controls: positive and negative reference sera, serially diluted and mixed with the sensitized erythrocytes, and two tubes containing buffered saline and sensitized cells.

The reaction mixtures are kept at 2 to 4° overnight and examined for the presence of agglutinated red blood cells by holding the hollowed racks over a source of fluorescent light. Agglutinated erythrocytes cover the entire bottom of tubes in a thin layer, whereas a red, smooth, and light disc is observed in the center of the tube bottom if red blood cells are not agglutinated. The test is regarded as positive if the hemagglutination occurs in at least two tubes of the first row of serum under test and also in the "positive" reference serum while no hemagglutination is seen in all the tubes of other rows.

7. *The Immunoconglutination Test*

The conglutination is an immunological phenomenon in which erythrocytes (or other cells), which have partially absorbed an antibody and complement, are agglutinated by a serum factor, the conglutinin. For example, guinea pig erythrocytes coated by a horse antierythrocyte serum and a horse complement clump in an ox serum; similarly the bacteria which have partially absorbed a specific antibody and complement agglutinate in a normal serum. The mechanism of the conglutination may depend on the absorption of the complement midpiece by antigen-antibody complexes, thus altering the surface of particulate antigens and increasing the tendency to collision. A serum or plasma factor termed "conglutinin" brings about the aggregation of red blood cells specifically sensitized with univalent antibodies.

An allied immunological phenomenon is the immunoconglutination (Streng, 1910). It depends on the agglutination of antibody-sensitized erythrocytes or bacteria by the antisera obtained through the immunization with cells, sensitized with an antibody, and exposed to complement. The immunoconglutinin seems to be specific for the complement adsorbed onto the sensitized cells.

Immunoconglutinin is an antibody against fixed complement which may be found in the sera of animals after a strong antigenic stimulation (Ingram, 1969). The immunoconglutinin acts as an antibody combining with a complement and displaying hemolysin activity in the presence of a hemolytic complement. Immunoconglutinin may be specifically absorbed from immune serum by using the antibody and complement present in the serum, which indicates that immunoconglutinin reacts with autologous complement. The function of immunoconglutinin is probably the enhancement of normal activities of complement. Immunoconglutinin arises in the course of bacterial and other diseases associated with strong antigenic stimulation of the host. Immunoconglutinin reacts with a bound complement but does not react with unfixed complement components in serum. It appears that immunoconglutinin is directed against antigenic determinants which are exposed upon fixation of complement to antigen-antibody complexes or to certain active surfaces.

Conglutinin does not occur in man, but the human serum contains a conglutinogen-activating factor which specifically reacts with C′3 and has a molecular weight of approximately 100,000.

Immunoconglutinin may be produced by Lachmann's (1962) or Ingram's (1969) method. According to Ingram's technique, rabbits are injected with bacteria, such as *Listeria monocytogenes* or *Proteus vulgaris,* using a dose ranging from 1×10^9 to 3×10^9 at 4-day intervals, after which the animals are bled 4 days after the last injection.

The immunoconglutinin assay is performed by Coombs' et al. (1961) or Lachmann and Müller-Eberhard's (1968) method, or by the conglutinating complement absorption test (Coombs et al., 1961).

Immunoconglutination Assay. The immunoconglutination test is most conveniently set up in plastic titration trays by diluting the serum with 0.025-ml transferring titration loops and adding 0.025 ml (or 1 drop) of

$\frac{1}{4}\%$ erythrocyte suspenson used as indicator cells (Lachmann and Müller-Eberhard, 1968).

The erythrocytes coated by a specific antibody can also be aggregated in the absence of complement by various serum components, by gum acacia or gelatin. This phenomenon is termed the "coagglutination" (Dean, 1911). Two techniques of the conglutination test, by Flick and Villafene (1952) and Hilleman et al. (1951), are presented here in detail, with preference given to the first method.

The Conglutination Test by Flick and Villafene (1952). A serum tested for conglutinins should be inactivated at 56° for 30 minutes, absorbed with sheep red cells, and diluted progressively in 0.1-ml volumes of saline. Equal amounts of an inactivated, serially diluted immune serum, for example, an antiserum of rabbit immunized with sheep or duck red blood cells, are added to each tube, followed by 0.1 ml of a suspension of sheep or duck red blood cells. Control tubes contain saline instead of the antiserum. The test should be conducted in duplicate. All tubes are agitated for 5 minutes on a shaker, then left at room temperature for 1 hour. One loopful of mixtures from each tube is examined by the hanging drop technique under the 40 × objective of microscope. The percentage of clumps is determined by counting at least 100 erythrocytes.

The Conglutination Test by Hilleman et al. (1951). The inactivated test serum is serially diluted in 0.2-ml amounts, and 0.2 ml of a horse serum complement in a dilution of 1:40 is added to each tube. The volumes are made up to 0.8 ml by adding a buffered saline, pH 7.1, followed by 0.2 ml of a 0.25% suspension of sheep red blood cells. The mixtures are incubated in a water bath at 37° for 30 minutes, then centrifuged at low speed, and read. The titer of the conglutinin is expressed in terms of the highest serum dilution showing complete hemagglutination.

8. The Conglutinating Complement-Absorption Test

This test has first been described by Streng (1910), developed by Hole and Coombs (1947), and modified by Hilleman et al. (1951). The test is based on the following principle: the antigen and a test serum are mixed together in the presence of a determined amount of a conglutinating complement. After a period of incubation, a conglutinating indicator system is added. It consists of sheep red blood cells and an inactivated bovine serum which contains an antibody to sheep erythrocytes and conglutinin. This indicator system permits unabsorbed complement to be determined.

In the Hilleman et al. technique, serum sample is inactivated and diluted serially in amounts of 0.2 ml. Each tube then receives 0.2 ml of a horse complement containing two hemolytic units and 0.2 ml of an "optimal dilution" of the antigen. The mixtures are incubated at room temperature for 30 minutes; 0.4-ml amounts of a conglutinin-sheep erythrocyte mixture are then added, which consists of 0.2 ml of 0.25% erythrocyte suspension and 0.2 ml of a solution of inactivated bovine serum containing four units of conglutinin. The test is read after final incubation at 37° for 30 minutes. The contents of tubes can be centrifuged at 2000 rpm for 1 minute and resuspended. The highest dilution of test serum giving complete absorption of complement is taken as the serum titer.

The amount of horse complement to be employed in the test proper must be estimated by titration in the following manner: to the graded amounts (0.08, 0.10, 0.12, etc., up to 0.20 ml) of a diluted fresh horse serum, 0.2 ml of the antigen solution is added, and the volume of fluid in each tube is made up to 0.6 ml with saline buffered at pH 7.0. The samples are left at room temperature (24 to 26°) for 30 minutes, and 0.4 ml of a mixture composed of equal volumes of 0.25% sheep erythrocyte suspension and a bovine serum solution containing four units of conglutinin in 0.2 ml are added to each tube.

After the incubation at 37° for 30 minutes, the tube with the smallest amount of complement giving complete agglutination is recorded. The conglutinin is titrated in a similar way as described above. The optimal dose of the antigen is estimated after a preliminary titration of the antigen against various dilutions of the test serum. The smallest amount of the antigen which gives the maximal serum titer is used in the test proper. A microtechnique of the conglutination test was published by Bier et al. (1957). Conglutination tests were used for the detection of antibodies to *Actinobacillus mallei* and *Brucella* and for certain investigations on rickettsiae and viruses (Hole and Coombs, 1947; Stoker et al., 1950; Hilleman et al., 1951).

IV. HEMAGGLUTINATION TESTS OF NONSENSITIZED ERYTHROCYTES

This class of serological tests depends on a reaction between "normal" or immune serum hemagglutinins and the erythrocyte antigens, which results in the clumping of erythrocytes. Hemagglutinins, involved in the individual types of hemagglutination of nonsensitized erythrocytes, exhibit their reactivity in different experimental conditions, to be presented in the following chapters. Some of these hemagglutinins, for example, isohemagglutinins, are present in normal sera; others, like cold hemagglutinins or conglutinins, are more characteristically and more frequently found in certain diseases, or like panhemagglutinins are produced directly by certain bacteria grown in the serum. Hemagglutinogens for most reactions of this class (isohemagglutinogens and heterophile antigen) are normally present in the cell walls of erythrocytes, but some other antigens, for example, certain Rh-agglutinogens or the T-hemagglutinogen, must be uncovered by digestion of erythrocytes with proteolytic enzymes.

1. The Cold Hemagglutination Test

The agglutination of red blood cells, which occurs at low temperatures ranging from 1 to 5° and is dissolved at higher temperatures, is caused by substances termed "cold agglutinins"; they function only in the cold. These antibodies can therefore be absorbed onto erythrocytes or their stromata at low temperatures and eluted at 37°. Cold hemagglutinins are globulins of a high molecular weight, with a sedimentation constant of S = 18 (Gordon, 1953). Cold agglutinins may be demonstrated in 48 to 100% of normal individuals, but are more frequently found in the sera from cases of primary atypical pneumonia, infectious mononucleosis, trypanosomiasis, tropical eosynophilia, hereditary spherocytosis, congenital hemolytic anemia, sickle cell and pernicious anemia, Raymond's syndrome, syphilitic liver cirrhosis, benzene poisoning, and in an extensive sulfa drug therapy. Substances similar to cold hemagglutinins which are able to aggregate human erythrocytes were found in soya beans (Bird, 1954).

The cold hemagglutination test can be carried out either with normal or trypsinized red blood cells. The albumin technique with normal erythrocytes seems to be the most sensitive procedure for incomplete cold agglutinins. Chief ingredients of the cold hemagglutination test are a serum sample to be tested and red blood cells. The serum to be examined for cold hemagglutinins must be collected on the same day or stored at −40°.

A 2% saline suspension of normal or trypsinized human group A, Rh-negative erythrocytes is used. The trypsinization of erythrocytes is carried out as follows: 1 ml of washed packed red blood cells is added to 1.5-ml volume of a 0.1% trypsin solution in saline, and incubated for 30 minutes at 37° with frequent agitation. The mixture is then centrifuged, and red blood cells are washed three times with cold saline.

The *cold hemagglutination test,* according to Bouroncle et al. (1951), is set up in a cold room at 4° in the following manner. Two rows of serial twofold dilutions of the serum under test are made in 0.1-ml volume of saline, and 0.07-ml aliquots of a 2% suspension of either normal or trypsinized red cells are added to each tube. The first row of tubes is incubated at 4° for 1 hour, whereas the other should be left at 37° for 30 to 60 minutes. All of the mixtures are then centrifuged at 800 × g for 1 minute. Tubes of the first row are examined in the cold room or in the ice water, whereas the other row of tubes is inspected at room temperature. The titer of cold hemagglutinins is expressed in terms of a final serum dilution in the first row showing definite agglutination, whereas no hemagglutination should be seen in tubes of the second row, incubated at 37°.

A similar technique, published by Gordon (1953), provides 1% suspension of type O Rh-human erythrocytes and 0.15 M solution of sodium chloride containing 0.2% of the human-plasma protein as diluent. Results of the test are read after the test mixture is left at 4° overnight.

The Albumin Technique for Incomplete Cold Hemagglutinins. This technique is applied if the standard cold hemagglutination test has been negative. The contents of all tubes are then centrifuged, the red cells are separated and resuspended in a 2% (w/v) solution of bovine albumin in saline. The mixtures are left for 5 to 10 minutes at room temperature, then centrifuged for 1 minute at 400 $\times$ g and examined for the presence of agglutinated red cells. Incomplete cold hemagglutinins can often be detected by the albumin test.

2. The Heterophile Hemagglutinin Test

The heterophile antibody is capable of reacting with a lipopolysaccharide hapten of erythrocytes, called the Forssman heterogenetic antigen (Brunius, 1936). It is immunologically related to the blood group A substance (Morgan and King, 1943; Bendich et al., 1946). It was detected in various organs of guinea pigs, horse, cat, mouse, chicken, tortoise, and carp, and in some bacteria, for example, in *Diplococcus pneumoniae* and *Shigella dysenteriae* (Landsteiner and Levine, 1927; Bailey and Shorb, 1933; Buchbinder, 1935; Brunius, 1936; Morgan and Partridge, 1941; Goebel et al., 1943). Another heterogenetic (enterobacterial) antigen was discovered by Kunin et al. (1962) in many species of enteric bacteria by means of the indirect bacterial hemagglutination test.

The original heterophile hemagglutination test (presumptive test), by Paul and Bunnell (1932), as modified by Melnick (1969), is performed as follows: the antigen preparation consists of a 1% suspension of sheep erythrocytes, washed with physiologic saline several times. The tested serum is heated at 56° for 30 minutes to inactivate normal sheep-erythrocyte lysins. Serial twofold dilutions from 1:2.5 to 1:1280 of the inactivated serum are then made in 0.5 ml; to each serum dilution, 0.5 ml of 1% sheep erythrocyte suspension are added yielding a final serum dilution ranging from 1:5 to 1:2560. Control tubes receive 0.5 ml of saline and 0.5 ml of the erythrocyte suspension. The mixtures are incubated at 37° for 2 hours and left at 4° overnight. Readings are made by shaking the tubes, and determining the highest serum dilution showing hemagglutination.

Titers of heterophile hemagglutinins which do not exceed the 1:40 serum dilution are regarded as normal, since these titers have been detected in about 10% sera of healthy individuals. Titers of heterophile hemagglutinins of 1:80 and preferably higher are observed in serum sickness, aplastic anemia, and after an administration of therapeutic horse serum. Higher titers, from 1:160 serum dilution upward, are regularly found in the sera obtained from patients with infectious mononucleosis. The reason for the occurrence of a high level of heterophile antibodies in cases of infectious mononucleosis is not yet known; however, it can depend on the presence of an assumed heterophile hapten among other antigens of the mononucleosis agent. Probably a similar hemagglutinin is responsible for the agglutination of rabbit erythrocytes in a majority of normal human sera. About 60% of human sera are able to agglutinate rabbit red blood cells at titers ranging from 1:8 to 1:64 (Kwapinski and Snyder, 1962).

An apparent relationship between titers of human heterophile hemagglutinins for sheep and rabbit erythrocytes was observed by Stuart et al. (1935).

Differential Absorption Hemagglutination Test. By means of this test, it is possible to distinguish between the hemagglutinins characteristic of infectious mononucleosis and other heterophilic antibodies or factors which agglutinate sheep red cells. It depends on the observation that the absorption of serum with antigens prepared from kidneys of guinea pigs removes heterophile antibodies of serum sickness, whereas heterophile hemagglutinins that are characteristically present in infectious mononucleosis and also in the serum sickness can be removed by an antigen preparation made of boiled beef blood corpuscles. These antigens are available as commercial preparations or can be prepared according to Davidsohn's method (1938).

The kidney reagent is prepared in the following way. Guinea pig kidneys are first disintegrated by repeatedly freezing and thawing, then washed with saline solution until the washings are free of blood. The tissues should be mashed into a fine pulp, and then suspended in saline to approximately 20% concentration, and boiled for 1 hour in the water bath. The boiled beef erythrocyte absorbent is prepared by boiling, for 1 hour in the water bath, washed beef red blood cells suspended in four volumes of saline. Phenol is added as preservative to 0.5 concentration.

Absorption with either of these preparations can be carried out by adding 0.5 ml of the kidney pulp or the erythrocyte absorbent per 0.1 ml of human serum, inactivated at 56°. The mixture is left for 1 hour at room temperature with occasional shaking, then centrifuged at 300 $\times$ g for 10 minutes. The supernatant fluid is used in the test to be performed as the ordinary heterophile hemagglutination test. A titer equal to, or higher than, 1:10 after the absorption with the guinea pig kidney is valid for the diagnosis of infectious mononucleosis. If hemagglutinins remain, the serum is further absorbed with bovine red blood cells as follows. Add 0.5 ml bovine red cells to 1 ml of the serum dilution absorbed with guinea pig kidney, mix, and incubate the mixture at 37° for 30 minutes. Centrifuge and collect the supernatant. Examine the double-absorbed serum with sheep erythrocytes in the same manner as the heterophile hemagglutinin test. Trypsinized red blood cells are recommended for the heterophile-hemagglutination test by Tomcsik (1960). In this procedure, 0.2 ml of 0.1% trypsinized and washed sheep erythrocytes are added to 0.1-ml volume of progressing dilutions of a human serum absorbed with a guinea pig kidney pulp.

Interpretation of the results of the differential absorption hemagglutination test are evident from Table 44.

Table 44. Absorption Reactions of Hemagglutinins in Human Serum

Absorption (+) of Hemagglutinins Attained By		Source of Serum
Guinea Pig Kidney	Bovine Erythrocytes	
−	+	Infectious mononucleosis
+	+	Serum sickness
+	−	Normal serum

3. The Immune Hemagglutinin Test

Immune hemagglutinin tests reveal serological reactions between certain antigens present in the surface layers of erythrocytes and homologous immune antibodies. Thus either whole red blood cells or the stromata may be employed as antigen preparations in these tests. Immune hemagglutinins, in contrast to the heterophile hemagglutinins or the isohemagglutinins, are heat-stable, show higher titers in the serum or in acacia gum solutions than in saline, and give a positive globulin test after the neutralization of the hemagglutinin titer.

i. *The Erythrocyte Test.* The test with whole erythrocytes is carried out either in tubes or on glass slides. In the first case, serial dilutions of a test serum, in 0.5-ml volumes, are mixed with an equal volume of 0.5 or 1% suspension of known red blood cells, and incubated at 37° for 1 to 2 hours, then centrifuged at 500 × g for 2 minutes, and read with the aid of a hand lens. The highest serum dilution showing a definite hemagglutination is taken as end point. Control tubes should contain series of dilutions of a known positive or negative serum mixed with the erythrocyte suspension. Additional control tubes receive 0.5 ml of saline and 0.5 ml of the erythrocyte suspension.

Table 45. Interpretation of the Rh Hemagglutination Test in Terms of
Phenotypes (Heiken and Rasmuson, 1966)

Reactions with Anti-

CC^w	C^w	c	D	E	e	Phenotypes	Genotypes	
−		+	−	−		rr	cde/cde	rr
−		+	+	−		R_0r	cDe/cde	R^0r
							cDe/cDe	R^0R^0
−		+	−	+	+	$r''r$	cdE/cde	$r''r$
−		+	−	+	−	$r''r''$	cdE/cdE	$r''r''$
−		+	+	+	−	R_2R_2	cDE/cDE	R^2R^2
							cDE/cdE	R^2r''
−		+	+	+	+	R_2r	cDE/cde	R^2r
							cDE/cDe	R^2R^0
							cDe/cdE	R^0r''
+	−	+	−	−		$r'r$	Cde/cde	$r'r$
+	−	+	+	−		R_1r	CDe/cde	R^1r
							CDe/cDe	R^1R^0
							cDe/Cde	R^0r'
+	+	+	+	−		R_1^wr	C^wDe/cde	$R^{1w}r$
							C^wDE/cDE	$R^{1w}R^0$
							C^wde/cDe	r'^wR^0
+	−	+	−	+	+	$r'r''$	Cde/cdE	$r'r''$
+	−	+	+	+	+	R_1R_2	CDe/cDE	R^1R^2
							CDe/cdE	R^1r''
							Cde/cDE	$r'R^2$
							CDE/cde	R^2r
+	−	+	+	+	−	R_zR_2	CDE/cDe	R^zR^0
							CDE/cDE	R^zR^2
+	+	+	+	+	+	$R_1^wR_2$	CDE/cdE	R^zr''
							C^wDe/cDE	$R^{1w}R^2$
							C^wDe/cdE	$R^{1w}r''$
+	+	+	−	+	+	r'^wr''	C^wde/cDE	r'^wR^2
+	+	+	−	−		R'^wr	C^wde/cdE	r'^wr''
+	−	−	−	−		$r'r'$	C^wde/cde	r'^wr
+	−	−	+	−		R_1R_1	Cde/Cde	$r'r'$
							CDe/CDe	R^1R^1
+	+	−	−	−		r'^wr'	CDe/Cde	R^1r'
							C^wde/Cde	r'^wr'
+	+	−	+	−		$R_1^wR_1$	C^wde/C^wde	$r'^wr'^w$
							C^wDe/CDe	$R^{1w}R^1$
							C^wDe/Cde	$R^{1w}r'$
							C^wDe/C^wDe	$R^{1w}R^{1w}$
							C^wde/CDe	R'^wR^1
+	−	−	+	+	+	R_zR_1	C^wde/C^wDE	r'^wR^{1w}
							CDE/CDe	R^zR^1
+	−	−	+	+	−	R_zR_z	CDE/Cde	R^zr'
+	+	−	+	+	+	$R_1^wR_z$	CDE/CDE	R^zR^z
							C^wDe/CDE	$R^{1w}R^z$
							C^wde/CDE	r'^wR^z

Table 46.   Numerical Notation of Rh
(Rosenfield et al., 1962; Race and Sanger, 1968)

	CDE[a]	Rh-Hr		CDE	Rh-Hr		CDE	Rh-Hr
Rh1	D	Rh_0	Rh10	V, ce^8	hr^v	Rh19		hr^8
Rh2	C	rh'	Rh11	E^w	rh^{w2}	Rh20	VS, e^8	
Rh3	E	rh''	Rh12	F	rh^G	Rh21	C^G	
Rh4	c	hr'	Rh13		Rh^A	Rh22	CE	
Rh5	e	hr''	Rh14		Rh^B	Rh23	Wiel, D^w	
Rh6	f, ce	hr	Rh15		Rh^C	Rh24	E^T	
Rh7	Ce	rh_i	Rh16		Rh^D	Rh25	LW	
Rh8	C^w	rh^{w1}	Rh17		Hr_0	Rh26		
Rh9	C^x	rh^x	Rh18		Hr	Rh27	cE	

[a] CDE and Rh-Hr notations are synonymous.

In the slide test, one drop of each serum dilution is mixed with one drop of 0.5% erythrocyte suspension. The mixtures are incubated at room temperature or at 37° for 2 to 5 minutes and observed under a magnifying glass.

ii. *The Erythrocyte-Stromata Test (Winn et al., 1953).* The erythrocyte stromata are prepared in the following manner: red blood cells are washed three times with saline solution and then sedimented by centrifugation, withdrawn, and resuspended in 40 volumes of cold distilled water and left in the cold for 1 to 6 hours. The fluid is then adjusted to pH 5.0 or 5.5 with hydrochloric acid, to sediment the stromata. The stromata should be centrifuged and resuspended in 10 ml of cold water at pH 4.0 to 4.5 and left for 2 hours. The fluid is then adjusted to pH 5.5 and centrifuged, and the supernatant is removed. The latter part of the preparation must be repeated until no hemoglobin is detected in the washings. The stromata are finally resuspended in saline containing 0.4% formalin, and they can be stored in the cold. This preparation should be washed prior to use.

In a more recent procedure, published by Klein (1960), the erythrocyte stromata are obtained by exposing red blood cells to a 10 to 12% aqueous solution of glycerin for 30 minutes at 37°. The erythrocytes thus treated are then centrifuged, washed in citrated saline (a 0.85% sodium chloride solution containing 0.03 *M* sodium citrate), and last in a buffered saline.

The test is set up by mixing equal volumes of the stromata suspension and various dilutions of the test serum and incubating the mixtures at 37° for 2 hours or at 4° for 18 to 24 hours, with frequent agitation. The tubes are then centrifuged at 500 to 800 × g for 45 minutes at 4°. The precipitates should be washed three times with a saline solution in the cold and analyzed for nitrogen contents. The results are expressed as milligrams of the antibody nitrogen. The antibody nitrogen is calculated from the difference between the total nitrogen in the test tubes and in the control tubes.

iii. *The Periodate-Erythrocyte Hemagglutination Test.* The periodate treatment of erythrocytes is carried out by incubating for 30 minutes at room temperature, a mixture of equal volumes of 50% suspension of washed human group O Rh+ or hen erythrocytes red blood cells, and *M/* 100 potassium periodate solution in a pH 7.4 phosphate-buffered saline. The cells are then spun down at 300 × g for 10 minutes and washed three times in PBS, pH 7.4, with centrifugation at 300 × g.

The hemagglutination test is set up by mixing equal volumes of a 5% suspension of periodate treated erythrocytes and serial dilutions of serum. The mixtures are left at room temperature for 30 minutes and read by examining the sediments with the aid of a hand lens.

The Panhemagglutination. Two related types of the panhemagglutination can be induced by certain alterations of either erythrocytes or serum. The first type of reaction is named the Thomson-Friedenreich or T-hemagglutination, and the other the bacteriogenic or the h-hemagglutination.

iv. *The T-hemagglutination Test.* The so called T-agglutinogen of erythrocytes is uncovered or activated by enzymes produced by some bacteria, for example, *Vibrio comma, Vibrio proteus, Clostridium perfringens, Diplococcus pneumoniae,* diphtheroids, and viruses of influenza, mumps, and Newcastle disease. The T-agglutinogen renders erythrocytes agglutinable by the T-agglutinin, a substance which occurs in the normal serum of many mammalian species. Apparently another antigen of human red blood cells can be revealed by digestion with animal proteolytic enzymes, which render the Rh-positive erythrocytes agglutinable in a solution of incomplete anti-Rh serum. This agglutinability of red cells can be observed after the digestion of erythrocytes with a crystalline trypsin or chymotrypsin used at 0.0025% concentration. The periodate treatment of erythrocytes also makes them susceptible to panagglutinins.

The T-agglutinin is distinct from the cold agglutinin, since it reacts optimally at 15 to 20°, is absorbable to the altered red blood cells and can be removed following an absorption with altered erythrocytes. The T-hemagglutination may cause erroneous results of blood grouping, if erythrocytes used in the test have been altered by microbial enzymes either *in vitro,* or *in vivo,* in cases of infections by the microorganisms ctied above. Although most of the slightly damaged red blood cells are eliminated by spleen, a number of altered erythrocytes can remain in the blood stream for a longer period, and these may be responsible for the T-hemagglutination.

The T-agglutinin is absent from newborns but occurs in all adults' sera at titers ranging from 1:128 to 1:256 (Stickl, 1953). Higher titers are found in the sera from primary atypical pneumonia (Lind and McArthur, 1947) and decreased levels are frequently found in the acute phase of an anthrax infection, which presumably depends on the alteration of cell receptors. The T-agglutinin titer returns to a normal level in the convalescence.

The T-agglutinogen can be uncovered by removing certain receptors of human, type O erythrocytes by the receptor-destroying enzyme (RDE), which occurs most abundantly in the culture filtrates of *Vibrio comma.* This enzyme may be used either in a crude form of a culture filtrate of *Vibrio comma* or as a purified preparation obtained by the Burnet et al. (1946) method.

The activity of the receptor-destroying enzyme can be estimated by Bial's method, measuring the release of *N*-acetylneuramic acid, which probably forms the virus receptors of red blood cells (Böhm et al., 1954).

The T-agglutinogen is prepared, according to the technique of Makinodan and Macris (1955), in the following manner: an 18-hour culture of *Vibrio comma* is filtered through a Seitz pad, and the salt contents in the filtrate is brought to 0.9%. A volume of this liquid is mixed with an equal volume of a 2% human or chicken erythrocyte suspension and incubated at 37° for 20 to 40 minutes. The cells are then centrifuged, washed twice with saline, resuspended at the original volume, and left at 4° for 12 hours.

The T-hemagglutination test by Wright and Slein (1957) is set up as follows. To serial, twofold dilutions of serum under test, made in 0.5-ml volumes of saline, are added 0.5-ml amounts of a 1% RED-digested erythrocyte suspension, and the mixtures are incubated at 37° for 30 minutes. The red cells are then resuspended by shaking, incubated for another half hour at 37°, left at room temperature for 30 minutes, and inspected for the presence of agglutinates. The titer is expressed as reciprocal of the final serum dilution showing definite hemagglutination. The test can also be set up on plastic or glass plates.

v. *The Bacteriogenic Hemagglutination Test.* This type of panagglutination, described by Davidsohn and Toharsky (1940, 1942), is due to some alterations in the human plasma and serum, caused by the growth of certain bacteria (*Corynebacterium* H, a strain similar to *Corynebacterium liquefaciens,* and a strain of *Pseudomonas aeruginosa*), resulting in the capacity of the plasma or serum of agglutinating any red blood cells. *Corynebacterium* H is capable of growth at a low temperature; therefore the bacterial hemagglutinins can be formed even in the sera stored in the cold.

The bacteriogenic hemagglutinin test is set up with the serum freed of bacteria by passing a sample of serum through a bacteriological filter. Two drops of undiluted and serially, from 1:2 to 1:32, diluted serum, are mixed with one drop of a 2% erythrocyte suspension. The mixtures are left at room temperature for 2 hours with occasional shaking, then observed by the aid of a low-power objective of the microscope, after agitating the tubes to suspend the sediment. The highest serum dilution causing a distinct clumping is recorded as the panagglutinating titer of the serum.

4. Isohemagglutination Tests

The isohemagglutination test depends on a reaction between the agglutinogens of erythrocytes and the corresponding hemagglutinins (Table 47)

Table 47. Blood Group Antigens in Human Erythrocytes
(Race and Sanger, 1968)

	Antigens Detected by	
System	Positive Reaction with Specific Antibody	Positive Reaction with One Antibody, Negative with Another
A_1A_2BO	A_1, B, H[b]	A_2, A_3, Ax, and other A and B variants
MNSs	M, N, S, s, M^g, M_1, Tm, M^k, Hu, He, Mi^a, Vw(Gr), Mur, Hil, Vr, Ri^a, St^a, Mt^a, Cl^a, Ny^a, Sul, Sj	M_2, N_2, M^c, M^a, M^v, S_2
P	P_1, p^k, Luke[b]	P_2
Rh	D, C, c, C^w, C^x, E, e, e^s, E^w, G, ce, ce^s(v), Ce, CE, cE, D^w, E^T, LW[b]	D^u, C^u, E^u, and other variants of D, C, c, e
Lutheran	Lu^a, Lu^b	
Kell	K, k, Kp^a, Kp^b, Js^a, Js^b	
Lewis	Le^a, Le^b	
Kidd	Jk^a, Jk^b	
Diego	Di^a, Di^b	
Duffy	Fy^a, Fy^b	
Yt	Yt^a, Yt^b	
I	I, i	
Xg	Xg^a	
Dombrock	Do^r	
Very frequent antigens	Vel, Ge, Lan, Co^a, Gy^a, At^a	
Very infrequent antigens	Levay, Wr^a, Be^a, By, Sw^a, Good, Bi, Tr^a, Wb, Bp^a, Rd, Ls^e, Box, Or, Ht^a, Gf, W^u	
Other antigens	Au^a, Sm, Bu^a, Bg, Cs^a, Sd^a, Ul^a, Go^a, Chido	

[a] Reproduced from *Blood Groups in Man* by Race and Sanger with the permission of Blackwell Scientific Publications.

[b] A genetically independent part of the system.

which may occur in a normal serum or after a natural or artificial immunization with certain hemagglutinogens. There are approximately 5×10^5 specific combining groups on an erythrocyte. As many as 4000 molecules of isohemagglutinins must combine with each single erythrocyte to bring about the agglutination. This is equivalent of 10^{-4} g of the hemagglutinin nitrogen per gram of the erythrocyte nitrogen (Filitti-Wurmser et al., 1954).

The determination of the blood group may be conducted by using the following serological systems for the hemagglutination test: (a) the red blood cells under test and standard blood group antisera containing iso-agglutinins anti-A and anti-B, anti-A alone, and anti-B alone; (b) the test serum and standard erythrocytes containing agglutinogens A, B, or AB.

Standard blood group antisera can be produced by the following procedure (Boyd, 1939): a 30% suspension of washed, packed erythrocytes of a required group (A, B, OM, or ON) is injected into rabbit three times a week, twelve injections in all. First injection is given intraperitoneally, followed by intravenous injections. One week after the last injection, the animals are bled. The sera are then inactivated, diluted in a ratio of 1:15 or 1:20 with saline, and absorbed at 37° with the appropriate cells, to remove nonspecific agglutinins. For example, the anti-A serum is absorbed with the B or O erythrocytes or with the BMN or OMN erythrocytes.

The anti-M sera should be absorbed with N cells such as ON, An, Bn, or ABN. The average titer of these sera is between 640 to 1280. The sera can be preserved for as long as 5 years by adding solutions of some dyes, for example, 1% aqueous solution of neutral acriflavine (0.01 ml of this solution to be added per milliliter serum) or 1% aqueous solution of brilliant green (0.02 ml/ml serum). These dyes not only preserve the sera but also color-label them.

Other methods of preparing standard group specific sera were published by Landsteiner (1928), and Wiener et al. (1934).

The isohemagglutination test may be set up either in the serological tubes, capillary tubings, or on glass slides. Techniques of this test in tubes, as described by Beiser and Kabat (1952), or by Wilkie and Becker (1955), are recommended. Older techniques can be found in the papers published by Landsteiner (1900), Landsteiner and Richter (1903), Lattes (1927), and Stuart et al. (1936).

   i. *The Beiser and Kabat (1952) Isohemagglutinin Test.* Progressing dilutions of the test serum are made in 0.2 ml of saline and mixed with the 0.1 ml of a 4% suspension of thrice washed A, B, or O human erythrocytes, and made up to 0.5 ml with saline. After the incubation at 37° for 1 hour, the mixtures are centrifuged at $300 \times$ g and the agglutination is observed with the aid of a hand lens. The titer of the serum is expressed in terms of the reciprocal of the highest dilution which produced a detectable hemagglutination.

The suspension of standard human red blood cells of the required group is made in buffered saline by cell-counting method to give totals of 12,500 to 14,500 cells/ml. The suspension can also be standardized spectrophotometrically, as described by Kabat et al. (1945). The test serum is diluted serially in duplicate, in 0.5-ml volumes, and mixed with 0.5 ml of erythrocyte suspension in serological tubes equipped with rubber stoppers, and left at room temperature for 10 minutes. Control tubes contain 0.5 ml of cell suspension and 0.5 ml of buffered saline. Before reading, the mixtures are centrifuged at $65 \times g$ for 1 minute. The cell deposits are agitated on the Kahn shaker for 2 hours at 120 oscillations/minute. Aliquots are then transferred by means of a capillary tubing into two chambers of a Bausch and Lomb phase-contrast hemocytometer. The number of free or nonagglutinated erythrocytes is counted either directly from the hemocytometer or from the photographic negatives taken with a microscope camera. Five large squares of the entire millimeter square are counted, and the number of single cells in the four chambers of each set of duplicates is averaged to calculate the number of free cells.

The number of free erythrocytes per milliliter given by the controls represents the number of erythrocytes agglutinated at this concentration of serum. The percentage of agglutinated cells is calculated by dividing the number of agglutinated cells per milliliter by the total number of cells per milliliter. The concentration of serum (milliliter per milliliter) is defined as the amount of undiluted serum contained in 1 ml of serum dilution.

The test, in which amounts of reagents as small as 0.1 ml are employed, was published by Young and Witebsky (1945).

In a simplified isohemagglutination technique (Kariher, 1944), the blood typing is performed on the individual's own skin. Blood drops, punctuated from two fingers, are mixed on the skin with group A or B serum and read under an adequate light.

ii. *The Absorption-Elution Isohemagglutination Assay.* In this test (Kind, 1960), the A and B isoagglutinogens in thick blood smears can be determined. Thus a dried blood smear made on a microscopic slide is first fixed by immersion in pH 7.4 McIlvaine buffer at 100° for 30 seconds. The denatured smear is then blotted dry and divided into separate cavities bounded by gum dammar per beeswax mixture.

Antiisoagglutinin sera are then dispensed into the cavities in excess of the amount required to saturate the antigen. The slide is left on a moist chamber for 3 hours with occasional gentle agitation, and rinsed with water and blotted dry.

A drop of 2% erythrocyte suspensions are subsequently added to the different cavities and the slide is incubated at 50° for 5 minutes in a moist chamber. The slide is then placed at room temperature and rotated gently. Agglutination of erythrocytes is observed in the cavities where the isoagglutinins were eluted by the elevated temperature. The same test may be used to determine isoagglutinogens in dried blood stains on fabrics (Kind, 1960).

iii. *The M and N Agglutinogen Test.* The assay after Wiener et al. (1934) is carried out by mixing in small test tubes one drop of a 3% citrate suspension of examined red blood cells and one drop of appropriate dilutions of absorbed antisera specific for M or N. The mixtures are left for 1 hour at room temperature, then examined for the presence of agglutinates above a small concave mirror. Centrifugation of test tubes at 300 × g for 2 minutes before reading is often advantageous.

A 1 to 2% cell suspension gives comparable results. Results are interpreted as shown in Table 48.

Table 48. Interpretation of the M and N
Agglutinogen Testing

Hemagglutination with the Serum		Agglutinogen Detected
Anti-M	Anti-N	
+	−	M
−	+	N
+	+	MN

iv. *The Isohemagglutination Test with Body Fluids.* Blood groups substances occur not only in the erythrocytes but also in the saliva, gastric juice, sweat, and the seminal fluid in most people known as "secretors." The test devised by Yamakami (1926) for the determination of blood group agglutinogens in saliva is carried out as follows. A standard group antiserum is diluted, on the basis of preliminary titration, to contain eight times the minimal amount of hemagglutinin needed to cause slumping of a 2.5% erythrocyte suspension containing homologous agglutinogen. Amounts of 0.5 ml of this serum dilution are added to 0.5 ml of varying dilutions of filtered specimens of saliva. The mixtures are shaken and left at 2° overnight; 0.2-ml volumes of each mixture are then transferred into three small test tubes containing one drop of a 2.4% suspension of erythrocytes belonging to groups O, A, and B, respectively. The samples are incubated for 30 minutes at 37° and examined for the presence of agglutinates.

A similar test can be used for detection of blood-group agglutinogens in other body fluids.

v. *The Capillary-Tube Isohemagglutination Test.* This assay (Chown, 1944) is more often used for the detection of Rh factor than for the ordinary grouping of blood. It is carried out in the following way.

A capillary tube (0.5 mm by 10 to 15 cm) is filled with an anti-Rh testing serum to the length of 2 cm, and then with a 10 to 20% suspension of a patient's red blood cells. After mixing the constituents, the tube is sealed at one end and placed in a rack at an angle of 45° to the base. The mixtures are incubated for 30 minutes at 37°, and read against a white background in a bright light above the concave side of a microscope mirror. If the Rh factor is present, a coarse agglutination along the tube is seen; and if it is absent, a smooth line of sedimented cells can be observed.

The Rh immune sera for the test can be produced by injecting human volunteers or guinea pigs with red blood cells containing the Rh factor. The Rh antigen occurs in the erythrocytes of the *Macacca rhesus* monkey and of a majority of human beings (Landsteiner and Wiener, 1940). Individuals with the blood cells containing no antigen Rh can be immunized artificially or following previous immunization by pregnancy or transfusion, and they often serve as donors of anti-Rh serum.

For experimental purposes, guinea pigs are injected with erythrocytes of *Macacca rhesus* or with human Rh+ cells (Carter, 1945). The animals should receive two intrabdominal injections of 1 ml of packed, washed erythrocytes, at 5-day intervals; and they are bled 1 or 2 weeks after the last injection.

The test according to the technique of Murray is set out on platforms of multiple-grooved 5-in. slides, and dilutions of sera for the titration are made in welled slides. Single drops of standard test sera are mixed with a 5 to 10% suspension of tested red blood cells. The slides are then put into flat plastic boxes, kept humid by a layer of damp blotting paper placed on the bottom. After 1 hour incubation at 37°, the slides are tilted and inspected with the naked eye for the presence of agglutinates of erythrocytes.

vi. *The Isohemagglutinin Slide Test.* The slide test is often used for the determination of the main group of erythrocytes and for detection of the Rh factor.

The *blood grouping* by slide test is carried out as follows. A blood from a finger is diluted in 1 ml of 0.9% sodium chloride, and a drop of this suspension is added to a drop of anti-A serum and anti-B serum placed on a divided glass slide. The serum and cells are mixed, and the slide is rocked to hasten the agglutination which occurs usually in 30 seconds to 2 minutes. The blood group is determined from the reactions in the standard sera as shown diagrammatically in Table 49.

Table 49.   Interpretation of the Isohemagglutinin Tests
Performed with Standard Antisera

Erythrocyte Reaction with Serum		Group Agglutinogen of Cells Detected
Anti-A	Anti-B	
−	−	O
+	−	A
−	+	B
+	+	AB

The group agglutinogen of cells should be confirmed by a "back typing" procedure, in which the serum of the individual being examined is tested for the presence of the appropriate isoagglutinin. For this purpose, 2% suspensions of standard group A and B cells are mixed with drops of serum of the examined individual and observed, after $\frac{1}{2}$ to 2 minutes, for the presence of agglutinates. The results can be interpreted by reference to Table 50.

Table 50.   Interpretation of the Isohemagglutinin Tests
Performed with Standard Erythrocytes

Serum Reaction with Erythrocyte Group				Antibodies against	Blood Group
A	B	O	AB		
−	+	−	+	B	A
+	−	−	+	A	B
+	+	−	+	A and B	O
−	−	−	−	−	AB

Both tests for blood grouping can be set up in tubes instead of glass slides. Each test should be accompanied by a control with a known anti-A and anti-B serum to check the sensitivity of the A and B cells. It is recommended that erythrocytes of the examined person be suspended in his own serum to exclude the possibility of an autohemagglutination which could be caused, for example, by cold hemagglutinins.

vii. *The Blood Grouping on Cellophaned Cards.*   The test, by Eldon (1956), is set up on cards covered with regenerated cellulose. Each of four panels on a card carries a serum reagent placed in an amount of 0.06 ml and dried. The reagent consists of 10 ml of a standard (anti-A, B, ABO, or anti-D) serum, 90 ml of 6% dextran, and 2 drops of 5% heparin solution. The reagents dried on a card are dissolved in water prior to the use and mixed with a drop of capillary blood tested or a saline suspension of blood cells. The card should be tilted slowly for 3 minutes at room temperature, then read for the presence of agglutinates. A similar test, set up in disposable plastic agglutination trays, was described by Sanders and Wright (1962). In this technique, one drop (approximately 0.03 ml) of 2% red blood cell suspension in Alsever's solution is added to a drop of absorbed sera in an appropriate dilution. The mixtures are agitated on a shaker for 15 minutes, left in the refrigerator for 1 hour, read, and left overnight in the refrigerator before final reading.

viii. *The Rh Factor Hemagglutination Test.* The assay after Simmons et al. (1944) is set up on glass slides, 4 × 3 in., divided into twelve rectangles by thick painted lines. One drop of a potent anti-Rh$_o$ serum, from which the anti-A and anti-B agglutinins were absorbed, is placed in one rectangle and mixed with one drop of a 5% suspension of the examined red blood cells suspended in the Rous-Turner solution.* Suspensions of known Rh-positive and Rh-negative red blood cells are mixed with the same anti-ORh serum in each of two other rectangles.

The slide is placed in a moisture chamber and left for 30 minutes at 37°. The slide is then gently rocked and examined for agglutinates by the naked eye. Larger or smaller aggregates of red blood cells are formed if the tested erythrocytes possess the Rh agglutinogen. In doubtful cases, the slide should be examined microscopically to distinguish between a fine granulation and the rouleaux formation. Other useful hemagglutination slide techniques for the Rh factor determination are those devised by Diamond and Abelson (1945) and Unger (1954). A similar procedure for the main agglutinogen was published by Gettler and Kramer (1936) and Murray (1952). A hemagglutination-inhibition test applied to the group substances is described on p. 529.

For a complete analysis of the Rh factors (Tables 45–46), it is necessary to examine the red blood cells being examined with the following antisera: anti-C (anti-Rh), anti-D (anti-Rh$_o$), and anti-E (anti-rh″), anti-c (anti-hr′), and possibly with anti-e (anti-hr″).

ix. *The Cross-Match (Direct Compatibility) Test.* The cross-match test is conducted to determine whether the blood of a donor is compatible with that of a recipient. This test can be set up either in tubes or on glass

---

* The Rous-Turner solution consists of 16 ml of 5.4% glucose solution and 6.6 ml of 3.8% sodium citrate solution, which are sterilized separately at 110° for 15 minutes, and then combined.

slides. Suspensions of red blood cells in 20 to 30% bovine albumin or saline, and sera of both the donor and recipient, are used for this test. In the tube technique, two drops of recipient's serum and two drops of donor's erythrocyte suspension are placed in one small tube, and two drops of recipient's erythrocytes and two drops of donor's serum are placed in another tube. Control tubes receive each serum and its own red blood cells. The tubes are centrifuged at a moderate speed for 3 minutes, then shaken to resuspend the cells and read. If no agglutination is observed in any tube, the donor's blood is regarded as compatible with that of the recipient individual.

The slide test is carried out by mixing one drop of donor's erythrocytes with one drop of recipient's serum on one half of a glass slide, and one drop of recipient's erythrocytes mixed with one drop of donor's serum on another half. The slide is placed in a Petri dish and read after 15 and 30 minutes.

Weak Rh antibodies may often be detected by the test with erythrocytes digested with papain or ficin (Stratton, 1953; Makinodan and Macris, 1955). Apart from these, several other animal and plant proteases, such as trypsin, chymotrypsin, bromelin, and erepsin, were found to render Rh-positive erythrocytes agglutinable by "incomplete" anti-Rh sera. Papainized cells are prepared by incubating mixtures consisting of equal volumes of washed packed erythrocytes and a solution containing equal parts of 1% papain and 0.2% L-cysteine hydrochloride for 10 minutes at 37°. Ficin can be used in the concentration of 1.5 mg/ml of packed cells. The erythrocytes, mixed with ficin at pH 4.7 to 7.8, should be incubated at 22 to 37° for 10 to 30 minutes (Makinodan and Macris, 1955).

The test may be carried out either on glass slides or in tubes, at room temperature or at 37°. Equal volumes of a 10% saline suspension of washed papainized erythrocytes and the serum under test, diluted 1:2, are mixed together. Control tubes receive papainized or ficin treated erythrocytes, suspended in either a normal, group AB serum, or in saline. The slides are rocked for 7 minutes, and examined for the presence of clumps of cells under the lower power of the microscope or through a hand lens.

x. *The Slide-Centrifuge Hemagglutination Test (Kwapinski, 1972)*

1. Arrange constituents of each plastic chamber in the cytocentrifuge in the following order: a glass slide, a cellulose-acetate strip (Serometrics), and a punched, water-absorbing filter-paper strip (Fig. 50).

2. Incubate for 1 to 2 minutes a mixture consisting of 0.1 ml of antiserum and 0.1 ml of 0.2% blood cell suspension in saline.

3. Transfer the mixture to a plastic chamber of the cytocentrifuge and spin the mixture at 1000 rpm for 5 minutes.

4. Wash off the noncombined material of the reaction mixture from the acetate strip in two changes of 1 M NaCl for 2 minutes.

5. View the cellulose strip against a fluorescent light through a $10\times$ magnifying glass.

The erythrocyte-antibody complexes appear in the form of red-stained disc, corresponding to the hole in the water-absorbing filter-paper strip. Similarly treated mixtures of erythrocytes and nonrelated hemagglutinins form no visible area of deposit on the cellulose-acetate membrane.

xi. *Determination of the Thermal Amplitude of Isohemagglutinins.* Only the isohemagglutinins which function readily at 37° may cause transfusion reactions, whereas the antibodies functioning at lower temperatures do not cause these reactions. Some warm isohemagglutinins, however, are able to act at a lower temperature, and occasionally a cold hemagglutinin gives a slight serological reaction at 37°.

The thermal amplitude of isohemagglutinins is determined by incubating parallel series of serum dilutions, mixed with an appropriate erythrocyte suspension at 40, 18, and 37° for 2 hours. The hemagglutination titers obtained at each temperature are then compared.

A practical scoring system (Dunsford and Bowley, 1955) depends on converting the recordings of reactions to numerical scores. Scores for the intensity of hemagglutination, recorded as $++$, $+$, $(+)$, gw, or w, are 8, 5, 3, 2, and 1, respectively. Scores estimated for each test tube are added to give a final numerical score.

xii. *The Forensic Blood-Group Determination.* The forensic isohemagglutinin test is used for determination of agglutinogens in dried blood stains. This assay should be preceded by a precipitin test with a human globulin antiserum, to prove that the stain contains human blood. Two assays are set up with a human blood stain, the test for group-specific absorptive power, and a modified isohemagglutinin test (Boyd and Boyd, 1937).

In the latter assay, samples of stained material are placed in 1-ml volumes of diluted anti-A and anti-B sera and left in an ice box for 24 hours. The supernatants are tested with the A and B group red blood cells. A negative result of hemagglutination test with either of these cells indicates that the corresponding isoagglutinins have been removed (aborbed) by the blood stain, and consequently the stain is classified as a group A or B, respectively.

Application of Isohemagglutinin Tests. Isohemagglutination tests are widely applied to the blood grouping before a transfusion, for medicolegal purposes (determination of relationships including the disputed fraternity), and for the study of the animal evolution and genetics.

xiii. *The Platelet Agglutination Test (Shulman, 1958).* Platelets are obtained from human blood mixed with an anticoagulent (1 part of 1.5% disodium ethylenediaminetetra-acetate, pH 7, to nine parts of blood). The blood is then centrifuged at 200 $\times$ g for 15 minutes.

The supertant plasma is withdrawn and centrifuged at 2500 $\times$ g for 30 minutes. The sediment containing platelets is washed in saline and resuspended in a saline solution to a concentration of 10^6/ml. The agglutination test is set up on siliconed slides or in siliconed tube by mixing equal volumes of a platelet suspension and serially diluted antiserum preheated at 56° for 40 minutes. Microscopic observations of clumps formed by agglutinated platelets are made at room temperature.

Chapter Ten

THE LYSIS ASSAYS

The common feature of reactions classified as the lysis assays is the destruction and dissolution of either blood cells (erythrocytes, leukocytes, platelets) or bacterial cells. In immunolytic tests, the immune reaction occurs on the surface of these cells, and it involves natural cell- or cell-absorbed antigens and corresponding antibodies. Immune complexes thus formed absorb complement which brings about the lysis of blood cells or gacteria. Reactions between the natural surface antigens of blood cells or bacteria, a specific antibody and complement, are placed in the group of direct or active immnunolytic tests. Indirect or passive immunolytic tests depend on immune reactions between the soluble antigens artificially attached to the cells and antibodies corresponding to the adsorbed antigen with the subsequent absorption of complement and the resulting lysis of antigen carriers. The immune hemolysis or bacteriolysis therefore provides an evidence for specific affinity and complementarity existing between the antigen and the antibody involved in this reaction.

The immunolytic assay must be distinguished from the nonimmune lysis of blood cells by hemolysins produced by certain bacteria, viruses, and microfungi. The microbial hemolysins are not antibodies but antigens which can be neutralized by specific antibodies, the antihemolysins. Microbial hemolysins participate as antigens in the immune hemolysis-inhibition tests (see p. 441).

I. IMMUNOLYTIC TESTS

Antigens used in the immunolytic tests are either cells or soluble preparations of antigens adsorbed onto erythrocytes or leukocytes. Immunolytic reactions were first described by Pfeiffer and Marx (1898) and Bordet (1898). Pfeiffer described an immune bacteriolytic test, and Bordet's paper dealt with a specific hemolysis caused by the immune serum hemolysin. The immune lysis of white blood cells was described by Wittkower (1923), and this test was further developed by Vaughan (1939), and Favour et al. (1949). The immunolytic test with blood platelets was introduced by Cruz (1953). The first technique of a passive hemolytic test was published in

1950 by Fisher and Keogh. Immunolytic tests may be divided into two major classes, the direct (active) and indirect (passive) immunolytic tests, with nine minor groups as follows:

I. *Direct (Active) Immunolytic Assays*

1. The immunohemolysin test.
2. The localized immunohemolysis test.
3. The autohemolysin test.
4. The isohemolysin test.
5. The heterophile-hemolysin test.
6. The blood platelet immunolysis test.
7. The leukocyte immunolysis test.
8. The immunobacteriolytic assays.
9. The ablastin test.

II. *The Indirect (Passive) Immunohemolysis Assay*

1. The passive immunohemolysin assays.
2. The indirect localized immunohemolysis assays.

Techniques of individual immunolytic tests, selected after numerous experiments, are presented below.

I. *Direct (Active) Immunolytic Assays*

Direct immune lytic tests depend on a reaction between the superficially situated normal or natural antigens of blood cells or bacteria and the corresponding antibodies. The absorption of complement by these immune complexes results in the lysis of blood cells or bacteria.

1. *The Immunohemolysin Test.* Antibodies that participate in the immune hemolysis test, as well as in the autohemolysin and isohemolysin tests, are immune hemolysins, autohemolysins, or isohemolysins. These immunoglobulins are directed against antigenic sites on the surface of erythrocytes and react with them in conjection with the complement to release hemoglobin from the red blood cells.

Immune hemolysins can be produced by immunizing rabbits with a suspension of human red blood cells. Autohemolysins are found in the human serum in paroxysmal hemoglobinuria, which is characterized by the destruction of erythrocytes and by hemoglobinemia at a lower body temperature. The autohemolysin is extremely thermolabile, and its action can only be demonstrated at low temperatures. Isohemolysins occur in normal sera.

(i). *The active immunohemolysin test.* The test according to Kwapinski's (1965) technique is conducted as follows: 1 ml aliquots of a suspension of erythrocytes, standardized to contain 5×10^8 cells/ml, are added to equal volumes of a 1:10 dilution of complement and equilibrated in a water bath at 37° for 10 minutes; 0.5-ml volumes of a series of dilutions of an inactivated antiserum are placed in each tube, and the mixture is incubated at 37° for 30 minutes. All dilutions are made in a saline buffered at pH 7.4 to 7.6. The tubes are then transferred into an ice water bath, cooled for a few minutes, and centrifuged in a refrigerated centrifuge at 112 × g for 3 minutes. The supernatants should be withdrawn for the determination of optical densities in a spectrophotometer at 545 nm. Results are calculated in terms of 50% hemolysis units, determined from a curve of standard hemoglobin dilutions. The degree of hemolysis is a function of the concentration of immune hemolysin and of complement.

(ii). *Quantitative chemical determination of serum hemolysins.* The quantification of immune hemolysins may be accomplished by substituting erythrocyte stromata for intact red cells in the reaction with the immune hemolysin.

According to the Heidelberger and Treffers technique (1942), the erythrocyte stromata are obtained by suspending packed, washed red cells in 20 volumes of distilled water. The stromata are then deposited by centrifugation, washed twice with water, twice with 0.9% sodium chloride at room temperature, and twice with saline, at 0°. The pale brown stromata should be resuspended in saline containing Merthiolate at 1:10,000 final dilution.

The immune-hemolytic test with the erythrocyte-stromata is set up at 0° in duplicate, by adding 1.0 ml of a stromata suspension to 1.0 ml of a serum diluted in 2.0 ml of saline. Control tubes contain 1.0 ml of the suspension stromata diluted in 3.0 ml of saline. The tubes are shaken and left in an ice box for 48 hours with occasional shaking, and inspected for the presence of agglutinates. The mixtures are then centrifuged in the cold and the sediments are washed three times with 0.9% saline at 0°. The supernatants should be collected and mixed with another 1.0-ml aliquot of the stromata suspension, and centrifuged. The sediments are washed several times with saline, and all the washings are pooled.

All supernatants and washings from the stromata blanks are analyzed separately for the contents of nitrogen. The antibody nitrogen in test tubes containing the reaction mixture (a serum and stromata) is calculated as the difference between the total nitrogen precipitated and the stromata nitrogen deposited in the stromata blanks. Antibody values obtained are usually slightly too high because of the antigen which has dissolved in the dilute serum.

2. *The Localized Immunohemolysis Test.* The localized immunohemolysis test, or the antibody-plaque technique, depends on a reaction between antibodies produced *in vitro* by lymphoid cells, obtained from the spleen or lymph nodes of animals preimmunized with a particulate or nonparticulate antigen. Technically, the cell suspensions obtained from im-

munized spleen or lymph nodes are mixed with the corresponding erythrocytes in a gel. After an incubation time, complement is applied, which reacts with the antibody adsorbed onto the corresponding cells and causes hemolysis, occurring in the form of a zone or plaque around the antibody-synthesizing cells. A single lytic zone, or plaque, represents one antibody-synthesizing cell.

The original localized immunohemolysis test (Jerne and Nordin, 1963) was used with the erythrocytes serving as a particulate antigen preparation and their antibodies (the direct test). The technique was modified so that polysaccharide- or protein-coated erythrocytes are employed for the detection of cells producing antipolysaccharide- or antiprotein immunoglobulins (the indirect test).

The number of antibody plaque-forming cells present in a spleen suspension prepared by ordinary methods is usually relatively small. The enrichment of antibody plaque-forming cells may be obtained by centrifugation in a sucrose gradient, equilibrium centrifugation in a protein gradient, and filtration through glass bead columns (Shortman et al., 1967; Plotz and Talal, 1967), but the most efficient enrichment method applies immunoadsorbents for this purpose (Mage et al., 1969).

Enrichment of Antibody-Forming Cells. According to Mage's et al. (1969) method, suspensions of immune mouse spleen cells are prepared on the third day after the second intraperitoneal injection of an antigen. The antibody-forming cells are enriched on an immunoabsorbent, rotating column equipped with a single foam disk (Evans et al., 1969). The foam disks are first incubated in Krebs-Ringer phosphate solution at pH 5, containing 2% gum arabic and 0.38% immune globulin obtained from rabbit antiserum specific for sheep or human erythrocytes, for 1 hour at 37°. After the incubation, the foam disks are washed three times in Krebs-Ringer phosphate, pH 7.4. The disk is then placed on top of the column, and a suspension of sheep or human erythrocytes (2×10^{10} cells in 4 ml) is pumped into the foam disk at 50 ml/hour while the column is being rotated at 60 revolutions/hour. After all the erythrocytes enter the column, the pump is stopped and the speed of rotation thereafter is adjusted to 13 revolutions/hour. The cell unbound to the foam disk are then pumped out of the column at 50 ml/hour while the column is being rotated at 60 revolutions/hour. The foam disk to which erythrocytes have been bound is incubated with suspensions containing approximately 2×10^8 mouse nucleated spleen cells for one hour at 4°. The unbound mouse spleen cells are then pumped out of the column and the column is disassembled. The disk bound cells are removed by squeezing the foam disk with Teflon forceps into a Hanks' solution containing 0.04% BSA. The cells are then used for localized hemolysis-in-gel test.

Guinea pig complement is optimal for the mouse-antisheep system, but rabbit complement is superior and the mouse-antirat system, and human complement is hemolytically most active in the mouse antihamster, hamster antimouse, and rat antimouse combination (Hübner and Gengozian, 1969). The number of plaques and the average size of plaque is dependent on the source and hemolytic activity. Each complement requires different ionic conditions and particularly adequate concentrations of calcium and magnesium irons in the gel. The optimal concentration of ions in a gel, when guinea pig complement is used, is 1.9×10^{-3} M Ca++ and 1×10^{-3} M Mg++. The presence of DEAE dextran in certain agar gels enhances the number of plaques but it is without effect in other agar media. Particular requirements of a system for the environmental conditions may be studied by the following immunohemolytic spot-testing.

(i). *The immune-hemolytic spot-assay.* The hemolytic spot-testing (Hübner and Gengozian, 1969) is conducted as follows: the gel consists of 0.7% Noble agar prepared in Eisen's medium, pH 7.4, containing 1 mg of DEAE dextran per 2 ml and calcium and magnesium ions at the final concentration of 1.9×10^{-3} and 1×10^{-3} M respectively. A Petri dish is coated with the agar in a thin layer, following which a top layer of the agar, cooled to 45° and mixed with 0.1 ml of 10% target RBC suspension per 2 ml of agar, and containing 0.15 M NaCl, which represents the top layer. After the top layer of gel has solidified, small drops of thoroughly diluted, heat-inactivated antisera are placed on the agar with the aid of a tuberculin syringe and a 26-gauge needle. The antisera are allowed to diffuse into the agar after which the plates are incubated at 37° in a water bath for 1 hour. The surface of agar is then flooded with 0.15 M NaCl, left for 10 minutes and the liquid being poured out thereafter. Complement at the chosen dilution is added to each plate and after 1 hour of incubation, the complement is poured off and the plates are examined microscopically and macroscopically to determine the degree of lysis caused by the hemolytic antibody placed in spots on the plates.

(ii). *The direct localized immunohemolysis test.* The following reagents are prepared for the test according to Dresser and Wortis (1967):

1. Spleen or lymph-gland cells, obtained from mice immunized by a single intraperitoneal injection of 0.5 ml of 20% suspension of sheep RBC (2×10^4 cells). The suspension of lymphoid or spleen cells is homogenized in Gey's solution by means of a very loose-fitting glass homogenizer. The cell suspension is then passed through a 150-μ hole stainless steel wire mesh, and the volume is adjusted to give 10×10^6 cells/ml, as counted by phase microscopy.

2. 1.2% (w/v) agarose in Dulbecco's phosphate buffer saline.

3. 0.6% agarose in Gey's solution.

4. Sheep erythrocytes, washed 3 times, and resuspended in Gey's solution at 2% concentration.

5. 10% dilution of fresh guinea pig serum.

6. Antimouse immunoglobulin rabbit serum.

Procedure. Pipette 2 ml of 0.6% warm agarose in Gey's solution to a tube held at 47°. Add 1 ml of 2% RBC suspension, and mix. Add 0.1 ml (1×10^6 cells) of the lymphoid cells and mix. Pour the suspension into a Perti dish, incubate the plate at 37° for 1 hour in a moist atmosphere of 5% CO_2 and 95% air. Pipette 2 ml of a diluted rabbit antimouse immunoglobulin serum on the surface of the plate and spread it gently. (The control plate receives 2 ml of normal rabbit serum in the same dilutions.) Incubate at 37° for 1 hour. Pour off the liquid from Petri plate, add 1 ml of 10% fresh guinea-pig serum in Gey's solution. Incubate at 37° for 30 minutes. Pour off complement. Invert plates. Count plaques with a dark-field illumination at a slight magnification.

Plaques may be counted under slide magnification using a conductivity type of colony counter, modified by the use of dark ground illumination. The plates can be stained with freshly prepared mixtures of 10 ml of a 2% benzidine solution in glacial acetic acid, containing 10 ml of 5% H_2O_2 and 80 ml distilled water. Plates can be fixed unstained by washing out protein overnight with Gey's solution, followed by pouring off the solution and adding 2% formalin in PBS. Statistical evaluation is conducted by calculating geometric means on transformed data using $\log (x + 1)$ transformation (Dresser and Wortis, 1967).

An improved direct localized-hemolysis test is based on the observation that peritoneal cells from nonimmunized mice incubated at 37° with sheep erythrocytes and complement on a film of carboxymethyl-cellulose gum produce plaques of hemolysis (Bussard, 1966).

(iii). *The plaque-slide technique (Bussard, 1966; Bendinelli, 1968).* Peritoneal cells are collected aseptically by rinsing the peritoneal cavity of a mouse with 5 ml of medium 199 containing 5–10 i.u./ml of heparin and antibiotics. The cells are centrifuged at 1000 rpm for 10 minutes in siliconized tubes, resuspended in a small amount of Tris-buffered Eagle's medium, counted and diluted to contain 10 to 15 $\times$ 10^6 cells/ml. Then 0.1 of the suspension is added to 0.95 ml of gum, together with 0.05 ml of packed sheep red blood cells and 0.1 ml complement. The mixtures are agitated and centrifuged to separate air bubbles, and 0.02-ml volumes of the mixture are placed on glass slides. A coverslip is then lightly pressed onto the gum to spread it in the form of a film and is sealed to the slide with melted vaseline. The slides are incubated at 37° for a few hours and inspected for the presence of hemolytic plaques at 80× magnification.

(iv). *The plaque-plate technique (Bendinelli, 1968).* Peritoneal cells are seeded in 3 ml of medium 199 in a plastic tissue culture Petri plate on the bottom surface of which a circle (10-mm diameter) has been marked. The amount of peritoneal cell suspension placed in each dish is approximately equivalent to 2×10^4 cells present in the marked area. The test is set in triplicate. The plates are incubated at 37° for 3 hours in a humidified atmosphere of 5% carbon dioxide in air. The supernatant is then removed and the cells adhering to a representative sample of the marked area of the plate are counted with phase-contrast illumination. A drop of carboxy-methyl-cellulose gum-sheep red blood cells and complement mixture is pipetted onto the centre of the marked area. The area is covered with a coverslip and sealed with vaseline. The plates are reincubated at 37°, and hemolytic plaques present in the marked area are counted at 80× magnification.

The carboxymethyl-cellulose gum medium is prepared by dissolving sodium salt of CMC (British Drug House, Poole) and sterilizing the solution by tyndallization. A five times concentrated Eagle's basal medium is added to this solution to produce an isotonic liquid. The buffering agent is Tris-buffer made in Hanks' solution consisting of Tris 15 g, HCl 5.8 ml, Hanks' solution 100 ml, and 0.2% phenol red 0.2 ml. Then 1 ml of this solution is added to 99 ml of the CMC solution. The final concentration in the carboxymethyl-cellulose gum medium is CMC 2.5%, Tris 0.1415%, penicillin 250 i.u./ml, streptomycin 50 μg/ml, pH 7.2. This mixture is used after standing at 4° for 24 hours.

In the conditions above, peritoneal cells form plaques of hemolysis after a latent phase of 15 to 20 hours. Plaques are not formed by lymph node, spleen, thymus, or bone marrow cells. Plaques are not formed at room temperature nor when the complement has been inactivated. The peritoneal cells display highest activity when the donor mice are about 10 weeks old. Plaque formation is suppressed by antimouse immunoglobulin serum.

3. *The Autohemolysin Test.* The autohemolysin test, by MacKenzie's (1929) technique, is set up according to the following pattern: 0.25 ml of a freshly obtained human serum being tested is added to 0.1 ml of 0.5% saline suspension of the individual's own erythrocytes and 0.1 ml of a guinea pig complement. The volume is made up to 0.5 ml with saline. A control tube receives normal serum instead of the tested serum. A further control consists of the serum being tested, complement, and a suspension of erythrocytes containing the same group hemagglutinogen obtained from a different individual. The mixtures are shaken and left on melting ice for 10 minutes and at 37° for 2 hours. A complete hemolysis in the test tube indicates the presence of autohemolysins.

4. *The Isohemolysin Test.* This test may be regarded as a modification of the immune lytic test which reveals a serological reaction between a natural hemolytic antibody (the isohemolysin) and a normal, characteristic group antigen of erythrocytes taken place in the presence of complement. The physical difference between the natural antigen of erythrocytes and the "sensitized erythrocyte antigens" is that the first is found normally in the walls of red blood cells, whereas the other is artificially absorbed onto the erythrocytes. Techniques for the passive hemolytic test with the cellular antigens were published by Bouroncle et al. 1951), Lazear and Ferguson (1953), and Elliott and Ferguson (1956). The technique proposed by Bouroncle et al. is simpler than the other procedures. In this assay, a number of test tubes receive 0.2 ml of serial dilutions of the heat-inactivated human sera, 0.2 ml of a guinea pig serum containing 2 hemolytic units of complement, and 0.1 ml of 2% suspension of normal O Rh-positive red blood cells. After the incubation at 37° for 1 hour, the tubes are inspected for the presence of hemolysis, and the isohemolysin titer is expressed in terms of the serum dilution in the last tube showing complete hemolysis.

The Lazear and Ferguson test requires the following components: an antiserum, a typing serum, absorbed with packed bovine red cells and inactivated, 3% suspension of bovine erythrocytes washed three times in buffered saline, a rabbit serum used as a source of complement, and a buffered saline, pH 7.3. Test tubes receive 0.05 ml (1.0 ml) of a 3% suspension of bovine erythrocytes, 0.05 ml (1.0 ml) of a rabbit serum (complement), and 0.10 ml (2.0 ml) of antiserum dilutions. Two control tubes are set, to contain:

(1) 0.05 ml (1.0 ml) of 3% erythrocyte suspension.
     0.15 ml (3 ml) buffered saline.
(2) 0.05 ml (1 ml) of 3% erythrocyte suspension.
     0.05 ml (1 ml) of a complement-containing serum.
     0.10 ml (2 ml) buffered saline.

The mixtures are left at room temperature and examined for the presence of hemolysis in 30 mintues, 90 minutes, and 3 hours.

Figures in parentheses represent volumes of components used in the test in which results are colorimetrically determined. In this case, 1-ml samples are withdrawn before the incubation, and at 30-minute intervals, then mixed with 4 ml of cold 3 $\frac{1}{2}$ solution of sodium citrate and centrifuged at 500 × g for 10 minutes. The supernatants are examined in a spectrophotometer at 545-nm wavelength, and the percentage of hemolysis is calculated according to a standard curve. This test can be applied to the study of group antigens of erythrocytes.

5. *The Heterophile-Hemolysin Test.* This test reveals an immunologic reaction between a heterogenous antigen (the Forssman antigen) of sheep erythrocytes and the heterophile antibody of human sera. The reaction in the presence of complement brings about the hemolysis. Results can be read either by the naked eye or photometrically.

According to the Gleeson-White et al. (1950) technique, the test is set by adding 0.1-ml volumes of progressing serum dilutions to equal volumes of 1% sheep red blood cells followed by 2 to 4 MHD of a guinea pig complement. The test mixtures are incubated at 37° for 30 minutes before being read.

Photometric determination of the hemolytic antibody by an adaptation of Mayer's (1961) method is conducted in the following manner: a series of 1.0-ml progressing dilutions of a serum tested are added to tubes containing 2.0 ml of a standardized sheep erythrocyte suspension (5×10^8 cell/ml) with constant mixing. After 15-minute incubation at 37°, 2-ml volumes of a diluted fresh guinea pig serum containing $12C'H_{50}$ are added, and the mixtures are held at 37° for exactly 15 minutes with occasional mixing. A 10.0-ml volume of a saline-citrate solution is then added to each tube, and the tubes are centrifuged. Contents of oxyhemoglobin in the supernatants are determined photometrically. The 50% hemolysis end point should be estimated and evaluated by the use of von Krogh equation (p. 502).

6. *The Blood-Platelet Immunolysis Test (Cruz, 1953).* Components of this test are 1.2 ml of suspension of blood platelets which can be separated by fractional centrifugation of blood collected in chilled sodium citrate, 0.1 ml of component, and 0.1 ml of an antiplatelet serum. The initial turbidity of this mixture and, subsequently, turbidities shown at 2- to 4-minute intervals are determined by the aid of a spectrophotometer. Decreasing values of optical density measured at the intervals indicate the presence of a platelet antibody which can be estimated by interpolation. This test may be applied for the investigations on antigens of platelets and for detection of the platelet antibody in human sera.

7. *The Leukocyte Immunolysis Test.* White blood cells mixed with a system of antigen and homologous antiserum in the presence of complement undergo a lysis. Polymorphonuclear leukocytes are predominantly affected by this immune lysis. The following reactants are used for the white-cell lysis test, as devised by Favour et al. (1949): (a) a test serum, which must not be inactivated, although its lytic capacity is not affected even at the temperature of 58°, (b) an antigen solution used at its optimum concentration, the antigen dilution which gives an optimum lysis can be estimated by titration in the presence of a constant amount of antiserum, and (c) normal blood used as a source of leukocytes.

The test tubes, siliconed with GE Drifilm 9987 to prevent blood clotting, are filled with 0.2-ml amounts of a normal blood, 0.2 ml of the test serum, and 0.1 ml of an antigen solution. The tubes are agitated for 3 minutes on an electric shaker. Leukocyte diluting pipettes are then filled with the mixtures withdrawn from individual tubes for the intial cell count. The tubes are stoppered and agitated in a rotator at 37°. After 5 minutes, the second and last samples are withdrawn with diluting pipettes for final count. A decrement of leukocytes is determined and compared with the number of white blood cells in the control tube.

The test should be carried out at least in duplicate, since the counts may vary by 10% above or below the probably true level. The immune leukocyte-lysis test may be applied to studies on antigens of white blood cells and to the detection of leukocyte antibodies in patients' sera. A quantitative lympholytic test was described by Terasaki and Rich (1964).

8. *The Immunobacteriolytic (Bactericidal) Assays.* The bacteriolytic test depends on the complement lysis of different Gram-negative bacteria in the presence of the appropriate specific antibody. The bacteriolysis, unlike the cytolysis by complement, is considerably accelerated by lysozyme. In the bacteriolysis, human complement acts on the outer lipoprotein-lipopolysaccharide layer of the bacterial cell wall and facilities the access of lysozyme to the deeper mucopeptide of the cell (Glynn, 1969).

Bacterial cells, which are brought into contact with a specific homologous antibody in the presence of complement, undergo lysis or destruction of certain vital function, which causes their death. These bacteria fail to multiply or grow when subsequently planted on a culture medium. About 700 to 860 molecules of the antibody and 1.5×10^7 molecules of complement are required to dissolve one cell of *Salmonella typhosa* at the 50% end point (Muschel and Treffers, 1956).

Complements of different animals vary considerably in the ability of activating bacteriolytic or bactericidal antibodies. Thus it is advisable to try out complements obtained from various animal species before deciding on the most suitable source of complement for a particular immunologic system. Various species of bacteria differ in their susceptibility to the immune lysis. Thus most of Gram-negative bacilli, and especially *Vibrio comma* and *Salmonella typhosa,* are readily killed and lyzed after the sensitization by a specific antibody in the presence of complement. In contrast, the Gram-positive bacteria, and particularly Gram-positive cocci, are insusceptible to the action of lysins and complement. Accuracy of results of a bacteriolytic or bactericidal test may be somewhat diminished by the agglutination of microorganisms caused by antibodies prior to the inoculation on culture media. Thus the test should be set up in triplicates for each antiserum.

Techniques of the immune bacteriolytic or bactericidal test designed by numerous investigators may be classified within the following types:

1. Assays depending on the determination of the number or quantity of surviving bacteria which have been exposed to different amounts of a serum in the presence of a constant amount of complement, as compared with the controls containing a heated normal serum (Gengou, 1899; Neisser and Wechsberg, 1901; Morris, 1943; Muschel and Treffers, 1952).

2. The immune bacteriolytic test in vivo (Pfeiffer, 1894).

3. Tests depending on the determination of the serum or plasma dilution capable of killing a given number of gacteria (Huddleson et al., 1945).

4. Determination of a bactericidal index, representing the difference between the reciprocal of the highest dilution of the control tube giving a growth of bacteria and the highest bacterial test dilution showing little or no growth (Irwin and Berman, 1950; Shrigley and Irwin, 1937).

5. The microcolony immune bactericidal test (Bienvenu et al., 1961).

The following four methods have been selected as the most suitable for the immunobacteriolytic test.

(i). *The bacteriolytic test in vivo.* In this assay, which was originally devised by Pfeiffer (1893, 1894), lethal doses of a bacterium, for example, *Vibrio comma,* are injected into the peritoneal cavity of normal and of the specifically immunized guinea pigs. Samples of the peritoneal fluid are withdrawn at intervals of a few minutes for microscopic examinations. Changes in shape, staining, and number of bacteria thus observed, as well as the survival rate of animals, are recorded. A "passive" bacteriolytic test in vivo can also be conducted in guinea pigs injected with a serum from immune animals and then challenged with a dose of corresponding bacteria.

(ii). *The Shrigley and Irwin bacteriolytic test.* Test mixtures in this test consist of 0.05-ml serial, differing by tenths, dilutions of a standardized suspension of 36-hour bacterial culture, 0.3 ml of a tested serum, and 0.2 ml of undiluted complement. (Young, 5- to 6-hour cultures of bacteria often prove to be more sensitive to bacteriolysins and more suitable for the bacteriolytic test than old cultures.) Control tubes also receive serial dilutions of the bacterial suspension and 0.2 ml of complement, but the serum is replaced by a diluent.

Test mixtures are incubated at 37° for 24 hours, and several samples from each tube are transferred on an adequate solid culture medium and incubated for 2 to 6 days. After the incubation, the number of colonies is counted on each plate. The presence of one colony on a plate denotes the end point. The index of the bacteriolytic (bactericidal) activity of an examined serum is calculated, as suggested by Mackie and Finkelstein (1932), by subtracting the last dilution of bacteria in the test mixture, at which the growth still occurred, from the highest dilution of bacteria in the control mixture, which yielded the growth on a culture medium. For example, if the serum mixture showed the growth of bacteria in the 10^{-4} dilution, the control mixture gave the growth in 10^{-7} dilution, the bacteriolytic (bactericidal) index is 3.

(iii). *The Morris bactericidal test.* Components of this test are (a) a young culture of bacteria; (b) immune serum or patient's serum; and (c) complement, represented by a normal rabbit serum absorbed with killed bacteria of the strain tested, to remove the natural bactericidal antibody.

The lytic activity of the complement is determined prior to the final test by adding different dilutions of a fresh normal rabbit serum to a 4% suspension of sheep erythrocytes sensitized with two units of a rabbit-anti-erythrocyte hemolytic serum. The amount of a rabbit serum which in 30 minutes at 37° has caused complete hemolysis of 0.2 ml of 4% sensitized erythrocytes, tested in a total volume of 1 ml of test mixture, is regarded as one unit of complement.

The qualitative bactericidal test is carried out by mixing varying amounts of an 18-hour bacterial culture diluted in broth with equal volume of varying dilutions of an antiserum. Control tubes receive a broth sample instead of the bacterial suspension. The mixtures are left for sensitization in an ice bath for 3 hours. A 0.5-ml volume is then withdrawn from each mixture and added to 0.5 ml of a saline solution containing one unit of complement. After 1-hour incubation in a water bath at 37°, samples of each test mixture are quantitatively mixed with a volume of melted culture medium and left for 48 hours at 37°.

Colonies are then enumerated by the aid of an electronic colony counter. The number of surviving bacteria is calculated by subtracting figures obtained from test mixtures from those of control tubes which did not contain any serum.

The titer of bacteriolysins can be expressed by the highest serum dilution, at which 50% or more of the starting population of bacteria were killed (Finkelstein, 1962).

(iv). *The photometric bactericidal test by Muschel and Treffers.* A standardized suspension of bacterial cells for this assay is prepared in the following manner: microorganisms are taken from a single colony and cultivated for 14 to 18 hours in an adequate liquid medium. Density of the culture grown is then adjusted spectrophotometrically at 650 nm to a desired optical density, for example, equal to 6×10^7 or 10^8, using the culture medium as blank. This bacterial suspension is kept in ice water until the test is carried out.

The antiserum used in the test must not be inactivated since the heat inactivation can partially destroy the antibody and its bactericidal power. The serum is measured in amounts of 1.35, 0.9, 0.6, and 0.4 ml, and the total volume is made up to 1.4 ml with the culture medium. Each tube then receives 0.3 ml of undiluted complement absorbed with the bacteria to be tested at 0° for 1 hour, and then filtered and 0.3 ml of the standardized suspension of microorganisms. The guinea-pig complement may be substituted by precolostrum calf serum (Evans and Mergenhagen, 1965). Three controls are set containing (a) 1.35 ml of antiserum made up to 1.7 ml with the culture medium, and 0.3 ml of the bacterium suspension; (b) 0.3-ml complement and 0.3 ml of the bacterium suspension made up to 2.0 ml with a diluent; and (c) 1.7 ml of the diluent and 0.2 ml of the bacterium suspension. Appropriate controls for the sterility of the antiserum, complement, and the diluent are also included.

All tubes are placed in a water bath at 37° for 1 hour, after which the reaction is stopped by adding 5.0 ml of a brain-heart infusion broth. The bactericidal process is thus terminated owing to the anticomplementary activity of this infusion and to the dilution of a serologic system.

To assay the growth, the tubes are reincubated in a water bath, with occasional shaking, until the growth in the complement-control tube (no. 2) is recorded at the optimum reading range, which corresponds to the optical density of 0.40 to 0.45. Tubes are then removed from the water bath and chilled in an ice-water bath to inhibit any further multiplication of microorganisms. Optical densities of suspensions in all tubes are examined in a photometer at 150-nm wavelength. The optical density of a reading standard, consisting of a nonincubated complement mixed with the culture medium, is taken as zero (100% transmission). Bactericidal activity is calculated by dividing the optical density of each tube by the optical density of the complement control tube. The resultant ratios are multiplied by 100, and these experimental quantities are called the percentage optical densities or the apparent (uncorrected) percentage survivals. These can be converted graphically to true (corrected) percentage survivals.

Bacteriolytic test was applied to the study on bactericidins in infected or immunized animals. For example, bactericidin in animals immunized with *Brucella* were investigated by Elberg et al. (1951). Bactericidal action of human serum against *Neisseria meningitidis, Diplococcus crassus, Haemophilus pertussis,* and *Salmonella typhosa* was studied by Wulff (1934), and Muschel and Treffers (1956).

(v). *The agglutination-lysis test.* The test, first described by Schuffner, depends on the lysis of a complex consisting of leptospires and antileptospire serum by the complement present in the noninactivated serum. The test is set up in depressions in porcelain or plastic plates or in tubes according to the schedule (Table 51).

Table 51.   A Schedule for the Agglutination-Lysis Test

Tube	(1)	(2)	(3)	(4)	(5)	(6)	(7)
1st row							
Saline (drops)	8	9	9				
Serum (drops)	2	1	1				
	From (1)	From (2)					
Serum dilution	1/5	1/50	1/500				
2nd row							
Leptospira culture	3	3	3	3	3	3	3 (drops)
Saline		2		2		2	
Serum 1/5	3	1					
Serum 1/50			3	1			
Serum 1/500					3	1	
Final dilution	1/10	1/30	1/100	1/300	1/1000	1/3000	

Procedure.   Incubate the mixtures at 32 to 37° for 3 hours and leave them at room temperature for 1 hour. (Alternatively, the test tubes may be left overnight at 4°.) Place a drop from each tube on a slide and examine with a 16-mm objective using dark-ground illumination. Lysis of the bacteria is indicated by a reduction of the number of live leptospires in the serum-antigen mixture when compared with a control possessing no serum (tube no. 7).

9. *The Ablastin Test.*   Antiblastic activity of the serum depends on the inhibition, by specific antibodies, of certain assimilative processes in the microorganisms, which prevents their reproduction.

Ablastins arise from an infection or immunization, and are found in the globulins of certain immune sera. In contrast to many other antibodies, the ablastins do not exhibit any marked affinity for the microorganisms in vitro, but they inhibit or reduce the reproduction of certain microorganisms, for example, *Trypanosoma lewisi* or *Trypanosoma duttoni,* without killing them.

The ablastin test, by Taliaferro and Pavlinova (1936), depends on determination of the rate of reproduction of microorganisms (trypanosomas) in animals injected with a species of *Trypanosoma.* This is accomplished by the estimation of the ratio between the dividing and short forms of these microorganisms in random samples of blood smeared on slides and stained with the Giemsa stain.

II. *The Indirect (Passive) Immunohemolysis Assay*

The principle of the indirect immune hemolysis test is a reaction that occurs in the presence of complement between a soluble antigen absorbed onto erythrocytes and the homologous antibody resulting in the dissolution of red blood cells. It is assumed that an immunologic complex formed on or near the surface of erythrocytes plays a passive part in the hemolytic test must be differentiated from "the microbial hemolysin test," in which the morphotic components of blood and especially the erythrocytes are dissolved by bacterial or viral lysins in the absence of a specific antibody (see p. 442).

The passive immune hemolytic test employs the following reactants: (a) a serum under study,(b) a solution or suspension of an antigen preparation; (c) erythrocytes coated by an antigen; (d) complement with estimated hemolytic titer, and (e) a buffered saline solution. The localized immunohemolysis test additionally requires a gel medium.

The serum to be titrated must be inactivated at 56° for 30 minutes or at 62° for 3 minutes, and absorbed with erythrocytes if sheep red blood cells are used in the test. The amount of an antigen preparation needed for the sensitization of erythrocytes should be determined prior to the test proper by using a hemagglutination or hemolytic test and a standard antiserum if available. It is desired that 1 mg of dry weight of an antigen preparation be sufficient for the sensitization of 1 ml of packed red blood cells. Erythrocytes of guinea pig or chicken can be used instead of sheep red blood cells, and in these cases no absorption of sera is required. Tanned erythrocytes are used as carriers of protein antigens, where as nonpretreated cells are adequate for the sensitization by other substances. To coat red blood cells with an antigen, a volume of 0.1 ml of packed cells is suspended in 10 ml of buffered saline, containing 1 mg of the antigen preparation. After a 60-minute incubation at 37°, the suspension is centrifuged, the sediment is washed twice or three times with a buffered saline, and resuspended to give 0.2 and 0.5% final concentration of erythrocytes. For greater accuracy, the suspension of red blood cells can be standardized by dilution, so that 0.2 or 0.5 ml of the suspension lyzed with 1.3 or 3.25 ml of distilled water gives a reading of 100% on the scale of a spectrophotometer, at 545-nm wavelength.

The complement is usually provided by a guinea pig serum. It must be absorbed twice with erythrocytes if sheep red blood cells are employed in the test. The absorption is carried out by mixing 15 volumes of guinea pig serum diluted 1:3 with 1 volume of packed sheep red blood cells. The mixture is left at 4° for 10 minutes, then centrifuged, and the supernatant is collected with a pipette. It should be used within 3 to 4 hours. Complement, at a certain concentration, may exert a nonspecific lytic activity toward the antigen-coated erythrocytes, and especially toward those pretreated with tannic acid, even in the absence of antiserum. This nonspecific lytic activity of complement must be tested by titration in the following manner. A guinea pig serum is serially diluted in duplicate from 1:25 to 1:320 with buffered saline, in a volume provided for the final test, for example, 0.25 ml, and supplemented with 0.25 ml of the Wallace buffer; 0.5% nonsensitized red blood cells are then added in 0.5-ml volume to the first row, whereas the tubes of the other row receive 0.5 ml of erythrocytes sensitized with an antigen. The mixtures are incubated at 37° for 1 to $1\frac{1}{2}$ hours.

The complement titer is estimated in terms of its dilution in the last tube of the second row, which shows a complete hemolysis. One half of this minimal hemolytic unit is employed in the hemolytic test; however, some authors, for example, Silverstein and Maltaner (1952), use two minimal hemolytic units.

Methods for the determination of serum hemolysins reacting with the erythrocyte-adsorbed soluble antigens, in the presence of complement, were designed by several scientists, for example, Fisher (1951), Wright and Feinberg (1952), Silverstein and Maltaner (1952), Neter et al. (1956), and Kwapinski (1959, 1965). Two recommended methods for this assay are presented below. Related tests are the modified lytic Coombs test for incomplete antibodies (Hall and Manion, 1951) and the isohemolysin test for group antigens of erythrocytes (Lazear and Ferguson, 1953; Bouroncle et al., 1951), see p. 448.

The indirect localized immunohemolysis assay depends on the reaction between the antibody-releasing lymphoid cells in gel and the antigen-coated erythrocytes, in the presence of complement. A number of techniques for the indirect localized immunohemolysis are presented below, since certain technical details of each of the subsequent procedures are helpful for the examination of different antigen-antibody systems and for different experimental aims.

1. *The Passive Immunohemolysin Assays*

(i). *Silverstein and Maltaner's immunohemolysin test.* The test serum is serially diluted in 0.1-ml volumes, and 0.2 ml of a 0.2% suspension of the antigen-coated erythrocytes are added to each tube. The samples are incubated at 37° for 10 minutes, then a volume of the complement solution is added which contains two hemolytic units, as determined by titration with sheep erythrocytes and a rabbit hemolytic serum. The volumes of tubes are made up to 0.5 ml with a saline solution. The test mixtures are incubated in a water bath at 37° for 15 to 30 minutes, with occasional shaking, and transferred into an ice-water bath, where they receive 1 ml of chilled saline. The tubes are then centrifuged, and the amount of liberated hemoglobin, or the percentag of hemolysis, is estimated in a Coleman Jr. spectrophotometer at 545-nm wavelength.

(ii). *Kwapinski's immunohemolysin test.* The pattern for this assay is presented in Table 52. After the final incubation, the test mixtures are centrifuged at 177 $\times$ *g* for 15 minutes, and the supernatant fluids are withdrawn and examined at 545 nm in a spectrophotometer. The 50% immune lysis point is determined by the application of the data to a standard o.d. curve drawn on the basis of prior examination of different hemoglobin dilutions at the same wavelength. The immune hemolysin titer is expressed by the antiserum dilution at the 50% hemolysis point of the highest antiserum dilution at which the sensitized erythrocytes were completely lyzed.

Table 52.   A Schedule to the Passive Immune Hemolytic Test (Kwapinski, 1959)

Reagents	Row 1	Row 2	Control 1	Control 2
Antiserum diluted from 1:10 to 1:1280 (ml)	0.25	0.25	—	—
Buffered saline, pH 7 (ml)	—	—	0.25	0.25
0.5% antigen sensitized erythrocytes (ml)	0.50	—	0.50	—
0.5% nonsensitized erythrocytes (ml)	—	0.50	—	0.50
Incubation at 37° for 30 minutes				
Complement, 0.5 hemolytic unit (ml)	0.25	0.25	0.25	0.25
Incubation at 37° for 30 minutes				

2.   *The Indirect Localized Immunohemolysis Assays*

(i). *Friedman's (1966) technique.* Sheep erythrocytes are first coated with antigen, using a 10% erythrocyte suspension and varying amounts of the antigen preparation ranging from 1 to 10 μg of dry mass. The mixtures are incubated at 37° for 1 hour to determine the optimal amount of antigen needed for sensitization.

In the indirect plaque assay, 0.1 ml of a freshly prepared 10% suspension of the antigen-coated erythrocytes is used in place of untreated erythrocytes. The 0.1 ml of the coated erythrocytes is added to a tube containing 2 ml of warm melted 0.7% Noble agar containing 1 mg of diethylaminoethyl-dextran prepared in Hanks' solution, 0.1 ml of the nucleated cells (10×10^6 cells/ml). This mixture is poured over a 3-m-thick layer of 1.5% Noble agar in Hanks' solution which has been previously prepared in the Petri plate. The plates are incubated at 37° for 1 hour after which 5 ml of a 1:10 diluted guinea pig serum as a source of complement is added. The plates are incubated at 37° for 30 minutes and observed for the presence of clear areas.

(ii). *The indirect localized immunolytic test by Parlett and Chu (1967).* The suspension of spleen cells in Eagle's medium is obtained by teasing of a spleen taken from an immunized animal into fragments and forcing the small splenic fragments through a microscreen fitted to a Sweeney filter syringe. The cells may be quantitated by means of a hemocytometer; 0.1 ml of the spleen suspension is added to 4 ml of molten 0.8% agar, prepared with Eagle's medium, containing 1 mg of diethyl-amino-ethylene (DEAE) dextran. To the above mixture, 0.1 ml of 50% (volume) sheep erythrocytes sensitized with an antigen and suspended in 0.8% molten agar are added. This mixture is rotated and poured into a Petri dish which has been coated with a layer of 1.6% agar prepared in Eagle's medium. The plate is left at 37° for 1 hour and then is flooded with 1 ml of reconstituted lyophilized guinea pig complement. The plates are observed after 30 minutes of incubation at 37°. The total number of clear zones (plaques) is determined.

The sensitization of erythrocytes with an antigen is obtained by exposing a 50% suspension of washed, packed sheep red blood cells in 0.01 M phosphate buffer, pH 6.4 to a soluble antigen in the ratio of 1:1 or 1:1.5 by volume. This mixture is left at 37° for 1 hour with occasional shaking. The antigen-coated erythrocytes are washed twice with phosphate buffer and resuspended to the final 50% suspension.

Dextran is added to the agar mixture to counter any anticomplementary action of agar.

(iii). *The indirect localized immunohemolysis test by Moore and Vas (1968).* In this technique, agarose in the medium 199 is the supporting medium. Sensitized erythrocytes or intermediate products are used as indicator cells in a final concentration of 2.5×10^7 cells/ml. The reaction plates are incubated at 37° in jars flushed with a mixture of oxygen and carbon dioxide. The details of the tests are as described underneath.

One volume of the immunized tissue cell suspension and one volume of erythrocytes, coated with an antigen, containing 1.5×10^9 cells/ml are added to three volumes of 0.7% agarose prepared in medium in 199. A drop of the mixture (0.02 ml) is placed in a plastic tissue culture dish leaving a thin film on the surface of the plate. The plates are immediately inverted, placed in a wet chamber, and left in a jar containing a mixture of 90% O_2 and 10% CO_2 at pH 6.8.

The R reagents, prepared from guinea pig serum by Mayer's (1961) method are then added to the plates before incubation or after incubation at 37°. The reagents are placed as drops (0.02 ml) directly over the agarose film. The R reagents are used in a dilution which are not lytic under these experimental conditions. After a suitable incubation time, the reagents are removed from the plates and the films are fixed with 10% formalin in Hanks' Buffered Salt Solutions (HBSS), washed with two changes of distilling water and air dried. The staining is performed with a 1:50 dilution of Giemsa dye for 5 minutes.

The antibody-producing tissue cells for this test are macrophages obtained from peritoneal exudates. The exudate is provoked by intraperitoneal injection of guinea pigs with casein. Three days later, the animals are bled out, and 15 ml of heparinized Hanks' BBS are injected into the peritoneal cavity. The peritoneal fluid content is aspirated with a pipette through an incision made through the abdominal wall. The collected cells are centrifuged and washed three times in HBSS containing 0.13% gelatin. An alternative cell source is the spleen or bone marrow. Suspensions of these cells are made as described by Siboo and Vas (1965). The washed cells are resuspended in medium 199, and viable cell counts are performed.

Agarose is used in preference to agar as supporting medium because it is not anticomplementary.

(iv). *Halliday and Webb's (1965) technique for the localized immuno-hemolysis test.* The following procedure has been designed for a test with the polysaccharide-coated erythrocytes. The spleen obtained from mice immunized by two intravenous injections of bacteria, 5 days apart, and sacrificed 4 days after the second injection, is cut up finely in Hanks' solution. The cells are dispersed by sucking them several times into a syringe; the suspension is filtered through a glass wood pad. The cells are then washed and resuspended to form 25% suspension which corresponds to about 1×10^8 nucleated cells/ml. A polysaccharide preparation obtained from the same strain of bacteria is used to sensitize sheep erythrocytes. For this purpose, a 5% sheep erythrocyte suspension is mixed with an equal volume of the polysaccharide solution, left for 2 hours at 37°, after which the cells are washed with saline and resuspended to 50% concentration in saline.

The plaque test is set up by layering a Petri plate with 1.4% agar made in Eagle's medium. The upper layer to be poured next contains 0.1 ml of spleen cells, 0.06 ml of sensitized erythrocytes, and 0.05 mg of DEAE-dextran, added to 1 ml of 0.7% agar made in Eagle's medium and melted and cooled to 45°. Control plates contain either normal sheep erythrocytes, normal spleen cells, or immune spleen cells and erythrocytes sensitized with an unrelated bacterial polysaccharide. The plates are left at 37° for 1 hour, after which complement (1ml of a fresh guinea pig serum diluted

1:3) is added and the plates are incubated for a further 30 minutes and then examined for the presence of clear areas around the cells (plaques).

The number of nucleated cells in the suspension is determined with a hemocytometer, and viability is estimated by Trypan blue staining technique. According to Friedman's (1966) modification, the plates are overlayered with 5 ml of 1:10 dilution of guinea pig serum as a source of complement and the plates are incubated at 37° for 30 minutes. Localized zones of hemolysis are observed as clear areas against a background of unlyzed erythrocytes. The plaques, however, may be made more distinct and the plates can be preserved for some time by staining with cold, freshly prepared benzidine-H_2O_2-acetic acid solution (Jerne et al., 1963). It is recommended to inspect the plates for nonspecific zones of hemolysis prior to the addition of the complement and using a number of control plates which have been incubated without the addition of complement. The number of hemolytic zones in the complement-free plates is subtracted from the number of plaques found in the plates treated with complement.

(v). *The hemolytic focus method.* According to the technique designed by Ceglowski and Friedman (1970), 6-μ-thick sections of spleens obtained from immunized mice are placed on the surface of previously prepared sheep-blood agar plates. After 1 hour, incubation at 37°, the plates are flooded with complement and incubated for 30 minutes. Discrete zones of hemolysis coinciding with individual lymphoid follicles representing clusters of hemolysis-forming cells, appear during this time.

iii. *Evauation and Application of Indirect Immunohemolysis Tests.* The passive hemolytic test, which can be regarded as a modification of the passive hemogglutination test by insertion of complement, is more sensitive than the later in respect to the serum titration; a relatively smaller amount of the antibody is able to produce a positive hemolytic reaction. Smaller amounts of antigens are required to sensitize erythrocytes for a hemolytic test than for the hemagglutination; and results of immune hemolytic tests are more clear cut.

Indirect hemolytic tests can be applied either for the detection or identification of antibodies and the determination of their titers, using erythrocytes coated by a known antigen, or to identify antigens and estimate their immunologic potency, by the aid of standard sera with known immunologic spectra. Here are some more detailed applications of hemolytic tests:

1. Detection and titration of antibodies in human sera, for example, antibodies in tuberculous sera which react with erythrocytes coated by **PPD** or by a nucleoprotein isolated from *Mycobacterium tuberculosis* (Kwapinski, 1959), antibodies in leprous sera reacting with red blood cells sensitized by methanol-phosphate extract of *Mycobacterium tuberculosis* (Fisher, 1951). A hemolytic modification of the Coombs test was success-

fully adopted for detection of incomplete tuberculous antibodies (Hall and Manion, 1951); and a hemolytic test by Bouroncle et al. (1951) was used for the determination of natural hemolysins.

2. Estimation of the activity and specificity of certain antigens, for example, of erythrocytes coupled with *p*-azophenylarsentea (Silverstein and Maltaner, 1952), or red blood cells coated with components of tuberculin or with boiled extracts of *Leptospira* (Cox, 1955). The hemolytic test by Lazear and Ferguson (1953) or a similar technique was used for the study of cellular antigens of erythrocytes.

The localized immunohemolysis test may be applied to different heterologous antibody-forming systems if the test is carried out in an appropriate physical chemical environment. A considerable modification of the original technique is the "free suspension method" (Zaalberg et al., 1966; Ingraham et al., 1967). This method is more sensitive than the original technique and is not limited to the detection of hemolysin-releasing cells, since it also allows observation of hemagglutination in the form of cell clusters clumped by hemagglutinin.

The localized immunohemolysis test has been applied for revealing an immune response by direct and indirect hemolysis, quantitation of antibody produced by individual cells, detection of precipitins against polysaccharides, synthetic polymers and immunoglobulins (Cunningham et al., 1966; Walsh et al., 1967; Barth and Merchant, 1967), autoradographic studies on hemolysin-forming cells (Berglund, 1964), and isolation of the antibody-forming cells for electronoptic observation (Bussard et al., 1965).

II. THE MICROBIAL HEMOLYSIN TEST

Some species of microorganisms secrete substances termed microbial hemolysins which possess enzymatic and antigenic activities and the ability of releasing the hemoglobin from erythrocytes. Bacterial hemolysins react with their specific antibodies, the antihemolysins. The following species of microorganisms are known to produce hemolytic substances: *Streptococcus pyogenes* (streptolysin), *Streptococcus zymogenes, Diplococcus pneumoniae, Staphylococcus aureus* (staphylolysin), *Leptospira pomona, Leptospira automnalis, Leptospira australis, Leptospira canicola, Leptospira hemolytica, Leptospira grippotyphosa, Clostridium tetani* (tetanolysin), *Clostridium welchii, Escherichia coli, Myxovirus influenzae,* Newcastle Disease virus, and *Poxvirus variolae.*

Some bacterial hemolysins, for example, streptolysin, theta hemolysin, were isolated in a state of considerable purity. Methods of producing pure preparation of a streptolysin were published by Smythe and Harris (1940), Herbert and Todd (1941), Pentz and Shigemura (1955), and Roth and Pillemer (1955).

Table 53. A Schedule to the Determination of Bacterial Hemolysins
(Kwapinski, 1965)

Tube Number	1	2	3	4	5	6	7	8	9	10	Control Tube
Hemolysin (ml)	0.5	0.45	0.4	0.35	0.30	0.25	0.20	0.15	0.10	0.05	0.0
Saline buffered at pH 6.5–6.2 (ml)[a]	1.0	1.05	1.1	1.15	1.20	1.25	1.30	1.35	1.40	1.45	1.5
5% suspension susceptible erythrocytes (ml)	0.5	0.5	0.5	0.5	0.5	0.5	0.5	0.5	0.5	0.5	0.5
Final volume (ml)	2.0	2.0	2.0	2.0	2.0	2.0	2.0	2.0	2.0	2.0	2.0

[a] The saline solution buffered at pH 6.5 to 6.7 contains 4.2 g of KH_2PO_4 and 1.81 g of $Na_2HPO_4 \cdot 12H_2O$ in 1000 ml of distilled water.

1. Technique of the Bacterial-Hemolysin Test

The aim of the bacterial-hemolysin test is to determine the activity of microbial hemolysins under standard experimental conditions. Either a crude culture filtrate or a purified preparation of hemolysins is employed in this assay, represented diagrammatically in Table 53 (Kwapinski, 1965).

Methods for the bacterial hemolytic test were also published by Roth and Pillemer (1955) and Russell (1956).

According to Russell's procedure, the culture filtrate is diluted serially in an isotonic, pH 7.2 to 7.4, buffered saline in 0.5-ml volumes. Equal volume of 5% suspension of washed sheep red cells in buffered saline is added to each filtrate dilution. Control tubes receive 0.5 ml of buffered saline and 0.5 ml of the erythrocyte suspension. The mixtures are incubated for 4 hours in a 37° water bath and for 12 hours at 4° and then centrifuged.

The percentage of hemolysis in the supernatant fluids is estimated by comparison with color standards prepared by mixing 5% suspension of sheep red blood cells and sheep hemoglobin in various proportions covering a range of hemolysis from 5 to 100%, as described by Gradwohl and Kouri (1948). The highest final dilution of the culture filtrate showing observable (5% or more) hemolysis denotes the hemolytic titer. Control tubes must not show any trace of hemolysis.

Alternatively, the 50% end point of hemolysis may be estimated colorimetrically, for example, by using a Klett-Summerson colorimeter with a green filter no. 54. The percentage of hemolysis is calculated from the following formula (Irwin and Seeley, 1959):

$$\% \text{ hemolysis } = \frac{\text{reading in Klett units of test tube} \times 100}{\text{reading in Klett units of the 100\% control}}$$

The 100% control consists of 5 ml of bacterial filtrate, 1 ml of the red blood cell suspension, and approximately 0.01 g of saponine added to lyze erythrocytes completely.

2. Technique of the Virus-Hemolysin Test

The virus-hemolysin test can be carried out according to the Morgan et al. (1948), Soule et al. (1959), or Kahnke (1951) technique. Kahnke's technique, as slightly modified by Kwapinski (1965), is conducted as shown in Table 54. The reaction mixtures are incubated for 1 to 2 hours at 37°.

Table 54.   A Schedule for Determination of Virus Hemolysins

Tube Number	1	2	3	4	5	Control Tube
Virus suspension						
diluted 1:	25	50	100	200	400	
(ml)	0.5	0.5	0.5	0.5	0.5	—
Buffered saline (ml)	—	—	—	—	—	0.5
2% chicken eryth-	0.5	0.5	0.5	0.5	0.5	0.5
rocyte in $M/15$						
phosphate buffer,						
pH 7.2 (ml)						

The highest final dilution of virus particles showing a complete or 50% hemolysis, determined spectrophotometrically after the sedimentation of erythrocytes, is used as titer of the test. The concentration of red cells per milliliter and the relative virus concentration should be carefully measured by Salk's technique (see p. 545).

According to Sagik and Levine's (1957) technique, results of the test are expressed by the number of cell equivalents of hemoglobin, liberated by virus action. This is recorded as percentage maximum hemolysis, which corresponds to the optical density given by the lysis of the same number of red cells in distilled water.

The active hemolytic assay is often used as a preparatory step to the hemolysis-inhibition test (see p. 532).

3. The Gel Chromatography of Microbial Hemolysins

The method (Kwapinski, 1968, unpublished) for the separation and detection of different microbial hemolysins by "gel chromatography" is carried out in the following manner: a bacterial or microfungal culture, or a fluid aspirated from the chorioallantoic cavity of embryos infected with a virus or rickettsia, is first liberated from the microorganisms by centrifugation and filtration through membranes with one appropriate porosity. The filtrate is dialyzed at 4° for 2 days against an 0.01 *M,* pH 7.2 phosphate buffer (small adjustments of pH must be made sometimes to attain complete solubility of the material). The dialyzate concentrated by partial lyophilization to contain approximately 10 μg/ml is then placed in the volume 0.05 ml on a strip or a larger sheet of Whatman no. 4 or 2 filter paper, while being dried on the stream of nitrogen. The paper is hung in a chromatography tank for the descending run in a pH 8.0 or pH 6.4, 0.1 *M* NaCl, 0.1 *M* EDTA, buffer for 5 hours, at 4°. The filter paper is then withdrawn, dried in the nitrogen stream, and placed flat on the surface of a 5% blood agar, contained in large plates. The plates are incubated at 37° for 3 to 6 hours, and then inspected for areas of hemolysis corresponding to the hemolytic components of the original dialyzates, separated on the filter paper.

Chapter Eleven

COMPLEMENT AND PROPERDIN ASSAYS

Complement, properdin, as well as opsonin, conglutinin, lysins, leukins, plakins, and C-reactive protein are factors of the nonspecific resistance or the innate immunity.

I. CHARACTERISTICS OF THE COMPLEMENT

Complement is a colloidal, heat-labile complex consisting of euglobulin combined with a carbohydrate and phospho-lipid. It is present in fresh plasma or serum and is able to combine with any antigen and antibody system, but its amount does not increase on immunization. Complement is antigenic and may induce the formation of specific antibody in animals (McKee and Jeter, 1956). Complement is inactivated at 51° in 35 minutes, at 55° in 12 minutes, and at 61° in 2 minutes, but it may regain a part of its hemolytic activity when left in temperatures between 7 and 37° for about 24 hours, or upon adding 10% of fresh complement. If a serum must be deprived of the complement activity prior to a test, it is usually heated either at 56° for 20 to 30 minutes or at 62° for 3 minutes. Decomplementation of a serum can be attained by absorption with the hemolysin-sensitized erythrocytestromata, as well as with casein, charcoal, Kieselguhr, or cells of bacteria, yeasts, and animal tissues. Violent agitations, for example, shaking a 1:10 diluted fresh serum for 20 to 24 minutes, the treatment with acids, alkali, alcohol, either, chloroform, soaps, bile salts, proteolytic enzymes, mustard gas, and some alkaloids, or exposure of the serum to ultraviolet rays or to alpha particles also inactivate the complement.

Complement absorbed onto a complex of antibody and a cell-surface antigen causes ultrastructural membrane lesions which lead to cell leakage and subsequent cell destruction. The complement activated by antigen-antibody complexes directs the migration of polymorphonuclear leukocytes. Complement is capable of attaching antigen-antibody complexes to the cells, and it can produce a split product that contributes actively to the release of histamine from most cells.

The human complement system consists of nine components which are designated C_1', C_4', C_2', C_3', C_5', C_6', C_7', C_8', and C_9' listed according to their sequence of action. The C_1' component is composed of three subunits which are termed C_{1q}', C_{1r}' and C_{1s}'. The macromolecular complex formed by the three subunits has a sedimentation rate of 18S, is calcium-dependent in action, and attaches to antigen-bound antibody. The C_3' component consists of at least four subunits, C_{3b}', C_{3c}', C_{3e}', and C_{3f}'. The components, originally classified as the third complement component, proved to consist of at least six different serum factors. These factors, deriving from a human serum, are designated as C_3', C_5', C_6', C_7', C_8', and C_9'. The C_6' and C_7' interact with the fifth component of complement forming a reversible protein-protein complex. Kinetic analysis shows that C_5', C_6', and C_7' function in this order, subsequent to the third component (C_3') and preceding the function of C_8'. A reaction of the component C_3', C_5', C_6', and C_7' with the complement-erythrocyte complex leads to the formation of a thermostable intermediate product, but the participation of components C_8' and C_9' in the second stage brings about the characteristic ultrastructural membrane lesions. The components C_5' and C_6' function interdependently in the immune hemolysis reaction, reacting with the complement-erythrocyte complex, designated as $EAC_{1a,4,2a,3}'$, where E stands for sheep erythrocytes, A is antibody and C_{1a}', C_4', C_{2a}', and C_3' are the activated components of complement. The reaction product is termed systematically $EAC_{1a,4,2a,3,5,6,7}'$. The C_1' bound to an antibody molecule on a cell surface acts as a catalyst for attachment of the C_4' component to the cell membrane and to its function as the acceptor for C_2'. The two components thus linked form a complex enzyme, designated C_3' convertase, which catalyzes the absorption of C_3' to the cell surface. The C_3' convertase and C_3' component act on the components C_5', and C_6', and C_7' which interact in the fluid phase to form a reversible complex interacting with the cell membrane as a single functional unit. Following this interaction, the cell membrane is susceptible to C_8' and C_9' and to ultrastructural lesions.

The first component of human complement (C_1') is a macromolecule possessing a sedimentation coefficient of approximately 18 to 19S. The molecular weight of C_{1a}' is about 10^6. The molecular weight of C_2' is 150,000; the molecular weight of C_4' is 180,000, but the C_1' molecule has a considerable larger weight. Molecular weights of the complement components are estimated by comparing the position of individual active fractions containing the individual components to the position of the 7S hemolytic antibody which is assumed to have a molecular weight of 160,000.

The hemolytic complement, composed of all components, is present in fresh serum of man, guinea pig, and frog. The nonhemolytic complement may be lacking of some components. The two-component complements, deficient in C_2' and C_4', are found in serum of mouse, sheep, cow, and horse, whereas a complement deficient only in C_2' occurs in the blood of carp. However, some of these complements are hemolytic in serological systems other than sheep red blood cells sensitized with a specific rabbit hemolysin. The function, for example, in systems consisting of ox red blood cells sensitized with cat hemolysin (Muir, 1911). Other examples follow: the bovine complement brings about the hemolysis of human erythrocytes coated by the rabbit, gunea pig, cat, or dog hemolysins (Noguchi and Bronfenbrenner, 1911); the sheep complement dissolves human erythrocytes coated by hemolysins of guinea pig or rabbit; and complement from the horse, cow, and sheep serum hemolyzes rabbit red blood cells sensitized with the sheep amboceptor.

These peculiarities of complements, erythrocytes, and hemolysins of various species of animals must be considered prior to the selection of an appropriate system of red blood cells sensitized with the amboceptor for the complement determination test.

II. ISOLATION AND PURIFICATION OF COMPLEMENT COMPONENTS

Individual components of complement may be isolated by gel filtration, ion exchange chromatography, and density-gradient centrifugation. Further purification is attained by a preparative electrophoresis method, for example, the block electrophoresis of acrylamide electrophoresis.

The C_1', C_2', and C_4' (the first, second, and fourth components of complement) may be separated by the filtration through a Sephadex G-200, using an isotonic veronal buffered saline and carrying out the filtration at 3 to 6° (Borsos and Rapp, 1965).

The C_1' alone may be isolated from guinea pig serum and from human serum by Nelson's et al. (1966) method, or by its modification (Cooper and Müller-Eberhard, 1968). According to the latter procedure, a fresh serum is first adjusted to pH 7.5 and diluted 1:3 with distilled water at 4°. The precipitate thus formed is centrifuged and washed with 5×10^{-2} M NaCl containing 7.5×10^{-4} M CaCl$_2$ and 0.006 M veronal buffer at pH 7.5. The precipitate is redissolved in an isotonic buffer containing 7.5×10^{-4} M CaCl$_2$. The preparation is purified by ultracentrifugation to remove floatable lipid, and it may be frozen in liquid nitrogen and stored at $-70°$.

The C_4' alone may be isolated by Müller-Eberhard and Biro's (1963) technique; C_{3e}' component can be obtained by Inoue and Nelson's (1965) method.

A very convenient method for the preparation of C_{1a}' is the technique of Colten et al. (1968). By the procedure, the guinea pig serum used as a source of C_{1a}' is first adjusted to pH 5.6 with 1 N HCl and dialyzed against distilled water at 0°. The resulting precipitate is collected by centrifugation, washed three times in 0.015 M NaCl, and resuspended in 20 ml of 0.15 M NaCl. This preparation is then placed on a 10 to 30% sucrose density gradient, made in veronal buffer saline (mμ = 0.065) containing 0.00015 M

Ca^{++} and 0.001 M Mg^{++}. The sample is spun down at 30,000 rpm at 10° for 16 hours after which the fraction showing high C'_{1a} are pooled.

The C'_4 component of hemolytic complement may be isolated from guinea pig serum by means of ion exchange chromatography, gel filtration, and electrophoresis, yielding an immunologically homogeneous protein (Chan and Cebra, 1968).

The C'_3 and C'_5 components of complement may be isolated by Nilsson and Müller-Eberhard's (1965) method, although the C'_3 component must be purified further by preparative block electrophoresis in barbital buffer, pH 8.6, ionic strength 0.05.

Relatively pure preparations of the C'_6, C'_7, and C'_8 components may be obtained by Nilsson's (1967) technique. According to this procedure, an euglobulin obtained from a fresh human serum is filtered through a DEAE-cellulose column utilizing the gradient elution procedure described by Nilsson and Müller-Eberhard (1965). Eluates obtained at the pH range of 8.1–6.9 are passed through a hydroxyl apatite column equilibrated with a pH 7.9 phosphate buffer, having a specific conductance of 6 mmho/cm. The fractions are eluted in the following order: C'_7, C'_6, and C'_8.

The sixth (C'_6), seventh (C'_7), and eighth (C'_8) components of human complement may also be separated by the chromatography on hydroxyl apatite and purified (Nilsson and Müller-Eberhard, 1967). The ninth component (C'_9) may be prepared by three preparative steps, consisting of filtration through DEAE-cellulose and Sephadex G-200 gels and electrophoresis (Hadding and Müller-Eberhard, 1967).

III. THE COMPLEMENT ASSAY

The amount of complement present in serum may be determined accurately by a chemical measurement of the nitrogen increase after the absorption of complement by a known quantity of an immune complex.

An approximate determination of the complement is based on the estimation of the final serum dilution effective in the lysis of erythrocytes sensitized with an antierythrocyte serum (the complement assay).

The complement assay is based on determination of the amount of serum, which under standard conditions brings about a complete hemolysis of erythrocyte suspension sensitized with antierythrocyte serum (hemolysin) in 30 to 45 minutes, at 37°. Techniques of the complement assay were described by Rutstein and Walker (1942), Ecker et al. (1943), Bier et al. (1945), Kabat and Mayer (1948), Vaughan et al. (1951), Kellett (1954), Hartmann (1955), McKee and Jeter (1956), Kwapinski (1962, 1965), and a microtechnique was devised by Raeder (1956). Methods of titrating complement components were published by Heidelberger and Mayer (1948) and Rice and Crowson (1950).

1. Kwapinski's Technique of the Complement Assay

Different amounts of a fresh serum under test, ranging from 0.01 to 0.5 ml, are distributed into nine tubes (Table 55) and the volumes are made up to 0.5 ml with 0.85% sodium chloride solution, buffered at pH 7.0. A control tube contains 0.5 ml of the buffered saline only. A 2% suspension* of sheep red blood cells sensitized with five minimal hemolytic doses of a rabbit anti-RBC hemolytic serum is added to each tube, in 0.5-ml volumes, and the test mixtures are agitated and incubated in a water bath at 37° for precisely 30 minutes. The last tube in the row, in which the red blood cells are completely lyzed, denotes the end. The volume of nondiluted serum in this tube is recorded, and the complement titer may be expressed by this amount of serum. However, it is more convenient to express the complement level in terms of "the complement percentage" (C'%). This can be calculated from the ratio of volumes of buffered saline in the end point tube (*Bs*) and in the control tube (*Bc*), multiplied by 100, as indicated by the formula

$$C'\% = \frac{Bs}{Bc} \times 100$$

For example, the complement percentage for tube 4 taken as end point is

$$C'\% = \frac{0.4}{0.5} \times 100 = 80\%$$

Complement percentage calculated for various effective volumes of human serum can be read from Table 55. Values between 90 and 94% are regarded as normal, whereas lower or higher titers are considered abnormal. The accuracy of the test may be increased by spectrophotometric determination of degrees of hemolysis in the reaction supernatants.

The determination of minimal hemolytic doses of a rabbit anti-RBC hemolytic serum is carried out as shown in Table 56.

The last tube showing complete hemolysis denotes the end point, and the amount of the anti-RBC hemolytic serum in this tube is equivalent to 1 MHD of the hemolysin.

The amount of anti-RBC hemolytic serum (*x*), in milliliters, to sensitize a certain volume (*a*) of 2% suspension of sheep erythrocytes is calculated according to the following formula:

$$x = \frac{5a}{T}$$

where T = the titer of amboceptor and a = the volume of 2% erythrocyte suspension to be sensitized.

*Concentration of erythrocytes is checked by a slide count, for more reproducible results.

Table 55. The Complement Titration Schedule, by Kwapinski (1965)

Tube Number	1	2	3	4	5	6	7	8	9	Control Tube
Human serum (ml)	0.5	0.4	0.3	0.2	0.1	0.05	0.03	0.02	0.01	0
Buffered saline (pH 7.0, ml)	0	0.10	0.20	0.30	0.40	0.45	0.47	0.48	0.49	0.5
2% sensitized sheep R.B.C. (ml)	0.5	0.5	0.5	0.5	0.5	0.5	0.5	0.5	0.5	0.5
				Incubation at 37° for 30 minutes						
"Complement percentage"	0	20	40	60	80	90	94	96	98	—

Table 56. Determination of Minimal Hemolytic Dose of Antisheep Erythrocyte Serum (Kwapinski, 1965)

Tube Number	1	2	3	4	5	6	7	8	Controls	
Hemolysin										
Diluted 1:	1000	2000	3000	4000	5000	6000	7000	8000	1000	—
Volume (ml)	0.2	0.2	0.2	0.2	0.2	0.2	0.2	0.2	0.2	—
Complement diluted 1:10 (ml)	0.2	0.2	0.2	0.2	0.2	0.2	0.2	0.2	—	0.2
Diluent (ml)	0.1	0.1	0.1	0.1	0.1	0.1	0.1	0.1	0.2	0.2
				Incubation at 37° for 60 minutes						
2% sheep erythrocytes (ml)	0.5	0.5	0.5	0.5	0.5	0.5	0.5	0.5	0.5	0.5
Final volume (ml)	1.0	1.0	1.0	1.0	1.0	1.0	1.0	1.0	1.0	1.0
				Incubation at 37° for 15 minutes						

2. *The Kabat and Mayer Technique of the Complement Determination*

The human complement is titrated by this technique, as arranged by Hederstedt (1961), in the manner presented in Table 57. The suspension of sheep erythrocytes is standardized to give a lyzate with the extinction of 0.34 at 545 mμ in the Coleman spectrophotometer, in 1:50 dilution with distilled water. Sensitized sheep erythrocytes consist of equal portions of the standardized erythrocytes suspension and a solution of anti-RBC serum containing four hemolytic units per milliliter.

Table 57.   The Complement Titration Schedule (Hederstedt, 1961)

Tube Number	1	2	3	4	5	6	7	8	9
Veronal-NaCl buffer (ml)	0.70	0.65	0.60	0.55	0.50	0.45	0.40	0.35	0.30
Complement dilution (ml)	0.05	0.10	0.15	0.20	0.25	0.30	0.35	0.40	0.45
Sensitized sheep erythrocytes (ml)	0.50	0.50	0.50	0.50	0.50	0.50	0.50	0.50	0.50

Reaction mixtures are incubated at 37° for 45 minutes, then centrifuged, and supernatants are withdrawn. Percentage of hemolysis in each supernatant fluid is determined in a spectrophotometer, and the 50% unit of complement is calculated graphically from the von Krogh's equation (see p. 502). Titers are expressed in log units.

3. *Hartmann's Technique of the Complement Assay*

Sheep red blood cells to be used in the test are washed four times in saline solution, and centrifuged at 800 to 1000 $\times$ g for 5 minutes. The sediment is suspended in saline to give an approximatete 2.8% concentration, which should be adjusted so that 1.0 ml of the erythrocyte suspension hemolyzed with 9 ml of distilled water shows an optimal density of 0.445 to 0.455, as measured in a spectrophotometer at 550 nm wavelength.

The minimum hemolytic dose of hemolysin is then estimated by titration in the following manner: a hemolytic rabbit serum is diluted 1:2, 1:4, 1:8, and 1:16 in 1-ml volumes in saline, and 0.85 ml of each dilution is transferred to cooled tubes. Each tube then receives 0.85 ml of 2.8% erythrocyte suspension, 3.8 ml of saline, and 3.0 ml of a saline solution containing complement in excess. The tubes are closed with rubber stoppers and left for 25 minutes in the water bath, at 37°. The last tube showing complete hemolysis is taken as end point, and the titer of amboceptor is calculated from the dilution in the tube. Erythrocytes are sensitized with four minimum hemolytic doses of hemolysin, by mixing one part of a dilute anti-erythrocyte serum containing 4 MHD and 1 part of sheep erythrocyte suspension. The mixture is incubated at 37° for 15 minutes and left in a refrigerator until used.

Human serum being tested is now diluted in the proportion of 1:100 with a veronal or phosphate buffer containing calcium and magnesium ions, and the test is set up as indicated in Table 58. The samples are then incubated for 40 minutes in a water bath at 37°, with frequent shaking, and transferred to the ice bath for 5 minutes. Contents of tubes are centrifuged, and optical densities of the supernatants are determined colorimetrically. Figures representing optical densities are proportionally altered into hemolysis percentages, and actual percentages are calculated by using a correcting scale of the photometer. The corrected hemolysis percentages are plotted against corresponding volumes of the serum, and a hemolysis curve is drawn from these data. The dose (K) of serum, in milliliters, which caused a 50% hemolysis, is read from the abscissa, and the activity of the complement is expressed in terms of 50% hemolytic units $(C'H_{50})$ per milliliter of nondiluted human serum. This is computed as the proportion between the coefficient of the original serum dilution, which is 100, as the serum was originally diluted 1:100, and the dose of serum (K), according to the following equation:

$$C'H_{50} = \frac{100}{K}$$

4. Small and Baxter's (1965) Complement Assay

According to this method, a standard sheep red cell suspension is sensitized with an equal volume of a 1:200 dilution of antiserum produced against boiled sheep red cell stroma, and the sensitized erythrocyte suspension is

Table 58. A Schedule of the Human Serum Complement Determination by Hartmann

Tube Number	1	2	3	4	5		6 (Control Tube)
Human serum diluted 1:100 (ml)	2.5	3.0	3.5	4.0	5.0		—
Buffered saline (ml)	4.3	3.8	3.3	2.8	1.8		3.8
Sensitized sheep erythrocytes (ml)	1.7	1.7	1.7	1.7	1.7	1.7	1.7
Guinea pig complement 1:20 (ml)	—	—	—	—	—	—	3.0
Total volume (ml)	8.5	8.5	8.5	8.5	8.5	8.5	8.5

diluted $1:30$ with a buffer to give a concentration of 1.67×10^7 cells/ml. A complement source, such as fresh plasma or a plasma stored at $-70°$, is then diluted serially at $0°$ in 1.6 ml of the buffer. Each complement dilution receives 0.8 ml of the sensitized erythrocyte suspension and the mixtures are incubated for 90 minutes, after which the absorbency of each tube is determined at 412-nm wavelength. The $C'H_{50}$ titer is determined from a von Krogh formula using the previously determined average hematocrit value of 50% according to Allen's et al. (1961) procedure.

IV. DETERMINATION OF COMPONENTS OF COMPLEMENT

Individual components of the complement can be determined by the use of a suitable serum reagent, which contains at a high concentration all components of the complement, except the one to be tested. Titers of individual complement components are determined by serial dilution, as in an ordinary complement assay. Here are details of the selected techniques: determination of the first C_1' component of complement according to Kornfeld and Weigle's (1965) method is conducted in the following manner. The C' reagent lacking C_1' consists of a guinea pig serum diluted $1:10$ and heated $56°$ for 30 minutes. An end piece (S) is prepared by dialysis and dilution with the serum. The EAC_1' or erythrocyte-antibody-C_1' complex is prepared by the sensitization of washed sheep cells (1×10^9 cells/ml) incubated wth an equal volume of a hemolysin preparation, diluted to contain twice the amount employed for $C'H_{50}$ titration. Reaction mixtures for titration of C_1' consists of 0.6 ml EAC_1', 0.1 ml of the C' reagent lacking C_1' (R_1), 0.1 ml S and 0.7 ml of veronal buffer containing 0.1% gelatine. The mixture is incubated at $37°$ in a water bath until partial hemolysis occurs. The tubes are then transferred to a $0°$ water bath, and 0.5 ml of 1 M sodium citrate and 5.0 ml cold buffer are added to each tube to stop further hemolysis. The contents of each tube is centrifuged. The supernatant is collected and optical densities are read at 541-nm wavelength. Appropriate controls are used to permit calculation of the percent lysis.

Molecular titration of C_2' and C_4' is carried out by methods designed by Borsos and Rapp (1963) and Cooper and Müller-Eberhard (1968). The molecular titration of C_4' is based on the specific interaction of EAC_{1a}' with different dilutions of C_4'.

The complexes EAC_{1a}', $EAC_{1a,4}'$, $EAC_{1a,4,2a}'$, $EAC_{1a,4,2a,3}'$, and $EAC_{1a,4,2a,3,5,6,7}'$ can be prepared by the methods described by Müller-Eberhard et al. (1966, 1967).

Hemolytic assays of C_5', C_6', C_7', and C_8' are conducted as follows: first, the substrate ($EAC_{1a,4,2a,3}'$) is prepared by exposing $EAC_{1a,4,2a}'$ to a purified C_3' per 1×10^8 cells. (The $EAC_{1a,4,2a}'$ complex is prepared by treating sensitized sheep erythrocytes with whole human serum in the presence of phlorid-zin, according to Nilsson and Müller-Eberhard's (1965) method). The $EAC'_{1a,4,2a,3}$ substrate is then exposed to mixtures of C'_5, C'_6, and C'_7 in 0.45-ml volume at 37° for 20 minutes, after which 0.05 ml of fresh, undiluted human serum are added. The mixture, which also contains EDTA at 0.01 M concentration, is left at 37° for 30 minutes. Each of the three components of complement are then assayed in reaction mixtures which were lacking the component in quesion. The usual quantity of the C'_5 component is 5 μg, whereas the other components are used in a moderate excess. The C'_8 is assayed employing 1×10^8 $EAC'_{1a,4,oxy2a,3}$ cells, 1.5 μg C'_5, and a moderate excess of C'_6, C'_7, and C'_9 in a total volume of 1 ml.

1. Hemolytic Plaque Assay for C'_1

According to Colten's et al. (1968) technique, a 1% agarose solution, melted and cooled to 42° and mixed with a solution containing 2.5 ml of an RL buffer and 2.5 ml of Medium 199 to 5.0 ml of the 1% agarose solution, represents the supporting medium. The RL buffer consists of Ringer's lactate solution containing 5% glucose, 50 units of penicillin, and 50 μg of streptomycin per milliliter.

To prepare a medium for the hemolytic plaques assay, the 0.5% agarose solution is mixed with EAC'_4 (1×10^9 cells) per milliliter (0.8 ml at 42°). Then $\frac{1}{10}$ ml of a cell suspension obtained from the kidney or spleen of immunized guinea pigs is mixed with 0.8 ml of the agarose-EAC'_4 mixture and poured into a Petri plate which has been coated with a thin layer of the agarose. After 40 minutes incubation at 30°, 2 ml of a C'_2 preparation (containing 7×10^{10} effective molecules per ml) are added, and the plates are reincubated at 30° for 30 minutes. The C'_2 is then poured off and replaced with 2.0 ml of C'EDTA and the plates are incubated at 36° for 60 minutes. The C'EDTA is then discarded. Control plates are treated in the same manner except that the C'_2 or C'EDTA is replaced with a buffer. After the incubation time, the plates are observed for the presence of clear zones around the antibody-producing cells. The plaques may also be stained with a nuclear fast red solution (0.1 g of nuclear fast red in 100 ml of aqueous 5% aluminum sulfate solution). Before the staining, the plates are flooded with 0.15 M saline solution and then the dye solution is added dropwise. The plates are kept at room temperature for 5 minutes and the excess dye is decanted. The plates are finally washed with several changes of 0.15 M saline solution and examined microscopically using a green filter.

V. EVALUATION AND APPLICATION OF THE COMPLEMENT ASSAY

Blood complement of healthy human beings and animals kept on balanced diet maintains at a relatively constant level. The titer of complement increases in parallel with the level of ascorbic acid in the blood serum of guinea pigs (Ecker et al., 1938). The decrease of complement in experimental conditions follows the injection of Indian ink, which absorbs the circulating complement and presumably blocks its hypothetical site of formation, the reticuloendothelial system (Jungeblut and Berlot, 1926). Similar conditions occur after the injection of carbon tetrachloride or chloroform and after a blockade of liver cells with gum acacia (Rice 1953). The complement level drops invariably during any strong reaction *in vivo* between an antigen and homologous antibody, for example, after the injection of streptococci or tubercle bacilli into sensitized animals (Bieling, 1930), or at the immunization and sensitization of animals with a species-foreign serum or erythrocytes (Stavitsky et al,, 1949). A similar reaction is provoked by the injection of a mixture of red blood cells and heated homologous plasma or acacia gum (Coca, 1914; Ecker and Reese, 1922, Wassermann, 1941), and it also occurs in the anaphylactic shock (Friedberger and Hartoch, 1909; Stavitsky et al., 1949; Schwab et al., 1950). Coburn and Pauli (1939) suppose that the decrease of complement is conditioned by the presence of an excess antigen and homologous antibody.

Complement titers in the sera of clinically healthy people vary between 0.03 and 0.05 ml of serum which corresponds to 90 to 94 complement percentage or to 80 to 150 C' units (Veil and Buchholz, 1932; Vaughan et al., 1951; Micheeveva, 1953; Kwapinski and Snyder, 1962). Increased complement levels have been observed in cases of x-ray treatment and neoplasmas. Decreased complement levels to between 0.06 and 0.2, equal to 88 to 60%, were found in 57.1 to 83.3% of rheumatic fever cases by Kwapinski (1962) and Rodenko (1954), and in 7.3 to 33% sera from rheumatoid arthritis (Kwapinski, 1962; Vaughan et al., 1951, respectively).

The complement determination test provides reliable and reproducible serological data which may inform of the existence of certain exceptionally vigorous immunological reactions *in vivo*. However, the practical significance of this test, which is immunologically nonspecific, must not be overestimated.

VI. THE PROPERDIN ASSAY

Properdin is a specific β-globulin which exists in the sera of human beings and other mammals.. Its isoelectric point is a pH 5.6, and the molecular weight is approximately one million. This substance constitutes less than 0.02% of total serum protein. It is stable between pH 7.8 and 8.4, at ionic strength of 0.15, but precipitates when dialysed at pH 5.5 at a low ionic strength, and is destroyed, partially at 50° and completely at 56° in 30 minutes. Properdin has an electrophoretical mobility of globulin and the sedimentation constant of 19S (Lepow et al., 1959).

Properdin plays an important part in the natural defence mechanisms of blood. In conjunction with complement and magnesium ions, the properdin system participates in the destruction of certain bacteria, protozoa, and abnormal mammalian cells. It also contributes to the neutralization and inactivation of certain animal and bacterial viruses. The maximum activity of the properdin system is at 37°, and it is practically inactive below 10°.

Properdin can be selectively removed from the serum either by zymosan or by antiproperdin rabbit serum. Combining with the zymosan in the presence of some additional serum factors, properdin forms a complex, which inactivates the third component of complement, that is a specific phospholipid or phosphoprotein, a heat-stable serum substance. The optimum temperature of this reaction is something between 30 and 37°. The characteristics of additional serum factor supporting properdin is not sufficiently known. However, they differ from the four components of complement. One of them is relatively heat stable, since it withstands the temperature of 56° for 30 minutes, but is destroyed by hydrazine; the other factor can be inactivated at 52° in 30 minutes, but not by hydrazine.

Serological estimation of the properdin level in the serum is based on a quantitative measurement of the reaction between properdin and certain polysaccharides of microbial, plant, or mammalian origin. This polysaccharide material, which occurs in abundance in the cell wall residue of yeasts, is termed zymosan. It combines with properdin at the temperature of 15°.

1. Methods of the Properdin Estimation

There are six quantitative methods of the properdin estimation:

1. The zymosan-complement assay, which depends on the inactivation by a polysaccharide-properdin complex of the third complement component, C_3' (Pillemer et al., 1956; Isliker and Linder, 1958).

2. Chemical method, based on determination of the nitrogen content of properdin, absorbed to the properdin-active polysaccharide. Nitrogen is estimated before and after incubation of the polysaccharide with the serum tested (Isliker and Linder, 1958).

3. Bactericidal properdin test, in which the number of properdin-sensitive bacteria, killed by the exposure of a certain amount of test serum, is determined (Wardlaw and Pillemer, 1956).

4. The bacteriophage inactivation test, based on the inactivation by properdin and its cofactors of the T2r bacteriophage. The criterion is provided by the number of cells of *Escherichia coli* lyzed by the residual bacteriophage particles, which were inactivated by the serum.

5. Cytolytic properdin test. Properdin is bound by certain pathologically altered cells, with subsequent lysis. For example, red blood cells of patients with paroxysmal nocturnal hemoglobinuria undergo lysis by properdin; the resulting hemolysis can be measured (Hinz and Pillemer, 1955; Martin and Voss, 1957).

6. A specific hemagglutination-inhibition test, which consists of the inhibition by a specific antiproperdin serum of the agglutination of the properdin-coated red blood cells. Here is the review of selected techniques of the properdin assay

7. *The Zymosan-complement assay of properdin.* The test is based on quantitative requirement of properdin for the inactivation of the third component of complement (C_3') by zymosan. Here are constituents of the Isliker and Linder technique: (a) a serum tested for the properdin level; (b) a buffer solution; (c) a zymosan preparation; (d) RP-reagent (a serum deficient in properdin); (e) RP-zymosan mixture; (f) R_3-reagent (a serum deficient in C_3'); (g) a suspension of sensitized erythrocytes.

All reagents must be carefully prepared and standardized in the following manner:

a. The serum to be tested should be fresh or stored frozen at $-30°$. A control standard serum is provided by twenty tested normal sera, which may be stored at $-30°$, in 0.5 ml samples.

b. A buffered saline (Mayer et al., 1946) which contains optimum concentrations of calcium and magnesium ions and is used for making dilutions and for washing. Its composition is as follows:

Sodium chloride	85.0 g
5,5-diethylbarbituric acid	5.75 g
sodium 5,5-diethylbarbiturate	3.75 g
1 *M* solution of magnesium chloride	5.0 ml
1 *M* solution of calcium chloride	1.5 ml

These ingredients are dissolved in a volume of 1500 ml of hot distilled water and the volume is increased to 2 liters with cold distilled water. This stock solution must be diluted with four parts of distilled water before use. The solution should be adjusted to pH 7.4.

c. *The zymosan preparation.* The 500 g of heat-denaturated and finely homogenized baker's yeast are extracted three times with 1 liter saline adjusted to pH 7.5 with 1 *N* NaOH. The mixture is centrifuged each time, and the sediment is washed three times with 200 ml of acetone and dried in a vacuum desiccator. This material is treated for 30 minutes at 75°, with 0.02 *N* HCl or with 50% phenol, using 10 ml of either solution per 1 g of dried material. The mixture is then centrifuged, and the sediment is washed three times with distilled water, twice with 96% alcohol, and once with absolute alcohol, and dried in a vacuum desiccator.

Another method of preparing zymosan employs the trypsin digestion of yeasts for 4 days, under constant stirring, at pH 8.0, at 37°. Trypsin is added daily up to 0.5% final concentration. The digestion may be expedited by adding urea to a final concentration of 3 moles/liter. At the end of digestion, the mixture is centrifuged, and the sediment is extracted with distilled water in a Soxhlet apparatus for 12 hours, then centrifuged. The sediment is dehydrated with 95% ethyl alcohol or acetone. A commercial preparation of zymosan can also be used for the properdin assay.

The activity of a zymosan preparation is tested by estimating the minimum amount required to remove properdin and C_3' from 1-ml volume of normal human serum in the following manner. A sample of zymosan is suspended in a buffer solution and dispersed in a ground glass homogenizer; 1 ml of this suspension is mixed with 1 ml of serum, in duplicate. One sample must be incubated at 17°, another at 37° for 1 hour. The amount of zymosan, in milligrams, which is sufficient to depress the C_3' and the properdin activity to about 80% of the original value is estimated.

d. Standard preparation of human properdin is manufactured according to the Pillemer et al. (1956) method, which is presented diagrammatically in Table 59.

e. The RP reagent is a serum, from which properdin has been removed in the following manner. A serum pooled from at least five donors is mixed with zymosan in a proportion of 1 ml/2 mg and incubated at 15 to 17° for 1 hour, with gentle stirring. The mixture is then centrifuged for 30 minutes at 15,000 $\times$ g. This procedure must be repeated to absorb and completely remove properdin from the serum.

The RP should have the following characteristics: it must maintain its C_3' above 80 units after the addition of 5 mg of zymosan per milliliter during an incubation at 37° (the third component of complement may be inactivated under those conditions only in the presence of properdin in the serum). The adequacy of a RP reagent may further be checked by conducting three properdin titrations of a standard serum with three different dilutions of the RP reagent. The undiluted RP must show a titer of 7 to 9 properdin units per milliliter.

f. The RP-zymosan mixture is used for properdin titration of examined sample of serum. To prepare a RP-zymosan mixture, 10 mg of zymosan are suspended in 1 ml of buffer solution and ground in a glass homogenizer. This is added to 1 ml of the RP reagent immediately before use.

g. The R_3 reagent is a serum, deficient in C_3' (third component of complement), but containing the C_1', C_2', and C_4' components in excess. To prepare this reagent, by the method of Pillemer et al. (1956), zymosan is mixed at 37° with a sample of fresh human serum in the ratio of 1 to 2 mg/ml. The mixture is agitated and incubated at 37° for 60 minutes, then centrifuged at 4000 rpm for 30 minutes at 1°. The clear supernatant must be stored at $-70°$, or it can be kept at 1° for use within 12 hours. The R_3 reagent should be standardized, for the following:

i. The lack of the hemolytic activity; 0.1 ml of the R_3-reagent must not lyze 2 ml of 0.4° red blood cells sensitized with an antierythrocyte (hemolysin) serum.

ii. The anticomplementary properties against small amount of fresh serum; 0.05 ml of R_3-reagent added to 0.1 ml of a fresh serum diluted 1:15 should increase the C′ titer of the serum by at least 200%.

iii. The ability to measure C_3' in a standard RP serum in the presence of zymosan and in the presence and absence of properdin; 0.05 ml of the R_3 reagent should be able to measure at least 120 units of C_3'/1ml of RP, and

Table 59. Preparation of Human Properdin (Pillemer et al., 1956)

100 ml of fresh human serum	
+ 4 ml of Zymosan susp. (50–57 mg/ml) stir 1 hr at 17°, adjust to pH 6.9, centrifuge	
Precipitate = PZ complex	Supernatant = RP
+ 50 ml of phosphate-saline buffer, pH 6.0, centrifuge, repeat washing two times	
Precipitate = washed PZ complex	
+ 36 ml of Michaelis buffer and 14 ml of $2M$ NaCl stir 1 hour at 37°, centrifuge	
Precipitate = eluted PZ complex	Supernatant = properdin eluate
	Dialysis against distilled water 3 days at 1°, adjust to ph 5.8, centrifuge
	Precipitate = crude properdin + 17 ml of barbital buffer, pH 7.4, at 1° centrifuge
Precipitate	Supernatant A = properdin extract
+ 8 ml of barbital buffer, pH 7.4 at 1°, centrifuge	
	Supernatant B = properdin extract
	Pool supernatants A and B, final pH 7.0-7.4

[a] All centrifugations are conducted at 400 rpm at 1° for 30 minutes. Phosphate-saline buffer contains one part of phosphate buffer (768.4 ml $M/10$ NaH₂PO₄ and 231.6 ml of $M/10$ Na₂HPO₄) and 19 parts of 0.15 M NaCl. Michaelis' buffer, pH 7.4, contains 9.714 g sodium acetate (3H₂O), 14.714 g sodium 5.5 g diethylbarbiturate, and 17.00 g NaCl dissolved in 1960 ml of distilled water, adjusted to pH 7.4.

not less than 90 units/ml of the RP previously treated with zymosan in the presence of 1 unit of properdin per milliliter of RP.

h. *The suspension of sensitized ertythrocytes.* Sheep red blood cells washed twice in saline and once with buffered saline are suspended in the buffer solution to give 5% concentration of cells. The concentration of erythrocytes must be checked by hemolyzing an aliquot sample and adjusting it to a constant extinction value (see p. 491).

The 5% erythrocyte suspension is now mixed with an equal volume of buffered saline containing four units of antierythrocyte serum per milliliter and incubated at 37° for 10 minutes, then diluted with six volumes of the buffer solution to give 0.4% suspension. The unit of hemolytic serum is previously determined by setting up 0.1-ml samples of a twofold serial dilution of hemolytic serum diluted 1:100 with 0.1 ml of a 5% erythrocyte suspension and 0.2 ml of 1:20 dilution of fresh guinea pig serum. After 30-minute incubation at 37°, the unit of hemolytic serum is determined by the highest dilutions giving complete hemolysis.

2. Determination of the Properdin Level

The serum to be tested is serially diluted from 1:1 to 1:64 in a volume of 0.1 ml. A volume of 0.1 ml of the buffer solution and 0.2 ml of the zymosan-RP mixture is added to each tube.

Control tubes contain: (a) 0.1 ml of a purified standard properdin preparation containing 10 PU (properdin unit)/ml, and 0.1 ml of buffer; (b) 0.2 ml RP reagent and 0.4 ml of buffer; and (c) 0.4 ml of the RP-zymosan mixture and 0.2 ml of the buffer.

After the incubation at 37° for 1 hour, with gentle stirring, the contents of tubes can be centrifuged to remove the particles of zymosan (or this step may be omitted). Two units of R_3 reagent in 0.05-ml volumes are then added to each tube, and the volumes are made up to 0.5 ml with a buffer solution. Each tube now receives 2.0 ml of a 0.4% suspension of sensitized erythrocytes. After reincubation at 37° for 30 minutes, the tubes are centrifuged for 5 minutes at 300 × g, and the hemolysis degrees of supernatant fluids are estimated spectrophotometrically.

The control tube c should show not less than 75% of the C_3' activity of the sample b. Reciprocal serum dilutions giving 50% hemolysis are arbitrarily designated as properdin units present in 1 ml of the original serum (PU ml). Extinctions of tubes giving more or less than 50% hemolysis are plotted as ordinate on a logarithmic scale against reciprocal serum dilutions. The properdin units are found, where a line between these two points intersects the extinction corresponding to 50% hemolysis.

Dilution of the tested serum giving 50° hemolysis may be conveniently determined by the procedure devised by Pillemer et al. (1956). In this technique, each tube is compared to a 50% hemolysis standard prepared by adding a trace of saponin to a mixture of 0.5 ml of sensitized sheep erythrocytes and 1 ml of the buffer. The number of properdin units ((PU) is calculated by multiplying the factor d of final dilution of the serum, giving a 50% hemolysis by the ratio v between the final volume of the fluid in this tube and the volume of diluted test serum, and by the dilution factor r of the RP serum, as employed in the test. For example, the final dilution of a serum giving 50% hemolysis is 1:24; thus $d = 24$. The final volume of the fluid is 1.0 ml, and the volume of diluted test serum $= 0.2$ ml; thus $v = 1.0/0.2 = 5$. The RP serum has been diluted threefold ($r = 3$); hence PU is calculated as follows: $24 \times 5 \times 3 = 360$ properdin units. If the samples show no trace of hemolysis, the C_3' titer is regarded as 0, and it is assumed that the C_3' in the RP serum has been completely inactivated.

Properdin levels in normal sera are as follows: 5 to 12 PU/ml in human sera, 12 to 15 PU/ml in mouse and dog sera, and 8 to 12 PU/ml in rabbit sera.

A simplified properdin assay was designed by Harm (1963).

Chapter Twelve

THE COMPLEMENT FIXATION TEST

I. PRINCIPLES OF THE COMPLEMENT FIXATION REACTION

Absorption of complement by specific immune complexes of antigen and antibody is the principle of the complement fixation test. Complement absorbed or combined in a sufficient quantity by red blood cells coated by, or sensitized with, a homologous antierythrocyte serum brings about the hemolysis. If, however, the complement has been previously absorbed by another nonhemolytic complex of an antigen and its homologous antibody and then added to a suspension of erythrocytes coated by an antierythrocyte serum, no hemolysis occurs since the complement cannot be easily released from the first serological complex. On the other hand, mixtures of noncorresponding antigens and antibodies do not absorb complement which remains free for the subsequent reaction with sensitized erythrocytes, leading to hemolysis. The immune hemolysis is a multiple-step process which is represented by the following formula:

$$E + A \rightarrow EA \xrightarrow[\text{Ca}^{++}]{C'_{1q,r,s}} EAC'_{1a} \xrightarrow[\text{Ca}^{++}]{C'_{4}} EAC'_{1a,4} \xrightarrow[\text{Mg}^{++}]{C'_{2}} EAC'_{1a,4,2a}$$

$$\xrightarrow{C'_{3}} EAC'_{1a,4,2a,3} \xrightarrow{C'_{5,6,7}} EAC'_{1a,4,2a,3,5,6,7} \xrightarrow{C'_{8}}$$

$$EAC'_{1a,4,2a,3,5,6,7,8} \xrightarrow{C'_{9}} E \text{ ghosts} + \text{hemoglobin}$$

Thus the erythrocyte first reacts with its antibody molecules to form a stable erythrocyte-antibody complex (EA). At the next stage, a complex of three substances present in the serum ($C'_{1q,r,s}$) either jointly or in the sequence, in the presence of calcium ions, interacts with the EA complex to produce $EAC'_{1q,r,s}$ or the intermediate E,A,C'_{1a} (where the designation a stands for an activated intermediate, susceptible to conversion to the succeeding state). The intermediate E, A,C'_{1a} is converted in the presence of C'_{4} component of complement to the intermediate $E,A,C'_{1a,4}$, and this in turn is coverted to the state $E,A,C'_{1a,4,2a}$ in the presence of magnesium ions. The intermediate

$E,A,C'_{1a,4,2a}$ is then converted to $EAC'_{1a,4,2a,3,5,6,7}$ by the participation of a C'_3 complex which consists of four constituents, termed C'_3, C'_5, C'_6, C'_7. This complex finally adsorbs C'_8 and C'_9, which results in the leakage of erythrocytes and the release of hemoglobin.

II. COMPONENTS OF COMPLEMENT FIXATION TEST

The complement fixation assay is a rather complex test procedure, which employs the following reactants:

1. The hemolytic system, composed of red blood cells and a homologous antierythrocyte serum (immune hemolysin).
2. A nonhemolytic system consisting of a microbial, cellular, or tissue antigen and a source of complementary antibodies.
3. The complement.
4. A buffered saline as diluent.

Activities of these constituents in a complement-fixation test and its products are functions of relative concentrations of all the components involved in this immunological reaction. The amount of erythrocytes, anti-RBC hemolysin, complement, and of either the tested serum or the antigen must be carelly predetermined and adjusted prior to the final test.

1. The Hemolytic System

The most popular hemolytic system consists of sheep red blood cells and a rabbit antisheep erythrocyte serum (anti-RBC hemolysin). However, certain techniques (e.g., of Rice and Boulanger's (1952) method) employ a system composed of rabbit red cells and a sheep antirabbit erythrocyte serum.

Erythrocytes should be obtained from a single animal; pooling of the blood from several animals must be avoided. Red blood cells are collected in an equal volume of sterile 2.5% sodium citrate or Alsever's solution* and centrifuged at a low speed. The cell-containing sediment is washed three times with Alsever's solution at 2 to 4° for a period not exceeding 2 weeks.

Sheep red blood cells contain at least two antigens capable of inducing the production of hemolytic antibodies, one of which is the heterogeneous Forssman antigen, a heat stable, lipopolysaccharide substance that is present in the stromata of erythrocytes. This antigen is mostly responsible for

---

* Alsever's solution consists of 2.05 g of dextrose, 0.8 g of trisodium citrate (dihydrate), and 0.42 g of sodium chloride in 100 ml of distilled water. This solution is adjusted to pH 6.1 with 10% citric acid and sterilized by filtration. Penicillin and streptomycin can be added to give a final concentration of about 50 units and 100 μg/ml, respectively.

inducing the production of sheep-erythrocyte antibodies. The erythrocyte stromata can be prepared according to Jaroslow and Taliaferro (1956) by gradual lysis of red blood cells suspended in the pH 7.4 buffered saline solutions of decreasing concentrations, followed by the removal of the hemoglobin by repeated centrifugation.

An antisheep erythrocyte serum (hemolytic serum, anti-RBC-hemolysin) can be produced in the following manner: a group of rabbits receives intravenously a total of seven injections, separated by 3-day intervals, of 1-ml doses of a 10% sheep erythrocyte suspension or an equivalent volume of stromata, suspended at the concentration of 1.6×10^9/ml. The sera are collected 2 weeks after the last injection. The average titer of hemolytic sera varies between 1:6000 and 1:10,000. These sera must be heated before use at 56° for 20 minutes or at 62° for 3 minutes to inactivate the complement.

2. The NonHemolytic System

The nonhemolytic system consists of an antigen prepared from microorganisms or tissues and a serum, the immunologic activities and spectra of both, or only one of the components being known. Particulate antigen preparations, for example, suspensions of bacterial cells, as well as soluble or insoluble constituents of microorganisms and higher organisms can be used as antigens in this immunologic reaction. By injection of, or infection with, a microorganism which possesses more than one antigen, two or several serologically distinct complement-fixing antibodies may be produced. For example, in the infection by mumps virus, antibodies against the soluble S antigen appear earlier and disappear sooner than the V-antibodies (Henle et al., 1948).

Immune sera of some animals, for example, horses, are usually incapable of fixing complement. Thus reactions of antibodies from these sera with homologous antigens cannot be detected by the complement fixation test (Zinsser and Parker, 1923; Stats and Bullowa, 1942).

Antisera to be used in the test should be transparent, and heated prior to the test at 56° for 30 minutes or at 62° for 3 minutes to destroy hemolytic complement that occurs at a particularly high level in fresh sera. Serum samples heated on a previous day must be reinactivated on the test day for 10 minutes at 56° or 1 minute at 62°.

3. The Complement

Complement is a complex, heat-labile serum substance essential for the lytic action of certain antibodies. The amount of complement required for immune hemolysis is appreciable, since about 6000 molecules of complement are needed to lyze a single erythrocyte (Haurowitz and Yenson,

1943; Heidelberger and Mayer, 1948). Complement occurs at varying concentrations in normal sera or different species of animals and even among members of a single species. The blood serum of guinea pigs kept on a proper diet, rich in ascorbic acid, contains the complement at the highest level. The complement is obtained from the blood, usually taken by a heart puncture and allowed to clot. The separated and centrifuged serum can either be used fresh or preserved in a frozen state at $-10°$ in which the complement remains active for several months. A lyophilized complement does not lose its potency for several years. Alternatively, the complement may be preserved for 2 to 3 weeks in Richardson's (1941) fluid, although this procedure is less commendable. Richardson's fluid consists of a mixture of three solutions, A, B, and C. Solution A is $M/4$ boric acid in saturated sodium chloride, prepared by dissolving 1.55 g of boric acid in a saturated solution of sodium chloride added up to a volume of 100 ml. Solution B consists of $M/2$ sorbitol and $M/8$ azide diluted in saturated sodium chloride (9.55 g of sorbitol and 0.81 g of sodium azide are made up to 100 ml with a saturated sodium chloride solution).

Eight volumes of a serum containing complement are mixed with one volume of solution A and one volume of an equal volume mixture of solutions B and C. The serum mixture is adjusted to pH 6.0 to 6.5 and diluted 1:7 with distilled water to bring the final dilution of complement to 1:10. Alternatively, eight volumes of serum are mixed with one volume of the solution and one volume of saturated sodium chloride solution. Guinea pig serum should be absorbed twice with sheep erythrocytes to remove the natural hemolytic antibody. For this purpose, 3 ml of packed washed sheep erythrocytes are used per 100 ml of an ice-cold guinea pig serum and held at 0° for 10 minutes and then centrifuged.

Maximum hemolytic activity of complement is at a pH value close to 6.8 (Ibe and Wardlaw, 1964) although the reaction in which the $EAC'_{1,4,2}$ is lyzed by C'_3 at 37° is scarcely affected by pH over the range 6.0 to 8.2. Adsorption of complement by antigen-antibody precipitates increases steadily as the pH rises from 6.15 to 8.5 but beyond pH 8.5 the complement itself is unstable. A fourfold increase in the sensitivity of the complement fixation test is obtained by raising the pH from 7.0 to 8.3.

4. The Diluent

The complement fixation test and its outcome are considerably influenced by the pH value and the composition of a diluent. Calcium is specifically required for the fixation of complement. Magnesium ions exert an enhancing influence on the lysis of sheep erythrocytes; it can be replaced by Co^{++} or Ni^{++} (Cernovodeanu and Henri, 1906; Levine et al., 1953).

An adequate diluent must not only maintain the required pH level but also enhance the sensitivity of the test. The buffered diluents of Wallace et al. (1950) Mayer et al. (1948), or Osler et al. (1952) are recommended. A stock solution of Wallace's diluent is prepared by dissolving 4.60 g of 5,5-diethyl barbituric acid in 500 ml of hot distilled water, and adding 3.0 g of sodium 5,5-diethyl barbiturate, 83.8 g of sodium chloride, 2.52 g of $NaHCO_3$, 0.2 g of $CaCl_2 \cdot 2H_2O$, and 1.0 g of $MgCl_2 \cdot 6H_2O$. The volume is made up to 2000 ml with distilled water prior to the test, and adjusted to pH 7.3 to 7.4.

The Mayer et al. buffer solution contains 42.5 g of sodium chloride, 2.875 g of 5,5-diethyl barbituric acid, 1875 g of sodium 5,5-diethyl barbiturate, dissolved in 900 ml of distilled water, mixed with 2.5 ml of a stock solution containing 1.0 M $MgCl_2$ and 0.3 M $CaCl_2$, and made up with distilled water to exactly 1000 ml. This diluent can be modified by adding an equal volume of 0.002% gelatin solution, which reduces the deterioration of complement and retards the spontaneous hemolysis (Stein and van Ngu, 1950). A colloidal solution of gelatin is made by dissolving 0.20 g of Bacto gelatin in 100 ml of boiling distilled water. The boiling solution is mixed with 200 ml of a starch solution, and made up to 1000 ml with distilled water.

Osler's et al. (1952) diluent consists of an isotonic veronal buffer (pH 7.4-7.8) containing 0.0005 M $MgCl_2 \cdot$ 0.00015 M $CaCl_2$, and 0.1% serum albumin.

III. TECHNIQUES OF THE COMPLEMENT FIXATION TEST

A great variety of qualitative and quantitative complement fixation techniques has been devised. Qualitative tests provide approximate data, whereas quantitative techniques of the complement fixation test permit a more accurate determination of the immunological potency of antigens or antisera. Quantitative complement fixation techniques can be based on one of these two principles:

1. The fixation or absorption of complement is regarded as a direct linear function of the amount of immune complex. This linearity can be attained by adjusting the amount of antigen to give maximum fixation while providing enough complement, in added graded amounts, to leave approximately one 50% unit of nonadsorbed complement. The titer is determined by extrapolation of the linear plot of complement versus the serum and expressed by the number of $C'H_{50}$ units which should be added to leave approximately one $C'H_{50}$ unit free in solution containing 0.05 ml of antiserum (Wadsworth et al., 1938).

2. The amount of complement absorbed in the presence of each quantity of the tested serum is determined. A constant amount of complement is employed with a serially diluted serum and an optimum dose of the antigen. At the end of the test, complement is plotted versus serum, and the titer is expressed as the reciprocal amount of serum required to fix 50 units from the 100 units of complement initially present (Mayer et al., 1948).

Both patterns of quantitative complement fixation test apply not only to the conditions when the amount of antigen is kept constant versus a series of serum dilutions but also to the reverse experimental conditions, in which the amounts of antiserum remain constant and dilutions of the antigen vary.

Complement fixation tests, in which the results are computed by plotting and extrapolation, provide the most accurate data. However, they may be found too complicated or time consuming for investigations involving large series of tests. In these cases, simplified quantitative techniques, and particularly those employing colorimetric estimation of the 50% hemolysis as end point, often bring satisfactory and comparable results. These tests are usually based on the second principle indicated above. The titer in these techniques is expressed by the reciprocal amount of antigen (in the presence of constant dose of antiserum), or by reciprocal amount of serum (if the antigen is employed in a constant dilution), by which enough complement is fixed to cause 50% or complete inhibition of hemolysis. The exact amount of antigen or serum, by which the titer should be expressed, is more practically substituted by the final dilution of antigen or serum in the end-point tubes. Microtechniques of complement fixation use minute amounts of constituents; and some procedures of the test are more specifically devised for certain microorganisms or antibodies. The large variety of complement fixation techniques can be divided into the following groups:

1. Qualitative tests; for example, the method of Torrey (1940) or Kolmer (1942).

2. Quantitative colorimetric methods, for example, techniques by Wadsworth et al. (1938), Mayer et al. (1948), Stein and van Ngu (1950), Osler et al. (1952), De Almeida (1956), Rapport and Graf (1957), and Wasserman and Levine (1960).

3. Simplified quantitative methods, for example, techniques by Casals and Palacios (1941), Kolmer et al. (1941), Brand (1955), and Kwapinski (1960).

4. Quantitative microtechniques, by Fulton and Dumbell (1949), Pike et al. (1954), and Takatsy (1955).

5. Individual techniques, devised for studies on: (a) animal viruses (Howitt, 1937; Hummeler, 1957) and serological diagnosis of viral infections (McKee et al., 1940; Blair, 1944; Svedmyr et al., 1944; Florman,

1945; Rice, 1947; Casals, 1949; Henle et al., 1947; Bedson et al., 1949; Wenner et al., 1950; Schlesinger et al., 1956), (b) bacteriophages (Rountree, 1951; Lanni and Lanni, 1953; Lanni, 1954), (c) rickettsiae and the diagnosis of rickettsioses (Castañeda, 1942; Plotz and Wertman, 1942; Plotz, 1943; Bengston, 1944; Varley and Weedon, 1945; Van der Scheer et al., 1947; Lennette et al., 1949), (d) bacteria (Thomson et al., 1935; Mayer and Eddie, 1948), (e) microfungi (Salvin, 1947; Tenenberg and Howell, 1948), and (f) isolated antigens and their antibodies (Pittman and Goodner, 1935; Kolmer et al., 1941; Chen et al., 1952; Kwapinski, 1960).

6. Indirect complement fixation method, for example, the techniques by Ciuca (1929), Hilleman et al. (1951), Rice and Brooksby (1953), and Rice and McKercher (1954).

Principles and rules of complement fixation test are observed in all techniques. However, technical details, such as concentrations of test components and time and temperature of incubation, may differ in various procedures of this test.

1. The concentration of the sheep erythrocyte suspension may vary between 2 and 5%, as shown in Table 60.

Table 60. Concentration of Sheep Erythrocytes in CFT

Concentration of Erythrocytes (%)	Authors
2	Castañeda (1936)
2.5	Howitt (1937), Henle et al. (1948), Rapport and Graf (1957)
3	Lush and Burnet (1937), Casals and Palacios (1941), Mikulaszek and Kwapinski (1954)
4	Witebsky et al. (1955)
5	Pittman and Goodner (1935)

2. The amount of the anti-RBC serum (hemolytic serum) used to sensitize erythrocytes can range from 2 to 5 minimal hemolytic doses (MHD); for example,

2 MHD (Witebsky et al., 1955).
$2\frac{1}{4}$ MHD (Howitt, 1937).
3 MHD (Casals and Palacios, 1941).
4 MHD (Kwapinski, 1960).
5 MHD (Lush and Burnet, 1937).

If the amount of hemolytic serum used for the erythrocyte sensitization is too small, no hemolysis in the presence of complement occurs. However, the hemolysis can also be retarded by an excess of the anti-RBC serum (the Neisser and Wechsberg phenomenon).

3. The amount of complement may vary from 1.25 to 2 MHD, as listed in Table 61.

Table 61. Amounts of Complement Used in CFT

MHD of Complement	Authors
1.25	Kwapinski, 1960
1.30	Van der Scheer et al. 1947
1.50	Henle et al., 1948; Seal, 1953; Portnoy and Magnuson, 1955; Kwapinski, 1960
1.75	Kwapinski, 1960
2.00	Pittman and Goodner, 1935; Castañeda, 1936; Howitt, 1937; Casals and Palacios, 1941; Plotz, 1943; Van der Scheer et al., 1947

4. The volume of reactants may vary between 0.1 and 1.0 ml, as examplified in Table 62.

Table 62. Volumes of Reactants Used in CFT

Volume (ml)	Authors
0.1	Castañeda, 1936; Lush and Burnet, 1937; Witebsky et al., 1955; Varley and Weedon, 1945; Rice, 1948; Hummeler, 1957
0.2	Aikawa and Miklejohn, 1949; Kwapinski
0.25	Casals and Palacios, 1941; Plotz, 1943; Seal, 1953
0.5	Pittman and Goodner, 1935
0.2 to 0.4 and 1.0	Brooksby, 1952

Time and temperature of the first incubation of samples may vary from 30 to 90 minutes at 37°, 2 hours at 20°, and 2 to 24 hours at 2 to 4°. In some microtests, the temperature of 50° provides more sensitive conditions than a lower temperature. More complement is often fixed at 2° overnight than at 37° in 1 to 2 hours, especially by cross-reacting antigen and antibody systems. The reincubation time after the addition of sensitized red-blood cells is usually 15 to 60 minutes at 37°. However, the reincubation of weak serological systems at 30° for 1 to 3 hours contributes to higher titers (Leon et al., 1955). The hemolytic activity of complement declines with the increase of pH, but it is enhanced under the influence of Mg^{++} at optimal concentration of about 0.0005 M (Cernovodeanu and Henri, 1906; Levine et al., 1953).

The $C'H_{50}$ unit of complement is defined as the amount, in milliliters of a fresh guinea pig serum, which lyzes 2.5×10^6 optimally sensitized erythrocytes out of a total of 5×10^8 cells, in the presence of optimal calcium and magnesium at an ionic strength of 0.147, in 1 hour's incubation at 37°, in a total volume of 7.5 ml (Mayer, 1961).

IV. GENERAL PATTERN OF THE COMPLEMENT FIXATION TEST

The whole procedure of adjustment of constituents of the complement fixation test is divided into five steps:

1. Preparation of the erythrocyte suspension.
2. Determination of hemolytic unit of the anti-RBC serum and the sensitization of erythrocytes.
3. Determination of hemolytic unit of complement.
4. Examination of the anticomplementary qualities of antiserum or antigen.
5. The complement fixation test proper.

In the first part of this chapter, a general pattern of the complement fixation method is described, whereas details of selected techniques are presented in the second part.

1. Preparation of the Erythrocyte Suspension

Suspensions of sheep erythrocytes, made in terms of the volume of packed red blood cells, are used in most of the complement fixation techniques. A 3% red blood cell suspension is prepared in the following manner: a 3-ml sample of erythrocytes is washed in buffered saline, sedimented by centrifugation at $500 \times$ g, and suspended in 97 ml of buffered saline or another diluent. Such a suspension is only roughly and conventionally regarded as 3%, but this is sufficient for qualitative tests and also for some quantitative techniques.

More accurate studies require a standardized concentration of red blood cells, determined by a chamber counting or spectrophotometrically.

A standard suspension of erythrocytes is prepared in the following manner: five different lots of sheep red blood cells are centrifuged, and the sediments are washed three times with a diluent, then packed at $1085 \times$ g in precisely 10 minutes. An approximately 3, 4, or 5% suspension (depending on the concentration required for the test proper) is made by volume from each sediment. The number of erythrocytes per milliliter should be determined by a chamber counting under a microscope, and all the specimens are adjusted to an average concentration, for example, 6.7×10^8 cells/ml in case of a 3% erythrocyte suspension. The concentration of erythrocytes can also be standardized according to the optical densities of lyzates. For this purpose, several 4-ml samples of the cell suspension are hemolyzed by rapid freezing and thawing, three times, or by adding 0.1% solution of anhydrous sodium carbonate or a minute drop of saponine. The hemolyzates are then diluted with distilled water in the proportion of 1:5, 1:10, 1:15, 1:20, and 1:30, and optical densities are measured in the photocolorimeter. Figures corresponding to the optical densities are plotted against the dilution of samples, and a calibration curve is drawn. The concentration of an unknown suspension of erythrocytes to be used in a complement fixation test is adjusted by referring to the optical density of hemolyzed samples of this suspension to the calibration curve and readjusting the concentration of erythrocytes accordingly. To prepare a more concentrated cell suspension from one too highly diluted, the red blood cells should be centrifuged and resuspended in a smaller volume of diluent according to the equation:

$$V_2 = V_1 \times \frac{OD}{0.453}$$

where V_1 and V_2 are the original and final volumes of erythrocyte suspensions, respectively, and OD is the original optical density of suspension.

By a simplified procedure, 1 ml of an approximately 5% erythrocyte suspension is lyzed with precisely 14 ml of 0.1% aqueous solution of anhydrous sodium carbonate, and optical density of the clear lyzate is determined in the spectrophotometer with a 1-cm cuvette, at a wavelength of 541 nm. The optical density (OD) of 0.7 corresponds approximately to 1×10^9 erythrocytes/ml of the erythrocyte suspension. If the optical density of lyzate prepared from a given erythrocyte suspension is greater than the standardization value of 0.7 ± 0.005, it must be adjusted by dilution, according to the following formula:

$$V_f = \frac{Vi \times OD}{0.7}$$

where OD is the optical density of the lyzate, Vi the aliquot of the approximate 5% red cell suspension, and V_f is the final volume, to which it should be adjusted with a diluent.

2. Determination of Hemolytic Unit of Anti-RBC Serum

The objective of this assay is to establish the minimum amount of antisheep RBC (hemolytic antiserum) which in the presence of a constant dose of complement, under standard experimental conditions, brings about the lysis of an amount of sheep red blood cells. The MHD (minimal hemolytic dose) of an antisheep RBC serum is determined by setting a double series of dilutions of a rabbit hemlytic serum, supplemented with two volumes of a buffered diluent (to replace the antigen and antiserum solutions employed in the final test) and with a constant dose of the diluted complement. After an incubation at 37° for 30 to 60 minutes, a volume of a red blood cell suspension is added, and the mixtures are reincubated for 15 to 30 minutes. The volume and concentration of each reactant and the incubation time are adjusted in accordance with the requirements of individual techniques.

The titer of the anti-RBC hemolysin is estimated in accordance with the end point of the 100% or preferably 50% hemolysis. In the first case, the last tube in a series of the anti-RBC serum dilutions showing complete hemolysis is taken as end point, and the amount of nondiluted antiserum in this tube represents the effective dose or 1 MHD of hemolysin. From this dose, the amount of anti-RBC serum required to sensitize a given volume of erythrocyte suspension is calculated. By a more accurate procedure, densities of the supernatants obtained after the centrifugation of all reaction mixtures are estimated against a reference sample of 100% hemolysis. The data are plotted against the corresponding amounts of the antiserum. The hemolysis percentage ($\%H$) is calculated according to the following formula:

$$\%H = \frac{OD}{OD_{H100}} \times 100$$

where OD and OD_{H100} are optical densities of a supernatant and of the 100% hemolysis reference sample, respectively.

From these data, the optimum amount of the anti-RBC hemolysin is calculated as the amount which has produced the 50% hemolysis in the presence of one $C'H_{50}$ unit of complement. This unit should be previously determined with the optimum amount of a reference anti-RBC hemolysin (Bier et al., 1952). Of two methods for titration of anti-RBC hemolysin, selected for presentation, Kwapinski's (1965) technique is shown diagrammatically (Table 72). In Van der Sheer's et al. (1947) method, an anti-RBC hemolytic serum to be tested is diluted serially in 0.2-ml volumes; a buffered saline solution is added to each tube in 0.4-ml amounts, followed by 0.2 ml of a fresh guinea pig serum diluted 1:10, and 0.2 ml of 6% suspension of washed sheep red blood cells. After an incubation at 37° for 30 minutes, the highest dilution of the antiserum showing complete hemolysis is selected as one hemolytic unit.

The sensitization of erythrocytes for the hemolysis in the presence of complement can be conducted in two ways. First, a desired dose of an anti-RBC serum is added to a suspension of red blood cells, in 50- to 200-ml volume, and incubated at 37° for 10 to 30 minutes before use. Alternatively, equal volumes, for example, 0.2 to 0.25 ml of the diluted anti-RBC hemolysin, and an erythrocyte suspension, are added separately to the whole series of preincubated mixtures of the antigen, antiserum, and complement. The erythrocyte concentration can vary from 2 to 5%, and the sensitizing dose of anti-RBC hemolytic serum may range from 2 to 5 MHD, subject to the individual CF technique.

The amount of undiluted anti-RBC hemolysin (X) required to sensitize a given volume of erythrocyte suspension (a) may be calculated from the following formula:

$$X = \frac{a \times c \times u}{10t}$$

where a = volume of the erythrocyte suspension required

c = the dilution coefficient representing relation of the amount of diluted antierythrocyte serum to the total volume of fluids

t = titer of the anti-RBC serum, represented by the factor of its effective dilution at the end point (e.g., 10,000 or 6000)

u = number of MHD units of the anti-RBC hemolysin to be employed for erythrocyte sensitization.

3. *Determination of Hemolytic Unit of Complement.*

The dose of a guinea pig serum capable of lyzing all, or a portion of red blood cells, in the presence of a constant amount of the hemolytic antiserum and of one component of the nonhemolytic system used in the test, is determined by titration. For this purpose, a series of progressing dilutions of a guinea pig serum is mixed with a double volume of the diluent, substituting the antigen and antiserum solutions in the test proper, or with one volume of a normal rabbit serum diluted 1:20 and one volume of the diluent. The samples are supplemented with a volume of the red blood cells suspension sensitized with the anti-RBC serum, or with a solution of hemolytic serum and a suspension of red cells added separately. After an incubation time ranging from 15 to 60 minutes, according to individual technique, the 100 to 50% hemolysis end point is determined. The titer is read in terms of the actual dilution of complement in the end point tube.

Three procedures for the complement titration are presented here in some detail. By Rice and Boulanger's (1952) method, the 100% hemolysis end point is determined, whereas by Bier's et al. (1952), and the modified Kwapinski's (p. 494) method, the 50% hemolysis end point is determined.

The Rice and Boulanger Technique of the Complement Titration. Ten different amounts of complement, 0.10, 0.09, 0.08, 0.07, 0.06, 0.05, 0.04, 0.03, 0.02, and 0.01 ml of undiluted or of a 1.2 or 1.5 dilution of guinea pig serum, are made up to 0.3 ml with 0.85% sodium chloride, and set up in duplicate. To each tube, a 0.2-ml volume of a mixture of equal parts of 3% suspension of rabbit red blood cells and a 1:18 solution of a homologous sheep antiserum is then added. The mixtures are incubated in a water bath at 37° for 60 minutes. The last tube in the series showing complete hemolysis is taken as end point.

Kwapinski's Method for Complement Titration. This assay is carried out as presented diagrammatically in Table 73. After the last incubation, the tubes are immediately centrifuged in a refrigerated centrifuge (Fig. 63), at $350 \times g$ for 5 minutes. The supernatant fluids are withdrawn, and the absorbancy is determined at 413 nm. The percentage of hemolysis corresponding to the absorbancy of each supernatant fluid is read from a standard graph (Fig. 64), constructed for different amounts of hemoglobin or erythrocyte-lysates. The lysates are made by exposing a suspension of 10^3/ml sheep erythrocytes sensitized with 5 MHD of an antierythrocyte serum, to different amounts of complement, as in Table 72. The data averaged from testing 20 different complement sources have been used to construct the standard graph. The tested supernatant fluid the absorbancy of which corresponds most closely to the 50% hemolysis value is selected as an end point for a complement titration. The dilution (and

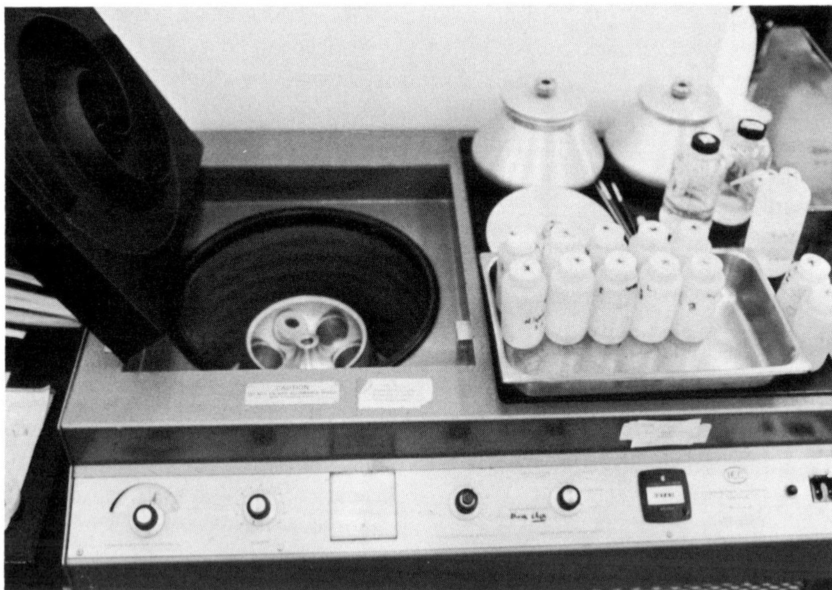

Figure 63.   A semiautomatic refrigerated centrifuge.

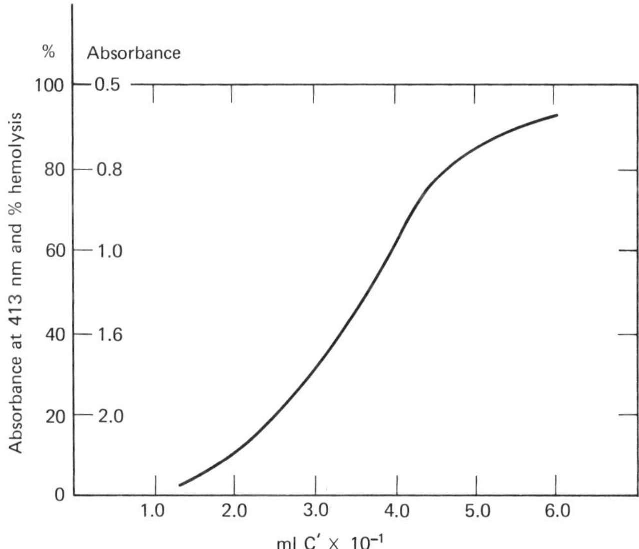

Figure 64. Determination of the C′H$_{50}$ dose of complement by the spectrophotometric measurement of the absorbance at 413 mm.

amount) of complement in the end point tube is noted as one 50% hemolytic unit (C′H$_{50}$) of the complement source.

Bier's et al. Method for Complement Titration. In this procedure, 2 ml of an adequate dilution of a guinea pig serum containing complement are mixed in the cold with 2 ml of saline and 1 ml of the erythrocyte antiserum-sensitized erythrocyte. The mixtures are incubated for 45 minutes, at 36 to 37° in a water bath; 2.5 ml of saline are added to each tube, which are centrifuged at 300 × g for 15 minutes. The percentage of hemolysis in the supernatants is determined spectrophotometrically at 550-nm wavelength, and the complement activity is expressed in terms of 50% units. One 50% unit (C′$_{50}$) is the amount of complement, by which approximately 50% of the red blood cells have been lyzed in a tube, under standard experimental conditions. This amount of complement may be read from a curve which is drawn from plotting percentages of the hemolysis corresponding quantities of the complement tested.

The amount of complement to be employed in the complement-fixation test must exceed 1 MHU or two C′H$_{50}$ units to overcome a nonspecific absorption of a certain amount of complement by the noncombined particles of the antigen or antiserum in the final test. The amount of the complement to be used varies between 1.25 and 2 MHU units or 4 to 5 C′H$_{50}$

units, depending on the species of origin of antibodies and complement, and above all on the size and physicochemical state of antigen particles and the antigen-antibody complexes. The complement is most powerfully fixed by particles large enough to cause an opalescence, but not visible to the naked eye.

More purified and less polymerized substances used an antigens in the test require a smaller amount of complement than crude extracts or more polymerized compounds. For example, 2 MHU or $5C'H_{50}$ must be used in a test with bacterial cells or with lecithin-cardiolipin emulsions, whereas only 1.25 or 1.50 MHU ($3C'H_{50}$) are needed for purified polysaccharide fractions. Based on a large series of immunochemical studies (Kwapinski, (1965), the following average amounts of complement are recommended: 1.25 MHU ($3C'H_{50}$) for polysaccharide fractions, 1.50 MHU ($4C'H_{50}$) for nucleoproteins, and 1.75 MHU ($5C'H_{50}$) for phospholipids, if the test is conducted at $37°$. If the test is set out at $2°$, the amounts of complement should be increased by one fifth in each case, since an overnight incubation in the cold causes a loss of about one fifth of the complement activity. A long incubation at a low temperature of an immune system containing complement often increases the sensitivity of a test without affecting its specificity.

4. *The Testing of Anticomplementary Properties of Antisera or Antigens*

Certain antisera or antigens incubated with a complement source absorb an amount of complement sufficient to inhibit immune lysis of sensitized erythrocytes. This nonspecific sorbing action of some antigen- or antiserum preparation depends greatly on the presence of lipids which produce aggregation and a change in the dispersion of other substances. This leads to a greater absorption of complement. The same phenomenon may be caused by a denaturation of serum globulins. Old or contaminated sera, or the sera possessing large concentrations of sterols, are regularly anticomplementary. The blood of animals recently fed often contains a large percentage of lipids; thus it is advisable to take blood samples long before feeding the animals. The anticomplementary action can also be induced by the presence of soaps, acid, alkali, oxalate, and by heating.

Anticomplementary sera were found to possess an extra component K, which migrates between β and γ-globulins in the electric field (Olhagen, 1949). The isolated, relatively thermostable anticomplementary pseudoglobulin has the molecular weight of about 170,000.

The anticomplementary substances may often be removed from antigens or sera by a careful extraction of lipids, by precipitation of the anticomplementary protein fraction with 8 volumes of 0.03% sodium chloride, or by absorption of serum with a delipidized mouse liver powder (Rapp et al.,

1955). Alternatively, the serum or antigen must be diluted above the non-specific inhibiting level. The nonspecific level is determined by titration of a serum in the absence of the antigen or of the antigen in the absence of antiserum, depending on whether the activity of the antigen or the antiserum is estimated in the final test. As another alternative, the amount of complement should be increased to satisfy the anticomplementary action.

Anticomplementary properties of an antigen can be examined in the following manner. A series of antigen dilutions, in duplicate, is added to a volume of buffered saline or to a normal, nonanticomplementary, inactivated rabbit serum diluted 1:10, supplemented by a constant volume of a guinea pig serum diluted to contain an adequate amount of complement. After 60 minutes of incubation at 37° in a water bath, the sensitized red blood cells are added to the tubes, and the mixtures are reincubated for 50 to 60 minutes. The end point is denoted by the tube showing a 50% or complete hemolysis, estimated by a simple comparison with a color standard, or spectrophotometrically. In the latter case, the tube contents are centrifuged, and supernatants are diluted 1:10 in a saline solution. The supernatant withdrawn from a control tube, containing saline instead of antigen solution, is used as zero hemolysis blank (Walton et al., 1957). The difference between the optical densities of each test dilution and that of the control tube of 100% hemolysis is expressed as percentage of the control reading. This represents the percentage inhibition of hemolysis shown at each concentration of the test substance. The antigen dilution in that tube is noted, and a twice higher dilution is employed in the test proper.

Certain antigen preparations, and especially some phosphatides, are hemolytic in low dilutions. This property is detectable by the test described above. If a preparation shows hemolytic activity in a dilution higher than 1:1000, it may prove unsuitable for the complement fixation test.

Anticomplementary properties of an antiserum are examined in the following manner. To a series of dilutions of an inactivated antiserum, ranging from 1:5 to 1:160, a volume of buffered saline is added to substitute antigen solution in the test proper, together with a constant volume of diluted guinea pig serum, containing an appropriate amount of complement. After the incubation at 37° for 60 minutes, the sensitized red blood cells, or a solution of anti-RBC hemolytic serum and an erythrocyte suspension are added, and the mixtures are reincubated for 50 to 60 minutes. The first tube in the series, showing a 50% or complete hemolysis is denoted as the end point. Alternatively, the amount of antiserum should be employed which contains a known amount of four combining units, determined in the presence of a known antigen. The combining unit is the amount of antibody which, when combined with its homologous antigen, fixes complement.

V. PROCEDURES FOR COMPLEMENT FIXATION TEST PROPER

The complement fixation test can be performed as either a qualitative or a quantitative assay. In the first instance, the activity of serum in the presence of an optimal concentration of the antigen is examined. In the quantitative test, immunologic potency of either the antigen or the antiserum is determined in the presence of constant or varying amounts of the other component of "the nonhemolytic system." The remaining constituents of the complement fixation test, that is, complement, erythrocyte antiserum, and red blood cells are added in the predetermined amounts. The sensitivity of the test may be increased by employing sera previously adsorbed with sheep erythrocytes to remove the natural antisheep hemolysins. A brief review of recommended techniques of complement fixation test is given below.

1. Qualitative Test

Techniques designed by Torrey (1940), Kolmer (1942), and Panton and Marrack (1945) are modifications of the routine Wassermann et al. (1906) test. These methods are as useful for diagnostic immunology as the more recent technique of Aprile et al. (1965), and the CDC standard complement fixation method.

i. *The Routine Test by Panton and Marrack (1945).* This is set up as shown in Table 63. Sensitized cells consist of equal parts of 5% sheep red blood cells and 0.5% buffered saline solution of a hemolytic serum. The test is regarded positive straightaway if a complete complement fixation (the hemolysis inhibition) is found in tubes 1 and 2 and a complete hemolysis in tube 3. If only a partial inhibition of hemolysis is observed, the tubes should be centrifuged and the supernatants compared with five standards made from control tubes which represent 100% hemolysis.

Table 63.   The Schedule for Panton and Marrack's Complement Fixation Test

Tube Number	Serum (ml)	Saline (ml)	Complement (3 MHD in 0.5 ml)	Antigen (ml)	Incubation time at 37° (minutes)	Sensitized red cells (ml)	Incubation time at 37° (minutes)
1	0.1	0.4	0.5	0.5	40	1.0	20
2	0.1	0.2	0.7	0.5	40	1.0	20
3	0.2	0.8	0.5	0	40	1.0	20

Standards are prepared by mixing 0.2, 0.4, 0.6, and 0.8 ml of the control supernatants with 0.8, 0.6, 0.4, and 0.2 ml of distilled water, respectively, obtaining standards of 20, 40, 60, and 80% hemolysis, or 80, 60, 40, and 20% fixation.

Table 64. A Schedule for the Torrey Complement Fixation Test

Tube Number	1	2	3	Control Tubes 4	5	6	7
Patient's serum (ml)	0.01	0.02	0.02	—	—	—	—
Antigen suspension (ml)	0.10	0.10	—	0.10	0.10	0.10	0.10
A known positive serum (ml)	—	—	—	—	0.02	—	—
A known negative serum (ml)	—	—	—	—	—	0.02	—
Pooled sera (ml)	—	—	—	—	—	—	0.02
Saline solution (ml)	0.19	0.18	0.28	0.20	0.18	0.18	0.18

Incubation at 37° for 35 minutes

Sensitized sheep erythrocytes (ml)	0.20	0.20	0.20	0.20	0.20	0.20	0.20

ii. *Torrey's Technique of the Qualitative Complement Fixation Test.* This is shown diagrammatically in Table 64. After the addition of sensitized sheep red cells and reincubation for 25 minutes at 37°, all the tubes, except those showing complete hemolysis, are centrifuged at low speed, and the degree of hemolysis and the amount of sedimented cells are noted. Results are evaluated as follows:

4+ if no hemolysis observed with 0.01 and 0.02 ml of patient's serum.

3+ if no hemolysis with 0.02 and a trace of hemolysis with 0.01 ml patient's serum.

2+ if a trace of hemolysis in the first and about 50% hemolysis in the second tube.

+ if about 50% hemolysis observed in the first and about 75% in the second tube.

iii. *Aprile's et al. (1965) Complement Fixation Technique.* The diluent used for the test is an 0.084 *M* NaCl barbital buffer, which due to the decreased molarity enhances the sensitivity of complement fixation test more than three times. The test is set up in 13 × 100 mm optically matched tubes. The test mixtures consist of 2.5 ml antigen dilution, 0.1 ml antiserum dilution, and 0.1 ml of complement dilution containing 4 to 5 HU_{50}. The mixtures are incubated at 5° for 18 hours and supplemented with 0.3 ml of 3% sheep red blood cells sensitized with two minimal hemolytic units of an antisheep erythrocyte serum. The mixtures are reincubated at 37° for 30 minutes. The tubes are then centrifuged, and the optical densities of supernatants are determined in a Coleman colorimeter with a green filter. Appropriate controls are included with each series of tests to provide checks for the potency and stability of complement and anticomplementary effect of antigen and antiserum. The complement-fixing activity of an antigen may be expressed in CF units per milliliter. (One CF unit is contained in such a volume of the antigen which when mixed with a suitable constant level of antiserum has reduced the hemolytic activity of the added complement to give 50% hemolysis.)

Sensitization of erythrocytes is accomplished by the incubation of a 6% suspension of washed sheep red blood cells mixed with an equal volume of a hemolytic antibody, diluted to provide $2HU_{100}$.

iv. *Standard Method of Complement Fixation.* The 50% end point complement fixation methods, recommended by the microbiologic diagnostic unit of Communicable Disease Center, is applied as follows: serum dilutions are made in 0.25-ml volume with barbital-buffered saline, pH 7.4. To each serum dilution, a standard concentration of antigen in 0.25 ml volume is added and followed by 0.5 ml of complement dilution containing five 50% hemolytic units. The mixtures are incubated from 15 to 18 hours at 5°. To each tube, 0.5 ml of sensitized 2% sheep erythrocytes are added and the mixtures are incubated at 37° for 30 minutes. The titers are recorded as the highest dilution of serum giving 3+ or 4+ reaction.

v. *A Three-Stage Method of Complement Fixation.* The standard, two-stage complement fixation test is conducted in the conditions in which antigen and antibody interact in the presence of complement, which sometimes leads to anticomplementary or procomplementary effects of antigen or antiserum thus creating difficulties in interpretation of results. Antisera absorbed with an antigen frequently become so anticomplementary that residual antibody content cannot be determined by an ordinary complement fixation test. The three-stage complement fixation technique (Rapp et al., 1965) obliviate these difficulties since the antigen and antiserum are incubated in the absence of complement, the aggregates are collected by centrifugation, washed, and then resuspended in a standard amount of complement. The modified, three-stage complement fixation test is performed as follows:

First Stage. The antisera, clarified by centrifugation at a minimum speed of $800 \times g$ for about 20 minutes, are diluted serially and added in equal volumes to different dilutions of an antigen. Controls contain antigen with a diluent, or an antiserum with diluent. This test may be set up with constant concentration of antigen and varying concentrations of antibodies or with a fixed concentration of antiserum and varying concentrations of antigen. The concentration selected for each reagent depends on the results of a checkerboard, or two-dimensional, titration in which the concentrations of both antigen and antiserum are varied.

The reaction mixtures and control tubes are capped and shaken overnight at 4° on an electric shaker so adjusted as to maintain particulate matter in suspension at 4°. The content of all tubes are then centrifuged in the cold at $800 \times g$ for 20 minutes and the supernatant fluid is discarded. Diluent (3 ml) is added to all tubes and to each of three additional test tubes which are to be used for complement titration. The tubes are then centrifuged and the supernatant is removed.

Second Stage. All the tubes, with the exception of three tubes to be used for complement titration, receive complement in such a volume that three $H'C_{50}$ units are present in the fluid remaining in the tubes after the removal of supernatant. One of the complement-titration tubes receives 0.55 ml of diluted complement ($2C'H_{50}$) and 0.18 ml of diluent, and the third tube receives 0.1 ml of diluted complement (one $C'H_{50}$) and 0.37 ml of diluent. The tubes are shaken overnight at 4°.

Third Stage. On the last day, 0.1 ml of sheep erythrocytes sensitized optimally with antierythrocytes serum are added to each tube and the mixtures are incubated at 37° for 1 hour. The degree of hemolysis is determined by visual inspection.

In the three-stage procedure, only the complement adsorbed onto antigen-antibody aggregates and not that due to nonspecific binding of anticomplementary material is measured. Although this technique sometimes gives lower titers than a two-stage technique, the results are more meaningful since anticomplementarity does not interfere. The three-stage procedure is particularly useful for titration of absorbed antiserum where the valid measurements of low level of antibody activity is needed.

2. Quantitative Methods of Complement Fixation

Quantification of the complement fixation may be accomplished in two ways: (a) by a chemical determination of the nitrogen increase following the adsorption of complement by a known quantity of an immune complex (Heidelberger and Mayer, 1942), and (b) by the determination of the amount of complement left free after the completion of a complement fixation reaction.

The latter procedure of the quantitative complement fixation test is used more frequently than the chemical analysis, because of its relative simplicity. The titration methods are based on the quantitative relationships between the degree of hemolysis and the amount of free complement.

Quantitative methods, introduced by Wadsworth et al. (1938) and Maltaner and Maltaner (1939) and developed by Heidelberger and Mayer

(1948), Mayer et al. (1948), Osler and Heidelberger (1948), Stein and Van Ngu (1950), De Almeida et al. (1952), and Wasserman and Levine (1961), depend on the spectrophotometric titration of the residual hemolytic activity of the fixation mixtures, which initially contained a large, constant amount of complement. The sorbing (fixing) potency of a system of antigen and antibody is determined in terms of 50% end point. This is reciprocal to the amount of antiserum or antigen, which in the presence of an optimally reactive dilution of the antigen or antiserum, respectively, fixes half of the $C'H_{50}$ units of complement employed in the test. The $C'H_{50}$ units are calculated from the percentages of the hemolysis either by a graphic method (Wadsworth, 1939) or by applying the conversion factors (Mayer et al., 1946), derived from the von Krogh formula, represented below in three forms:

$$\log x = \log K + \frac{1}{n} \log \left(\frac{y}{1-y} \right),$$

$$x = K \left(\frac{y}{1-y} \right)^{1/n}, \qquad \text{or} \qquad x = \left(\frac{y}{1-y} \right)^{0.2}$$

in which x = the amount, in milliliters, of complement (a diluted guinea pig serum) used in the test

y = the resulting degree of hemolysis or the degree lysis expressed as a fraction of 1; for example, $y = 0.80$ indicates 80% hemolysis

n and K = parametric constants for the test conditions.

The constant K is the 50% unit of complement since at this point $y = 0.5$, and the term $y/1 - y$ equals unity, and therefore $x = K$. The values of x for the range of $y = 0.10$ ot 0.190 are shown in Table 65.

The amount of $C'H_{50}$ (50% units of complement) left after fixation in the tubes containing nonhemolytic system determined at 545 nm is subtracted from the number of units present in the controls containing complement and either an antigen or antiserum. This yields the number of $C'H_{50}$ fixed specifically by the interaction of the antibody with antigen. According to De Almeida et al. (1952), the reaction of complement with the immune complex can be expressed by the formula:

$$\frac{(F - W) \times (C - W)}{W} = K$$

in which C = total amount of complement added

F = the total immune complex present

W = the amount of complement fixed

K = the dissociation constant of the hypothetical reaction.

Table 65. The Conversion Factor Values of $1/n$ in Von Krogh's
Formula, for $1/n = 0.2$ (Wadsworth, 1939)

Hemolysis Degree	Conversion Factor	Percentage Hemolysis	Conversion Factor
0.10	0.644	5	0.62
0.12	0.671	10	0.69
0.14	0.696	15	0.75
0.16	0.718	20	0.79
0.18	0.738	25	0.83
0.20	0.758	30	0.87
0.25	0.803	35	0.89
0.30	0.844	40	0.93
0.35	0.884	45	0.96
0.40	0.912	50	1.00
0.45	0.961	55	1.03
0.50	1.000	60	1.07
0.59	1.041	65	1.10
0.60	1.084	70	1.15
0.65	1.132	75	1.19
0.70	1.185	80	1.25
0.75	1.211	85	1.32
0.80	1.320	90	1.44
0.82	1.354		
0.84	1.393		
0.86	1.438		
0.88	1.490		
0.90	1.550		

If the complement and antigen are added in a constant volume to each tube containing antiserum in varying amounts, the quantitative relationship between the complement fixed and the antiserum can be graphically estimated. The graph shows an almost linear interdependence of the amount of antiserum and complement fixed.

The international reagin unit was estimated by the Expert Committee for Biological Standardization of W.H.O., and is kept in the State Serum Institute in Copenhagen, Denmark. The reagin titer of any test serum can be calculated by comparison with the titer of standard serum set up in parallel according to the formula (Heymann, 1960):

$$U_w = U_a \times \frac{S_a{}^t}{S_w{}^t}$$

where U_w = the value of test serum, in reagin units per milliliter

U_a = actual geometric mean titer of the test serum

$S_a{}^t$ = actual geometric mean titer of the standard serum

$S_w{}^t$ = the value standard serum in reagin units per milliliter.

i. *The Stein and Van Ngu Complement Fixation Technique.* The test is set up in Kahn's tubes of 10-mm inside diameter, standardized by calibration with a solution of hemolyzed sheep erythrocytes.

Titration of the anti-RBC hemolysin is conducted by adding different solutions of an inactivated rabbit antisheep erythrocyte serum to equal amounts of 2% suspension of sheep erythrocytes and exposing these mixtures to constant amounts of complement. The 2% suspension of sheep erythrocytes is prepared by spectrophotometric adjustment of an originally 2.5% suspension to the desired optical density, as follows: a 0.2-ml sample of a roughly 2.5% erythrocyte suspension in buffered saline is mixed with 1.8 ml of distilled water and centrifuged. Optical density (OD) of the supernatant fluid is determined in a spectrophotometer at 550-nm wavelength against distilled water as reference zero. From the reading figure, the amount of diluent (Vd) should be calculated which must be added to adjust a volume (Vo) of erythrocyte suspension to the optical density (OD) = 0.400± 0.01 according to the following formula.

$$Vd = Vo \times \frac{OD - 0.400}{0.400}$$

Seven dilutions of the erythrocyte antiserum (1:500, 1:1000, 1:2000, 1:4000, 1:666, 1:1338, 1:2666) are made, and 1 ml of each solution is slowly added, at 20°, to 1 ml of 2% erythrocyte suspension. A further step of the procedure is presented in Table 66.

The whole set is incubated for 30 minutes at 37°, then centrifuged at 500 × g for 10 minutes, and the optical density of each supernatant fluid is measured in a spectrophotometer at 550 nm, using the supernatant fluid of the last control tube as reference zero. Figures representing optical densities are plotted on a graph against amounts of the erythrocyte antiserum, and the percentage of hemolysis (*%H*) is calculated according to the formula:

$$H\% = \frac{OD}{OD_{H100}} \times 100$$

in which OD is the optical density of the supernatant from an individual tube, and OD_{H100} is the average optical density of the 100% hemolysis reference sample. From these data, the amount of erythrocyte antiserum giving a 50% hemolysis in the presence of a certain amount of complement is calculated. The titration of complement is set up as shown in Table 67.

The samples are incubated for 30 minutes at 37°, and centrifuged at 500 × g for 10 minutes. Optical densities of the supernatant fluids are

Table 66.   Titration of the RBC-Antiserum by the Stein and Van Ngu Technique

First Row	1	2	3	Tubes 4	5	6	7
Complement 1:800 (ml)	1.2	1.2	1.2	1.2	1.2	1.2	1.2
Erythrocyte sensitized with anti-RBC serum							
Diluted	500	666	1000	1338	2000	2666	4000
ml	0.8	0.8	0.8	0.8	0.8	0.8	0.8
Second row							
Complement 1:600 (ml)	1.2	1.2	1.2	1.2	1.2	1.2	1.2
Erythrocytes sensitized with anti-RBC serum							
Diluted	500	666	1000	1338	2000	2666	4000
ml	0.8	0.8	0.8	0.8	0.8	0.8	0.8
Control rows							
Complement 1:20 (ml)	0.4	0.4	0.4	0.4	0.4	0.4	—
Complement 1:600 (ml)	—	—	—	—	—	—	1.2
Diluent	0.8	0.8	0.8	0.8	0.8	0.8	—
Erythrocytes sensitized with anti-RBC serum							
1:500 (ml)	0.8	0.8	0.8	0.4	0.4	0.4	—
Supernatant of sensitized erythrocytes (ml)	—	—	—	0.4	0.4	0.4	—
Hemolysis percentage	H_{100}				H_{50}		H_0

Table 67. Titration of the Complement in the Stein and Van Ngu Test

Reagent	Tube Number								Ref. H_{100}			Ref. H_{50}		Ref. H_0	
	1	2	3	4	5	6	7	8	9	10	11	12	13	14	15
Complement 1/20 (ml)									0.4	0.4	0.4	0.4	0.4		0.4
Complement 1/200 (ml)	0.2	0.25	0.30	0.35	0.40	0.50	0.55								
Diluent (ml)	1.0	0.95	0.90	0.85	0.80	0.75	0.70	0.65	0.80	0.80	0.80	0.80	0.80	0.80	0.80
Erythrocytes sensitized with an optimal amount of anti-RBC hemolysin	0.80	0.80	0.80	0.80	0.80	0.80	0.80	0.80	0.80	0.80	0.80	0.40	0.40	0.40	0.40
Supernatant of sensitized cells (ml)												0.40	0.40	0.40	

measured using H_0 as reference zero. The percentage of hemolysis ($H\%$) is calculated according to the formula

$$H\% = \frac{OD}{OD_{H100}} \times 100$$

The percentage of hemolysis for each titration placed on abscissa is plotted against an appropriate volume of the complement diluted 1:200 on ordinate, and a straight line is fitted to the plotted points. One and two 50% units of complement in 0.4-ml volume are employed in the antigen titration and in the test proper.

Titration of the antigen is carried out in the following manner. Two series of antigen dilutions in the geometric 1:5 time progression are made in 0.4-ml volumes of a buffered diluent. Each tube of the first row receives 0.4 ml of a solution containing two complement units whereas the other row receives 0.4 ml of a solution containing one complement unit. An inactivated serum diluted 1:100 to 1:800, in 0.4-ml volume, is added to all tubes. The samples are left at 4° overnight then supplemented with 0.8 ml of a mixture of equal parts of 2% red blood cells and the erythrocyte antiserum at its optimum dilution. After a 30-minute incubation at 37°, the contents of tubes are centrifuged at 500 × g for 10 minutes, and optical densities of supernatants are estimated spectrophotometrically at 5400 Å against a reference zero, consisting of 0.4 ml of diluent and 0.4 ml of a solution containing one complement unit. Percentages of hemolysis are assigned to the ordinate and antigen dilutions on the abscissa, and the values for each tube in both rows are plotted. The optimal dilution of the antigen is that giving minimal hemolysis in the neighborhood of the 50% zone. The test proper is set out in two rows, as indicated in Table 68.

Table 68.	The Schedule for the Complement Fixation Test by Stein and Van Ngu

Tube Number	1	2	3	4	5	6	7	8	9	10
Antiserum (0.4 ml)	4	8	16	32	64	128	256	512	1024	2048
Complement, 1 unit (ml)	0.4	0.4	0.4	0.4	0.4	0.4	0.4	0.4	0.4	0.4

The other row is set out in a similar way, with the exception of replacing the antigen solution by 0.4 ml of diluent. All the samples are left at 4° overnight. Then 0.8 ml of a mixture consisting of equal parts of a 2% sheep erythrocyte suspension and an erythrocyte antiserum solution are added to each tube. The tubes are shaken and incubated at 37° for 30 minutes, and centrifuged. Optical densities of supernatants are measured against a reference zero sample containing one complement unit in 0.8 ml of diluent. The percentage of hemolysis is calculated by applying the formula

$$H\% = \frac{\text{OD}}{\text{OD}_{H100}} \times 100$$

The titer can be expressed by an amount of a dilution of the serum showing 50% hemolysis or less. The 100% hemolysis is given by optical densities of supernatants from tubes 9 and 10.

ii. *The Wadsworth et al. (1935) Complement Fixation Test.* Progressive serum dilutions are made in two amounts of 0.05 and 0.02 ml and mixed with 0.1 ml of the antigen solution and 0.1 ml of the complement containing 2 MHD. The mixtures are incubated for 4 hours at 3 to 6°; 0.2 ml of sensitized sheep red blood cells are then added to each tube, and these are incubated for 15 minutes at 37 to 38°. The percentage of hemolysis inhibition in each tube is then determined by comparison with color standards. The reaction is evaluated by the use of this formula:

$$\frac{(IS + A) - C/(IS - C)}{(NS + A) - C/(NS - C)}$$

where $(IS + A)$ and $(NS + A)$ are amounts of complement required to give 50% hemolysis in the presence of an immune serum and an antigen, and of a normal serum and antigen, respectively; C, the amount resulting in this degree of hemolysis, when complement is titrated alone; IS and NS, the amounts giving 50% hemolysis in the presence of immune serum and normal serum alone.

The quotient obtained by the use of this formula is regarded as an index of the specific antibody titer of an immune serum.

iii. *The Mayer et al. Method (1948) of the Complement Fixation Test.* In this test, 2.5-ml volumes of a dilution of antiserum are mixed in the cold with 5.0-ml volumes of a diluted guinea pig serum containing varying amounts of $C'H_{50}$ units of complement, and with 2.5-ml volumes of an antigen solution. After the incubation at 37° for 90 minutes, or at 2 to 4° overnight, the tubes are chilled in the ice water to retard any further fixation of the complement.

Hemolytic activity of the remaining amount of free complement is estimated by testing 3.0, 3.5, and 4.0 ml portions of tenfold dilution of the reaction mixtures with 1.5 ml of sensitized red blood cells, standardized spectrophotometrically. A chilled isotonic buffer is added to make a final volume of 7.5 ml. The tubes are shaken, incubated at 37° for 1 hour, and centrifuged. The amount of hemoglobin in the supernatants is determined spectrophotometrically to estimate the degree of lysis. The hemolytic activity is expressed in terms of the $C'H_{50}$ calculated with the aid of the conversion factors, obtained for $1/n = 0.2$ in the Von Krogh equation (see p. 502).

This test was slightly modified and adjusted to a smaller volume of reactants, by Wasserman and Levine (1961). In this technique (Table 69), 0.1 ml of the diluent, 0.1 ml of antiserum, 0.1 ml of complement, and 0.1 ml of varying concentrations of an antigen are solution placed into a series of 13 × 100-mm test tubes in an ice-water bath. Controls of the antigen, the antibody, and the complement are included. The isotonic veronal buffer by Osler et al. (1952) is used as diluent.

Table 69. A Schedule for Microcomplement Fixation by Wasserman and Levine (1961)

Tube Number	1	2	3	4	5	6	7	8	9	10	11	12
Diluent (ml)	0.3	0.3	0.3	0.3	0.3	0.3	0.3	0.4	0.4	0.5	0.4	0.6
Antiserum (ml)	0.1	0.1	0.1	0.1	0.1	0.1	0.1	0.1				
C' (ml)	0.1	0.1	0.1	0.1	0.1	0.1	0.1	0.1	0.1	0.1	0.2	
Antigen increments (ml)	0.1	0.0	0.1	0.1	0.1	0.1	0.1		0.1			
Incubation at 2 to 4° for 18 hours												
Sensitized erythrocytes (5 × 10⁷/ml) (ml)	0.1	0.1	0.1	0.1	0.1	0.1	0.1	0.1	0.1	0.1	0.1	0.1
Incubation at 37° for 1 hour												

The dilution of complement to be used in the test is estimated by a complement titration under the same conditions as in the test proper; between 1.1 and 1.2 $C'H_{50}$ of complement is employed as determined graphically by plotting volumes of a complement containing serum against the percentage of hemolysis. The quantity of antiserum is chosen for the final test as the amount which, after fixation, is sufficient to yield partial hemolysis on addition of the sensitized erythrocytes.

After the incubation at 2 to 4° for 18 hours, 0.1 ml of the indicator system is added. The indicator contains 5 × 10⁷ erythrocytes sensitized with the anti-RBC hemolysin per milliliter. The total reaction volume is 0.7 ml. The tubes are reincubated at 37° for 60 minutes, and then immersed in an ice bath to stop a further hemolysis, and centrifuged for 10 minutes to separate nonlyzed erythrocytes. The supernatant fluids are decanted and analyzed spectrophotometrically for the presence of hemoglobin at 413 nm. The results of the complement fixation are calculated from a difference in optical densities obtained in the presence of antigen and antibody, when the hemolysis in the C' control is equal to, or less than 90%.

3. Simplified Quantitative Methods

In these techniques, 50 or 100% end point of the hemolysis inhibition is determined either photocolorimetrically (Kwapinski, 1960, 1965) or by the naked eye (Casals and Palacios, 1941; Kolmer et al., 1951; Witebsky et al., 1955). Titers of the antigen or serum are expressed in terms of their actual dilutions in the end point tube. The 50% hemolytic unit of complement designated $C'H_{50}$ is the quantity of a complement-containing serum required for the 50% lysis of a quantity of sensitized erythrocytes. Estimation of the 50% hemolysis as end point has an advantage over the 100% end point since the degree of lysis of the optimally sensitized erythrocytes in the central region of the hemolysis curve is more sensitive to small changes in the amount of complement than near the zone of complete hemolysis. The 100% hemolysis procedure does not provide a sharply defined end point.

i. *The Casals and Palacios (1941) Complement Fixation Technique.* This technique is used for determination of the antibody contents in a serum. Prior to the test proper, complement is titrated in two sets, one in the absence and the other in the presence of an antigen, as shown in Table 70.

Erythrocytes are sensitized by mixing equal volumes of a 3% suspension of sheep red blood cells and a solution of rabbit hemolysin containing 3 MHD/0.25 ml, that is, 12 MHD/ml. The last tube showing complete hemolysis is considered end point, from which the titer of complement can be determined. The test proper is set out by mixing a constant solution of antigen, in 0.25-ml volume, with equal volumes of serial dilutions of antiserum, and with 0.5 ml of a complement solution containing 2 MHD/ml. After an incubation at 37° for 30 minutes or at 20° for 18 hours, a 0.5-volume of sensitized red cells is added, and the mixtures are reincubated for 30 minutes at 37°. The titer is determined by the last dilution of serum showing a 2 plus or better fixation (about 50% hemolysis).

The method of complement fixation test by Witebsky et al. (1955) requires smaller volumes of reagents, that is,

    0.1 ml of serum dilutions
    0.1 ml of the antigen solution
    0.1 ml of the complement solution

The samples are incubated at 4° for 3 hours and at 37° for 1 hour, then 0.2 ml of sensitized red cells is added to each tube and left at 37° until the

Table 70.   The Complement Titration by Casals and Palacios

Preliminary Titration

Tube Number	1	2	3	4	5	6	7	8	9	10
Complement diluted 1:20 (ml)	0.04	0.1	0.15	0.2	0.25	0.3	0.35	0.4	0.45	0.5
Diluent	0.5	0.5	0.5	0.5	0.5	0.5	0.5	0.5	0.5	0.5
3% sheep erythrocytes sensitized with 3 MHD of anti-RBC serum (ml)	0.5	0.5	0.5	0.5	0.5	0.5	0.5	0.5	0.5	0.5

Incubation at 37° for 1 hour

Final Titration

Tube Number	1	2	3	4	5	6	7	8	9	10	Control
Complement (ml)	0.05	0.1	0.15	0.2	0.25	0.3	0.35	0.4	0.45	0.5	0.05
Diluent (ml)	0.70	0.65	0.60	0.55	0.50	0.45	0.40	0.35	0.30	0.25	0.95
Antigen Solution	0.25	0.25	0.25	0.25	0.25	0.25	0.25	0.25	0.25	0.25	—

Incubation at 37° for 30 minutes or 2° for 18 hours

| 3% sensitized sheep erythrocytes (ml) | 0.25 | 0.25 | 0.25 | 0.25 | 0.25 | 0.25 | 0.25 | 0.25 | 0.25 | 0.25 | 0.25 |

Incubation at 37° for 30 minutes

controls are hemolyzed. The test tube in the main row showing no trace of hemolysis denotes end point.

ii. *The Kwapinski (1965) Complement Fixation Technique.* In this method, anti-RBC hemolytic serum titer is determined in terms of 100% hemolytic units, the complement is evaluated preferably by 50% hemolytic units (or by 100% hemolytic units), whereas readings of final complement fixation test are always made by the spectrophotometric determination of 50% hemolysis end point, prior to the calculation of the antigen or antibody titer.

The hemolytic potency of an anti-RBC serum is carried out according to the schedule presented in Table 71.

After the final incubation, the last tube showing complete hemolysis is taken as end point. The titer of the anti-RBC serum is expressed by the dilution factor in the end point tube. The amount of nondiluted immune hemolysis in this tube is equivalent to 1 MHD of anti-RBC serum.

Red blood cells should be sensitized with 4 MHD of the immune hemolysin prior to the titration of complement. The amount of hemolytic serum (x), in milliliters, needed for the sensitization of a certain volume (a) of 3% suspension of sheep erythrocytes is calculated according to the following formula:

$$x = \frac{a \times u}{T}$$

where T = the estimated titer of immune hemolysin
       a = the amount of erythrocyte suspension, to be sensitized
       u = the amount of MHD of the anti-RBC serum to be used for sensitization.

The sensitization of red blood cells is carried out as follows. The amount of diluent required to obtain a certain volume of 3% sensitized erythrocyte suspension and the corresponding amount of packed red cells and anti-RBC serum needed to sensitize a desired amount of 3% red cells are measured separately. The diluent is now divided in two parts, and each part is mixed either with the red cells or with the anti-RBC serum. The anti-RBC serum solution is then slowly added to the erythrocyte suspension and left at 37° for 10 minutes. The titration of the complement is set out as indicated in Table 72.

The last tube in the series showing 50% or complete hemolysis is taken as the end point, and the complement titer is expressed in terms of its original dilution. One $C'H_{100}$ of complement is present in the volume of the guinea pig serum serving as complement's source. The number of hemolytic doses of complement employed in further stages of the test varies between

Table 71.   The Anti-RBC Hemolysin Titration by Kwapinski's Method

Tube Number									Controls	
Anti-RBC serum										
Diluted 1:	1000	2000	3000	4000	5000	6000	7000	8000	1000	
Volume (ml)	0.2	0.2	0.2	0.2	0.2	0.2	0.2	0.2	0.2	—
Complement diluted 1:10 (ml)	0.2	0.2	0.2	0.2	0.2	0.2	0.2	0.2	—	0.2
Diluent (ml)	0.2	0.2	0.2	0.2	0.2	0.2	0.2	0.2	0.4	0.4
				Incubation at 37° for 60 minutes						
3% sheep erythrocytes (ml)	0.4	0.4	0.4	0.4	0.4	0.4	0.4	0.4	0.4	0.4
				Incubation at 37° for 15 minutes						

Table 72. A Schedule for Complement Titration by Kwapinski's Method

Complement	Diluted 1:	10	15	20	30	40	50	Control
	Volume (ml)	0.2	0.2	0.2	0.2	0.2	0.2	—
Normal inactivated rabbit serum diluted 1:10 (ml)		0.2	0.2	0.2	0.2	0.2	0.2	0.2
Wallace's buffered diluent, pH 7.3 (ml)		0.2	0.2	0.2	0.2	0.2	0.2	0.4
Incubation at 37° for 60 minutes or at 2° for 16 hours								
3% erythrocytes sensitized with 4 MHD (ml) of anti-RBC serum		0.4	0.4	0.4	0.4	0.4	0.4	0.4
Incubation at 37° for 15 minutes								

1.25 and $2C'H_{100}$, or between 3 and $5C'H_{50}$, depending on the physico-chemical characteristics of individual antigens (see p. 496).

Prior to the test proper, the anticomplementary activity of antiserum should be estimated in the manner presented diagrammatically in Table 73. The first tube showing complete hemolysis is taken as end point, and a double antiserum dilution of the end point tube is used for the final test.

Table 73. A Schedule for Testing the Anticomplementary Property of Antiserum

Inactivated Antiserum	Diluted 1:	5	10	20	30	40	Control
	Volume (ml)	0.2	0.2	0.2	0.2	0.2	—
Saline buffered at pH 7.0 (ml)		0.2	0.2	0.2	0.2	0.2	0.4
Complement (1,25 to 1,5 $C'H_{100}$) or 3 to 5 $C'H_{50}$		0.2	0.2	0.2	0.2	0.2	0.2
Incubation at 37° for 1 hour or at 2° for 16 hours							
3% erythrocytes (ml) sensitized with 4 MHD of anti-RBC serum		0.4	0.4	0.4	0.4	0.4	0.4
Incubation at 37° for 15 minutes							

The final complement fixation test is set up as indicated in Table 74. After the second incubation at 37° for 15 minutes, the tubes are centrifuged at 350 × *g* for 5 to 10 minutes. The supernatant fluids are collected, diluted with an equal volume of the diluent, and their optical den-

Table 74. The Schedule for Antigen Titration by Kwapinski's Complement Fixation Test

Tube Number	1	2	3	4	5	6	7	8	9	10	Control Tubes		
											A	B	C
Antigen													
Dilution 1:	1000	2000	4000	8000	16000	32000	64000	125000	250000	500000	1000	0	0
ml	0.2	0.2	0.2	0.2	0.2	0.2	0.2	0.2	0.2	0.2	0.2	—	—
Antiserum (1:20) (ml)	0.2	0.2	0.2	0.2	0.2	0.2	0.2	0.2	0.2	0.2	0.	0.2	0
Complement (1.6 to 2.0) $C'H_{100}$ or 3 to 5 $C'H_{50}$	0.2	0.2	0.2	0.2	0.2	0.2	0.2	0.2	0.2	0.2	0.2	0.2	0.2
Buffered saline, pH 7.2 (ml)	0	0	0	0	0	0	0	0	0	0	0.2	0.2	0.4

Incubation at 37° for 1 hour or at 5° for 16 hours

| 3% sheep erythrocytes sensitized with 4 MHD of anti-RBC serum (ml) | 0.4 | 0.4 | 0.4 | 0.4 | 0.4 | 0.4 | 0.4 | 0.4 | 0.4 | 0.4 | 0.4 | 0.4 | 0.4 |

Incubation at 37° for 15 to 30 minutes

sities are measured in a spectrophotometer at 545-nm or, for a greater extinction, at 413-nm wavelength, against a buffered diluent used as reference zero. The data obtained are applied to a graph carrying optical densities of the color standards plotted against percentages of hemolysis; the corresponding percentages of hemolysis are calculated from the curve.

The last supernatant with the hemolysis percentage equal to, or lower than, 50 is taken as end point, and the antigenic activity of the examined preparation is expressed in terms of its final dilution in this tube or preferably in micrograms of dry mass.

iii. *The Two-Dimensional Complement Fixation Test.* The two-dimensional procedure or the "chessboard" (Box) titration is mainly used for determination of the optimal amount of an antigen preparation to be employed for studying a series of sera. In this technique (Hoyle, 1945), progressing dilutions of an antigen preparation, placed vertically, are added to progressing twofold dilutions of antiserum, added in the horizontal direction (Table 75). Complement (5 $C'H_{50}$ or 2 $C'H_{50}$) is added to each tube, including control series of separate antigen and serum solutions. After an incubation time, the highest antigen dilution bringing about the comparatively highest titer of antiserum is recorded. The antigen in this optimal dilution is employed for the series of tests. (In the example shown in Table 75, the antigen dilution to be selected has been encircled.)

Table 75.   The Diagram of Two-Dimensional Complement Fixation Test

Antigen Dilutions 1:

Antiserum Dilutions 1:	5	10	20	40	80	160	320	690	Saline
5	4	4	4	4	4	3	2	1	0
10	4	4	4	4	3	2	1	0	0
20	4	4	4	4	2	1	1	0	0
40	4	4	(4)	3	1	1	0	0	0
80	3	3	3	2	0	0	0	0	0
160	2	1	1	1	0	0	0	0	0
320	0	0	0	0	0	0	0	0	0
0	0	0	0	0	0	0	0	0	0

4. Microtechniques of the Complement Fixation Test

The advantages of microtechniques of the test are the economical use of antigen preparations and antisera, simplification of the test, and a greater speed of diluting antigens and sera. Two techniques by Fulton and Dumbell (1949) and Wasserman and Levine (1961), and the rapid slide-immunocentrifuge complement fixation test (Kwapinski, 1971), are recommended.

The Fulton and Dumbell (1949) Technique of the Complement Fixation Test. The test is carried out on Plexiglass plates, $\frac{1}{4}$-in. thick and 12 in. square, with 100 1-in. squares marked on the surface. Drops of liquids are distributed by means of 19-gauge needles fitted to Wintrobe pipettes. The tips of needles should be slightly lubricated with petroleum jelly, and calibrated to deliver a uniform volume of fluid. Spiral loops devised by Takatsy (1955) for transferring exact amounts of reactants are very useful in preparing dilutions of the serum or antigen directly on plates.

Prior to the test proper, the antigen should be standardized against a homologous antiserum in the following way. Eight complement dilutions and five antigen dilutions are prepared in tubes. Antiserum diluted 1:2 is distributed by drops along six rows of the first eight columns. One drop of each complement dilution is then added to the first three rows in the rectangular direction. The distribution of the complement solution starts in rows 4 to 7 with the third column, and in rows 8 to 12 with the fifth column. Finally, a drop of one of the five antigen dilutions are added to rows 2 to 6, the first row acting as the serum control. After the incubation at 4, 37, or 50° overnight, the hemolytic system is added, consisting of equal parts of a 0.4% sheep erythrocyte suspension and a solution of anti-RBC hemolysin, which has produced maximal sensitization. The plates are reincubated at 37° for 1 or 2 hours, and left at room temperature or in a refrigerator for 1 hour. The antigen concentration required to give a fixation of 1.0 ml of complement is made from a graph, on which antigen dilutions (on abscissa) are plotted against the volume (ml) of complement-log (on ordinates).

The final part of complement fixation is carried out in the following way. Eleven serial dilutions of the serum examined, made in tubes, are distributed by drop, each to one of eleven rows of hollows. The control row receives one drop of the diluent. A series of complement dilutions is then distributed in the rectangle direction. This set is made in duplicate, on two plates. One drop of the antigen solution or suspension in the standardized concentration is added to all rows of one plate, whereas the other row receives one drop of the diluent. The plates are placed in a moist chamber (a box saturated with water vapor from cotton wool left in the bottom). The mixtures are incubated at 4, 37, or 50° overnight, and upon addition of the hemolytic system are reincubated at 37° for 1 or 2 hours, and then left at room temperature or in the refrigerator for 1 hour.

Results are read by placing the sheets flat on a white background with a strong light overhead. The nonhemolyzed red blood cells collect in a central dot. The end point is taken as that square on each sheet which shows half the cells hemolyzed, as judged by the density of the dot. Amounts of complement required for 50% hemolysis in the presence and absence of the antigen are recorded. By subtracting the second value from the first, the amount of complement fixed in the antigen-antibody reaction is obtained. The minimal amount of complement needed to produce 50% hemolysis in the presence of a given volume of the antigen (e.g., 0.05 ml if one drop of antigen has been added) is regarded as unit. The volume in cubic millimeters of the complement fixed is divided by the volume of the antigen solution added to obtain the number of units fixed at each serum dilution.

5. The Slide Centrifuge Complement Fixation Test (Kwapinski, 1972)

1. Incubate for 3 minutes a mixture consisting of 0.1 ml of a test antigen solution, 0.1 ml antiserum, and 0.1 ml of a fresh guinea pig serum, serving as a complement source, diluted 1:5 in PBS.

2. Add 0.2 ml of a 1% suspension of washed sheep red blood cells sensitized with a 4 MHD of an antisheep cell serum, used in a volume dependent on its titer.

3. Spin the mixture at 500 rpm in the cytocentrifuge for 5 minutes.

4. Remove the cellulose strip from the centrifuge and examine it in a fluorescent light through a 4× magnifying glass. The formation of an antigen-antibody complex is indicated by the presence of clumped red blood cells in the middle of the cellulose strip which correspond to the opening in the absorbing paper whereas controls show hemoglobin stains spread in and around the central area (Fig. 65).

6. Special Techniques of the Complement Fixation Test

Although any technique of the complement fixation test presented above can be adapted to a large variety of investigations, including the detection and examination of various antigens and antibodies, sometimes a little rearrangement of the experimented conditions, doses, and volumes of reac-

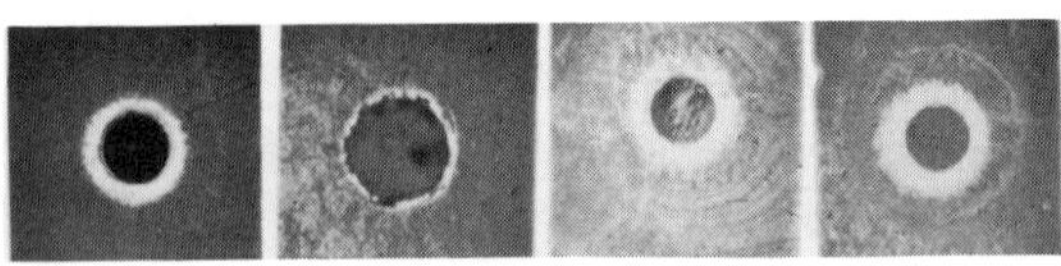

Figure 65. An example of the slide centrifuge CFT; examination of an antiserum, used in two different dilutions, against an antigen; left to right: complete and partial inhibition of hemolysis, and complete lysis of sensitized erythrocytes in the last two, control sections.

tants may result in a greater sensitivity or accuracy. This applies more specifically to some methods used for studies on viruses and rickettsiae and their antibodies, whereas the technique by Kwapinski (see p. 512) proved to be useful in the investigations on the antigenic structure of microorganisms.

i. *Complement Fixation Tests for Viruses.* The complement fixation, by Melnick (1969) is run as follows: a series of twofold dilutions of an antiserum, inactivated at 60° for 20 minutes, are made in 0.25 ml of a phosphate-buffered saline; 0.25 ml of an antigen, pretitrated by a chessboard titration, and 0.5-ml volume of saline containing 2 units of complement are then added to each tube. The mixtures are incubated at 37° for 1 to 2 hours and at 2 to 4° for 18 hours. After the incubation, each tube receives the hemolytic system, consisting of 0.25 ml of a 3% suspension of packed sheep blood erythrocytes and 0.25 ml of rabbit antisheep hemolysin diluted to provide 3 minimal hemolytic doses. The tubes are incubated at 37° for 20 minutes and inspected for the absence of hemolysis. The tube with the highest antiserum dilution showing no hemolysis denotes the end point.

In the technique developed by Rice, all reactions are expressed in terms of the number of complement units (K') required for 50% hemolysis. The values of K' can be determined by referring to the tables of results from a large series of tests with a particular viral antigen.

Titers of tested sera are expressed as the ratio $(S + A)':S$ where $(S + A)'$ corresponds to the number of complement units needed for 50% hemolysis with 0.05 ml of serum in the presence of antigen, and S represents the number of units required for this degree of hemolysis with 0.05 ml of serum alone, as indicated by the following formula:

$$\frac{(S + A)'}{(S)} = \frac{K' \text{ for a test of 0.05 ml serum with antigen}}{K' \text{ for a test of 0.05 ml serum alone}}$$

ii. *The Phage Complement Fixation Test.* The assay, according to Rountree's (1951) technique, is set up using 0.1-ml volumes of progressing dilutions of a phage suspension and antiserum, together with 2 MHD of complement. After the incubation at 37° for 1 hour, 0.2-ml volume of sheep red blood cells sensitized with $2\frac{1}{2}$ MHD rabbit hemolysin is added to give a final concentration of 1% cells (Table 76).

iii. *The Complement Fixation Test for the Diagnosis of Rickettsioses.* The antigen used in this test developed by Castañeda (1936) consists of a suspension of rickettsial bodies containing about 1000 organisms per oil-immersion field. The volume of the suspension employed in the test proper is estimated by the minimal amount which, if mixed with a homologous

Table 76.   Diagram of the Phage Complement-Fixation Test (Rountree, 1951)

Serum serial dilution	0.1 ml
Antigen suspension	0.1 to 0.4 ml (depending on results of the antigen titration)
Complement (2 MHD)	0.1 ml
Saline solution	up to 0.6 ml
	Incubation at 37° for 1 hour
1% sensitized red blood cells	0.4 ml
	Incubation at 37° for 1 hour

immune serum, gives a definite inhibition of hemolysis, not being anti-complementary in the control serum.

The optimal amount of rickettsiae is determined by titrating the antigen suspension in volumes varying from 0.1 to 0.4 ml, made up to 0.5 ml with saline, and mixed with 0.1 ml of an inactivated antirickettsial serum, and 0.1 ml (2 MHD) of a complement solution. A similar set is placed with a control normal serum. All tubes are incubated at 37° for 1 hour, and then 0.4-ml volumes of a 2% suspension of sensitized sheep erythrocytes are added, and incubated at 37° for 1 hour. The test proper is set up as presented in Table 76. Results can be read against a color standard, and the complete inhibition of hemolysis, or a 50% hemolysis, is taken as end point.

iv. *Kolmer's Complement Fixation Test.* The antigen for the test is either an acetone extract from beef heart powder, an emulsion consisting of 0.03% cardiolipin, 0.05% lecithin, and 0.6% cholesterol, or a Reiter protein antigen prepared by the D'Allessandro and Dardanoni (1953) method.

Cardiolipin is a nitrogen-free, carbohydrate-containing phospholipid (Pangborn, 1942). Eight tubes, set up for each serum, receive the following volumes of saline: 0.3, 0.2, 0.2, 0.2, 0.2, 0.2, 0.2, and 0.1 ml, respectively. A 0.2-ml volume of an inactivated serum is added to tubes 1, 2, and 8; 0.2 ml of the content of tube 2 is then transferred to tube 3, and so on to tube 7, from which 0.2 ml is discarded; 0.1 ml of an antigen solution is added to the first seven tubes, followed by 0.1 ml of diluted complement containing 2 MHD, added to each tube. The mixtures are left at 6 to 8° for 15 to 18 hours. The test is then supplemented with 0.1 ml of a rabbit hemolytic antiserum (2 MHD) and 0.1 ml of sheep erythrocyte suspension. The mixtures are shaken and incubated in a water bath at 37° for 1 hour.

The degree of the complement fixation in each tube is determined by comparison with reading standards, and expressed in a number of plusses. Results are reported in Kolmer units, according to the formula $S = 4D$, which corresponds to the sum of all 4+ reactions shown.

Examples. If the first two tubes or first three tubes show 4+ reactions, results are read 8 or 16, respectively. If the first tube shows less than 4+ reaction, for example, 1+, 2+, or 3+, the results are 1, 2, or 3 units, respectively. Alternatively, results of Kolmer test can be reported by listing all numbers corresponding to the intensity of complement fixation; for example, positive (4432−) or positive (31−).

The test with the spinal fluid is set in a similar manner, using 0.5-ml volumes of nondiluted spinal fluid and twofold dilutions ranging from 1:2 to 1:32 (Table 77).

Table 77. A Schedule of the Qualitative Kolmer Test with the Spinal Fluid

Tube Number	Spinal Fluid (ml)	Saline Solution	Incubation for 10 to 15 minutes at room temperature	Complement 2 Hemolytic Units	Incubation at 6° for 15 to 18 hours and 10 minutes at 37°	Hemolytic Antiserum 2 MHU	Sheep Erythrocyte, 2% Suspensions
1	0.1	0.1		0.2		0.1	0.1
2	0.1	—		0.2		0.1	0.1
Controls							
3	0.2	0.1		0.2		0.1	0.1
4	0.3	—		0.2		0.1	0.1
5	0.0	—		—		—	0.1

In a simplified Kolmer's test, a single 0.2-ml dose of serum is used to which 0.2 ml of 50% egg-white solution and 0.5 ml of an antigen dilution is then added. Other details of the test, including control tubes, are unchanged. Reading standards are prepared from the hemoglobin solution, obtained from control tubes of the day's tests or from the titration of test components. The hemoglobin should be heated at 56° for 5 minutes and distributed into five tubes together with a 2% sheep erythrocyte suspension diluted 1:6. The amounts placed in the individual tubes and the mode of recording are shown in Table 78.

Table 78. Kolmer's Reading Standards

Erythrocyte Suspension (ml)	Hemoglobin Solution (ml)	Equivalent Fixation (%)	Complement Report
0.7	0.0	100	4+
0.35	0.35	50	3+
0.175	0.525	25	2+
0.07	0.63	10	1+
0.035	0.665	5	
—	0.7	0	

v. *The Native Complement Fixation Test.* The test, devised by Gradwohl (1956), utilizes the native complement and native antisheep hemolysin which are present in practically all human bloods. By this procedure, both the thermostable and thermolabile factors of reagins are saved in the unheated examined serum to react with the antigen. The test is set up as presented in Table 79.

Table 79.   Diagram of the Native Complement Fixation Test

Tubes	1	2	3	4	5	6	7	8	9	10	11	12	13	14
Serum examined	0.1	0.1	0.1	0.1	0.1	0.1	0.1	0.1	0.1	0.1	0.1	0.1	0.1	0.1
Saline	1.0	0.9	0.8	0.7	0.6	0.5	0.4	0.3	0.2	0.1	0.2	0.15	0.1	0.3
Antigen	—	—	—	—	—	—	—	—	—	—	0.1	0.15	0.2	—
6% sheep erythrocytes	0.1	0.2	0.3	0.4	0.5	0.6	0.7	0.8	0.9	1.0	—	—	—	—

The mixtures are incubated at 37 to 40° for 30 minutes and examined for the presence of hemolysis. Hemolytic activity of the serum and the amount of 6% sheep erythrocytes to be added to tubes 11 to 14 is estimated from the following index. If the complete hemolysis is observed in any number of tubes up to 4, 0.1 ml should be added; if the hemolysis is recorded in tubes 5, 6, or 7, 0.15 ml should be added; and 0.2 ml of the sheep erythrocyte suspension is added when the hemolysis occurs in tube 8, 9, or 10. However, in the last case, when all samples are hemolyzed, the test is reincubated after the addition of an extra 1.0 ml of 6% sheep red blood cells to all the first ten tubes. According to the occurrence of hemolysis in the 4, 7, and 10 tubes, the corresponding amounts of the erythrocyte suspension for tubes 11 to 14 are 0.25, 0.3, or 0.35. These tubes should now be incubated at 37 to 40° for 30 minutes and read. The tube 14 must always show hemolysis. The intensity of the complement fixation is evaluated from the inhibition of hemolysis in tubes 11 to 13, and expressed in +, ++, +++, depending on whether one, two, or three tubes show the hemolysis inhibition.

vi. *The Indirect Complement Fixation Test.* Certain mammalian and bird antisera fail to absorb complement in the presence of a homologous antigen, although they are reactive in other immunological tests. The presence of these antibodies can be indirectly revealed by employing an additional standard antiserum (a serum reagent) known to react with a particular antigen in the complement fixation test. If the first antiserum contains specific antibodies, these combine with the antigen, and the serum reagent cannot react with the antigen. Consequently, the complement added will remain free, and the hemolysis of sensitized erythrocytes will occur, especially in tubes containing a higher concentration of the original antiserum. The hemolysis may be inhibited toward the greater dilution, since a portion of free antigen can react with the standard antiserum. The inhibition of hemolysis occurs in all the tubes if the original serum did not contain specific antibodies at all. Two similar techniques of the indirect complement fixation test have been described (Hilleman et al., 1951, and Rice and Brooksby, 1953).

Hilleman's et al. Technique. The complement and the hemolytic system are standardized in the usual manner. The inactivated serum being tested is serially diluted in 0.2-ml amounts; 0.2-ml volumes of a guinea pig serum containing two units of complement and 0.2 ml (two units) of an antigen suspension are then added. After the incubation at 37° for 1 hour, 0.2-ml volumes of an immune standard serum (the serum reagent) containing two units of an antibody specific for the antigen are added, and the mixtures are reincubated at 37° for 1 hour. Finally, the hemolytic system, consisting of 0.1 ml of a 4% suspension of sheep red blood cells and 0.1 ml of a solution containing two units of the anti-RBC serum in this volume are added. The tubes are left at 37° for 30 minutes, and the end point of reaction should be determined by the highest dilution of the test serum which has bound the antigen completely, hence causing the hemolysis.

The Rice and Brooksby Technique. The assay is set up as shown in Table 80. Four controls are inserted containing:

1. The complement alone.
2. The antigen and 2 units of complement.
3. The antigen and 3 units of complement.
4. A standard complement-fixing antiserum, antigen, and 3, 6, and 12 units of complement.

Table 80.   Diagram of the Indirect CFT, by Rice and Brooksby

0.10 ml of twofold dilutions of the test serum	Incubation at 37° for 1 hour
0.05 ml of a constant dilution of antigen	
0.10 ml of complement solution, with 3 $C'H_{50}$ units	Incubation at 36° for 30 to 60 minutes
0.05 ml of a "standard" complement-fixing guinea pig antiserum, diluted 1:20	
0.20 ml of 2.5% sensitized red blood cells	Incubation at 37° for 30 minutes

The titer is estimated in terms of the highest dilution of test serum, at which at least 50% hemolysis or more is observed in the presence of the antigen and a standard complement-fixing antiserum.

The indirect complement fixation test can also be set out with varying amounts of antigen and a constant amount of antiserum, as first published by Ciuca (1929).

7. *Evaluation of the Complement Fixation Test*

The complement fixation test is a very sensitive serological test, since it permits the detection of as little as 0.05 μg of the antibody nitrogen with an accuracy of 5%. Although the estimated titer of an antigen or antiserum provides valuable information with regard to their serological potency, the titer of an antiserum must not be regarded as a direct measure of its antibody content. The complement giving activity per microgram of antibody nitrogen may vary with the length and intensity of the immunization (Wallace et al., 1950). The complement fixation test may fail to demonstrate antibodies present in the antisera produced in certain mammalian and avian species, especially after the inactivation of a complement-containing serum. For example, reactions of antibodies present in horse antisera with the homologous antigens are seldom detectable by the complement fixation tst. Similarly, pneumococcal antisera from man, goat, cat, dog, and mouse, as well as certain bacterial and viral antisera of avian origin, combined to the homologous antigens, fail to absorb sufficient complement to cause visible inhibition of hemolysis. These antibodies, however, can be demonstrated by an indirect complement fixation test. The effect of anticomplementary bodies, simulating the inhibition of hemolysis, the multiplicity of constituents required for complement fixation, and difficulty in standardization of the complements are factors responsible for a more recent decrease in the popularity of the complement fixation test in many facets of immunological research.

8. *Applications of the Complement Fixation Test*

The complement fixation test is used for detection, identification, and evaluation of antibodies as well as for the identification and quantification of antigens and antigen preparations present in the serum and in other body fluids or in feces (Koshland, 1953). A major application of the complement fixation test has remained the immunological diagnosis of infections, assessment of the progress of infectious diseases, and measurement of the antibody-response after a vaccination.

This test provides valuable data on the content and range of the antibody immunoglobulins in the sera, on the specificity of antibodies, the potency and specificity of antigens, and the immunological relationships between the antigenic structure of microorganisms and different microbial animal and plant species.

Some examples of the application of the complement fixation test follow.

Detection of Antibodies

1. In the sera of individuals infected with *Treponema pallidum, Neisseria gonorrhoeae, Haemophilus pertussis* (Parfentjev and Virion, 1948), *Mycobacterium tuberculosis,* poliomyelitis virus (Neustaedter and Benzhaf, 1917), measles virus (Bech, 1959), variola, mumps, influenza, parainfluenza, encephalitis, herpes, dengue, rubella viruses, adenoviruses, West Nile fever virus, Rift Valley fever virus, rickettsiae (Castaneda, 1936), ornithosispsittacosis, and lymphogranuloma venereum chlamydiae, *Blastomyces* (Martin, 1953), and such.

2. In the sera of clinically health persons, the detection of antpoliomyelitis and anti-Coxsackie virus antibodies (Horstmann and Kraft, 1955; Melnick, 1950; Kraft and Melnick, 1952).

3. In the sera of animals infected naturally or experimentally with the rickettsiae, the vesicular stomatitis virus (Rice and McKercher, 1954), yellow fever virus (Perlowagora and Hughes, 1948).

4. In the sera of immunized people, to study the response after the vaccination with Cox-type vaccine of *Rickettsia prowazeki* (Murray et al., 1952), poliomyelitis vaccine (Lennette et al., 1961), as well as in the sera of monkeys immunized with mixtures of poliomyelitis virus and serum (Kolmer and Rule, 1935).

The Detection and Evaluation of Antigens.

1. The qualitative and quantitative estimation of antigens of leptospiras (Rothstein and Hiatt, 1956; Terzin, 1956), fractions isolated from *Treponema pallidum* (Portnoy and Magnuson, 1955), the Vi antigen of *Enterobacteriaceae* (Landy et al., 1954), antigens of *Salmonella typhosa* (Landy et al., 1955), fractions of *Corynebacterium* (Kwapinski, 1956), *Mycobacterium* (Mikulaszek and Kwapinski, 1954; Kwapinski, 1956), *Streptococcus* (Kwapinski, 1959), PPLO (Coriell et al., 1962), *Rickettsia burnetti* (Colter et al., 1956), herpes simplex virus (Hayward, 1950; Womack and Hunt, 1954; Halonen and Tarpila, 1961), the psittacosis-lymphogranuloma group of viruses, and bacteriophages (Lanni, 1954), *Actinomyces* and *Nocardia* (Kwapinski, 1960, 1964), *Streptomyces* (Kwapinski and Merkel, 1957), *Trichophyton* (Merkel, 1959), *Diplococcus* (Kwapinski and Snyder, 1961), as well as the blood group substances (Glynn et al., 1956), and thyroid glands extracts (Witebsky et al., 1955).

2. The classification of bacteria, for example, of *Salmonella* strains (Seligman, 1945), or *Nocardia* strains (Kwapinski and Seeliger, 1964).

3. The detection and identification of species origin of foreign proteins in blood stains.

Chapter Thirteen

IMMUNE INHIBITION ASSAY

Immune inhibition assays are attributed to the formation of soluble immune complexes so that no free antibody or antigen molecules are available for combining with a related, particulate antigen or bivalent antibody. Consequently, the products that would normally be elicited by the latter combination of antigen and antibody are not seen. The following categories of the immune inhibition assays have been distinguished (Kwapinski, 1965):

I. Immune inhibition tests.
   1. The immune hemagglutinin-inhibition test.
   2. The isohemagglutinin-inhibition test.
   3. The Gm-hemagglutination-inhibition test.
   4. The hemagglutination-blocking test.
   5. The enhanced hemagglutination-inhibition test.
   6. The immune hemolysis-inhibition test.
   7. The automated passive hemolysin-inhibition test.
   8. The complement fixation-inhibition test.
   9. The agglutination-inhibition test.
   10. The virus-cell agglutination-inhibition test.
   11. The agglutination-blocking test.
   12. Flocculation-inhibition tests.
   13. The precipitin-inhibition test.
   14. The immunodiffusion-inhibition test.
   15. The bactericidin (vibriocidin)-inhibition test.
   16. The immunofluorescence-inhibition test.
II. Active hemagglutination-inhibition tests.
   1. The virus hemagglutination-inhibition test.
   2. The virus hemagglutinin-absorption test.
   3. The immune adherence-inhibition test.
   4. The bacterial hemagglutinin-inhibition test.
III. Immunobiochemical inhibition test.
   1. The active hemolysis-inhibition tests.
      i. The antistreptolysin test.
      ii. The antistaphylolysin test.

      iii. The leptospira hemolysin-inhibition test.
      iv. The hemolysin diffusion-inhibition test.
   2. The antileukocidin test.
   3. The protease-inhibition tests.
      i. The antistreptokinase test.
      ii. The antiproteinase test.
      iii. The anticoagulase test.
   4. The carbohydrase-inhibition tests.
      i. The antihyluronidase test.
   5. The antinuclease test.
IV. The immunoimmobilization test.

I. IMMUNE INHIBITION TESTS

Any immune reaction between an antigen and a complementary antibody can be prevented by exposing either the antigen to an antibody possessing appropriate combining sites, or the antiserum to an antigen containing determinant groups for the antibody. If the antigen or antibody thus neutralized has been combined by a complementary, heterologous immunologic partner, and then it has been brought into contact with a homologous immune partner, no immunologic reaction is observed. The lack of normal reaction products indicates that both antigens are immunologically related, or both antibodies possess certain identical combining sites. The simplest procedure for the inhibition reaction is the absorption of an antiserum by the saturation with a corresponding antigen, or the absorption of an antigen with an appropriate antiserum.

1. The Immune Hemagglutination-Inhibition Test

The hemagglutination-inhibition test depends on the neutralization of serum hemagglutinins by an antigen which renders the serum so pretreated unable to agglutinate erythrocytes carrying a homologous antigen. In this procedure, the antiserum in a constant amount is added to a series of progressing dilutions of a soluble antigen preparation. After an incubation period, the erythrocytes sensitized with the same or a related antigen are suspended in the serum. No hemagglutination occurs if both the substances added to the serum and the sensitizing antigen are immunologically related. If the antigen added to the antiserum has no determinative groups for these antibodies, the noncombined antibodies react with the antigen adsorbed onto red blood cells causing agglutination.

The inhibition of hemagglutination is a sensitive reaction, since as little as 0.001 μg of an antigen can be detected by this technique (Wright and Feinberg, 1952).

Techniques of the hemagglutination-inhibition test were published by Boyden (1950), Meynell (1954), Stavitsky (1954), Boyden and Sorkin (1955), Chun et al. (1957), Stevens and McKenna (1958), Kwapinski (1965), and Whang and Neter (1962). Of the selected methods for presentation, the technique of Meynell employs various amounts of the "blocking" antigen and a constant dilution of antiserum, whereas procedures by Boyden and Sorkin and by Kwapinski use various dilutions of antiserum versus constant amount of the "blocking" antigen. The hemagglutination-inhibition test is used for the detection and evaluation of the potency and specificity of antigens, for the identification of microoranisms, and for the detection of specific antibodies in certain infectious diseases.

Meynell's Method for the Hemagglutination-Inhibition Test. The antigen, in twofold, progressing dilutions made in 0.4-ml saline or in 1% normal rabbit serum is mixed with 0.05-ml amounts of an antiserum. This volume of the serum should contain four minimum hemagglutinating units of antibody, determined by a preceding hemagglutination test with the homologous, erythrocyte sensitizing antigen preparation. A control tube receives 0.05 ml of the antiserum and 0.4 ml of 1% rabbit-serum diluent.

The tubes are incubated at 37° for 45 minutes. Each tube then receives 0.05 ml of a 1.7% erythrocyte suspension sensitized with an antigen homologous to the antiserum used. The mixtures are left at room temperature for 2 to 3 hours, and read. The titer of the hemagglutination-inhibition test is expressed as the dilution of the antigen in the last tube showing no agglutination of erythrocytes.

The Cross-Inhibition Test. The test can be set up with varying dilutions of either the antigen or the serum. Here are some details of the cross-inhibition technique by Boyden and Sorkin (1955). Twofold progressing dilutions of an antigen are made in 1-ml volumes of buffered saline. Two control tubes receive buffered saline alone. An equal volume of antiserum, diluted to contain four hemagglutinating doses, is added to each tube. A 0.1-ml amount of each mixture is then transferred to small (45 × 3.5-mm) tubes and left at 4° overnight; 0.1-ml volumes of 0.5% tanned cells, sensitized with an appropriate antigen preparation, are then added. The tubes are incubated at 37° for 2 to 4 hours, read, left at 4° overnight, and read again. The end point is indicated by the tube, in which no hemagglutination is observed at the highest dilution of antigen. Control tubes should show hemagglutination. Titer of the hemagglutination-inhibition test is expressed in terms of final dilution of the antigen end point tube.

The Cross-Inhibition Technique by Chun et al. (1957). In this test, the antigen in a constant dilution is added to an equal volume of serial dilutions of a serum. The mixtures are incubated at 37° for 15 minutes, and left overnight in the refrigerator; 0.1 ml of 0.25 to 0.5% erythrocyte suspension, sensitized with another antigen, is then added to 0.2-ml volume of each test mixture. The tubes are incubated at 37° for 2 hours before reading.

Control tubes contain (a) a saline solution of normal rabbit serum and sensitized tanned erythrocyte suspension; and (b) dilution of a normal serum and nonsensitized tanned red blood cells. If the two antigens tested are serologically related to each other, no hemagglutination is observed.

Kwapinski's Method for the Hemagglutination-Inhibition Test. Constituents of this test are as follows.

1. 0.2% suspension of normal or tanned chicken erythrocytes, or human O Rh-negative red blood cells, coated by an antigen homologous to the antiserum.

2. 0.2% control suspension of nonsensitized erythrocytes.

3. A solution or suspension of another antigen to be tested for its serological relationship with the first antigen.

4. A heat-inactivated antiserum, used in a dose of five hemagglutinating units.

The technique of preparation and sensitization of erythrocytes for this hemagglutination test is described on p. 407. The minimum hemagglutinating unit of antiserum is determined as follows. Two series of dilutions of antiserum, ranging from 1:10 to 1:1280, are made in 0.2-ml volumes of a phosphate-buffered saline, pH 7.3. Each tube receives an additional 0.2-ml volume of the buffered saline. The 0.2% suspension of antigen-coated erythrocytes is then added to the first row in 0.4-ml amounts, whereas the other row obtains non sensitized cells. Additional control tubes receive 0.4 ml of buffered saline and 0.4 ml of either the sensitized or nonsensitized erythrocytes.

After an incubation at 37° for 2 hours and at 2° for 3 to 16 hours, the titer of hemagglutination is estimated in terms of the highest final dilution of the antiserum showing agglutination of the antigen-coated erythrocytes, whereas no hemagglutination should be observed in all control tubes. The amount or dilution of serum in the end-point tube denotes one hemagglutinating unit. Five units are employed in the hemagglutination-inhibition test, which is set up with two series of twofold antigen dilutions according to the schedule in Table 81.

2. The Isohemagglutinin-Inhibition Test

This test, devised by Beiser and Kabat (1952) for measuring the relative activity of different blood group A or B substances, is conducted in the following manner. An antiserum, produced by immunizing human beings with a purified blood group preparation, is distributed to a number of

Table 81.   The Schedule of the Hemagglutination-Inhibition Test (Kwapinski, 1965)

Reactant	First Row	Second Row	Control 1	Control 2
Antigen dilutions, from 1:500 to 1:64,000 ml	0.2	—	0.2	—
Buffered saline, pH 7.4 (ml)	—	0.2	0.2	0.4
Antiserum (five hemagglutinating units) (ml)	0.2	0.2	—	—
Incubation at 37° for 30 minutes				
0.2% antigen-sensitized erythrocytes (ml)	0.4	0.4	0.4	0.4
Hemagglutination after 2-hour incubation at 37° and 3 to 16 hours at 2°	–	+	–	–

tubes in 0.1-ml volume, containing four to eight hemagglutinating units. The minimum hemagglutinating unit of serum should be determined according to a technique of isohemagglutination tube test (see p. 432). At the same time, varying amounts of a solution of purified blood group A or B preparation (obtained by the Beiser and Kabat method, 1952) are incubated with 0.1 ml of a 4% suspension of washed group A or B erythrocytes. These mixtures are transferred to tubes containing the solution of the blood group antiserum. After a short period of incubation, the minimum amount of each blood group preparation which completely inhibited the hemagglutination, is determined.

The isohemagglutinin-inhibition test, as modified by Gibbs et al. (1961), is set up with the following amounts of reactants: 0.25 ml of a dilution of group A substance; 0.5 ml of a suspension of red blood cells, group A; 0.25 ml of an anti-serum, diluted to contain 5 HD_{50} (hemagglutinating dose 50) units of antibody. The tubes are stoppered and rotated on a 10-rpm rotator for $2\frac{1}{2}$ hours to achieve an equilibration of the system. The number of free erythrocytes is then determined by the hemacytometer counts, and the percentage of agglutinated cells is calculated. The probit corresponding to the percentage of agglutination is obtained from a statistical table of probability units (Fisher and Yates, 1953) and plotted against the logarithm of the A substance concentration.

3.   *The Gm-Hemagglutination-Inhibition Test*

The test depends on inhibition of the agglutination of erythrocytes coated by the Gm(*a*) factor, normally caused by their reaction with anti-Gm(*a*) antibodies, due to the prior neutralization of these antibodies. Sensitization of antigen carrier (O Rh-positive erythrocytes) with an anti-Rh serum is carried out as follows (Prokop and Uhlenbruck, 1969): 0.1 ml of an anti-Rh+ serum containing Gm(*a*)-gamma globulin diluted with saline to make 1 ml is mixed with 0.1 ml of washed O Rh-positive erythrocytes, and incubated at 37° for 1 to 2 hours. The coated red cells are then washed and resuspended in saline to a desired concentration.

The Gm-hemagglutination-inhibition test is set up in small tubes or on glass or porcelain plates. A microtest is preferred. In this test, a tiny drop of a serum to be examined, diluted 1:4 and 1:8, is placed on a plate. A micro-drop of a suitably diluted anti-Gm(a) serum is added and, after a few minutes, a small drop of the O Rh+ erythrocytes, coated with an anti-Rh serum (see above) is added to the mixture of the two sera. The reaction mixture is shaken and left in a refrigerator for 1 to $1\frac{1}{2}$ hours. Before the reading, the plate is shaken slightly to reveal the presence of clumped cells.

Clumping of erythrocytes occurs if the tested serum does not contain a Gm(a) factor, since a free anti-Gm(a) antibody is required to agglutinate the sensitized cells.

4. The Hemagglutination-Blocking Test

The hemagglutination-blocking test is based on the following observation: if the reactive groups of an antigen are saturated by incomplete antibodies or by immune substances responsible for the "prozone" phenomenon, the antigen is rendered inactive in any test with the corresponding complete antibody. The blocking test by Wiener (1944) is used for the detection of incomplete isohemagglutinins, especially the Rh antibodies (see p. 437).

An adaptation of the test for *Brucella* blocking antibodies was devised by Zinneman et al. (1959).

5. The Enhanced Hemagglutination-Inhibition Test

A factor inhibiting the hemagglutinating activity of rheumatoid sera occurs in a majority of normal sera but not in the rheumatoid arthritis sera. The inhibition test (Ziff et al., 1956) is set up in the following manner.

A serum or, preferably, the immunoglobulins, isolated from the serum by the procedure described on p. 268, is serially diluted from 1:7 to 1:56 in 0.25-ml volumes of saline.

Each tube receives an equal amount of a standard rheumatoid serum diluted to contain eight units of hemagglutinating activity, as estimated by Heller's test (see p. 417). Control tubes receive 0.5 ml of saline solution alone, or 0.25 ml of a diluted positive serum and 0.25 ml of saline. Each tube then receives 0.5 ml of 0.25% suspension of sheep erythrocytes sensitized with $\frac{1}{10}$ agglutinating unit of a hemolytic serum (erythrocyte antiserum). The tubes are left at 2 to 4° overnight and read, with the aid of a hand lens, by agitating the tubes in front of a light source.

The inhibition titer is expressed as the highest dilution of a serum euglobulin fraction showing no hemagglutination. The inhibition of hemagglutination at a final euglobulin dilution of 1:14 or higher is regarded as significant. Negative results of the enhanced hemagglutination inhibition test are characteristic of the rheumatoid arthritis sera.

6. The Immune Hemolysis-Inhibition Test

The test is conducted in two stages. First, the antiserum used in a constant volume is incubated with varying amounts of an antigen preparation. In the second stage, a suspension of erythrocytes coated with an antigen homologous to the serum and complement are added to the first system. No hemolysis of coated red blood cells occurs if the antibody has combined with determinant groups of the tested antigen. This reaction indicates that both antigens are serologically related to each other. Two techniques of the immune hemolysis inhibition test, by Neter et al. (1956) and Kwapinski (1965), are presented here in detail.

The Neter et al. Hemolysis-Inhibition Test.   Twofold dilutions of the tested antigen, in 0.1-ml volumes, are mixed with 0.2 ml of an antiserum, containing three to four minimal hemolysing units, and incubated at 37° for 30 minutes. A 2.5% suspension of sheep red cells coated with two to three sensitizing units of the respective antigen is then added, in 0.2-ml volumes, followed by 0.1 ml of complement, diluted 1:20. The samples are reincubated at 37° for 30 minutes and checked for the inhibition of hemolysis.

Kwapinski's Hemolysis-Inhibition Test.   This employs the following constituents:

1. The tested antigen, diluted serially from 1:500 to 1:64,000.

2. An antiserum, inactivated at 62° for 3 minutes and used in a dose of four hemolytic units predetermined by an immune hemolytic test (p. 442).

3. 0.5% suspension of normal or tanned sheep erythrocytes, coated with an antigen homologous to the antiserum as described on p. 455–457.

4. A guinea pig serum, absorbed with sheep red blood cells, as the source of complement, used in a dose of two minimal hemolytic units.

A minimal hemolytic unit of complement is determined in the presence of the tested antigen, as follows. Two parallel series of twofold dilutions of complement are made in 0.2-ml volumes of buffered saline, pH 7.2; 0.2 ml of the initial dilution of the tested antigen and 0.2 ml of buffered saline are added to each tube. The first series of complement dilutions then receives 0.4 ml of 0.5% suspension of sensitized red cells, whereas the second, control series obtains unsensitized cells. After a 30-minute incubation at 37°, the titer of complement is estimated in terms of the dilution in the last tube with sensitized erythrocytes, in which a complete hemolysis was observed. This complement dilution corresponds to its minimal hemolytic unit.

The minimal hemolytic unit of antiserum is determined in the usual manner, as in the hemolytic test. Thus 0.2 ml of various dilutions of an antiserum in the presence of two minimal units of complement are exposed to 0.2-ml amounts of 0.5% suspension of sheep erythrocytes, coated with a homologous antigen. After a 30-minute incubation a 37°, the last tube showing complete hemolysis is taken as end point; one hemolytic unit of the antiserum is expressed in terms of its dilution in the end-point tube.

The hemolysis-inhibition test is set up according to the diagram shown in Table 82. After the reincubation at 37° for 30 minutes, the titer of hemolysis inhibition is recorded in terms of the final antigen dilution in the first series dilution, at which the hemolysis has not occurred.

Table 82.　Diagram of the Hemolysis-Inhibition Test (Kwapinski, 1965)

	Series 1	Series 2	Control 1	Control 2
Antigen diluted 1:500 to 1:64,000 (ml)	0.2	—	0.2	—
Antiserum (4 MHU) (ml)	0.2	0.2	—	—
Buffered saline (ml)	—	0.2	0.2	0.4
Incubation at 37° for 30 minutes				
0.5% antigen sensitized erythrocytes (ml)	0.4	0.4	0.4	0.4
Complement (2 MHU) (ml)	0.2	0.2	0.2	0.2
Hemolysis after 30 minutes incubation at 37°	—	+	—	—

7.　*The Automated Passive Hemolysin-Inhibition Test*

A method for automated immunochemical quantitation of the passive hemolysin-inhibition test (Sturgeon et al., 1969) depends on a combination of the light scattering and electronic systems. The apparatus is a single-channel, fully automated, continuous flow system (AutoAnalyzer) which consists of a sampler, sample changer, the proportioning pumps, the manifolds, a continuous flow colorimeter to measure hemoglobulin content, and an optical erythrocyte counter and pen recorder as detection devices.

The automated method has been applied to measurements of ferritin, transferrin, fibrinogen, and immunoglobulins. It has a maximum sensitivity in the range of 0.1 to 0.4 μg/ml of these substances. Results are available in 30 minutes, and the productivity may be more than 200 tests per day. This automated method is particularly useful in mass screening programs for epidemiological and diagnostic purposes and in research work requiring numerous, accurate, quantitative determinations of complex biological materials, such as antigen and antibody occurring in concentrations of 0.2 μg/ml or greater.

The apparatus used is a standard AutoAnalyzer (Technicon Instruments Corp., Chauncey, N. Y.) incorporated into a manifold trough which passes a continuous flow hemolytic system as shown in Fig. 66.

In the test, the sheep cells sensitized or conjugated with an antigen are mixed with an appropriate antiserum and a complement source and incubated at 37° until hemolysis occurs. An aliquot of the hemolysate is withdrawn and diluted approximately thirtyfold with saline and passed through the detector. The hemoglobin is ignored in the detector but if as the result of inhibition of the hemolysis or hemolytic system, unlyzed red blood cells have remained, the cells set up in the detector a counting rate which is traced on the recorder chart. A direct proportion exists between the amplitude of the signal and the degree of inhibition of hemolysis which has resulted from the soluble antigen introduced to the sample line into the antiserum.

The system has maximal sensitivity for the detection of soluble antigens in the reaction sample if the reagent (antigen) concentration has been reduced to the lowest level possible, that is, one that gives a slightly submaximal scale tracing on the recorder chart with the detector set at its near maximum sensitivity. In these conditions, a minimal concentration of erythrocytes permits the use of the minimal concentration of antibody to attain complete hemolysis.

Phosphate buffer saline (pH 7.3) used for the test is made from a concentrated, stock PBS solution, prepared by dissolving 180 g NaCl, 17.6 g Na_2HPO_4, and 3.8 g of $NaHPO_4 \cdot H_2O$ in 1 liter of distilled water. The concentrated stock solution is diluted 1 to 20 for use.

Complement is in the form of a guinea pig serum which may be preserved −70° for a few weeks. Prior to use, the complement source is absorbed with 1 to 4 volume of washed packed sheep erythrocyte at 4° for 15 minutes.

Conjugated (sensitized red blood cells) are prepared by suspending washed packed sheep cells in an antigen solution, in the ratio of 1 ml packed cells to 1 to 2 mg/ml of antigen for most systems. The DBD (bis-diazo-benzidine) conjugated cells are obtained by exposing the erythrocyte-antigen mixture used in varying concentrations to three different amounts of BDB. The mixture is rotated gently for 9 to 10 minutes after which the reaction is stopped by the addition of veronal buffer saline containing 1.5 g/liter bovine serum albumin (VBSA). The mixture is centrifuged and washed two to three times with VBSA. The conjugated and washed cells are made up to an 0.5 to 0.25% suspension and filtered through a "C"

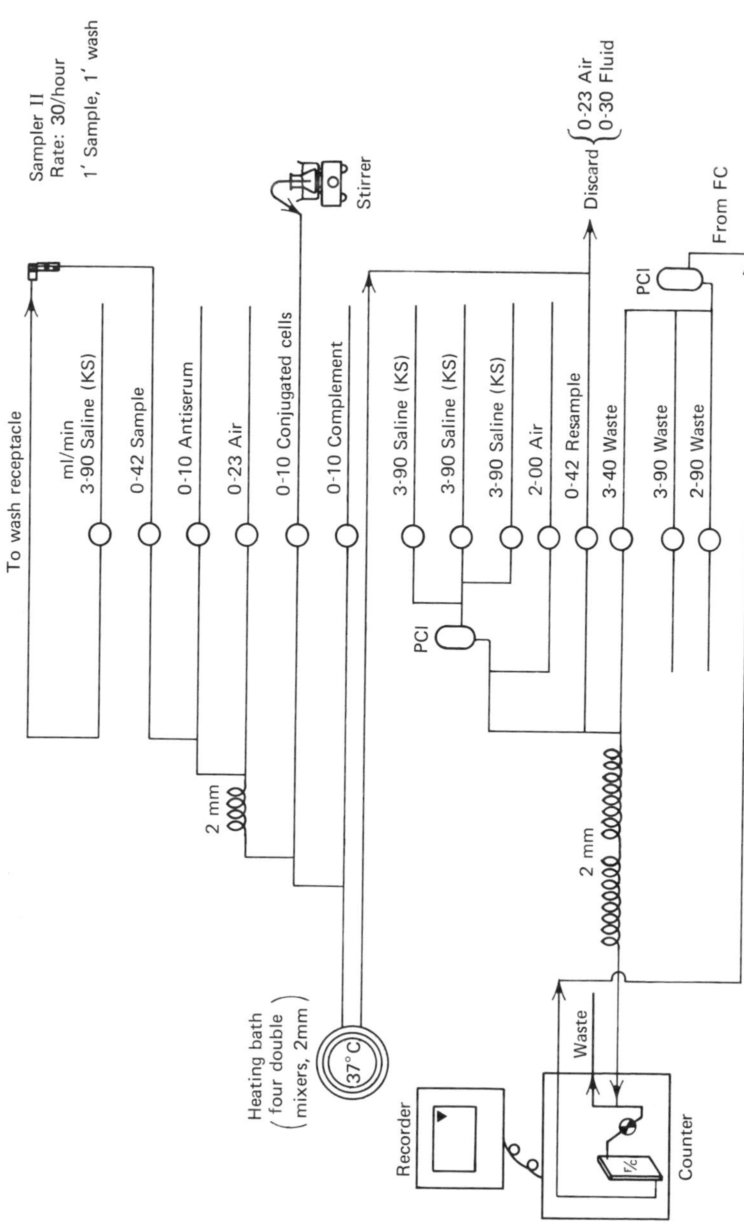

Figure 66. The flow diagram for automated passive hemolysis-inhibition system (Sturgeon et al., 1969).

535

sintered glass Büchner filter. In this way, optimal concentration of antigens and BDB for cell sensitization is estimated. The quantity of antigen and BDB which have given the maximal specific hemolysis without nonspecific hemolysis is selected for preparation of the reagent cells as described above.

The next step in the automated immunochemical quantitation is adjustment of serological conditions for optimal machine sensitivity (Sturgeon et al., 1969) in the following manner.

The minimal concentration of conjugated cells giving a signal of 90 on the recorder chart when the counter is set at near maximal sensitivity is continuously drawn through the reagent cell line, which usually requires 0.5 to 0.25% cells. Complement diluted 1:2 is drawn next. Set the sample probe in the wash position and the antiserum line in a beaker containing VBS - Alb. Manually transfer the antiserum line through twofold serial dilutions of antiserum and back into the VBS - Alb, starting with the greatest dilution of antiserum. The titration of antiserum should be repeated with the varying concentrations of complement ranging from 2 to 1:20. The concentration of complement for the final test is selected as the concentration which permits with the lowest concentration of antiserum complete hemolysis (the lowest hemolytic base).

Standardization, Calibration, and Replication. Prepare a standard antigen solution in a concentration of 10 μg/ml, and prepare twofold serial dilution ending with a concentration of 0.15 μg/ml, using volumetric equipment. Transfer 2 ml of the 10 μg/ml standard and each of the serial dilution to sample cups. Set in the apparatus in operation and holding the sample probe in the wash position introduce the reagents, adjusted to their optimal concentrations as indicated above. To establish the "cell" or 100% inhibition phase introduce conjugated cells and complement for a few minutes. Introduce antiserum next until the maximal hemolysis or "hemolytic" base has been established. Start sampling with the least concentrated standard first at the rate of 30 samples per hour with 1 minute of sampling and 1 of wash.

Quantitation of Antibody in Unknown Antiserum. The final test follows determination of optimal concentrations of all the reagents and establishment of the hemolytic phase and calibration completed. In this procedure, 1 to 2 ml of the unknown antigen preparation diluted 1:1000, 1:100, and 1:10 are placed in the sampling cups which are to be loaded on the sampler. The sampling rate for calibration curve and the unknowns can be increased to 50/hour to save time and reagents.

The AutoAnalyzer has also been used for hemagglutination-inhibition methods applied for quantitation of blood group substances (Sturgeon and McQuiston, 1965), and it probably can find application for counting bacterial cells.

8. The Complement Fixation-Inhibition Test

Kwapinski's Technique of the Complement Fixation-Inhibition Test. This is conducted as presented in Table 83. Amounts of a hemolytic serum and complement to be used in this test must be predetermined as described on pp. 492 and 504. The serum inactivated at 62° for 3 minutes is employed at the 50% nonanticomplementary amount. The antigen A should be diluted to contain eight minimal complement fixing units, as determined by a complement fixation test (see p. 514). Results of the CFT-fixation test can be read as either 100 or 50% hemolysis end point, by spectrophotometric examination of supernatants at 545 nm.

The quantitative complement fixation inhibition assay by Wasserman and Levine (1961) is carried out similarly to the complement fixation test described on pp. 509–510, except that one antigen is kept constant and the diluent now contains various quantities of the inhibitor. The antigen is used in a quantity which reacts with the antibody in a slight antigen excess.

The test arranged by Kwapinski is presented in Table 84. The complement is used in the amount equivalent to 4 $C'H_{50}$ units, predetermined by the titration of complement in the presence of the inhibitor. After the final incubation, the tubes are immersed in an ice bath, to stop further hemolysis and centrifuged for 10 minutes at $400 \times g$. The supernatant fluids are collected and examined at 413 nm. The end point is denoted by the first tube in the inhibitor-dilution series, showing 50% hemolysis. The inhibitor's titer is expressed by its dilution or amount present in the preceding tube.

9. The Agglutination-Inhibition Test

According to the Castellani (1902) technique, as slightly modified by Seligman (1945), the serum is diluted progressively in 0.5-ml volumes approximately up to a half of its agglutinating titer and mixed with 0.5-ml solution of an antigen preparation, such as bacterial cells, extracts or solutions of fractions isolated from the microorganisms. A control series of serum dilutions receives 0.5 ml of saline instead of the antigen solution.

The mixtures are left at room temperature for a period which may vary between 15 minutes and 24 hours, without any influence on results of the reaction. A suspension of bacterial cells, related with the antigen preparation employed in the test, is then added to each tube in 0.5-ml volume, and the mixtures are left at room temperature for 2 hours. The tubes are inspected for the presence of agglutinates. If the antigen preparation was related with these bacteria, the agglutination in the first row is inhibited completely or at least in the higher serum dilutions. The agglutinin titer estimated in this row should be compared with the agglutinin titer in the control row.

Table 83.   The Schedule for Kwapinski's (1965) Complement Fixation-Inhibition Test

Antigen B	Dilution 1:	1000	2000	4000	8000	16000	32000	64000	128000	Controls 1	2	3	4
	Volume (ml)	0.2	0.2	0.2	0.2	0.2	0.2	0.2	0.2	0.2	—	—	—
Antiserum A, diluted in complement containing 2.5–3.0 MHD/ml		0.2	0.2	0.2	0.2	0.2	0.2	0.2	0.2	—	—	—	—
Phosphate-buffered saline, pH 7.0 (ml)		—	—	—	—	—	—	—	—	—	—	0.2	0.2
Antiserum A, diluted in saline (ml)		—	—	—	—	—	—	—	—	0.2	0.2	0.2	—
Complement 2.5–3.0 MHD/ml		—	—	—	—	—	—	—	—	0.2	0.2	0.2	0.2
Incubation at 37° for 1 hour													
Antigen A (ml)		0.2	0.2	0.2	0.2	0.2	0.2	0.2	0.2	—	0.2	—	0.2
Incubation at 37° for 1 hour and at 2° for 16 hours													
3% erythrocytes sensitized with 4MHD antierythrocyte serum (ml)		0.4	0.4	0.4	0.4	0.4	0.4	0.4	0.4	0.4	0.4	0.4	0.4

Table 84. Schedule of Micro Complement-Inhibition Test

Inhibitor		1000	2000	4000	8000	16000	32000	64000	Controls		
	Dilution 1:	1000	2000	4000	8000	16000	32000	64000	1000	—	
	Volume (diluent)	0.3	0.3	0.3	0.3	0.3	0.3	0.3	0.3	0.4	0.4
Anti-Ag 1 serum/ml		0.1	0.1	0.1	0.1	0.1	0.1	0.1	0.1	—	0.1
Complement (4 $C'H_{50}$) (ml)		0.1	0.1	0.1	0.1	0.1	0.1	0.1	0.1	0.1	0.1
				Incubation at 2° for 10 hours							
Antigen A (constant) (ml)		0.1	0.1	0.1	0.1	0.1	0.1	0.1	0.1	0.1	—
				Incubation at 37° for 3 hours							
Erythrocytes (5 $\times$ 10^7/ml) sensitized with 3 MHD of antierythrocyte serum (ml)		0.1	0.1	0.1	0.1	0.1	0.1	0.1	0.1	0.1	0.1
				Incubation at 37° for 1 hour							

The test can be applied for studies on immunologic relationships between various bacteria and to the classification of bacterial species. For example, this technique was used in studies on the classification of *Salmonellae.*

10. The Virus-Cell Agglutination-Inhibition Test

This test depends on the inhibition by an immune serum of the agglutination of mammalian cells by adsorbed virus particles. Thus the mechanism of this reaction is identical with the inhibition of the virus dependent hemagglutination. The procedure of this immune inhibition reaction, published by Mayyasi et al. (1959), is as follows.

First, the agglutinating unit of virus must be determined, by incubating a virus suspension in progressing dilutions with a constant amount of cells. Cells such as fibroblasts are obtained from a 24 to 72 tissue culture, digested with 0.2% trypsin in Hanks' BSS, pH 7.4. The dispersed cells are then resuspended in the medium to give 2 to 3 million cells/ml; 0.1 ml of this suspension is added to each virus dilution. Mixtures are shaken and incubated at 37° for 24 hours. The tubes are then inspected for the presence of clumped or agglutinated cells under the 200 to 400 magnification. The result is regarded as positive if at least half of fields examined have shown cell agglutination. The highest dilution of virus causing the clumping of at least 50% cells observed is taken as its titer. Ten virus agglutinating units are employed in the inhibition test.

In this test, 0.5 ml of the virus suspension (ten agglutinating units) is added to a series of twofold serum dilutions, made in 0.5-ml volumes of the Hanks' BSS medium. The tubes are incubated at 37° for 1 hour, then 0.1 ml of a cell suspension, containing 200,000 to 300,000 cells, is added to each tube. After a 24-hour incubation, each mixture is examined microscopically for the presence of clumped cells. The titer is expressed as the reciprocal of the highest serum dilution inhibiting the agglutination of cells.

11. The Agglutination-Blocking Test (Zinneman et al., 1959)

As indicated before, blocking tests depend on the saturation of reactive groups of antigens by incomplete antigens or by serologic substances responsible for the "prozone" phenomenon. In this test, a serum which shows no agglutination of a particulate antigen or gives a prozone phenomenon in the agglutination test is diluted progressively in 0.5-ml volume of saline; 0.5 ml of suspension of heat-killed bacteria is added to each tube, followed by 0.03 ml of diluted antiserum homologous to these microorganisms. Control tubes receive 0.5 ml of saline instead of the first serum. The tubes are incubated at 37° for 48 hours and examined immediately against a black background. "Blocking" of the reaction is indicated by a lower titer or no agglutination in the test row, as compared with the control tubes.

12. *Flocculation-Inhibition Tests*

Any flocculation reaction can be converted into a flocculation-inhibition test by first exposing the flocculating serum to a nonflocculating antigen or another combining substance, and then testing this serum against the homologous antigen.

i. *The Latex Flocculation (Fixation)-Inhibition Test.* A factor inhibiting the flocculation of latex particles is found most normal, but not in rheumatoid, sera. Thus a negative latex fixation-inhibition test is regarded as characteristic of rheumatoid arthritis. The test (Jeffrey, 1959) is carried out as follows. The serum euglobulin fraction, prepared according to Ziff's procedure (see p. 418), is diluted in the ratio of 1:7, 1:14, and 1:28 in 1-ml volumes of saline. Each tube receives 1 ml of a reference positive rheumatoid serum, diluted eight times the highest dilution causing the agglutination of latex particles "sensitized" with a γ-globulin preparation, and 1 ml of a later γ-globulin reagent. (The latex γ-globulin reagent is prepared by incubating at 37° for 60 minutes a mixture consisting of 0.1 ml of polystyrene latex suspension with 0.5 ml of 0.5% solution of an antipoliomyelitis immune globulin, diluted with 9.5 ml of the borate buffered saline.) The test samples are incubated at 56° for 2 hours, then centrifuged at 600-800 $\times$ g for 3 minutes, and examined for the presence of latex floccules. The last tube showing a complete inhibition of flocculation is taken as end point, and the titer is expressed in terms of the euglobulin dilution in this particular tube.

Inhibition of the flocculation by an euglobulin dilution of 1:14 or more is regarded as normal. The euglobulin isolated from a normal serum shows either an increased flocculation with dilution, as the inhibitor is consequently diluted, or an equal grade of agglutination in all tubes. In contrast, a rheumatoid euglobulin usually shows the strongest agglutination in the first tube, decreasing in the next tubes are the concentration of euglobulin containing "rheumatoid factor" drops gradually.

ii. *The Resin Flocculation-Inhibition Test (Segre, 1957).* The technique of preparing resin particles and titrating the virus are described on p. 390. The highest agglutinating dilution is considered one agglutinating unit of virus. Four units, contained in a volume of diluent, are added to equal volumes of twofold serial dilutions of a serum being examined, diluted in 2% solution of normal calf serum. One drop of each virus-serum mixture is then added on a glass plate to one drop of the resin particles suspension, sensitized by an antiserum γ-globulin. The plate is then rotated for a few minutes and read. The highest dilution of serum being examined, at which no clumping of resin particles is observed, is taken as end point and titer.

iii. *The Toxin Flocculation-Inhibition Test.* The test, designed by Kwapinski (1965), for the study of antigenic relationships between immunochemical fractions of bacteria and their exotoxins, is conducted in the following manner. Two series of progressing, twofold dilutions of a flocculating, antitoxic serum are prepared in 0.2 ml of buffered saline, pH 7.2. One series then receives 0.2-ml volumes of an active dilution of the antigen fraction being tested, while the other row receives 0.2 ml of saline. Controls are also set containing 0.2 ml of fraction solution and 0.2 ml of saline. All tubes are incubated at 40° for 1 hour. A homologous toxin solution containing 10 Lf* doses/ml is then added to each tube, in 0.2-ml volumes. The tubes are returned to the water bath at 40° and observed at 5-minute intervals for the occurrence of flocculates. The time in which the flocculates have been noticed in any tube are also recorded. Inhibition of the reaction, a lower flocculating titer of antiserum, or by a longer flocculation time. All figures recorded with the first row are subtracted from those of the control series.

13. The Precipitin-Inhibition Test

This test depends on the inhibitory action of tested substances on serum precipitins. Thus solutions of inhibitory substances are used as diluents in place of a saline or buffered saline. The precipitin-inhibition test is carried out in the following way (Kwapinski, 1965).

The tested substance for the inhibitory effect is diluted 1:25,000 or 1:100,000 and used for making serial dilutions of antiserum, in 0.2-ml volumes. A similar row of antiserum dilutions is made in 0.85% saline. The antigen known to react with the antiserum is added to each tube of both series of dilutions. Control tubes contain (a) 0.2 ml of antigen and 0.2 ml saline; (b) 0.2 ml of antigen and 0.2 ml solution of an inhibitory substance; (c) 0.2 ml of antiserum and 0.2 ml of the inhibitory substance solution; and (d) 0.2 ml of antiserum and 0.2 ml of saline.

The reaction mixtures are incubated for 2 hours at 38° and left overnight at 2 to 4°, then examined for the presence of precipitates. All controls must not show any precipitate. The first tube in the row containing the inhibitory substance and the last tube in the other row which show precipitations are selected, and the corresponding dilution factors of antiserum in these tubes are noted. The precipitin-inhibition titer is calculated by dividing the dilution factor in the end-point tube of the second row by that of the first row.

Culbertson's neutralization assay (1932) can be included in this class of tests, since it permits detection of the inhibition of precipitation. In this

---

* The amount of toxin corresponding to one unit of antitoxin in the mixture which shows optimal flocculation.

procedure, constant amounts of antiserum are added to varying amounts of antigen. After a period of incubation, the contents of tubes are centrifuged, and supernatants are divided in two aliquots. These are tested for the uncombined antigen or antibody, by using a homologous serum or antigen, respectively. If no visible reaction now occurs it indicates that both reactants were completely saturated in the first reaction. Culbertson's test was originally devised for the determination of optimal proportions of the antigen and antibody.

14. The Immunodiffusion-Inhibition Test

The immunodiffusion-inhibition test, designed by Ray and Shay (1965) and arranged by Kwapinski, consists of two parts: (a), the determination of minimal reacting dilution of antigens and antibody, and (b) the determination of the serum dilution which completely inhibits the formation of a visible line or precipitate.

The minimal reacting dilution of antigen and antibody is determined by block titration of antigen-antibody systems. Serial twofold dilutions of an antigen and antiserum are made in saline. Three rows of wells are cut in the agar layer contained in a Petri plate; the outer wells are parallel to each other whereas the wells of the central row, which possess a smaller diameter than the other, fall between the spaces occupied by outer walls. The middle row is filled with sequential dilutions of an antiserum and incubate at room temperature for 30 minutes. After the incubation, each of the two outer rows of wells is filled sequentially and in duplicate with different antigen dilutions. The plates are left 23 to 27° for 24 hours and observed with the agar diffusion reading lamp. The final reading is performed after 48 hours. The antigen-antibody end point is determined as that combination of the highest dilution of antigen and antibody which produces a visible line of precipitate in 48 hours. This end point reading is taken as representative of a minimal reacting dilution of antigen and a minimal reacting dilution of antibody.

The immunodiffusion-inhibition test is set up as follows: the inhibiting antigen preparation is diluted serially in a 0.2-ml volume of saline. The antiserum, previously titrated, is added to each dilution of the antigen in a twofold concentration in relation to the minimal reacting dilution, in 0.2-ml volume. The mixtures are agitated for 30 seconds and incubated at 37° for 30 minutes to permit antigen-antibody combination to proceed to completion. The wells of the center row of agar immunodiffusion plates are filled with a test antigen used in the strength corresponding to a minimal reacting dilution of antigen, and the plates are incubated at room temperature for 1 hour. Outer rows of wells are now filled sequentially and in duplicate with the incubated mixtures of inhibiting antigen and antibody.

The plates are incubated at room temperature for 48 hours and observed at 24- and 48-hour incubation. The end point of the immunodiffusion-inhibition reaction and the corresponding titer is determined by the dilution of the inhibiting antigen which has completely inhibited the formation of a visible precipitation band with the test antigen in the agar-gel plates.

The immunodiffusion-inhibition test possesses a higher degree of sensitivity than the capillary tube-precipitin inhibition test.

According to Björklund's technique (1952), all basins in an agar plate are first filled with one component of the tested serological system, for three consecutive days; alternatively, the antigen can be incorporated into the melted agar. The antiserum and two other antigen solutions are then placed in separate basins in the main and in a control agar plate. Both plates are left at room temperature for a few days, the basins being refilled three times. If the number of precipitation bands in the main agar plate is reduced in comparison with the regular gel-precipitation pattern on the other plate, it is indicative of an inhibition cause by the examined fraction.

15. *The Bactericidin (Vibriocidin)-Inhibition Test*

According to Finkelstein's (1962) technique, the inhibiting antigen, for example, an endotoxin preparation, a culture filtrate, or a chemical fraction, is serially diluted in 0.25-ml amounts of a suspension of vibrios or other test bacteria made in a sterile 0.1% solution of peptone in normal saline. Each tube then receives 0.25 ml of a serum diluted to contain 10 to 100 bactericidal doses for the test strain as estimated by the preceding bactericidal or vibriocidal test (see p. 452). These mixtures are incubated at 37° for 1 hour, and transferred into an ice bath. Each tube then receives 0.25 ml of a complement diluted 1:20 and 0.25 ml of a bacterail suspension two times the concentration used in the vibriocidal test. After a further incubation for 1 hour at 37°, 0.1-ml amounts of each mixture are planted on an appropriate medium starting with the highest dilution of antigen, and incubated at an adequate temperature. The number of colonies is then calcuated. The end point is determined by the highest dilution (or the smallest amount) of antigen which protects 25% or more of the bacteria against the bactericidal activity of the serum. Controls contain equivalent mixtures of a serum dilution, complement, and bacteria. A control of the viability of bacteria is also set up.

16. *The Fluorescent Antibody-Inhibition Test*

In this assay (Moody et al., 1956; Goldman, 1957), smears of bacteria are treated with mixtures of unlabeled antiserum and fluorescent globulin (p. 609) of the same type. If the intensity of fluorescence is hence reduced or abolished, the result of reaction is considered positive. Goldman's technique, as modified by Kaufman et al. (1962), depends on a comparison of the fluorescence of microorganisms stained with a mixture of equal (0.1-ml) volumes of labeled antiglobulins and unlabeled normal serum with the fluorescence of microorganisms stained with a mixture of equal volumes of labeled antiglobulins and unlabeled test serum. Smears of formalin killed microorganisms are made and heat fixed, then covered with a mixture of the conjugate and a serum, and incubated in a moist chamber at 37° for 30 minutes. Stained preparations are examined under the fluorescent microscope. The inhibition is manifested by a distinct reduction of the staining intensity. It is recommended to determine the optimum concentration of labeled antibody prior to test properties.

According to Möller (1961), the serum titer corresponds to the last serum dilution in which the fluorescence is visually as bright as the normal serum control slide.

II. ACTIVE HEMAGGLUTINATION-INHIBITION TESTS

The agglutination or red blood cells by virus, bacterial, or fungal hemagglutinins can be prevented by neutralizing the hemagglutinins with specific antisera prior to the contact with erythrocytes. Particular serological assays were devised for each group of microbial hemagglutinins.

1. The Virus Hemagglutination-Inhibition Test

Techniques of the test, by Salk (1944), Green and Wooley (1947), Hilleman et al. (1950), Horsfall and Tamm (1953), Chanock and Sabin (1953), and Fazekas de St. Groth et al. (1958) are essentially alike although devised originally for different viruses, for example, influenza viruses, Columbia-SK, St. Louis, or polyoma virus. The original Salk method, the technique devised by the Committee of Standard Procedure in Influenza Studies (1950), and the spectrophotometrically standardized test (Hierholzer *et al.* 1969) are recommended.

Micromethods for the virus hemagglutination-inhibition test have been designed by Smith and Mirick (1951), Fazekas de St. Groth et al. (1954), and Sever (1962). The microtechniques are useful when economical use of the immunological reagents is essential.

i. *Salk's Hemagglutination-Inhibition Test.* Serial twofold dilutions of an inactivated test serum are made directly in 0.5-ml volumes of 0.25% chicken erythrocyte suspension; 0.5 ml of a virus suspension containing two hemagglutinating units are added to each tube. Control tubes receive (a) 0.5 ml of virus and 0.5 ml erythrocyte suspension; (b) 0.5 ml of erythrocyte suspension and 0.5 ml of a known negative serum, diluted 1:8; and (c) 0.5 ml of saline and 0.5 ml of erythrocyte suspension.

All tubes are incubated at room temperature for 2 hours. Results are read by viewing tubes from the bottom of rack and observing pattern of sedimented erythrocytes. The highest serum dilution causing complete inhibition of the hemagglutination is taken as end point, and the titer is expressed in terms of the reciprocal of final serum dilution.

ii. *The CSSPIS Hemagglutination-Inhibition Test.* Reactants of the test are a 0.5% chicken erythrocyte suspension in saline solution, virus suspensions made from cultures in the allantoic fluid of strains PR8, Fm-1, and Lee, and diluted to contain one hemaggalutinating unit in 0.25-ml volume, and the inactivated serum being examined. The virus hemagglutinating unit is determined in the following manner. Two series of twofold virus dilutions are made in 0.25-ml volumes of saline. Each tube then receives 0.25 ml of saline and 0.25 ml of 0.5% chicken erythrocyte suspension. The erythrocyte control contains 0.5 ml of saline and 0.5 ml of erythrocyte suspension. The mixtures are shaken and left for 1 hour at 22 to 24° and for 90 minutes at 4°. Results are read by observing pattern of sedimented erythrocytes. A 0.25-ml quantity of the highest dilution of virus particles, which completely agglutinated the erythrocytes, denotes one hemagglutinating unit.

The inhibition test is conducted by setting up a few series of twofold progressing dilutions of serum, made in 0.25-ml volumes, one series for each antigen. Each series, except one, receives 0.25-ml amounts of different virus and 0.5 ml of 0.5% erythrocyte suspension.

The last series receives saline instead of the antigen. The mixtures are left for 60 minutes at 22 to 24°, and then read by observing the pattern of settled cells. The titer is expressed in terms of the highest initial serum dilution (i.e., the dilution before addition of the antigen and erythrocytes) which brought about a complete inhibition of hemagglutination.

iii. *Standardized Viral Hemagglutination-Inhibition Test.* Standardization of components for a hemagglutination-inhibition test and of the methods for testing antibodies is important for accuracy and reproducibility of data, since titers depend considerably on the test procedure and components. Standardization must apply to all the arbitrary constants which make up the test, such as volume and concentration of red blood cells, volume of antigen, composition of the diluent, serum treatment, relative volume of antigen, serum and erythrocyte, and incubation time. Here are the details for standardization of the reagents (Hierholzer and Suggs, 1969).

RBC Suspension Preparation. Blood collected from sheep, guinea pigs, rhesus and velvet monkeys, albino rats, white mice, geese, chickens, or type "O" humans is stored in Alsever's solution. Alsever's solution, pH 6.1, sterilized by membrane filtration, contains:

Dextrose	20.5 g
Trisodium citrate dihydrate	8.0 g

Citric acid monohydrate	0.55 g
Sodium chloride	4.2 g
Distilled water	1000 ml

The Alsever solution is used in the proportion of 4 to 1 with blood. Before use, the red blood cells are washed and resuspended in phosphate buffered saline (PBS), pH 7.2.

Phosphate-buffered saline (PBS), 0.171 *M,* pH 7.2, is supplemented with bovine albumin, fraction V (BAFV).

Disodium phosphate anhydrous	1096 g
Monosodium phosphate monohydrate	0.315 g
Sodium chloride	8.5 g
BAFV	10 g
Distilled water	1000 ml

Standardization of RBC Suspensions by Spectrophotometry (Hierholzer and Suggs, 1969). Here 0.4% mammalian and 0.5% chicken cells standardized spectrophotometrically are used.

The spectrophotometric standardization of RBC suspension is far superior to the conventional procedure in which red blood cell suspensions are prepared by reading the packed RBC volume in a conical centrifuge tube after the third wash and diluting the packed cells to the desired concentration.

The determination of an adjustment of standardized RBC suspension depends on the calculation of target OD values of a cell suspension on the photometer from a standard curve of 0.280 mg of cyanmethemoglobin per 100 ml, followed by computation of the "factor." By means of this factor, the target OD for each self-suspension to be used is calculated as follows:

$$\text{target OD} = \frac{\text{target milligrams of cyanmethemoglobin per 100 ml}}{\text{factor (milligrams of cyanmethemoglobin per 100 ml/OD)}}$$

The target OD calculated and recorded for each of the four possible RBC suspensions are employed for all subsequent cell standardization on the same spectrophotometer. The standardization of red cells is then performed as follows:

Red cells preserved in Alsever's solution are centrifuged and washed three times in PBS, and after each wash the buffy coat is carefully removed. Read the packed cell volume after the last wash and dilute it to an approximate 4% suspension with PBS. The cells are washed three times in conical graduated centrifuge tubes at approximately 1500 $\times$ *g* for 5 minutes at room temperature. Mix and transfer 1.0 ml of the suspension into a 25-ml volumetric flask. Fill to the mark with a cyanmethemoglobin reagent and mix carefully allowing the solution to stand for about 30 minutes at room temperature.

Check the calibration of the spectrophotometer by reading the absorbence of the 1:2 standard consisting of 40 mg of cyanmethemoglobin per 100 ml and checking this reading with that on the previous standard curves. Transfer an aliquot of the cell suspension to incubate and read the OD at 540 nm against reagent blank.

The dilution needed (DN) for desired suspension is calculated as follows:

$$DN = \frac{\text{OD of test suspension} \times \text{volume of test suspension}}{\text{target OD}}$$

Preparation of Cyanmethemoglobin Standard Curve. Cyanmethemoglobin is obtained by lyzing erythrocytes in a hypertonic solution following which the liberated hemoglobin is oxidized to cyanmethemoglobin which has a strong adsorption band at 540 nm. (A cyanmethemoglobin reagent may be obtained in powder form from Hycel Inc., Houston, Tex.) The reagent is used at one half strength and it can be stored at room temperature.

The cyanmethemoglobin standard curve is prepared by diluting the Hycel standard to contain 80, 60, 40, 20, and 0 mg of cyanmethemoglobin per 100 ml. The absorbence is read at 540 nm to calculate a factor by which the OD of unknown samples is converted to milligrams of cyanmethemoglobin per 100 ml. The factor can be calculated by dividing the sum of concentrations of the standards (at 60, 40, 20, and where the 0 standard is the reagent blank) by the sum of the OD readings of the standards.

The average of five OD readings for each sample is converted to grams of hemoglobulin or milligrams of cyanmethemoglobin per 100 ml by multiplication of the OD by the factor calculated from the appropriate standard curve as follows.

grams of hemoglobin or milligrams of cyanmethemoglobin per 100 ml of suspension x = OD of suspension x × factor

Antisera should be treated by adsorption with the erythrocytes to be used in the test, by kaolin extraction, or by the RDE of *Vibrio comma*. The adsorption is carried out using 0.1 ml of the appropriate 50% RBC suspension per milliliter of starting serum dilution at 4° for 1 hour. The cells are removed by centrifugation. The kaolin extraction is conducted by exposing a volume of 1–5 serum dilution to an equal volume of 25% acid washed kaolin in PBS, the mixture being incubated at room temperature for 20 minutes. This is followed by centrifugation and withdrawal of the serum.

The RDE treatment involves 1 volume of undiluted serum and 4 volumes of RDE (100 units/ml), incubated overnight in a water bath at 37°. Three volumes of 2.5% trisodium citrate (dihydrate) is then added; the mixture by addition of PBS. These treatments cause the removal or inactivation of the nonspecific inhibitors and natural hemagglutinins from the sera.

iv. *Viral Hemagglutination Inhibition Test.* The diluent for most systems in which viral hemagglutinin and antibody is 0.1 M pH 7.2 PBS with two exceptions: the testing of the group III adenoviruses requires a PBS-HS mixture consisting of PBS containing 1% heterotypic serum, usually adenovirus 6 antiserum, and polyoma virus which requires a PBS/BSA diluent consisting of PBS containing 0.1% bovine serum albumin fraction V.

The standardized HA microtest employs 0.05 ml of virus dilutions and 0.05 ml of RBC suspension per well. After the incubation at a required temperature for 1 to 2 hours, the end point of hemagglutination is determined. The temperature for most viruses, such as reoviruses, myxoviruses, PVM, and Coxsackie viruses is 24°; but the temperature of 37° is required for adenoviruses and some types of Coxsackie B viruses, whereas optimal temperature for Coxsackie A viruses, as well as for polyoma and K virus, is 4°.

Standardized hemagglutination-inhibition microtest is performed as follows: a serum from which nonspecific inhibitors have been removed with kaolin is diluted starting at 1:10 to a desired final dilution in a volume of 0.025 ml. Each dilution of serum receives equal volume of virus suspension containing 4 HA units per well. The mixtures are incubated at room temperature for 40 to 60 minutes after which 0.05 ml of RBC suspension is added, and the reaction mixtures are incubated for 1 to 2 hours at the temperature indicated above. The end point of inhibition of hemagglutination is read and the corresponding final dilution of serum is recorded as the titer. An HI macrotest is performed in tube tests with $10\times$ larger volumes of components of the test.

If a twofold dilution scheme is used and if serial specimens from one individual are employed fourfold or greater changes in the titer are considered as diagnostically and clinically significant.

v. *The Capillary Hemagglutination-Inhibition Test by Smith and Mirick (1951).* The test is carried out in capillary tubes of a standard bore of 1.2 and 76 mm long. The internal wall of tubes is coated with a heparin solution containing 10 mg of heparin per milliliter of isotonic saline to prevent blood clotting. Equal volumes of the blood sample being examined and a virus suspension containing eight hemagglutinating units are introduced into tubes by capillary attraction. The tubes are placed in a plasticene block and incubated at room temperature or at 37° for 15 to 30 minutes. The hemagglutination, in a negative case, is shown by red blood cells being sedimented in the lower third or quarter part of the tube. Nonagglutinated cells remain uniformly distributed throughout the tube. Nonspecific inhibitory substances present in certain sera can be removed by treatment with filtrates of *Vibrio comma* at 37°, for 15 to 18 hours, using 0.5 ml of filtrate per 0.1 ml of serum (Appleby and Stuart-Harris, 1950). A technique of the hemagglutination-inhibition test set up on plastic trays was published by Fazekas de St. Groth et al. (1954) and by Sever (1962).

The virus hemagglutination-inhibition tests have been used mostly for the detection of antibodies against myxoviruses, poxviruses, adenoviruses, enteroviruses, reoviruse, rubella virus, and some murine viruses.

2. The Virus Hemagglutinin-Absorption Test

According to Walker and Horsfall technique (1950), as modified by Hamre et al. (1958), a virus antiserum diluted to contain about 64 hemagglutination-inhibition units per 0.2 ml is absorbed twice with pellets of a virus at 4°, left overnight each time. The mixture is then centrifuged at $40,000 \times g$. Excess virus should be removed from the supernatant fluid with packed, washed chicken erythrocytes by incubation at 4° for 90 minutes, followed by centrifugation at $500 \times g$ for 10 minutes. The supernatant fluid is tested by a hemagglutination-inhibition test set up against another virus. The virus hemagglutinin-absorption test can be used for the study on antigenic relationships among viruses.

3. The Immune Adherence-Inhibition Test

The absorption of erythrocytes by tissue culture cells infected with the influenza virus can be prevented by exposing an infected monkey-kidney cell monolayer to a homologous immune serum before the erythrocytes are added. The characteristic aggregation of erythrocytes over the cell monolayer is hence abolished. Undiluted or serially diluted serum can be used. The control, virus-infected cells must not be pretreated with the antiserum and should show the characteristic aggregation of absorbed red blood cells of guinea pig or chicken.

The immune adherence-inhibition test, according to Irie *et al.* (1969), is conducted in the following manner.

The antigen diluted in GVB diluent (0.3 ml) is added to 0.2 ml of an antiserum dilution and incubated at 37° for 30 minutes and at 0° for 60 minutes. The reaction mixture is centrifuged at $1000 \times g$ for 15 minutes. To the supernatant is added 0.1 ml of a suspension of tumor cells 10^5 (ml/ 0.1 ml of GVB diluent), and the mixture is incubated at 37° and 0° for 20 minutes; 7 ml of cold diluent are added and the mixture is centrifuged at $600 \times g$ for 8 minutes. To the deposited tumor cells are added 0.4 ml of complement (120 C'IA50) absorbed with the target cells and indicator erythrocytes. Finally, 0.1 ml volume of human type O, Rh+ erythrocytes (2 × 10⁷ cells) is added, and the mixture is incubated at 37° for 10 minutes and at 20° for 10 minutes. The immune adherence pattern is read under a microscope.

Inhibition of immune adherence is signified by the absence of clumps of erythorcytes attached to the tumor cells. If more than two erythrocytes are attached to more than 25% of target cells, the adherence-inhibition test may be regarded as negative. The GVB diluent is a gelatin veronal buffer containing 0.02% KCl and 0.1% glucose.

The dose of complement for the immune adherence-inhibition by the immune adherence test, and it is expressed by C'IA50 (50% immune-adherence) units (Nishioka, 1963).

4. The Bacterial Hemagglutinin-Inhibition Test

In the test devised by Kwapinski (1965), the following reactants are used: 1% suspension of chicken erythrocytes, an inactivated serum being examined, a buffered saline solution, pH 7.2, and a preparation of bacterial or fungal hemagglutinins. The hemagglutinating unit of this preparation is determined as described on p. 400.

The test is set up as follows. Serial twofold dilutions of a serum are made in 0.2-ml volumes of buffered saline, pH 7.0. Each tube receives 0.2 ml of hemagglutinin containing four hemagglutinating units. Control tubes receive 0.2 ml of saline and 0.2 ml of hemagglutinin solution or 0.2 ml of the lowest serum dilution and 0.2 ml of saline. All mixtures are incubated at 37° for 30 minutes. Then 4% erythrocyte suspension is added, in 0.2-ml volumes, to each tube which should be reincubated at 37° for 60 minutes. Results are read by observing patterns of sedimented red blood cells. The highest dilution of serum, at which no hemagglutination occurs, is taken as end point, and the titer is expressed by the reciprocal final solution.

The test can be used for the identification of antigens or antibodies, and for studies on antigenic relationships among microorganisms.

Dolby's (1958) Bacterial Hemagglutinin-Inhibition Test. Twofold serial diluitons of antiserum in 0.2-ml volumes are mixed with 0.2 ml of a hemagglutinating suspension of bacteria containing sixteen hemagglutinating units per milliliters. The mixtures are incubated at 37° for 1 hour, and 0.2 ml of 1% sheep red blood cells are added to each tube. The tubes are left at 37° for 1 hour and at room temperature for 2 hours, then read.

The bacterial hemagglutinin-inhibition test can also be set up on a porcelain tile with depressions. In this technique (Gillies and Duguid, 1958), one drop of undiluted serum is first mixed with one drop of 3% guinea pig red blood cells. This is followed by one drop of a preparation of bacterial hemagglutinins, used in the strength which gives a strong hemagglutination in the controls containing no serum.

III. IMMUNOBIOCHEMICAL INHIBITION TESTS

The principle of all the immunobiochemical inhibition tests is the abolition by an immunologically specific inhibitor of a characteristic chemical reaction, which is normally shown by a biochemically and antigenically active substance acting on an appropriate substrate. The following tests depend on the immune inhibition of biochemical reactions:

1. Tests based on the immunological inhibition of active hemolysis: the anstreptolysin test, antistaphylolysin test, and the virus hemolysis-inhibition test.

2. Tests involving inhibition of active hemagglutination.

3. Tests based on the neutralization of specific proteolytic enzymes: the antistreptokinase test, antistaphylolysin test, antiproteinase test, anticoagulase test.

4. Tests based on the inhibition of specific carbohydrases, the antihyaluronidase assay.

5. Tests depending on specific inhibitions of nucleases, e.g., the antistreptoribonuclease assay.

1. The Active Hemolysis-Inhibition Tests

Hemolysins produced by certain microorganisms are able to destroy red blood cells, which results in the release of hemoglobin. Most hemolysins are antigenic, thus inducing the formation of antihemolysins in the host. These specific inhibitors neutralize homologous hemolysins, rendering them incapable of causing the lysis of erythrocytes.

Thus bacterial or virus hemolysin-inhibition tests involve three principal components: a hemolysin as antigen, a serum containing specific antihemosin as antibody, and red blood cells as substrate of the specific biochemical reaction and an indicator of the immunological action.

i. *The Antistreptolysin Test.* In this test, the volume or dilution of serum is determined, which in the presence of a constant dose of the streptolysin O prevents the hemolysis of an amount of erythrocytes.

Methods for the obtaining and the purification of preparations of the streptolysin O were published by Smythe and Harris (1940), Herbert and Todd (1941), and Pentz and Shigemura (1955). The combining activity of a streptolysin O preparation is determined prior to the test proper by testing it versus a standard antiserum supplied by the Serum Institute, Carshalton, Surrey, Great Britain, or Statens Serum Institut, Copenhagen.

For estimation of the combining dose of a streptolysin O preparation, the standard antiserum must be diluted in an isotonic saline solution, pH 6.4,* to contain one unit of antistreptolysin per milliliter solution.

Determination of the combining unit of streptolysin O is conducted as indicated in Table 85. End point of the titration is indicated by the last tube in the series showing a complete inhibition of hemolysis. The amount of streptolysin O in this tube denotes one combining unit. The combining unit can be determined more precisely by repeating the titration with amounts of streptolysin used at 0.01-ml increments between the tube showing complete inhibition of hemolysis and the next in the series. The antistreptolysin O test was originally published by Todd (1932) and modified by Hodge and Swift (1933), Coburn and Pauli (1939), Smythe and Harris (1940), Herbert and Todd (1941), Robinette (1952), Rantz et al., (1956), Crawford and Robinson (1954), and Kwapinski (1965). Economical microtechniques were published by van der Veen (1955), Rappaport and Stark (1955), and Jablon et al. (1958). A method of the antistreptolysin O titration in the capillary blood was published by Crawford and Robinson (1954). Robinette's technique (1952) is shown diagrammatically in Table 86.

The ASO titer is represented by the serum dilution in the last tube showing complete inhibition of hemolysis.

The Microtechnique of the Antistreptolysin O Test by Jablon et al. The test serum is diluted 1:10, 1:100, and 1:500 in buffered saline; 0.05 ml of each dilution is mixed with an equal volume of Difco streptolysin O solution made as indicated by the producer. The tubes are gently shaken and incubated at 37° for 15 minutes; 0.05 ml of 5% human group O erythrocyte suspension as added; the mixtures are reincubated at 37° for 15 minutes, and then centrifuged at 300-400 × g for 1 minute, and read for inhibition of hemolysis.

The antistreptolysin test is very specific and sensitive, although its "experimental error" varies between 20 and 30% of the actual titer. The test is widely used for the immunological diagnosis of acute streptococcal infections and particularly of rheumatic fever (see Kwapinski and Snyder, 1962).

Rapid Antistreptolysin O Slide Test. A rapid test for determination of antistreptolysin O (Blum and Ellner, 1970) is carried out as follows: 0.1 ml of the tested serum is added to 0.3 ml of freshly reconstituted standard streptolysin O solution and the mixture is left at room temperature for 15 minutes. Then 0.05 ml or one drop of this serum dilution and an equal volume of an ASO latex reagent (Behring Diagnostics, Woodbury) are

---

* Isotonic saline solution buffered at pH 6.4 to 6.6 contains in 1000 ml of distilled water 4.5 g of NaCl, 9.0 g of KH_2PO_4, and 23.3 g of $Na_2HPO_4 \cdot 12H_2O$.

Table 85. Estimation of the Combining Dose of Streptolysin O

Tube Number	1	2	3	4	5	6	7	8	9	10	Control Tube
Todd's standard antiserum (1 unit/ml) (ml)	1.0	1.0	1.0	1.0	1.0	1.0	1.0	1.0	1.0	1.0	1.0
Streptolysin O solution (ml)	0.50	0.45	0.40	0.35	0.30	0.25	0.20	0.15	0.10	0.05	0.0
Isotonic saline solution (ml)	0.0	0.15	0.10	0.15	0.20	0.25	0.30	0.35	0.40	0.45	0.50

Incubation at 37° for 15 minutes

Tube Number	1	2	3	4	5	6	7	8	9	10	Control Tube
5% suspension of rabbit erythrocytes (ml)	0.50	0.50	0.50	0.50	0.50	0.50	0.50	0.50	0.50	0.50	0.50
Final volume of fluid (ml)	2.0	2.0	2.0	2.0	2.0	2.0	2.0	2.0	2.0	2.0	2.0

Incubation at 37° for 60 minutes

Table 86. Robinette's (1952) Antistreptolysin O Test

Tube Number	1	2	3	4	5	6	7	8	9	10	11	12	13
1 ml of the serum diluted 1:	50	100	150	200	250	300	350	400	450	500	600	800	1000
Streptolysin O (2 units/ml)	0.5	0.5	0.5	0.5	0.5	0.5	0.5	0.5	0.5	0.5	0.5	0.5	0.5

Incubation at room temperature for 15 minutes

| 5% suspension of rabbit erythro-cytes or 10% suspension of human group O erythrocytes (ml) | 0.5 | 0.5 | 0.5 | 0.5 | 0.5 | 0.5 | 0.5 | 0.5 | 0.5 | 0.5 | 0.5 | 0.5 | 0.5 |

Incubation at 37° for 60 minutes

mixed on a glass slide. The mixture is rotated 10 times and examined microscopically for the presence of flocculates, which usually occur within a few seconds of rotation. Specimens showing no flocculates after 10 revolutions are regarded as having ASO titers of 166 units or less.

The antistreptolysin S test was originally devised by Todd et al. (1939), and its spectrophotometric modification was described by Robinson (1951).

ii. *The Antistaphylolysin Test.* The principle of this test is the reaction between a *Staphylococcus* specific hemolysin and corresponding antibody, detected by erythrocytes, employed as indicator. Erythrocytes, normally susceptible to the staphylolysin, are not lyzed if the staphylolysin has combined with its antibody. The pattern of antistaphylolysin test is shown in Table 87.

Table 87.   A Schedule for Antistaphylolysin Determination

Tube Number	1	2	3	4	5	6	7	8	9	10
0.1% gelatin saline	—	0.5	0.5	0.5	0.5	0.5	0.5	0.5	0.5	0.5
Serum (inactivated at 56° for 30 minutes)	0.5	0.5	0.5	0.5	0.5	0.4	0.5	0.5	0.5	—
Staphylolysin (2 units/ml)	0.5	0.5	0.5	0.5	0.5	0.5	0.5	0.5	—	0.5

Incubation at room temperature for 30 minutes

| 10% rabbit red cells in 0.1% gelatin saline | 0.1 | 0.1 | 0.1 | 0.1 | 0.1 | 0.1 | 0.1 | 0.1 | 0.1 | 0.1 |

Incubation at 37° for 1 hour

| Saline (ml) | 3.0 | 3.0 | 3.0 | 3.0 | 3.0 | 3.0 | 3.0 | 3.0 | 3.0 | 3.0 |

Centrifuge all tubes and read the degree of hemolysis. The tube showing 50% hemolysis is the end point. The reciprocal of this dilution is expressed as the titer in units per milliliter.

iii. *The Leptospira Hemolysin-Inhibition Test.* A test for determination of the serum inhibition of hemolysis produced by leptospiras was published by Russell (1956). In this test, the sera of animals immunized with cultures of leptospiras are serially diluted in 0.5-ml volumes of a buffered saline. An equal volume of the antigen (a culture filtrate of leptospiras) is added to each tube, and these mixtures are incubated for 25 to 30 minutes at 37°. Each tube then receives 0.5 ml of a 5% suspension of sheep red blood cells. These mixtures are incubated for 4 hours at 37° and left overnight at 4°. End point of the neutralization is estimated by the highest serum dilution showing no hemolysis.

iv. *The Hemolysin Diffusion-Inhibition Test (Russell, 1956).* Two filter paper strips (20 × 4 mm) are saturated with 0.1 ml of the antigen or a filtrate and placed parallel on a 5% sheep blood agar plate. A larger (26 × 11 mm) paper strip, saturated with the antiserum, is placed perpendicularly at the bottom of the other two paper pieces. Control plates may contain a standard positive serum or a "negative" serum. The plates are incubated at 37° for 48 hours and left at 4° for 24 to 48 hours.

Diffusing hemolysin produces a clear zone around the two strips impregnated with the hemolytic antigen except of the area bordering paper saturated with the antiserum. In this area, the hemolysis zone is either reduced or abolished altogether following the serological reaction.

v. *The Viral Hemolysin-Inhibition Test.* In the technique devised by Kahnke (1951), 1-ml volumes of a standard virus suspension are added to two series of dilutions of an inactivated serum tested. Dilutions of the serum are made in 1-ml volumes of $M/15$ phosphate buffer, pH 7.2. Three control tubes receive; (a) 1 ml of the virus suspension and 1 ml of buffer; (b) 2 ml of the buffer alone; and (c) 0.5 ml of a hyperimmune serum diluted 1:100, 1 ml of the virus suspension, and 0.5 ml of the buffer.

The mixtures are incubated at 37° for 30 minutes. Each tube then receives 2 ml of 2% chicken erythrocytes, and all mixtures are reincubated at 37° for 2 hours. The contents of tubes should be centrifuged, and supernatants pooled from two parallel tubes are read against the supernatants of blank control tubes.

2. The Antileukocidin Test

Two methods of the antileukocidin assay are distinguished: one is based on determination of the inhibition of the leukocyte respiration; in the other, the death of leukocytes is determined by microscopic observation of characteristic morphological changes in the cells. The first test was devised by Neisser and Wechsberg (1900) and modified by Jensen and Maaloe (1950) and Woodin (1959). The second method of the antileukocidin test was published by Panton and Valentine (1932) and modified by Gladstone and Heyningen (1957) and Gladstone et al. (1962).

Constituents of the Gladstone et al. (1962) test are (a) a leukocidin preparation; (b) a test serum, inactivated at 56° for 30 minutes; (c) leukocytes; and (d) a gelatin diluent (0.5% gelatin solution in saline).

Leukocytes are obtained from human blood in the following manner. Fresh human blood is mixed with an equal volume of ice-cold Hanks' solution or balanced salt solution in a siliconed tube. The diluted blood is dropped onto a number of glass areas of a Parafilm slide preparation, placed into a moist Petri dish, and incubated at 37° for 30 minutes. The clot is then removed with fine forceps, and red cells are washed away with 0.5% solution of gelatin in saline. Leukocytes remain adhered to the glass. (Parafilm slides are made by cutting 0.5-cm-diameter holes through a Parafilm, which is then placed on a glass slide to be heated at 60 to 70° until the film melts and firmly adheres to the glass.)

The leukocidin preparation should be standardized against a standard antitoxin. For this purpose, 0.2 ml of serial dilutions of a leukocidin preparation at 20% increments is added to an equal volume of a standard antileukocidin containing one unit and left at room temperature for 15 minutes; 0.2 ml of each mixture is then added to one compartment of the leukocyte slide, placed in a moist Petri dish. After 30-minute incubation at 37°, the slide is scanned with 10× objective on a dark field.

The end point is denoted by a preparation containing the smallest amount of leukocidin in which the leukocytes have become spherical and show nuclei. The L+ dose of leukocidin is determined by the amount of the leukocidin preparation which, when mixed with one unit of antitoxin and added to the leukocytes, is just sufficient to cause morphological changes characteristic of the death of leukocytes.

The antileukocidin test is set up as follows: 0.02-ml volumes of serial dilutions of a leukocidin preparation are mixed on a waxed welled slide with equal volumes of an inactivated test serum diluted 1:5, 1:10, or 1:25. The mixtures are left at room temperature for 15 minutes; 0.02 ml of each mixture is then added to one compartment of the leukocyte slide incubated at 37° for 30 minutes, and examined microscopically with 10× objective and a dark field. Dead leukocytes occur in the form of spherical cells with visible nuclei and granules showing the Brownian movement. In contrast, living leukocytes show an irregular shape and a brighter outline; the nuclei are nonvisible.

The end point is determined by the lowest dilution of leukocidin, at which the leukocytes are killed. The L+ volume of this tube multiplied by the serum dilution gives the antibody contents in units per milliliter.

3. The Protease-Inhibition Tests

i. *The Antistreptokinase Test.* The antistreptokinase test depends on a reaction between the streptokinase and its specific serological inhibitor, which brings about the inhibition of fibrinolysis, normally catalyzed by the free streptokinase.

Methods of the antistreptokinase titration were published by Garner and Tillett (1934), Massel et al. (1939), Christensen (1949), and Kwapinski and Snyder (1962). The latter two methods are recommended.

Christensen's Method for Antistreptokinase Test. The assay is performed in four steps, which involve the streptominase titration, determination of the antistreptokinase unit in a standard antiserum, the standardization of streptokinase against a standard antiserum, and determination of the antistreptokinase titer in an unknown serum.

The sreptokinase titration is carried out in the following manner. Serial dilutions of a streptokinase preparation in 0.1-ml volumes of a gelatin buffer are added to the substrate containing 0.4 ml of a 0.25% suspension of beef plasma fibrinogen diluted in a borate buffer, 0.5 ml of a 0.25% solution of the third plasma fraction (as the source of plasminogen), and 0.1 ml of a hemostatic globulin diluted 1:3 in a borate buffer (as the source of thrombin). The mixtures are incubated at 35°, and the time of the fibrin clot lysis is measured. The dilution or the amount of streptokinase, at which the fibrin clot has been dissolved within 10 minutes, is taken as one unit of streptokinase. The antistreptokinase unit (1 ASK unit) is estimated by the highest dilution of a standard serum (or of the second fraction of human serum containing γ-globulin), at which the biochemical activity of one unit of streptokinase is inhibited. For this purpose, a series of dilutions of a lyophilized preparation of human serum fraction II is made in 0.5-ml volumes. Each tube then receives 0.5 ml of a streptokinase solution containing one unit of streptokinase in this volume. The test mixtures are incubated at 35° for 10 minutes. Each tube now receives 0.5 ml of 0.25% solution of human scrum fraction III, 0.5 ml of 0.5% beef fibrinogen suspension, and either 0.1 ml of a hemostatic globulin diluted 1:3 in saline or 0.1 ml of a thrombin solution. The tubes are incubated at 35° for 30 minutes.

The highest dilution of standard serum is then recorded, at which the lysis of fibrin clot has been prevented. One ASK unit is present in this dilution or amount of antiserum.

Standardization of a streptokinase preparation against a standard immune serum is carried out as follows. A series of dilutions of streptokinase is made in 0.5-ml volumes of gelatin buffer, pH 7.6 to 7.8. Each tubes receives 0.5 ml of a solution of standard antiserum containing two units of ASK in 1 ml. The serum should be slightly preheated at 56° for 30 to 45 minutes to destroy a small amount of plasminogen and the nonspecific streptokinase inhibitor. The test mixtures are incubated at 35° for 30 minutes, and supplemented with 0.5 ml of 0.25% solution of serum fraction III, 0.5 ml of 0.50% suspension of beef fibrinogen, and 0.1 ml of hemostatic globulin diluted 1:3 or a thrombin solution. After another incubation in a water bath at 35°, the first tube in the row in which the fibrin clot is not dissolved is recorded. The unit of streptokinase corresponds to the dilution and amount of streptokinase preparation in this tube.

Determination of the antistreptokinase titer is carried out as follows. The serum being examined is inactivated for 30 minutes at 56° and serially diluted in 0.5-ml volumes of saline. Each tube then receives 0.5 ml of a streptokinase solution containing approximately one to two units of streptokinase in this volume. The samples are incubated at 35° for 30 minutes and supplemented with three other ingredients of the test, that is, 0.5 ml of 0.25% solution of serum fraction III, 0.5 ml of 0.5% suspension of fibrinogen, and 0.1 ml of a hemostatic globulin or thrombin solution. After another incubation in a water bath at 35° for 35 minutes, the highest dilution of the test serum is recorded, which prevented the lysis of fibrin clot. Results are expressed in terms of the ASK units.

Kwapinski's Method of the Antistreptokinase Test. This assay is divided into three steps: (a) titration of the thrombin; (b) estimation of the streptokinase titer; and (c) determination of the antistreptokinase titer.

Titration of the thrombin is performed to estimate the minimum dose of a thrombin preparation needed to transform the fibrinogen to fibrin, under the experimental conditions. If a purified lyophilized preparation of human or horse thrombin is available, the titration is carried out only once in 1 or 2 months, in the manner presented in Table 88.

The streptokinase titer should be estimated a day prior to a series of antistreptominase tests. In this titration, the minimal fibrinolytic dose of streptokinase (DFM) is determined, that is, the dilution of streptokinase bringing about a complete lysis of fibrin under conditions of the experiment. It is carried out as shown in Table 89.

The antistreptokinase test determines the highest dilution of test serum, at which the minimal fibrinolytic dose of streptokinase is neutralized so that lysis of the fibrin clot does not occur. The serum being examined should be inactivated at 62° for 3 minutes or at 56° for 30 minutes to destroy fibrinogen and nonspecific inhibitors of the antistreptokinase. Thus the inactivated serum is serially diluted from 1:20 to 1:2560 in 0.5-ml volume of a saline solution or a phosphate, pH 7.4, buffer. Two or three control tubes receive 0.5 ml of a streptokinase solution containing one minimal fibrinolytic unit in this volume. After the incubation for 30 minutes in a water bath at 37°, the substrate is added. The substrate consists of 0.5 ml of 2% suspension of fibrinogen and 0.2 ml of a thrombin solution containing one unit in this volume of fluid. The substrate for streptokinase is a fibrin clot formed by the thrombin activation of fibrinogen. The fibrinogen suspension consists of 2.0 g of a purified horse fibrinogen preparation, 0.2 g of lyophilized human plasma, and 98 ml of phosphate buffer, pH 7.4. Each series of tests is accompanied by a control row of dilutions of a "negative" serum, tested simultaneously.

Table 88.   A Schedule for Thrombin Titration

Tube Number	1	2	3	4	5	6	7	8	Control 9
Thrombin									
Dilution 1:	100	200	400	800	1600	3200	6400	12800	—
ml	0.2	0.2	0.2	0.2	0.2	0.2	0.2	0.2	—
Phosphate buffer, pH 7.4 or saline solution (ml)	1.0	1.0	1.0	1.0	1.0	1.0	1.0	1.0	1.2
2% activated fibrinogen (ml)	0.5	0.5	0.5	0.5	0.5	0.5	0.5	0.5	0.5
Final volume (ml)	1.7	1.7	1.7	1.7	1.7	1.7	1.7	1.7	1.7

Incubation for 5 to 10 minutes at room temperature or at 37°

Table 89.   A Schedule for Streptokinase Titration

Tube Number	1	2	3	4	5	6	7	8	Control
Streptokinase									
Dilution 1:	1000	2000	4000	8000	16000	32000	64000	128000	—
ml	0.5	0.5	0.5	0.5	0.5	0.5	0.5	0.5	—
Saline solution (ml)	0.5	0.5	0.5	0.5	0.5	0.5	0.5	0.5	1.0
2% activated fibrinogen (ml)	0.5	0.5	0.5	0.5	0.5	0.5	0.5	0.5	0.5
Thrombin diluted at its titer (ml)	0.2	0.2	0.2	0.2	0.2	0.2	0.2	0.2	0.2
Final volume (ml)	1.7	1.7	1.7	1.7	1.7	1.7	1.7	1.7	1.7

Incubation for 5 minutes at room temperature and for 45 minutes in a water bath at 37°

All mixtures are left for 5 minutes or longer at room temperature at 37° until the fibrin clot is formed, and then incubated at 37° for about 30 minutes, until the fibrin clot in the control tubes containing no serum dissolves completely. The titer of antistreptokinase is determined by the highest serum dilution, at which the clot fills over half the tube. The result can be expressed in terms of the number of ASK units, which corresponds to the serum dilution and is equivalent to one unit of streptokinase present in each tube.

ii. *The Antiproteinase Test.* Three techniques can be used for titration of the antiproteinase test: (a) the milk-clotting inhibition test; (b) the complement fixation test; and (c) the erythrocyte absorption-agglutination test. The last assay as regarded as most sensitive.

The Antiproteinase Milk-Clotting Inhibition Test. This test, devised by Ogburn et al. (1958) for the antistreptoproteinase determination, is based on the neutralization of the proteinase by a specific serum inhibitor which prevents the milk proteolysis and clotting. The test is carried out as follows.

A series of twofold dilutions, in 0.4-ml volumes of a saline solution containing 0.1% of normal serum, receives 0.2 ml (two units) of a proteinase preparation. One control tube is set up with 0.4 ml of diluent and 0.2 ml of proteinase preparation, and another tube with 0.4 ml of the first dilution of serum and 0.2 ml of diluent. The tubes are left at 37° for 30 minutes; 0.6 ml of skimmed milk with sodium thioglycollate is then added to each tube. Contents of the tubes are examined for the presence of clots after 18 hours of incubation at 37°. The highest serum dilution, at which no clot is observed, is taken as titer of the antiproteinase.

The Antiproteinase Complement-Fixation Test. This test can be set up either with a constant amount of serum and varying dilutions of a specific proteinase or with a constant amount of proteinase and serial dilutions of the serum.

In the first pattern of the test, twofold dilutions of a proteinase preparation in 0.4-ml volume of saline are mixed with 0.1 ml of test serum diluted to its optimum concentration, and with 0.1 ml of a guinea pig serum containing 1.3 units of complement. After a 30-minute incubation at 37°, all tubes receive 0.1-ml volumes of 4% washed sheep erythrocytes and 0.1 ml of a rabbit antisheep-erythrocyte serum diluted to the optimum concentration of this system. The tubes are left at 37° for 30 minutes and overnight at 4°, and then the degree of hemolysis in each tube is recorded.

In the assay with constant amount of proteinase, the inactivated serum is serially diluted in 0.4-ml volumes, and mixed with 0.1 ml (two units) of a proteinase solution and 0.1 ml (1.3 hemolytic units) of a guinea pig serum. After an incubation at 37° for 30 minutes, 0.1 ml of 4% suspension of sheep red cells and 0.1 ml of rabbit antisheep-erythrocyte serum, diluted to the optimal concentration for this system, are added. The tubes are reincubated at 37° for 30 minutes and left at 4° overnight. The last tube showing a complete inhibition of hemolysis is chosen as end point. The final dilution of serum in this tube denotes the titer of specific antiproteinase.

The Antiproteinase Erythrocyte Absorption-Agglutination Test. This hemagglutination test, after Ogburn et al. (1958), is carried out with tanned erythrocytes, coated by a proteinase preparation in the following manner. A 2 to 5% suspension of fresh sheep erythrocytes in isotonic buffered saline is treated with an equal volume of 5.0 mg % tannic acid solution, and incubated at 37° for 10 minutes. The erythrocytes are then centrifuged, washed twice with saline, and resuspended to the original volume; 5 ml of this suspension is mixed with 0.5 ml of a specific proteinase preparation at its optimal sensitizing concentration, and incubated at 37° for 30 minutes. The red blood cells are then centrifuged and washed three times with an isotonic saline solution containing 1% normal rabbit serum, and resuspended in this diluent in the original volume. The suspension is diluted 1:10 in 1% normal rabbit serum prior to use in the hemagglutination test.

The serum being examined is serially diluted in twofold steps, in 0.2-ml volumes of an isotonic saline solution containing 1% normal rabbit serum. Each dilution receives 0.2 ml of 0.25% suspension of sensitized erythrocytes, and the tubes are left at room temperature for 30 minutes, then centrifuged for 4 minutes at 800 rpm, shaken, and read. The highest dilution of serum showing definite hemagglutination is taken as the titer of antiproteinase.

iii. *The Anticoagulase Test.* The coagulase is a protetolytic enzyme which promotes the clotting of fibrinogen activated by a substance occurring in the plasma and tissue globulins, termed the coagulase activator, coagulase reacting factor, or coagulase globulin (Smith and Hall, 1944; Tager, 1948). This activator can be precipitated from the plasma at 60% saturation with ammonium sulfate. Coagulase is produced by some bacteria, and particularly by pathogenic strains of *Staphylococcus aureus*. It is antigenically active.

A specific inhibitor which occurs in human sera in infections with coagulase-producing bacteria inhibits *in vitro* the clotting of plasma or another substrate suitable for the action of coagulase. This is the principle on which the anticoagulase test depends. Thus ingredients of the anticoagulase test are an appropriate substrate for the function of coagulase, a preparation of coagulase, and serum to be examined for the presence of anticoagulase.

A substrate for the coagulase assay is provided by a diluted human or rabbit plasma, a mixture of human and bovine plasma (Illés, 1964), a solution of bovine fibrinogen activated by minute amounts of 0.1% human serum, or 0.1% human fibrinogen containing 5% rabbit plasma as a activator. The rabbit plasma can be stored for months at 20° without any loss of the activator.

Coagulase can be produced by the method of Duthie and Lorenz (1952) or Tager (1948). According to the Duthie and Lorenz technique, a 12-hour infusion broth culture of an active producer of coagulase, for example, the strain "Newman" (NCTC 8178) of *Staphylococcus aureus,* is mixed with "Filter cel" and passed through a filter paper.

The filtrate is cooled at 4° and treated with cadmium sulfate, added to a final 0.5% concentration. The mixture should be adjusted to pH 5.8 and left at 4° overnight, then centrifuged. The flocculant precipitate is collected and dissolved in $N/1$ HCl, added to obtain pH 2.0. This solution must be dialyzed, centrifuged to remove the insoluble material, and lyophilized. The Tager technique of the coagulase preparation is as follows. A culture filtrate of *Staphylococcus aureus* is adjusted to pH 3.8 with 4 $N/$HCl. The resultant precipitate is dissolved in distilled water, and this liquid is adjusted to pH 7.0. Coagulase is precipitated from this solution with three volumes of ethyl alcohol at $-5°$. The precipitate is dissolved in $M/100$ phosphate buffer, pH 7.0, and centrifuged. The coagulase is reprecipitated from the supernatant with ethanol as before, then suspended in distilled water and lyophilized.

Determination of the Coagulase Activity. The activity of a coagulase preparation can be measured by the method of Lominski and Roberts (1946), Tager and Hales (1949), Kaplan and Spink (1948), Rammelkamp et al. (1949), Duthie and Lorenz (1952), or Barber and Wildy (1958).

The Duthie and Lorenz Method of the Coagulase Determination. A coagulase preparation is serially diluted in 0.2-ml volumes of saline, and 0.2 ml of 0.1% human fibrinogen solution containing 5% rabbit plasma as an activator is added to each tube. The mixtures are incubated for 1 hour at 37°, then 0.02 ml of 1% suspension of Supercel are added to each tube, and the mixtures are left in a refrigerator for 20 to 30 minutes, and then read. The Supercel particles, added to facilitate the reading of results, occur in different degrees of dispersion, depending on the amount of coagulation. The end point is taken from the tube showing visible flocculation of particles. The minimum clotting dose is defined as the amount of coagulase per milliliter which, when mixed with 1 ml of plasma fibrinogen and incubated for 1 hour at 37° under the conditions specified, gives just visible flocculation of particles. Activity of a given preparation should be compared to the activity of a standard coagulase preparation tested in the same experiment.

Techniques of the Anticoagulase Test. Methods of the anticoagulase test were published by Lominski and Roberts (1946), and modified by Tager and Hales (1949), Barber and Wildy (1958), and Duthie and Lorenz (1952).

The Duthie and Lorenz Technique of the Antigoagulase Test. The serum being examined must not be inactivated, but incubated with heparin for a few minutes to destroy thrombin, since this enzyme acts on a similar substrate and can interfere. The serum is diluted progressively from 1:2 to 1:256 in 0.1 ml of saline buffered at pH 7.0. Equal volumes of a coagulase solution, containing 20 minimum clotting doses per milliliter, are added to each tube, and the mixtures are left for 30 minutes at room temperature; 0.2 ml of 0.1% suspension fibrinogen, containing 5% (v/v) rabbit plasma, is then distributed to all tubes, and the mixtures are incubated for 1 hour at 37°. Finally 0.02 ml of 1% Supercel suspension is added, and the tubes are left for 30 minutes at 4°. The reciprocal of serum dilution just sufficient to allow minimum clotting is taken as the titer and expressed in units of anticoagulase. For comparison, a serum with a known anticoagulase titer should be simultaneously treated in the same manner.

4. The Carbohydrase-Inhibition Tests

i. *The Antihyaluronidase Test.* Antistreptohyaluronidase, a specific enzyme antibody, neutralizes the immunochemical activity of streptococcal hyaluronidase, rendering this enzyme unable to hydrolyse hyaluronic acid. This specific biological inhibitor of streptococcal hyaluronidase is relatively heat resistant, since it cannot be damaged at 56° for several hours, whereas a nonspecific serum inhibitor of hyaluronidase is destroyed in 30 to 45 minutes at this temperature. Similar enzyme antibodies can be formed by the host in response to specific hyaluronidases of other bacteria, for example, of clostridia or corynebacteria. Three methods are used for estimation of the antihyaluronidase: the turbidimetric, the mucin clot preventing, and the viscosimetric methods.

The turbidimetric method, originally devised by Kass and Seastone (1944) for study of the activity of hyaluronidase, was adapted for the antihyaluronidase titration by Meyer (1947), Harris and Harris (1949), Faber (1953), MacLennan (1956), and Kwapinski (1965). Techniques by Meyer or Kwapinski involve a constant concentration of antigen, whereas the others employ a constant concentration of the test serum.

Kwapinski's Antihyaluronidase Test. Prior to the test proper, the activity of a specific hyaluronidase preparation is estimated by a viscosimetric assay. In this assay, 4-ml amounts of 0.4% hyaluronate solution are placed in three tubes, and upon the addition of 1 ml of phosphate acetate buffer, pH 7.0, equilibrated at 38° in a water bath. The first tube then receives

0.1 to 0.5 ml of a hyaluronidase preparation being examined, the second 0.1 to 0.5 ml of a standard hyaluronidase preparation, and the third an equal volume of the culture medium. The contents of the tubes are immediately transferred to three Ostwald viscosimeters, which are placed in an ultrathermostat at 37.5°.

The initial viscosity of the fluids should then be estimated. The fluids are first drawn to the upper mark over the bulb of the viscosimeter. The time is then measured for the fluid to flow down to the lower mark beneath the bulb. Each measurement is taken twice. Similar estimates are repeated in 5-minute intervals up to 30 minutes of incubation. The time of flow in minutes is plotted against the time of sampling on a graph for the standard and unknown hyaluronidase preparation and, from the data corresponding to the point where both curves cross, the relative activity of the streptococcal hyaluronidase preparation can be calculated. If necessary, the test should be repeated by using various amounts of the preparation of hyaluronidase under test. A unit of hyaluronidase is the amount of the enzyme preparation which, under the specific conditions of the reaction, reduces by half the initial time of the flow of the reactant fluid through the viscosimeter.

The antihyaluronidase test is set up in this way. Two series of dilutions of an inactivated serum ranging from 1:25 to 1:6400 are made in 0.25-ml volumes of 0.2 M, pH 6.0, phosphate buffer. The first row receives 0.25 ml of an aqueous solution of a specific hyaluronidase solution containing 4 TRU in this volume; 0.25 ml of phosphate buffer is added to tubes of the second row. Three control tubes are set to contain (a) 0.25 ml of phosphate buffer, and 0.25 ml of the specific hyaluronidase, (b) 0.5 ml of phosphate buffer, and (c) 0.75 ml buffer.

The tubes are agitated on an electrical shaker for 15 minutes at room temperature to allow the enzymatic antigen to combine with the specific antibody. After this time period, 0.5 ml of substrate is added to each tube, except the last control tube, which receives 0.25 ml of hyaluronate solution alone. During the second incubation at 37° for 30 minutes, the hyaluronate is decomposed in these tubes, where hyaluronidase is not, or only partly, fixed by antihyaluronidase.

A protein solution is added as an indicator system. This solution can be prepared from normal rabbit serum "aged" by storage at 2 to 4° for 10 days. It must be centrifuged and diluted 1:10 in saline, prior to the test. Rabbit serum can be replaced by 1% solution of beef serum albumin. The protein indicator is added in 0.25-ml volumes to all tubes cooled in an ice-water bath, followed by 0.25 ml of a 10% acetic acid. Protein in an acid environment forms a complex with nonhydrolyzed hyaluronate to give a turbid colloidal suspension. Its density depends on the amount of the non-decomposed hyaluronate in the test mixtures.

The rate of turbidity is measured in a spectrophotometer. The titer of the serum antihyaluronidase is estimated by comparing the optical densities given by fluids in the first row to optical densities of samples in the control row which contains corresponding serum dilutions but no hyaluronidase. The tube of the first row showing a comparative optical density with a parallel tube of the control row represents the end point, since in that tube the specific hyaluronidase is present at an effective concentration. The ASH titer is expressed in terms of the number corresponding to effective dilution of the tested serum. Titers equal to, or higher than, 200 are regarded as abnormal.

The MacLennan Antihyaluronidase Test. Two series of a specific hyaluronidase solution are made in a gelatin buffer containing 0.5, 1.0, 1.5, 2.0, 3.0, or 4.0 TRU (turbidity recuding units) in 0.8-ml volumes. The first row receives 0.2 ml of an inactivated test serum diluted in water, while 0.2 ml of distilled water is added to the other series. After an incubation for 30 minutes at room temperature, all tubes receive 0.8 of a 0.08% hyaluronate solution and are left for 30 minutes in a water bath at 37°, then cooled and supplemented with 0.2 ml of a solution of acidified serum. Results are read immediately and expressed in terms of the turbidity-reducing units of hyaluronidase, neutralized by 1 ml of nondiluted serum.

The Mucin Clot Prevention Test. Of a number of techniques (Friou and Wenner, 1947; Quinn, 1948; Harris and Harris, 1949) the method of Friou and Wenner is recommended. The test is carried out as follows. A specific hyaluronidase is diluted in tenfold difference in 0.5-ml volumes, in two series. The test serum diluted 1:10 in the Sørensen, pH 6.4, phosphate buffer is then added to the first row in 0.25-ml volume. The second control row receives 0.25 ml of saline solution. After an incubation for 15 minutes at room temperature, the tubes are placed in an ice-water bath, and 1 ml of ice-cooled hyaluronate solution is added. The samples are then left in the water bath at 37° for 20 minutes, and transferred into ice water for 5 minutes; 0.5 ml of 2 *N* acetic acid is finally added to each tube, and the results read immediately. Effective concentrations of hyaluronidase which prevented the formation of mucin clot in both rows are determined. Results of the test are calculated according to the equation:

$$\text{ASH} = \frac{\text{the highest effective enzyme dilution in the control row}}{\text{the highest effective enzyme dilution in the serum tested}}$$

Viscosimetric Method of the Antihyaluronidase Estimation. Viscosimetric ASH titration depends on the estimation of a serum concentration, at which an activity of 50% unit of specific hyaluronidase is inhibited in a system composed of one unit of the hyaluronidase, a test serum, and hyaluronate, within 10 minutes, at 25°, at pH 7.2 (Hadidian and Murphy,

1955). The hyaluronidase unit corresponds to the amount of enzyme preparation which brings about a complete lysis of the substrate in half the time period of 100 (± 10) seconds.

5. *The Antinuclease Tests*

The antinuclease assay depends on the inhibition, by a specific antibody, of a characteristic biochemical reaction of the depolymerization of nucleic acids or breakdown of nucleotides by NASase (-DPase) or DNase. The chemically defined substrate for NADase activity is nicotinamide-adenine-dinucleotide. Inhibition of the specific action of nucleases by antibodies (the antinuclease) can be determined by a viscosimetric technique (Hazlehurst, 1950), by optical density measurements (McCarty, 1949; Hazlehurst, 1950; Kaplan et al., 1951), or by a plate test (Olitzky et al., 1962). The antigen for this test can be prepared by the Kellner et al. (1956) method.

The Viscosimetric Technique (Hazlehurst, 1950). Twofold serial dilutions of a serum under test are made in 0.2-ml volumes of $M/40$ veronal buffer, pH 7.4. Control tubes contain 0.2 ml of buffer alone. Each tube receives 0.2 ml of a nuclease solution containing exactly 50 units of the enzyme per milliliter, that is, 10 units in 0.2 ml. The samples are incubated for 30 minutes in a water bath at 30° and then kept at 2 to 4° to prevent any deterioration of the enzyme. The volume of fluid in each tube is now made up to 1.0 ml by adding 0.6 ml of 20% neopeptone solution, and the residual activity of nuclease is estimated after the method of McCarthy (1948), as partially modified by Christensen (1949), in the following way. The contents of each tube is mixed in the proportion of 0.1:2.4 with the substrate consisting of 0.2% solution of ribonucleic or deoxyribonucleic acid made in a veronal buffer. Viscosities of these fluids are measured in an Ostwald viscosimeter at the beginning of recation and after 10 and 20 minutes incubation at 30°. The viscosity given by 0.1 ml of the control reaction mixture, containing nuclease but no serum, refers to one unit of the enzyme.

In the presence of a nuclease inhibitor, the relative viscosity is decreased. The serum dilution causing a decrease of the relative viscosity between 0.20 and 0.80 is recorded. The decrease of relative viscosity is subtracted from 1.0 to determine the amount of the antinuclease present. This figure is multiplied by five (the original serum dilution), by ten to make up the amount of antibody per 1 ml, and by the serial dilution factor. This denotes the number or antinuclease units per milliliter of serum, one unit being that amount of antinuclease which neutralizes one unit of nuclease.

The Alcohol Precipitation Technique of the Antinuclease Test. The technique of McCarty (1949), modified by Hazlehurst (1950), consists of alcohol precipitation of residual desoxyribonucleate, which has not been depolymerized by the nuclease.

The test is set up as follows. Serial twofold dilutions of serum in 0.2-ml volumes of $M/40$ veronal buffer, pH 7.5, are mixed with 0.2 ml of a nuclease solution containing 50 units of the enzyme per milliliter of 20% neopeptone, which functions as a stabilizer. The tubes are incubated for 30 minutes at 30°, then 0.6 ml of a deoxyribonucleate solution is added, and the mixtures are reincubated for another 30-minute period. Finally, 1.0 ml of 95% ethyl alcohol is added to each tube. The tube with the highest serum dilution showing characteristic fibrous precipitate denotes the end point. The dilution factor of this tube, multiplied by 50, expresses the number of antinuclease units per milliliter of serum.

The Kaplan et al. (1951) Technique of the Antidiphosphopyridine Nucleotidase Estimation. The general pattern of this assay, modified by Kellner et al. (1958), is this. The test serum, in serial twofold dilutions, is mixed with equal 0.5-ml volumes of diphosphopyridine nucleotidase containing 100 units of the enzyme. Control tubes receive DPNase with buffer. The mixtures are incubated in a water bath at 37° for 30 minutes. The amount of residual DPNase activity is then estimated by adding 0.2 ml of each mixture to 0.3 ml of a solution containing 0.4 mg of diphosphopyridine nucleotidase. After a $7\frac{1}{2}$-minute incubation, 3.0 ml of 1 M sodium cyanide is added to each tube, and optical densities are measured in a spectrophotometer at 340 nm, using 1.0-cm convex cuvettes. The anti-DPNase titer of serum is calculated from the reduction of nucleotidase activity to the level corresponding to the optical density between 0.400 and 0.600. The unit of the anti-DPNase activity is the amout of antibody per milliliter of serum which neutralizes 100 units of diphosphopyridine nucleotidase.

The Antinuclease-Plate Test. This test, devised by Olitzky et al. (1962), depends on the incubation of a serum tested for the content of the antiribonuclease with a preparation of deoxyribonuclease and the detection of residual active enzyme in a solid medium containing deoxyribonucleic acid. Thus the serum is first heated at 65° for 30 minutes to destroy the serum nuclease activity, and then it is serially diluted in 0.2-ml volumes. An equal volume of a deoxyribonuclease preparation, adjusted to a predetermined concentration, is added to each tube, and these are incubated at 37° for 30 minutes to allow the neutralization to proceed. After this time, a drop or 0.05 ml of each mixture was placed on an agar medium plate containing deoxyribonucleic acid, which is commercially available. The plates are then incubated at temperatures ranging from 22 to 37° for a few hours. Zones of clearing caused by the nonneutralized deoxyribonuclease are demonstrated by flooding the plates with 1 N HCl. Plates are viewed on a black background.

The end point is denoted by the greatest dilution of serum which has completely neutralized the enzyme, thus showing no clear zone on the plate. The titer of the antideoxyribonuclease is expressed by the reciprocal of this dilution.

The enzyme concentration to be used in the deoxyribonuclease test is adjusted by estimation of the highest dilution of a deoxyribonuclease preparation which still produce a completely clear zone on the deoxyribonucleic acid containing agar medium, under the incubation condition stated above. The deoxyribonuclease preparation is used in two times this concentration in the antiribonuclease test.

6. *The Urease Inhibition Test.*   This metabolic inhibition test depends on the inhibition by a specific antibody of ammonia production which is formed by microorganisms possessing the ability to metabolize urea (Purcell et at., 1966).

The urease inhibition test is performed in disposable plastc microtiter plates with U-shaped cups. Hyperimmune rabbit serum is diluted 1:5 in a culture medium containing 1% urea, and inactivated at 56° for 30 minutes. To set up the test, 0.025 ml of the culture medium is placed in each cup of the microtiter plate, and twofold serum dilutions are made in this medium. Two drops of 0.05 ml of a suspension of microorganisms are added to all cups except a medium control cup. All cups then receive 5 drops or 0.125 ml of the culture medium whereas the medium control cup receives an additional 0.05 ml to bring the volume of fluid in all cups to a total 0.2 ml. The plates are sealed with a cellophane tape and incubated at 34°. The antibody titers of serum are recorded when the pH of medium in cups containing microorganisms but no antiserum had changed by approximately 0.5 pH unit as determined by comparison of color with the medium containing phenol red and adjusted to known pH values. The end point corresponds to the highest serum dilution which prevented a change of approximately 0.25 pH unit or greater (i.e., greater than 50% suppression). One color-changing unit (CCU) is described as the highest dilution of a microbial suspension which has produced a color change equivalent to 0.5 pH unit or greater in a culture medium supplemented by 1% crystalline urea and 0.002% phenol red.

IV. THE IMMUNOIMMOBILIZATION TEST

1. *The Treponema-Immobilization Assay*

The immobilization test (*Treponema pallidum* Immobilization Test), introduced by Nelson and Mayer (1949), is based on the observation that treponemal antibodies, in the presence of complement, inhibit the ordinarily active movements of homologous or related spirochetes, for example,

Treponema pallidum. The immobilizing antibody which occurs in syphilitic sera is similar to, if not identical with, the spirocheticidal substances described by Eberson (1921), but is not related to the syphilis reagins.

The immobilization test requires the following reactants: a culture of *Treponema pallidum,* antiserum or test serum, complement, and diluent. The Nichols strain of *Treponema pallidum* is commonly used as antigen in the test. It is maintained by regular transfer in male rabbits weighing 2.5 to 3.5 kg, at approximately 2-week intervals. Testicular emulsions containing *Treponema pallidum* are employed for quantitative skin inoculations (Magnuson et al., 1948). Each rabbit is inoculataed intracutaneously at six different sites on the back, in tenfold dilution steps ranging from 2×10^5 to 2 organisms. Sites of the inoculation are examined twice weekly for a 3-month period. The inoculation is regarded as positive if motile treponemas are observed on dark-field examination. Three months after the first inoculation, the rabbits are injected daily for 4 days with 16,000 units/kg of penicillin emulsified in peanut oil and beeswax. After 6 weeks, the animals are reinoculated with the emulsion of *Treponema pallidum,* and they receive six injections of doses ranging from 2×10^5 to two microorganisms. Sites of the inoculation are observed for another period of 2 to 3 months.

Treponemas are then eluted from tissues by shaking, for 5 to 6 hours or overnight, pieces of syphiloma suspended in 20 ml of the medium cited below, in the atmosphere of 1% carbon dioxide and 99% nitrogen. The eluate is then centrifuged in the cold for 10 minutes at $200 \times g$ to remove erythrocytes and spermatozoa. The supernatant is recentrifuged for 50 minutes in the cold at $3000 \times g$ to concentrate treponemas. The supernatant is withdrawn, mixed with 0.71 g of sodium bicarbonate, and warmed to 35°. Composition of the medium, in which the treponemas are eluted and maintained outside the body, under an atmosphere of 95% nitrogen and 5% carbon dioxide, is given in Table 90.

The immobilization test according to Magnuson et al. (1951) is carried out in small tubes, 13×100 mm (for 0.5-ml test mixture) or 12×125 mm (for 1.0 ml), with plugs fitted loosely into the mouth of tube, to facil-tate equilibration of the medium with the gaseous atmosphere.

Serial, twofold dilutions of an inactivated tested serum, ranging from 1:2 to 1:256, are made in saline, and 0.05-ml amount of each dilution is added to test mixtures, which consist of 0.4 ml *Treponema* suspension and 0.05 ml of a 1:10 diluted guinea pig complement. In these circumstances, final dilutions of the serum are tenfold of original dilutions. Controls contain 0.05 ml of a normal rabbit serum, with and without complement, and 0.4 ml of the *Treponema* suspension.*

* The antigen is available from Sylvana Chemical Co., Orange, N.J.

Table 90.   Composition of the Maintaining Medium for *Treponema Pallidum*

Constituent	Stock Solution (%)	Amount Used for 20 ml (ml)	Final Concentration (%)
Crystalline bovine albumin or a fraction of bovine plasma	5.0	10.0	2.00
Na_2HPO_4	3.58	2.50	0.36
Phosphate buffer			
KH_2PO_4	2.00	0.63	0.05
Sodium thioglycollate	1.50	0.60	0.03
Glutathione	1.23	0.63	0.03
Cysteine·HCl	0.63	0.63	0.02
Sodium pyruvate	1.00	0.31	0.01
Sodium bicarbonate	1.26	1.13	0.06
Sodium chloride	0.85	2.32	—
Ultrafiltrate of undiluted beef serum	—	1.25	5.00

Motility determinations are carried out after 18 hours by the dark-field microscope under high dry magnification ($550\times$). A total of 50 treponemas are examined, and percentages of motile microorganisms in the test sample and in control tubes are recorded. The percentage of immobilized treponemas %IT is calculated according to the formula:

$$\%IT = \frac{\text{percentage motile in C'-free control less percentage in C' test sample}}{\%\text{ motile in C'-free control}}$$

The residual complement in test mixtures should be determined at the end of test, in the manner recommended by Mayer et al. (1948). In this technique, 0.1 ml of 5% suspension of sheep erythrocytes sensitized with an antisheep hemolysin and 0.15 ml of isotonic veronal buffer containing magnesium and calcium chloride are added to 0.5 ml of the test mixtures. The complement-free test mixtures containing the sensitized erythrocytes and buffer are used as control. All tubes are incubated for 30 minutes at 37°, and the degree of hemolysis is determined by the naked eye. If less than 2 plus (++) activity of complement is observed, the immobilization test must be regarded as invalid and should be repeated with another preparation of treponemas. The 50% immobilization end point can be estimated by placing the percentages of treponemas immobilized in particular test mixtures on an arithmetic scale (ordinate) against reciprocals of serum dilutions graphed on the logarithmic scale (abscissa). The 50% end point and the immobilization titer are calculated from graphic plots by linear interpolation.

The *Treponema* immobilization test is highly specific for treponematoses. Reactive antibodies are found only in the sera from syphilis, yaws, pinta, and bejel. The test is a reliable means of differentiating true positive reaction, characteristic of syphilis, from false positive reactions.

2. The Disk Immunoimmobilization Technique. The disk immunoimmobilization method (Mohit, 1968) is based on the principle that motile bacteria inoculated into a motility agar containing a specific antiserum directed against the flagella become immobilized. Thus if a motile bacterium has been inoculated in the center of a motility agar plate and a paper disk impregnated with a specific antiflagella antiserum is placed in the periphery of the plate, the bacteria growing during the incubation time are spread in a widening circle toward the disk. When the motile bacterium encounters an antiserum reacting with its flagella, they are immobilized, and a semicircular line of immobilization occurs around the reactive antiserum disk.

The actual procedure is as follows: melted motility medium containing 0.3% agar in addition to the required nutrients is poured into Petri plates. Blank filter paper disks are impregnated with 0.02 ml of approprite dilutions of antiserum in a sterile Tris-albumin buffer, pH 7.4.

The buffer consists of 8.16 g sodium chloride, 1.21 g *Tris*-(hydroxymethyl)-amino methane, 0.66 ml of concentrated HCl and 500 ml distilled water, supplemented with 3.3 ml of 0.15 M MgSO$_4$ − 7H$_2$O and 0.5 ml of 0.1 M CaCl$_2$ and distilled water adjusted to 1 liter. One gram of bovine serum albumin is added to the solution to protect diluted antisera from possible denaturation.

The antiserum disks are placed in a circle near the edge of the agar on the surface of the plate. The bacteria are inoculated in the center of the plate by stab inoculation, after which the plates are incubated at room temperature for 18 hours. During this time, antisera diffuse around each disk in a decreasing concentration gradient and the motile bacteria move uniformly to the agar periphery from the stab inoculation in the center. The bacteria encountering the specific flagella antibody are agglutinated and immobilized, forming a line of immobilization discernible around a disk containing appropriate antiserum. Nonagglutinataed and nonimmobilized bacteria continue their growth toward the disk and no discernible line of immobilization is observed.

Antigenic relationships between the different bacteria may be studied by the immunoimmobilization methods, using antisera produced against each of the test organisms to impregnate disks. If an indicator bacterium reacts with both or more antisera, the immobilization lines fuse to form an identity line between the disks.

The method above is used for the study of surface antigens of live bacteria and to study relatedness of surface antigens of motile bacteria. The method is much superior to those that require solubilization of the antigens and thus carry the risk of structural alteration resulting from the extraction procedure. The antiserum disk is prepared by dilution of antisera and impregnated filter paper disks are stable for at least 5 months at 4° which contributes to the reproducibility of larger series of tests.

3. The Immune Growth-Inhibition Test.   The test depends on the inhibition of growth of a microorganism in the proximity of an area where a specific, corresponding antiserum has been deposited. The most convenient method for immunological growth inhibition test has been described by Stanbridge and Hayflick (1967). In this technique, sterile filter-paper disks (4.35-mm diameter) are impregnated with 0.02 ml of undiluted antiserum. Smaller disks can be saturated with 0.01 ml of antiserum. The disks are dried in a Petri dish at 5° over anhydrous calcium chloride and silica gel for 3 days, and may be stored at $-20°$. The test bacteria are inoculated on the surface of a solid medium by the push-block method on which single disks impregnated with the antiserum or a ring containing 8 disks is placed. The plates are incubated at 37° for a desired period of time after which the surface area adjacent to each disk is examined microscopically for zones of inhibition.

4. The Bacterium-Immobilization Test.   In this test (Nossal, 1959), serial twofold dilutions of an antiflagella serum are made in dilute motile bacterial suspension. The effect of the antiserum on bacterial motility is observed microscopically.

The flagellar antigen activity assay, by Ada's et al. (1964) modification of Nossal's test is carried out in two steps: (a) determination of immobilization dose of antiserum. Two volumes of a fresh preparation of flagellated bacteria, adjusted to a standard turbidity, are added to four volumes of heart infusion broth and 94 volumes of 1% fetal calf serum saline. (The final concentration of bacteria in this suspension is about 10^6 cells/ml.) A volume of the suspension is then exposed to an equal volume of a serially diluted antiserum, and observing the effect of serum in a drop of the mixture, placed on a microscope slide (under paraffin). An 80% immobilization of the bacteria is taken as the end point of the titration. The reciprocal of this antiserum dilution is termed the immobilization titer. Five immobilizing units per 0.25 ml are employed for determination of the flagellar antigen activity. (b) In this test, 0.25 ml of serial dilutions of flagellated bacteria are added to 0.25 ml of the antiserum containing five immobilizing units. The mixtures are shaken at room temperature for 30 minutes and then examined microscopically. The final antigen dilution at which immobilization of bacteria has occurred is determined.

Chapter Fourteen

IMMUNE NEUTRALIZATION TESTS

The principle of immune neutralization tests is the abolishment of the toxicity or virulence of microorganisms due to the saturation of the toxicity or virulence factor(s) by specific antibodies. The immune neutralization is detected and measured by exposing susceptible animals or tissue cultures, or bacteria to the mixtures consisting of a serum and a toxin or virulent microorganisms, and recording the death time and rate, the degree of tissue destruction, or the lysis of bacteria.

I. THE TOXIN-ANTITOXIN NEUTRALIZATION TESTS

The mechanism of the detoxification by specific antitoxins of toxins produced by microorganisms and animals has not been sufficiently elucidated. According to Arrhenius and Madsen (1904), the combination of toxin and antitoxin with the formation of a nontoxic complex may be regarded as a reversible chemical reaction, to which the mass-action law can be applied. The toxin-antitoxin interaction was regarded by Bordet (1898) as a simple absorption phenomenon. Eagle (1937) found that both reagents were multivalent with respect to each other. He proved with experiments that in the excess toxin, the antitoxin binds several times as much toxin as is indicated by its neutralizing activity, and the resulting compound itself is toxic. In the presence of excess antitoxin, the toxin combines with more than the neutralizing quantity of antitoxin, to form a detoxified compound. The toxin-antitoxin neutralization test may be carried out with a constant amount of either the antiserum (Jawetz and Meyer, 1944; Ender, 1944) or the antigen (Miles and Wilson, 1955).

1. The Toxin-Antitoxin Neutralization Test with Constant Amount of Toxin

According to the Jawetz and Meyer technique (1944), 0.5-ml amounts of antiserum diluted 1:4, 1:8, and 1:16 in a saline solution are injected intraperitoneally into a group of white mice. This is followed in 30 minutes by the injection of 0.3 ml of a tested culture filtrate, undiluted or diluted 1:5 with saline. A control group of mice should receive the same dose of the toxin mixed with 0.5-ml amount of a normal serum. The mice are observed for 48 hours, and the time of deaths is recorded. Results of the test are expressed in terms of the number of mice surviving over the total number of mice used per serum, for example, $\frac{3}{10}$, or by the survival index as compared with the surviving rate or index of the control groups. The minimum effective dose of the antiserum, which secures either a 100 or a 50% (ED_{50}) surviving rate, or the survival index of mice should be estimated. The ED_{50} can be determined graphically by plotting the dose of antiserum against the mortality of animals challenged with a fatal dose of a toxic agent. The survival index is calculated from the following formula:

$$\text{survival index} = \frac{\text{number of surviving animals}}{\text{number of all animals}} \times 100$$

2. The Toxin-Antitoxin Neutralization Test with Constant Amount of Serum

Increasing amounts of a toxin preparation are mixed with one unit of a standard antitoxin and injected into guinea pigs weighing 250 g, on average. The minimal volume of toxin which causes death of guinea pigs in 4 days is taken as end point and called the L_+ dose. The amount of toxin which has been sufficiently neutralized by one unit of the antitoxin is termed the L_0.

3. The Intradermal Toxin Neutralization Test

The test may be carried out with progressive dilutions of either the antiserum or the antigen. In the Enders test, 1 ml of serial, progressing dilutions of an antitoxic serum is mixed with 1 ml of a constant dilution of the toxin and held for 30 minutes at room temperature; 0.1 ml of each mixture is then inoculated intradermally into the dorsal skin of white rabbits. Control injections contain the antigen or serum alone. A standard antitoxin or toxin preparation may be included, if available. The highest dilution of an antitoxic serum, at which no skin reaction was observed after 72 hours, is taken as the end point and the neutralization titer.

In the assay by Lepow and Pillemer (1952), progressing dilutions of an antigen preparation made in a saline buffered at pH 7.4 are mixed with an equal volume of the antitoxic serum diluted 1:5 or 1:10. These reaction mixtures are injected into the skin of 250-g guinea pigs. The L_0 dose of the antigen preparation is estimated from the concentration that did not produce any skin reaction when combined with a given amount of antiserum.

II. THE BACTERIUM-NEUTRALIZATION TEST

Procedures for testing protective activity of antibacterial sera were devised by Heidelberger and·Kendall (1930), Mishulov et al. (1939), Staub and Grabar (1943), Watson et al. (1947), and Kwapinski (1965). The test, according to Watson et al. (1947), is conducted by injecting 1 ml of an immune or test serum intraperitoneally into guinea pigs, and challenging them after 24 hours with a lethal dose of microorganisms, injected intracutaneously. Control animals receive intraperitoneally a normal serum and the same dose of bacteria.

In Kwapinski's (1965) technique, the antiserum is injected intramuscularly in various doses, ranging from 0.5 to 2.0 ml, to a group of mice or guinea pigs, 2 to 15 hours prior to the injection of a minimum fatal dose of the freshly cultivated microorganisms. A control group receives 1.0 ml of normal serum and the same dose of microorganisms.

Animals are under observation until all, or 50%, of animals from the control group die. Survival times of animals in each are then summed, and the survival coefficient is calculated by multiplying the figure obtained from the antiserum treated group by that of the control group.

III. THE VIRUS-NEUTRALIZATION TEST

The neutralization or inactivation of the virus infectivity by a homologous antibody appears to depend on a first-order reaction between virus particles and antibody molecules. A constant proportion of infective particles is inactivated per a time unit. The rate of inactivation is proportional to the antibody concentration and the temperature. The inactivation *in vitro* is never complete, since approximately one particle in a thousand escapes the neutralization. Neutralization reaction is sometimes reversible by simple dilution under physiological conditions, or by extreme pH values of the environment.

The virus-neutralization test may be carried out in the tissue culture, chick embryo, or in experimental animals. The route of injection of test mixtures into animals can be intracutaneous, intraperitoneal, intravenous, or intranasal. The most accurate virus-neutralization test is the kinetic neutralization test.

1. The Kinetic Neutralization Assay

Two, generally similar techniques for the kinetic neutralization test were published, by Hahon (1969) and Wheeler *et al.* (1969).

The Kinetic Neutralization Technique by Hahon (1969). This is applied as follows: a virus suspension containing an estimated number of particles per milliliter (e.g., 5×10^8 CIU), and an appropriately diluted antiserum are first prewarmed at the temperature to be employed for incubation of the immunological system (e.g., 35°). The two reactants are then mixed in equal volume and incubated. At time intervals during the incubation, 1-ml aliquots of the mixture are withdrawn and placed immediately in a capped tube held in ice-water, to stop the neutralization reaction. Test samples are diluted in a cold phosphate-buffered saline (PBS), pH 7.1, free of calcium and magnesium ions, and tested for unneutralized virus. A control tube contains the same virus dilutions and a normal serum used at the same concentration as in the main tube. The amount of active virus particles remaining after the incubation time is determined from the ratio of unneutralized virus in the reaction tube to the virus titer in the control tube, estimated at time intervals during the incubation period.

The Kinetic Neutralization Test by Wheeler et al. (1969). The virus preparation is diluted in phosphate-buffered saline (PBS), pH 7.1, free of calcium and magnesium ions, to contain 10^4 plaque-forming units (PFU)/ 0.1 ml. Serial doubling dilutions of an antiserum in 0.1-ml volumes are made. The two preparations are prewarmed to 35° in a constant temperature room. Then 0.1-ml samples of each reaction mixture are withdrawn at zero time and at 5 to 15 minutes thereafter and transferred to 9.9 ml of a modified maintenance medium (Syverton et al., 1954), kept in ice water. After thorough mixing, 0.2 ml aliquots are placed in 4 to 6 HeLa cultures.

The percentage survival of virus against time is plotted, and inactivation curves are drawn through the corresponding points on the graph. From these curves, the time required for neutralization of 50% of the initial virus amount is determined. Normalized 50% neutralized times (NT) are calculated according to the following formula for comparison of the required time for 50% neutralization of homologous virus with the time needed for 50% neutralization of heterologous virus:

$$\text{NT} = \frac{\text{time for neutralization of 50\% of heterologous virus}}{\text{time for neutralization of 50\% of homologous virus}} \times 100$$

The NT values exceeding 100 are expected to be found with heterologous virus. The neutralization rate constant may also be determined according to the following equation:

$$K = \frac{D}{t} 2.3 \log \frac{V_0}{V_t}$$

where K is the neutralization rate constant, V_0 the concentration of active virus at time zero, V_t the concentration of active virus at time t, and $D = 1/c$ − dilution of antiserum. Normalized K values are calculated by assigning a value of 100 to the K value of the homologous virus-antiserum. It is expected that NK values for heterologous virus would be under 100 (Wheeler et al., 1969).

2. The Multiplicity Neutralization Test

This test, designed by Wheeler et al. (1969), is performed by the following procedure: equal, 0.5-ml volumes of serial doubling dilutions of antiserum are added to a constant volume of virus containing between 100 and 400 plaque-forming units, and the mixture is incubated at 35° for 1 hour. Aliquots of 0.2 ml of the virus-serum mixtures are then transferred to four HeLa cultures and left at 35° for 2 hours. After this initial incubation, 1 ml of Syverton's et al. (1954) maintenance medium containing 10 μg of hydrocortisone is added to each tube. The cultures are reincubated at 35° and refed at 24 hours. Plaque counts are made at 48 to 50 hours after the cultures have been fixed and stained with Paragonformalin (Wheeler et al., 1968) and observed at 8× magnification.

The 50% neutralization titer of an antiserum is expressed as the reciprocal of the serum dilution which has caused reduction of the plaque count by one-half. This serum concentration is determined by plotting the percentage of neutralized virus on a linear scale on the ordinate against antiserum concentration on a logarithmic scale of the abscissa. In order to calculate normalized titers, a figure of 100 is assigned to 50% neutralization titer when the homologous virus-antiserum combination was employed and the normalized titer (NT) is calculated according to the following equation:

$$NT = \frac{50\% \text{ neutralization titer of heterologous virus-antiserum mixture}}{50\% \text{ neutralization titer of homologous virus-antiserum mixture}} \times 100$$

The neutralizing potency (pN) values may be calculated according to the following formula:

$$pN - \log A + \log \log \frac{V_0}{V_s}$$

where A is the antiserum dilution expressed in terms of final volume, V_0 the initial virus concentration, and V_s the surviving virus concentration. The pN values should be calculated for three to five antiserum concentrations and the final pN value represents the mean of all the determinations. The pN values for homologous and heterologous viruses are compared by calculating normalized pN values according to the formula:

$$\text{normalized pN (NpN)} = \frac{\text{pN value of heterologous virus-serum mixture}}{\text{pN value of homologous virus-serum mixture}} \times 100$$

Heterologous virus should give normalized pN values below 100.

The multiplicity neutralization test can be performed with constant virus amount and varying antiserum dilutions, and with combined constant virus-varying serum and constant serum-varying virus amounts and with constant virus amount and varying antiserum dilutions using a mixture of two different viruses. These modifications of the neutralization may be employed for the study of immunological relationships between different viruses. The most recommended test is the multiplicity neutralization test with 50% plaque reduction and small pN value determination, although the neutralization test which employs artificial mixtures of two different viruses and constant amount tested against varying dilutions of antiserum against one or the other type, is useful in detecting antigenic differences and similarities.

3. The Immunofluorescence-Neutralization Test

The immunofluorescent-neutralization test is a combination of a neutralization test in tissue culture and a direct immunofluorescent technique by which the residual nonneutralized particles of a particulate antigen preparation are quantitatively determined.

In this test, designed by Hahon and Cooke (1965), a constant quantity of psittacosis agent is added to an equal volume of serial twofold dilutions of an antiserum made in phosphate buffered saline (PBS). The quantity of the antigen used is 2×10^4 cell-infecting units (CIU). The mixtures are incubated at 35° for 2 hours after which 0.2 ml of each mixture is placed in three cover-slip cultures of McCoy cells. The unneutralized agent is allowed to adsorb onto the cells during the centrifugation at $500 \times g$ at 21 to 23° for 15 minutes. For this part of the procedure, vials containing cover-slip cultures are placed in slotted cups containing tube adapters. After the centrifugation, the cover-slip cultures are rinsed twice with maintenance medium, and 1 ml of the medium is added to each vial for further incubation at 35° for 20 to 22 hours. Cover-slip cultures are rinsed twice with cold PBS and then fixed with cold ($-60°$) acetone and either layered with fluorescein-tagged antiserum or stored at $-60°$ for subsequent examination.

The monolayers are washed three times with PBS and layered with an immunoglobulin conjugate for 30 minutes. The cover-slip cultures are then rinsed in three changes of PBS to remove excess conjugate and finally mounted in 10% glycerol in PBS. Fluorescent cell counts are made at $645 \times$ magnification in a microscope equipped with a Fluorolume illuminator, the no. 5840 and BG-13 exciter filters, and an E.K. no. 2A barrier filter. Fifty microscopic fields for each cover-slip culture are examined and totalled. The percentage reductions in counts incurred by the first serum, as compared to the controls containing a nonrelated or normal serum, are calculated. The 50% serum-neutralizing end point is determined by the interpolation from a plot of the logarithm of serum dilutions against the percent reduction of counts stradding the 50% value.

4. Deinhardt and Henle's Virus-Immunoneutralization Test

In this procedure, first a series of twofold dilutions of an inactivated serum, made in 0.2 ml of sterile Hanks' balance salt solution, are made. The solutions are added to equal volumes of a virus suspension containing $10^{3.1}$ hemagglutinatinating units and $10^{5.7}$ egg infectious doses (EID_{50}). The control row receives a standard serum mixed with the virus suspension. All tubes are shaken, covered with sterile aluminum foil, and incubated for 1 hour at 37° and for 12 to 18 hours at 4°. A suspension of mature HeLa cells is made to contain 60,000 cells/0.6 ml of a pH 7.3 to 7.4 buffer. This amount is added to the serum-virus mixture, which should be left at 37° for 3 days.

The percentage of cells showing cytolysis and degeneration is then evaluated. The serum dilution preventing the destruction of about half the HeLa cells is considered as end point. The titer is expressed as reciprocal of the serum dilution. In a similar technique by Dulbecco et al. (1956), the neutralizing power of a serum is determined by counting of infective virus in a monolayer tissue culture.

5. The Metabolic Neutralization Test

This test is based on the following principles. Metabolizing cell cultures produce acids which can change phenol indicator in the medium from red to yellow whereas the inhibition of cellular metabolism by a cytopathic effect of viruses is manifested by red color of the indicator. If the virus has been neutralized by a serum, its cytopathic effect is abolished, and the metabolizing cells show red color of the medium. Two metabolic tests, by Melnick and Opton (1956) and by Schmidt et al. (1962), are recommended.

The metabolic neutralization test by Schmidt et al. (1962) is set up as follows. Series of antiserum dilutions in 0.25-ml volumes are mixed with an equal amount of the virus, diluted to contain approximately 100 TCD_{50}, as estimated by the preceding titration. After an hour's incubation at room temperature, each test mixture receives 0.25 ml of the HeLa cell suspension (50,000 cells) and 0.25 ml of the metabolism medium. The cell control consists of four tubes containing 0.25 to 0.50 ml of metabolism medium and 25,000 to 100,000 cells. All tubes are sealed with 0.5 ml of sterile mineral oil and incubated at 36° until the pH of control tubes is lowered to at least 7.2. A pH 7.2 or lower is considered indicative of the virus neutralization, whereas a pH 7.4 or higher is regarded as evidence of the viral cytopathogenesis.

The metabolism medium consists of 5% heat inactivated rabbit or horse serum, 1.5 or 20% glucose solution, 2.5% of an 8.8% $NaHCO_3$ solution, and 91% of the mixture 199 (in Earle's balanced salt medium). Antibiotics are added to give a final concentration of 250 units of penicillin, 250 μg of streptomycin, and 2.5 units of bacitracin per milliliter of the medium.

6. *The Neutralization Test in the Chick Embryo*

The neutralization test by Hilleman and Horsfall (1950) is carried out in the following way: 0.5-ml amounts of serial, twofold serum dilutions are mixed with equal volumes of allantoic fluid from embryonated eggs infected with a virus, diluted in Pfansthiel's peptone broth to contain approximately 1000 EID_{50} (egg infectious doses) of the virus in 0.2 ml. Controls contain either a normal serum and virus, or virus dilutions alone. The mixtures are left for 15 minutes at room temperature and then placed in an ice bath. A 0.2-ml amount of each serum-virus mixture is injected into the allantoic fluid or four embryonated, 9-day-old eggs, and incubated for 48 hours at 35°.

After this time period, the eggs are chilled, and the allantoic fluid is withdrawn and tested for the presence of hemagglutinating virus. This is carried out by mixing 0.1 ml of allantoic fluid with 0.1 ml of 1% suspension of human group O erythrocytes on a porcelain test plate. The effective serum dilution preventing the hemagglutination is determined. Alternatively, the 50% mortality in the presence of a 1:10 (final) dilution of a serum is estimated by an adequate statistical method.

The interpretation of results is facilitated by computing the serum titer ratios, diving the heterologous titer by homologous titer (Archetti and Horsfall, 1950).

Similar neutralization tests in chick embroys were published by Burnet et al. (1937), Golub (1948), Gottlieb et al. (1953), Bashe et al. (1953), and Boulanger and Bannister (1960).

The neutralization titer of a serum, according to the Burnet et al. technique, is determined by counting characteristic lesions, for example, pocks, on the chorioallantoic membrane. Each lesion corresponds to one infective virus particle. The serum tested by a virus-neutralization procedure *in vitro* should be heated at 56° for 30 minutes, to remove a heat-labile inhibitor, present in the sera of human beings and of various experimental animals.

7. *The Immunoneutralization Tests in Animals*

The test is usually performed in mice (Hahon and Cooke, 1965; Smithburn, 1942), although other small animals, notably guinea pigs and hamsters, as well as rabbits and frogs (Kwapinski, 1970), and sometimes higher animal species, for example, monkeys (Kolmer and Rule, 1935; Smithburn, 1942) are employed.

Hahon and Cooke's (1965) immunoneutralization test, designed for experiments with psittacosis agent, may also be applied to other infectious agents. According to this method, serial dilutions of an antiserum, made in a phosphate-buffered saline are added to an equal volume of a constant quantity of the agent used in the concentration of 2×10^4 cell-infecting units (CIU)/ml. The mixtures are incubated at 35° for 2 hours after which 0.02 ml of each mixture is injected intracerebrally into Swiss mice weighing 10 to 14 g each. A control mouse receives the amount of agent alone or the antiserum alone. The animals are observed daily for 14 days and the survivors are noted. The results are reported by plotting the logarithm of serum dilutions against the number of survivors and determining the 50% antiserum-neutralizing end point by interpolation (Kwapinski, 1970).

Smithburn's (1942) Immunoneutralization Test. Test mixtures containing 0.4 ml of serum inactivated at 56° for 1 hour and 0.4 ml of a virus suspension diluted in 0.75% solution of Armour's fraction V of bovine plasma albumin to contain 50 LD_{50} or more in this volume are incubated for 1 to 2 hours at 37°. The test mixtures are then injected into mice either intraperitoneally or intracerebrally in respective doses of 0.1 or 0.2 ml. In a similar test by Fong and Bernal (1953), various twofold dilutions of serum are mixed with a virus suspension and incubated for 1 hour at room temperature; 0.05-ml amounts of these mixtures are inoculated intranasally into 3-week-old mice. The serum dilution, which gives the protection in 50% mice, is calculated and computed by statistical methods.

A *serum-neutralization test in monkey* was described by Kolmer and Rule (1935). A similar test can be adopted to studies on the serum neutralization of the virulence of bacteria by a liquid culture or washed bacteria, standardized to contain two million of fatal doses per milliliter.

Arbitrarily, one mouse protective unit can be defined as that fraction of cubic centimeter of antiserum which protects a certain proportion of mice against one million fatal doses of an 18-hour liquid culture of bacteria of such virulence that 1 to 10 cells cause death of the animals in 48 hours when injected by an appropriate route (Felton, 1928, slightly modified).

8. The Intradermal Neutralization Test

This assay is carried out by injecting 0.1-ml amounts of mixtures of antigen and antibody in various ratios into the skin of albino rabbits. Controls containing antigen alone are injected into an adjacent area. The zones of erythema observed are to be measured by the aid of a planimeter after 12 to 24 hours. The highest serum dilution, at which no redness of the skin is noticed, represents the neutralization titer. Veldee (1932) recommends the injection of reaction mixtures into ears of rabbits, as a more accurate procedure.

Several other techniques of the virus neutralization test in animals were devised: for example, the method of titrating the foot-and-mouth disease virus by inoculating mixture of serial serum dilutions with a constant amount of the virus into five sites on calf's tongue. The neutralization titer is calculated by estimating the number of lesions observed in 20 to 28 hours after injections (Brooksby, 1949). The accuracy of the virus-neutralizing test can be improved by applying the "chess-board" procedure, in which different amounts of the virus are added to varying amounts of the serum.

9. *The Cross-Neutralization Test*

This test, published by Smithburn (1942), is carried out as follows: a suspension of the virus infected tissue is diluted serially in 10% normal monkey serum; 0.3-ml amounts of varying virus dilutions are placed in three rows and mixed with 0.2-ml volumes of either the test serum, a heterologous or a normal control serum. The virus-serum mixtures are incubated for 3 hours at 37.5° and injected intracerebrally into normal white mice, to be observed for 15 days. The results are evaluated by an adequate statistical method.

10. *The Cross-Immunity (Cross-Resistance) Test*

The cross-immunity test (Koprowski, 1950) is based on a reaction of the host, immunized actively with a virus or recovering from a given viral disease, to the challenge by a heterologous viral agent. The immunization is attained by means of inoculation with an inactivated or live vaccine. The conferred immunity should be verified, if possible, through artificial exposure to the homologous virus. The immunized host is then exposed to a heterologous virus and observed for a time period. A nonimmune host of the same species is used as a control.

IV. THE BACTERIOPHAGE-NEUTRALIZATION TEST

The phage neutralization phenomenon depends on the adsorption of antibody molecules on the phage surface and the interference with the phage infectivity. The inactivation of bacteriophage by antibody proceeds according to the first-order inactivation constant. The rate of the immunological reaction at a constant temperature may be expressed by the following equations (Adams, 1959):

$$\frac{-dp}{dt} = \frac{Kp}{D}$$

$$K = 2.3 \frac{D}{t} \times \log_{10} \frac{P_0}{p}$$

$$\frac{P}{P_0} = \frac{e^{-Kt}}{p}$$

where P_0 is the phage assay (phage count) at zero time, p the phage assay at time t minutes, K the velocity constant, D — final dilution of antiserum expressed by a number like 200, 400, and so on, and t the time required to obtain 99% *phage neutralization.*

The K value is a characteristic of the individual rates of antiserum. Determination of K value of an antiserum, tested with different phages, can be used for estimation of the degree of antigenic relationships between the viruses. A more accurate test employing the determination of activation constant has been published by Attardi et al. (1964), but the simpler assays of Burnet and Freeman (1937) and of Jerne and Avegnol (1956) are practically useful.

Burnet and Freeman's (1937) assay is set up by mixing equal 0.05-ml volumes of serial dilutions of antiserum and the bacteriophage at a standard dilution. Control tubes receive the phage suspension and saline. The standard phage dilution is made to give an easily countable number of plaques, for example, 100 to 250, when 0.02-ml volume of the control tube contents is planted. The mixtures are incubated at 37 or 45° for 4 hours. Duplicate 0.02-ml lots from each tube are then titrated on 1% agar plages, inoculated previously with a young broth culture of sensitive microorganisms. The plates are incubated at 37° overnight, and the number of plaques formed is estimated. The end point is determined by a plate showing 80% reduction of the control plaque count.

Jerne and Avegnol's (1956) test employs equal amounts of an undiluted or diluted serum and a bacteriophage suspension at the concentrations ranging from 10^4 to 10^8 particles per milliliter are incubated at 24° for a period of 3 hours. At 30-minute intervals, samples of mixtures are withdrawn, diluted with sterile distilled water to stop the inactivating action of the antiserum, and assayed for survivors by direct planting. Inactivation curves are drawn by plotting the logarithm of the survivor fraction against time, in minutes, at which the inactivation was stopped by dilution. About 5000 antibody molecules are absorbed by one phage particle.

Attardi's et al. (1964) Test. The test consists in the incubation of a bacteriophage mixture with a cell suspension of the immunized lymph nodes cell suspension at 37° and assaying the bacteriophage activity at various times. The kinetics of disappearance of bacteriophage is determined by the kinetics of appearance of antibody activity in the cell suspension and by kinetics of neutralization of bacteriophage by antibodies. An average inactivation constant $(\overline{K}_{Ab})$ is determined according to the following equation:

$$\overline{K}_{Ab} = -\frac{1}{t} \ln \frac{P_{Ab}}{P_0}$$

where the parameter K_{Ab} represents at any time t, the inner activation constant the suspension could have at $t = 0$ to give the observed inactivation; P_0 is the bacteriophage titer at t = 0, P_{Ab} is the bacteriophage titer after t minutes of exposure to antibody.

V. THE IMMUNE BACTERIUM-NEUTRALIZATION TEST IN TISSUE CULTURE

The test (Diena et al., 1971) depends on the specific inhibition by antiserum of infective and destructive action of bacteria on a TC monolayer.

The source of cells is monkey kidney cells (RE2), passaged in M199 medium containing 10% fetal calf serum and 1% glutamine. The tissue culture is trypsinized, and the monolayers are dispersed and dispensed at 2-ml aliquots (about 2.5×10^4 cells/ml) in tissue culture tubes and incubated upright at 37°.

Determination of $TCID_{50}$ (50% tissue culture infecting dose of bacteria). Four to 5-day-old tissue cultures are infected with dilutions of various bacteria, suspended in 0.1 ml of 199 medium and incubated at 37° for 24 to 40 hours, depending on the species of bacteria. The fluid medium is replaced after the incubation with 2 ml of agar overlay possessing the following composition: 3% agar and double strength M199 (1:1), without phenol red, 5% calf serum, 0.2% skim milk, 100 IU of penicillin/ml, 100 μg streptomycin per milliliter, and 1:30,000 neutral red.

The tubes are reincubated for 72 hours and observed microscopically.

Viability of cells is indicated by the presence of neutral red at the bottom of the tubes, whereas the agar layer remains clear. Destruction of the monolayer is shown by the inability of the tissue culture to take up neutral red, resulting in the agar layer becoming yellowish-brown. The infection by bacteria causes considerable degeneration of the cytoplasm and nuclei, with final destruction of the monolayer. The dose of bacteria causing complete destruction of the monolayer is noted and determined as ITCID unit. Half the amount represents $ITCD_{50}$ unit.

The bactericidal test is set up by adding aliquots of antiserum to an equal volume of $TCID_{50}$s of bacteria, incubating the mixture at 37° for 30 minutes, and inoculation of the mixture into a series of RE2 cultures using five tubes per each antiserum dilution. The tubes are incubated at 37° for 24 to 40 hours, following which the overlay agar is added, and the tubes are reincubated for 72 hours. The tubes are then inspected for color and destruction of the monolayer. The lowest antiserum dilution producing complete inhibition of the monolayer destruction is considered as the neutralization end point and the titer is expressed in terms of the antiserum dilution. This test is very reliable and specific.

VI. STATISTICAL APPRAISAL OF NEUTRALIZATION TESTS

Only a brief account of a procedure suggested by Boyd (1956) for computing data obtained from the neutralization and other immunological tests may be given here; for more information consult Boyd's monograph.

The actual results obtained from a series of tests should be compared with those to be expected on the basis of pure chance. Since in most experiments the true exception is unknown, the standard deviation must be estimated from the data of actual experiments. The significance of any difference in the mortality rate between the antiserum treated and control animals is measured by the χ^2 test may be estimated from experimental data in the following manner. First, the numbers of deaths to be expected in the treated and untreated group are calculated, assuming that the injection of the serum did not confer any change. These numbers are taken from marginal totals.

Example.   Total number of animals 40.
             Total serum treated group 20.
             The control group 20.
             Deaths in the control group 5.

Thus the total of dead is 20/40 of all animals in the experiment. If the antiserum were ineffective, the number of expected deaths would be 20:40 times the total number of animals obtaining the antiserum, that is, $20/40 \times 20 = 10$. Similarly, the expected number of dead in the control group would be $20/40 \times 20 = 10$. Each expected number must be subtracted from the deaths actually recorded, or vice versa, depending on which volume is larger. Remaining figures are deviations (d). Thus in the example quoted, the deviations are, for the treated group, $10 - 5 = -5$; for the control group, $15 - 10 = +5$.

The χ^2 is now computed by squaring each deviation, dividing the expected value of that category, and adding results so obtained; $\chi^2 = (d^2/m)$, where m is the value expected in each case. The probability of values recorded from the results may be taken from tables published by Pearson (1930) or Fisher (1936).

Calculation of 50% Neutralization Unit of Serum. The 50% neutralization titer in terms of LD_{50} (the dose killing 50% of mice, or TCD_{50} (the dose producing cytopathic changes in 50% of inoculated tissue culture) may be calculated by Reed and Muench's (1938) method or by Kärber's (1931) method. According to Reed and Muench's method, the data on animal mortality are first tabulated as shown in Table 91. Accumulated data (Table 92) and mortality percentages are obtained by (a) adding the

Table 91.   Tabulation of Animal Mortality and Survival Data

Virus Dilution	Dead/Live Mice	Dead Mice	Survived Mice
10^{-1}	10/10	10	0
10^{-2}	10/10	10	0
10^{-3}	8/10	8	2
10^{-4}	3/10	3	7
10^{-5}	1/10	1	9
10^{-6}	0	0	10

Table 92.   Calculation of Mortality Factors by Reed and Muench's Method

Virus Dilution	Died	Survived	Mortality	
			Ratio	Percentage
10^{-1}	32	0	32/32	100
10^{-2}	22	0	22/22	100
10^{-3}	12	2	12/14	86
10^{-4}	4	9	4/13	31
10^{-5}	1	18	1/19	5
10^{-6}	0	28	0/28	0

figures representing numbers of dead animals from the bottom of the second last column to the level of a serum dilution being considered, and (b) adding the figures in the last column, starting at the top and ending at the level parallel to the dilution in question. From Table 92, two borderline serum dilutions are noted, one showing the mortality above 50%, and the other dilution representing mortality below 50% of animals. The proportionate distance (PD) between the two dilutions, wherein the 50% end point lies, is calculated thus:

$$PD = \frac{\text{percentage mortality above } 50 - 50\%}{\text{percentage mortality above } 50\% - \text{percentage mortality below } 50\%}$$

Negative logarithm of LD_{50} titer is then calculated as being equal to negative log of dilution above 50% mortality plus proportionate distance.

According to Kärber's method, the LD_{50} (or TCD_{50}) value is determined as:

$$\log LD_{50} = 0.5 + \log \text{ of highest concentration}$$

$$\frac{\text{of virus used} - \text{sum of \% of dead animals}}{100}$$

The neutralization index (NI) is expressed by the ratio of the virus control LD_{50} titer to the LD_{50} titer of the serum-virus mixtures where the virus has been added to undiluted scrum (Melnick, 1969), as shown in the formula:

$$\log NI = \log LD_{50} \text{ of virus control} - \log LD_{50} \text{ of serum-virus mixture}$$

The antilogarithm of this difference represents the neutralization index. A neutralization index of less than 10 is considered as insignificant.

VII.　APPLICATION OF THE IMMUNE NEUTRALIZATION TEST

The most important application of neutralization tests for research and diagnostic purposes are as follows.

1. Detection of specific antibodies in the sera of people or animals.
2. Identification and differentiation of the causative agent (toxin, virus).
3. The study of antigenic relationships among different viruses and among toxins.
4. Determination of the potency of antitoxins and antiviral neutralizing or protective sera, and the standardization of therapeutical antisera.
5. Determination and comparison of the immunogenicity of toxoids and virus vaccines.

Chapter Fifteen

IMMUNOHISTOCHEMICAL TESTS

Immunological techniques, classified within the category of the immune histochemical tests, are used to reveal antigens or antibodies present in or adsorbed onto tissues or cells. Foreign antigens can be detected in individual organs of the host either by their isolation from tissues, or by locating them in ultrathin sections by means of specific antibodies. In the first case, microbial toxins, polysaccharides, or other materials are extracted with appropriate solvents, and the extracts are tested against microbial antisera by the neutralization, precipitation, or bacterium-adherence test. This group of assays is only partially connected with the true immune histochemical tests in that all of them are devised to detect foreign antigens or adsorbed (sessile) antibodies in cells or tissues. The true immune cytochemical tests permit direct detection of antigens or antibodies adsorbed onto cells or tissues in either of three ways: (a) by revealing chemical characteristics of natural or artificially coupled antigens (the cytochemical technique), (b) by tracing in tissues the radioactivity of isotope labeled antigens or antibodies (the isotope technique), or (c) by detecting the fluorescence of the fluorescent dye-labeled antigens or the reaction of ordinary antigens with specific, labeled antibodies (the immunofluorescence technique).

I. THE TOXIN FIXATION TECHNIQUE

This test, one of the earliest in immunology, has been designed for tracing soluble antigens in tissues. The fixation of toxins of *Bacillus tetani* and *Corynebacterium diphtheriae* in tissues of chickens, rabbits, or guinea pigs was studied by determining the toxicity in adequate biological assays (Metchnikoff, 1897; Wolff-Eisner, 1908; Bieling and Gottschalk, 1923).

II. THE HISTOPRECIPITATION TEST

By this test, the presence of soluble antigens in tissues may be revealed. Thus soluble, partially purified constituents of bacteria, extracted from infected tissues, were used as antigens in the precipitation tests with specific antisera. A soluble polysaccharide antigen of *Diplococcus pneumoniae* was detected in extracts from lungs, liver, kidneys, and spleen, obtained from fatal cases of pneumonia, by a precipitation reaction with type-specific antiserum (Nye and Harris, 1937; Frisch et al., 1942). Similar extracts injected into mice showed a specific antigenic action and could be revealed in the tissues by a precipitation test (Felton, 1949). Extracts from various organs of animals that died of anthrax show a precipitation reaction with a specific antiserum (the Ascoli test).

III. THE FIXED ANTIBODY-NEUTRALIZATION TEST

This test, devised by Pfeiffer and Marx (1898), is carried out by injecting susceptible laboratory animals with the mixtures consisting of small portions of ground organs obtained from rabbits immunized with bacteria and living homologous microorganisms. The surviving rate is then computed by comparison with a control group which received mixtures consisting of ground organs of nonimmunized animals and living bacteria.

IV. THE TISSUE ANTIBODY-ADHERENCE TEST

This test depends on microscopic observation of the adherence of homologous bacteria to plasma cells or lymphocytes isolated from lymph nodes of immunized animals. Particulate antigens, for example, live cells of *Salmonella typhosa* or *Brucella,* are injected into the hind footpad of rabbits. After a period of time, the popliteal lymph nodes, which drain the site of injection, are extirpated and ground in a mortar. Saline suspensions of cells should be mixed with washed homologous microorganisms on glass slides. If the antibodies adsorbed to tissue cells react with the bacteria, the bacteria adhere to the surface of plasma cells or large lymphocytes, and can be observed microscopically (Hayes et al., 1951; Moeschlin and Demiral, 1952).

V. CYTOCHEMICAL ASSAYS

Two immune cytochemical techniques can be differentiated: one is used for the detection of antigens in host cells by means of selective dyes, whereas the other has been employed for tracing dye- or metal-conjugated antigens in cells or tissues of the host by microscopic observations or by chemical tests.

An example of the first type of cytochemical techniques is the detection of certain wax-like substances of tubercle bacilli by the Ziehl-Neelsen staining, which reveals the acid fastness. In a slightly different method, malachite green "combined" with the antipneumococcus serum is used for the detection of pneumococcus polysaccharides in tissues of animals, to which it was previously injected (McClintock and Friedman, 1945).

The other group of cytochemical techniques employs colored protein conjugates or chemically labeled antigens which are injected into experimental animals and traced in smears and sections of tissues, either microscopically or by appropriate chemical tests. Some examples of the dye-conjugated antigens are R-salt-azo-diphenyl-azo-crystalline egg albumen; a protein coupled to R-salt-azo-benzidine (Heidelberger and Kendall, 1930); and the alum-precipitated dye protein conjugated to proteins through carbamide linkage (Hopkins and Wormall, 1933). Examples of chemically labeled antigens are proteins diazotized with atoxyl or *p*-aminobenzoic acid; proteins combined with arsenic, iron, or uranium; and iodinated proteins (Haurowitz and Breinl, 1932; Rous and Beard, 1934; Pressman et al., 1949). These labeled antigens are injected into animals, and after a period of time the amounts of metals or combined compounds in tissues are chemically estimated.

Specific, metal-combined antisera are used to localize antigens in tissues. For instance, an antipneumococcal serum "combined" with uranium was used to localize a pneumococcus polysaccharide in tissues of guinea pigs (McClintock and Friedman, 1945). A somewhat different reaction was described by Marrack (1934), where a bidiazotized benzidine antityphoid serum agglutinated typhoid bacilli, turning them red.

VI. THE RADIOISOTOPE TECHNIQUE

The use of radioisotopes to trace antigens in tissues was introduced by Stanley (1942), and Libby and Madison (1947). Isotopes ^{32}P and ^{131}I are commonly used whereas ^{35}S is employed less frequently for the labeling of antigens or antibodies (Warren and Dixon, 1948; Pressman and Keighley, 1948; Crampton and Haurowitz, 1952; Crampton et al., 1953; Masouredis, 1957). Antibodies can be radiolabeled *in vivo,* by incorporation of the label in the antibody as it is formed, or *in vitro* by coupling a radioactive substance to the antibody of an antiserum. The labeling *in vivo* is attained by feeding animals with radioactive amino acids, or precursors of the amino acids, containing radioactive carbon or sulfur. Antibodies produced by animals fed with these radioactive substances become naturally labeled; however, only low levels of radioactivity can be incorporated. In the *in vitro* methods, radioactive iodine or sulfur is usually employed for labeling the antigens or antibodies. Iodine is incorporated by direct iodination of proteins, and sulfur as *p*-azobenzene sulfonate groups.

Autoradiography techniques have been applied to the following immunological investigations: the detection of labeled antigens or haptens in tissues and cells involved in the immune response, the localization of labeled antibody to reveal the distribution of antigenic material, and the specific identification of reactants in gel diffusion or immunoelectrophoresis. Autoradiography is more sensitive for certain immunological tests than the methods depending on detection of dye markers. The method is more useful for precise localization of antigens or antibodies than the techniques employing fluorescent labels.

Labeling may be attained externally by adding a radioactive tag to a protein by covalent bonds, or internally, accomplished either by an *in vivo* biosynthesis involving small molecular radioactive precursors, or by *in vitro* synthesis using smaller radioactive reactants. Internal labeling is recommended if the synthesis is feasible utilizing ^{14}C or ^{3}H because of their long half-life and relatively low energies of emission. However, the ^{32}P, ^{35}S, and ^{131}I shorter-lived isotopes have greater energies of emission and therefore cause much faster registration on photographic film.

Ultrathin, 1 μ-thin, sections for autoradiography are prepared by Salpeter and Bachmann's (1964) method. Tissue sections are mounted on chemically clean slides previously dipped in a solution, consisting of 0.5 g gelatin and 0.5 g chrome alum dissolved in 1 liter of distilled water. The slides are dried over a hair dryer and either applied directly to a photographic plate so that the two glass slides are held tightly together by metal clips, or the gelatin sheets are stripped from coated glass slides and then applied to the photographic plate.

Another method utilizes liquid photographic emulsion such as nuclear track emulsion (emulsions of gelatin and AgBr). The emulsion is applied with a camel hair brush using emulsions warmed to 50° and diluted in 0.05% Duponol-C (one to seven parts of emulsion) for more uniform flow. Alternatively, the slides may be dipped in the emulsion solution, allowed to drain vertically, and placed horizontally on a level rack for 10 to 15 minutes until the emulsion has gelled. The slides are then placed in light-proof boxes saturated with KNO_2 to maintain relative humidity at 47%.

The exposure time for ^{14}C is about 30 days; the exposure time for ^{3}H (e.g., ^{3}H-thymidine) varies from 20 to 60 days but sometimes it must be prolonged to 130 days (Nossal and Mäkelä, 1962). The autoradiographs are developed in total darkness with time and temperature rigidly controlled and developed according to the manufacturer's guide accompanying the film. The slides are then examined for photographic registration preferably by phase contrast microscopy accomplishing the grain counting with high-dry objectives and a reticule in the objective. After the preliminary examination, the slides should be stained and mounted for histological detailed photography and preservation.

The Iodination Technique. Iodination techniques were described by Pressman and Keighley (1948), Warren and Dixon (1948), Talmage et al. (1954), McFarlane (1958), and Webster et al. (1962). A radio-immunoelectrophoretic test was devised by Yagi et al. (1962) and Onoue et al. (1964).

The Warren and Dixon Method. This method, modified by Korngold et al. (1953), is used as follows: 2 mc (millicuries) of ^{131}I are pipetted into a solution of 13 mg of sodium iodide in 2 ml of distilled water. The iodide is oxidized to iodine with an excess of nitrous acid, by adding 1 ml of a solution containing 16 mg of $NaNO_2$ and 0.06 ml of concentrated hydrochloric acid. These reactions lead to the generation of iodine, as shown by these formulas:

$$2NaNO_2 + 2HCl \rightarrow 2HNO_2 + 2NaCl$$

$$2NaNO_2 + 2NaI + 2HCl \rightarrow I_2 + 2H_2O + 2NO + 2NaCl$$

Immediately after the iodine is generated, a solution of antigen (or antibody globulin) is added to the fine iodine suspension, and the resulting mixture is left at 25 to 28° for 1 hour. It is then dialyzed against distilled water at 7 to 8° for 48 hours.

Nucleic acids, for example, the nucleic acid portion of a virus molecule, can be tagged by cultivating the virus in a medium containing sodium phosphate with the radioactive phosphorus ^{32}P in a final concentration of 15 to 20 mg of $Na_2HPO_4/1000$ ml. This corresponds to about 300 μc of $P^{32}/1000$ ml.

The Webster et al. Iodination Method (1962). The carrier 0.001 *M* KI (0.25 ml) is mixed with a carrier-free radioiodide. Distilled water is added up to 3.5 ml and acidified with 0.2 ml of 1 *N* sulfuric acid. The iodine is liberated by the addition of 0.2 ml of hydrogen peroxide. The reaction mixture should be shaken with 2.0 ml of carbon tetrachloride at intervals of 30 minutes to extract the free iodine into the organic phase. The aqueous phase is then removed, and carbon tetrachloride washed twice with 10 ml of water. The globulin fraction which was dissolved in a 0.1 *M* bicarbonate buffer at pH 8.9 is added to the washed carbon tetrachloride. The solution is mixed immediately, and agitated for 10 minutes. The two phases are separated by centrifugation, and the aqueous phase is dialyzed against tap water for 12 hours, and then against saline for 1 hour. The iodinated globulin thus prepared remains biologically unaltered.

The isotope-labeled antigens or antibodies are detected in tissues or cells by measuring their radioactivities with the aid of a bell-shaped Geiger-Müller counter tube, or a scintillation apparatus (Fig. 67).

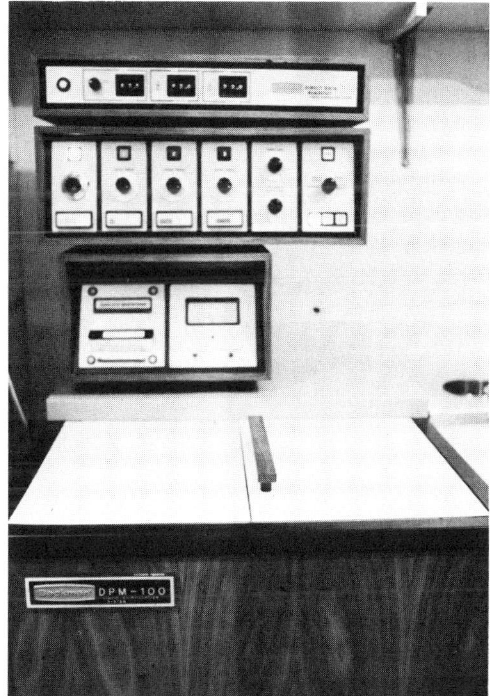

Figure 67. A scintillation apparatus.

The tissue sample to be tested for the radioactivity can be prepared by digestion in the following manner (Pressman and Keighley, 1948). The tissue sample is at first macerated in a small (10 ml) volume of water; 1 ml of 0.1 N potassium iodide solution is added to this mixture as carrier, followed by 3 ml of 1 N silver nitrate solution, 10 ml of concentrated nitric acid, and 5 ml of 30% hydrogen peroxide solution. This mixture is heated at 80° for 30 minutes, after which another 5-ml volume of 30% hydrogen peroxide is added. This is heated for another 30 minutes. The mixture should then be cooled, and filtered through a paper disk. The precipitate is then washed with distilled water and acetone, air-dried, spread uniformly with a spatula on a filter paper disk, and mounted on aluminum holders. The sample is hence ready for the radioactivity counting.

The Talmage et al. (1954) Iodination Technique. A dialyzed globulin preparation (0.5 ml) is first diluted with an equal volume of 0.2 M carbonate buffer, pH 10, and added to a ^{131}I solution. The ^{131}I solution is made by adding one or two drops of freshly prepared 0.01 N solution of KI, one drop of 0.5 *N* HCl, and one drop of 0.1 *N* NaO$_2$ to 6 MC of ^{131}I in a volume less than 0.5 ml. The ^{131}I-globulin mixture is left for 3 minutes, and then filtered through a column of Amberlite IR-4B resin, to be washed with 9 ml of distilled water. The eluate is collected, made isotonic with 8.5% sodium chloride, buffered to pH 7.0 with Merthiolate, added to 1:10,000 concentration.

This method was adapted by Powell (1961) for obtaining and measuring *specific labeled virus antibody*. In this procedure, a 50% suspension of virus-coated red cells is mixed 1:10 with a ^{131}I labeled globulin. This mixture is agitated at 4° overnight, and then the red cell-virus labeled antibody complex is centrifuged and washed fifteen times in large volumes of saline and 0.15% potassium iodide.

The antibody can be released from the red cell-virus-labeled antibody complex by suspending this mixture in a small volume of normal saline and adjusting the pH to 3.5 with 0.2 *M* citric acid. After 15 minutes the suspension is centrifuged, and the supernatant, which now contains more specific labeled antibody, is adjusted to pH 7.0 with 0.5 *N* sodium hydroxide. A further purification of the labeled antibody is attained by a repetition of the adsorption of the supernatant and elution, as described above.

The isotope-labeled antigens or antibodies were used in various immunological investigations, for example, in studies on the mechanism of antibody response, the formation and localization of antibodies in organs and tissues, the retention of antigens at the injection sites, the localization in other organs and elimination from the host, the uptake of antibodies by host cells, and the antigen-antibody molecular ratios (Libby and Madison, 1947; Pressman et al., 1949; Korngold et al., 1953; Masouredis, 1957; Weigle and Maurer, 1957; Ritts and Cutting, 1955). Radiolabeled antisera were applied to certain immunological tests *in vitro,* the precipitation test (Cohen, 1951; Gerloff et al., 1962), and a hemagglutination test (Roberts and Haurowitz, 1962).

1. *The Radioisotope Precipitation Test*

The first, direct radioisotope precipitation (flocculation) test has been described by Cohen (1951) and later by Askonas and Rhodes (1965). The method has been modified as indirect test by Gerloff et al., (1962) and Tabert and Lackman (1965). The indirect radioisotope precipitation test depends on the measurements of radioactivity in a radiolabeled antigen which has combined with a specific immunoglobulin to form a complex precipitable by an anti-γ-globulin.

i. *Direct Radioisotope Precipitation Test.* In order to relate specific radioactivity of one of the constituents of an antigen-antibody precipitate to the antibody nitrogen, the following procedure may be used (Minden and Farr, 1969).

Quadruplicate precipitates, obtained at the equivalence point, are divided in two portions; one portion is used for nitrogen determination, and the other two precipitates are employed for determination of radioactivity. The precipitates in which radioactivity is to be estimated are first dissolved with two or three drops of 0.1 N NaOH and transferred quantitatively with 2 ml of distilled water to an aluminum pan. The liquids are evaporated underneath a heat lamp, and the residues are employed for counting the radioactivity of antibody in an end-window GM counter.

Usually no correction factor is needed for self-absorption of the radioisotope as may be determined by the following procedure: a constant amount of the radioisotope is added to varying amounts of precipitates, which are then dissolved and counted. If the residues in a test series do not exceed a few milligrams, a correction for self-absorption is unnecessary.

Antibody nitrogen is determined by subtracting from the total nitrogen in the equivalence precipitate, the antigen nitrogen which has been added to form the equivalence precipitate.

A similar radioprecipitation procedure can be used to determine the capacity of serum immunoglobulins to bind an antigen. This capacity can be measured by precipitating a labeled antigen, for example, a complex consisting of an ^{131}I-labeled antigen and antibody, with 50% saturated ammonium sulfate. In this procedure, 0.5-ml aliquots of different antiserum dilutions made in duplicate, incubated with an equal volume of an ^{131}I-labeled antigen at 4° for 18 hours. The mixture then receives 1 ml of 50% saturated ammonium sulfate, is incubated and centrifuged, and the precipitates are collected and washed with the 50% ammonium sulfate solution. The radioactivity in the precipitates is determined in a radioactivity counter. Results are expressed as the percentage of iodine-labeled antigen specifically bound by a 1:10 dilution of a test antiserum. Alternatively, results may be expressed as micrograms of iodine-labeled antigen N bound per milliliter of undiluted antiserum (Minden and Farr, 1969).

The test described by Askonas and Rhodes (1965), as modified by Ada and Williams (1966) is conducted in the following manner. Iodination of proteins with ^{131}I is performed by Ada's et al. (1964) method. The extract containing antigen is mixed in the ratio of 20:1 with a 10% aqueous solution of freshly prepared sodium deoxycholate solution and with one tenth of the volume of a rabbit antiserum. The mixture is incubated at 37° for 1 hour and left at 2° overnight. Goat antirabbit γ-globulin serum is then added in an approximate volume of one fifth of the volume of mixture and the mixture is incubated at 37° for 1 hour and left overnight at 2°. The mixture is then centrifuged at 2000 $\times$ g for 15 minutes while the supernatant is rejected and the radioactivity is estimated in the deposit. The amount of radioactivity which reacted specifically with antiserum is thus calculated. An allowance should be made for the amount of radioactivity mechanically trapped in the precipitate which usually amounts to 3% of that occurring in the supernatant. Radioactivity is estimated in a scintillation counter.

The direct radioisotope precipitation test by Cohen (1951) is set up as follows. The ^{131}I-labeled antiserum, for example, a diphtheria antitoxin, is serially diluted, in 1-ml volumes, in triplicate. Series of dilutions of noniodinated antiserum are made parallelly. Varying amounts of antigen are added to the first two or three antiserum dilutions (1:2, 1:3), incubated for 1 hour at 37 to 40°, and left in the refrigerator for 3 days. The precipitates are washed three times with cold saline, dissolved in 1 ml of 0.1 N sodium hydroxide, and diluted to 10 ml with distilled water. Then 1 ml of this solution is dispensed in triplicate on metal cup planchetes; one drop of 10% gelatin is added to the mixture, and it is dried overnight under an end-window Geiger-Müller tube. Corrections should be made for the background count and decay.

ii. *Indirect Radioisotope Test.* The antigen is labeled with ^{131}I by persulfate oxidation as described by McKeil and Millar (1968). Then 1 ml of a suspension of particulate antigen is mixed with 0.1 ml of 1.7×10^{-4} M KI made in 0.05 M pH 7.4 phosphate buffer; 5 mC of 131/NaI is added, followed by one volume of 10% ammonium persulfate in 0.05 M phosphate buffer, sufficient to make 2.5% final concentration of the oxidizing agent. The mixture is incubated at room temperature for 2 hours and then filtered through a Sephadex G-25 short column to remove the unbound iodine. The particulate material is eluted from the column with 0.02 M, pH 7.4 phosphate buffer, centrifuged at $17,000 \times g$ for 20 minutes and resuspended in the same buffer to which a trace of ether has been added as a preservative. Specific activity of the antigen preparation is expressed in millicuries/per milliliter. The antigen can be stored in a lead container at 4°.

The amount of antigen to be used for the radioisotope precipitation test should correspond to 1500 to 2000 counts per minute/25 μl.

The labeled antigen is washed four times to remove iodine excess and resuspended to an estimated concentration in 0.02 M, pH 7.1 phosphate-buffered saline. The labeled antigen may be diluted further depending on the amount of radioactivity. The 0.04 ml of the diluted antigen and an equal volume of serial, twofold dilutions of antiserum are combined. Dilutions of both the antigen and antiserum are made in 0.01 M, pH 7.1 phosphate-buffered saline, containing 1:25 parts of 0.05 M ethylene diaminetetra-acetic acid. The mixtures are rotated at 37° for 1 hour. Each tube then receives 0.2 ml of an appropriate anti-γ-globulin, diluted according to its specific immunological strength. The tubes are rotated again at 37° for

1 hour and left overnight at 4°. To each tube, 0.5 ml of the diluent is then added and the mixtures are shaken vigorously with a cyclomixer and centrifuged at $175 \times g$ for 10 minutes in a centrifuge with a horizontal head. The 0.5 ml of the supernatant fluid is removed from each tube with a constriction pipette and placed in a planchet. The planchets are dried, and the radioactivity is determined by a Nucelar-Chicago Gas Flow Counting Apparatus. The indirect radioisotope precipitation test has been employed for measuring Q-fever antigen-antibody reactions (Tabert and Lackman, 1965) and for serodiagnosis in Q-fever (McKeil and Millar, 1968).

2. The Radioisotope Immunoelectrophoresis Test

This test (Onoue et al., 1964) is a combination of the immunoelectrophoresis and the iodination techniques. Thus an antigen preparation is first partitioned in the agar gel on a microscope slide submitted to the electrophoresis for 30 to 60 minutes. An ^{131}I-labeled antigen or a mixture of horse antirabbit globulin serum and a ^{131}I-labeled hapten is diffused overnight from the central trough. Arcs of specific precipitates are formed. The slide is then washed with buffered saline, pH 8, for 8 to 24 hours to remove remaining soluble proteins, dried, and stained with nigrosin.

Autoradiographs are obtained by placing an x-ray film in contact with the dry stained slide wrapped with a plastic film (Saran or Handiwrap). The exposure factor is defined as the product of the average specific radioactivity (mc/mg) of the test antigen during exposure and the length of time of contact (hour). In most cases, films are exposed to the extent of an exposure factor of 35 to 40.

VII. THE IMMUNOFLUORESCENCE METHOD

The immunofluorescent method depends on the detection in tissues of homologous antigen-antibody complexes, in which one of the components has been conjugated with a fluorescent dye. These complexes are detected as fluorescent microprecipitates by means of an ultraviolet microscope. There are two types of fluorescent antibody techniques, the direct and the indirect. In the direct method, the specific antiserum is itself conjugated to a fluorescent dye and applied to the material tested. In the indirect or layering technique, first the unconjugated specific antiserum is applied to a test specimen to allow a combination between antibody and antigen. The specimen is then washed free of excess serum and treated with a fluorescein-labeled antibody which is directed against the species of the antiserum. For example, a conjugated goat antirabbit globulin is employed if the specimen was treated with a nonlabeled rabbit antiserum. This labeled antibody adsorbs onto the serological complex, which becomes fluorescent thereby.

Protein antigens or antibodies in this method are labeled with certain fluorescent pigments, for example, isocyanates of higher aromatic hydrocarbons (Creech and Jones, 1941; Miller and Stanley, 1941), giving green or blue fluorescence, 1-dimethyl-amino-5-sulphonylchloride-naphthalene (Coons and Kaplan, 1950), to give a yellow fluorescence, benzaldehyde-6-nitro-nitro-2-sodium-diazotate, the nuclear fast red, giving brilliant orange fluorescence (Chadwick et al., 1958), or aminorosamine B giving an orange fluorescent dye (Borek and Silverstein, 1960). Both the labeled and unlabeled antigens reacting with the specific labeled antibodies may be detected by means of the ultraviolet microscopy.

The main ingredients of the direct technique are (a) microtome tissue sections or slide smears, made from a specimen containing a specific antigen, (b) globulin fractions isolated from an appropriate standard antiserum and from a control serum, and (c) a fluorescent dye.

The indirect technique requires, in addition, a standard antiglobulin serum.

1. Sectioning and Ultrasectioning

Adequate techniques for making ultrathin tissue sections were designed by Coons and Kaplan (1950) and Coons, Leduc, and Kaplan (1951), both being modifications of the Linderstrøm-Lang and Mogensen (1938) technique. According to the modified Linderstrøm-Lang and Mogensen technique, pieces of tissue, 4 to 5 mm in their dimension, are dipped in a freezing mixture of dry ice and alcohol, and placed in a refrigerated cabinet, where several frozen sections, 400–700 Å thick, are cut by the aid of a microtome (Fig. 68). The tissue sections are transferred on glass slides, previously coated with formalized gelatin as adhesive, then thawed and dried rapidly in a current of warm air. Most sections require treatment with a suitable fixative selected according to the chemical characteristic of an antigen to be found in the tissue section. Thus for proteins 95% v/v ethanol at 37° or formalin-dioxane can be used. For viruses, acetone is most widely used. Sections should be labeled with fluorescent isothiocyanate as soon as possible, since the grey-blue autofluorescence of tissue proteins increases during the following few hours, which hampers microscopic observations.

Ultrathin (4–10 mμ) tissue sections may be prepared by Luft's (1961) or Conti and Naylor's (1959) method. The most satisfactory medium for imbedding of tissue for cutting sections or ultrasections is a combination containing Epon 812, which is a glycerol-based epoxy resin of low viscosity and has a rapid penetration force. Blocks prepared in this medium are cut easily and sections show greater contrast in the electron microscope than sections prepared in other resins (Luft, 1961). Sufficient contrast is obtained with this resin to permit the use of tetroxide fixation alone without additional staining. Details of the method are as follows.

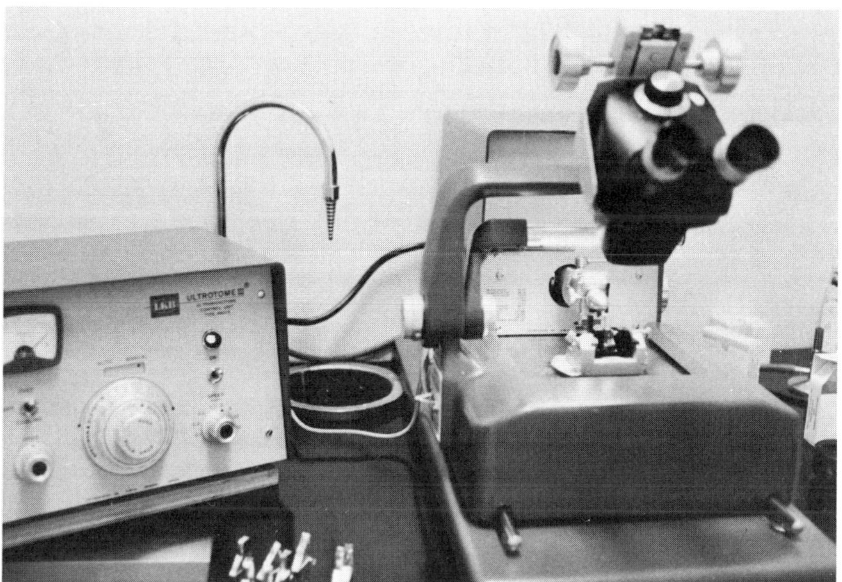

Figure 68.   The microtome.

The tissue sample is fixed and dehydrated in one change of absolute
ethyl alcohol. The tissues can subsequently be put through a propylene
oxide although this step is not essential. The tissue block is then immersed
in an equal quantity of the complete mixed resin containing accelerator
and the mixture is swirled. The tissue is left to stand for 1 hour. Gelatin
capsules are filled nearly full with the complete resin mixture and each tissue block is sucked up into a pipette, allowed to settle to the tip and transferred with a minimum of liquid to the surface of resin in the capsule. The
tissue block slowly settles to the bottom of the capsule losing most of its
solvent. The resin is cured overnight at 60°. Sections or ultrathonsections can
be cut from the block following completion of polymerization, although
cutting is easier when the polymerization time has been extended. One of
the following mixtures may be applied as resin mixture: mixture A contains 62 ml of Epon 812 (Shell) and 100 ml DDSA (dodecenyl succinic
anhydride). Mixture B contains 100 ml of Epon 812 and 89 ml of MNA
(methyl endomethylene tetrahydrophthal anhydrate). Immediately before
use, the DMP-30 (2,4,6-tri dimethyl aminomethyl phenol) accelerator is
added to the selected resin mixture to the final concentration of 1.5 to 2%
(v/v) and stirred thoroughly. This mixture constitutes the complete resin
mixture used for embedding of tissue.

Ultrathin (4–10 mμ) sections are cut in a cryostat at $-15°$. The sections are placed on a 0.1% gelatin-coated slide, and may be stored at $-70°$. Cells or tissues, fixed in 1.5% aqueous solution of potassium permanganate for 40 minutes at 4°, are treated with partially polymerized *n*-butyl methacrylate, placed in gelatin capsules, and centrifuged at 2000 $\times$ *g* for 2 minutes. The gelatin capsules are left at 60° for 8 to 12 hours, and then at room temperature for 3 days. Sections are cut with a Porter-Blum microtome, equipped with a glass knife. Ultrathin sections are picked up on a 200-mesh copper grid, on which a thin collodion membrane has been mounted and dried.

Ultrasectioning of bacteria are made most conveniently by Kellenberger's et al. (1958) technique. In this technique, the fixative in the form of 1% OsO_4, dissolved in the Michaelis' acetate veronal buffer, pH 6.1, is added to a suspension of bacteria (1:10) and centrifuged at once for 5 minutes at 2000 $\times$ g. The pellet is resuspended in 1 ml of the fixative, sometimes supplemented by 0.1 ml of the growth medium, which may be omitted or supplemented by 0.1 ml of distilled water. The suspension is left at room temperature overnight and then diluted into 8 ml of acetate veronal buffer, pH 6.1, and centrifuged at 2000 $\times$ g for 5 minutes. The pellet is resuspended in about 0.03 ml of a 2% melted agar, cooled to 45°. The suspension is mixed and placed as a drop on a microscope slide. After cooling and gelation, the gel is cut into little cubes, which are immersed for 2 hours in 0.5% uranise acetate solution made in the acetate-veronal buffer.

The little cubes are dehydrated in acetone (25, 50, and 75% for 15 minutes, 90 and 100% for 30 minutes) and embedded in vestopal W by 30 minute immersions in four different vestopal mixtures: (a) vestopal acetone, 1:3; (b) vestopal acetone, 1:1; (c) vestopal acetone, 3:1; and (d) vestopal:benzoyl peroxide, 1:1 + 0.5% cobalt naphthenate. The cubes are finally placed in gelatine capsules filled with the last mixture and polymerized at 60° for 12 to 24 hours. Ultrathin sections are cut using a Porter-Blum ultramicrotome with a diamond knife. The sections are floated off the knife edge onto distilled water, picked up on acid cleaned 200 mesh copper grids and examined in an electron microscope.

2. *Reagents for Immunofluorescence*

Smears of tissues may be made on cover slips, which should be air-dried for 30 minutes before staining (Moulton and Brown, 1954). Smears of other materials, for example, sputum, pus, and saline suspensions of bacteria, may be prepared either on nonfluorescing cover slips or on microscope glass slides. Living bacteria or bacteria killed with 0.5% formalin can be used. A drop of suspension is placed on a slide and air-dried. It is then fixed gently with heat, methanol, or formalin. The heat-fixation is the simplest, and quite satisfactory, method.

The antisera against microorganisms are obtained by ordinary techniques of immunization of rabbits or guinea pigs with increasing doses of microorganisms. The antiglobulin serum is produced by injecting a human being, a rabbit, or a guinea pig, serum, an isolated serum globulin, or a γ-globulin into another species of animals, for example, in a goat* or a horse. A goat is conventionally immunized by injecting every second or third day, increasing amounts of normal rabbit γ-globulin, for example, 20, 30, 40, 50, 60, 70, 70, 80, 80 mg. According to the often-used Proom's (1943) technique, goats are injected intramuscularly with potassium-alum serum precipitates. Three fourth-nightly injections of 5 to 10 ml of precipitate are given in one or two legs, and the fourth dose, consisting of 10 ml of the whole serum, is injected subcutaneously, 1 month later. In 2 weeks after the last injection, the blood is collected and centrifuged, and the serum is separated and stored. The γ-globulin preparation, emulsified in Freund's complete adjuvant, is injected subcutaneously into the flank of goats (24 mg of protein per animal). The injection is repeated in 2 months and the animal is bled 1 month later.

Isolation of immunoglobulins from a serum may be accomplished by column chromatography, by dilution-dialysis or by ammonium sulfate precipitation.

According to Ada and Williams' (1966) method, rabbit γ-globulin is prepared by dialyzing normal rabbit serum against 0.01 M, pH 7.5 phosphate buffer and passing the dialyzate through a DEAE-cellulose column equilibrated against the same buffer, which is also used for the elution of fractions. The first protein peak in the effluent is γ-globulin.

According to the dilution-dialysis procedure, the euglobulin fraction may be obtained from a serum by adjusting to pH 6.0 and then dialyzing against 25 volumes of a 0.01 M, pH 6.0 phosphate buffer for 24 hours at 5°. The resulting euglobulin precipitate is separated by centrifugation and reconstituted in a phosphate-buffered saline, pH 7.2 to one-half the original serum volume. If ammonium sulfate is used, globulins from immune or control sera may be prepared by precipitation of the globulin fractions in 18% sodium sulfate, using two volumes of 27% sodium sulfate to one volume of sera at 15° to 30° and leaving the mixture for 5 to 6 hour after which the precipitate is collected by centrifugation at 800 $\times$ g for 20 minutes. The precipitate containing globulins is then dissolved in a 0.01 M, pH 8.5 phosphate buffer, dialyzed against this buffer at 4° until no sulfate can be detected in the dialyzate with barium chloride. The globulin preparation is then reconstituted with a pH 9.0 buffer to the original volume of serum or preferably, to the protein concentration of 1%. If the protein con-

---

* The goat antihuman globulin is commercially produced by Difco Laboratories, Detroit, Mich.

centration is lower than 1%, the volume of solution should be reduced by pervaporation through a dialysis tank. Equal volumes of the antiserum and a saturated solution of neutral ammonium sulfate are mixed and left at 0 to 4° overnight. The arising precipitate is collected, dissolved in distilled water, and dialyzed again in saline solution until free from sulfate, as tested with barium hydroxide.

The supernatant must be reprecipitated several times, until it ceases to show any coloration. The sediment containing globulin and ammonium sulfate is collected, dissolved in distilled water, and dialyzed against 0.85% sodium chloride solution. The dialysis is completed when no sulfate can be detected in the fluid with barium chloride. Globulins are reconstituted with distilled water to the original volume of serum. However, to provide a suitable medium for labeling, the protein concentration must not be less than 1%. If the protein concentration is lower, the volume of solution should be reduced by pervaporation through a dialysis sac.

The intensity of fluorescence of labeled solutions can be measured in the Coleman photofluorometer (model 12C), using Corning no. 3389-4308 (primary), and 5874 (secondary) filters (Kaufman and Cherry, 1961).

Fluorescein isothiocyanate can be synthesized according to the method of Coons and Kaplan (1950), or Riggs (1957), which partially follows a technique described in 1905 by Bogert and Wright. The synthesis procedure consists of the following steps. First, the 4-nitrophthalic acid is heated with two equivalents of resorcinol to produce nitrofluorescein; this being refluxed with acetic anhydride forms nitrofluorescein diacetate, which is then subjected to fractional crystallization. Isomeric acetates thus separated are saponified, and a pure isomer of nitrofluorescein is recovered. By a catalytic hydrogenation, fluorescein amine is produced which converts to fluorescein isocyanata in the presence of phosgene. In Riggs' technique, a solid preparation of fluorescein isothiocyanate is made from the fraction II of fluorescein amine.

Adequate labeling techniques for various dyes were devised by Coons and Kaplan (1950), Marshall et al. (1958), Chadwick et al. (1958), Borek and Silverstein (1960), Del Giudice et al. 1967), Caldwell et al. (1966), and Shifrine et al. (1968), and a rapid labeling technique was designed by Peacock et al. (1971).

3. The Rapid Fluorescent-Antibody Conjugation

According to Peacock et al. (1971), an IgG globulin preparation obtained by Baumstark's et al. (1964) method, is mixed with the Cl⁻ form of DEAE-Sephadex, A-50 (0.5 g) equilibrated with 0.01 M phosphate buffer, pH 6.5. The slurry is stirred slowly in an ice bath for 1 hour, and then placed into two centrifugal devices (Centrifugal Filter Holder, Cat.

no. 4305, Gelman Instr. Co.) and spun down in a horizontal head at $450 \times g$ for 10 minutes. The residues in the upper cup are then washed with cold 0.01 M, pH 6.5, phosphate buffer and recentrifuged as above. The eluates collected in the lower cup are pooled and mixed with more DEAE-Sephadex, A-50, Cl⁻ form. The resultant slurry is treated as above. To the collected, and ice-cooled final eluates (24.5 ml) are added 5 ml of 0.5 M bicarbonate buffer, pH 9.0, and 0.1 ml (1 mg) of a freshly prepared solution of fluorescein isothiocyanate. The mixture is stored for 5 minutes, left at 37° for 45 minutes with occasional stirring, and filtered through a 45-μm membrane filter and rapidly passed through a 2- $\times$ 21-cm Sephadex G-25 (coarse) column equilibrated with $M/15$ phosphate-buffered saline, pH 7.35. The purified conjugated globulin passes rapidly down the column, whereas unconjugated dye remains at the top of the column. The colored conjugated globulin fraction is collected and absorbed with acetone-extracted normal yolk-sac powder (10 mg/ml) at room temperature for 1 hour. After the centrifugation at 20,000 $\times$ g for 15 minutes, the supernatant fluid is filtered through a 0.2-μm membrane filter. The conjugate is preserved with 0.05% sodium azide and stored at 4°.

4. *The Fluorescein-Labeling Technique of Coons and Kaplan*

As the first step, 10.5 ml of 0.15 M sodium chloride and 3.0 ml of acetone are mixed together in a 50-ml Erlenmeyer flask, placed in an ice bath, and stirred mechanically. When the temperature of this mixture falls to 0 to 2°, a volume of 3 ml of a globulin solution containing about 350 to 400 mg of protein is added. A volume of 1.5 ml of a stain solution, which consists of 17 to mg of fluorescein isothiocyanate, 1 ml of acetone, and 0.5 ml of dioxane, is added dropwise. This brings the ratio between fluorescein isothiocyanate and protein to 0.05/1 mg of 1:20. (However, lower dye-to-protein ratios may occasionally be preferred, since they reduce the nonspecific fluorescence.)

A yellow precipitate which appears in the meantime dissolves almost completely during 18 hours of stirring at 0 to 2°. Simultaneously, the fluid becomes more fluorescent. This fluid should be dialyzed against a buffered saline, usually for 5 to 7 days, until the fluorescence outside the dialysis sac is less than that given by a 1:20,000 solution of fluorescein. According to Del Giudice's et al. (1967) technique, labeling of the antibody globulin is carried out by adding one part of fluorescein isothiocyanate to 70 parts of the globulin dissolved in a phosphate buffer, pH 8.8, and leaving the mixture overnight at 4 to 10°. Unbound fluorescein is removed by molecular filtration through a Sephadex G-25 column, adjusted to pH 7.2–7.4 with 0.01 M phosphate-buffered saline. The conjugate is dialyzed overnight against the same buffer.

Conjugation of the globulins with fluorescein isothiocyanate is conducted by Caldwell's et al.(1966) method in the following manner. The globulin solution is added to a dry mixture of one part of fluorescein isothiocyanate (0.025 mg of FITC protein) and nine parts of cellulose powder (Celite), and the mixture is shaken for 5 minutes. The cellulose powder is removed by centrifugation, and the unbound dye is removed by filtration through a small (2 × 5 cm) Sephadex G-25 column, using a 0.1 M, pH 7.5 phosphate buffer containing 0.1 M sodium chloride. The conjugated globulin preparation may be freeze-dried or concentrated in liquid form and stored at −25°.

A more efficient technique for removal of excess dye is the gel filtration, which is a much faster procedure as it only requires 10 to 15 minutes (Killander et al., 1961). In this technique, the fluorescein-treated material is put on a 2 × 5 cm column, made of Sephadex G-25 (AB Pharmacia, Uppsala, Sweden), or Amberlite CG 400, washed with a saline-phosphate buffer, pH 7.0 to 7.5. The same buffer is used for elution. The fast-moving yellow zone, containing the conjugated protein, is collected, whereas the unbound dye migrates at a much slower rate. The eluate is concentrated by lyophilization or by water absorption on Carbowax 20 M at 5°, and then reconstituted to the original or one-half antiserum volume, dialyzed against PBS to remove the excess salts, and relyophilized (if the preparation is to be stored).

The crude globulin preparation may be fractionated on diethylamino-ethyl (DEAE)-cellulose columns according to Wood's et al. (1965) method. Rabbit γ-globulin fractions may be obtained by elution of the DEAE-cellulose column with 0.01 M phosphate followed by 0.05 M NaCl in 0.01 M phosphate buffer. These liquids containing globulin fractions are concentrated by positive pressure (Finegold et al., 1968).

Any stained and fluorescent but nonspecific material must be removed from this fluid with liver powder, cardiac powder (National Biochemical Corporation), and blood cells of the animal species whose tissues have been used for sectioning. Tissue powders prepared from kidney and gut are used occasionally. Liver powder can be prepared in the following manner (Coons and Kaplan, 1950). Fresh, frozen liver suspended in an equal volume of 0.15 M sodium chloride is homogenized in a Waring blender. The homogenate is first extracted with 4 volumes of acetone for a few minutes, then centrifuged, and washed with several changes of saline solution, until the supernatant remains clear and unstained. The washed precipitate is suspended in saline and treated with four volumes of acetone, and centrifuged after a few minutes. The sediment is separated and treated again with four volumes of acetone, then filtered through a Büchner funnel, washed with acetone, and dried. It can be stored at 4°.

The absorption of a fluorescein labeled antibody solution is conducted by mixing this solution with the liver powder in a proportion of 1 ml:100 mg. The mixture is left at room temperature for 1 hour, with occasional stirring, and centrifuged in the cold at about 40,000 × g. The absorption of the supernatant is repeated by increasing the amount of liver powder to 300 mg/ml. The twice absorbed serum is collected and preserved with Merthiolate added to a final concentration of 1:10,000. Sodium azide at 0.3% final concentration can be used alternatively.

A very rapid procedure for *labeling of antigens* with fluorescein isothiocyanate absorbed on Celite was described by Rinderknecht (1962). The absorbent, Celite containing about 10% fluorescein isothiocyanate is used in the ratio of 1:10 in respect to protein antigen. The fluorescent proteins are freed from the unconjugated dye by filtration through a Sephadex G-25, at pH 6.5 in a 0.02 *M* phosphate buffer.

A simplified procedure for the coupling of isocyanate to protein was described by Goldman and Carver (1957). Fluorescein isocyanate dried on thick filter paper is used in this technique. An appropriately sized piece of this paper is simply added to stirred, buffered antibody solution, but no organic solvent is required.

5. *The Marshall et al. Conjugation Technique (1958)*

Whole serum (5.0 ml), diluted with 0.15 *M* NaCl (8.2 ml) and 0.5 *M* carbonate bicarbonate buffer, pH 9.2 (3.4 ml), is first cooled by stirring at 2° in a cold room. It is then treated with an acetone solution of fluorescein isothiocyanate (40 mg/2 ml of acetone), added dropwise to the serum solution, and stirred continuously at 2° for 18 hours. The resultant fluorescein solution is dialyzed at 2° against 0.15 *M* NaCl buffered to pH 7.0 with 0.01 *M* phosphate until no further fluorescence is detected by ultraviolet rays. The dialyzed conjugate solution should be cleared by a high-speed centrifugation.

6. *The Rhodamine Conjugation of Globulins*

The recommended procedure for conjugation of globulins with rhodamine is the method of Cebra and Goldstein (1965), although an earlier method designed by Chadwick et al. (1958) is also useful. The conjugation of globulins to rhodamine isothiocyanate (Baltimore Biological Laboratories, Baltimore, Md.) is performed as follows: tetramethyl rhodamine isothiocyanate is added to a γ-globulin preparation in a ratio of 0.04 to 0.02 mg/mg protein. The reagents and mixture are kept at 4° while the pH is maintained at 9.5 for the first hour of conjugation, after which the mixture is stirred at this temperature for 18 hours. In order to remove the nonconjugated dye, the mixture is filtered through a Sephadex G-50 column, equilibrated with 0.14 *M* NaCl in 0.01 *M* phosphate buffer, pH 7.4.

The absorption at 280 and 515 mμ is determined on all eluted fractions, and the fractions in which the ratios of OD 280:OD 515 are two or more are collected and pooled.

The rhodamine-globulin conjugates are then absorbed with a mouse liver powder (Baltimore Biological Laboratories) using 100 mg of powder per 1 ml of conjugate, followed by centrifugation and filtration through a 0.2-μ pore size filter. The filtered conjugate may be used either full strength or diluted 1:5 or 1:10 in a phosphate buffered saline.

Layering with the Rhodamine Conjugate. A suspension of cell or a cell culture to be used as the source of antigen should be first washed in Hanks' balanced salt solution and then resuspended in the solution containing 30% (w/v) bovine albumin. The cell suspension is smeared on the cover slips, air-dried, and fixed in absolute methanol, left at 4° for 10 minutes. The smears are washed in PBS, pH 7.2. The rhodamine-conjugated globulin is then applied to the smears for 1 to 2 hours or longer, followed by washing in PBS and mounting in 50% glycerol in PBS or in DPX. If an indirect immunofluorescence test is used, the smear is layered with unconjugated specific antiserum, followed by washing with PBS and by the application of a rhodamine-conjugated goat antirabbit antiserum.

According to the earlier Chadwick et al. (1958) method, the dye for globulin labeling is prepared by grinding one gram of Lissamine Rhodamine B 200 (Imperial Chemical Industries Ltd. of England) with 2 g of PCl_2 and suspending in 10 ml of dry acetone. After 15 minutes, the dye solution should be filtered. A volume of 1.5 ml of this dye is added drop by drop to the immune globulin preparation, dissolved in 15 ml of 0.5 M carbonate-bicarbonate buffer, pH 10, with constant stirring in the cold. The stirring should be continued for about 16 hours. The conjugate is then dialyzed against buffered saline and absorbed with fresh liver powder prior to use.

7. The Aminorosamine B Labeling of Immunoglobulins

The 4′-aminorasamine B can be prepared by condensation of 2 moles of m-diethylaminophenol with 1 mole p-nitrobenzaldehyde, followed by catalytic reduction of the nitro group (Borek and Silverstein, 1960). The dye is conjugated with the serum proteins in the following manner: 5.2 mg (1.2×10^{-2} millimole) of 4′-aminorosamine B, dissolved in 0.48 ml of 0.1 N hydrochloric acid and 0.32 ml of water, is mixed in the cold with a solution of sodium nitrate (1.1 mg or 1.5×10^{-2} millimole) in 0.4 ml of water. After standing in the cold for 10 minutes, the resultant solution of diazonium salt is added dropwise to a cold solution of 1 ml of antiserum in 5 ml of 0.15 M sodium chloride and 1 ml of 0.5 M bicarbonate-carbonate buffer at pH 9.1. The mixture is stirred overnight and dialyzed for 4 days against 0.15 M saline made in 0.01 M phosphate buffer, at pH 7.2.

8. Techniques of Staining with Fluorescent Antibody

i. *The Direct Immunofluorescence Technique.* The most adequate direct fluorescent antibody techniques were published by Caldwell et al. (1966) and earlier methods are those of Coons et al. (1942), Moody et al. (1956, 1959), and Masiga and Stone (1968). These procedures are applied in the following manner.

According to Caldwell's et al. (1966) method, the bacteria, washed from constituents of the culture medium, are sedimented, resuspended in 5% formaldehyde and left for 15 minutes. The formalinized cells are then spun down and suspended in 0.01 M, pH 7.5 phosphate buffer to a desired final concentration. The bacterial suspension is then added in equal volume to the labeled globulin preparation diluted 1:10 in the same phosphate buffer, and the mixture is incubated at 37° on a rotary shaker for 10 minutes. After the incubation, the suspension is diluted with 10 times larger volume of the buffer solution, shaken thoroughly and centrifuged at 1000 × g for 15 minutes. The sediment is washed two to three times with a buffer, and finally resuspended in 0.2 to 0.5 ml of buffer. A drop or 0.05 ml of this material is transferred to a glass slide, air-dried, and mounted under a cover slip in a drop of buffered glycerol, pH 8.5, and sealed with lacquer. The buffered glycerol is prepared by mixing one part bicarbonate buffer, pH 8.5, to nine parts of glycerol. The conjugate is filtered through a Sephadex G-25 column equilibrated with the buffer. The ratio of absorption at 280 to 495 nm is determined on all collected fractions. A drop of nondiluted or 1:10 diluted conjugate (a fluorescein labeled immune globulin) is put on a section or smear to be examined for the presence of an antigen, and left for 15 to 30 minutes in a small plate containing a piece of moist filter paper, to prevent evaporation. The preparation is then washed for 10 minutes in a saline buffered to pH 7.0 to 8.0 and blotted carefully. Finally, a drop of glycerol reagent, containing one part of glycerol in 10 parts of buffered saline (pH 7 to 8), is placed on the section and covered with a cover slip. Smears from a source of infection are made in much the same way by the use of sterile cotton applicator sticks. The swabs are usually incubated in a broth or a similar culture medium for 24 to 48 hours at 37°, and smears are made from cultures thus obtained and overlayered with the conjugate. Nonfluorescent mountant (Hartman-Leddon) may be used for mounting cover slips on smear slides.

Control sections or smears should be prepared simultaneously from the same material and stained with a labeled normal globulin and with a labeled heterologous antiserum. Additional controls consist of sections made from tissues of normal animals, treated with the conjugated antiserum globulin. All the control tests must be negative.

A similar technique was adopted for treponemal antibodies by Deacon et al. (1957). Complement techniques of the fluorescent antibody method were published by Goldwasser and Shepard (1958) and Hinuma and Hummeler (1961).

ii. *The Indirect Immunofluorescence Technique.* The procedures devised by Deacon et al. (1957) and Carter and Leise (1958) were slightly modified by Montgomery et al. (1960). According to the Carter and Leise method, a section or a smear carrying the antigen is first treated for 10 to 15 minutes with a specific, nondiluted or 1:10 diluted, nonlabeled antiserum, and then washed for 10 minutes with a saline buffered at pH 8. Several drops of fluorescent antiglobulin serum, diluted 1:5, are now placed on the preparation and left in a Petri dish for 10 minutes at room temperature. The preparation is then washed with buffered saline, wiped, and mounted in a drop of buffered glycerol under a cover slip. Control sections or smears are treated in a similar manner, first with an unlabeled normal globulin and next with a fluorescent antiglobulin serum.

Each direct or indirect test must be accompanied by two control tests: (a) a test on the specific inhibition with an unconjugated homologous serum; and (b) the test on the removal of antibody from the conjugate by precipitation with the antigen.

Details of the indirect fluorescence technique for the diagnostic detection of antibodies follow. Smears of bacteria prepared on microscope slides and gently heat-fixed are first covered with a test serum, left for 30 minutes at 37°, and washed with a buffered saline, pH 8. One drop (0.03 ml) of a fluorescein labeled horse antihuman globulin is then dispensed onto smears, which are rotated for 30 minutes at 37°. The slides are rinsed with a buffered saline (one part of buffered saline pH 7.2 and nine parts of C.P. glycerin), and examined for the presence of fluorescent precipitates.

iii. *The Polyimmuno Fluorescent Technique.* In this technique, devised by Clayton (1954), a mixture of globulins isolated from several antisera of different specificity is used. With the aid of the immunoglobulin preparations each labeled by a different dye, a number of unrelated antigens may be detected if present in a tissue section or a smear.

Thus individual immunoglobulin preparations are labeled with a different fluorescent dye, for example, fluorescein isothiocyanate, 1-dimethyl-amino-5-sulfonylchloride-naphthalene, or benzaldehyde-6-nitro-2-sodium-diazotate, which give a green, yellow, or red fluorescence, respectively. Alternatively, tetramethylrhodamine isothiocyanate and fluorescein isothiocyanate or a combination of fluorescein and rhodamine labels can be used (Hiramoto et al., 1961). The sequential staining with two or more different immunofluorescent conjugates or reagents is carried out as follows. First one conjugate, for example, a fluorescein-conjugated globulin preparation is applied to the cover slip carrying a smear of particulate antigen for 1 to 2 hours, and then the smear is washed with PBS and subjected to the second fluorochrome conjugate, for example, a rhodamine-globulin conjugate for another period of 1 to 2 hours. The smear is finally washed in PBS and mounted in 50% glycerol in PBS and DPX.

9. *Histochemical Fluorescent Test for Tissue-Fixed Antibodies*

The principle of the histochemical technique, devised by Coons, Leduc, and Connolly (1955), for the detection of antibodies in tissues, is the reaction between an antibody fixed in the tissue and a homologous antigen deposited over an antibody-containing sera. The antigen deposited over the antibody-containing section serves as a bridge joining the sought tissue-fixed antibody and another labeled indicator antibody, which is homologous to that antigen.

This technique involves the following reactants: (a) frozen sections of tissues of immunized, hyperimmunized, and nonimmunized animals to be tested. The sections may be prepared by the method of Linderstrøm-Lang and Morgensen (1938), as modified by Coons et al. (1951), or by Balfour's (1961) freeze-substitution (wax embedding) method. (b) The antigen to be used for the immunization of animals. (c) The fluorescent conjugate antibody, which is homologous to the immunizing antigen.

To prepare the conjugate, the γ-globulin or globulin should be isolated from an antiserum and coupled to the fluorescein isothiocyanate by one of the procedures presented on pp. 603–607. The conjugate must be absorbed with a liver powder to remove the nonspecific fluorescence (see p. 606).

The preparation of tissue sections by Balfour's (1961) technique is carried out as follows. Small 1- to 2-mm pieces are cut (most conveniently by an automatic Sorvall tissue sectioner, see Fig. 3) and are plunged into liquid propane for freeze substitution. This is then transferred into a small tube containing absolute ethyl alcohol and a small amount of anhydrous sodium sulfate as a drying agent, and left in a freezing cabinet for 3 days. The wax for embedding the tissue is prepared by melting together a 99% polyester wax and 1% cetyl alcohol, and pouring this liquid into brass cups in a vacuum embedding oven at 40.5°. The freeze-substitution tubes are now warmed to room temperature, and the blocks are transferred to fresh dry alcohol for 1 hour before the infiltration with wax. The tissues are infiltrated twice for 20 minutes, under vacuum. The blocks are then allowed to solidify overnight, at room temperature.

Serial sections, 3-μ thick, are cut on a microtome from the polyester block which should be cooled in the refrigerator before sectioning, since the wax has a low melting point. The sections are collected on glass slides, to which they adhere firmly owing to the presence of unfixed proteins. It is advisable to float sections on 18% sodium sulfate, prior to the fluorescent staining. This procedure improves the staining. After the sections have been floated, the slide is tilted and dried off; the wax is removed with xylol, and the slide is rinsed in alcohol and in buffered saline. The wax-embedded blocks can be kept for 3 months at room temperature in a state suitable for the fluorescent assay.

The procedure of the histochemical technique is as follows. Frozen sections of tissues are fixed for 15 minutes in 95% ethanol (v/v) at 37°, dried at this temperature for 30 minutes, and rinsed with a 0.8% saline buffered to pH 7.0. The sections are then covered with a drop of an antigen solution, diluted 1:2000 in the buffered saline. The glass slides are left for 30 minutes in a moist chamber, then rinsed off, and washed in the buffered saline for 10 minutes. Excess of the moisture is removed by wiping dry the slide around the area of the section, which is then covered with a drop of an absorbed fluorescent antibody conjugate, and left for 30 minutes in a moist chamber, at room temperature. The sections treated are now washed with the buffered saline for 10 minutes, wiped dry, and mounted in a buffered glycerol, which consists of nine parts of glycerol and one part of buffered saline.

Control preparations, made from organs of nonimmunized animals, are processed in a similar manner. Additional control preparation is provided by a section made from organs of immunized animals, and exposed to a heterologous antibody.

Areas in the tissue sections, where fluorescent precipitate has been formed, show a yellow, green fluorescence in a fluorescent microscope. This fluorescent precipitate results from a serological reaction between a complex formed by the cell-adsorbed antibody and a corresponding antigen, and the fluorescent γ-globulin conjugate, which is homologous to the antigen. The cell-adsorbed antibodies can be most easily found in plasma cells of the red pulp of spleen, in medullary areas of lymph nodes, and in the connective tissues of the liver portal. Particular attention must be paid to the differentiation between the true immunological fluorescent reaction and a "nonspecific" fluorescence of certain components of the tissue. The nonspecifically fluorescing tissues components appear as large amorphous aggregates or clusters.

10. *Microscopic Examination of Fluorescent Preparations*

Sections or smears, treated with a fluorescent antibody conjugate, are examined by the aid of a microscope with ultraviolet light source. A 150-W, high-pressure mercury vapor bulb (e.g., a Leitz-Phillips Cs 150 lamp or Osram HBO 200-W lamp), mounted in a fluorescence lamp and possibly attached to a good microscope such as Zeiss GF425 microscope (Fig. 69), serves as an adequate ultraviolet light source. The microscope for the immunofluorescence studies must be equipped with a set of ultraviolet excitation filters, BG 12, UG 1, UG 2, or UG 5 or a combination of Corning 5850 and BG 12 and EK barrier filters. The ocular barrier system consists of an ultraviolet excluding eyepiece, the OG 4, or OG 1 filter alone, or a combination of OG 1 with GG 4 or a Wratten 2A filter. The filters exclusively allow the excitation light to reach the object but only absorb the remaining ultraviolet light, thus preventing short length waves reaching the eyes of the observer. An alternative apparatus recommended for the immunofluorescence observation is Leitz Ortholux UV fluorescence microscope equipped with a BG 38 heat filter, BG 12 exciter filter and OG 9 barrier filter.

The optical system consists of a 2-mm oil immersion objective or an Apochromat 40/1.0 oil objective and a 10–15× ocular. Intensity of the fluorescence can be approximately estimated by the eye, and recorded in plus symbols; but is more adequately determined by taking photomicrographs on a film Super Ektachrome or Anscochrome 500 color film (ASA 100), and passing the film through a microphotometer. Microphotographs may be taken on a high speed Kodak Tri X film.

A special apparatus for quantitative, as well as qualitative, immunofluorescence microscopy was recently devised by Hovnonian et al. (1964). Results of investigations are regarded as satisfactory if the fluorescence has been shown only by tested sections or smears coupled with the reagent of a labeled homologous antiserum globulin; control preparations should emit

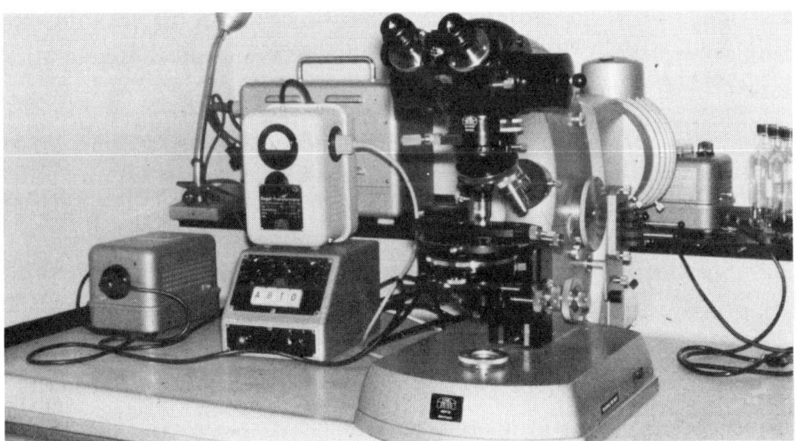

Figure 69.   The fluorescence microscope.

none or only very faint traces of fluorescence in the localized areas. It is sometimes advisable to check results by examining other sections treated with the antiserum globulin at differing concentrations, so as to demonstate inhibition of the reaction.

11. *The Slide Centrifuge Immunofluorescence Test (Kwapinski, 1972)*

Incubate 0.1 ml of antigen preparation with 0.1 ml of a fluorescein-labeled antiserum or globulin preparation for 3 to 5 minutes. Transfer the mixture to a plastic compartment of the cytocentrifuge and spin the mixture at 1000 rpm for 5 minutes. Wash off the noncombined material from the cellulose strip with 1 *M* NaCl for 2 minutes. View the strip in a UV light.

Antibody-antigen complexes show a fluorescent central areas, whereas no fluorescence is displayed by control samples.

12. *Soluble Antigen Immunofluorescence Technique*

The direct immunofluorescence technique relies on the following principle: particulate antigens can be represented as cells possessing a number of functional antigens on the surface which function as a natural matrix; antibody reacts with a functional antigen present in the matrix, and the reaction is detectable when the complex is exposed to a fluorescein-labeled antiserum and visualized on microscope.

An individual type of antigens cannot be selected objectively from among the constituents of a particulate antigen preparation so that the reading of the test results are highly subjective. This problem of the immunofluorescence method can be overcome by the use of selected soluble antigens fixed onto an artificial matrix, such as a glass microscope slide, a paper strip, or agar gel (Friou, 1962; Paronetto, 1963), by the application of the indirect immunofluorescence technique devised by Toussaint and Anderson (1965). The indirect immunofluorescence test involves two antigen-antibody systems. The secondary system consists of the washed primary system and the fluorescein-conjugated antiglobulin serum, directed against globulins of the species which provided the first antiserum. The most suitable matrix consists of $\frac{1}{4}$-in. disks of a cellulose-acetate paper, possessing 0.45-mμ porosity. The minor, nonspecific fluorescence of the cellulose acetate paper is effectively reduced by the incorporation of 1% bovine serum albumin into the system. Maximum fluorescence is obtained in a 0.05 *M* Tris (hydroxymethyl) amino-methane (Tris) buffer, pH 8.0, made in 0.85% NaCl used as diluent. Details of the procedure are described underneath.

The cellulose acetate paper disks are soaked in a solution of antigen diluted to an optimal concentration in Tris-buffered saline containing 1%

bovine serum albumin. Control disks are soaked in Tris-buffered, 1% BSA solution. The liquid is allowed to penerate the paper from underneath after which the disks are submerged and allowed to soak for approximately 30 seconds. The disks are then removed from the fluid, permitted to drain of excess fluid and placed on a flat, clean glass surface to dry for approximately 2 hours. The antigen disk is then placed in a tube containing 0.2 ml of an antiserum diluted 1:2 and incubated at 3° to 6° for 18 hours, after which the fluid is aspirated from the tubes by suction and the disks are washed in Tris-buffered saline three times for 10 minutes each time. The washed disks are submerged in 0.2 ml of a fluorescein-conjugated antiserum, diluted to an optimal concentration in Tris-buffered saline, containing 2% Tween 80. Addition of the Tween 80 to the conjugate facilitates the removal of the excess fluorescein from the disks. After the incubation at room temperature for 30 minutes, the disks are washed three times with Tris-buffered saline and finally blotted and mounted on the adhesive side of a 2-in. masking tape. As many as 32 disks can be mounted on a single strip of tape to be read in the fluorometer with the filters. The tape is mounted on a chromatogram doom of a fluorometer (Model 111 (GK), Turner Associates, Palo Alto, Calif.).

The fluorometer is equipped with a 4-W far UV lamp, possessing a major emission wave length of 254 nm, a primary filter (no. 7-54) transmitting 254 to 420 nm, and a secondary filter system consisting of a no. 2A-12 sharp cut filter passing over 510 nm and 1% neutral density filter. The fluorescence dial reading is obtained with a fluorometer set at 0 with appropriate blank. The titer is expressed as the reciprocal of the highest serum dilution showing a strong fluorescence.

The reproducibility obtained by this method is well within the ranges normally accepted for an immunological test. The test has a great advantage over a complement fixation test since a smaller amount of antigen is required for the immunofluorescence test and it is not influenced by anticomplementarity of antigens or antisera. The method has been applied successfully for immunological detection of infections.

13. The Immunofluorescence Kinetics Assay

The immunofluorescence method is a direct immunological study of biologically important macromolecular reactions occurring in a serological test. By means of a fluorescence polarization technique, the equilibrium measurement of antigen-antibody systems can be attained directly. Changes in the fluorescence polarization occurring in an immunological system as it develops can be measured directly as a function of time for reaction mixtures at $1.5 \pm 0.5°$ in a neutral buffer with the use of a specially designed fluorescence polarometer. The initial stage of antigen-antibody combination corresponds to the empirical rate law, which is represented by the following equation:

$$\text{rate} = k(\text{Ab})(\text{Ag})$$

This empirical rate law is applicable over a wide range of the initial antibody and antigen concentrations ranging from 5.5×10^9 to 1.8×10^{-7} M and 8.0×10^{-10} to 8.0×10^{-8} M, respectively. The antigen and antibody molecules are combined reversibly as a bimolecular system. The rate constant for association and dissociation of the system in the case of oval albumin and antioval albumin is 2×10^5 M/second and approximately 1×10^{-3} M/second, respectively (Dandliker and Levison, 1967).

The macromolecular kinetics may be studied by an immunofluorescence technique (Dandliker et al., 1964). In this method, one reactant is tagged with a small fluorescent molecule and is subsequently used as the detecting and measuring agent for the secondary corresponding reactant. The extent of antigen-antibody combination is related to changes in either the polarization or intensity of fluorescence (enhancement or quenching). The instrument used for kinetic studies is a fluorescent polarometer which permits direct reading of the fluorescent intensity and polarization.

14. *The Indirect Immunofluorescence Method with Absorption and Diffusion*

In this method (Gordon and Al-Doory, 1965), one-third of a small steel cylinder is packed with cellulose powder, made into a paste with 1 N saline buffered at pH 7.4 with phosphate. The second one-half part of the cylinder is packed with a paste consisting of 1:1 mixture of cellulose powder and cellulose powder-absorbing antigen. An antigen smear is then prepared for the fluorescent antibody staining on a glass slide, and the smear is covered with a square pad of Whatman no. 3 MM electrophoresis paper (2×2 cm), moistened with the buffered saline. The cylinder packed with cellulose powder and cellulose powder-absorbing antigen mixture is placed on top. The remaining one-third of the cylinder is filled with the antiglobulin to be absorbed. The cylinder is then covered with a Petri dish and left at room temperature for 1 hour and at 4° overnight. The cylinder and pad are then removed; the smear is washed in buffer saline, and the indirect immunofluorescence staining method is thus completed. If two or more different antigen are to be compared by the test with an antiglobulin and absorbing antigen, smears of two or three antigens are made on the same slide in parallel and are exposed simultaneously to the same filled cylinder combination.

15. *Automated Immunofluorescence Technique*

The automated instrument for immunofluorescence test was developed by Binnings et al. (1969). The instrument, termed Sero-Matic system, consists of a processor and a microscope attachment as the major parts. The processor is an electropneumatically controlled test instrument which automates the performance of about 30 test specimens per hour. Specimens are processed sequentionally at approximately 2-minute intervals in the following manner.

The antigen slide is inserted at the load station via loader mechanism into one of fifty slide-holding positions. In about 4 minutes thereafter, the slide is positioned under the serum-sorbent applicator where the saline-sorbent mixture is forced onto the antigen spot on the slide. The slide is then indexed to the first incubator at 37° for about 30 minutes. After the incubation, the slide is washed in PBS, pH 7.2, for 10 seconds, rinsed with distilled water at an appropriate station to remove the PBS and the particulate matter not related to the antigen-serum reaction, and air-dried to remove all distilled water from the top surface of the slide cover glass. A conjugate is applied to the antigen spot on the slide cover glass, and the slide is incubated for about 30 minutes. The slide is then washed in distilled water, dried with a blower, and ejected from the rotating table onto a unload platform and onto a slide unload magazine. The slide is now ready for examination with a fluorescence microscopy equipment.

The microscope attachment is installed onto a dark-field fluorescence microscope, and it permits the ready slide to be visually examined. The illumination system consists of an Osram HBO-200 UV light source and 6-V 30-W tungsten light source, excitation filter KG 1 (heat adsorption filter), the 2-mm thick BG-12 and BG-38 excitation filters, and the OG-1 barrier filter. The slide is accurately positioned under the objective lens of the microscope by the operator, but the attachment provides a very easy slide adjustment necessary to obtain fine focus and a sharp filled image. If special READI-FIX lights are used, the slides are placed in the attachment in an inverted position so that the reacted antigens are on the lower side of the slide. Installing of a cover glass over the specimen is thus eliminated.

16. *Quantitation of Fluorescent Antibody*

Fluorescent precipitates are quantitatively determined most precisely by photofluorometric measurements in solutions (Tengerdy, 1963). Less accurate, but convenient, techniques for quantitative immunofluorescence titration rely on the measurement of relative intensity of fluorescent antibody, shown by preparations stained with fluorescent antibodies by means of a microfluorometer mounted on a microscope (Goldman, 1960), or by the photometric measurement of fluorescence intensity (DeRepentigny et al., 1963). Semiquantitative methods (Montgomery et al., 1960; Sonea et al., 1961) depend on the determination of the lowest, effective dilution of a fluorescein-labeled immunoglobulin preparation, giving observable reaction with the corresponding antigen.

The quantitative method for quantitative determination of immuno-fluorescence, described by Tengerdy (1963), is based on measurement of the excess fluorescent antibody in the supernatant of a fluorescent precipitin reaction mixture. In this method, 0.1 ml of different dilutions of a gamma globulin preparation labeled with fluorescein isothiocyanate are added to a constant amount of an antigen (0.1 ml) and incubated at 4° for 16 hours. The precipitates are centrifuged at $8000 \times g$ and washed with a saline buffered at pH 7.2. An aliquot of the clear supernatant is then diluted 1:20 with an 0.01 M, pH 8.5 borate buffer. The fluorescence of this solution is measured in a Turner chamber M 110 fluorometer. The fluorescence measurements are made against a fluorescence reaction blank, which is prepared by precipitating all active fluorescent antibody from the antiserum with excess homologous antigen. The method is basically a differential fluorometric measurement since the difference between two readings is equal to the amount of fluorescent antibody reacted with an antigen. The procedure is practically independent of the amount of the fluorescent, non-antibody materials present in the solution. To enhance the fluorescence intensity and selectivity for the fluorescein label, a primary filter with 436-nm sharp peak and the secondary filter to pass wavelength greater than 510 nm are used.

A fluorescence calibration curve is prepared with a pure preparation of a fluorescent rabbit anti-human-gamma globulin and a fluorescent rabbit antibovine gamma globulin.

The fluorescence measured in the Turner spectrofluorometer is plotted against the protein concentration of the conjugate as determined by an appropriate chemical method, for example, the Folin-Ciocalteu method. In the fluorescent-precipitate reaction, the values for fluorescent antibody protein are obtained directly from this curve. Since a close agreement has been found between the antibody antigen ratios determined by chemical and fluorometric methods, Heidelberger and Kendall's (1935) equation for precipitate (FAg reacted % = FAg unreacted/FAg can be employed in the following form:

$$\frac{\text{FAb pptd}}{\text{Ag pptd}} = a - b \text{ (Ag pptd)}$$

where a and b are empirical constants; FAg pptd = FAb added − FAb excess. The a and b values are established from a calibration curve and used for series of measurements. The FAg unreacted is calculated from fluorescence measurements in the supernatant.

Quantitative Determination of Immunofluorescence by DeRepentigny's et al. (1963) Method. This depends on the evaluation of immunofluorescence quantitatively by photometric measurement of the fluorescence intensity of antibody-treated bacteria as compared to an equal volume of untreated bacteria. Results are expressed as the difference between the intensity given by the antibody-treated and nontreated bacteria. The intensity of the specific fluorescence is expressed in 0.0001 microlumens as calculated according to the following equation:

$$\frac{\text{total fluorescence after staining}}{\text{total primary fluorescence}} \times 100$$

17. The Fluorescence Quenching Method

The spectrofluorometric method depends on the fluorescence quenching of a purified antibody and is applied to measure antigen-antibody reactions, measured in solution by a change in the intensity or polarization of fluorescence. The fluorescence is derived from tryptophane residues of the antibody molecule.

The equipment for fluorescence quenching consists of a spectrofluorophotometer equipped with monochromers and emitted beam. The antibody solution is activated at 290 nm and fluorescence is measured in arbitrary units at 350 nm. Filter fluorometers with an adequate light source and suitable filters can be used instead of spectrofluorophotometer. The fluorometer should be equipped with a shutter to protect the protein and hapten from incident ultraviolet radiation.

In the test, 1.0-ml antibody solution made in 0.15 M NaCl $-$ 0.01 M Tris or phosphate buffer is used. Fluorescence readings are made in arbitrary units after the instrument setting has been adjusted so that the initial readings of about 70 to 80 are obtained. After the temperature equilibration, a stable fluorescent value is obtained, after which a hapten solution is added in the volume increasing from 0.01 to 0.2 ml. Fluorescence measurements are made after each addition, and a solvent fluorescence blank is measured after each titration.

To calculate binding constants, it is first required to determine the diminution in antibody fluorescence when essentially all antibody sites are occupied by haptens which require titrations of the hapten at high concentration of the substance. The antibody quenching must be compared to that obtained with normal globulin or tryptophane. Fluorescent values are corrected for dilution and the solvent length and related to the initial fluorescence value which is taken to be 100%. At a given total hapten concentration, the ratio of the observed quench to Qmax is regarded as the fraction of antibody sites occupied by the haptens. The association constant K_a is represented by the following equation:

$$K_a = \frac{Ab - H}{(ab_f)(c)}$$

where AB − H is bound hapten or occupied antibody sites, c is unbound hapten, and ab_f are free antibody sites.

The fluorescent quenching method is very accurate, easy, and rapid. The fluorescent quenching is applied for the study of kinetics of the antibody-hapten reaction (Day et al., 1963). The method has been most frequently used for studies of interactions between haptens and antibodies. The amounts of antibody required for tests are minute.

In the test described by Montgomery et al. (1960), the serum being examined is first heated at 56° for 30 minutes and diluted serially; 0.03 ml, or one drop, of each serum dilution is then placed on smears containing the antigen. Slides are put into a plastic container with a piece of moistened filter paper in its top. The container is rotated at 1000 rpm for 30 minutes, at 37°. Slides are rinsed with buffered saline and gently blotted.

18. *The Fluorescent Treponemal-Antibody Test*

The following reagents are required for this test, devised by Deacon et al. (1957, 1960):

1. The antigen, a Nichols strain of *Treponema pallidum,* extracted from rabbit testicular tissue (see p. 19), suspended to contain approximately 50 microorganisms per microscopic field at 450× magnification.

2. A fluorescent reagent, for example, a fluorescein-labeled antihuman globulin which is commercially available. This globulin must be diluted in a buffered saline containing 2% Tween 80 to the optimum dilution ranging from 1:5 to 1:320.

3. A phosphate buffered saline, pH 7.2.

4. A mounting medium consisting of one part buffered saline and nine parts glycerin.

The test is carried out as follows. Approximately 0.01 ml of an antigen suspension is smeared in two circles on a glass slide, and dried in the air. The slides are then immersed in acetone for 10 minutes and air-dried. The test serum, inactivated and diluted in the ratio of 1:10 and 1:100 with a buffered saline, is placed in 0.03 ml amount on the antigen smears. The slides should be rotated for 30 minutes at 37°, rinsed with buffered saline and distilled water, and blotted with a filter paper. Each smear is then covered with 0.02 ml of diluted fluorescein conjugate and mounted with the mounting medium under a cover glass. Slides should be examined under

450 magnification of a fluorescent microscope. A definite fluorescence of serological complexes is indicative of positive reaction and of the presence of *Treponema* antibodies. Fluorescence can be measured by the aid of a spectrophotometer, at the emission wavelength of the maximum intensity of 525 nm.

19. The Immunofluorescence Enumeration of Rickettsiae

The assay according to Hahon and Cooke's (1966) method is set in triplicate. A rickettsial suspension is diluted in a maintenance medium, and 0.2-ml aliquot is introduced into a vial containing coverslip cell cultures. The absorption is enhanced and expedited by centrifugation of the vials at $500 \times g$ for 15 minutes at 23 to 25°. Cover-slip cell cultures are then rinsed twice with the maintenance medium; 1 ml of the medium is added to each vial, and the cultures are rinsed twice with cold phosphate-buffered saline, pH 7.2 and with cold acetone, and then subjected to the immuno-fluorescent antibody in the following manner.

The coverslip cell cultures washed three times with PBS are stained with a fluorescein conjugate for 30 minutes, and then rinsed in two changes of PBS to remove excess conjugate and mounted in 20% glycerol in PBS. The slides are examined in a fluorescent microscope at 600 to 700 × magnification. The enumeration of infected cells on immunofluorescent staining proved to be much more rapid than enumeration of infected cells on yolk sac inoculation. The method is also less variable and gives a slightly higher mean titration value than the method of holk sac inoculation. Coverslip cultures made for the fluorescein staining can be stored at $-60°$ for a few weeks if necessary.

20. The Immunofluorescence Method for Viral Antibodies

The antigen preparation for immunofluorescence test for viruses may be in the form of cell films prepared when the cytopathic effect of a virus has appeared as moderate or strong but cell sheets are still intact. The cells are washed in PBS, pH 7.6, and spread on glass slides and dried in air. The cells are then fixed in acetone for 10 minutes and repeated in fresh acetone. The cell films are left at room temperature for 30 minutes and may be stored at minus 60°. The cell films are then layered with a fluorescein-labeled antibody preparation (Cohen et al., 1968).

21. The Complement Method of the Immunofluorescence Technique

In this test, complement is first absorbed by a homologous antigen-antibody sytem in cells or tissues. Sites at which the complement is fixed are then visualized by a fluorescent antiglobulin versus guinea pig serum. The C_1', C_2', and C_4', components of complement are necessary for a staining reaction, but the C_3', component does not participate.

In the test by Hinuma and Hummeler (1961), a normal guinea pig serum is employed as a source of complement. This serum diluted 1:10 with a phosphate-buffered saline is used to prepare dilutions, from 1:16 or 1:64 of an antiserum tested. The diluted antiserum is placed in a smear made of cells containing an antigen and incubated at 37° for 30 minutes. The treated smears are then washed twice with a $M/100$ phosphate-buffered saline, and layered with a fluorescein-isothiocyanate conjugated anti-complement antibody at an approximate concentration of 0.5 mg of protein per milliliter.

After standing at 37 minutes, the smears are washed twice for 10 minutes with the buffered saline and mounted with a semipermanent mounting medium.

22. *The Mixed Antiglobulin Immunofluorescence Test*

In the test (Beutner et al., 1965), immunoglobulins conjugated with fluorescein are used as primary antigens. The mixed immunofluorescence test is carried out as follows.

A series of dilutions of human sera containing tissue antibodies are applied to frozen tissue sections and incubated for 20 minutes, after which the sections are washed in a phosphate buffered saline. The sections are then layered with antihuman immunoglobulin, preheated at 56° for 30 minutes and diluted to contain 1–4 agglutinating units. After 20 minutes, the sections are washed in a phosphate buffered saline for 1 hour and exposed for 20 minutes to a fluorescein-labeled human immunoglobulin, diluted at the strength of 1 to 2 units/ml in a heated normal rabbit serum used in a 1:15 dilution. The preparation is then washed in a phosphate buffered saline for 2 hours and mounted in glycerine diluted 9:10 in the buffer. Washing minimizes nonspecific staining. The specimen is examined in a fluorescent microscope.

23. *The Colony-Immunofluorescence Technique*

Two tests are designed for the detection of antigens in bacterial colonies by Deddish and Slade (1969) and Del Giudice et al. (1967).

In the first version of the test, a suspension of bacteria spread over the surface of an agar medium, supported by glass slides, is incubated in a Perti plate at 37° for 24 to 48 hours to yield bacterial colonies. The slides are overlayered with a fluorescein-conjugated antiserum, diluted 1:10 in 0.8% purified, melted agar. These slides are incubated at room temperature for 3 hours, covered with saline, and left at room temperature for another 1 hour to detect unbound antiserum. The saline is decanted, a second volume of saline is added, and the slides are held for 1 hour. The slides are finally dried at room temperature and inspected at a magnification of 100 on a fluorescence microscope, equipped with a BG 12 filter.

The colonies possessing antigen(s) against which the antibody was directed are easily visible as shiny, fluorescent areas.

According to the other version of the microcolony immunofluorescence test, microscopically detectable colonies grown on a solid medium are flooded with 5 ml of a saline buffered at pH 7.2 and washed in this solution for 20 to 30 minutes after which the liquid is decanted. The washed culture is then layered with a fluorescein globulin conjugate and left at room temperature for 30 minutes. The unbound conjugate is decanted, and the agar surface is rinsed three times with buffered saline. The colonies are examined for fluorescence in an ultraviolet microscope.

24. *Fluorescence Enhancement Methods for Quantitative Determination of Hapten-Antibody Interaction*

The fluorescence enhancement method depends on the observation that a number of polycyclic aromatic compounds which are nonfluorescent in aqueous solution become highly fluorescent when bound by certain proteins, such as antibody globulins. In this phenomenom, fluorometric methods for the quantitative determination of serum antibodies are based. The following ligands show fluorescence when bound by antibody globulins: 5-toluidinyl-naphthalene-1-sulfonate, 8-anilinonaphthalene-1-sulfonate and 5-dimethylaminonaphthalene-1-sulfonate, 4-anilinonaphthalene-1-sulfonate, and 6-anilinonaphthalene-2-sulfonate. Antibodies directed against a ligand react with the corresponding hapten producing fluorescence which is measured with an Aminco-Bowman spectrofluorometer according to Yoo's et al. (1967) methods. The maximum fluorescence of each ligand occupying sites on the homologous antibody is about $600\times$ the fluorescence shown by the ligand in the presence of normal immunoglobulins (Yoo, 1970).

A quantitative method for the determination of hapten-antibody interaction relying on the fluorescence enhancement of the ligand when bound to a corresponding antibody has been described by Nakamura et al. (1970).

25. *The Immunofluorescent Plaque Method*

According to Spendlove and Lennette's (1962) technique, the test is set up in the following manner. Cover slips placed in the bottom of a Petri plate are coated with 0.2 ml of an appropriate agar medium, such as that described by Adams and Imagawa (1957), containing 2 to 4 $\times$ 10^5 of HeLa cells. The slips are left for 1 to 2 hours at room temperature to allow the cells to attach to the glass, then 5 ml of the outgrowth medium containing serum is added. The cultures are incubated to an atmosphere of 5% CO_2 at 35° for 24 hours. The medium is then removed from the Petri plate, and the cover slips are washed with 5 ml of a yeast extract—lactalbumin hydrolyzate medium. A suspension of the virus is added in an amount of 0.02 to 0.04 ml on each cover slip, and incubated for 4 hours in a moist chamber at 35° to allow for the infection of cells. After the incubation, the cover slips are inverted on an agar medium in a Petri plate, to be sealed with the agar, and incubated at 35°. When foci of infection are formed, the cover slips are removed from the agar by softening it by heating the plate for 2 to 3 minutes on a hot plate at 65 to 70°.

The cover slips are fixed for 10 minutes in cold acetone, dried, and treated for 30 minutes with a fluorescein-labeled serum globulins according to the direct technique of Coons and Kaplan (1950). The cover slips are mounted in buffered glycerol and examined in the fluorescence microscope.

26. Evaluation of Immunofluorescence Technique

The immunofluorescent technique is a very sensitive and reliable procedure for the detection of antigens in cells and tissues. Soluble protein antigens or antibodies can be detected at a concentration of 100 to 200 μg/ml. A good optical definition provided by the fluorescence makes the fluorescein-antibody conjugates easily visible. The fluorescent antibody technique allows the direct testing of insoluble antigens in tissues, whereas other, indirect methods are subjected to various interfering factors.

The antigenic analysis of microorganisms by the immunofluorescence technique has not always been satisfactory. However, very interesting results were obtained by this method in studies on sites of the antibody formation in tissues or cells, and in the analysis and identification of unknown serum antibodies by means of labeled standard species of microorganisms.

The immunofluorescence technique has been found to be superior than culture methods and precipitation tests for diagnostic purposes. The immunofluorescence test proved to be more specific and sensitive than any other serological tests used for detection of syphilis. A rapid and reliable presumptive diagnosis of diphtheria and detection of microorganisms causing bacterial meningitis, such as *H. influenzae* and *N. meningitidis* can be made by the immunofluorescence technique. The method is less suitable for detection of typhoid bacteria in carriers.

The factor that interferes rather often with the fluorescent antibody test is the autofluorescence of host cells and tissues and of some species of bacteria. For example, mycobacteria and certain species of microfungi contain a fair concentration of riboflavin which is a fluorescent compound. The nonspecific autofluorescence of host cells and tissues can be abolished, or at least diminshed, by the absorption of conjugates with a human or rabbit liver powder or with the acetone-dried bone marrow powder.

27. Applications of Immunofluorescence Technique

The fluorescent antibody method was successfully employed for the detection and identification of a great variety of antigens in tissues, for example:

1. Capsular polysaccharides of *Diplococcus pneumoniae* and *Klebsiella pneumoniae,* injected intravenously into mice, detected in cells of the reticulo-endothelial system and in other organs (Coons et al., 1942; Kaplan et al., 1950).

2. Cells of *Actinobacillus pseudomallei, Bacillus anthracis, Shigela, Listeria monocytogenes, Pasteurella pestis,* or *Brucella sp.,* detected in impression smears made from tissues or other host materials (Moody et al., 1956; Thomason et al., 1956; Meysel et al., 1957; Smith et al., 1960; Moody and Winter, 1959; Moody et al., 1961), *Neisseria gonorrhoeae* (Deacon et al., 1959; Lind, 1967).

3. Detection of bacteria in the cerebrospinal fluid (Biegeleisen et al., 1965), and *Leptospira hemorrhagiae* in sections of muscles of a patient infected with this microorganism (Sheldon, 1953).

4. Identification of *Enterobacteriaceae, Bordetella* pertussis and grouping of *Shigella, Brucella, Bacillus anthracis, Listeria,* and *Leptospira* (Cherry and Moody, 1965).

5. Detection of *Rickettsia prowazeki, Rickettsia rickettsii,* and *Coxiella burnetii,* detected in smears and sections prepared from peritoneal or pericardial exudates, the liver and spleen of artificially infected cotton rats, and from cultures in yolk sac or infected mice (Coons et al., 1950; Burgdorfer, 1961; Hahon and Cooke, 1966; Kordova and Kovačova, 1968).

6. Detection of Miyagawanella (Hahon and Nakamura, 1964) and *Mycoplasma* (Masiga and Stone, 1968).

7. Localization of tetanus toxin (Fedinec, 1962).

8. Detection of mumps virus in sections of parotid glands of artificially infected monkeys and in infected tissues of chick embryos (Watson, 1952), other myxoviruses (Wheelock and Tamm, 1961), adenovirus (Philipson, 1961), West Nile virus, herpes zoster virus found in the cytoplasm of cells (Noyes and Watson, 1955; Weller and Coons, 1954), herpes virus (Goodheart and Jaross, 1963), poxviruses (Carter, 1965).

9. Detection of influenza virus in white blood cells (Boand et al., 1956) and other viruses, for example, poliomyelitis virus (Buckley, 1956, 1957), herpes simplex virus, vaccinia virus, and enteroviruses in the tissue culture cells (Loh and Riggs, 1961; Riggs and Brown, 1962).

10. Detection of inclusion bodies of canine infectious hepatitis virus (Coffin et al., 1953), mouse hepatitis virus (Starr et al., 1960), canine distemper virus (Moulton and Brown, 1954), mumps virus (Coons et al., 1950; Watson, 1952), adenoviruses (Boyer et al., 1959), measles virus (Cohen et al., 1955), and elementary bodies of trachoma virus (Nichols and McComb, 1962).

11. Detection of microfungi, for example, *Candida, Histoplasma,* and *Blastomyces* (Gordon, 1958; Vogel and Padula, 1958; Kaufman and Kap-

lan, 1963; Kaufman and Brandt, 1964), *Aspergillus* in soil (Schmidt and Bankole, 1962), and diagnosis of histoplasmosis and blastomycosis (Porter et al., 1965).

12. Detection of protozoa, *Endamoeba histolytica, Endamoeba coli,* and *Toxoplasma gondii* (Goldman, 1953, 1954, 1956, 1957).

13. The Forssman antigen, its distribution in tissues of various animals (Tanaka and Leduc, 1956).

14. Detection of specific tissue or plasma protein and polysaccharide antigens, for example, homologous plasma proteins in tissues of infants and children (Gitlin et al., 1953), protein antigens from the lens and muscles of mice (Clayton, 1954), a rat connective tissue antigen (Cruickshank and Hill, 1953), and other tissue protein antigens (Marshall, 1951), crystalline hen's egg albumin, crystalline bovine plasma albumin, and human plasma γ-globulin (Coons et al., 1951; White et al., 1955; Coons et al., 1955).

15. Demonstration of antibodies, for example, the *Treponema, Brucella* and malaria antibodies (Deacon et al., 1959; Montgomery et al., 1960; Pillot and Borel, 1961; Moody et al., 1961; Biegeleisen et al., 1962; Niel and Fribourg-Blanc, 1962), by the indirect reaction with a labeled anti-human globulin, demonstration of adrenal antibodies in sera of patients suffering from Addison's disease (Bigazzi et al., 1968). Positive results of the fluorescent treponemal antibody-absorption test proved to be correlated in 95% with firm diagnosis of syphilis.

The immunofluorescence technique was adopted for the detection, identification, and antigenic analysis of microorganisms, for example, *Actinobacillus mallei, Actinobacillus pseudomallei* (Moody et al., 1956), *Diplococcus* (Coons et al., 1942), *Streptococcus pyogenes* (Moody et al., 1958), *Neisseria* (Deacon et al., 1959), *Staphylococcus aureus* (Cohen and Oeding, 1962; De Repentigny et al., 1963), *Salmonella typhosa* (Thomason et al., 1957 and 1959), *Shigella* (La Brec et al., 1958), *Streptomyces* (Arai et al., 1962), *Actinomyces* (Slack et al., 1961), *Dermatophilus* (Kwapinski, 1969), *Erysipelothrix insidiosa* (Dacres and Groth, 1959), and *Sendai* virus (Hinuma et al., 1963), in sections and smears made either directly from an infected material, or indirectly from isolated cultures.

VIII. THE IMMUNOELECTRON ASSAY

This category of immunological assays depends on the detection of antigen-antibody complexes by means of immunoglobulins labeled with substances which absorb electrons. Electron-absorbing substances, the ferritin, para-aminophenyl-mercury, and uranium (Singer, 1959; Morgan et al., 1961; Zhdanov et al., 1962; Kul'berg and Azadova, 1964; Sternberger et

al., 1963) have been employed for labeling of the immunoglobulins to be
detected in the electron microscope on reaction with the corresponding
antigens.

1. The Immunoferritin Test

Direct immunoferritin test depends on the reaction between the ferritin-
labeled antibodies and the particulate antigens, revealed by electron
microscopy.

The indirect immunoferritin test depends on two sequential reactions, the
combination of an antigen with the antibody globulins and the reaction of
the globulins with the ferritin conjugated globulin antibodies. The indirect
test may be used to examine a number of antigen-antibody systems utilizing a single ferritin conjugate directed to the serum species which was used
for production of various nonlabeled antibodies.

The identification of bacteria in pathological materials by the use of
labeled antisera has the advantage of being quick and reliable, since it is
based on an observable, specific immunological reaction. However, it is
sometimes difficult or even impossible to differentiate by this method between closely related species of microorganisms, due to cross reactions with
labeled antibodies.

Commercial horse spleen ferritin is first recrystallized eight times with
cadmium sulfate and reprecipitated four times with ammonium sulfate
(Granick, 1946), and finally purified by passage through Sephadex G-200
in 0.1 M NaCl and 0.1 M Tris, pH 8.0 buffer. The ferritin concentration
in the effluent is measured at 255-nm wavelength which is the maximal
absorption area for ferritin (Patterson et al., 1965).

Ferritin aggregates of 2000 to 3000 atoms confer high electron density
so that ferritin particles are easily seen in the electron microscope and exhibit a characteristic micellar arrangement. Ferritin can be isolated from a
horse spleen and purified by Rifkind's et al. (1964) and Hsu (1967)
method. Purified ferritin is a crystalline protein with the molecular weight
of about 460,000, containing about 23% iron in ferric hydroxide-phos-
phate micelles.

Purification of Ferritin. Although commercial preparations of ferritin
are useful for many immunoferritin tests, clearer and optimal experimental
results are obtained when purified ferritin is used.

According to Hsu (1967), the commercial ferritin is first recrystallized
by diluting the ferritin preparation to 1 to 2% solution with 2% ammonium
sulfate, pH 5.85, and recrystallizing it from this solution in 5% cadmium
sulfate. The recrystallization procedure is repeated until only typical
orange-brown ferritin crystals are seen on the electron microscope examination of a sample.

The crystalline ferritin is redissolved on 2% ammonium sulfate, and amorphous ferritin is precipitated three times with ammonium sulfate at 50% saturation.

The amorphous ferritin is collected, dissolved in a small amount of distilled water and dialyzed, first against cold running water until salt free, and then against 0.05 M, pH 7.5, phosphate buffer overnight. The solution is sterilized by filtration and stored at 4 to $-20°$.

Before use, the ferritin preparation ought to be centrifuged at 100,000 × g for 2 hours. The upper three-fourths of the fluid is then discarded from a centrifuge tube. The remaining suspension is collected and added, in an ice bath, to 0.05 M, pH 7.5 phosphate buffer and 0.3 M, pH 9.5 borate buffer, so as to obtain final concentration of 20–25 mg of ferritin per milliliter in 0.1 M borate buffer.

Ferritin conjugates with the immunoglobulin or antigens by the mediation of a coupling agent, forming linkages through one of the two NCO groups of a coupling agent reacting with amino groups of the protein envelope of ferritin. The following coupling agents have been used for obtaining ferritin-antibody conjugates: xylylene m- diisocyanate (XMDIC), toluene-2,4-diisocyanate, meta-xylylene-diisocyanate (XC), p,p'-difluoro-m,m'-dinitrophenyl and glutaraldehyde.

Ferritin-globulin conjugates are best prepared according to Sri Ram's et al (1963) or Howe's et al. (1969) method, although the original Singer's method is still useful.

Linking of Ferritin to a Coupling Agent. According to Howe et al. (1969), a coupling agent (e.g., XMDIC of XC) is added to a ferritin solution in the proportion of 0.1 ml of the coupling agent per 100-mg ferritin. The mixture is stirred vigorously in an ice bath for 45 minutes, and then centrifuged at 4° at 1500 × g for 30 minutes. The supernatant fluids, containing the coupled ferritin, are collected and left in ice bath for 1 hour.

Conjugation of Ferritin to Antibody (or Antigen). According to Sri Ram et al. (1963) and Hsu (1967), the immunoglobulin- or antigen-preparation is added to the ferritin linked to a coupling agent in the ratio of one part of antibody (or antigen) to four parts of ferritin, by weight. Borate buffer is added to attain 0.1 molarity and pH 9.5. The mixture is stirred gently at 4° for 48 hours, and then dialyzed in cold first against 0.1 M ammonium carbonate overnight, and secondly against 0.05 M, pH 7.5, phosphate buffer for 4 hours.

Coupling of ferritin to the antibody globulin according to Singer (1959), is carried out as follows: 5 ml of 1.6% solution of crystalline horse spleen ferritin made in a sodium borate buffer, pH 9.5, are cooled at 0° mixed with 0.1 ml of *m*-xylylene diisocyanate, and stirred at 0° for $\frac{3}{4}$ hour, then centrifuged. The supernatant is added to 5 ml of a 1.6% buffered saline solution of the rabbit γ-globulin containing a specific antibody. The mixture should be stirred at 6° for 2 days, and then dialyzed against 0.1 *M* ammonium carbonate and against phosphate buffer, pH 7.5.

The ferritin-globulin conjugates can be purified by means of a continuous flow paper electrophoresis, or by ultracentrifugation removing the uncoupled ferritin and the uncoupled globulin. The continuous flow paper electrophoresis, according to Borek and Silverstein (1961), is conducted in a Spinco electrophoresis apparatus, model CP, with a 50-mA current, in a medium of 0.025 *M* barbital buffer, pH 8.6, at 4 to 5°, for about 20 hours. The protein content of the effluent fractions is measured optically at 280 nm after the dialysis against a buffered, pH 7.0 saline.

The unlabeled immunoglobulin may be separated from the ferritin-labeled immunoglobulins by sequential centrifugation of a ferritin-reacted antibody preparation, after dialysis, at 100,000 × *g* for 4.5 hours (Hsu et al., 1963). The heavier ferritin-conjugated protein and unconjugated ferritin form a pellet, which should be collected, resuspended in 0.01 *M* PBS, pH 7.5 and recentrifuged at the same speed. The final pellet is resuspended in 0.05 M phosphate buffer, pH 7.5, filtered through a 0.45-μ membrane and stored at 4°, or preferably at −20°. Ferritin may be stored for a year or so. The unconjugated ferritin may be removed by starch-block or continuous flow electrophoresis.

The iron content in the ferritin conjugates can be determined by the ferrocyanide method of Snell and Snell (1949).

The test with the ferritin-labeled globulin preparations may be conducted by a direct or indirect method.

i. *The Direct Immunoferritin Method (Sri Ram et al., 1963).* The material to be stained and examined is smeared onto a slide and flooded with the ferritin labeled antibody. If bacteria are used, they are pretreated with 10% formalin for at least 1 hour and washed in saline. The preparations are then placed on copper grids (200 mesh, coated with collodion and carbon), dried in air, and examined with an electron microscope. In the indirect method, the antigen preparation is preincubated in unlabeled globulin preparation, centrifuged, washed with saline, and incubated with a homologous ferritin labeled globulin. The preparation is then placed on a copper grid for electron microscopic observations.

According to Morgan's et al. (1961) technique, the test is conducted as follows: tissue culture cells or chorio-allantoic membranes, fixed in formalin, frozen, and sectioned in a cryostate, are thawed in a ferritin-conjugated antibody globulin. The sections should be fixed with osmium tetroxide, dehydrated, embedded, and cut for the electron microscope. Sections studied in the electron microscope show electron-dense, punctiform zones around virus particles which react with the antibody.

ii. *The Indirect Immunoferritin Test.* This is carried out in the following manner: the washed antigen preparation, for example, a tissue culture infected with a virus, is centrifuged, and the cell pellet is resuspended in 0.2 ml of the test antiserum globulin. After an incubation at room temperature for 90 minutes, the antigen-antibody complex is spun down and washed three times in a phosphate buffer containing 1% sucrose. The pellet is resuspended in 0.1 ml of a ferritin-conjugated antiserum globulin, obtained from an antiserum produced against the serum's species which provided the first antiserum. Controls consist of the antigen and a normal serum globulin, subsequently exposed to the same ferritin-conjugate. After a 90-minute incubation at room temperature, the mixture is centrifuged, washed in phosphate buffer, and fixed in 1% glyceraldehyde and 1% osmium tetroxide dehydrated, and embedded in Epon 812 (Luft, 1961). Ultrathinsections are cut, mounted on a grid, and observed in an electron microscope. Complexes with the ferritin conjugate appear in the form of dark crystals formed in or outside cells.

iii. *The Hybrid Immunoferritin Method.* This technique (Hammerling et al., 1968) depends on the hybridization of the antiferritin antibody with an anticell antigen immunoglobulin or antiserum, and it utilizes the ability of ferritin to combine with antiferritin antibodies. The hybridization technique is rather laborious and time consuming but it proves advantageous in the investigations of surface antigen structures. By the direct or indirect hybrid ferritin-antibody method, the surface antigen present on the cell is more easily detected and visualized than by other immunoferritin techniques since the ferritin particles form a uniform layer around the site of antigen in contrast to the rather randomly distributed ferritin granules frequently observed around the antigen site when an ordinary immunoferritin procedure is applied. One of the chief applications of the hybrid immunoferritin method is the detection of histocompatibility antigens on the surface of blood cells.

iv. *Differential Immunoferritin Test.* The differential immunoferritin test has been designed by Kwapinski to differentiate between the immunological specificities of different anatomical components of bacteria by applying ferritin labeled antisera to the ultrathinsections of bacterial cells. For this assay, antisera are produced against the bacteria, the purified cell wall, and cytoplasm and other anatomical constituents, as required. Euglobulins are separated from the other serum proteins by three, successive precipitations with ammonium sulfate at 33% saturation, followed by the dialysis against saline at 4° for 5 days. The globulins are then concentrated by lyophilization and labeled with ferritin according to Sri Ram's et al. (1963) method.

A portion of the nonlabeled anticell wall and anticytoplasm globulin preparations are cross-absorbed with 100 μg of the cell wall or cytoplasm preparation per milliliter, maintaining the mixtures at 37° for 2 hours and at 4° for 6 hours on an electric shaker. After the incubation, the mixtures are centrifuged at 14,000 $\times$ g for 10 minutes, and the supernatants are collected and recentrifuged for 5 minutes at 23,500 $\times$ g. The absorbed globulin preparations are then conjugated with ferritin as above.

Ultrathinsections of bacteria are made by Kellenberger's et al. (1958) method and are placed on collodion-coated grids. The grid with the ultrasection side down is then floated on one of the nonabsorbed or cross-absorbed, ferritin-labeled globulin solutions. The grid is incubated for 15 minutes and then is washed with three drops of distilled water, blotted carefully with filter paper, and mounted into an electron microscope.

Depending on the specificity of the labeled antibody, and its reactivity with an anatomical part or the whole body of bacterium, the following patterns of ferritin deposition are observed:

1. A dotted ferritin ring, as a product of reaction between the cell-wall and the ferritin-labeled immunoglobulin.

2. A round or oval cytoplasm of bacterium filled with the ferritin granules, resulting from a reaction between the cytoplasm and the anticytoplasm ferritin-labeled immunoglobulin.

3. A round or oval area, larger than the cytoplasm zone, filled with the ferritin, deposited over the whole ultrasection of a bacterium, due to the lack of immunological discrimination between the cell wall and the cytoplasm.

v. *Double (Fluorescein-Ferritin) Labeling of Antibodies.*   Antibodies may be doubly labeled with ferritin and fluorescein according to Hsu's et al. (1963) method using either of the labels first. If ferritin is employed first, the immunoglobulins are conjugated with purified ferritin recrystallized five to seven times with cadmium sulfate followed by three precipitations with ammonium sulfate and ultracentrifugation. The ferritin conjugation is carried out by a modification of Singer's (1959) method employing xylylene metadiisocyanate. The ferritin-conjugated antibodies are subsequently labeled with fluorescein. The double-labeled conjugate is dialyzed against 0.5 M, pH 7.5 phosphate buffer until no fluorescence is found in the dialyzing fluid in ultraviolet light. The nondialyzable conjugate is ultracentrifuged at 100,000 $\times$ g for 4 hours and the pellet is redissolved in one-third the volume of the same buffer. The fluid containing reconstituted ferritin-fluorescein conjugated globulin is filtered through a Millipore filter and stored at 4°.

In case of the application of fluorescein as the first label, the fluorescein labeled globulin is passed through a Sephadex G-25 column to eliminate unbound fluorescein and is labeled with ferritin xylylene metadiisocyanate. The doubly labeled fluorescein-ferritin conjugate is ultracentrifuged twice, reconstituted, and sterilized by membrane-filtration.

The doubly conjugated immunoglobulins are employed for the following immunological technique: smears of bacteria are made on slides, fixed in 95% ethanol for 30 seconds and incubated at room temperature for 30 minutes with twofold serial dilutions of the doubly labeled specific or non-specific conjugates. The excess immunoglobulins are washed off with buffer and the slides are examined in ultraviolet light, and then in an electron microscope.

The electron microscopic studies are carried out as follows: the microorganisms are washed in ice-chilled, 0.5% formalin in buffered saline and recentrifuged in the cold. Sediment of the bacteria is resuspended in 0.2 ml of formalinized buffered saline and added to 0.2 ml of either ferritin-conjugated or doubly labeled specific immunoglobulins. The mixtures are incubated at room temperature for 15 to 30 minutes and then centrifuged and washed with 0.01 M, pH 7.2 phosphate-buffered saline and recentrifuged.

The blocking test is employed by overlaying the bacterial smears with unconjugated specific antibody for 30 minutes before the specific doubly labeled conjugate is applied. For homologous blocking experiments, the bacterial suspensions are incubated with the unconjugated specific antibody for 15 minutes and washed with formalinized buffered saline and subjected to specific conjugates for 30 minutes. An additional control consists of the bacteria incubated with heterologous conjugates. The pellets are finally treated with phosphate-buffered osmium tetroxide and embedded in methacrylate.

vi. *Evaluation of Immunoferritin Assay.* The immunoferritin test is perhaps the most suitable procedure for the identification and detection of locality of an antigen in the structure of cells or tissues due to apposition of characteristic granules of ferritin conjugated to the immunoglobulin molecules. However, a difficulty encountered rather frequently with the ferritin-labeled immunoglobulins is the random distribution of ferritin particle as a background which may obscure the specific immunoferritin reaction. It is therefore mandatory to reduce the amount of nonspecific globulin and un-coupled ferritin in the preparative procedure by using such methods of electrophoretic purification of a crude ferritin-globulin conjugate, poly-acrylamide-gel filtration or electrophoresis, and extensive washing of antigen preparations exposed to the ferritin-labeled antibody preparation.

An immunohistochemical reaction observed in the electron microscope or in a fluorescent microscope can only be regarded as reliable if the immunoglobulin conjugate has been adsorbed specifically to certain antigen bearing sites and not randomly throughout the cell or tissue. Furthermore, the adsorption of the conjugate with a specific antigen preparation should be proved to abolish the capacity of the conjugate to react subsequently with the antigens in a section with specific antigens in the section or a smear. Finally, the antigen preparation preexposed to an unconjugated specific immunoglobulin- or antiserum-preparation should be able to suppress or abolish the intensity of a specific physicochemical reaction given by the immunoglobulin conjugate.

vii. *Applications of the Immunoferritin Technique.* The main applications of the immunoferritin test have been as follows:

1. The detection and recognition of viral antigens, such as influenza virus, polyoma virus, Herpes simplex virus, papova viruses and foot-and-mouth disease virus (Morgan et al., 1961, 1962; Duc-Nguyen et al., 1966; Oshiro et al., 1967; Shalla and Amici, 1967; Breese, 1970).

2. Localization of antigens in microbial cells, for example, in *Paramecium* (Mott, 1965) and *Coxiella* (Cracea et al., 1970).

3. Investigations on structural antigen relationships of microorganisms, for example, Herpes simplex virus, Epstein-Barr virus, and African swine fever virus (Hampar et al., 1970).

4. Determination of blood group in blood stains by means of anti-A and anti-B globulin preparations conjugated with ferritin (Suzuki, 1970).

5. Immunological diagnosis of diseases (Andres et al., 1963; Seegal et al., 1965).

2. The Immunomercury Assay

The following procedures are used in the mercury-conjugate antibody technique designed by Kul'berg and Azadova (1964):

To prepare *p*-aminophenyl mercury acetate (PAPMA) used in this technique, 7.7 g of mercury acetate dissolved in 40 ml of distilled water is added to a solution containing 12.5 ml of distilled aniline and 17.5 ml of 90% ethyl alcohol. PAPMA crystallizes in 1 to 3 hours.

The crystalline sediment is collected by centrifugation, washed on a no. 4 glass filter with distilled water, and dried in the air. PAPMA thus obtained occurs in the form of fine crystalline powder with a melting point of 105°.

Labeling of globulins is conducted in the following manner. Globulins are first pretreated with an excess of monoiodacetate at pH 7.5 at 25° in 2 hours to eliminate side reactions, and then dialyzed against 1 M veronal buffer, pH 8.6. The protein concentration should be brought to 15 to 20 mg/ml.

PAPMA is diazotized by dissolving 50 mg of PAPMA in 1 ml of 50% acetic acid and adding to it 10 mg of sodium nitrate. This mixture is kept at 30° for 2 hours. The solution of diazotized PAPMA is then adjusted to pH 4 to 5 with alkali and added dropwise, with stirring to the chilled globulin solution; pH 8.5 to 9.0 should be maintained during the labeling.

The amount of the mercury derivative added to the protein solution should correspond to 1.5% of the protein concentration. The labeled protein is kept at 2° for 24 hours, then it is dialyzed in the cold for 48 hours against physiological saline buffered at pH 8.2.

Viruses to be tested with the mercury-labeled antibody can be first adsorbed onto chick erythrocyte stromata according to Powell's (1961) method. Thus erythrocyte stromata, treated with 30% formalin for 24 hours and then washed with four volumes of physiological saline, are loaded with a virus, processed with 0.04 M potassium periodate. This preparation is washed with a large quantity of saline and added to the labeled globulin solution in a proportion of 0.1 ml of the stromata-virus complex per 1 ml of the labeled globulin. This mixture is left at 4° for 5 to 6 hours, and then it is washed with five to six volumes of cold saline, and two to three times with an ammonium acetate solution. The stromata-virus-globulin complex should finally be dried briefly and examined in the electron microscope.

3. *The Immunouranium Test*

The immunouranium test (Sternberger et al., 1963) depends on the visualization of an antigen-antibody complex in tissue- or cell-sections upon their reaction with an uranium-labeled immunoglobulin preparation as observed through an electron microscope. The test may be conducted directly, indirectly, and quantitatively.

The labeling of immunoglobulins with uranium is conducted as follows: the immunoglobulin preparation for an antiserum is added at 1° to a uranyl acetate solution in the amount sufficient to yield a final concentration of 147 to 256 uranium atoms per immunoglobulin molecule. The concentration of uranyl acetate solution to be used for this purpose may vary in a wide range from 0.0122 to 0.122 M uranyl acetate. After a short time of incubation at 1°, the mixture is dialyzed against saline and then against borate buffer, pH 8.0, and centrifuged at 1000 $\times$ g at 1° for 20 minutes. Following the centrifugation, the supernatant fluid is collected.

Uranium contents in the labeled immunoglobulin preparation is estimated by the radioactivity determinations using a gamma-scintillation spectrometer which has been standardized so that 2.0 ml of 0.01 M uranyl acetate solution yielded 300 counts per minute with a background count of 14.6.

i. *The Direct Immunouranium Test.* The direct immunouranium test is set up in the following manner: the bacteria are placed on a grid by floating a carbon celloidin copper grid for 1 hour on a drop of a bacterial suspension of a density predetermined colorimetrically. The bacteria adhering to the grid are then exposed for formalin vapor at 23° for 30 minutes or to air at 65° for 1 hour. The grid is subsequently floated on a drop of the uranium labeled immunoglobulin- or antiserum preparation for 30 minutes. After this step, the grid is washed twice in saline for 10 minutes and dried on a piece of filter paper. Controls, consisting of the same bacteria exposed to unconjugated immunoglobulins or to saline, or to normal serum, are set up concurrently.

If the immunouranium test is to be conducted with ultrasections of bacteria, the bacteria are first suspended in 10% formalin made in veronal buffer, pH 7.5 to 7.8 at 23° for 30 minutes. The mixture is subsequently centrifuged, and the sediment is washed several times with saline or distilled water. The bacteria are then brought to graded alcohols at 22° and embedded at 60° in a 3:1 mixture of n-butyl alcohol and methylmethacrylate to which benzoyl peroxide has been added to the concentration of 2%. Thins sections are cut with a glass knife in a Porter-Blum microtome and placed on a carbon colloidin copper grid. Further steps in the immunouranium procedure follow those described above.

Micrographs are taken on Kodak lantern slide contrast plates.

The particulate antigens reacting with the uranium-labeled immunoglobulin appear in the electron microscope as cells or sections of bacterial cells surrounded by or filled with the fine, homogeneous intransparent particles of uranium so that the contrast appears as if directly conferred in the manner of a specific stain in the cytoplasm and/or cell wall.

ii. *The Indirect Immunouranium Test (Sternberger et al., 1966).*
This depends on the coupling of antiimmunoglobulin antibodies with uranyl acetate in much the same way as described above and applying this reagent to the antigen or antigen-site pretreated with the antiantigen antibodies. The uranium labeled antiimmunoglobulin antibodies adsorbed onto the site or complexes of antigen and corresponding antibody and may be visualized in an electron microscope. One of the most convenient methods for isolation of immunoglobulin-antibodies from an antiserum is the absorption on the immunoglobulins used as antigen insolubilized by coupling it with diazotized *p*-aminobenzyl cellulose.

The indirect immunouranium technique seems to be adequate for the localization of virus antigens in infected cells but is less efficient for studies on structural antigens of bacteria.

The contrast between an antigen site reacting with the uranium labeled antibodies and the background may be enhanced when a tissues or tissue-

or cell-section subjected to the uranium-labeled antibody has been exposed to osmium tetroxide vapor. The latter treatment causes a deposition of osmium black on the sites where a uranium-labeled antibody complexed with the antigen.

iii. *The Quantitative Immunouranium Method.* The quantitative immunouranium technique (Sternberger, 1969) utilizes the densitometry study of electron micrographs taken on six successive sections made from one tissue block treated with the uranium-labeled antibodies.

4. *The Immunoenzyme Assays*

The principle of the immunoenzyme assay is the immunological reaction between antibody-immunoglobulins, coupled to a relatively stable enzyme, and a corresponding antigen, which yields characteristic products of the immunoenzymatic interaction. The enzyme most commonly used for immunoenzyme assays is peroxidase. Enzymes used less frequently for immunoenzyme assays are glucose oxidase (prepared from *Aspergillus niger*), acid phosphatase, alkaline phosphatase of *E. coli,* and tyrosinase (prepared from mushrooms, Avrameas, 1969, 1970).

The enzymes are coupled to antibodies by one of the bifunctional reagents, such as *p,p'*-difluoro-*m,m'*-dinitrodiphenyl sulfone, tetrazotized benzidine, toluene-2,4-diisocyanate, and meta-xylylene diisocyanate, but the most successful coupling agents seem to be 1-ethyl-3-(3-dimethylaminopropyl) carbodiimide and possibly glutaraldehyde.

The Immunoperoxidase Test. For this histiotropic test (LeDuc and Avramas, 1968), the antibody globulin is first coupled with peroxidase and tissue sections are flooded with this labelled immunoglobulin. After a short time of incubation, the tissue section is exposed to paradiaminodibenzidine, which is converted by the active peroxidase, in the presence of hydrogen peroxide, to an osmiophilic chelating agent. Subsequently, the postfixation of the thus treated tissue section in osmium tetroxide for electron microscopy yields a heavy deposition of osmium at the site where the immunoglobulin-peroxidase complex has been bound.

The coupling of peroxidase to antibody molecules (Nakane and Pierce, 1967) is conducted as follows.

To a mixture consisting of 100 mg of gammaglobulin preparation dissolved in 4 ml of 0.5 *M* cold carbonate buffer, pH 10, and 100-mg horse radish peroxidase are added 0.5 ml of 0.5% 1-ethyl-3-(3-dimethylaminopropyl) carbodiimide or *p,p'*-difluoro-*m,*m'-dinitrodiphenyl sulfone in acetone. The mixture is agitated gently for 6 hours at 4° and dialyzed against PBS.

If glutaraldehyde is used as a coupling agent, the following procedure is recommended (Avrameas, 1969).

To 1 ml of a solution containing 5 mg of an antibody globulin dissolved in 0.1 M phosphate buffer, pH 6.8, are added 12 mg of peroxidase. The mixture is stirred gently and to it 0.05 ml of 1% aqueous solution of glutaraldehyde is added dropwise. The reaction mixture is left at room temperature for 2 hours and then dialyzed against a large volume of PBS 4° overnight. Any precipitate thus formed is removed by centrifugation at 45,000 × g for 30 minutes. The stock solution of peroxidase-labelled antibodies may be stored at 4° and used within 3 months without noticeable loss of its catalytic and immunological activity.

Purification of the Enzyme-Labeled Antibodies. The enzyme-labeled antibodies may be purified by gel filtration on Sephadex G-200 and collection of the solutions containing labelled antibodies alone, but the antibodies may be purified more efficiently by electrophoresis. Unbound peroxidase may also be removed at 50% saturation by ammonium sulfate, but this procedure sometimes causes the inactivation of antibodies. The precipitate of labelled and unlabelled immunoglobulins is then separated, resuspended in PBS, and dailyzed.

A combined technique of immunoenzyme and autoradiography procedures was described by Wicker and Avrameas (1970).

Methods for the Immunoenzyme Assay. The following techniques have been designed for the immunoenzyme assay.

These are mixed antbody immunoenzyme technique (Avrameas, 1969), used for the demonstration of cell-bond immunoglobulins, the immunoglobulin-enzyme bridge method (Mason et al., 1969), the hybrid-antibody method (Avrameas, 1969), the amplification antibody method (Avrameas, 1969), the indirect immunoenzyme method, and the combined technique of the immunoenzyme and autoradiography procedure (Wicker and Avrameas, 1970).

The Indirect Immunoenzyme Technique. In this method, the antigen preparation is first subjected to an unlabeled antibody and the complex is then exposed to the enzyme-labeled antiimmunoglobulin serum directed against the donor of the first antiserum. The antigen is identified by the catalytic reaction of peroxidase on hydrogen peroxide in the presence of 3,3′-diaminobenzidine, after the peroxidase-labeled antiimmunoglobulin antibodies have combined to the antiantigen immunoglobulin. The osmium tetroxide treated preparations are then examined in an electron microscope.

The 3,3′-diaminobenzidine is used as oxidable substrate for peroxidase. The substrate is oxidized to an indamine polymer which is altered by oxidative cyclization by a phenazine polymer yielding a brown and strongly osmiophilic product.

All the controls required for the assessment of specificity of the immunoenzyme reaction are the same as used for the assessment of specificity of immunofluorescence and immunoferritin tests.

The immunoenzyme assays have been applied for the demonstration of antibodies, and soluble and insoluble antigens, to include antigens present in cells and tissues.

Chapter Sixteen

IMMUNOPHYSICAL ASSAYS

Certain physical changes, such as adsorption, aggregation, sedimentation, and loss of solubility and dispersion, accompany most immune reactions occurring between complete antibodies and antigens or haptens. Similar physical phenomena probably occur in reactions between incomplete antibodies and corresponding antigens, but are not strong enough to form visible reaction products. Other changes in the physical state of solutions or suspensions containing soluble complexes of incomplete antibodies and antigens, for example, alterations of the diffusion or the surface fixation coefficients and changes in the optical rotation, viscosity, and thickness of monolayers, can be more readily detected by appropriate physical measurements.

I. IMMUNOCHROMATOGRAPHIC METHODS

Immunological techniques, classified in the immunochromatographic category, are based on the principle of "the surface fixation," by which complexes of an antigen and a complementary antibody are strongly adsorbed on a filter paper, so that they cannot be eluted as are the noncombined reactants. These complexes are then detected on staining UV irradiation or by another suitable method. Thus samples of an antigen and antibody or a mixture of these reactants are first placed on a filter paper strip and then are exposed to the flow of a buffer through the paper. If an immune reaction takes place between the antigen and antibody, the precipitate or agglutinate formed remains absorbed at the starting point. If no serological reaction occurs, the noncombined antibody and antigen are carried away by the buffer, leaving "a tail" on the strip of filter paper. The paper strips are then colored by a stain and rinsed, revealing the position of reactants. Alternatively, the position of some reactants may be determined by an impression culture.

The immunochromatographic reactions can be studied either qualitatively or quantitatively. Quantitative data are obtained either by the estimation of the highest reactive dilution of a serum or an antigen, or by the spectrophotometric determination of proteins accumulated at the site of immune reaction and eluted from the paper.

Methods which reveal precipitation or agglutination by the aid of a chromatographic technique were devised by Castañeda (1950), Hess and Roepke (1951), Spalding and Metcalf (1954), Stöss (1957), Ito 1958), Miguel et al. (1960), and Kwapinski (1965). In the two first techniques, bacterial cells are used as antigens, whereas the other procedures may be applied to the nonparticulate, soluble antigens. Related techniques, which employ "impression culture procedure," were published by Friedberger and Putter (1920), Vajda and Bakhausz (1954), and Hodes et al. (1957). Immune paper electrophoresis methods were devised by Gurvicz (1955) and Lang et al. (1955).

1. The Spalding and Metcalf Technique

Bacterial cells, killed with 10% formalin, washed, centrifuged, and resuspended in water at a ratio of 1 ml of packed cells to 5 ml of water, are mixed with 1 ml of a fresh filtered solution of Delefield's hematoxylin. Hematoxylin may be substituted by tolouidin blue. This mixture is left at room temperature for 24 hours, and then centrifuged. The deposited cells are washed three times with a saline solution. The stained antigen should be resuspended in three volumes of saline, and 0.01 ml of this suspension is placed on a strip of Whatman filter paper no. 1, 2, or 4. The drop of the antigen is dried, and 0.001 ml of a serum under test is deposited on top of the dried antigen by means of a wire loop or by a micropipette, and dried. The paper strip is hung so that the distant part remains immersed in a saline solution buffered at pH 7.0 and left for 15 minutes. This strip is then dried in the air, and photographed. The descending chromatography can also be applied. Three controls, containing the antigen alone, antigen and normal serum, and the antigen and a heterologous antiserum, are set and processed in a similar manner.

A complex of homologous antibody and antigen, remaining at the starting point, appears as a violet dot, whereas the controls form columns ascending or descending the paper strip. However, short tails or columns arising from the dots may sometimes be observed if the concentration of antibody has not been sufficient to combine the whole amount of the antigen.

2. The Miguel et al. Technique

Components of the reaction, that is, 0.01 ml of antiserum and 0.01 ml of an antigen solution, are mixed in calibrated blowout micropipettes. One control pipette contains 0.01 ml of the antigen solution and 0.01 ml of saline buffered at pH 7.4. Another control consists of 0.01 ml of the antiserum and 0.01 ml of buffer. The contents of each pipette are mixed and left for half an hour in an incubator at 37° and for a few days at 4° (or for 12 to 18 hours at room temperature), then transferred, by means of a Spinco sample applicator, on strips of Schleicher-Schüll 2043A paper. The strips should be 3.0-cm wide by 30.6-cm long and wet with a pH 7.4 buffer solution, the excess being removed by pressing the strip between two sheets of filter paper. The mixtures from the capillary tubes may be transferred directly by pressing the polished ends of pipettes against the filter paper (Stöss, 1957). A descending chromatography is conducted for 30 minutes in a 0.01-M sodium phosphate buffer, pH 7.4, containing 0.15 M NaCl. Stöss recommends the ascending chromatography in a pH 8.6 veronal buffer, with 0.1 M ionic strength. The strips are then dried at 37°, stained in a bromophenol blue solution for 20 minutes, and washed for 2 to 5 minutes in three changes of 5% acetic acid . If the antibody has reacted with the antigen, a sharply demarcated, narrow blue zone is seen at the site of application of reactants. Otherwise, a diffuse coloration extending from this zone is observed.

The staining solution consists of 0.05 g of bromophenol blue, 70.0 ml of ethyl alcohol (95%), 5.0 ml of glacial acetic acid, and 30.0 ml of distilled water. (Amido-black 10B is used in the Stöss technique.)

For quantitative studies, 0.5-cm-wide segments of the stained zone are cut off with scissors. They are pressed between two sheets of filter paper to remove the excess of fluid and eluted for 30 minutes in 2 ml of a solution consisting of 10 ml of 1 molar sodium hydroxide, 70 ml of ethyl alcohol (95%), and 20 ml of distilled water. The eluates are examined in a spectrophotometer at 595-nm wavelength, with an eluate from a paper strip containing a control serum used as a blank. Calibration curves are prepared in the following way. A solution of bovine γ-globulin fraction II, containing an ascertained concentration of protein, which is equal to 10 μg of nitrogen per 0.01 ml, is diluted with a buffer to contain amounts of protein corresponding to 1, 3, 5, and 7 μg of nitrogen per 0.01 ml. Samples of 0.01 ml of each solution are placed on paper strips, dried, stained, and eluted as described above.

A similar technique is applied to the fluorescent antibody. In this procedure, a mixture of antiserum labeled with a fluorescent marker according to Coons and Kaplan (1950) and unlabeled antigen is placed on a filter paper strip. Position of the precipitate at the end of the chromatography can be revealed with the aid of ultraviolet light.

In the radioautographic technique by Bennington (1960), a mixture of radioactive ^{131}I labeled antigen and corresponding antibodies is applied to a filter paper strip and run for 20 hours in the electrophoresis apparatus, in the medium of a pH 8.6 barbiturate buffer. The paper strip is then dried, and a radioautograph is prepared by tightly pressing Dupont 508 x-ray film against the filter paper strip, and leaving it for 48 hours. The film is then developed, and autographs are scanned in a densitometer.

3. Kwapinski's Two-Dimensional Immunochromatography Technique

This test depends on a specific absorption reaction on a filter paper between antigens and antibodies which migrate from opposite directions in an adequate solvent. The stock solvent solution consists of 5 ml of 1% boric acid, 3 ml of glycerol, 2 ml of 20% phenol, and 110 ml of 1% sodium chloride. This solution is diluted 2:1 in 1% sodium chloride prior to use.

One microdrop of each antigen solution at 1:200 to 1:500 concentration is placed on a piece (6 x 11 in.) of Whatman no. 3 filter paper, $1\frac{1}{2}$ in. apart and $1\frac{1}{2}$ in. from the edge. Microdrops of undiluted or 1:2 diluted sera are put at the opposite end to antigens, at 3 in. distance between the two components of the test. The drops are dried at 37° for 10 minutes. Edges of the paper strip are then immersed in the solvent contained in narrow plastic cuvettes, and left at room temperature or at 37° for 20 to 24 hours. Paper strips are then removed from the solvent, dried at 100° in a hot air oven for 3 to 4 minutes, sprayed with 0.12% of alcoholic solution of ninhydrin, and heated at 100° for 3 to 5 minutes.

A positive reaction is indicated by a violet halo zone formed by the antiserum around a central, oval-shaped, orange-colored spot of the antigen preparation. Diameters of spots produced by antigen-antibody complexes vary from 5 to 20 mm, depending on the potency of components and the strength of a serological reaction. A negative result is indicated by an orange-colored, oval spot, surrounded occasionally by a violet tail on the approximate site of a noncombined serum.

This test can be used as a qualitative or quantitative procedure with series of serum or antigen dilutions.

4. The Surface-Fixation Technique

One test, devised by Dunsford and Bowley (1955), is used for the selection of high titer blood donors. In this technique, two drops of a serum being examined are placed on a strip (26 x 6 cm) of blotting paper, followed by one drop of an appropriatae red blood cell suspension. After 30 to 45 seconds, one or two drops of saline are placed, at 2- to 5-second intervals, in the center of erythrocyte-serum mixtures to expedite the spreading.

A positive reaction is marked by a sharply defined and limited area, while uniform spreading and coloring of a wider area are observed in the case of a negative result.

Another procedure for the surface-fixation technique, described by Ito (1958), can be used for screening the results of the complement fixation or hemolysin tests. In this simple procedure, chromatographic filter paper strips (1 × 20 cm) are dipped gently into test tubes upon completion of an immunologic test. The nonlyzed red blood cells show a little movement on the paper and form a red band on one end of the strip, whereas the lyzed erythrocytes rise with the ascending fluid to give homogenous coloration of the filter paper.

5. *The Immune Paper-Electrophoresis Technique*

In the procedures devised by Gurvicz (1955) and Lang et al. (1955), the antigen and the antibody placed on a filter paper strip migrate toward each other and react in the electric field. The antigen is placed on a filter paper strip in front or behind the antiserum, depending on their speed of migration in the electric field. During the 16- to 24-hour electrophoresis in a veronal or phosphate buffer, pH 9.2, the antiserum and the antigen pass each other and react at the site where they meet in an optimal concentration ratio. The position of an antigen-antibody complex is discovered by a staining or radiography technique and may be compared with the positions of various serum proteins, revealed on a parallel electrophoregram.

6. *Evaluation of Immune Chromatographic Methods*

The immune chromatographic techniques are simple, demonstrative, and fairly sensitive. As little as 1.2 μg of protein or about 0.2 μg of nitrogen present in a precipitate on a filter paper can be detected by these procedures (Miguel et al., 1960), diphtherial toxoid, and the chemical fractions of *Streptococcus pyogenes* (Kwapinski, 1965).

II. THE CAPILLARY-RISE TEST

This test, originally devised by Friedberger and Putter (1920), modified by Vajda and Bakhausz (1954), and adopted to virus-antibody systems by Hodes et al. (1957), differs from the techniques presented above in that the soluble antigens are replaced by bacterial cells or viruses, and positions of serological systems on filter paper strips are indicated by impression culture techniques instead of staining.

1. *The Bacterium-Rise Test*

In the technique adopted by Vajda and Bakhausz, the serum examined is serially diluted in 10- or 15-ml volumes, and 10-ml aliquots are mixed in sterile Petri dishes with 1 ml of a suspension containing 500 million bacterial cells per milliliter. Control tubes receive 10 ml of a saline solution and 1 ml of a bacterial suspension. Sterile strips of the Whatman filter paper no. 1 or 4, 20-cm long and 2-cm wide, are immersed with one end into each plate to the depth of 0.5 cm. Any kind of filter paper which permits the solution to rise up by 14 to 16 cm in 30 minutes may be used. After 20 minutes, portions of the filter paper which have been soaked by the suspension of bacteria are cut off and placed flat on the surface of a nutrient agar plate to make an impression culture. The plates are incubated for 24 hours at 37°.

The strips of the filter paper are then removed from the surface, and the zone occupied by colonies is measured in centimeters. The diameter of this zone is reciprocal to the height to which bacterial cells had originally risen.

The "capillary rise" of bacteria differs from species to species. For example, *Escherichia coli, Salmonella,* and *Shigella* rise up to 10 to 12 cm in 20 minutes, whereas Gram-positive cocci rise only 1 to 2 cm. Homologous antisera reduce the capillary rise by one fifth to one tenth.

The bacterium-rise test was used for the differentiation of various strains and species of bacteria (Friedberger and Putter, 1920; Vajda and Bakhousz, 1954) and for the study of protective substances (Castañeda, 1950; Hodes et al., 1957).

2. The Virus-Rise Test

According to the Hodes et al., technique (1957), a filter paper strip should be first impregnated with a certain amount of antiserum, dried, and immersed in the upright position into a virus suspension. The virus wanders upward to the edge of the paper strip with the flow of dispersing medium, if it does not meet the corresponding antibody. If an immune reaction occurs, the virus is "blocked" and remains close to the starting point. Position of the virus is revealed on the paper strip by a tissue culture plate technique.

III. DETECTION OF IMMUNE REACTIONS BY DETERMINATION OF THE OPTICAL ROTATION

When two or more antibody molecules are attached to a molecule antigen, the optical rotation in an immune system increases. According to Ishizaka and Campbell (1959), the most likely causes of this change are the formation of salt linkage and hydrogen bonds which participate in the specific antigen-antibody combination and the electrostatic interactions around asymmetric carbon atoms of the antigen and/or antibody surface. Another reason for the increase of the optical rotation may be a slight denaturation of protein, presumably as a result of combination between an antigen and antibody.

Optical rotation can be measured at room temperature with the photoelectric polarimeter at wavelength of 650 nm, using sodium light. Each complex of antigen and antibody is measured at three different concentrations and read ten times. Specific rotations $(\alpha)_D$ obtained are averaged. Experimental error in the specific rotation values is between 0.4 and $1.0°$.

IV. DETECTION OF IMMUNE REACTION BY VISCOSITY MEASUREMENTS

Two varieties of the viscosity test, the direct and indirect, may be distinguished. In the direct test, the increase of viscosity is observed, resulting from the formation of antigen-antibody complexes which are more highly polymerized than single components. In the indirect test, which is used to determine enzyme-antienzyme reactions, the viscosity depending on the antigen-antibody complexes reacting in a substrate is compared with the viscosity of controls, in which the substrate was depolymerized by the enzyme.

1. The Direct Viscosity Test

Antiserum, diluted 1:5, is added in an equal amount to a 1:100 solution of a purified antigen or to a culture filtrate, diluted 1:5 in a phosphate buffered saline, pH 7.0. Controls receive (a) buffered saline alone, (b) a normal serum instead of antiserum, and (c) a 1:100 solution of glycogen or albumin instead of the antigen, depending on the chemical character of the antigen. The reactants should be heated at 37° and mixed together prior to the introduction into three identical viscosimeters, to the upper mark. The viscosimeters are placed in an automatic water bath at 37°, and the first measurement of viscosities is taken immediately, and then in 10 to 15 minute intervals over a period of 2 hours, by taking times of flow between marks of a viscosimeter.

Results are calculated according to this formula for the differential viscosity (Dv):

$$\mathrm{Dv} = \frac{2t_0 \times m_0}{t_1 \times m_1 \times t_2 \times m_2}$$

where t_0, t_1, and t_2 are times in which the antibody-antigen mixture and controls 1 and 2 pass the lower mark of viscosimeters m_0, m_1, m_2, which are the corresponding densities or relative densities.

Results of viscosity tests can be confirmed by measuring refractometric indexes of the antigen-antibody mixtures.

Similar direct viscosity tests were described by Lecomte de Nouy and Hamon (1936), Faillie et al. (1938), and Loiseleur et al. (1946).

2. The Indirect Viscosity Test

By this test, immune reactions are revealed through the determination of (a) the highest antiserum dilution which has prevented the depolymerization of a viscous substrate by an active bacterial enzyme (Hadidian and Murphy, 1955), or (b) the estimation of residual enzyme activity after the incubation with an antiserum (Hazlehurst, 1950). Techniques of this test were presented on p. 368.

V. THE FALLING DROP ASSAY

The test is based on the measurement of a specific gravity of a dissolved antigen-antibody precipitate. In this assay, the time is measured in which a drop of the dissolved antigen-antibody precipitate falls and traverses a given distance in an organic solution composed of xylene and chlorobenzene, in which it is immiscible. This test was devised by Barbour and Hamilton (1926) who used bromobenzene for the reaction and improved by Lipton (1948).

Here is a brief description of the assay. The precipitate, obtained by adding an antigen to the antiserum, is centrifuged, washed in saline, and dissolved in 0.5% sodium hydroxide solution. Falling drop tubes (bottom opening closed with a cork) are filled with a xylene-chlorobenzene solution to the level just below the surface of water in a constant temperature bath, at 25, 35°. The solution of the antigen-antibody system is drawn into a delivery pipette to the top graduation mark; 0.01 ml of this solution is then delivered into the falling drop tube. The time in which the drop traverses a distance of 15 cm to the second graduation mark is recorded with the aid of a stopwatch. The falling drop times for control solutions of a serum, antigens, and the diluent are determined in parallel.

Figures obtained from the measurement of falling drop times may be converted to assigned density differences. The conversion table is prepared by assigning the falling drop times to hypothetical solutions in a hypothetical falling drop fluid at a temperature of 25.34°. The assigned density difference of the diluent (0.5% sodium hydroxide solution) should be subtracted from the values of the solution of the dissolved antigen-antibody precipitate. The resulting data are regarded as being due to the antigen-antibody precipitate.

VI. SPECTROFLUOROMETRIC DETECTION OF IMMUNE REACTIONS

Spectrofluorometric method described by Velick et al. (1960) utilizes purified antibodies which, due to their tryptophane contents, emit a fluorescence maximal in the region of 340- to 360-nm wavelength. The method is especially useful for detection and determination of soluble antigen-antibody complexes. The reaction between antibody and hapten is determined quantitatively by measurement of the diminution of the antibody fluorescence when the antibody interacts specifically with a hapten which absorbs intensely in the region of the fluorescence emission. The bound hapten exerts its quenching effect by dissipating the energy responsible for the excitation of fluorescence.

The test is carried out as follows: 0.1 ml of a solution of purified antibody is activated with the ultraviolet light at 280 or 290 nm, and intensity of the antibody fluorescence is measured in arbitrary units at or near 350 nm. Univalent hapten is then added in 0.01- to 0.02-ml increments, and the fluorescence is measured after each addition of the hapten preparation.

The hapten preparation must be used in such a concentration that no more than 0.20 volume hapten will be required to complete titration.

Another useful method for measurement of the interaction of simple haptens or simple organic determinants with a specific antibody in an entirely soluble system is the equilibrium dialysis (Marrack and Smith, 1932). This method, however, requires relatively large amount of antibody.

VII. DETERMINATION OF IMMUNE REACTIONS BY MEASURING THE THICKNESS OF ANTIGEN-ANTIBODY MONOLAYERS

Immunophysical techniques designed by Chambers (1941), Rothen and Landsteiner (1942), and Ogata et al. (1952) depend on the absorption of antibody from an antiserum placed on the antigen monolayer film. In the technique devised by Ogata et al. (1952), antigen films are first prepared on filter paper strips thoroughly washed in benzene. These paper strips are then held vertically, brought into close contact with the water surface, and lifted just above it. A drop of the antigen solution is now dripped on the strip with a capillary pipette, so that the antigen solution spreads over the water surface. After 5 minutes, the surface film is compressed to 15 dynes/ cm² with the use of castor oil as piston oil and transferred onto a narrow chromium plated slide, previously coated with barium stearate by dipping the coated slide into the antigen film spread.

To carry out the immunophysical test, the slide covered by an antigen film is wetted with distilled water and immersed into undiluted antiserum, poured into a test tube just big enough to allow the slide to enter. The slide carrying an antigen-antibody film is left at 0° for 15 to 20 hours, and the thickness of the film is measured optically by using polarized sodium light (Blodgett and Langmuir, 1937). The plates are viewed through a Nicol analyzer adjusted to transmit only the Rs rays. The increase of thickness, indicative of an immune reaction, may range from 10 to 270 Å (Chambers et al., 1941; Rothen and Landsteiner, 1942; Ogata et al., 1952). The apparent thickness (T) of protein can be calculated from the formula (Bateman et al., 1941):

$$T = \frac{\lambda}{4\sqrt{u^2 - \sin^2 i}} - (N + 4.3)t$$

where λ = the wavelength of the incident light
     u = index of the refraction
    N = layers of the stearate
    t = the thickness of barium stearate
    i = the angle of incidence, at which the reflected intensity is mini-
       mal with added layer of protein.

VIII. IMMUNOSTRUCTURAL REACTIONS

This group of immunophysical tests depends on the reactions of different structural constituents of microorganisms, particularly capsules and cell walls, with the corresponding antibodies, bringing about an enlargement or intensification of contours of these structures. Antibody molecules are absorbed or bound by the surface antigens of cells in these reactions, which are greatly facilitated by the permeability of superficially situated structures. Adequate sites of microorganisms for specific structural reactions are capsules, sporangia, and exosporium, and, to a lesser extent, cell walls.

The following types of specific structural reactions were devised: the capsular reaction (Neufeld, 1903; Ettinger-Tulczynska, 1933; Evans, 1950); the cell wall reaction (Baumann-Grace and Tomcsik (1957, 1958).

1. The Specific Capsular Reaction

The test, originally described by Ettinger-Tulczynska (1933) and modified by Evans (1950), is carried out as follows. One drop of the antiserum diluted 1:8 is mixed with one drop of a cell suspension on a microscope slide, under a cover slip.

A control slide contains normal serum instead of the antiserum. The cells are examined at 440 magnification after 10-minutes incubation at room temperature.

A dye, for example, India ink, may be added to facilitate the observation. If an immunological reaction occurs, outlines of capsules become more contrasting. The test may be carried out directly with a diagnostic material, for example, a sputum sample. In this procedure a small fleck of the sputum is placed on a cover slip and mixed with a typing serum added in a four to five times greater amount. The cover slip is inverted on a glass slide and examined after 5 minutes through the oil immersion objective.

The specific capsular test was used for the immunological classification of pneumococci, meningococci (Little, 1938), and *Cryptococcus neoformans* (Evans, 1950), and for the C-reactive protein test (Löfström, 1944).

2. The Immune Cell-Wall Reaction

The test (Baumann-Grace and Tomcsik, 1957; Tomcsik and Baumann-Grace, 1958) is carried out with the cell walls obtained by the disintegration of bacteria and purified by physical and chemical methods. Thus one loopful of the cell wall suspension is mixed with a small drop of a non-diluted antiserum, on a glass slide under cover slip. A control slide contains the bacteria without antiserum. The mixtures are examined through a phase-contrast microscope or preferably by a phase-interference microscope. Cell walls that have not reacted with the antiserum are thin and pale but visible, whereas the contours of reactive cell walls are thicker and dark and the cross-walls are intensified.

The immune cell-wall reaction was used successfully by the authors for immunological classification of *Bacillus megatherium* and *Bacillus cereus*.

3. The Immune Sporangium Reaction

The sporangium shows a marked swelling when mixed with a homologous antivegetative polysaccharide serum (Tomcsik and Baumann-Grace, 1958; Tomcsik et al., 1959). The "swelling" results from the depolymerization, by sporangiolytic enzymes, of the mother cell wall during the antigen-antibody reaction. The depolymerized cell wall is made microscopically observable through the immunologic reaction. A similar "swelling" reaction is observed when the exosporium, prepared from spores disintegrated in an electromagnetic or sonic vibrator, are exposed to an antispore serum. The exosporium thus freed from the inner contents of the spore and reacting with the homologous antibody occurs as a capsule-like layer.

4. The Immune Exosporium Reaction

Spores are freed from the residues of vegetative bacteria by centrifugation of sporulating cultures in Grelet's (1961) sporulating medium. The sediment is resuspended in $M/30$ phosphate buffer, pH 7.0, and treated with an equal volume of crystalline lysozyme diluted 1:10,000 in a buffer solution. This mixture is incubated at 37° for 30 minutes, or until no vegetative remains are detectable microscopically. The spore suspension is chilled immediately and washed five times with distilled water, in the cold.

The immune exosporium reaction, by Tomcsik and Baumann-Grace (1959), is set up as follows. One loopful of undiluted antispore serum is applied to the edge of the cover slip of a set amount of unstained spores and allowed to flow under the cover slip by the capillary action. Alternatively, one loopful of the spore suspension is mixed with the antiserum on a slide and covered with a cover slip.

The reaction is observed by a phase-contrast microscope for several hours, while the reaction mixtures are maintained in a moist chamber. Positive reaction is manifested by the aggregation of black ovoid bodies (spores).

IX. THE IMMUNE L.E.-CELL TEST

The L. E. phenomenon (Hargraves et al., 1948) is caused by the "L.E.-cell factor," a specific substance which is found in cases of systemic *lupus erythematosus disseminatus*. This factor acts first on the nuclei of whole blood cells or bone marrow cells; and it reacts in the second stage with the white cells which have phagocytized the altered nuclear material, bringing about the formation of characteristic L.E.-cells. The second step involves a heat labile substance present in any serum. The L.E.-factor is regarded as an autoantibody, whereas nucleoprotein or deoxyribonucleic acid participates as the antigen. The L.E.-cells are predominantly polymorphonuclear neutrophilic leukocytes which engulfed a large mass of amorphous material filling the cytoplasm and pushing the nucleus to the margin of the cell. Another characteristic feature of the reaction is the "rosette" formation.

Several methods of the L.E.-cell test were described by Eppes and Ludovic (1951), Zinkham and Conley (1956), Kievits and Schuit (1957), Fallet and Ziff (1958), and Aisenberg (1959).

Aisenberg's Technique of the L.E.-Cell Test. Buffy coat cells are obtained from a sample of heparinized normal human blood by the addition of bovine fibrinogen. The pellets are centrifuged, resuspended in saline solution of a γ-globulin under test, and to this 0.05 ml of a 0.1 *M*, pH 7.4 phosphate buffer and 0.15 ml of a saline solution are added. Two glass beads are added to the tube, and it is agitated on an Eberbach shaking machine for 50 minutes at room temperature. The tube is then centrifuged and the pellets are smeared on cover slips, stained with Wright's stain, and the number of the L.E.-cells per 100 leukocytes is counted.

X. THE IMMUNE LONG-CHAIN REACTION

This reaction depends on the formation of long chains by bacteria grown in the presence of a homologous antibody, as a result of the end-to-end agglutination. This phenomenon, observed by Stollerman and Ekstedt (1957) in cultures of streptococci Group A grown in the presence of homologous anti-M antibody, is believed to be specific. This type of reaction can be expected to occur in other systems of bacteria and homologous antibodies.

The test (Stollerman et al., 1959) is set up in the following manner: 0.2 ml of a serum to be tested for the specific antibody is mixed with 0.05 ml of a 10^{-2} broth dilution of a 16- to 18-hour broth culture of bacteria. Control tubes receive either a strong homologous antiserum and bacteria, or a normal rabbit serum and bacteria. Dilutions should be preferably made in a heat-inactivated, pooled normal rabbit serum instead of broth, since the lowering of protein concentrations causes some long chaining.

The tubes (9.0 × 100 mm) are closed with sterile rubber stoppers and incubated at 37° for 3 to 4 hours. The contents of tubes are then mixed by gentle inversion. A drop from each tube is placed on a microscope slide, covered with a glass slide and examined immediately under the oil immersion of the dark-phase contrast microscope. The number of cocci in each of 50 chains, selected at random from several representative fields, is counted and the mean chain length of cultures grown in the tested serum is divided by the mean chain length of bacteria grown in a normal control serum, to obtain the "long chain index."

The results of long chain reactions can be more precisely evaluated by an analysis of the frequency distribution of chain lengths formed in the test and control sera (Hahn and Cole, 1962).

XI. THE IMMUNOADHERENCE ASSAY

The immunoadherence test is based on the phenomenon of adhesion of antigens to human and primate red cells or platelets sensitized with an antibody in the presence of complement, which results in the enhanced phagocytosis and aggregation of these morphotic blood elements. To this category also belongs the immunological erythrocyte-adherence test. The immune adherence is a highly sensitive immunological reaction. The mechanism of this reaction probably involved the absorption of C_1' and C_4' components of complement in the first stage, the reaction with the C_2' component in the second stage, and finally the reaction with C_3'; but the exact sequence of these and further components of complement in this reaction has not been thoroughly investigated. The microorganisms sensitized by a specific antibody and altered through the absorption of complement components attach themselves to the red blood cells, causing clumping of these cells.

The immune adhesion reaction, involving trypanosomas, was first described by Duke and Wallace in 1930, although the adhesion of trypanosomas to animal platelets was observed as early as 1917 by Rieckenberg.

Microorganisms and antigens undergoing the immune adherence are trypanosomas, *Staphylococcus aureus, Diplococcus pneumoniae, Mycobacterium tuberculosis, Salmonella typhosa, Shigella paradysenteriae, Treponema pallidum, Leptospira, Rickettsia,* vaccinia virus, T2 bacteriophage, toxoid of *Corynebacterium diphtheriae,* polysaccharides isolated from *Shigella flexneri, Salmonella typhosa* and *Streptococcus* (Brown and Broom, 1938), and *Treponema pallidum* (Nelson, 1953, 1956, 1957; Olansky et al., 1954; Turk, 1958; Kiraly and Porganyi, 1960), as well as Moloney virus (Tachibana and Klein, 1970).

Turk's (1958) Immunoadherence Test. This assay is carried out as follows. The antiserum is serially diluted in 0.2-ml volumes, in a veronal buffered saline containing bovine albumin. The complement is diluted to produce the maximal immune-adherence hemagglutination with the optimal antigen-antibody mixture and added to each tube in 0.2-ml volume. Each tube subsequently receives 0.5 ml of a suspension or solution of an antigen, and the mixtures are shaken and incubated at 37° for 20 minutes. Finally, 0.1 ml of 0.5% human group A erythrocyte suspension is added to all tubes, which are left for 60 to 70 minutes at 37° and examined for the presence of agglutinates on the bottom of tubes.

Negative results are indicated by a compact button or ring of cells with no visible agglutination. In case of a positive result, a layer of red cells covering the bottom of the tube or at least flakes of agglutinated cells surrounding the central button are observed.

Kiraly's and Porganyi's Technique of the Treponema-Adherence Test. Components of the test are (a) a suspension of Treponema pallidum, containing 2.5 to 5×10^6 of treponemas per milliliter, (b) washed and packed human erythrocytes group O, and (c) a guinea pig complement. The test is set up in the following way: the serum being examined is added in 0.05-ml volume to 0.3 ml of a *Treponema* suspension and 0.2 ml of complement. Control tubes receive (a) 0.3 ml of antigen alone, (b) 0.3 ml of antigen and 0.2 ml of an inactivated guinea pig serum, (c) 0.3 ml of antigen and 0.2 ml of complement (the spontaneous adherence, SA control), and (d) 0.3 ml of the antigen solution and 0.05 ml of the examined serum. All mixtures are incubated at 35° for 18 hours. In the second phase of the assay, 0.05 ml of human group O Rh+ erythrocytes and 0.3 ml of veronal buffer, pH 7.2, are added. The mixtures are left at 37° for 30 minutes and centrifuged for 5 minutes at 500 rpm. The quantity of treponemas in 0.005-ml volumes of the supernatant is then estimated under a 600 magnification of a microscope. Reduction of the number of treponemas in the test sample, as compared with the serum control, is expressed in percentage. The percentage adherence can be calculated according to the following formula (Miller et al., 1959):

$$\% \text{ adherence} = \frac{\text{count in SA control} - \text{count in the test tube}}{\text{count in SA control}} \times 100$$

The decline of the number of treponemas by 21 to 50% or more is regarded as a significant result.

A similar test was published earlier by Nelson (1953) and by Olansky et al. (1954).

The Immunoadherence on Monolayer Cells. The test originally designed by O'Neill (1968) and modified by Tachibana and Klein (1970), employs monolayers of cells transformed with a tumor virus, and possessing surface antigens of the histocompatibility or tumor-specific nature. The cells are seeded into wells on Falcon plastic "Microtest" plates by placing one drop (about 20 μl) of cell suspension containing approximately 5 × 10^4 cell/ml. The plate is covered and incubated for 18 to 24 hours at 37° in CO_2 atmosphere. The cells attach and grow on the well surface. When reasonably confluent monolayers are obtained, they are washed three times in GVB diluent (see below). To wash the monolayer, the wells are filled with the diluent, the plate is inverted, and the fluid is sucked off by touching its surface with a trumpet-shaped glass capillary tube. The washing is then repeated twice.

Antiserum (10 μl) (possessing virus-antibodies) used in two or three-fold dilutions is then introduced to each well. The plate is incubated at 37° for 60 minutes, and then the cells are washed again. The indicator system consisting of 10 μl of a suspension of human group O erythrocytes (2 × 10^7 cells/ml) containing 1 to 2% adsorbed guinea-pig complement are added to each well. Controls consist of: (a) dilutions of normal serum used instead of the antiserum, (b) a control lacking complement and antiserum, and (c) a complement control possessing no antiserum or normal serum. The systems are incubated at 37° for 30 minutes. The plate is then inverted and left at 37° for 60 minutes. The reaction patterns are read under the microscope without washing. The antiserum titer is expressed as the reciprocal of the greatest dilution at which aggregation formation and attachment of erythrocytes to the monolayer cells have been observed.

The strength of the immune adherence is scored as follows: heavy rosette formation or attachment to all target cells, 4; moderate rosette formation and attachment of erythrocytes to 75 to 85% of target cells, 3; three or more erythrocytes attached to 50 to 75% of target cells, 2; two or more erythrocytes attached to less than 50% of target cells, 1; one or two erythrocytes attached to 25% or less target cells, 0.5.

The complement source (guinea pig serum) must be absorbed successively with the target cells and human erythrocytes at 0° for 3 to 10 minutes. Natural antibodies against human erythrocytes are absorbed from the antiserum by an equal volume of packed erythrocytes at room temperature for 60 minutes.

XII. THE IMMUNOHEMADSORPTION ASSAY

1. *The Mixed Hemadsorption Test*

The test may be set up on mammalian target cells grown in wells of a plastic "microtest" plate (Tachibana and Klein, 1970) or on cells grown on cover slips (Watkins and Grace, 1967). The mixed hemadsorption test

(Tachibana et al., 1970) is initially set up identically to the immunoadherence test (Tachibana and Klein, 1970; see above). For this part, human group O erythrocytes are used as indicator whereas the indicator for the second part of the mixed hemadsorption consists in sheep erythrocytes. After the incubation with an antiserum, the target monolayer cells are washed three times with PBS. One drop of an 0.5 to 1% indicator erythrocyte suspension is then added to the target cells, in a plastic "microtest" plate. The plate is left for 60 minutes at room temperature to allow the indicator cells to settle. The plate is then shaken by knocking its sides against a hard object and washed by immersion into PBS. The plate is inverted and read under the microscope. The aggregation of human and sheep erythrocytes is observed and expressed as above.

The $C'IA_{50}$ (50% unit of immune adherence activity) is determined in two steps (Nishioka, 1963, as arranged by Kwapinski).

1. Estimation of the optimal amount of antgien-antibody complex: 0.2 ml of a suspension of bacteria, for example, *Brucella* or *Salmonella* adjusted to optical density of 0.1 to 650 nm are added to the serial dilutions of a rabbit antibody to be used for the immune adherence test. The test mixtures are incubated at 37° for 30 minutes. The patterns of erythrocytes are observed under a microscope, and the reaction mixture showing a diffused deposit is noted as optimal amount of the antigen-antibody complex.

2. The optimal Ag-Ab amount is then tested against varied dilutions of complement; and the highest complement dilution giving 2+ hemagglutination is determined. The corresponding volume of complement, divided by 2 represents one $C'IA_{50}$ unit. The dilution factor multiplied by 2 represents the amount of $C'IA_{50}$ units in the volume of complement, at the end point well.

2. The Immunoadherence Hemagglutination Test

The reaction (Nishioka, 1963) is set up by mixing different dilutions of a particulate or nonparticulate antigen, a constant antibody amount (or *vice versa*), an optimal complement amount (or 1 $C'HA_{50}$ unit) at a total volume of 0.9 ml. To each tube is then added 0.1 ml of 0.2% human type O Rh+ erythrocytes (standardized spectrophotometrically so that 1 ml of the suspension lyzed by dilution with distilled water to 10 ml gave an O.D. of 0.395 at 541 nm). The tubes are shaken at 37° for 10 minutes and left for an additional 55 minutes. The pattern of settled erythrocytes is recorded.

Nonagglutinated cells collect in a central button or ring whereas the erythrocytes agglutinated due to the adherence through an antigen-antibody complex form an even and diffuse deposit. The end point may be determined, in doubtful cases, by dark-field microscopy.

The antigen or antibody titer is expressed by the reciprocal dilution giving a distinct, diffuse deposit.

3. The Immunocytoadherence Test

The immunocytoadherence phenomenon depends on the aggregation of erythrocytes around lymphoid cells secreting a specific antibody. This assay is used for the detection of antibodies produced by single cells and for enumerating the antibody-synthesizing cells.

Antibody producing cells are obtained from the spleen of a mouse injected with a test antigen. The cells are finally minced and strained through steel wire mesh into a balanced salt solution containing 30% fetal calf serum. After 10 minutes allowed for sedimentation of clumps of cells, the suspension is removed, and the cells are mixed with a capillary pipette. The cells are centrifuged at $500 \times g$ for 7 minutes and washed in 4 ml of the medium. After the second wash, the cells are resuspended in 1 ml of medium to which 0.2 ml of a suspension of a bacteria in a liquid culture medium, containing approximately 85×10^6/ml, is added. This mixture is left at room temperature for 20 minutes to allow the adherence of bacteria to the cells secreting specific antibody. Then 0.1-ml aliquots of the incubated mixture, and controls containing 0.1 ml of normal cells and 0.1 ml of the bacteria are transferred to 3 ml of a liquid nutrient agar medium, melted at $42°$. Each of these mixtures is immediately poured into Petri plates. The cultures are incubated at $37°$ for 2 to 3 hours after which the plates are investigated under a dissecting microscope at a magnification of $20\times$ using semitransmitted light through frosted glass. Colonies derived from single bacterium are thus identified. When the colonies are observed on a control plate, all the plates are removed from the incubator and flooded with 0.25% chlorhexidine gluconate containing 0.5% methanol blue to stop further growth and to stain the colonies. The colonies are then examined under low power magnification in semitransmitted light. Colonies derived from bacterial clumps formed on antibody-forming cells (adherence colonies) stand out clearly from single refractile cells and the much smaller colonies which have derived from single nonadherent bacteria.

The formation of adherence colonies is abolished by pretreatment of the immune cells with an antimouse gamma globulin for 59 minutes prior to, and after the addition of bacteria to the suspension of immune cells (Diener, 1968).

The bacterial immunocytoadherence inhibition test may be employed for the study of all major phenomena of immunity at the cellular level.

4. The Immune Erythrocyte-Clustering Test

According to Zaalberg's (1964) method, the potentially antibody forming cells are derived from spleens obtained from mice immunized with sheep red cells by intraperitoneal injections of 10^9 cells twice a week for three consecutive weeks. Six days after the last injection, the spleen is removed and a homogenous suspension of cells is prepared. The washed spleen cells are suspended in a test tube, at 10^7 cells/ml of a tissue culture medium containing 1% washed sheep erythrocytes. The test tubes are incubated at 37° in a roller tube apparatus for 2 hours. The cells are then pipetted into a hemacytometer and counted under a microscope. It is observed that nucleated, antibody-producing spleen cells are surrounded by agglutinated sheep erythrocytes and the number of agglutinated erythrocytes clustered around a cell appears to reflect the amount of antibody produced by that cell.

This method is suitable for the determination of the number of antibody-forming cells in a lymphoid tissue after different routes of immunization, as well as for the determination of antibodies produced after immunization with two different antigens, such as sheep and fowl erythrocytes. The use of the erythrocytes possessing different morphology makes it possible to decide whether the cell cluster around a single lymphoid cell consists of a mixture of the two red cell types or a single type. The two different types of cells can be coated with various antigens.

Potassium cyanide at 0.01 molar concentration added to the culture medium containing immunized lymphoid cells stops cellular antibody formation.

Chapter Seventeen

ASSAYS FOR INCOMPLETE
ANTIBODIES AND ANTIGENS

Incomplete, univalent antibodies are able to adsorb onto the corresponding antigens but incapable of producing visible reactions in ordinary serological tests. Incomplete antibodies are classified within the following four varieties, beginning with the least and ending with the most incomplete: blocking antibodies, agglutinoids (albumin agglutinins), cryptagglutinoids, and aggloids. Blocking antibodies prevent the complete or saline agglutinating antibodies from clumping corresponding complete antigens. They may be detected by the agglutination in protein (plasma, serum, albumin), media, in the blocking test, the antiglobulin test, and the hemagglutination test with proteinase treated erythrocytes. Agglutinoids are detectable by all these assays, except the blocking test; cryptagglutinoids may be detected only by indirect antiglobulin test, and aggloids by collidone or trypsin tests.

Other reactions between incomplete antibodies and antigens can be revealed by detecting alterations of some physical properties, such as the viscosity or optical rotation. Particulate antigens, and especially erythrocytes, can be rendered agglutinable by incomplete antibodies, if pretreated with, or suspended in, solutions of trypsin, papain, ficin, or exoenzymes of *Vibrio comma.*

I. THE BLOCKING TEST

The blocking test of incomplete antibodies depends on the saturation of antigen by incomplete antibodies, which makes the antigen unable to react with a complete antibody. Incomplete blocking antibodies occur in the serum, usually a free state. However, in some cases they may be firmly adsorbed onto red blood cells *in vivo;* this condition is found more commonly in the blood of infants than in adults. The adsorbed antibodies can be eluted from erythrocytes and detected by a test with trypsinized (Rh-positive) red cells.

Wiener's (1944) test is usually employed for the detection of free incomplete blocking antibodies in the serum; and the procedure devised by

Sussman and Pretshold (1954) is suitable for the elution and testing of blocking antibodies absorbed *in vivo*.

Wiener's Blocking Test.   The serum being tested is incubated for 30 minutes at 38° with an equal volume of a 2% suspension of appropriate (O Rh-positive) red blood cells. The erythrocytes are then centrifuged, washed with saline, suspended in a diluted standard antiserum which possesses a complete homologous antibody for the red blood cells, and incubated at 38° for 30 to 60 minutes. If no agglutination occurs or if the agglutination is observed at a greatly reduced level, as compared to the test with erythrocytes not pretreated with the test serum, this indicates that reactive groups of the antigen have been blocked by incomplete antibodies present in the examined serum.

The test may be carried out either in tubes, with measured amounts of reagents, or on glass slides, by a drop technique.

Sussman and Pretshold's (1954) Blocking Test.   Incomplete antibodies which have adsorbed onto erythrocytes *in vivo* are eluted in the following manner. The blood sample is first centrifuged and the erythrocytes are washed off from the serum with six to eight portions of a saline solution, at room temperature. The washed cells, packed to form a nearly dry button, are suspended in two drops of a fresh saline solution, incubated at 56° for 15 minutes, and centrifuged.

The test is set up by using one drop of eluate and one drop of a 2% suspension of freshly trypsin-digested (Rh-positive) erythrocytes. Appropriate controls of elution, containing known Rh-positive or Rh-negative cells and an anti-Rh_0 serum, are inserted. After a 30-minute incubation at 38°, the tubes are examined for the presence of clumped red blood cells. The agglutination indicates that erythrocyte eluates contain hemagglutinins.

II. ENZYME TESTS FOR INCOMPLETE ANTIBODIES

Pickles (1946) was the first to show that the anti-D serum containing an incomplete antibody was able to agglutinate D-positive red cells, if they were pretreated with a culture filtrate of *Vibrio comma*. It was later found that trypsin, papain, a *Streptomyces* lysin (Morton and Pickles, 1947, 1951; Kuhns and Bailey, 1950; Wheeler et al., 1950), and ficin (Wiener and Katz, 1951) alter red blood cells, rendering them agglutinable by incomplete antibodies.

1. The Trypsinized Cell Agglutination Test

According to the Morton and Pickles' (1951) technique, red blood cells are trypsinized by suspending them in four volumes of a solution containing 0.1 g of a crystalline or 2 g of a commercial trypsin preparation in 10 ml of 0.05 *N* HCl, diluted with nine parts of 0.1 *M* phosphate buffer, pH 7.7.

This mixture is incubated at 37° for 30 to 60 minutes. Red blood cells are then sedimented by centrifugation, washed with saline, and resuspended to a 5% concentration.

The test is carried out by mixing 0.1-ml volumes of an examined serum, perwarmed in the water bath at 37°, with 0.1 ml of warmed suspension of appropriate trypsinized red blood cells. (Reactans are warmed prior to the test to prevent a nonspecific agglutination.) After 30- to 60-minutes incubation at 37°, the contents of tubes are examined for the presence of agglutinated cells which produce a characteristic pattern with ragged edge on the bottom of the tubes. The test may be standardized by a parallel titration of a standard antiserum containing the incomplete antibody.

A slightly modified technique of this test was described by Race and Sanger (1958) and Unger (1951).

In Unger's (1951) modification of the original test, the trypsinized cell method is combined with, or followed by an antiglobulin test, performed on the cells used with each serum dilution which failed to produce clumping in the first test. The trypsinized cell indirect antihuman globulin method permits the detection of antibodies occurring in very low concentrations, below the threshold of other methods designed for incomplete antibodies and is especially useful for detecting Rh_0 antibodies occurring in extremely low titers.

2. The Papainized Erythrocyte Agglutination Test

Two techniques, by Berthier tand Woo (1942) and by Low (1955), are briefly presented.

The papainization of erythrocytes, after Berthier and Woo (1942), is conducted by means of a 0.1% papain solution made in 0.9% NaCl dissolved in a 0.15-*M*, pH 7.4, Sørensen buffer. A 2-ml volume of this papain solution is added to 1 ml of saline washed human red blood cells of an appropriate group, packed to a constant volume. This mixture is incubated at 37° for 45 minutes, with periodical agitation. The cells are then washed three times in a saline solution to remove the enzyme, and suspended in the saline to a 3% concentration. This reagent is stable for at least 5 days.

The test is conducted by adding 0.1 ml of the 3% papainized erythrocytes to 0.1 ml of an undiluted or progressively diluted serum to be tested. The tubes are shaken and incubated for 10 minutes at 37°, then centrifuged at 150 × g for 2 minutes, and examined for the presence of agglutinates with the aid of a 7× stereoscopic microscope. The titer of hemagglutination is estimated according to the highest serum dilution showing a 1+ agglutination.

In the Low technique (1955), a 3% erythrocyte suspension is added in equal volume to a serum-papain solution which consists of a fresh mixture of three parts of 1% papain solution and one part of the test serum. The mixture is incubated at 37° for 2 hours, then examined microscopically for the presence of agglutinated cells.

The papain solution is made by grinding 2 g of papain (Papayotin Merck 1:350) with 100 ml of $M/15$ phosphate buffer, pH 5.4. After filtration, 10 ml of 0.5 M cysteine solution, used as an activator, is added. This solution is made up to a 200-ml volume and incubated at 37° for 1 hour.

3. The Ficin-Hemagglutination Test

In the Haber and Rosenfield (1957) technique, as adjusted by Race and Sanger (1958), nine parts of 2% erythrocyte suspension are added to one part of 1% ficin solution prepared in Hendry's buffer, pH 7.3 to 7.5. After a 15-minute incubation at 37°, the mixture is centrifuged; red blood cells are resuspended in the saline to 2% concentration, and left at 4° for a few hours or longer before being read.

Hendry's buffer consists of one part of a NaH_2PO_4 solution (0.514 g/ 100 ml of water) and four parts of Na_2HPO_4 solution (0.445 g/100 ml of water).

4. The Absorption-Elution Test

A particulate antigen, which failed to show a visible reaction with an antiserum in the ordinary serological test, may prove to possess adequate determinants for these antibodies, when the serum is absorbed by this antigen and eluates are tested versus another, standard antigen preparation.

Techniques of the absorption-elution test were described by Landsteiner and Miller (1925), Kidd (1949), Vos and Keisall (1956), and Weiner (1957), the last being recommended.

Weiner's Absorption-Elution Test. Cells sensitized with an antibody are washed four to six times with a cold saline, centrifuged, and frozen and thawed several times. Five volumes of a 1:1 mixture of ethyl alcohol and distilled water precooled at $-20°$ are added to the packed cells. This suspension is left at $-20°$ for 30 to 60 minutes, then centrifuged at 3000 rpm for 5 minutes. The sediment is washed twice with distilled water. The deposit is then suspended in one to three volumes of a normal serum or in a 20% bovine albumin, incubated at 37° for half an hour or longer, then sedimented. The supernatant containing the eluted antibody is tested against a particular antigen in the agglutination test.

The Landsteiner and Miller Technique. In this assay, packed test cells are mixed with a homologous antiserum, incubated at room temperature for 30 minutes, then centrifuged. The absorbing cells are washed three times in saline to free them from the surrounding serum, and resuspended in half the original volume of the cell suspension. This mixture is agitated continuously in a water bath at 56° for 5 minutes. The tube containing the eluted cell suspension is now transferred quickly to centrifuge cups containing an adequate amount of water heated to 56°. After the centrifugation, the supernatant, which contains the eluted antibody, is removed as quickly as possible and employed in a suitable test to reveal the presence of this antibody.

III. THE AUGMENTATION ASSAYS

The augmentation tests, devised for the detection of incomplete antibodies or reagins, consist of two consecutive immune reactions superimposed on each other. An incomplete or "weak" antibody, which is unable to exhibit visible products of the reaction, is first allowed to combine with the homologous particulate antigen. This complex of an incomplete antibody firmly absorbed to a particulate antigen ("the sensitized antigen") is then coated with a complete antiglobulin antibody or suspended in another protein, for example, albumin, or in a nonprotein colloid menstruum, such as gum acacia or polyvinyl alcohol, which results in a visible aggregation.

The first augmentation test, the anti-γ-globulin test, was described by Moreschi (1908), but it was independently devised by Coombs et al. (1945) for the study on incomplete Rh-agglutinins, and subsequently adjusted for testing either weak erythrocyte antibodies or incomplete bacterial antibodies (Sturgeon, 1952, 1954).

The group of augmentation tests should include also some other aggregation reaction, for example, the Waaler-Rose hemagglutination test, the albumin agglutination test, the precipitative aggregation test, and tests with trypsinized cells.

1. The Antiglobulin Test

There are two types of the antiglobulin test, the direct and the indirect. In the direct test, red blood cells coated by an incomplete homologous antibody clump on the addition of the antiglobulin serum, since most antibodies are globulins. This reaction is chiefly used in studies of erythrocyte antigens and isohemagglutinins.

In the indirect antiglobulin test, the "unknown" serum tested for the presence of an incomplete antibody is first incubated with a preparation of a particulate antigen, for example, bacterial cells, to allow the incomplete antibody to adsorb onto cells. The sensitized cells are then washed and added to a solution of the anti-γ-globulin serum which reveals the presence of the adsorbed incomplete antibody.

The antihuman globulin reagent is prepared by immunization of rabbit with human serum or, preferably, with a purified human γ-globulin prepared by Proom's (1943) method. In this method, a 25-ml volume of the group-O serum is first diluted with 80 ml of distilled water, mixed with 90 ml of 10% aqueous solution of potassium alum, and adjusted to pH 6.5 with 5 N sodium hydroxide. The mixture is centrifuged, and the precipitate is washed twice with a 1:10,000 saline solution of Merthiolate. The precipitate is now made up to a volume of 100 ml by adding saline solution in 1:10,000 Merthiolate.

The most potent antiserum can be produced by the aid of adjuvants (Emmerson et al., 1951). A serum-adjuvant mixture consists of 3 ml of a fresh, normal human blood serum, group O Rh_0-negative, 4.5 ml of sterile Falba, and 7.5 ml of dried, heat-killed cells of *Mycobacterium butyricum* suspended in 7.5 ml of sterile mineral oil. Doses of 1 ml of this mixture are injected subcutaneously at weekly intervals, for 9 weeks. The antiserum thus obtained is absorbed for 1 hour at 37° with pooled, washed human blood cells, which include A, B, O, M, N, and the Rh factors C, D, E, c, d, e, to remove antibodies against normal human erythrocytes, according to the method of McDuffie and Kabat (1956) or Dunsford and Grant (1959). In the latter technique, the antihuman globulin serum is, first, mixed with an equal volume of group-O washed packed cells and left overnight at 4°. The mixture is then centrifuged and the supernatant mixed with packed, washed A, B (or A_1 + B) erythrocytes, left overnight at 4° and recentrifuged.

The supernatant fluid containing the absorbed antiglobulin serum is tested for reactions against A, B, and O cells by an isohemagglutination technique. No reaction should be observed.

i. *The Direct Antiglobulin Test.* In the technique by Dunsford and Grant (1959), the red blood cells with incomplete antibody molecules adherent to their surfaces are centrifuged and washed thoroughly in a saline solution. The tets is set up on a glass slide divided in four squares. Squares 1 and 2 receive one drop of test cells and a drop of either the antiglobulin serum or saline, respectively. Squares 3 and 4 receive one drop of the antiglobulin serum and a drop of either nonsensitized red blood cells or cells sensitized with a known anti-D serum, respectively. The contents of each square is mixed thoroughly and rocked gently for 3 to 4 minutes, then left for another 5 to 6 minutes before being read. The test is read microscopically.

ii. *The Indirect Antiglobulin Test.* Techniques of the indirect antiglobulin test were devised by Gleeson-White et al. (1950), Coombs et al. (1951), Dunsford and Grant (1959), and McDuffie and Kabat (1956). Although the first two assays were originally used for detection of incomplete heterophile hemagglutinins and the other two for incomplete anti-D antibodies, each procedure can be adapted for studies on the erythrocyte and bacterial incomplete antibodies. An antiglobulin test with sensitized tanned erythrocytes was published by Mathewes (1959).

Here are compiled details of Gleeson-White's et al. and Coombs' et al. techniques: 0.1- or 0.4-ml volumes of twofold, progressing serum dilutions are added to equal volumes of 1.2% suspension of sheep or bovine red blood cells. The tubes are incubated at 37° for 30 to 60 minutes, then centrifuged lightly. The cells are washed twice in saline and resuspended in 0.1- or 0.4-ml saline. One drop of suspensions from each tube is then mixed with a single drop of 1:20 dilution of a rabbit antihuman globulin serum. Single drops of a diluted normal serum are added to another drop from each cell suspension for control purposes. After the incubation at 37° for $1\frac{1}{2}$ hours and a light centrifugation for 30 seconds, one drop of deposited cells is placed on a glass slide and observed under the microscope. If no agglutination is noticed at this stage, another volume of a rabbit antihuman globulin serum is added to the remaining cells in tubes, and the whole procedure is repeated. If no agglutination is observed at the second stage, the deposited cells are washed twice and resuspended in saline. The procedure is now repeated, using 0.14% solution of human-γ-globulin instead of the antiglobulin serum. In this way, inagglutinable bovine red blood cells may be rendered agglutinable by weak antibodies.

The Dunsford and Grant Method of the Indirect Antiglobulin Test. Four drops of a serum suspected to contain incomplete anti-D antibody are mixed in a test tube with two drops of a 50% suspension of standard group O, D-positive red blood cells. Control tubes receive: (a) standard group O, D-positive cells suspended in a serum known to contain incomplete anti-D antibodies; and (b) the same cells and a serum known to contain no D-antibodies. The tubes are incubated for $1\frac{1}{2}$ hours at 37°; small drops of each mixture are examined microscopically for any agglutination which would show the presence of complete antibody. If no agglutination is observed, the content of each tube is centrifuged, the sediment is washed, and further processed as in the direct antiglobulin test.

The McDuffie and Kabat (1956) Technique of the Indirect Antiglobulin test. The test is set up in six rows consisting of five to ten dilutions for testing each anti-A or anti-B serum (Table 93).

Each tube of the first row receives 0.1 ml of saline, whereas the second row receives 0.1 ml of an appropriate dilution of the serum examined. Next higher twofold serial dilution of the antiserum in 0.1-ml volume is added to each succeeding row. Each tube then receives 0.1 ml of a 4% suspension of washed group A cells, and the total volume is made up to 0.5 ml with 0.9% saline. The tubes are shaken and incubated at 37° for 1 hour, and then centrifuged at 150 × g for $1\frac{1}{2}$ minutes. The agglutina-

Table 93.   The Schedule of the Antiglobulin Test (McDuffie and Kabat, 1956)

Dilution of the Test Serum	Dilution of Anti-γ-Globulin Serum					
	1:50	1:100	1:200	1:400	1:800	1:1600
1:200						
1:400						
1:800						
1:1600						
1:3200						

tion is read with the aid of a lens, and results are expressed in terms of the original 0.1 ml of the antiserum added.

The contents of tubes are then recentrifuged; the supernatant is discarded, and cells are washed three times with saline. An anti-γ-globulin serum is added in 0.5-ml volume to each sediment present in the first tube of all six or ten rows (vertically). The same volume of a series of twofold dilutions of the anti-γ-globulin is added to each consecutive vertical row. The contents of tubes are mixed and left for 10 minutes at room temperature, then centrifuged at 150 × g for 1 $\frac{1}{2}$ minutes, and examined for the presence of agglutinates. The highest dilution of serum showing clumped cells is considered as the anti-γ-globulin titer.

The antiglobulin test was applied for the detection of incomplete antibodies and for the study on antigen-antibody reactions of various cellular elements. It is widely used for immunological diagnosis of hemolytic disease and in the identification of species specificity of blood stains for forensic medicine.

2. The Antiglobulin Compatibility Test

In this test, the indirect procedure by Dunsford and Grant (1959) is used. Washed donor's blood cells are mixed with a double volume of recipient's serum and incubated for 1 $\frac{1}{4}$ hours at 37°, then examined for the presence of agglutinates. If no agglutination occurs, the mixture is centrifuged, and sedimented cells are thoroughly washed in saline.

Washed cells are mixed with a "wide spectrum" antiglobulin serum on a glass slide, rocked for 3 to 4 minutes, and left for another 5- to 6-minute period before being examined microscopically for the presence of agglutinates. If the agglutination occurs, the donor's blood is unsuitable for transfusion.

3. The Antiglobulin Augmentation Test

The test, according to Sturgeon's (1954) technique, is carried out as follows. The serum to be investigated for the presence of an incomplete antibody is diluted serially in 0.5-ml volume of saline solution; 0.1-ml amounts of each serum dilution are transferred to a second parallel row of tubes. The tubes of the first row, containing 0.4 ml of serial serum dilutions, receive 0.1 ml of 2 to 4% suspension of test cells, whereas the second row obtains 0.4 ml of this suspension. Test mixtures of the latter row are incubated for 1 hour at 37°, then centrifuged lightly, and examined for the presence of agglutinates. The highest serum dilution giving an observable agglutination is recorded.

The first row of tubes is incubated at 37° for 30 minutes; the contents of tubes are centrifuged, and sediments are washed three times with 0.9% saline to remove nonabsorbed serum proteins. Washed sediments are resuspended in 0.5 ml of fresh saline, and one drop of each suspension is placed on two parallel glass slides. One drop of saline is added to each drop of the suspension on the first slide, whereas one drop of a rabbit antihuman globulin serum is given to the second row of drops. This part of the test may also be set up in small tubes with 0.1- to 0.2-ml volumes of reagents. It is advisable to absorb the antiglobulin serum with the antigen used in the augmentation test. The slides or tubes are gently rotated and left for 5 minutes, then observed against a background light by rotating the mixtures. If cells in the first, saline row clumped spontaneously, it indicates that they combined with a complete homologous antibody. The clumping of cells in the second, antiglobulin row is caused by the antiglobulin antibody reacting with the antibody globulin combined with the homologous antigen. The highest titer of the antiglobulin serum is regarded as a positive test. The augmentation titer may be expressed by subtracting the saline agglutination titer from that of the antiglobulin agglutination.

4. The Antiglobulin Consumption Test

The test devised by Steffen (1954) for detection of autoantibodies depends on the following principle. A tissue preparation is first incubated with a tested human serum, then washed and transferred into an antiglobulin serum which should react with the antibody attached to the tissue. If the antiglobulin serum has not reacted, it is withdrawn by centrifugation and examined in the Coombs test with sensitized red blood cells. However, if an autoantibody was present in the human serum and adsorbed onto the tissue, the antiglobulin serum is "consumed" by this autoantibody, and the resulting titer of agglutination is lower than in the control.

The tissue antigen is prepared by grinding a piece of tissue with an equal volume of buffered saline, pH 7.2, in a mechanical homogenized (omnimixer) for 30 seconds. The tissue should then be centrifuged, washed, and rehomogenized. Homogenization and washing are repeated until the supernatant is free of detectable serum protein. The tissue sediment may then be lyophilized.

The antiglobulin consumption test, according to Kite et al. (1962), is conducted in the following manner. First, 10 mg of a lyophilized tissue are incubated with 0.5 ml of a heat inactivated, undiluted or serially diluted patient's serum at 37° for 10 minutes, then washed down with 1 ml of saline and centrifuged at 500 × g for 5 minutes. The tissue sediment must be washed eight times with 5-ml volume of saline. The washed tissue sediment is then mixed with 0.5 ml of a diluted Coombs' serum diluted to contain six times minimal hemagglutination titer. This suspension is agitated for 45 seconds, and then centrifuged at 500 × g for 30 seconds; the supernatant should be collected.

The supernatant is serially diluted in 0.1-ml amounts, and 0.1 ml of 30% suspension of group O Rh-(D) positive erythrocytes, sensitized with an equal volume of a suitable dilution of the Rh-antibody (chest fluid), is added to each tube. The mixtures are shaken and centrifuged at 500 × g for 10 seconds, and examined for the presence of agglutinated cells.

Control tubes should contain a normal human serum instead of patient's serum.

5. *The Tanned Erythrocyte-Antiglobulin Test*

According to Mathewes' (1959) technique, human red blood cells of group O Rh-negative are first washed with saline and suspended to 2% concentration in a saline buffered at pH 7.2. This suspension is added to an equal volume of a 1:20,000 solution of tannic acid, incubated for 10 minutes at 37°, and then centrifuged and washed with the buffered saline.

These blood cells are subsequently sensitized with an antigen by suspending them at 2% concentration in a solution of the antigen, and incubating for 15 minutes at 37°. The sensitized erythrocytes should be washed with 0.1% solution of bovine albumin.

The sensitized and nonsensitized cells, washed with 0.1% bovine albumin, are then suspended in two volumes of a heat-inactivated normal rabbit serum diluted in the ratio of 1:2 or 1:4 with a saline buffered at pH 6.4. These suspensions are in cubated for 15 minutes at 37°, and then washed in saline and resuspended in 0.1% bovine albumin at 2% concentration.

The test is set up as follows. First 1-ml amounts of sensitized and control cell suspensions are added to 1-ml volumes of examined human antisera, which were inactivated with heat or zymosan and serially diluted. These test mixtures are then incubated for 30 to 60 minutes at 37°, and centrifuged. The sedimented cells should be washed three times with 0.1% bovine albumin, and resuspended in a 0.05-ml volume of this diluent.

To determine whether the antibody has been bound by the antigen-carrying erythrocytes, the following slide test is set up. One drop of each suspension is added to a drop of a rabbit antihuman globulin serum on a glass slide; another drop is mixed with a heat inactivated normal rabbit serum diluted 1:40 in 0.1% bovine serum. The slide is tilted for 2 minutes and inspected for hemagglutination. The presence of clumped cells in the test with the antiglobulin serum denotes a positive result, which is characteristic of incomplete hemagglutinins in the sera which failed to react in a direct hemagglutination test with sensitized, tanned red blood cells.

6. The Radio-Labeled Anti-IgG Technique

The quantitative I-labeled anti-IgG technique (Hughes-Jones, 1967) is suitable for the estimation of incomplete antibody content. The method depends on the calibration of ^{125}I-labeled anti-IgG which depends on the quantitative determination of molecules of ^{125}I-labeled anti-IgG that will combine with a ^{131}I-labeled anti-D (anti-Rh$_0$) antibody molecule, bound to the erythrocyte surface. The estimation of specific antibody content of an unknown sample is conducted by absorbing the unknown antibody or antiserum on to the Rh-positive red cells and determining the amount thus absorbed using the previously calibrated ^{125}I-labeled anti-IgG. By this method, the value of the equilibrium constant, which is important in assessing potency of an antiserum, can be estimated.

7. The Incomplete Isohemagglutinin Fluorescence Test

The test by Konda et al. (1960) depends on the reaction of a fluorescein-labeled antihuman globulin serum with incomplete isohemagglutinins, adsorbed onto red blood cells *in vivo*. A 2% suspension of examined washed red blood cells is used in the test, and the reaction mixtures are incubated at 37° for 1 hour.

Agglutinates of erythrocytes should be washed with saline and observed under a fluorescent microscope.

8. The Reagin-Augmentation Test

This test, described by Kritzman (1958), probably depends on an aggregation of the γ-globulin coated erythrocytes in the presence of rheumatoid reagins. The assay is conducted in the following way: 0.5 ml of 50% washed human group O cells are suspended in 2.5 ml of 1% γ-globulin solution. One milliliter of a 0.005 *M* chromic chloride solution is added to this suspension to allow the globulin to adsorb onto red blood cells. The suspension is shaken for 4 minutes, then the cells are centrifuged, washed repeatedly with saline, and finally resuspended to a 25% concentration.

Two drops of this suspension are mixed on a slide with two drops of a serum or an euglobulin fraction under test and are inspected for the presence of agglutination over a light source. After the completion of the assay, the slide may be dried in air at room temperature and kept as a permanent record.

9. The Albumin-Agglutination Test

Certain incomplete antibodies, the agglutinoids, adsorbed to homologous particulate antigens (e.g., to red blood cells), are able to produce clumps when suspended in the bovine serum albumin or in other protein solutions, including normal human serum. Albumin appears to be most effective in providing nonspecific linkage of aggregation, leading to clumping. However, albumin can be effectively replaced in some cases by other colloidal substances, for example, gum acacia, galatin, dextran, or polyvinyl pyrrolidone (Fisk and McGee, 1947; Grubb, 1949; Jones, 1950; McNeil et al., 1952).

The albumin-agglutination test devised originally by Diamond and Denton (1945), and adjusted by Wiener (1948), is preceded by an ordinary saline agglutination test. Cells that have not been agglutinated by the antiserum are sedimented by centrifugation, washed with saline, and resuspended in a 7 to 20% albumin solution. The occurrence of agglutinates in the albumin medium is indicative of the presence of incomplete, univalent antibody adsorbed to the particulate antigen. Titer of an incomplete antibody may be determined according to the Diamond and Denton (1945) technique by serially diluting the test serum in 20% albumin and adding an equal volume of 4% suspension of appropriate red blood cell suspension made in albumin. After incubation for 1 to 2 hours at 37°, the tubes are examined for the presence of agglutinates.

The albumin test according to Grove-Rasmussen and Soutter (1953) is set up by mixing in a tube two drops of an antiserum (e.g., anti-Kell serum) with a small amount of red blood cells being tested, to make approximately a 2% suspension. Two drops of 30% bovine albumin are added to this test tube. The suspension is immediately centrifuged at 200 × g for 2 minutes, and any agglutination observed is recorded. The test tube should then be shaken, incubated at 37° for 20 to 30 minutes, and recentrifuged before the final reading is made.

The Albumin-Hemagglutination Test for Incomplete Antibodies This can be carried out by adding 0.5-ml amounts of 0.5% erythrocyte suspension, sensitized with an antigen, to an antiserum or a test serum, diluted progressively in 15% bovine serum albumin. A control series of the serum diluted in saline should be tested against the sensitized erythrocytes. After a 2-hour incubation at 37°, the reaction mixture is left at 2° overnight, then read.

The presence of clumped cells in the albumin series, in the absence of a hemagglutination in the saline series, is indicative of incomplete hemagglutinins.

An albumin-hemagglutination test has been successfully used by Gaines et al. (1960) and Kwapinski (1965) for studies on incomplete anti-Vi and *Mycobacterium* antibodies, respectively.

10. The Precipitate-Adherence Test

Certain materials of a mucopolysaccharide or protein nature, which characteristically occur in rheumatoid arthritis sera, can adsorb onto various antigen-antibody complexes. This adsorption causes a clumping of enlarged complexes or yields a higher amount of precipitates.

The precipitation test, devised by Vaughan (1956) for detection of the adherence reaction, is carried out as follows. At first, specific precipitates are prepared in the region of a maximal antibody precipitation, that is, in the zone of equivalence or a slight antigen excess. This is done by incubating a mixture of a purified precipitinogen, for example, a crystalline egg albumen, and homologous rabbit antiserum at 37° for 1 hour and at 4° for 2 to 7 days. Precipitates are washed twice with chilled saline. A rheumatoid arthritis serum is then added to the precipitate and left overnight at 4°. The precipitate is washed again with chilled saline and analyzed for the nitrogen and protein contents.

Amount of nitrogen absorbed by the specific precipitate is calculated by subtracting the nitrogen content of a specific precipitate from that of the aggregated precipitate.

Chapter Eighteen

IMMUNE CELLULOTROPIC AND HISTIOTROPIC REACTIONS

Cellulotropic and histiotropic (Amano, 1948) tests depend on the interaction between antibodies or allied substances adsorbed onto tissue cells (e.g., leukocytes, HeLa cells); tissues, or organs (skin, lung, kidney, testicle, heart, brain), and the corresponding particulate or soluble antigens or haptens, added *in vitro* or injected into tissues.

The cellulotropic reaction *in vitro* results in the enhanced absorption and digestion of particulate antigens by cells. The best-known cellulotropic reaction is the phagocytosis that depends on the reaction of polymorphonuclear leukocytes and other cells activated by serum opsonin, a thermolabile serum substance inactivated at 55°, similar or identical with the complement; it promotes the action of phagocytes through its adsorption onto bacterial cells (Wright and Douglas, 1903). The promoting activity of various sera differ considerably in respect to the species of bacteria. For example, bovine fetal serum is more effective than horse or chicken serum in influencing the phagocytosis of mycobacteria (Shepard, 1960). The heat inactivation or adsorption of opsonins on zymosan causes a partial reduction of the opsonizing activity of a serum. The phagocytosis-promoting factor seems to be bound to the β-globulin and to a rapidly migrating albumin fraction (Tullis and Surgenor, 1956).

Histiotropic reactions in vivo apparently damage tissues, particularly the vascular endothelium. As a result, a proteolytic enzyme is released within cells or tissues, in which the antigen-antibody reaction occurs. This enzyme liberates a physiologically highly active substance, for example, histamine or acetylocholine. This substance is transported into the circulating blood to sensitize tissues, which are hence stimulated to elicit local or general anaphylactic symptoms. The release of histamine from the anaphylactic organs is inhibited by sodium salicylate (Trethewie, 1959).

I. IMMUNE CELLULOTROPIC REACTIONS

The following types of immune cellulotropic reactions may be differentiated: the opsonophagocytic test which can be conducted with either white blood cells or HeLa cells, the opsonin assay, and the bacteriotropin assay. The last two assays are used to estimate effective amounts of antibodies quantitatively.

Assay for Opsonizing Factors. The procedure originally described by Benacerraf and Miescher (1960) and modified by Evans and Mergenhagen (1965) is as follows. The test bacteria are grown overnight in a culture medium containing uniformly labeled ^{14}C dextrose. After the incubation, the cells are collected by centrifugation and washed in saline until radioactivity present in the supernatant is negligible. The washed cells are resuspended in saline to an optical density of 2.0. The serum or other fluid to be tested for the presence of opsonizing factors is then added to the cells at a final concentration of 125 to 250 $\mu l/0.1$ ml of bacterium suspension. Controls receive the saline suspension of radioactive cells alone. The mixtures are incubated for 30 minutes at 37°, following which 0.1 ml aliquots are withdrawn and injected into the tail vein of female mice. Blood is then drawn from the mice at 1, 2, 4, and 8 minutes after the injection and 0.1 ml of blood obtained from each mouse is counted for 2 minutes in a low background gas-flow counter or a radioactivity counter.

Results are expressed by K values of the average counts in the blood samples from five mice for each time interval, according to the following formula:

$$K = \frac{\log C_1 - \log C_2}{t_2 - t_1}$$

where C_1 and C_2 are the counts at 0 time and at 4 minutes, and t is the time in minutes.

1. Opsonophagocytic Tests

The phagocytic system consists of leukocytes, bacteria, and an opsonin-containing serum. Leukocytes may be obtained most conveniently from peritoneal exudates induced by the injection of either a sterile saline containing 1 mg/ml of glycogen or a starch-aleuronat mixture. The latter consists of 1 g of starch and 1 g of aleuronat, mixed with saline to form a thick paste. The paste is diluted to a volume of 20 ml prior to the peritoneal injection into rabbits or guinea pigs. In 16 to 20 hours after the injection of either mixture, the exudate is withdrawn by the aid of a syringe containing a 3 to 5% sodium citrate solution, and centrifuged. The cells are pipetted from beneath the oil and washed with saline. Leukocytes may also be separated from the citrated human blood by centrifuging at a moderate speed and carefully collecting the top layer of sedimented cells. The sedimentation of erythrocytes is accelerated by dextran. A plastic tube centrifugation technique of separating blood leukocytes was published by Juhlin and Shelley (1961).

Leukocytes can be preserved in the medium proposed by Tullis (1953). This medium consists of two stock solutions and some substances to be added directly before the use. Stock solution 1 contains 0.12 g of $Na_2HPO_4 \cdot 2H_2O$, 0.12 g of KH_2PO_4, 7.5 g of NaCl, 0.75 g of KCl, 0.05 g of K_3PO_4, and 100 ml of distilled water. Stock solution 2 is a 4% $NaHCO_3$. Both solutions should be autoclaved separately mixed in the proportion 100:2 and adjusted to pH 7.4 by bubbling them in carbon dioxide. The following substances are added separately at final concentrations indicated in parentheses: sodium acetate (0.2 g %), dextrose (0.4 mg %), ascorbic acid (0.33 mg %), veridase (10 SK units/ml), phenol red (0.004 g %), and 8.6% sterile gelatin solution (1.0%).

Several methods of measuring the extent of phagocytosis have been described since the early procedures devised by Leishman (1902), and Wright and Douglas (1903). Techniques recommended are presented below.

i. *Hanks' (1940) Technique of the Opsonophagocytic Test.* In this procedure, a mixture of equal 0.2-ml volumes of a serum and a leukocyte suspension is added to 0.2 ml of bacterial suspension, in 10×75-mm tubes, which are then sealed with paraffinized cork stoppers and rotated for 30 to 60 minutes at 37°. The amounts of bacteria and leukocytes must be standardized to obtain reproducible results. Smears from these mixtures are made before and after the incubation, dried with a hot air drier, and stained with the Wright or Giemsa stain, or tolouidin blue or pyronin solution (Lucke et al., 1933). The tolouidin blue and pyronin staining are probably most effective. The latter stain consists of a mixture of three solutions, A, B, and C. Solution A contains 2.5 g of pyronin, 3 g of methyl green, 50 ml of ethyl alcohol, and 100 ml of glycerin in 1000 ml of 2% aqueous phenol. Solution B contains 0.5 g of pyronin, 10 ml of ethyl alcohol, and 40 ml of glycerin in 200 ml of 2% aqueous phenol. Solution C consists of 250 ml of glycerin and 750 ml of 2% aqueous phenol. Two parts of the solution A are mixed with one part of solution B and three parts of solution C. The fixed smears are stained for 3 to 6 minutes, then rinsed with water.

One hundred polymorphonuclear leukocytes should be examined under the high power of the microscope; the number of active leukocytes and the total number of bacteria found in 100 leukocytes are recorded.

Results of the test are expressed in terms of the percentage of leukocytes participating in the phagocytosis ("percentage phagocytosis" or the phagocyte index), according to the following formulas:

$$\text{percentage phagocytosis} = \frac{\text{number of granulocytes containing bacteria}}{\text{total number of granulocytes counted}} \times 100$$

$$\text{phagocyte index} = \frac{\text{total number of bacteria in 100 granulocytes}}{100}$$

The opsonophagocytic index is computed for some investigations according to the following formula:

$$\text{opsonophagocytic index} = \frac{\text{phagocytic index with the test serum}}{\text{phagocytic index with control serum or saline}}$$

Normal percentage phagocytosis is about 40, the normal phagocyte index is 1.0, and the opsonophagocytic index varies between 0.8 and 1.2. Figures above or under these normal averages are regarded as abnormal. However, the experimental error of the phagocytic test is between 20 and 30%. Limits of the error must not exceed the coefficient of variation $v\sqrt{2\%}$, where $v\ \%$ is the coefficient of variation of the mean number of bacteria ingulfed by one leukocyte per slide (Davies, 1951).

Relative number of bacteria and leukocytes, the number of each per unit volume, as well as the age of microorganisms and temperature of incubation should be controlled in the phagocytic test to obtain uniform results. Concentrations of leukocytes ranging from 3000 to 5000 and of bacteria between 200 and 300 million/ml seem to satisfy the optimal conditions of the test (Ecker et al., 1942). The percentage-phagocytosis values vary according to the logarithm of the number of bacteria whereas the bacteria-per-leukocyte values change as a linear function of the number of bacteria. If the number of bacteria increases against a constant number of leukocytes, the percentage-phagocytosis and bacteria-per-leukocyte values increase. With a considerable increase of the concentration of bacteria, the effectiveness of a phagocytic system decreases; also an increase of the leukocyte number against a constant concentration of bacteria lowers both the percentage-phagocytosis and the bacteria-per-leukocyte values. A parallel increase in the absolute numbers of both the bacteria and the leukocytes without any change of the relative ratio of these components is accompanied by higher values for the percentage-phagocytosis and bacteria-per-leukocyte number (Hanks, 1940). Young and especially encapsulated bacteria are resistant to the phagocytosis. Thus fully grown 24-hour cultures are generally employed for this test. The rate of phagocytosis usually increases with rising temperature to 40°, and the temperature around 38° seems to be optimal for the phagocytosis test with most bacteria.

ii. *Castañeda's (1942) Opsonophagocytic Test.* In this test, devised mostly for the diagnosis of brucellosis, 1 ml of formalin-killed bacteria is mixed with 1 ml of a whole, citrated blood of a patient, and incubated at 37° for 30 minutes; the tubes are shaken gently at 10-minute intervals. Thick smears are then made on slides and stained by the Illodi method. Cells of *Brucella* stain blue, the nuclei of leukocytes stain purplish, and the

cytoplasm stain reddish. The number of bacteria in each of 25 polymorphonuclear leukocytes is counted. The intensity of phagocytic reaction is estimated as follows:

+ when the average number of bacteria is less than 10.
++ when the average number of bacteria is less than 20.
+++ when the average number of bacteria is 20 to 30.
++++ when leukocytes are full of bacteria.

A similar test with the heparinized fresh blood (eight units of heparin per
milliliter) and dead staphylococci was described by Argenton et al. (1961).

iii. *The Phagocytic Test Based on Counting Undigested Bacteria.* This
test devised by Fenn (1921) and adjusted by Maaløe (1947) is conducted
by incubating an estimated number, for example, 30,000 bacterial cells
with a standardized saline suspension of washed leukocytes. The leukocytes
which have ingested bacteria are separated from nonphagocyted bacteria by
a moderate centrifugation. The supernatant is quantitatively planted on
suitable culture media to determine the number of nondigested bacteria.
The number of phagocytized bacteria is calculated from these data in comparison with the number of bacteria determined by a culture method in
control samples, which do not contain leukocytes.

iv. *The HeLa Cell Phagocytosis Test.* In this test described by Shepard
(1960), HeLa cells grown on cover slips in Leighton tubes are washed,
and then placed in a suitable infection medium, for example, Eagle's medium containing 20% of the serum being studied. A bacterium inoculum is
introduced into this medium and left at 37° overnight. The fluid is then
changed to the growth medium, which consists of 40% human serum and
60% Hanks' balanced salt solution. To determine the amount of phagocytosis, the cover slips are washed, fixed, and stained. The number of cells
containing the bacteria is counted in standard representative areas.

The opsonophagocytic test was used for various investigations, for example, in studies on the virulence of streptococci and mycobacteria (Mudd
et al., 1938), on toxic metabolites of staphylococci (Pike, 1934), for the
toxicity of antiseptics and antibiotics, as a diagnostic tool for the identification of bacteria (Castañeda et al., 1942), and to study the immune response to vaccines (Kendrick et al., 1937).

v. *The Phagocytosis Inhibition Test.* The test devised by Merchant
and Chamberlain (1952) depends on the inhibition of phagocytosis of
bacteria in the presence of an immune system composed of a nonrelated
antigen and its homologous antibody. This test can be used for studies on
antigenic relationships of various antigens. The phagocytosis inhibition
test is set up by adding 0.1 ml of an antigen solution diluted 1:500 or
1:1000 to 0.3 ml of a homologous antiserum, and 0.1 ml of a leukocyte
suspension.

In the control tubes the soluble antigen is replaced by 0.1 ml of a buffer. All tubes are incubated for 15 minutes at 37°, and then 0.1 ml of a homogenized suspension of an antigenically nonrelated bacteria is added. These mixtures are reincubated for 15 minutes, with occasional shaking.

After the second incubation, a sample is taken from each tube to make smears on glass slides, which are fixed and stained with the Wright and Giemsa stain.

Phagocytic index of the main (PI) and the control tubes (CPI) is then determined, and the opsonophagocytic index (OI) is calcuated in percentages according to the following equation:

$$OI = \frac{PI}{CPI} \times 100$$

To evaluate the inhibition of phagocytosis, the percentage thus calculated must be subtracted from 100% (i.e., from the 100% control opsonophagocytic index).

vi. *The Opsonin Test.* Opsonic activity of the blood plasma can be determined either by a phagocytosis test with the plasma *in vitro,* or by studying the bacterium-clearance effect *in vivo.*

Titration of the opsonin *in vitro,* by the method of Victor et al. (1952), is carried out by conducting a phagocytosis test with a serially diluted test plasma. Red-blood cells obtained from a heparinized human blood are washed six times with tenfold volumes of the Krebs gelatin solution, and mixed with equal (0.1 ml) volumes of plasma dilutions and a suspension of bacteria. Tubes containing these mixtures are slowly rotated for 30 minutes at 37°; smears are then made from the contents of each tube, stained, and examined microscopically to determine the percentage of active neutrophiles which have digested bacteria or rickettsiae. In the latter case, the smears are colored with the Macchiavello stain. Fifty or 100 polymorphonuclear neutrophiles should be viewed.

A unit of the opsonin is expressed by the amount of the plasma which promoted phagocytosis by 94 to 100% of neutrophile leukocytes. An opsonin titer of 1000 is regarded as diagnostic of an active infection whereas titers as low as 1.0 are often found in noninfected individuals.

Determination of the opsonic effect in vivo, by the Biozzi et al. (1961) technique, is conducted by the use of radiolabeled bacteria. Mice, with average weight of 20 g, receive intravenously 5×10^8 of ^{131}I labeled bacteria. This is preceded by an injection of 5 mg of heparin, 10 minutes before the introduction of bacteria. Blood samples are taken before and after the injection, in 3- to 5-minute intervals. In 8 to 10 minutes after the introduction of bacteria, 0.1 ml of the serum tested for contents of opsonins is injected, and further samples of the blood are withdrawn during subsequent 5 to 20 minutes.

Each blood sample is added to 3 ml of 0.1% sodium bicarbonate, and the radioactivity is measured in a well-type scintillating counter. The blood reactivity is plotted against time on a semilogarithmic scale, and the constant rate of the blood clearance before (K) and after (K_1) the injection of serum is estimated graphically. The values of K and K_1 are calculated from the following equation:

$$\frac{\log C - \log C'}{t' - t} = K$$

where C and C' are blood radioactivities at times t and t', respectively. The opsonic effect of injected serum is determined by the difference $K_1 - K$, and the opsonic titer of the serum is expressed by the "opsonizing unit." The opsonizing unit corresponds to the amount of serum which gives $K_1 - K = 0.010$.

The serum opsonic titer is calculated according to the formula:

$$1000 \, (K_1 - K) \times D = \frac{\text{OpU}}{\text{ml}} \times D = \text{the reciprocal of the serum dilution}$$

vii. *Determination of Delayed Hypersensitivity by Inhibition of Cell Migration in Vitro.* The migration *in vitro* in an appropriate medium of cells taken from animals with delayed hypersensitivity is inhibited by specific, corresponding antigen (Rich and Lewis, 1932). This reaction has been employed for studies on delayed hypersensitivity *in vitro* although the specificity and reproducibility of the reaction is not always satisfactory. The method for determination of inhibition of cell migration by antigens, described originally by George and Vaughan (1962) and modified by David et al. (1964) is applied as follows.

The cells for the test are obtained from hypersensitive and normal control guinea pigs by producing peritoneal exudates produced through the intraperitoneal injection of 30 ml of sterilized light mineral oil (Bayol F). The animals are bled completely in 72 hours to reduce erythrocyte contamination of the peritoneal exudates. Cold Hanks' balanced salt solution (100 ml) is then injected intraperitoneally and the contents of the peritoneal cavity is drained into a separatory funnel with a cannulated trocar and plastic tubing. The aqueous phase is separated from the oil and centrifuged at 300 × g for 10 minutes at 4°. The collected cells are washed and resuspended to 10% by packed volume in minimum essential Eagles' medium containing 15% normal guinea pig serum. Small capillary tubes (1.5 mm in diameter, 75 mm long) are then filled with the cell suspension and sealed at one end with warm paraffin wax. The capillaries are centrifuged at 900 rpm for 5 minutes and then cut at the cell-fluid interphase. The portion containing the cells is placed on the bottom cover slip of Mackaness-type chambers of 1-ml capacity. Two capillaries may be put in each chamber, held in place by a small amount of silicone. The top cover slip is sealed in place with paraffin, and the chambers are filled through the side holes. At least two chambers are filled with Eagles' medium containing 15% normal serum and at least two chambers are filled with the same medium to which the appropriate antigen has been added. (The average concentration of antigens is 15 to 30 μg/ml.) The chambers are placed in an incubator at 37° and examined at 24 and 48 hours. The extent of migration of cells from the peritoneal exudate is determined by the following formula:

$$\frac{\text{average area of migration with antigen}}{\text{average area of migration without antigen}} \times 100 = \text{of migration with antigen}$$

The average area is calculated with at least four capillary tubes. The area of migration is measured by projecting the microscopic image of cell growth from each capillary onto drawing paper with a Bausch and Lomb projecting prism. The outline of the migration is drawn and measured by planimetry.

Cells obtained from guinea pigs producing precipitating antibody are not inhibited by antigen.

viii. *The Bacteriotropin Test.* The bacteriotropin is a specific, thermostable substance which occurs in immune sera and promotes the phagocytosis (Neufeld and Rimpau, 1904). The test, by Hughes (1933), is carried out in the following manner. Equal 0.05 volumes of a serially diluted antiserum, the leukocyte suspension, and a bacterial emulsion are mixed and incubated in the water bath at 37° for 15 minutes. Contents of tubes are then withdrawn by the aid of fine capillary pipettes and spread on cover slips, dried, and fixed with methyl alcohol for 10 minutes.

The smears may now be stained by the Gram or Ziehl-Neelsen method, depending on the species of bacteria used in the test. Stained preparations are dried, and cover slips are mounted on glass slides and examined microscopically.

One hundred polymorphonuclear and mononuclear leukocytes must be counted, and the degree of phagocytosis is determined with each serum dilution. The bacteriotropic strength of a serum is evaluated by the highest dilution with which the percentage of leukocytes containing bacteria exceeds that with the normal serum.

II. IMMUNE HISTIOTROPIC REACTIONS

The main anaphylactic antibodies are the IgE antibody immunoglobulins. These antibodies do not fix complement, and are heat labile, cytophilic for granulocytic cells, and able to induce passive cutaneous anaphylaxis. Antibodies responsible for cutaneous anaphylaxis are presumably identical in molecular character with those that produce true anaphylaxis.

Histiotropic tests may be employed in the form of either local or generalized, active or passive reactions. Local histiotropic or allergic reactions display on a limited area of deposition of antigens in tissues, usually in the skin or mucous membranes. They may be conducted as active or passive tests. Active allergic reactions are based on either the Arthus or the Shwartzman phenomenon, whereas the passive test depends on the Prausnitz-Küstner phenomenon. Allergic reactions may be of the "immediate" ("early") or "delayed" type. The early reaction occurs in a few minutes, whereas the delayed reaction is evident only after several hours or more. Specificity of histiotropic reactions is similar to that of serological reactions *in vitro*.

Generalized histiotropic reactions involve one or many tissues and organs and provoke vigorous pathophysiological symptoms which often cause the death of experimental animals. The generalized histiotropic test may be arranged as an active or passive anaphylactic reaction.

1. Local Histiotropic Antigen-Antibody Reactions

i. *The Arthus Allergic Test.* The Arthus phenomenon is elicited by repeated injections of an antigen under an area of the skin in albino rabbits or guinea pigs. After an appropriate number of injections, a local infiltration arises, which later develops into the necrosis and an abscess at the site of inoculation.

A technique of the active allergic skin test, devised by Kwapinski (1965) is applied as follows. Albino rabbits are sensitized by one or two intravenous injections of 1- to 5-mg doses of intact or disintegrated bacteria, or isolated antigenic fractions. After 3 to 6 weeks, 0.1- to 0.2-ml samples of fivefold serial dilutions of individual fractions ranging from 1:1000 to 1:100,000 are introduced into the skin of these animals; 0.1 ml of a buffered saline and 0.1 ml of the culture medium diluted 1:50 to 1:100 should be injected as controls.

A positive allergic reaction is manifested by an erythema and swelling at the site of the skin injection. It has been estimated that for the occurrence of Arthus phenomenon, antibody of a titer in excess of 1:10,000,000 is required.

ii. *The Allergic Shwartzman (1937) Test.* In this test, a sample (e.g., 0.2 to 0.3 mg) of the tested material is injected into rabbits intracutaneously, followed in 24 hours by an intravenous injection of 1.0 mg of the same or another antigen preparation. A positive test is manifested by an inflammatory and necrotic reaction at the site of intracutaneous implantation of the material.

iii. *The Allergic Tissue-Culture Test.* The test, devised by Heilman et al. (1958), depends on the specific inhibition by an antigen of the *in vitro* migration of motile cells (macrophages), derived from an animal with delayed hypersensitivity. The extent of migration of wandering cells in cultures of tissues obtained from animals with delayed hypersensitivity and control animals in the presence and absence of the antigen. Cultures maintained in D5 Carrel flasks consist of 0.5-ml plasma, 1.0 ml of chick embryo extract, and explants of spleen placed in the medium before clotting occurred. The antigen, for example, a suspension of bacteria inactivated at 70° for 45 minutes, in a standard concentration is added to each flask, which should be incubated for 24 to 96 hours at 37°.

The average radius of the migration zone of small or large wandering cells is then determined for each explant with an ocular micrometer at a magnification of 60, and expressed in ocular micrometer units. Statistical analysis is performed by the method published by Treloar (1951).

The results are expressed in terms of a cytotoxic index according to the formula:

$$\text{Cytotoxic index} = \frac{\text{average migration extent in test cultures} + \text{antigen}}{\text{average migration in controls with no antigen}}$$

A value less than 0.90 is usually indicative of the toxicity of the antigen. The relative effect of the antigen on normal tissues and on the tissue of infected animals is expressed in terms of a comparative cytotoxic index. A value less than 0.90 is usually indicative of the toxicity of an antigen.

The relative effect of the antigen on normal tissue and on the tissue of infected animals is expressed in terms of a comparative cytotoxic index.

iv. *The Passive Allergic Test.* The Prausnitz-Küstner test is performed by injecting a small amount of a test serum into the skin of a normal person, and followed in 24 to 48 hours by injection of an allergen at the same site and into an untreated control sera. A cutaneous evanescent reaction is elicited in 10 to 15 minutes by a homologous serologic system, consisting of a reagin and an allergen. The control area must now show any symptom.

In the test by Ramsdell (1928), 0.05 to 2.0 ml of antiserum is introduced intraperitoneally into guinea pigs. After 24 hours, a freshly prepared 0.2% trypan blue solution is injected intravenously in the ratio of 0.15 ml/100 g weight, followed immediately by an intracutaneous injection in the lower portion of ear of 0.1- to 0.2-ml amount of a 1:10,000 antigen solution. Positive reaction is marked by bluish coloration of the injection site, due to the oedem and diffusion of trypan blue from the circulation into the inflammatory area.

Passive cutaneous allergic test by Ovary and Biozzi (1954) or Salvin and Smith (1960) is carried out by injecting 0.1 ml of the test serum intradermally in the flank of guinea pigs or other animals. Three or four hours later, 0.5 ml of an antigen preparation and 0.5 ml of 1% Evans blue saline solution are introduced intravenously. After 30 minutes, areas of pigmentation in the skin around the site of the intradermal injection of serum should be measured and recorded.

The passive cutaneous anaphylaxis test is performed by injecting serial dilutions of antibody intracutaneously, followed after an incubation period of 12 hours by the intravenous injection of antigen mixed with a solution of Evans blue (which is a high molecular-weight dye combining with serum albumin). The passive cutaneous anaphylaxis is characterized by increased permeability of small blood vessels of the skin; thus the dye-albumin complex escaping during such reaction through the damaged vessels makes the outlines of the reaction site clearly visible. The reaction occurs within a few minutes, develops the greatest erythema and edema within 20 minutes, and then fades rapidly. By this test, as little as 0.003 μg of antibody nitrogen may be detected. The reaction is apparently due to the local release of mediators presumably from mast cells and recovery of resensitizability results from restoration of mediators.

The test originally described by Ovary (1958), as slightly modified by Parker et al. (1965), is applied as follows: 0.1 ml of different antisera or sera are injected intradermally into guinea pigs weighing about 250 g on the ventral surface. Six hours later, 0.5 mg of an antigen or a hapten-albumin conjugate in a volume of 1.0 ml of 0.5% Evan's blue in saline is injected intravenously. Sites at the antiserum or serum injections are observed by bluing 20 to 30 minutes after injection. Each serum should be injected in duplicate or triplicate animals. Reactions are best read from the inside of the skin (Ishizaka and Campbell, 1959; Almeida and Kwapinski, unpublished).

A passive modification of the Arthus test performed in the rabbit eye was devised by Waksman and Bullington (1956).

2. Generalized Immune Histiotropic Reactions

Two types of generalized histiotropic reactions may be differentiated, the anaphylactic (active and passive) test and the modified Schultz-Dale test.

i. *The Active Anaphylactic Test.* The test by Carpenter (1955) is performed by sensitizing guinea pigs with the antigen introduced intraperitoneally and injecting, after 3 weeks, an amount ten times higher of the same antigen by intravenous or cardiac route.

ii. *The Passive Anaphylactic Test.* The test by the Lancefield (1928) technique, as slightly modified, is carried out as follows. Guinea pigs are passively sensitized by intraperitoneal injection of a 0.5 to 1.0 ml of the antiserum. In 12 to 24 hours, 0.5 to 1.0 ml of an antigen or isolated fraction diluted 1:500 to 1:1000 is introduced intravenously. If the serum and antigen are homologous to each other, an anaphylactic convulsive shock is elicited. The minimum anaphylactic dose of the antigen which regularly causes the death of passively immunized guinea pigs should be determined.

iii. *The Modified Schultz-Dale Test.* In the technique by Sulzberger (1932), as adopted by Jadassohn et al. (1937), virgin guinea pigs are first injected with bacteria or with an isolated fraction of microorganisms. Strips of the extirpated uterus (or a terminal 4-cm-long part of small intestine) are then suspended in the Tyrode fluid containing 0.05 g of Ca Cl_2 in the Ringer-Locke* balanced solution, contained in a tissue bath. The antigen preparation is added to the physiological solution. Control tubes contain strips of a nonpretreated uterus horn or small intestine. Anaphylactic reaction, which is observed as a contraction of the uterus or intestine muscles, results from the interaction of an antigen and homologous antibody adsorbed onto the uterus or the intestine tissues. The contractions are graphically recorded on a kymograph or measured by an isometric muscle tension apparatus. Another technique of the Schultz-Dale test was devised by Mehlman and Seegal (1934).

By means of allergic and anaphylactic cross tests, useful information may be obtained about antigenic relationships existing between different biomolecules and superstructures.

Very useful cytotropic techniques, especially applicable for studies on the cell-mediated immunity and delayed hypersensitivity, have been designed by Fauve and Dekaris (1968) and Lolekha et al. (1970). The Fauve and Dekaris test depends on the observation that the macrophages taken from animals with delayed hypersensitivity have a markedly decreased ability to spread in the presence of specific antigen, in contrast to the peritoneal macrophages obtained from normal guinea pigs or mice. The macrophages are observed in a counting chamber after incubation with an antigen for 30 minutes. The spreading is noticed when the cytoplasm is clearly visible under microscopic observation and shows an irregular border, whereas the whole macrophage becomes darker. The percentage of spread macrophages in terms of the total 100 macrophages counted is thus estimated.

The test of Lolekha's et al. depends on the aggregation of peritoneal exudate cells from sensitive animals in the presence of specific antigen. The

---

* The Ringer-Locke solution contains 0.9% NaCl, 0.023% $CaCl^2$, 0.02% KCl, and 0.01 to 0.03% $NaHCO^3$.

antigen solution is added to the tube containing a suspension of the macrophages. The supernatant fluid from sensitive lymphoid cells cultured with the antigen also has an ability to aggregate nonsensitive peritoneal exudate cells. The release of the macrophage aggregation factor is correlated with cutaneous delayed hypersensitivity. (Ref. *Science* **160**:795, 1968; *J. Immunol.* **104**:296, 1970).

BIBLIOGRAPHY

AALUND, O., J. W. OSEBOLD, and F. A. MURPHY. Isolation and characterization of ovine gamma globulins. *Arch. Biochem. Biophys.* **109**:142, 1965.

ABEL, K., H. DESCHMERTZING, and J. I. PETERSON. Classification of microorganisms by analysis of chemical composition. I. Feasibility of utilizing gas chromatography. *J. Bacteriol.* **85**:1039 1963.

ABELEV, B. L., *Biull. Eksptl. Biol. Med.* **49**:310, 1960.

ABELEV, G. T., and V. S. ZVETKOV. The immunofiltration method for the elution of a tranplantable mouse hepatoma. *Vop. Onkol.* **6**:67, 1967.

ABELL, C. W., L. A. ROSINI, and M. R. RAMSEUR. Resolution of ribosomal complexes and RNA isolated from bacterial and mammalian sources. *Anal. Biochem.* **18**:305, 1967.

ABELL, L. L., B. B. LEVY, B. B. BRODIE, and F. E. KENDALL. A simplified method for the estimation of total cholesterol in serum and demonstration of its specificity. *J. Biol. Chem.* **195**:357, 1952.

ABERNATHY, R. S., and D. C. HEINER. Precipitation reactions in agar in North American blastomycosis. *J. Lab. Clin. Med.* **57**:604, 1961.

ABRAMOFF, R. S., and H. WOLFE. Precipitin production in chickens. XIII. A quantitative study of the effect of simultaneous injection of two antigens. *J. Immunol.* **77**:94, 1956.

ACHER, R., and C. CROCKER. Réactions colorées spécifiques de l'arginine et de la tyrosine réalisées aprés chromatographie sur papier. *Biochim. Biophys. Acta*, **9**:704, 1952.

ADA, G. L., and B. T. PERRY. Influenza virus nucleic acid: relationship between biological characteristics of the virus particle and properties of the nucleic acid. *J. Gen. Microbiol.* **14**:623, 1956.

ADA, G. L., G. J. V. NOSSAL, J. PYE, and A. ABBOT. Antigens in immunity. I. Preparation and properties of flagellar antigens from *Salmonella adelaide. Aust. J. Exp. Biol. Med. Sci.*, **42**:267, 1964.

ADA, G. L., and J. M. WILLIAMS. Antigen in tissues. I. State of bacterial flagella in lymph nodes of rats injected with isotopically-labelled flagella. *Immunology*, **10**:417, 1966.

ADAMS, E. T., Jr., and D. L. FILMER. Sedimentation equilibrium in reacting systems. IV. Verification of the theory. *Biochemistry*, **5**:2971, 1966.

ADAMS, G. A., T. G. TORNABENE, and M. YAGUCHI. Cell wall lipopolysaccharides from *Neisseria catarrhalis. Can. J. Microbiol.* **15**:365, 1969.

ADAMS, J. M., and D. T. IMAGAWA. Immunological relationship between measles and distemper viruses. *Proc. Soc. Exper. Biol. Med.* **96**:240, 1957.

ADESNIK, M., and C. LEVINTHAL. Synthesis and maturation of ribosomal RNA in *Escherichia coli. J. Mol. Biol.* **46**:281, 1969.

ADLER, F. L. Studies on the bactericidal reaction. *J. Immunol.* **70**:79, 1953.

AIKAWA, J. K., and G. MILKEJOHN. The serologic diagnosis of mumps. A comparative study of three methods. *J. Immunol.* **62**:261, 1949.

AISENBERG, A. C. Studies on the mechanism of the lupus erythematosus (L.E.) phenomenon. *J. Clin. Invest.* **38**:325, 1959.

AKASHI, S., and K. SAITO. A branched saturated C^{15} acid (sarcinic acid) from *Sarcina* phospholipoids and a similar acid from several microbial lipids. *J. Biochem.* **47**:222, 1960.

AKIYA, S. Bacterial components of *Bacillus pyocyaneus.* VI. Studies on polysaccharides. *Jap. J. Med. Sci. Biol.* **5**:1, 1953.

ALADJEM, F., and M. LIEBERMAN. The antigen-antibody reaction. I. Influence of sodium chloride concentration on the quantitative precipitin reaction. *J. Immunol.* **69**:117, 1952.

ALBERSHEIM, P., D. J. NEVINS, P. D. ENGLISH, and A. KARR. A method for the analysis of sugars in plant cell-wall polysaccharides by gas-liquid chromatography. *Carbohydrate Res.* **5**:340, 1967.

ALDERTON, G., and H. L. FEVOLD. Direct crystallization of lysozyme from egg white and some crystalline salts of lysozyme. *J. Biol. Chem.* **164**:1, 1946.

ALDERTON, G., W. H. WARD, and H. L. FEVOLD. Isolation of lysozyme from egg white. *J. Biol. Chem.* **157**:43, 1945.

ALEXANDER, H. L., M. B. JOHNSON, and J. H. ALEXANDER. A method for quantitating the precipitation test. *Science*, **101**:547, 1945.

ALEXANDER, M., G. G. WRIGHT, and A. C. BALDWIN. Observations on the agglutination of polysaccharide-treated erythrocytes by tularemia antisera. *J. Exper. Med.* **91**:561, 1950.

ALLEN, F., and E. McDANIEL. A study of the relation of temperature to antibody formation in cold-blooded animals. *J. Immunol.* **39**:143, 1937.

ALLEN, J. C., J. H. BAXTER, and H. C. GOODMAN. Effects of dextran, polyvinylpyrrolidone and gamma globulin on the hyperlipidemia of experimental nephrosis. *J. Clin. Invest.* **40**:499, 1961.

ALLEN, P. Z., and E. A. KABAT. Studies on the capacity of some polysaccharides to elicit antibody formation in man. *J. Exper. Med.* **105**:383, 1957.

ALPER, C. A., and A. M. JOHNSON. Immunofixation electrophoresis: A technique for the study of protein polymorphism. *Vox Sang.* **17**:445, 1969.

ALSEVER, J., and R. AINSLIE. A new method for preparation of dilute blood plasma and the operation of a complete transfusion service. *N.Y. State J. Med.* **4**:126, 1941.

ALTGAUZEN, V. P., *Zhur. Mikrobiol. Epidermiol. Immunobiol.* **30**:65, 1959.

AMANO, S. *Fundamentals of Hematology.* Maruzen Ltd., 1948.

AMES, B. N., and D. T. DUBIN. The role of polyamines in the neutralization of bacteriophage deoxyribonucleic acid. *J. Biol. Chem.* **235**:769, 1960.

AMIES, C. R. The envelope substance of *Pasteurella pestis. Brit. J. Exper. Pathol.* **32**:259, 1957.

AMINOFF, D. Methods for quantitative estimation of N-acetyl-neuraminic acid and their application to hydrolysates of sialomucoids. *Biochem. J.* **81**:384, 1961.

AMOS, D. B., and M. PEACOCKE. *Proc. 9th Conf. European Soc. Haematol.* Karger, Basel, 1963. p. 1132.

ANACKER, R. L., D. B. LACKMAN, E. G. PICKENS, and E. RIBI. Antigenic and skin-reactive properties of fractions of *Coxiella burnetii. J. Immunol.* **84**:145, 1962.

ANDERSON, H. C., and M. McCARTY. Determination of C-reactive protein in the blood as a measure of the activity of disease process in acute rheumatic fever. *Amer. J. Med.* **8**:445, 1950.

ANDERSON, N. G. The development of zonal centrifuge introduction. *Nat'l. Cancer Inst. Monograph*, **21**:1, 1966.

ANDERSON, N. G. An introduction to particle separations in zonal centrifuges. *Nat'l. Cancer Inst. Monograph*, **21**:9, 1966.

ANDERSON, N. G., W. W. HARRIS, A. A. BARBER, C. T. RANKIN, JR., and E. L. CANDLER. Separation of subcellar components and viruses by combined rate- and isopycnic-zonal centrifugation. *Nat'l. Cancer Inst. Monograph*, **21**:253, 1966.

ANDERSON, R. J. The separation of lipoid fractions from tubercle bacilli. *J. Biol. Chem.* **74**:525, 1927.

ANDERSON, R. J. Chemistry of lipoids of tubercle bacilli; concerning phthioic acid; preparation and properties of phthioic acid. *J. Biol. Chem.* **83**:505, 1929.

ANDERSON, R. J. The chemistry of the lipids of tubercle bacilli. *Harvey Lectures*, **35**:271, 1939–1940.

ANDERSON, R. J. Structural peculiarities of acid fast bacterial lipides. *Chem. Rev.* **29**:225, 1941.

ANDERSON, R. J., and E. CHARGAFF. The chemistry of the lipoids of tubercle bacilli. V. Analysis of the acetone soluble fat. *J. Biol. Chem.* **83**:703, 1929.

ANDERSON, R. J., and M. M. CREIGHTON. The composition of the polysaccharide of the firmly bound lipids of the leprosy bacillus. *J. Biol. Chem.* **131**:549, 1939.

ANDERSON, R. J., M. M. CREIGHTON, and R. L. PECK. The chemistry of the lipids of tubercle bacilli. *J. Biol. Chem.* **133**:675, 1940.

ANDO, K., and T. KOMIYAMA. Purification of diphtheria toxin and anatoxin. *J. Immunol.* **29**:439, 1935.

ANDO, K., T. KOMIYAMA, and K. MANAKO. Alum precipitation of diphtheria toxoid (improvement of diphtheria alum-toxoid). *J. Immunol.* **31**:355, 1936.

ANDRES, G. A., C. MORGAN, K. C. HSU, R. A. RIFKIND, and B. C. SEEGAL. Electron microscopic studies of experimental nephritis with ferritin-conjugated antibody. *J. Exper. Med.* **115**:929, 1962.

ANDRES, G. A., B. D. SEEGAL, K. C. HSU, M. S. ROTHENBERG, and M. L. CHAPEAU. Electron microscopic studies of experimental nephritis with ferritin conjugated antibody. Localization of antigen-antibody complexes in rabbit glomeruli following repeated injections of bovine serum albumin. *J. Exper. Med.* **117**:691, 1963.

ANGLE, F. E., W. H. ALGIE, and D. MORGAN. Brucellosis: studies emphasising strain variation in serologic testing. *J. Lab. Clin. Med.* **27**:1259, 1942.

APGAR, J., R. W. HOLLEY, and S. H. MERRILL. Purification of the alanine-, valine-, histidine-, and tyrosine-acceptor ribonucleic acids from yeast. *J. Biol. Chem.* **237**:796, 1962.

APPLEBY, J. C., and C. H. STUART-HARRIS. The use of filtrates of *Vibrio cholerae* in the classification of influenza virus strains. *Brit. J. Exper. Pathol.* **31**:797, 1950.

APRILE, M. A., K. M. VIJH, and A. C. WARDLAW. Increase in sensitivity of the complement fixation test by use of low ionic strength buffers; Studies with heat-aggregated gamma globulin and with poliomyelitis vaccines. *J. Lab. Clin. Med.* **66**:146, 1965.

ARAI, K. and H. W. WALLACE. Electrophoretic determination of glycoprotein: An improved method with cleared cellulose acetate membrane. *Anal. Biochem.* **31**:71, 1969.

ARAI, T., S. KURODA, and M. ITO. Possible utility of fluorescent antibody technique in the serological identification of antagonistic streptomyces. *J. Bacteriol.* **83**:20, 1962.

ARCHETTI, I., and F. L. HORSFALL. Persistent antigenic variation of influenza viruses after incomplete neutralization in ovo with heterologous immune serum. *J. Exper. Med.* **92**:441, 1950.

ARCHIBALD, W. J. A demonstration of some new methods of determining molecular weight from the data of the ultracentrifuge. *J. Phys. Colloid. Chem.* **51**:1204, 1947.

ARGENTON, H., H. BECKER, H. FISCHER, J. OTTO, R. THIEL, and O. WESTPHAL. Ueber die resistenzsteigernde Wirkung von Lipoid A. beim Menschen. *Deutsche Med. Wochenschr.* **86**:774, 1961.

ARJONA, E., J. DIAZ, J. M., SEGOVIA, and A. ORTEGA. Technique actuelle de la réaction microprécipitine. *Acta Allergol.* **7**:215, 1954.

ARMSTRONG, J. J., J. BADDILEY, J. G. BUCHANAN, and B. CARSS. Nucleotides and the bacterial cell wall. *Nature*, **181**:1692, 1958.

ARMSTRONG, J. J., J. BADDILEY, J. G. BUCHANAN, B. CARSS, and G. R. GREENBERG. Isolation and structure of ribitol phosphate derivatives (teichoic acids) from bacterial cell walls. *J. Chem. Soc.* 4344, 1958.

ASKONAS, B. A., and J. M. RHODES. Immunogenicity of antigen-containing ribonucleic acid preparations from macrophages. *Nature*, **205**:470, 1965.

ARONOFF, S. Carbohydrates. In *Techniques of Radiochemistry*. Iowa State College Press, 1956, pp. 100–101.

ARRHENIUS, S. *Immunochemie*. Akademishe Verlagsgesellschatt, 1907.

ARRHENIUS, S., and T. MADSEN. Toxines et antitoxines. Le poison diphtérique. *Centralbl. Bakteriol.* **36**:612, 1904.

ASCOLI, A. *Münch. Med. Wochenschr.* **49**:1409, 1902.

ASCOLI, A. Die Präzipitindiagnose bei Milzbrand. *Centralbl. Bakter. I. Orig.* **58**:63, 1911.

ASHBY, W. The determination of the length of life of transfused blood corpuscles. *J. Exper. Med.* **29**:267, 1919.

ASKONAS, B. A., and R. G. WHITE. Sites of antibody production in the guinea-pig. The relation between in vitro synthesis of anti-ovalbumin and gamma-globulin and distribution of antibody-containing plasma cells. *Brit. J. Exper. Pathol.* **37**:61, 1956.

ASSELINEAU, J. Lipides due bacille tuberculeux. Constitution chimique et activité physiologique. *Advanc. Tuberc. Res.* **5**:1, 1952.

ASSELINEAU, J. Sur la composition des lipides de *Corynebacterium diphtheriae*. *Biochim. Biophys. Acta*, **54**:359, 1961.

ASTROWE, P. *J. Amer. Med. Assoc.* **79**:1511, 1922.

ATTARDI, G., M. COHN, K. HORIBATA, and E. S. LENNOX. Symposium on the biology of cells modified by viruses or antigens. II. On the analysis of antibody synthesis at the cellular level. *Bacteriol. Rev.* **23**:213, 1959.

ATTARDI, G., M. COHN, K. HORIBATA, and E. S. LENNOX. Antibody formation by rabbit lymph node cells. I. Single cell responses to several antigens. *J. Immunol.* **92**:335, 1964.

AUBERT, E. A., K. BOORMAN, and B. E. DODD. Agglutinin-inhibiting substance in human serum. *J. Pathol. Bacteriol.* **54**:89, 1942.

ATFIELD, G. N., and C. J. O. R. MORRIS. Analytical separation by high-voltage paper electrophoresis. Amino acids in protein hydrolysates. *Biochim. J.* **81**:606, 1961.

AUBERT, E. A., V. PAVILANIS, and D. H. STARKEY. Virus antibody titrations using latex suspension. *Canad. J. Publ. Health*, 206, 1962.

AUSGUSTIN, R. Fundamental aspects of single versus double diffusion methods for immunological assays. *Intern. Arch. Allergy Appl. Immunol.* **11**:153, 1957.

AUGUSTIN, R., and B. HAYWARD. Standardisation of pollen extracts by gel diffusion. *Intern. Arch. Allergy Appl. Immunol.* **6**:154, 1955.

AVERY, O. T. A further study on the biologic classification of pneumococci. *J. Exper. Med.* **22**:804, 1915.

AVERY, O. T., and W. F. GOEBEL. Chemoimmunological studies on soluble specific substance of pneumonocci; isolation and properties of acetyl polysaccharide of pneumococcus type I. *J. Exper. Med.* **58**:731, 1933.

AVERY, O. T., and M. HEIDELBERGER. Immunological relationships of cell constituents of pneumococcus. *J. Exper. Med.* **42**:367, 1925.

AVERY, O. T., M. HEIDELBERGER, and W. F. GOEBEL. The soluble substance of Friedlander bacillus. *J. Exper. Med.* **42**:708, 1925.

AVERY, R., and F. BLANK. On the chemical composition of the cell walls of the Actinomycetales and its relation to their systematic position. *Canad. J. Microbiol.* **1**:140, 1954.

AVRAMEAS, S., and J. URIEL. A method of preparative electrophoresis in horizontal gels. *Nature*, **202**:1005, 1964.

AVRAMEAS, S. Coupling of enzymes to proteins with glutaraldehyde. Use of the conjugates for the detection of antigens and antibodies. *Immunochemistry* **6**:43, 1969.

AVRAMEAS, S. Indirect immunoenzyme techniques for the intracellular detection of antigens. *Immunochem.* **6**:825, 1969.

BABA, T. Analytical Serology of Bacillaceae. In *Analytical Serology of Microorganisms* (J. B. G. Kwapinski, Ed), Vol. 1. Interscience, New York, 1969, pp. 600–642.

BACHMAN, B. A. *A Study of Brucellicidal Antibody Production*. M. A. Thesis. University of Texas Library, Austin, Tex., 1949.

BACON, J. D., and J. EDELMAN. The carbohydrates of Jerusalem Artichoke and other compositae. *Biochem. J.* **48**:114, 1951.

BAER, H., J. BRINGAZE, and N. MCNAUREE. The immuno-chemistry of blood group O. *J. Immunol.* **73**:87, 1954.

BAER, R. L., and Y. MEYER. Skin tests in various infections and parasitic diseases. *Arch. Derm.* **62**:491, 1950.

BAGULEY, B. C., P. L. BERQUIST, and R. K. RALPH. Fractionation of amino acid acceptor ribonucleic acids on diethylaminoethyl-cellulose columns. *Biochim. Biophys. Acta*, **95**:510, 1965.

BAILEY, G. H., and M. S. SHORB. Chemical and immunological properties of pneumococci and other heterophile antigens. *Amer. J. Hyg.* **17**:329, 1933.

BAIN, R. V. S., and K. W. KNOX. The antigens of *Pasteurella multocida* Type I. II. Lipopolysaccharides. *Immunology*, **4**:122, 1961.

BAIRD, G. D., P. ALBERSSON, and B.V. HOFSTEN. Separation of bacteria by counter distribution. *Nature*, **192**:236, 1961.

BAKER, E. E., H. SOMMER, L. E. FOSTER, E. MEYER, and K. E. MEYER. Studies on immunization against plague. The isolation and characterization of the soluble antigen of *Pasteurella pestis*. *J. Immunol.* **68**:131, 1952.

BAKER, E. E., and R. E. WHITESIDE. Vi antigens of the *Enterobacteriaceae*. IV. Purification and properties of Vi antigen of *S. parahyphi C. Proc. Soc. Exper. Biol. Med.* **105**:328, 1960.

BAKER, E. E., R. E. WHITESIDE, R. BASCH, and M. A. DEROW. The Vi antigens of *Enterobacteriaceae*. I. Purification and chemical properties. *J. Immunol.* **73**:680, 1954.

BAKER, P. J., M. BERNSTEIN, V. PASANEN, and M. LANDY. Detection and enumeration of antibody-producing cells by specific adherence of antigen-coated bentonite particles. *J. Immunol.* **97**:767, 1966.

BALFOUR, B. M. Immunological studies on a freeze-substitution method of preparing tissue for fluorescent antibody staining. *J. Immunol.* **86**:206, 1961.

BANTISTA, G., C. JUNGEBLUT, and H. KODZA. Experiments on adsorption in vitro of Type II poliomyelitis virus on red cells. *J. Immunol.* **82**:242, 1959.

BANZHAF, E. J. The distribution of the immune bodies occurring in types O, II, and III antipneumococcus serum. *Proc. Soc. Exper. Biol. Med.* **22**:329, 1925.

BARBER, M., and P. WILDY. A study of antigenic specificity of staphylococcal coagulase in relation to bacteriophage group. *J. Gen. Microbiol.* **18**:92, 1958.

BARBOUR, H. G., and U. F. HAMILTON. The falling drop method for determining specific gravity. *J. Biol. Chem.* **69**:625, 1926.

BARKSDALE, W., and A. GHODA. Agglutinating antibodies in serum and feces. *J. Immunol.* **66**:395, 1951.

BARKULIS, S. S., and M. F. JONES. Studies of streptococcal cell walls. I. Isolation, chemical composition and preparation of M protein. *J. Bacteriol.* **74**:207, 1957.

BARNES, L. A., and E. C. WIGHT. Serological relationship between pneumococcus type I and an encapsulated strain of *Escherichia coli. J. Exper. Med.* **62**:281, 1935.

BARROLIER, J., J. HEILMAN, and E. WATZKE. Polychrome Sichtbarmachung von Aminosäuren auf Papierchromatogrammen und-elektrophoregrammen. Hoppe-Seuler's Zeitschr. *Physiol. Chem.* **304**:22, 1956.

BARRY, G. T., V. ABBOT, and T. TSAI. Relationship of colomic acid (poly-N-acetyl-neuraminic acid) to bacteria which contain neuraminic acid. *J. Gen. Microbiol.* **29**:335, 1962.

BARRY, G. T., F. CHEN, and E. ROARK. Isolation of N-acetyl-neuraminic acid and 4-oxynorleucine from a polysaccharide obtained from *Citrobacter freundii. J. Gen. Microbiol.* **33**:97, 1963.

BARRY, G. T., J. D. HAMM, and M. G. GRAHAM. Evaluation of colorimetric methods in the estimation of sialic acid in bacteria. *Nature*, **200**:806, 1963.

BARTH, R. F., and B. MERCHANT. Adaption of the hemolytic plaque technique for enumeration of immune cells responding to heterologous immunoglobulin antigens. *Proc. Soc. Exper. Biol. Med.* **125**:307, 1967.

BARTH, W. F., C. L. McLAUGHLIN, and J. L. FAHEY. The immunoglobulins of mice. VI. Response to immunization. *J. Immunol.* **95**:781, 1965.

BARTLETT, G. R. Phosphorus assay in column chromatography. *J. Biol. Chem.* **234**:466, 1959.

BARWELL, C. F. Some observations on the antigenic structure of psittacosis and lymphogranuloma venereum viruses. I. Preparation and use in complement fixation tests of antiserum from different study. *Brit. J. Exper. Pathol.* **33**:258, 1952; II. Treatment of virus suspensions by various reagents and the specific activity of acid extracts. *Brit. J. Exper. Pathol.* **33**:28, 1952.

BASHE, W. J., G. HENLE, and W. HENLE. Studies on prevention of mumps. VI. The relation of neutralizing antibodies to the determination of susceptibility. *J. Immunol.* **71**:76, 1953.

BASSETT, E. W., S. M. BEISER, and S. W. TENENBAUM. Purification of antibody to galactosylprotein conjugates. *Sciences*, **133**:1475, 1961.

BATEMAN, J., H. CALKINS, and L. CHAMBERS. Optical study of the reaction between transferred monolayers of Lancefield's "M" substance and various antisera. *J. Immunol.* **41**:321, 1941.

BATHURST, N. O., and K. J. MITCHELL. The effect of light and temperature on the chemical compositions of pasture plants. *N.Z. J. Agric. Res.* **1**:540, 1958.

BATSON, H. C. Statistical methods in immunology. *J. Immunol.* **66**:737, 1951.

BAUMAN, N. S., and B. D. Davis. Selection of auxotrophic bacterial mutants through diaminopimelic acid or thymine deprival. *Science*, **126**:170, 1957.

BAUMANN-GRACE, J. B., and J. TOMCSIK. The surface structure and serological typing of *Bacterium megaterium*. *J. Gen. Microbiol.* **17**:227, 1957.

BAUMANN-GRACE, J. B., and J. TOMCSIK. Elektronenmikroskopische Utersuchung der komplexen Kapselstruktur bei *B. megaterium*. *Schweiz. Zeitschr. Allgem. Pathol. Bakteriol. Sep.* **21/5**:906, 1958.

BAUMSTARK, J. S., R. J. LAFFIN, and W. A. BARDOUILE. A preprarative method for the separation of 7S gamma globulin from human serum. *Arch. Biochem. Biophys.* **108**:514, 1964.

BAUR, E. W. A thin layer starch-gel electrophoresis and plastification method. *J. Lab. Clin. Med.* **61**:166, 1963.

BEACHEY, E. H., and R. M. COLE. Cell wall replication in *Escherichia coli*, studied by immunofluorescence and immunoelectron microscopy. *J. Bact.* **92**:1245, 1966.

BEALE, A. J., and P. J. MASON. The measurement of the D-antigen in polio-virus preparations. *J. Hyg.* **60**:113, 1962.

BECH, V. Studies on the development of complement fixing antibodies in measles patients. *J. Immunol.* **83**:267, 1959.

BECHHOLD, H. *Zeitschr. Physiol. Chem.* **52**:185, 1905.

BECKER, E. L. The molecular weight of an antigen-antibody complex. *J. Immunol.* **70**:372, 1953.

BECKER, E. L. Antigen-antibodies reactions in gel. *Feder. Proc.* **12**:717, 1953.

BECKER, E. L. Concerning the mechanism of complement fixation. *J. Immunol.* **77**:462, 1956.

BECKER, E. L. Concerning the mechanism of complement action. IV. The properties of activated first component of guinea pig complement. *J. Immunol.* **82**:43, 1959.

BECKER, E. L. Mechanism of complement action. V. Early steps in immune hemolysis. *J. Immunol.* **84**:299, 1960.

BECKER, E. L., and J. MUNOZ. Multiplicity of antigens in extracts as demonstrated by the technic of Oudin. *Proc. Soc. Exper. Biol. Med.* **72**:287, 1949.

BECKER, E. L., J. MUNOZ, C. LAPRESLE, and L. LE BEAU. Antigen-antibody reactions in agar. II. Elementary theory and determination of diffusion coefficients of antigen. *J. Immunol.* **67**:50, 1951.

BECKER, E. L., and J. C. NEFF. Antigen-antibody reactions in agar. IV. Concerning the measurement of antibody concentration. *J. Immunol.* **83**:571, 1959.

BEDSON, S., C. F. BARWELL, E. KING, and L. BISHOP. The laboratory diagnosis of lymphogranuloma venereum. *J. Clin. Pathol.* **2**:241, 1949.

BEHRING, VON, E. Untersuchungen über das Zustandekommen der Diphtherie-Immunität bei Tieren. *Deutsche Med. Wochenschr.* **16**:1145, 1890.

BEHRING, VON E., and Y. KITASATO. Ueber das Zustandekommen der Diphtherie-Immunität und der Tetanus-Immunität bei Tieren. *Deutsche Med. Wochenschr.* **1**:1113, 1890.

BEISER, S. M., and E. A. KABAT. Immunochemical studies on blood groups. *J. Immunol.* **68**:19, 1952.

BEISER, S. M., E. A. KABAT, and J. M. SCHOR. Immunochemical studies on the specific polysaccharide of type II pneumococcus. *J. Immunol.* **69**:297, 1952.

BEKKER, J. Studies on staphylocoagulase. II. Antistaphylocoagulase on human serum. *Ant. van Loewenhoek, J. Microb.* **13**:128, 1947.

BELCHER, R., A. J. NUTTEN, and C. M. SAMBROOK. The determination of glucosamine. *Analyst,* **79**:201, 1954.

BELJANZKI, M., and S. OCHOA. Protein biosynthesis of cell-free bacterial system. *Proc. Natl. Acad. Sci. U.S.* **44**:494, 1958.

BELL, D. J., and M. Q.-K. TALUKDER. Thin-layer quantitative chromatography of arabinose, ribose and xylose in the presence of other sugars. *J. Chromatog.* **49**:469, 1970.

BELYAVIN, G. Influenza complement-fixation. A simple quantitative micro-method. *J. Hygiene,* **51**:492, 1953.

BENACERRAF, B., and P. MIESCHER. Bacterial phagocytosis by the reticuloendothelial system in vivo under different immune conditions. *Ann. N.Y. Acad. Sci.* **88**:184, 1960.

BENDICH, A. A., E. KABAT, and A. BEZER. Immunochemical studies on blood groups. III. Properties of purified blood group A substances from individual hog stomach linings. *J. Exper. Med.* **83**:485, 1946.

BENDINELLI, M. Haemolytic plaque formation by mouse peritoneal cells, and the effect on it of friend virus infection. *Immunology,* **14**:837, 1968.

BENEDICT, A. A., and S. S. ELBERG. Cutaneous hypersensitivity in brucellosis. *J. Immunol.* **70**:152, 1953.

BENEDICT, A. A., and E. O'BRIEN. Antigenic studies on the psittacosis-lymphogranuloma venereum group of viruses. II. Characterization of complement-fixing antigens extracted with sodium lauryl sulfate. *J. Immunol.* **76**:293, 1956.

BANESCH, R., and R. E. BENESCH. Thiolation of proteins. *Proc. Natl. Acad. Sci. U.S.* **44**:848–853, 1958.

BENGTSON, I. A. Complement fixation in rickettsial diseases-technique of test. *Publ. Health Rep.* **59**:402, 1944.

BENGTSSON, S., and L. PHILIPSON. Countercurrent distribution of poliovirus type I. *Virology,* **20**:176, 1963.

BENJAMIN, H., and J. SLUKA. Antikörperbildung nach experimenteller Schädigung des hämopoetischen Systems durch Röntgenstrahlen. *Wiener Klin. Wochenschr.* **10**, 1908.

BENNETT, C. W. *Clinical Serology.* C. C Thomas Publishing, Springfield, 1964.

BENNETT, I. L., Jr. Observations on the fever caused by bacterial pyrogens. *J. Exper. Med.* **88**:267, 1948.

BENNINGTON, J. L. Radioautographic analysis of soluble antigen-antibody complexes separable by paper electrophoresis. *Proc. Soc. Exper. Biol. Med.* **104**:148, 1960.

BERAN, M., and J. DAUSSET. The use of the inverted microscope in leuco-agglutination. *Vox. Sang.* **8**:371, 1963.

BERCKS, R. Methodische Untersuchunger über den serologischen Nachweis pflanzen-pathogener Viren mit dem Bentonit-Flockungstest, dem Latex-test und dem Bariumsul-fat-Test. *Phytopath. Z.* **58**:1, 1967.

BERG, G., W. FRENGER, and F. SCHEIFFARTH. Die Agglutinationselektrophorese. (Eine Methode zum Nachweis von Antikörpern und deren Lokalisation in den Serum-Protein-fraktionen). *Klin. Wochenschr.* 767, 1955.

BERGDOLL, M. S., J. L. KADAVY, M. J. SURGALLA, and G. M. DACK. Partial purification of staphylococcal enterotoxin. *Arch. Biochem. Biophys.* **33**:259, 1951.

BERGER, J. A., and A. G. MARR. Sonic disruption of spores of *Bacillus cereus*. *J. Gen. Microbiol.* **22**:147, 1960.

BERGLUND, K. A micro-slide method permitting autoradiography of haemolysin-producing cells. *Nature*, **204**:89, 1964.

BERGMAN, S. Culture of human fibroblasts on glass plates. *Acta Path. Microbiol. Scandinav.* **59**:279, 1963.

BERGMAN, S., and S. B. NILSSON. Effect of endotoxin on embryonal chick fibroblasts cul-tured in monolayer. *Acta Path. Microbiol. Scandinav.* **59**:161, 1963.

BERGMAN, S., and C. WEIBULL. Effects of endotoxin on tissue culture cells. *Acta. Path. Microbiol. Scandinav.* **77**:698, 1969.

BERGOLD, G., and L. PISTER. The quantitative microdetermination of desoxy and ribonucleic acids. *Z. Naturforsch.* **3b**:406, 1948.

BERNER, J. J., J. KING, and A. REICH. Evaluation of the Reiter protein complement-fixation (RPCF) test for syphilis. *Cleveland Clin. Quart.* **27**:162, 1960.

BERNHEIMER, A. W., and M. E. FARKAS. Hemagglutinins among higher fungi. *J. Immunol.* **70**:197, 1953.

BERTHELOT, M. P. E. *Rep. Chim. Appl.* **284**, 1909.

BERTHIER, M. G., and J. L. WOO. Detection of atypical antibodies in erythrocytes. *Amer. J. Clin. Pathol.* **24**:1419, 1942.

BESON, P. Tolerance to bacterial pyrogens. I. Factors influencing its development. *J. Exper. Med.*, **86**:29, 1947.

BETTS, A., and E. L. SEWALL. Identification of blood stains by immunodiffusion in agar gel. *Amer. J. Clin. Pathol.* **43**:535, 1965.

BEUTNER, E. H., E. J. HOLBOROW, and G. D. JOHNSON. A new fluorescent antibody method: Mixed antiglobulin immunofluorescence or labelled antigen indirect immunofluorescence staining. *Nature*, **208**:353, 1965.

BEYER, H. G., and A. L. REAGH. *J. Med. Res.* **12**:319, 1904.

BIBERFELD, P., and N. RINGERTZ. The application of immune electron microscopy to the demonstration of polyoma virus antigen in cultured mouse embryo cells. *J. Nat. Cancer Inst.* **37**:451, 1966.

BIDE, R. W. An automated method for the estimation of total phosphate in biological material. *Anal. Biochem.* **29**:393, 1969.

BIEGELEISEN, J. Z., B. R. BRADSHAW, and M. D. MOODY. Demonstration of *Brucella* anti-bodies in human serum. *J. Immunol.* **88**:109, 1962.

BIEGELEISEN, J. Z., Jr, M. S. MITCHELL, B. B. MARCUS, D. L. RHODEN, and R. W. BLUM-BERG. Immunofluorescence techniques for demonstrating bacterial pathogens associated with cerebrospinal meningitis. II. Growth, viability, and immunofluorescent staining of *Hemophilus influenzae*, *Neisseria meningitidis*, and *Diplococcus pneumoniae* in cerebrospinal fluid. *J. Lab. Clin. Med.* **65**:976, 1965.

BIELING, R. Herdinfektion und Immunität. *Verhandl. Deutsch. Gesellsch. Inn. Med.* **42**: 438, 1930.

BIELING, R. Die view Arten von kompletten und inkompletten Antikörpern. *Deutsche Med. Wochenschr.* **465**, 1952.

BIELING, R., and A. GOTTSCHALK. Die VERTEILUNG der Toxine im Körper. *Zeitschr. Hyg. Infektionskr.* 99:125, 1923.

BIENVENU, R. J., JR., L. J. RODE, and V. T. SCHUHARDT. Microcolony brucellacidal test. *J. Bacteriol.* **81**:684, 1961.

BIER, O. G. Observations préliminaires sur l'hémagglutination, l'hémolyse et la conglutination "passive." *Ann. Inst. Pasteur*, **81**:650, 1951.

BIER, O. G., R. FURTADO, and E. CISALPINO. A plate technic for the conglutinative complement fixation test. *Proc. Soc. Exper. Biol. Med.* **95**:335, 1957.

BIER, O. G., G. LEYTON, M. M. MAYER, and M. HEIDELBERGER. A comparison of human and guinea pig complements and their component fractions. *J. Exper. Med.* **81**:449, 1945.

BIER, O. G., M. SIQUEIRA, and R. S. FURLANETTO. Amboceptor titration as a statistically controlled assay. *J. Immunol.* **69**:241, 1952.

BIGAZZI, P. L., J. A. ANDRADA, E. C. ANDRADA, E. H. BEUTNER, and E. WITEBSKY. Immunofluorescence studies on Addison's disease. *Int. Arch. Allergy*, **34**:455, 1968.

BILLINGHAM, R. E., L. BRENT, and P. B. MEDAWAR. The antigenic stimulus in transplantation immunity. *Nature*, **178**:514, 1956.

BINAGHI, R. A. Production of 7S immunoglobulin in immunized guinea pigs. *J. Immunol.* **97**:159, 1966.

BINNINGS, G. F., M. J. RILEY, M. E. ROBERTS, R. BARNES, and T. C. PRINGLE. Automated instrument for the fluorescent treponemal antibody-absorption test and other immunofluorescence tests. *Appl. Microbiol.* **18**:861, 1969.

BIOZZI, G., C. STIFFEL, B. N. HALPERN, L. LEMINOR, and D. MOUTON. Measurement of the opsonic effect of normal and immune sera on the phagocytosis of *Salmonella typhi* by the recitulo-endothelial system. *J. Immuno.* **87**:296, 1961.

BIRD, G. W. G. Observations on suppressed or "latent" haemagglutinins. *Brit. J. Haematol.* **1**:375, 1954.

BIRKBECK, T. H., and J. STEPHEN. Specific removal of host-cell or vaccinia-virus antigens from extracts of infected cells by polyvalent disulphide-linked immunosorbents. *J. Gen. Virol.* **8**:133, 1970.

BISHOP, B. S. Digital computation of sedimentation coefficients in zonal centrifuges. *Natl. Cancer Inst. Monograph*, **21**:175, 1966.

BJÖRKLUND, B. Specific inhibition of precipitation as an aid in antigen analysis with gel diffusion method. *Proc. Soc. Exper. Biol. Med.* **79**:319, 1952.

BJÖRKLUND, B. Qualitative analysis of gel precipitates with the aid of chemical color reactions. *Proc. Soc. Exper. Biol. Med.* **85**:438, 1954.

BLAIR, J. The complement fixation reaction with the antigen of lymphogranuloma venereum. *J. Immunol.* **49**:63, 1944.

BLAKE, F. *Arch. Int. Med.* **27**:519, 1935.

BLIX, G., A. TISELIUS, and H. SVENSON. Lipids and polysaccharides in electrophoretically separated blood serum proteins. *J. Biol. Chem.* **137**:485, 1941.

BLIX, U., C. M. ILAND, and M. STACEY. The serological activity of deoxypentose nucleic acids. *Brit. J. Exper. Pathol.* **35**:241, 1954.

BLOCH, K. J., and J. J. BUNIM. Simple, rapid diagnostic test for rheumatoid arthritis: bentonite flocculation test. *J. Amer. Med. Assoc.* **169**:302, 1959.

BLODGETT, K. B., and I. LANGMUIR. Built-up films of barium stearate and their optical properties. *Phys. Rev.* **51**:964, 1937.

BLUM, G., and P. D. ELLNER. Evaluation of a rapid slide test as a screening procedure for antistreptolysin O. *Amer. J. Clin. Pathol.* **53**:936, 1970.

BLUMER, M., T. CHASE, and S. W. WATSON. Fatty acids in the lipids of marine and terrestrial nitrifying bacteria. *J. Bacteriol.* **99**:366, 1969.

BOAKE, W. Antistaphylocoagulase in experimental *Staphylococcus* infections. *J. Immunol.* **76**:89, 1956.

BOAND, A., J. KEMP, and R. HANSON. Phagocytosis of influenza virus. *J. Immunol.* **73**:416, 1957.

BOAS, N. F. Method for determination of hexosamines in tissues. *J. Biol. Chem.* **204**:553, 1953.

BODANSKY, A. Phosphatase studies. I. Determination of inorganic phosphorus. *J. Biol. Chem.* **99**:197, 1932.

BODIAN, D. Simplified method of dispersion of monkey kidney cells with trypsin. *Virology*, **2**:575, 1956.

BODMAN, J. The separation of serum glyco-proteins by continuous electrophoresis. *Lab. Practice*, part 1, p. 517, 1957.

BOELL, E. J., and S. C. SHEN. An improved ultramicro-Kjeldahl technique. *Exper. Cell Research*, **7**:147, 1954.

BOGER, W. P., J. W. FRANKEL, and J. J. GAWIN. Detection and titration of *Staphylococcus aureus* agglutinins in serum. *Proc. Soc. Exper. Biol. Med.* **104**:639, 1960.

BOGERT, M., and R. WRIGHT. Some experiments on the nitro-derivates of fluorescein. *J. Amer. Chem. Soc.* **27**:1310, 1905.

BÖHM, P., S. DAUBER, and L. BAUMEISTER. Ueber Neuraminsäure, ihr Vorkommen und ihre Bestimmung im Serum. *Klin. Wochenschr.* **289**, 1954.

BOIVIN, A., and L. MESROBEANU. Résearches sur les antigénes somatiques et sur les endotoxines des bacteries. *Immunology* **1**:533, 1935.

BOIVIN, A., and L. MESROBEANU. Résearches sur les antigénes somatiques du bacille typhique. Sur la nature chimique des antigénes "O" et "V," *Compt. Rend. Soc. Biol.* **128**:5, 1937.

BOJALIL, L. F., and A. ZAMORA. Precipitin and skin tests in the diagnosis of mycetoma due to *Nocardia brasiliensis*. *Proc. Soc. Exper. Biol. Med.* **113**:40, 1963.

BONNELYCKE, B. E., K. DUS, and S. L. MILLER. *Analyt. Biochem.* **27**:262, 1969.

BORDET, J. *Ann. Inst. Pasteur*, **9**:462, 1895.

BORDET, J. Sur l'agglutination et la dissolution des globules rouges par la sérum d'animeaux injectes de sang defibrine. *Ann. Inst. Pasteur*, **12**:688, 1898.

BORDET, J. Agglutination et dissolution des globules rouges par le sérum. *Ann. Inst. Pasteur*, **13**:273, 1899.

BORDET, J. *Traite de l'Immunité*. Masson and Co., Paris, 1920.

BORDET, J., and F. P. GAY. Sur les relations des sensibilisatrices avec l'alexine. *Ann. Inst.* **20**:67, 1906.

BORDET, J., and F. P. GAY. *Studies in Immunity*. Wiley, New York, 1909.

BORDET, J., and O. GENGOU. Sur l'existence des substances sensibilatrices. *Ann. Inst. Pasteur*, **15**:289, 1901.

BORDET, J., and O. GENGOU. Le microbe de la coqueluche, *Ann. Inst. Pasteur*, **20**:731, 1906.

BORDET, J., and O. STRENG. Les phénomenes d'absorption et la conglutinine du sérum de boeuf. *Z. Bakteriol. Orig.* **49**:260, 1909.

BOREK F., and A. M. SILVERSTEIN. A new fluorescent label for antibody proteins. *Arch. Biochem. Biophys.* **86**:293, 1960.

BOREK, F., and A. M. SILVERSTEIN. Characterization and purification of ferritin-antibody globulin conjugates. *J. Immunol.* **87**:555, 1961.

BOREL, E., R. F. HOSTATTLER, and H. DEVEL. Quantitative Zuckerbestimmung mit 3,5-Dinitrosalicilsäure und Phenol. *Helv. Chim. Acta.* **35**:115, 1952.

BOREL, Y., E. C. FRANKLIN, and P. A. MIESCHER. The effect of unaggregated bovine γ-globulin and γM and γG antibody formation. *Immunology* **14**:899, 1968.

BORN, H., A. LANG, G. SCHRAMM, and K. ZIMMER. Versuche zur Markierung von Tabak-mosaik-virus mit Radiophosphor. *Naturwissenschaft.* **29**:222, 1941.

BOROFF, D. Specific aggregation of streptococcal proteins adsorbed on oil droplets. *Proc. Soc. Exper. Biol. Med.* **43**:294, 1938.

BOROFF, D., and L. TRIPP. Specific aggregation of streptococcal proteins on oil droplets. *J. Immunol.* **57**:369, 1947.

BORSOS, T., H. J. RAPP, and M. M. MAYER. Studies on the second component of comple-ment. I. The reaction of immune hemolysis and determination of C′2 on a molecular basis. *J. Immunol.* **87**:310, 1961.

BORSOS, T., and H. J. RAPP. Chromatographic separation of the first component of comple-ment and its assay on a molecular basis. *J. Immunol.* **91**:851, 1963.

BORSOS, T., and H. J. RAPP. Estimation of molecular size of complement components by Sephadex chromatography. *J. Immunol.* **94**:510, 1965.

BOSSAK, H. N., W. P. DUNCAN, W. P. HARRIS, and V. H. FALCONE. Evaluation of Tpcf-50 and other TPCF tests for syphilis. *Publ. Health Rep.* **75**:130, 1960.

BOULANGER, P., and G. L. BANNISTER. A modified direct complement fixation test for the detection of antibodies in serum of cattle previously infected with vesicular stomatitis virus. *J. Immunol.* **85**:368, 1960.

BOURONCLE, B., M. DODD, and C. WRIGHT. A study of cold hemagglutinins for normal and trypsinized red blood cells in the cerum of normal individuals and of hemolytic anemias. *J. Immunol.* **67**:265, 1951.

BOVARNICK, M. R., J. C. MILLER, and J. C. SNYDER. The influence of certain salts, amino acids, sugars, and proteins on the stability of rickettsiae. *J. Bacteriol.* **59**:509, 1950.

BOWEN, H. E. The homogeneity of purified diphtheria toxins as investigated by the semi-solid precipitation technic. *J. Immunol.* **68**:429, 1952.

BOWEN, H. E., and L. WYMAN. The flocculation reaction of rabbit antibody. *J. Immunol.* **71**:86, 1953.

BOYD, W. C. Production and preservation of specific antisera for blood-group factors A, B, M, and N. *J. Immunol.* **37**:65, 1939.

BOYD, W. C. Hemagglutinating substances for human cells in various Egyptian plants. *J. Immunol.* **65**:281, 1950.

BOYD, W. C. *Fundamentals of Immunology*, 3rd ed. Interscience, New York, 1956.

BOYD, W. C., and H. BERNARD. Quantitative changes in antibodies and globulin fractions in sera of rabbits injected with several antigens. *J. Immunol.* **33**:111, 1937.

BOYD, W. C., and L. BOYD. Blood grouping in forensic medicine. *J. Immunol.* **33**:159, 1937.

BOYD, W. C., and S. HOOKER. Influence of molecular weight antigen on proportion of anti-body to antigen in precipitates. *J. Gen. Physiol.* **17**:341, 1934.

BOYDEN, S. V. Adsorption by erthrocytes of antigens of *Pfeifferella mallei* and *Pf. whitmori.* *Proc. Soc. Exper. Biol. Med.* **73**:289, 1950.

BOYDEN, S. V. Fixation of bacterial products by erythrocytes treated with tannic acid and subsequent hemagglutination by anti-protein sera. *J. Exper. Med.* **93**:107, 1951.

BOYDEN, S. V. Serological reactions dependent upon the fixation of antigens and subsequently their antibodies onto erythrocytes. *Atti. VI Congr. Int. Microb.* **2**:159, 1953.

BOYDEN, S. V., E. BOLTEN, and D. GEMEROY. Precipitin testing with special reference to the photo-electric measurement of turbidity. *J. Immunol.* **57**:211, :947.

BOYDEN, S. V., and E. SORKIN. A study of antigens active in the tannic acid hemagglutination test present in filtrates of culture of *Mycabacterium tuberculosis*. *J. Immunol.* **75**:15, 1955.

BOYDEN, S. V., and E. SUTER. Stimulating effect of tuberculin upon production of circulating antibodies in guinea pigs injected with tubercle bacilli. *J. Immunol.* **68**:577, 1952.

BOYER, G. S., F. W. DENNY, JR., and H. S. GINSBERG. Intracellular localization of type 4 adenovirus. II. Cytological and fluorescein labeled antibody studies. *J. Exper. Med.* **109**:85, 1959.

BOYNS, A. R., and J. HARDWICKE. Immunological responsiveness following the continuous circulation of soluble antigen-antibody complexes. *Immunology*, **15**:263, 1968.

BOZICEVICH, J., J. J. BUNIM, J. FREUND, and B. W. STANLEY. Bentonite flocculation test. *Proc. Soc. Exper. Biol. Med.* **97**:180, 1958.

BOZSOKY, A. Antikörperbestimmung im Kammerwasser mittels Mikroverfahren. *Docum. Ophtalmol.* **14**:65, 1960.

BRADFIELD, A., and A. E. FLOOD, Soluble carbohydrates of fruit plants. *Nature*, **166**:264, 1950.

BRAKKE, M. K. Density gradient centrifugation: a new separation technique. *J. Amer. Soc.* **73**:1847, 1951.

BRAKKE, M. K. Zonal separations by density-gradient centrifugation. *Arch. Biochem. Biophys.* **45**:275, 1953.

BRAKKE, M. K. Estimation of sedimentation constants of viruses by density-gradient centrifugation. *Virology*, **6**:96, 1958.

BRAND, F. C., and W. M. SPERRY. The determination of cerebrosides. *J. Biol. Chem.* **141**: 545, 1941.

BRAND, G. Erfahrungen bei der Durchführung und Ablesung quantitativer Komplementbindungsreaktion im Hinblick aug due Reproduktion. *Zentralbl. Bakt. Orig.* **163**:549, 1955.

BRANDTZAEG, P., I. FJELLANGER, and S. T. GJERULDSEN. Adsorption of immunoglobulin A onto oral bacteria in vivo. *J. Bacteriol.* **96**:242, 1968.

BRANDZAEG, P., I. FJELLANGER, and S. T. GJERULDSEN. Immunoglobulin A deficienty. *Science*, **160**:789, 1968.

BRECHER, G., E. F. JAKOBEK, M. A. SCHNEIDERMAN, G. Z. WILLIAMS, and P. J. SCHMIDT. Size distribution of erythrocytes. *Ann. N.Y. Acad. Sci.* **99**:242, 1962.

BREESE, S. S. An indirect ferritin-tagged antibody system for a foot-and-mouth disease virus. *J. Gen. Virol.* **8**:153, 1970.

BREESE, S. S., S. S. STONE, C. J. DEBOER, and W. R. HESS. Electron microscopy of the interaction of swine fever virus with ferritin-conjugated antibody. *Virology*, **31**:508, 1967.

BREINL, F., and P. HAUROWITZ. Chemische Untersuchungen des Präzipitates aus Hämoglobin und Anti-Hämoglobin-Serum und Bemerkungen über die Natur der Antikörper. *Z. Physiol. Chemie.* **192**:45, 1930.

BREWER, C. R., W. G. McCULLOGH, R. C. MILLS, W. G. ROESSLER, and E. J. HERBST. Application of nutrition studies for development of practical culture media for *Bacillus anthracis*. *Arch. Biochem.* **10**:77, 1946.

BRODHAGE, H., and H. FREY. Beobachtungen bei Hamagglutinationreaktion auf Bang und Tuberkulose mit menschlichen und tierischen Sera. *Z. Hyg. Infektionskrankh.* **141**:76, 1955.

BRONFENBRENNER, R. H. Changes in viscosity during lysis of bacteria by bacteriophage. *Proc. Soc. Exper. Biol. Med.* **23**:635, 1926.

BROOKS, J. B., and W. E. C. MOORE. Gas chromatographic analysis of amines and other compounds produced by several species of *Clostridium. Can. J. Microbiol.* **15**:1433, 1969.

BROOKS, J. B., V. R. DOWELL, D. C. FARSHY, and A. Y. ARMFIELD. Further studies on the differentiation of *Clostridium sordellii* from *Clostridium bifermentans* by gas chromatography. *Can J. Microbiol.* **16**:1071, 1970.

BROOKSBY, J. B. Differential diagnosis of vesicular stomatitis and foot-and-mouth disease. Examination of virus from Mexico with special reference to complement fixation. *J. Hygiene,* **47**:384, 1949.

BROOKSBY, J. B. The technique of complement fixation in foot-and-mouth disease research. *Agric. Res. Counc. Rep. Ser.,* No. 12, London, 1952.

BROWN, E., and L. P. HALL. Separation of carboxylate ions on the paper chromatogram. *Nature,* **166**:66, 1950.

BROWN, F., and J. CRICK. Specific precipitin reactions with the viruses of foot-and-mouth disease and vesicular stomatitis. *Nature,* **179**:316, 1957.

BROWN, F., and J. CRICK. Application of agar-gel diffusion analysis to a study of the antigenic structure of inactivated vaccines prepared from the virus of foot-and-mouth disease. *J. Immunol.* **82**:444, 1959.

BROWN, H. C., and J. C. BROOM. Studies in trypanosomiasis. II. Observations on the red cell adhesion test. *Trans. Roy. Soc. Trop. Med.* **32**:209, 1938.

BROWN, J. B., and D. K. KOLB. Applications of low temperature crystallization in the separation of fatty acids and their compounds. *Progr. Chem. Fats Lipids,* **3**:57, 1955.

BROWN, M. R. W., J. H. S. FOSTER, and J. R. CLAMP. Composition of *Pseudomonas aeruginosa* slime. *Biochem. J.* **112**:521, 1969.

BROWN, R. Chemical and immunological studies of the pneumococcus. V. The soluble specific substances of type I-XXXII. *J. Immunol.* **37**:445, 1939.

BRUNIUS, F. E. Chemical studies on the true Forssman-hapten, the corresponding antibody and their interaction. *Ark. Kem. Mineral.* **12**:18, 1936.

BUCHBINDER, L. Heterophile phenomena in immunology. *Arch. Pathol.* **19**:841, 1935.

BUCHNER, H. Ueber die bakterientötende Wirkung des zellenfreien Blutserums. *Centralbl. Bakteriol. Parasit.* **VI**:817, 1889.

BUCHNER, H. Ueber Bakteriengifte und Gegengifte. *Munch. Med. Wochenschr.* **24**:25, 1893.

BUCKLEY, S. M. Visualization of poliomyelitis virus by fluorescent antibody. *Arch. Ges. Virusforsch.* **6**:388, 1956.

BUCKLEY, S. M. Cytopathology of poliomyelitis virus in tissue culture. Fluorescent antibody and tincturial studies. *Amer. J. Pathol.* **33**:69, 1957.

BUKANTZ, S., C. REIN, and J. KENT. Studies in complement fixation. II. Preservation of sheep's blood in citrate dextrose mixtures (modified Alsever's solution) for use in the complement fixation reaction. *J. Lab. Clin. Med.* **31**:394, 1946.

BULLOCK, W. E., and F. S. KANTOR. Hemagglutination reactions of human erythrocytes conjugated covalently with dinitrophenyl groups. *J. Immunol.* **94**:317, 1965.

BUNN, C. R., B. B. KEELE, JR., and G. H. ELKAN. A technique for improved thin-layer chromatography of phospholipids. *J. Chromatog.* **45**:326, 1969.

BUNNEY, W., and M. MIAMIL. The speed of flocculation of diphtheria toxin. *J. Immunol.* **20**:433, 1931.

BURGDORFER, W. Evaluation of the fluorescent antibody technique for the detection of Rocky Mountain spotted fever rickettsiae in various tissues. *Pathol. Microb.* **24**, Suppl., 27, 1961.

BURGDORFER, W., and D. LACKMAN. Identification of the virus Colorado tick fever in mouse tissues by means of fluorescent antibodies. *J. Bacteriol.* **80**:131, 1960.

BURGDORFER, W., and D. LACKMAN. Identification of *Rickettsia rickettsii* in the wood tick, *Dermacentor andersoni*, by means of fluorescent antibody. *J. Infect. Dis.* **107**:241, 1960.

BURGER, M. Microscopic observation of collodion particles as indicators of type specific meningococcus immune reaction. *J. Lab. Clin. Med.* **28**:1128, 1943.

BURNET, F. M. Growth of influenza viruses in the allantoic cavity of the chick embryo. *Austral. J. Biol. Med. Sci.* **19**:291, 1941.

BURNET, F. M. Vaccinia hemagglutinin. *Nature,* **158**:119, 1946.

BURNET, F. M. *Enzyme Antigen and Virus.* Cambridge University Press, Cambridge, 1956.

BURNET, F. M. A modification of Jerne's theory of antibody production using the concept of clonal selection. *Austral. J. Sci.* **20**:67, 1957.

BURNET, F. M. *The Clonal Selection Theory of Acquired Immunity.* Vanderbilt University Press, Nashville, Tenn., 1959.

BURNET, F. M. Auto-immune disease: some general principles. *Postgraduate Med.* **30**:91, 1961.

BURNET, F. M., and S. G. ANDERSON. Modification of human red cells by virus action. II. Agglutination of modified human red blood cells by sera from cases of infectious mononucleosis. *Brit. J. Exper. Pathol.* **27**:236, 1946.

BURNET, F. M., and S. G. ANDERSON. The "T" antigen of guinea pig and human red blood cells. *Austral. J. Exper. Biol. Med. Sci.* **25**:214, 1947.

BURNET, F. M., and F. FENNER. *The Production of Antibodies,* 2nd ed. Macmillan, New York, 1949.

BURNET, F. M., and M. A. FREEMAN. Comparative study of the inactivation of a bacteriophage by immune serum and by bacterial polysaccharide. *Austral. J. Exper. Biol. Med. Sci.* **15**:48, 1937.

BURNET, F. M., E. V. KEOGH, and D. LUSH. The immunological reactions of filterable viruses. *Austral. J. Exper. Biol. Med. Sci.* **15**:226, 1937.

BURNET, F. M., and D. LUSH. Influenza strains isolated from the Melbourne, 1939, epidermic. *Austral J. Exper. Biol. Med. Sci.* **18**:49, 1940.

BURNET, F. M., J. MCCREA, and J. STONE. Modification of human red blood cells by virus action. I. The receptor gradient for virus action in human red blood cells. *Brit. J. Exper. Pathol.* **27**:228, 1946.

BURROWS, W., M. ELLIOTT, and I. HAYENS. Studies on immunity in Asiatic cholera. The excretion of coproantibody in experimental enteric cholers in the guinea pig. *J. Infect. Dis.* **81**:261, 1947.

BURTON, K. A study of the conditions of mechanism of the diphenylamine reaction for the colorimetric estimation of deoxyribonucleic acid. *Biochem. J.* **62**:315, 1956.

BURTON, R. M., and A. SAN PIETRO. The paper chromatography of oxidized and reduced pyridine nucleotides. *Arch. Biochem. Biophys.* **48**:184, 1954.

BUSSARD, A. E., and J. L. BINET. Electron micrography of antibody-producing cells. *Nature,* **205**:675, 1965.

BUSSARD, A. E. Antibody formation in nonimmune mouse peritoneal cells after incubation in gum containing antigen. *Science,* **153**:887, 1966.

BUTEAU, G. H., JR., and J. E. SIMMONS. Determination of nucleoside composition of deoxyribonucleic acid by thin-layer chromatography. *Anal. Biochem.* **37**:461, 1970.

BUTLER, E. C. B., and F. C. O. VALENTINE. Further observation on acute staphylococcal infection. *Lancet,* **1**:194, 1943.

CALDWELL, W. J., C. S. STULBERG, and W. D. PETERSON, JR. Somatic and flagellar immunofluorescence of *Salmonella*. *J. Bacteriol*. **92**:1177, 1966.

CAMPBELL, D. H., and N. BULMAN. Some current concepts of the chemical nature of antigens and antibodies. *Fortschr. Chem. Org. Naturstoffe*, **9**:443, 1952.

CAMPBELL, D. H., and L. FAUST. Immunochemistry of catalase. *J. Biol. Chem*. **129**:385, 1939.

CAMPBELL, D. H., J. S. GARVEY, N. E. CRAMER, and D. H. SUSSDORF. *Methods in Immunology*, 2nd ed. W. A. Benjamin, New York, 1970.

CAMPBELL, D. H., E. LUESCHER, and L. S. LERMAN. Immunologic absorbents. I. Isolation of antibody by means of a cellulose-protein antigen. *Proc. Natl. Acad. Sci. U.S*. **37**:575, 1951.

CAMPBELL, L. L., JR. Bacterial spore germination-definition and methods of study. In *Conference on Bacterial Spores*. University of Illinois Press, Urbana, Ill., 1957.

CANN, J. R., R. A. BROWN, and J. C. KIRKWOOD. Application of electrophoresis-convection to the fractionation of bovine gamma-globulin. *J. Biol. Chem*. **181**:161, 1949.

CANN, J. R., D. H. CAMPBELL, R. A. BROWN, and J. C. KIRKWOOD. Fractionation of rabbit antiserum by electrophoresis convection. *J. Amer. Chem. Soc*. **73**:4611, 1951.

CANNEFAX, C. R., and W. CARSON. Reiter protein complement fixation test for syphilis. *Publ. Health Rep*. **72**:335, 1957.

CANNON, P. R., and C. E. MARSHALL. An improved serologic method for the determination of the precipitative titers of antisera. *J. Immunol*. **38**:365, 1940.

CANNON, P. R., and C. E. MARSHALL. Studies on the mechanism of the Arthus phenomenon. *J. Immunol*. **40**:127, 1941.

CANTOW, M. J. R. (Ed.) *Polymer Fractionation*. Academic Press, New York, 1967, Chapter B-1, B-2, B-3, and B-4.

CAREY, W. F., and L. S. BARON. Comparative immunologic studies of cell wall structures isolated from *Salmonella typhosa*. *Bacteriol. Proc*. **74**:1958; *J. Immunol*. **83**:1517, 1959.

CARLISLE, H. N., V. HINCHLIFFE, and S. SASLAW. Immunodiffusion studies with *Pasteurella tularensis* antigen-rabbit antibody systems. *J. Immunol*. **89**:638, 1962.

CARNAGIE, P. R., and G. PACHECO. Immunochromatography: A combination of chromatography and immunodiffusion on a micro-scale. *Proc. Soc. Exper. Biol. Med*. **117**:137, 1964.

CARPENTER, C. M. Brucellosis. In Hull, *Diseases Transmitted from Man and Animals*, Thomas, Springfield, Ill., 1955.

CARPENTER, C. M., M. FUKUDA, and C. L. HEISKELL. Cytometric assay of toxicity of *Brucella* antigens for sensitized and non-sensitized cells from the guinea pig. *J. Exper. Med*. **115**:613, 1962.

CARPENTER, P. L. *Immunology and Serology*. Saunder, Philadelphia and London, 1958.

CARREL, L., and R. INGEBRIGTSEN. The production of antibodies by tissues living outside of the organism. *J. Exper. Med*. **15**:287, 1912.

CARRERE, L., and I. ROUX. Hémagglutination passive d'hématies sensibilisées par antigenes brucelliques on des substances soluble spécifiques. *Ann. Inst. Pasteur*, **83**:810, 1952.

CARTER, B. B. The production of Rh antiserum in guinea pig through inoculation with human red blood cells. *Amer. J. Clin. Path*. **15**:278, 1945.

CARTER, C. H., and J. M. LEISE. Specific staining of various bacteria with a single fluorescent anti-globulin. *J. Bacteriol*. **76**:152, 1958.

CARTER, G. B. The rapid detection, titration, and differentiation of variola and vaccinia viruses by a fluorescent antibody-coverslip cell monolayer system. *Virology*, **25**:659, 1965.

CARTER, R. O., and J. HALL. The physical chemical investigation of certain nucleoproteins. I. Preparation and general properties. *J. Amer. Chem. Soc*. **62**:1194, 1940.

CASALS, J. Acetone-ether extracted antigens for complement fixation with certain neutropic viruses. *Proc. Soc. Exper. Biol. Med.* **7**:339, 1949.

CASALS, J., and L. V. BROWN. Hemagglutination with arthropod-borne viruses. *J. Exper. Med.* **99**:429, 1954.

CASALS, J., and J. FREUND. Sensitization and antibody formation in monkeys injected with tubercle bacilli in paraffin oil. *J. Immunol.* **36**:399, 1939.

CASALS, J., and R. PALACIOS. The complement fixation test in the diagnosis of virus infections of the central nervous system. *J. Exper. Med.* **74**:409, 1941.

CASPER, W. The preparation of the type-specific carbohydrates of gonococci. *J. Immunol.* **32**:421, 1937.

CASTAÑEDA, M. R. Studies on the mechanism of immunity in typhus fever. *J. Immunol.* **31**:285, 1936.

CASTAÑEDA, M. R. Selective agglutination. A possible substitute for the absorptive test in the classification of *Brucella* saccharides and their antisera. *J. Immunol.* **43**:203, 1942.

CASTAÑEDA, M. R. Differentiation of typhus strains by slide-agglutination test. *J. Immunol.* **50**:179, 1945.

CASTAÑEDA, M. R. Preparation and purification of rickettsial suspensions. *J. Immunol.* **58**:283, 1948.

CASTAÑEDA, M. R. Surface fixation. *Proc. Soc. Exper. Biol. Med.* **73**:46, 1950.

CASTAÑEDA, M. R., and R. SILVA. Immunological relationship between spotted fever and exanthematic typhus. *J. Immunol.* **42**:127, 1942.

CASTAÑEDA, M. R., R. SILVA, and A. MONNIER. Diagnostica expesifical y na especificio del tifa exantematico. *Revista Med. Hosp. Gener.* **2**:382, 1940.

CASTAÑEDA, M. R., R. TOVAR, and R. VELEZ. Studies on brucellosis in Mexico. Comparative study of various diagnostic tests and classification of isolated bacteria. *J. Infect. Dis.* **70**:97, 1942.

CASTAÑEDA, M. R., and S. ZIA. The antigenic relationship between Proteus X-19 and typhus rickettsiae. A study of the Weil-Felix reaction. *J. Exper. Med.* **58**:55, 1933.

CASTELLANI, A. Die Agglutination bei gemischter Infektion und die Diagnose der letzteren. *Z. Hygiene*, **40**:1, 1902.

CAVELTI, P. A. The technic of collodion particle agglutination. *J. Immunol.* **58**:141, 1948.

CAWLEY, L. P., L. EBERHARDT, and D. SCHNEIDER. Simplified gel electrophoresis. II. Application of immunoelectrophoresis. *J. Lab. Clin. Med.* **65**:342, 1965.

CAYEUX, P. Étude immunologique de l'antigene précipitant specifique du type 24 de Streptococcus pyogenes (groupe A). *Ann. Inst. Pasteur*, **103**:24, 1962.

CEBRA, J. J., D. GIVOL, and E. KATCHALSKI. Soluble complexes of antigen and antibody fragments. *J. Biol. Chem.* **237**:751, 1962.

CEBRA, J. J., and G. GOLDSTEIN. Chromatographic purification of tetramethyl rhodamine-immune globulin conjugates and their use in the cellular localization of rabbit γ-globulin polypeptide chains. *J. Immunol.* **95**:230, 1965.

CEBRA, J. J., and J. B. ROBBINS. γA immunoglobulin from rabbit colostrum. *J. Immunol.* **97**:12, 1966.

CEGLOWSKI, W. S., and H. FRIEDMAN. Immunosuppression by leukemia viruses. IV. Effect of Friend leukemia virus on antibody-precursors as assessed by cell transfer studies. *J. Immunol.* **105**:1406, 1970.

CEPELLINI, R., and M. DE GREGORIO. Emagglutinazione ed emolisi condizionate mediante gli antigeni della *Sallmonella typhi*. *Bol. Ist. Sieroterap. Milan.* **32**:429, 1953.

CERIOTTI, G. A microchemical determination of desoxyribonucleic acid. *J. Biol. Chem.* **198**:297, 1952.

CERNOVODEANU, P., and V. HENRI. Activation du povoir hémolytique de certain sérums par les sels de magnesium. *Compt. Rend. Soc. Biol.* **60**:571, 1906.

CHADWICK, C. S., M. G. MCENTEGART, and R. C. NAIRN. Fluorescent protein tracers. A trial of new fluorochromes and the development of an alternative to fluorescein. *Immunol.* **1**:315, 1958.

CHAMBERS, L. A., J. P. BATEMAN, and H. E. CALKINS. Further studies of the orientation of reactive sites in thin films of streptococcal antigens. *J. Immunol.* **41**:483, 1941.

CHAMBERS, L. A., and E. W. FLOSDORF. Sonic extraction of labile bacterial constituents. *Proc. Soc. Exper. Biol. Med.* **34**:631, 1936.

CHAN, P. C. Y., and J. J. CEBRA. Isolation and purification of the fourth component of guinea-pig complement. *Immunochemistry*, **5**:17, 1968.

CHANARIN, T. An investigation of *Neisseria gonorrhoeae* by a red cell sensitization technique. *J. Hygiene*, **52**:425, 1954.

CHANG, R. S. A serologically active erythrocyte-sensitizing substance from typhus rickettsiae. *J. Immunol.* **70**:212, 1953.

CHANG, R. S. and D. MCCOOMB. Erythrocyte sensitizing substances from five strains of leptospirae. *Amer. J. Trop. Med.* **3**:481, 1954.

CHANG, R. S., E. S. MURRAY, and J. C. SNYDER. Erythrocyte-sensitizing substances from rickettsiae of the Rocky Mountain spotted fever group. *J. Immunol.* **73**:8, 1954.

CHANOCK, R. M., and A. B. SABIN. The hemagglutinin of St. Louis encephalitis virus. *J. Immunol.* **70**:271–285, and 302–316, 1953.

CHANOCK, R. M., and A. B. SABIN. The hemagglutinin of Western Equine encephalitis virus: recovery, properties and use for diagnosis. *J. Immunol.* **73**:337, 1954.

CHANOCK, R. M., and A. B. SABIN. The hemagglutinin of West Nile virus: recovery, properties and antigenic relationships. *J. Immunol.* **73**:352, 1954.

CHAPLIN, H., S. COHEN, and E. M. PRESS. Preparation and properties of the peptide chains of normal 19s γ-globulin (IgM). *Biochem J.* **95**:256, 1965.

CHAPPLE, P. J., E. T. W. BOWEN, and N. D. LEWIS. Some observations on the use of the Ouchterlony gel diffusion technique in the study of myxomatosis. *J. Hyg. Camb.* **61**:373, 1963.

CHARKES, M. D. Hemagglutination test in tularemia. *J. Immunol.* **83**:213, 1959.

CHASTEL, C., and J. VIRAT. Essai d'interprétation de certaines de faillances de la réaction de fixation du complément dans la poliomyelité au moyen de la réaction d'inhibition de la fixation du complément. *Ann. Inst. Pasteur*, **101**:505, 1961.

CHATTAWAY, F. W., M. R. HOLMES, and A. J. E. BARLOW. Cell wall composition of the mycelial and blastospore forms of *Candida albicans. J. Gen. Microbiol.* **51**:367, 1968.

CHEN, P. S., JR., T. Y. TORIBARA, and H. WARNER. Microdetermination of phosphorus. *Anal. Chem.* **28**:1756, 1956.

CHEN, T. H. Studies on immunization against plague. The method of the hemagglutination test and some observations on the antigen. *J. Immunol.* **69**:587, 1952.

CHEN, T. H., and K. F. MEYER. A hemagglutination test with the protein fraction of *Pasteurella pestis. J. Immunol.* **72**:282, 1954.

CHEN, T. H., and K. F. MEYER. An evaluation of *Pasteurella pestis* fraction. I. Specific antibody for the confirmation of plague infections. *Bull. Wld. Hlth. Org.* **34**:911, 1966.

CHEN, T. H., and K. F. MEYER. Studies on immunization against plague. Specific precipitation of *Pasteurella pestis* antigens and antibodies in gels. *J. Immunol.* **74**:501, 1955.

CHEN, T. H., S. QUAN, and K. F. MEYER. Studies on immunization against plague. II. The complement-fixation test. *J. Immunol.* **68**:147, 1952.

CHERRY, W. B., and M. D. MOODY. Fluorescent-antibody techniques in diagnostic bacteriology. *Bacteriol. Rev.* **29**:222, 1965.

CHIDLOW, J. W., J. STEPHEN, and H. SMITH. Further studies on the specific quantitative aspects of antigen adsorption by disulphide-linked antibody immunosorbents. *Immunochemistry*, **7**:505, 1970.

CHOWN, B. Rapid, simple and economical method for Rh agglutination. *Amer. J. Clin. Path. Techn. Sect.* **14**:194, 1944.

CHRISTENSEN, L. R. Methods for measuring the activity of components of the streptococcal fibrinolytic system, and streptococcal desoxyribonuclease. *J. Clin. Invest.* **28**:163, 1949.

CHRISTIAN, C. L., R. MENDEZ-BRYAN, and D. L. LARSON. Latex agglutination test for disseminated lupus erythematosus. *Proc. Soc. Exper. Biol. Med.* **98**:220, 1958.

CHU, C. M., and R. R. A. COOMBS. Modification of human red cells by virus action. Agglutination by "incomplete" Rh antibodies. *Lancet*, **I**:484, 1947.

CHUN, D., and R. HOYT. Reaction of T Vi and ballerup Vi haptens with antisera against Vi-coated erythrocytes. *J. Hygiene*, **52**:100, 1954.

CHUN, D., and B. PARK. Demonstration of *Shigella flexneri* antigens by means of hemagglutination. *J. Infect. Dis.* **98**:82, 1956.

CHUN, D., Y. T. YOUNG, and H. R. PARK. A study of tannic acid hemagglutination test with antigenic substances of *Shigella flexneri. J. Infect. Dis.* **100**:241, 1957.

CIANCIARULO, J., and W. MALCOLM. Hemolytic streptococcus toxins and antitoxins. IV. The concentration of scarlet fever streptococcus antitoxin. *J. Immunol.* **28**:47, 1935.

CITROL, J. Die Serodiagnostik der Syphilis. *Berl. Klin. Wochenschr.* **44**:1370, 1907.

CIUCA, A. The reaction of complement fixation in foot-and-mouth disease as a means of identifying the different types of virus. *J. Hygiene*, **28**:325, 1929.

CLARK, H. W., J. S. BAILEY, R. C. FOWLER, and T. P. BROWN. Identification of *Mycoplasmataceae* by the fluorescent antibody method. *J. Bacteriol.* **85**:111, 1963.

CLAYTON, G. D. Improvement of M.S.A. electrostatic precipitator. *J. Indust. Hyg. Toxicol.* **29**:400, 1947.

CLAYTON, R. M. Localization of embryonic antigens by antisera labelled with fluorescent dyes. *Nature*, **174**:1059, 1954.

CLEGHORN, R. H., and L. JENDRASSIK. Photometrische Stickstoffbestimmung. *Biochem. Zeitschr.* **274**:189, 1934.

CLOUGH, M. C., and I. M. RICHTER. A study of an autoagglutinin occurring in a human serum. *Bull. Johns Hopkins Hosp.* **29**:86, 1918.

CLYDE, W. A., JR., F. W. DENNY, and J. H. DINGLE. Fluorescent-stainable antibodies to the Eaton agent in human primary atypical pneumonia transmission studies. *J. Clin. Investig.* **40**:1638, 1961.

COBURN, A. F., and E. M. KAPP. The effect of salicylates on the precipitation of antigen with antibody. *J. Exper. Med.* **77**:173, 1943.

COBURN, A. F., and R. H. PAULI. Studies on the immunological response of the rheumatic subject and its relationship to activity of the rheumatic process. I. The determination of antistreptolysin titer. *J. Exper. Med.* **62**:129, 1935.

COBURN, A. F., and R. H. PAULI. Significance of prolonged streptococcal antibody development in rheumatic fever. *J. Clin. Invest.* **18**:141, 1939.

COCA, A. The site of reaction in anaphylactic shock. *Z. Immunitätsforsch.* **20**:622, 1914.

COFFIN, D. L., A. H. COONS, and V. J. CABASSO. A histological study of infectious canine hepatitis by means of fluorescent antibody. *J. Exper. Med.* **38**:13, 1953.

COHEN, C. Blood group factors in the rabbit. *J. Immunol.* **74**:432, 1955.

COHEN, C., and L. FERGUSON. Quantitative studies on the hemolytic test. *J. Immunol.* **71**:15, 1953.

COHEN, J. O., and P. OEDING. Serological typing of staphylococci by means of fluorescent antibodies. I. Development of specific reagents for seven serological factors. *J. Bacteriol.* **84**:735, 1962.

COHEN, S., and A. G. COOPER. Chemical differences between individual human cold agglutinins. *Immunology*, **15**:93, 1968.

COHEN, S., and R. R. PORTER. Heterogeneity of the peptide chains of γ-globulin. *Biochem. J.* **90**:278, 1964.

COHEN, S. M. Determination of antibody through the use of I[131] label; experiments with equine diphtheria antitoxin. *J. Immunol.* **67**:339, 1951.

COHEN, S. M., C. P. DUCHARME, C. A. CARPENTER, and R. DIEBEL. Rubella antibody in IgG and IgM immunoglobulins detected by immunocluorescence. *J. Lab. Clin. Med.* **72**:760, 1968.

COHEN, S. M., I. GORDON, F. RAPP, J. C. MACAULEY, and S. M. BUCKLEY. Fluorescent antibody and complement-fixation test of agents in tissue culture from measles patients. *Proc. Soc. Exper. Biol. Med.* **90**:118, 1955.

COHN, E. J., J. L. ONKLEY, L. E. STRONG, W. L. HUGHES, and S. H. ARMSTRONG, JR. Chemical, clinical and immunological studies on the products of human plasma fractionation. I. The characterization of the protein fractions of human plasma. *J. Clin. Invest.* **23**:417, 1944.

COHN, E. J., L. E. STRONG, W. L. HUGHES, D. I. MULFORD, J. N. ASHWORT, M. MELIN, and H. L. TAYLOR. Preparation and properties of serum and plasma proteins. IV. A system for the separation into fractions of the protein and lipoprotein components of biological tissues and fluids. *J. Amer. Chem. Soc.* **68**:459, 1946.

COHN, M., and A. M. PAPPENHEIMER, JR. A quantitative study of the diphtheria toxin-antitoxin reaction in the sera of various species including man. *J. Immunol.* **63**:291, 1949.

COLE, L., and V. FARRELL. A method for coupling protein antigens to erythrocytes. *J. Exper. Med.* **102**:631, 1955.

COLE, R. M. Cell wall replication in Salmonella typhosa. *Science*, **143**:820, 1964.

COLEMAN, G. E., and J. B. GUNNISON. Serologic types of *Clostridium tetani*. *J. Infect. Dis.* **43**:184, 1928.

COLLI, W., and M. OISHI. A procedure for gene purification: The purification of ribosomal RNA genes of *Bacillus subtilis* as DNA-RNA hybrids. *J. Mol. Biol.* **51**:657, 1970.

COLLIER, W., and M. JACOBS. Experiments with a haemagglutinating strain of *E. coli*. *Ant. van Loewenhoek*, *J. Microbiol.* **21**:113, 1955.

COLON, J. I., and J. W. MOULDER. Folic acid in purified preparations of members of psittacosis group of micro-organisms. *J. Infect. Dis.* **79**:741, 1960.

COLTEN, H. R., T. BORSOS, and H. J. RAPP. Reversible loss of activity of the first component of complement (C'1) as a function of ionic strength. *J. Immunol.* **100**:799, 1968.

COLTEN, H. R., J. M. GORDON, H. J. RAPP, and T. BORSOS. Synthesis of the first component of guinea pig complement by columnar epithelial cells of the small intestine. *J. Immunol.* **100**:788, 1968.

COLTER, J. S., R. A. BROWN, H. H. BIRD, and H. R. COX. The preparation of a soluble immunizing antigen from Q fever rickettsiae. *J. Immunol.* **76**:270, 1956.

COMBIESCO, D., E. SORU, and C. COMBIESCO. Immunological properties of glucidelipide complexes extracted from typhoid bacilli. *Compt. Rend. Soc. Biol.* **129**:1003, 1938.

COMBIESCO, D., E. SORU, and S. STAMATESCO. Les substances solubles specifiques de la bacteridie charbonneuse. Proprietes chemique et biologiques. *Compt. Rend. Soc. Biol.* **102**:124, 1929.

Committee on Standard Serological Procedures in Influenza Studies. An agglutination-inhibition test proposed as a standard of reference in influenza diagnostic studies. *J. Immunol.* **65**:347, 1950.

CONSDEN, R., and J. KOHN. Immunodiffusion on cellulose acetate. *Nature*, **183**:1512, 1959.

CONSDEN, R., and W. M. STANIER. Ionophoresis of sugars on paper and some applications to the analysis of protein polysaccharide complexes. *Nature*, **169**:793, 1952.

CONSTANTOPOULOS, G., A. S. DEKABAN, and W. R. CARROLL. Determination of molecular weight distribution of acid mucopolysaccharides by Sephadex gel filtration. *Anal. Biochem.* **31**:59, 1969.

CONTI, S. I., and H. B. NAYLOR. Electron microscopy of ultrathin sections of *Schizosaccharomyces octosporus*. I. Cell Division. *J. Bacteriol.* **78**:868, 1959.

COOK, R. J. Titration of *Clostridium oedematiens* antitoxin by reversed passive haemagglutination. *Immunology*, 9:249, 1965.

COOMBS, R. R. A., D. BEDFORD, and L. F. ROUILLARD. The A and B group antigens on human epidermal cells demonstrated by mixed agglutination. *Lancet*, 1:461, 1956.

COOMBS, R. R. A., A. M. COOMBS, and D. G. INGRAM. The serology of conglutination and its relation to disease. Blackwell Scientific Publications, Oxford, England, 1961.

COOMBS, R. R. A., M. R. DANIEL, B. W. GURNER, and A. KELUS. Recognition of the species of origin of cells in culture by mixed agglutination. I. Use of antisera to red blood cells. *Immunology*, 4:55, 1961.

COOMBS, R. R. A., and B. DODD, Possible application of the principle of mixed agglutination in the identification of blood stains. *Med. Sci. Law*, 1:359, 1961.

COOMBS, R. R. A., and M. FISET. Detection of complete and incomplete antibodies to egg albumen by means of sheep red cell egg albumen antigen unit. *Brit. J. Exper. Pathol.* 35:472, 1954.

COOMBS, R. R. A., M. H. GLEESON-WHITE, and J. G. HALL. Factors influencing the agglutinability of red cells. *Brit. J. Exper. Pathol.* 31:195, 1951.

COOMBS, R. R. A., A. HOWARD, and L. MYNORS. A serological procedure theoretically capable of detecting incomplete or non-precipitating antibodies to soluble protein antigens. *Brit. J. Exper. Pathol.* 34:525, 1953.

COOMBS, R. R. A., A. HOWARD, and E. WILD. Titration of antisera to soluble proteins on the basis of an agglutination reaction. *Brit. J. Exper. Pathol.* 33:390, 1952.

COOMBS, R. R. A., and A. E. MOURANT. On certain properties of antisera against human serum and its various protein fractions, their use in detection of sensitization of human red cells with incomplete Rh antibody and on the nature of this antibody. *J. Pathol. Bacteriol.* 59:105, 1947.

COOMBS, R. R. A., A. MOURANT, and R. RACE. A new test for detection of weak and "incomplete" Rh agglutinins. *Brit. J. Exper. Pathol.* 26:255, 1945.

COONS, A. H. Histochemistry with labeled antibody. *Int. Rev. Cytol.* 5:1, 1956.

COONS, A. H. The application of fluorescent antibodies to the study of naturally occurring antibodies. *Ann. N.Y. Acad. Sci.* 69:658, 1957.

COONS, A. H. The cytology of antibody formation. *J. Cellul. Comp. Physiol.* 52, Suppl. 55, 1958.

COONS, A. H. Fluorescent antibody method. In *General Cytochemical Methods*, J. F. Danielli, Ed. Vol. 1. Academic Press, New York, 1958, p. 399, 400.

COONS, A. H., H. J. CREECH, and R. N. JONES. Immunological properties of an antibody containing fluorescent groups. *Proc. Soc. Exper. Biol. Med.* 47:200, 1941.

COONS, A. H., H. J. CREECH, R. N. JONES, and E. BERLINER. The demonstration of pneumococcal antigens in tissues by means of fluorescent antibody. *J. Immunol.* 45:159, 1942.

COONS, A. H., and R. N. JONES. The conjugation of horse serum albumin with 1,2 benzathryl-isocyanates. *J. Amer. Chem. Soc.* 62:1970, 1940.

COONS, A. H., and R. N. JONES. Conjugates synthesized from various proteins and the isocyanates of certain aromatic polynuclear hydrocarbons. *J. Amer. Chem. Soc.* 63:1661, 1941.

COONS, A. H., and M. H. KAPLAN. Localization of antigen in tissue cells. II. Improvement in a method for the detection of antigen by means of fluorescent antibody. *J. Exper. Med.* 91:1, 1950.

COONS, A. H., E. H. LEDUC, and J. M. CONNOLLY. Studies on antibody production. I. A method for the histochemical demonstration of specific antibody and its application to a study of the hyperimmune rabbit. *J. Exper. Med.* 102:49, 1955.

COONS, A. H., E. H. LEDUC, and M. H. KAPLAN. Localization of antigen in tissue cells. VI. The fate of injected foreigh proteins in the mouse. *J. Exper. Med.* 93:173, 1951.

COONS, A. H., J. C. SNYDER, F. S. CHEEVER, and E. S. MURRAY. Localization of antigen in tissue cells. IV. Antigens of rickettsiae and mumps virus. *J. Exper. Med.* **91**:31, 1950.

COOPER, N. R., and H. J. MÜLLER-EBERHARD. A comparison of methods for the molecular quantitation of the fourth component of human complement. *Immunochemistry*, **5**:155, 1968.

CORDEN, M. E. Paper chromatography of galacturonic acids to determine polygalacturonase activity. *Biochim. Biophys. Acta*, **83**:124, 1964.

CORIELL, L., D. P. FABRIZIO, and S. R. WILSON. Comparison of PPLO strains from tissue culture by complement fixation. *Ann. N.Y. Acad. Sci.* **79**:574, 1962.

CORRIGAN, M. Antibody response to large and small doses of multiple and of single antigens, and restimulation of specific antibody formation by heterologous antigens. *J. Infect. Dis.* **37**:549, 1925.

CORVAZIER, P. Etude de l'antigene Vi a l'aide d'une téchnique d'hémagglutination passive. *Ann. Inst. Pasteur*, **83**:173, 1952.

COSTLOW, R. D. Lecithinase from *Bacillus anthracis*. *J. Bacteriol.* **76**:217, 1958.

COTA-ROBLES, E. H., A. G. MARR, and E. H. NILSON. Submicroscopic particles in extracts of *Azotobacter agilis*. *J. Bacteriol.* **75**:243, 1958.

COX, C. D. Hemolysis of sheep erythrocytes sensitized with leptospiral extracts. *Proc. Soc. Exper. Biol. Med.* **90**:610, 1955.

COX, C. D., and S. D. VERMILLION. Preservation of sheep erythrocytes and their use in a rapid plate titration of heterophilic antibodies in infectious mononucleosis. *J. Lab. Clin. Med.* **48**:299, 1956.

COZAD, G. C., and H. W. LARSH. A capillary tube agglutination test for histoplasmosis. *J. Immunol.* **85**:387, 1960.

CRĂCEA, E., R. VOILESCU, G. ZARNEA, M. IONESCU, and D. BOLEZ. Electron microscopic study of phase I and II *C. burnetii* in the chick yold sac by use of ferritin conjugated antibody. *Z. Immun. Forsch.* **140**:358, 1970.

CRADDOCK, C. G., JR., and J. S. LAWRENCE. The effect of Roentgen irradiation on antibody formation in rabbits. *J. Immuniol.* **60**:241, 1948.

CRAIG, L. C. In *A Laboratory Manual of Analytical Methods of Protein Chemistry*. (P. Alexander and R. J. Block, eds.), **1**:211, Pergamon Press, Oxford, 1960.

CRAIG, L. C., and D. CRAIG. *Technique of Organic Chemistry*, 2nd ed., 1956.

CRAIG, L. C., and W. H. KONIGSBERG. Dialysis studies. III. Modification of pore size and shape in cellophane membranes. *J. Phys. Chem.* **65**:166, 1961.

CRAIG, L. C., and K. STEWART. Thin-film countercurrent dialysis. *Biochemistry*, **4**:2712, 1965.

CRAIGIE, J. Studies on the serological reactions of the flagella of *B. typhosa*. *J. Immunol.* **21**:417, 1931.

CRAIGIE, J. Application and control of ethyl-ether-water surface effect to separation of *Rickettsia* from yolk sac suspensions. *Canad. J. Res.* **23**:104, 1945.

CRAIGIE, J., and W. TULLOCH. *Spec. Rep. Ser. Med. Res. Counc. London*, No. 156, 1931.

CRAMER, R. Zone electrophoresis of Rous sarcoma. *Nature*, **183**:195, 1959.

CRAMER, R., and S. E. STEWART. Zone electrophoresis studies on hemagglutinin of hemagglutinating and masked strain of pyeloma virus. *Proc. Soc. Exper. Biol. Med.* **103**:697, 1960.

CRAMER, R., and H. SVENSSON. Density gradient electrophoresis as a new tool in virology. *Experientia*, **17**:49, 1961.

CRAMPTON, C. F., and F. HAUROWITZ. Deposition of small doses of injected antigen in rabbits. *J. Immunol.* **69**:457, 1952.

CRAMPTON, C. F., H. H. RELLER, and F. HAUROWITZ. Deposition of beef serum gamma-globulin in rabbit organs and subcellular fractions. *J. Immunol.* **71**:319, 1953.

CRAWFORD, Y. E., and J. J. ROBINSON. Method for determining antistreptolysin O titer using capillary blood. *Amer. J. Clin. Pathol.* **24**:1103, 1954.

CREECH, H. J., and R. M. JONES. The conjugation of horse serum-albumin with isocyanates of certain polynuclear aromatic hydrocarbons. *J. Amer. Chem. Soc.* **63**:1661, 1941.

CREIGHTON, M. M., and R. J. ANDERSON. The chemistry of the tubercle bacillus (H37) cultivated on dextrose-containing medium. *J. Biol. Chem.* **154**:509, 1944.

CROWLE, A. J. A simplified micro double-diffusion agar precipitation technique. *J. Lab. Clin. Med.* **52**:784, 1958.

CROWLE, A. J. Immunizing constituents of the tubercle bacillus. *Bacteriol. Rev.* **22**:183, 1958.

CROWLE, A. J. Interpretation of immunodiffusion tests. *Ann. Rev. Microbiol.* **14**:161, 1960.

CROWLE, A. J., and D. C. LUEKER. Microimmunoelectrophoresis: Comparison of template with nontemplate methods. *J. Lab. Clin. Med.* **59**:697, 1962.

CRUICKSHANK, B., and A. R. CURRIE. Localization of tissue antigens with the fluorescent antibody technique: application to human pituitary hormones. *Immunology*, **I**:13, 1958.

CRUICKSHANK, B., and A. G. S. HILL. The histochemical identification of a connective-tissue antigen in the rat. *J. Pathol. Bacteriol.* **66**:283, 1953.

CRUICKSHANK, J., and G. FREEMAN. Immunizing fractions isolated from *Haemophilus pertussis*. *Lancet*, **II**:507, 1937.

CRUMPTON, M. J., and J. M. WILKINSON. Amino acid compositions of human and rabbit γ-globulins and of the fragments produced by reduction. *Biochem. J.* **88**:228, 1963.

CRUZ, W. Quantitative method of titrating anti-platellet serum in vitro. *J. Immunol.* **71**:346, 1953.

CULBERTSON, J. A quantitative study of the precipitin reaction with special reference to crystalline egg albumen and its antibody. *J. Immunol.* **23**:438, 1932.

CUMLEY, R. G., and M. IRWIN. Individual specificity of human serum. *J. Immunol.* **46**:63, 1941.

CUMMINS, C. S. Some observations on the nature of the antigens in the cell wall of *Corynebacterium diphtheriae*. *Brit. J. Exper. Pathol.* **35**:166, 1954.

CUMMINS, C. S., O. GLENDENNING, and H. HARRIS. Composition of the cell wall of *Lactobacillus bifidus*. *Nature*, **180**:337, 1957.

CUMMINS, C. S., and H. HARRIS. The chemical composition of the cell wall of the *Staphylococcus-Micrococcus* group as shown by their cell wall composition. *Int. Bull. Bact. Nomen. Taxon.* **6**:111, 1956.

CUMMINS, C. S., and H. HARRIS. The chemical composition of the cell wall in some Gram-positive bacteria and its possible value as a taxonomic character. *J. Gen. Microbiol.* **14**:583, 1956.

CUMMINS, C. S., and H. HARRIS. Studies in the cell composition and taxonomy of *Actinomycetales* and related groups. *J. Gen. Microbiol.* **18**:173, 1958.

CUNNINGHAM, A. J., J. B. SMITH, and E. H. MERCER. Antibody formation by single cells from lymph nodes and efferent lymph of sheep. *J. Exper. Med.* **124**:701, 1966.

CURNEN, E. C., and F. L. HORSFALL, JR. Properties of pneumonia virus of mice (P.V.M.) in relation to its state. *J. Exper. Med.* **85**:39, 1947.

CURPHEY, T. Susceptibility to pneumococcus infection as measured by species-specific agglutinins. *J. Immunol.* **28**:55, 1935.

CURTAIN, C. C. Concentrating protein solutions. *Nature*, **203**:1380, 1964.

CUSHING, J. E. A comparative study of complement. II. The interaction of components of different species. *J. Immunol.* **50**:75, 1945.

CUSHMAN, W., E. BECKER, and G. WIRTZ. Concerning the mechanism of complement action. *J. Immunol.* **79**:198, 1957.

CZISMAS, L. Preparation of formalinized erythrocytes. *Proc. Soc. Exper. Biol. Med.* **103**: 157, 1960.

DACRES, W., and W. GROTH. Identification of *Erysipelothrix insidiosa* with fluorescent antibody. *J. Exper. Pathol.* **72**: 198, 1959.

DAFAALLA, E., and M. SOLTYS. Studies on agglutination of red cells by clostridia. *J. Exper. Pathol.* **32**: 510, 1951.

DALE, H. H. The anaphylactic reaction of plain muscle in the guinea pig. *J. Pharmac. Exper. Pathol.* **4**: 167, 1913.

D'ALLESSANDRO, G., and L. DARDANONI. Isolation and purification of protein antigen of Reiter treponeme, study of its serologic reaction. *Amer. J. Syph.* **37**: 137, 1953.

DAMMIN, G., and F. BILLINGS. The Weil-Felix reaction in patients with *Proteus* and *Pseudomonas aeruginosa* infections. *J. Immunol.* **47**: 241, 1942.

DAMON, D., Y. MARKOVSKY, A. FUREDI, and I. OHAD. *Biochim. Biophys. Acta.* **104**: 281, 1964.

DANDLIKER, W. B., and V. A. DE SAUSSURE. Fluorescence polarization in immunochemistry. *Immunochemistry*, **7**: 799, 1970.

DANDLIKER, W. B., S. P. HALBERT, M. C. FLORIN, R. ALONSO, and H. C. SCHAPIRO. Study of penicillin antibodies by fluorescence polarization and immunodiffusion. *J. Exper. Med.* **122**: 1029, 1965.

DANDLIKER, W. B., and S. A. LEVISON. Investigation of antigen-antibody kinetics by fluorescence polarization. *Immunochemistry*, **5**: 171, 1967.

DANDLIKER, W. B., H. C. SCHAPIRO, J. W. MEDUSKI, R. ALONSO, G. A. FEIGEN, and J. R. HAMRICK. Application of fluorescence polarization to the antigen-antibody reaction. *Immunochemistry*, **1**: 165, 1964.

DANIEL, T. M., J. G. M. WEYAND, and A. B. STAVITSKY. Micromethods for the study of proteins and antibodies. IV. Factors involved in the preparation and use of a stable preparation of formalinized, tannic acid-treated, protein-sensitized erythrocytes for detection of antigen and antibody. *J. Immunol.* **90**: 741, 1963.

DANYSZ, J. *Ann. Inst. Pasteur*, **16**: 331, 1902.

DAOD-NATHAO, F. A., A. DODIN, and E. R. BRYGGAS. Récherches sur les antigenes de *Pasteurella pestis*. I. Antigenes de la souche E. V. étudié par précipitation en geliose. *Arch. Inst. Pasteur, Madagascar*, **27**: 9, 1959.

DARK, F. R., and R. E. STRANGE. Bacterial protoplast from *Bacillus* species by the action of autolytic enzymes. *Nature*, **180**: 759, 1957.

DATE, R. A., and A. M. DECKER. Minimal antigenic constitution of 28 strains of *Rhizobium japonicum*. *Can. J. Microbiol.* **11**: 1 1965.

DAVID, J. R., S. AL-ASKARI, H. S. LAWRENCE, and L. THOMAS. Delayed hypersensitivity in vitro. I. The specificity of inhibition of cell migration by antigens. *J. Immunol.* **93**: 264, 1964.

DAVIDSOHN, I. Heterophile antibodies in serum sickness. *J. Immunol.* **16**: 259, 1929.

DAVIDSOHN, I. Further studies on heterophile antibodies in serum sickness. *J. Immunol.* **18**: 31, 1930.

DAVIDSOHN, I. Isoagglutinin titers in serum disease, in leukemias, in infectious mononucleosis and after blood tranfusion. *Amer. J. Clin. Pathol.* **8**: 529, 1938.

DAVIDSOHN, I. Test for infectious monoucleosis. *Amer. J. Clin. Pathol. Tech. Suppl.* **2**: 56, 1938.

DAVIDSOHN, I., and B. TOHARSKY. The production of bacteriogenic hemagglutination, *J. Infect. Dis.* **67**: 25, 1940.

DAVIDSOHN, I., and B. TOHARSKY. Bacteriogenic hemagglutination. *J. Immunol.* **43**: 273, 1942.

DAVIDSON, J., J. MATHIESON, and A. W. BOYNE. The use of automation in determining nitrogen by the Kjeldahl method, with final calculations by computer. *Analyst*, **95**:181, 1970.

DAVIDSON, J. N., and R. M. S. SMELLIE. Phosphorus compounds in the cell. II. The separation by ionophoresis on paper of the constituent nucleotides of ribonucleic acid. *Biochem. J.* **52**:594, 1952.

DAVIES, D. A. L., M. J. CRUMPTON, T. D. MACPHERSON, and A. M. HUTCHISON. The absorption of bacterial polysaccharides by erythrocytes. *Immunology*, **1**:157, 1958.

DAVIES, D. A. L., W. T. J. MORGAN, and N. MOSIMAN. Studies in immunochemistry. 13. Preparation and properties of the "O" somatic antigen of *Shigella dysenteriae* (Shiga). *Biochem. J.* **56**:572, 1954.

DAVIES, D. E. A method for obtaining accurate and reproducible results in experiments on phagocytosis. *J. Pathol. Bact.* **63**:149, 1951.

DAVIS, B. Disk electrophoresis. II. Method and application to human serum proteins. *Ann. N.Y. Acad. Sci.* **121**:404, 1964.

DAVIS, B. D., D. H. MOORE, E. A. KABAT, and A. HARRIS. Electrophoretic, ultracentrifugal, and immunochemical studies of Wassermann antibody. *J. Immunol.* **50**:1, 1945.

DEACON, W. E., V. H. FALCONE, and A. D. HARRIS. A fluorescent test for treponemal antibodies. *Proc. Soc. Exper. Biol. Med.* **96**:477, 1957.

DEACON, W. E., E. W. FREEMAN, and A. HARRIS. Fluorescent treponemal antibody test. A modification based on quantitation. *Proc. Soc. Exper. Biol. Med.* **103**:827, 1960.

DEACON, W. E., J. B. LUCAS, and E. V. PRICE. Fluorescent treponemal antibody-absorption (FTA-ABS) test for syphilis. *J. Amer. Med. Assoc.* **198**:624, 1966.

DEACON, W. E., W. L. PEACOCK, E. M. FREEMAN, and A. HARRIS. Identification of *Neisseria gonorrheae* by means of fluorescent antibodies. *Proc. Soc. Exper. Biol. Med.* **101**:322, 1959.

DE ALMEIDA, J. O. Isofixation curves as a method of standardizing quantitative complement fixation tests. *J. Immunol.* **68**:567, 1952.

DE ALEMEIDA, J. O., A. M. SILVERSTEIN, and F. MALTANER. Principles governing the practical application of complement fixation tests. *J. Immunol.* **68**:567, 1952.

DEAN, H. R. An experimental inquiry into the nature of the substance in serum which influences phagocytosis. *Proc. Roy. Soc.* **76**:506, 1905.

DEAN, H. R. The relation between the fixation of complement and the formation of precipitate. *Proc. Roy. Soc. Med.* **5**:62, 1911.

DEAN, H. R. The influence of temperature on the fixation of complement. *J. Pathol. Bacteriol.* **21**:193, 1916.

DEAN, H. R., and R. A. WEBB. The influence of optimal proportion of antigen and antibody in the serum precipitation reaction. *J. Pathol. Bacteriol.* **29**:473, 1926.

DE BRUJIN, J. H. A simplified method for the preparation of Reiter protein antigen. *Antonie van Loewenhoek J. Microb.* **26**:317, 1960.

DEBURGH, P. M., P. C. YU, C. HOWE, and M. BOVARNICK. Preparation from human red cells of a substance inhibiting virus hemagglutination. *J. Exper. Med.* **87**:1, 1948.

DEDDISH, P. A., and H. D. SLADE. Detection of polysaccharide, teichoic acid, and protein antigens in bacterial colonies on an agar surface. *J. Bacteriol.* **97**:1352, 1969.

DEDEKEN- GRENSON, M., and R. H. DEDEKEN. Elimination of substances interfering with nucleic acid determination. *Biochim. Biophys. Acta*, **31**:195, 1959.

DE GARA, P., S. BUKANTZ, and J. BULLOWA. Pneumococcal capsular polysaccharide in urine; detection by precipitation and centrifugation. *J. Immunol.* **37**:305, 1939.

DE GREGORIO, M. Fissazione di antigen sulla superficie cellulare. *Boll. Ist. Sieroter. Milan*, **34**:118, 1955.

DEICHER, H. H., H. R. HOLMAN, and H. G. KUNKEL. The precipitin reaction between DNA and a serum factor in systemic lupus erythematosus. *J. Exper. Med.* **109**:97, 1959.

DEINHARDT, F., and G. HENLE. Determination of neutralizing antibodies against mumps virus in HeLa cell culture. *J. Immunol.* **77**:40, 1956.

DEL GIUDICE, R. A., N. F. ROBILLARD, and R. CARSKI. Immunofluorescence identification of mycoplasma on agar by use of incident illumination. *J. Bacteriol.* **93**:1205, 1967.

DELORY, G. E., and E. J. KING. A sodium carbonate-bicarbonate buffer for alkaline phosphatases. *Biochem. J.* **39**:245, 1945.

DELVES, E. J. *J. Infect. Dis.* **60**:55, 1937.

DENT, C. E. A study of the behaviour of some sixty amino acids and other nin-hydrin-reacting substances on phenol "cllidine" filter-paper chromatography, with notes as to the occurrence of some of them in biological fluids. *Biochem. J.* **43**:169, 1948.

DENYS, J., and J. LECLEF. Sur le méchanisme de l'immunité chez le lapin vaccine contre le streptocoque pyogene. *La Cellule,* **11**:175, 1895.

DEREPENTIGNY, J., S. SONEA, and A. FRAPIER. Comparison of quantitative immunofluorescence and immunodiffusion for the evaluation of antigenic materials from *Staphylococcus aureus. J. Bacteriol.* **86**:1348, 1963.

DEUTSCH, H. F. Separation of antibody-active proteins from various animal sera by ethanol fractionation techniques. *Methods Med. Res.* **5**:284, 1952.

DIAMOND, L. K., and W. ABELSON. Demonstration of anti-Rh agglutinins accurate and rapid slide test. *J. Lab. Clin. Med.* **30**:204, 1945.

DIAMOND, L. K., and R. DENTON. Rh agglutination in various media with particular reference to value of albumin. *J. Lab. Clin. Med.* **31**:621, 1945.

DIENA, B. B., R. WALLACE, C. P. KENNY, and L. GREENBERG. A tissue culture technique for the assay of antibacterial immune sera. *Canad. J. Microb.* **17**:13, 1971.

DIENER, E. A new method for the enumeration of single antibody-producing cells. *J. Immunol.* **100**:1062, 1968.

DIFERRANTE, N. M. The measurement of urinary mucopolysaccharides. *Anal. Biochem.* **21**:98, 1967.

DI NARDO, J. Fissazione di antigeni batterici sulla superficie di leucociti epiastrine. *Boll. Ist. Sieroter. Milan,* **37**:527, 1958.

DINGLE, J. H., and L. D. FOTHERGILL. The isolation and properties of the specific polysaccharide of type B *Hemophilus influenzae. J. Immunol.* **37**:53, 1939.

DINTER, H., and T. WESSLEN. Antikörperreaktion bei Rindern, vakziniert gegen Maul- und Klauenseuche. *Zentralbl. Bakt. I. Orig.* **171**:157, 1957.

DISCHE, Z. Über einige neue charakterischen Farbreaktionen der Thymus-nukleinsäure und eine Methode zur Bestimmung derselben in tierischen Organen mit Hilfe dieser Reaktionen. *Mikrochemie,* **2**:4, 1930.

DISCHE, Z. A new specific color reaction of hexuronic acids. *J. Biol. Chem.* **167**:189, 1947.

DISCHE, Z. A modification of the carbazole reaction of hexuronic acids for the study of polyuronides. *J. Biol. Chem.* **183**:489, 1950.

DISCHE, Z. Qualitative and quantitative colorimetric determination of heptoses. *J. Biol. Chem.* **204**:983, 1953.

DISCHE, Z. New color reactions for the determination of sugars in polysaccharides. In *Methods of Biochemical Analysis,* D. Glick, Ed., Vol. 2. Interscience, New York, 1955, p. 313.

DISCHE, Z. α-naphto measurement of carbohydrates.

DISCHE, Z., and E. BORENFREUND. A spectrophotometric method for the microdetermination of hexosamines. *J. Biol. Chem.* **184**:517, 1950.

DISCHE, Z., and E. BORENFREUND. A new spectrophotometric method for the detection and determination of keto sugars and trioses. *J. Biol. Chem.* **192**:583, 1951.

DISCHE, Z., and L. B. SHETTLES. A specific color reaction of methyl pentoses and a spectrophotometric micromethod for their determination. *J. Biol. Chem.* **175**:595, 1948.

DITTERBRANDT. M. Application of Weichselbaum Biuret reagent to the determination of spinal fluid protein. *Amer. J. Clin. Pathol.* **18**:439, 1948.

DIXON, F., R. MAURER, and M. DEICHMILLER. Primary and specific anamnestic antibody responses of rabbits to heterologous serum protein antigens. *J. Immunol.* **72**:179, 1954.

DIXON, F. J., and P. H. MAURER. Immunologic unresponsiveness induced by protein antigens. *J. Exper. Med.* **101**:245, 1955.

DOCHEZ, A., and O. AVERY. *Proc. Soc. Exper. Biol. Med.* **14**:126, 1917.

DODD, M. C., C. S. WRIGHT, B. A. BOURONCLE, J. A. BAXTER, H. J. WINN, and A. E. BRUNNER. The immunologic specificity of antiserum for trypsin-treated red blood cells and its reactions with normal and hemolytic anemia cells. *Blood*, **8**:640, 1953.

DOGGOTT, R. G., G. M. HARRISON, R. N. STILLWELL, and E. S. WALLIS. Enzymatic action on the capsular material produced by *Pseudomonas aeruginosa* of cystic fibrosis origin. *J. Bact.* **89**:476, 1965.

DOLBY, J. M. The separation of histamine-sentizing factor from the protective antigen of *Bordetella pertussis*. *Immunology* **1**:328, 1958.

DOLEZEL, J., and J. BIENENSTOCK. Immunoglobulins of the hamster. 3. Immunofluorescent localization of γA, γ1, and γ2 in various tissues. *Can. J. Microbiol.* **16**:727, 1970.

DORNBUSCH, S. The value of the gel-precipitation method for the study of autoimmunological problems. *Int. Arch. Allergy*, **11**:206, 1957.

DOWNIE, A. W. The immunological relationship of the virus of spontaneous cowpox to vaccinia virus. *Brit. J. Exper. Pathol.* **20**:158, 1939.

DOWNS, C., J. FEVURLY, and M. MEYER. Studies on hemagglutination inhibition phenomena. *J. Immunol.* **75**:35, 1955.

DRAKE, C. Natural antibodies against yeast-like fungus as measured by slide-agglutination. *J. Immunol.* **50**:185, 1945.

DRESCHER, J., A. V. HENNESSY, and F. M. DAVENPORT. Photometric methods for.the measurement of hemagglutinating viruses and antibody. I. Further experience with a novel photometric method for measuring hemagglutinins. *J. Immunol.* **89**:794, 1962.

DRESSER, D. W., and H. H. WORTIS. Use of an antiglobulin serum to detect cells producing antibody with low haemolytic efficiency. *Nature*, **208**:859, 1965.

DRESSER, D. W., and H. H. WORTIS. Localized Haemolysis in Gel. In *Handbook of Experimental Immunology*, D. M. Weir, Ed. Blackwell Science Publishers, Oxford, 1967, p. 1054.

DREYWOOD, R. *Ind. Eng. Chem. Anal. Ed.* **18**:499, 1946.

DRIMMER-HERRENHEISER, H. Hemagglutination by pseudomonas of faecal origin. *Bull. Res. Counc. Israel.* **2**:445, 1953.

DUBOIS, M., K. A. GILLES, J. K. HAMILTON, P. A. REBERS, and F. SMITH. Colorimetric method for determination of sugars and related substances. *Anal. Chem.* **28**:350, 1956.

DUBOS, R., and O. AVERY. Decomposition of the capsular polysaccharide of pneumococcus type III by a bacterial enzyme. *J. Exper. Med.* **54**:51, 1931.

DUC-NGUYEN, H., H. M. ROSE, and C. MORGAN. An electron microscopic study of changes at the surface of influenza-infected cells as revealed by ferritin-conjugated antibodies. *Virology*, **28**:404, 1966.

DUFF, J. T., G. G. WRIGHT, J. KLERER, D. E. MOORE, and R. H. BIBLER. Studies on immunity to toxins of *Clostridium botulinum*. I. A simplified procedure for isolation of type A toxin. *J. Bacteriol.* **73**:42, 1957.

DUGUID, J. P., and R. R. GILLIES. Fimbriae and adhesive properties in dysenteriae bacilli. *J. Pathol. Bacteriol.* **74**:397, 1957.

DUGUID, J. P., I. W. SMITH, G. DEMPSTER, and P. N. EDMUNDS. Non-flagellar filamentous appendages ("fimbriae") and haemagglutinating activity in *Bacterium coli. J. Pathol. Bacteriol.* **70**:335, 1955.

DUKE, H., and J. WALLACE. Red cell adhesion in trypanosomiasis of man and animals. *Parasitology*, **22**:414, 1930.

DULBECCO, R., M. VOGT, and A. G. R. STRICKLAND. A study of the basic aspects of neutralization of two animal viruses. Western equine encephalitis virus and poliomyelitis virus. *Virology*, **2**:162, 1956.

DUNSFORD, I., and C. C. BOWLEY. *Techniques in Blood Grouping.* Oliver and Boyd, Edinburgh, 1955.

DUNSFORD, I., and J. GRANT. *The Anti-globulin (Coombs) Test in Laboratory Practice.* Oliver and Boyd, London, 1959.

DURRUM, E. L. Continuous electrophoresis and ionophoresis on filter paper. *J. Amer. Chem. Soc.* **73**:4875, 1951.

DURRUM, E. L., and S. R. GILFORD. Recording integrating photoelectrophoresis and radioactive scanner for paper electrophoresis and chromatography. *Rev. Sci. Instr.* **26**:51, 1955.

DURRUM, E. L., M. H. PAUL, and E. R. B. SMITH. Lipid detection in paper electrophoresis. *Science*, **116**:426, 1952.

DUS, K., S. LINDROTH, R. PABST, and R. M. SMITH. Continuous amino acid analysis: Elution programming and automatic column selection by means of a rotating valve. *Anal. Biochem.* **14**:41, 1966.

DUTHIE, E., and L. LORENZ. Staphylocoagulase: the nature of plasma activator in the clotting process. *Nature*, **165**:729, 1950.

DUTHIE, E., and L. LORENZ. Staphylocoagulase: mode of action and antigenicity. *J. Gen. Microbiol.* **6**:95, 1952.

DUTTON, R. W., and J. D. EADY. An *in vitro* system for the study of the mechanism of antigenic stimulation in the secondary response. *Immunology*, **7**:40, 1964.

DZULYNSKA, J., and E. MIKULASZEK. Chromatographic studies on sugars of some strains of bacteria. *Acta Biochim. Pol.* **3**:191, 1954.

EAGLE, H. On the mutual multivalence of toxin and antitoxin. *J. Immunol.* **32**:119, 1937.

EAGLE, H. The minimum vitamin requirements of the L and HeLa cells in tissue culture, the production of specific vitamin deficiencies, and their cure. *J. Exper. Med.* **102**:595, 1955.

EBERSON, F. *Arch. Derm. and Syphil.* **4**:490, 1921.

EBINA, T., M. MOTOMIYA, K. MUNAKATA, and O. SATAKE. Pigments of unclassified mycobacteria. *Amer. Rev. Resp. Cis.* **86**:740, 1962.

ECKER, E. E., and L. PILLEMER. Complement. *Anal. N.Y. Acad. Sci.* **43**:63, 1942.

ECKER, E. E., L. PILLEMER, and S. SEIFTER. Immunochemical studies on human serum. I. Human complement and its components. *J. Immunol.* **47**:18, 1943.

ECKER, E. E., L. PILLEMER, D. WITHEIMER, and H. GRADIS. Ascorbic acid and complement function. *J. Immunol.* **34**:19, 1938.

ECKER, E. E., and A. REESE. Effect of hemorrhage on complement of blood. *J. Infect. Dis.* **31**:361, 1922.

ECKER, E. E., A. WEISBERGER, and L. PILLEMER. The opsonins of normal and immune sera. *J. Immunol.* **43**:227, 1942.

EDEBO, L. A new press for the disruption of micro-organisms and other cells. *J. Biochem. Microbiol. Technol. Engin.* **2**:453, 1960.

EDEBO, L., and T. HOLME. Preparation of biologically active fractions from *Salmonella typhi-murium*. 2. Disintegration of pathogenic microorganisms. *Acta Pathol. Microb. Scandinav.* **51**:173, 1961.

EDELMAN, G. M. The covalent structure of a human immunoglobulin. XI. Functional implications. *Biochem.* **9**:3197, 1970.

EDWARDS, P. *J. Bacteriol.* **17**:339, 1929.

EEGRIVE, E. Reaction and reagents for the detection of organic compounds. *Z. Anal. Chem.* **110**:22, 1937.

EGGERS, H. J., and A. B. SABIN. A phase contrast microprecipitin test with polio-virus antigens. I. Properties of the antigens and antibodies and optimum conditions for reaction. *Arch. Virusforsch.* **11**:120, 1961.

EHRLICH, P. Die Wertbemessung des Diphtherieheilserums und deren theoretische Grundlagen. In *Klin. Jahrbuch*, Vol. VI. Fischer, Jena, 1897.

EHRLICH, P. *Proc. Roy. Soc. (London)*, **66**:424, 1900.

EISELE, C. W., N. B. McCULLOUGH, and G. A. BEAL. Discrepancies in the agglutination test for brucellosis as performed with various antigens as reported from different laboratories. *J. Lab. Clin. Med.* **32**:847, 1947.

EISEN, H. N. Ultraviolet absorption spectroscopy of immune precipitates. *J. Immunol.* **60**:77, 1948.

EISEN, H. N. The significance of "valence" in antibody interactions. *J. Allergy*, **20**:393, 1949.

EISEN, H. N., S. BELMAN, and M. E. CARSTEN. The reaction of 2,4 dinitrobenzenesulfonic acid with free amino groups of proteins. *J. Amer. Chem. Soc.* **75**:4583, 1953.

EISEN, H. N., and F. KARUSH. The interaction of purified antibody with homologous hapten. Antibody valence and binding constant. *J. Amer. Chem. Soc.* **71**:353, 1949.

EISEN, H. N., and A. KESTON. The immunologic reactivity of bovine serum-albumin labeled with trace-amounts of radioactive iodine (I^{131}). *J. Immunol.* **63**:71, 1949.

EISEN, H. N., and D. PRESSMAN. The zone of localization of antibodies. VIII. Some properties of the antigen responsible for the renal localization of anti-kidney serum. *J. Immunol.* **64**:487, 1950.

EISENBERG, P., and R. VOLK. Untersuchungen über die Agglutination. *Zeitschr. Hyg.* **40**:155, 1902.

EISLER, D. Influence of collodion particles on the visible end-point in antibody titrations. *J. Immunol.* **41**:405, 1941.

EJELLSTRÖM, K. E. Preparation of complement reagents by means of gel filtration. *Acta Pathol. Microb. Scandinav.* **54**:439, 1962.

ELBERG, S., M. HERZBERG, P. SCHNEIDER, S. J. SILVERMAN, and K. F. MEYER. Studies on the immunization of guinea pigs and mice to *Brucella* infection by means of the "native antigen." *J. Immunol.* **67**:1, 1951.

ELDERING, G., W. C. EVELAND, and P. L. KENDRICK. Fluorescent antibody staining and agglutination reactions in *Bordetella pertussis* cultures. *J. Bacteriol.* **83**:745, 1962.

ELDERING, G., C. HORNBECK, and J. BAKER. Serological study of *Bordetella pertussis* and related species. *J. Bacteriol.* **74**:133, 1957.

ELDON, K. Experience with ABO and Rh-blood grouping cards (Eldon Cards). *Brit. Med. J.* **11**:1219, 1956.

ELEK, A., and H. SOBOTKA. The Kjeldahl-Pregl method applied to nitro-compounds. *J. Amer. Chem. Soc.* **48**:501, 1926.

ELEK, S. D. The recognition of toxigenic bacterial strains in vitro. *Brit. Med. J.* **1**:493, 1948.

ELEK, S. D. The plate virulence test for diphtheria. *J. Clin. Pathol.* **2**:250, 1949.

ELEK, S. D. *Staphylococcus Pyogenes and Its Relation to Disease*. Livingstone, Edinburgh, 1959.

ELLENBOGEN, E., and E. BRAND. Determination of neutralization equivalents by titration in alcohol. *Anal. Chem.* **27**:2007, 1955.

ELLIOTT, R., and L. FERGUSON. The incidence of antigen I in cattle and the production of autoimmunization. *J. Immunol.* **76**:78, 1956.

ELLIOTT, S. D. Group and type-specific polysaccharides of group D streptococci. *Nature*, **184**:1342, 1959.

ELLIOTT, S. D. Type and group polysaccharides of group D streptococci. *J. Exper. Med.* **111**:621, 1960.

ELLIS, H., and K. WALTON. Variations in serum complement in the nephrotic syndrome and other forms of renal disease. *Immunology*, **1**:234, 1958.

ELLNER, P. D., and S. S. GREEN. Serological grouping of the pathogenic clostridia. *J. Bacteriol.* **86**:1098, 1963.

ELSON, L. A., and W. T. J. MORGAN. A colorimetric method for the determination of glucosamine and chondrosamine. *Biochem. J.* **27**:1824, 1933.

EMMERSON, C., W. FRANKLIN, and F. LOWELL. The production of potent antihuman globulin (Coombs reagent) in rabbits immunized with serum-adjuvant mixtures. *J. Immunol.* **63**:323, 1951.

ENDERS, J. F. Chemical, clinical and immunological studies on the products of human plasma fractionation. X. The concentration of certain antibodies in globulin fractions derived from human blood plasma. *J. Clin. Invest.* **23**:510, 1944.

ENDERS, J. F., and A. PAPPENHEIMER. Specific carbohydrate of type I pneumococcus. *Proc. Soc. Exper. Biol. Med.* **31**:37, 1933.

ENTEL, H. J., and E. WEINHOLD. Zur Blutentnahme beim Meerschweinchen. *Zentralbl. Bakteriol. I. Orig.* **171**:523, 1957.

EPPES, W., and E. LUDOVIC. Demonstration of LE-cell without use of anticoagulants. *Blood*, **6**:466, 1951.

EPSTEIN, L. A., and E. CHAIN. Some observations on the preparation and properties of the substrate of lysozyme. *Brit. J. Exper. Pathol.* **21**:339, 1940.

EPSTEIN, N. H. *Z. Bakteriol. Orig.* **87**:533, 1922.

EPSTEIN, W., E. ENGLEMAN, and M. ROSS. Quantitative studies of the precipitation and agglutination reactions between serum of patients with "connective tissue disease" and a preparation of human globulin. *J. Immunol.* **75**:441, 1951.

EPSTEIN, W., A. JOHNSON, and C. RAGAN. Observations on a precipitin reaction between serum of patients with rheumatoid arthritis and a preparation (Cohn fraction II) of human gamma globulin. *Proc. Soc. Exper. Biol. Med.* **91**:235, 1950.

ETTINGER-TULCZNSKA, R. Bakterienkapseln und Quellungsreaktion *Zeitschr. Hyg.* **114**:769, 1933.

EVANS, A. Serological studies on infectious mononucleosis and viral hepatitis with human erythrocytes modified by different strains of Newcastle disease virus. *J. Immunol.* **64**:44, 1950.

EVANS, A. The interaction of serum with erythrocytes modified by Newcastle disease virus. *J. Immunol.* **74**:391, 1955.

EVANS, A., and E. CURNEN. Serological studies in infectious mononucleosis and other conditions with human erythrocytes modified by Newcastle disease virus. *J. Immunol.* **58**:323, 1948.

EVANS, D. G., and H. B. MAITLAND. Agglutination as diagnostic test for whooping cough. *J. Pathol. Bacteriol.* **48**:468, 1939.

EVANS, E. The antigenic composition of *Cryptococcus neoformans.* I. A serologic classification by means of capsular agglutination reaction. *J. Immunol.* **54**:423, 1950.

EVANS, E., and R. F. HAINES. The agglutination of ion exchange resin particles coated with polysaccharide. *J. Bacteriol.* **68**:130, 1954.

EVANS, E. E., L. J. SORENSEN, and K. W. WALLS. The antigenic composition of *Cryptococcus neoformans*. *J. Bacteriol*. **66**:287, 1953.

EVANS, R. T., and S. E. MERGENHAGEN. Occurrence of natural antibacterial antibody in human parotid fluid. *Proc. Soc. Exper. Biol. Med*. **119**:815, 1965.

EVANS, W. H., M. G. MAGE, and E. A. PETERSON. A method for the immunoadsorption of cells to an antibody-coated polyurethane foam. *J. Immunol*. **102**:899, 1969.

EWING, W. H., K. E. TANNER, and D. A. DENNARD. The Providence Group—an intermediate group of enteric bacteria. *J. Infect. Dis*. **94**:134, 1954.

FABER, V. Anti-streptococcal hyaluronidase. I. The turbidimetric method for determination of antistreptococcal hyaluronidase (ASH) in serum. *Acta Pathol. Microb. Scandinav*. **32**: 147, 1953.

FAHEY, J. L. E. C. FRANKLIN, R. S. NEGLIN, and T. WEBB. Antibody purification on insoluble adsorbent and purification and characterization of immunoglobulin. *Bull Wld. Health Organig*. **35**:779, 1966.

FAHEY, J. L., and E. M. MCKELVEY. Quantitative determination of serum immunoglobulins in antibody-agar plates. *J. Immunol*. **94**:84, 1965.

FAILLIE, R., R. JONNARD, and F. ZUCKERKANDL. Étude du pouvoir réactionelle du sérum sanguin par la methode refractométrique. *Biol. Med. Paris*, **28**:129, 1938.

FAIRBARN, N. Modified anthrone reagent. *Chem. Ind*. **86**:1953.

FAKUHARA, Y. Über hämagglutinierende Eigenschaften der Bakterien. *Zeitschr. Immunitätsforsch*. **2**:313, 1909.

FALCONE, R., and A. HARRIS. Comparison of several serologic tests for syphilis. *Amer. J. Clin. Pathol*. **28**:91, 1957.

FALK, C. R., and E. APPELBAUM. Type specific meningococcic agglutinins in human serum. I. Description of method. *Proc. Soc. Exper. Biol. Med*. **57**:341, 1944.

FALLETT, G. H., and M. ZIFF. Leucocyte disc method for LE-cell test in serum fractions. *Arthrit. Rheumat*. **1**:70, 1958.

FANTES, K. H. Concentration and partial purification of poliomyelitis viruses. *J. Hygiene*, **60**:123, 1962

FARSHTCHI, D., and C. W. MOSS. Characterization of bacteria by gas chromatography: Comparison of trimethylsilyl derivatives of whole-cell hydrolysate. *Appl. Microbiol*. **17**: 262, 1969.

FASTLER, L. B. Studies on the hemagglutinin of infectious canine hepatitis. *J. Immunol*. **78**:413, 1957.

FAVOUR, C. R. Autohemagglutinins-cold agglutinins. *J. Clin. Invest*. **23**:891, 1944.

FAVOUR, C., P. FREMONT-SMITH, and J. MILLER. Factors affecting the in vitro cytolysis of white blood cells by tuberculin. *Amer. Rev. Tuberc*. **60**:212, 1949.

FAZEKAS DE ST. GROTH, S. Quick test for the early diagnosis of influenza. *Nature*, **167**:43, 1957.

FAZEKAS DE ST. GROTH, S., and D. M. GRAHAM. The production of incomplete virus particles among influenza strains: experiments in eggs. *Brit. J. Exper. Pathol*. **35**:60, 1954.

FAZEKAS DE ST. GROTH, S., R. G. WEBSTER, and A. DATYNER. Two new staining procedures for quantitative estimation of proteins on electrophoretic strips. *Biochim. Biophys. Acta*, **71**:377, 1963.

FAZEKAS DE ST. GROTH, S., J. WITHELL, and K. J. LAFFERTY. An improved assay method for neutralizing antibodies against influenza viruses. *J. Hygiene* **56**:415, 1958.

FEDER, N., and R. L. SIDMAN. Methods and principles of fixation by freeze-substitution. *J. Biophys. Biochem. Cytol*. **4**:593, 1958.

FEDINEC, A. A. Localization of tetanus toxin with fluorescent antibody technique. *Anatom. Record*. **142**:304, 1962.

FEINBERG, J. G. A new quantitative method for antigen-antibody titration in gels. *Nature*, **177**:530, 1956.

FEINBERG, J. G. Identification, discrimination and quantification in Ouchterlony gel plates. *Int. Arch. Allergy*, **11**:129, 1957.

FEINBERG, R., J. DAVISON, and J. FLICK. The detection of antibodies in hay fever sera by means of haemagglutination. *J. Immunol.* **77**:279, 1956.

FELGENHAUER, K. Microelectrophoresis on polyacrylamide gel. *Biochim. Biophys. Acta*, **133**:165, 1967.

FELGENHAUER, K. Immunological techniques following microelectrophoresis on polyacrylamide gel. *Biochim. Biophys. Acta*, **160**:267, 1968.

FELIX, A. The qualitative serum diagnosis of enteric fevers. *Lancet*, **I**; 505, 1930.

FELIX, A. *J. Hygiene*, **38**:750, 1938.

FELIX, A., and H. BENSTED. Proposed standard agglutinating sera for typhoid and paratyphoid A and B fevers. *Bull. World Health Org.* **10**:919, 1954.

FELL, N., and D. RODNEY. Histamine-protein complexes: synthesis and immunological investigation. *J. Immunol.* **47**:237, 1943.

FELSENFIELD, O., N. FREEMAN, and V. MOORING. Tube and slide technic in hemagglutination of *Vibrio comma. Amer. J. Trop. Med. Hyg.* **4**:318, 1955.

FELTON, L. D. Concentration of pneumococcus antibody. *J. Infect. Dis.* **43**:543, 1928.

FELTON, L. D. The use of ethyl alcohol as precipitant in the concentration of antipneumococcus serum. *J. Immunol.* **21**:357, 1931.

FELTON, L. D. The significance of antigen in animal tissues. *J. Immunol.* **61**:107, 1949.

FELTON, L. D., and G. BAILEY. Biologic significance of the soluble specific substances of pneumococci. *J. Infect. Dis.* **38**:131, 1926.

FELTON, L. D., G. KAUFMANN, B. PRESCOTT, and B. OTTINGER. Studies on the mechanism of the immunological paralysis induced in mice by pneumococcal polysaccharides. *J. Immunol.* **74**:17, 1955.

FELTON, L. D., and C. R. McMILLON. Chromatographically pure fluorescein and tetramethylrhodamine isothiocyanate. *Ann. Biochem.* **2**:178, 1961.

FELTON, L. D., B. PRESCOTT, G. KAUFMANN, and B. OTTINGER. Studies on immunizing substances in pneumococci. XIV. The distribution of specific polysaccharides in mouse tissues after injection of a paralyzing dose. *Proc. Fed. Assoc. Exper. Biol.* **6**:427, 1947.

FELTON, L. D., B. PRESCOTT, G. KAUFMANN, and B. OTTINGER. Pneumococcal antigenic polysaccharide from human tissues. *J. Immunol.* **76**:69, 1956.

FENN, W. D. The phagocytosis of solid particles. I. Quartz. *J. Gen. Physiol.* **3**:439, 1921.

FENNER, F. Studies on *Mycobacterium ulcerans;* cross-reactivity in guinea pigs sensitized with *Mycobacterium ulcerans* and other mycobacteria. *Austr. J. Exper. Biol. Med. Sci.* **30**:11, 1952.

FERRARI, A. Nitrogen determination by a continuous digestion and analysis system. *Ann. N.Y. Acad. Sci.* **87**:792, 1960.

FERRARI, A., E. CATANZARO, and F. RUSSO-ALESI. Nitrogen analysis by a continuous digestion system. *Ann. N.Y. Acad. Sci.*, **130**:602, 1965.

FILITTI-WURMSER, S., Y. JACQUOT-ARMAND, G. AUBEL-LESURE, and R. WURMSER. Physicochemical study of isohemagglutination. *Ann. Eugenics*, **18**:183, 1954.

FINEGOLD, I., J. L. FAHEY, and T. F. DUTCHER. Immunofluorescent studies of immunoglobulins in human lymphoid cells in continuous culture. *J. Immunol.* **101**:366, 1968.

FINGER, I., and C. HELLER. Gel diffusion analysis of cross-reactions of a protein-hapten conjugate. *J. Immunol.* **85**:332, 1960.

FINGER, I., and E. A. KABAT. A comparison of human antisera to purified diphtheria toxoid with antisera to other purified antigens by quantitative precipitin and gel diffusion techniques. *J. Exper. Med.* **108**:453, 1958.

FINK, K., and R. FINK. Application of filter paper partition chromatography to qualitative analysis of volatile and organic acids. *Proc. Soc. Exper. Biol. Med.* **70**:645, 1949.

FINK, R. M., R. E. CLINE, C. McGAUCHEY, and K. FINK. Chromatography of pyrimidine reduction products. *Anal. Chem.* **28**:4, 1956.

FINKELSTEIN, R. A. Vibriocidal antibody inhibition (VAI) analysis: a technique for the identification of the predominant vibriocidal antibodies in serum and for the detection and identification of *Vibrio cholerae* antigens. *J. Immunol.* **89**:264, 1962.

FINKELSTEIN, R. A., P. Z. SOBOCINSKI, P. ATTHASAMPUMA, and P. X. CHARUMUNNA. Pathogenesis of experimental cholera: identification of choleragen (procholeragen A) by disc immunoelectrophoresis and its differentiation from cholera mucinase. *J. Immunol.* **97**:25, 1966.

FINLAND, M. Cold agglutinins. VI. Agglutinins for an indifferent streptococcus in primary atypical pneumonia and in other conditions and their relation to cold isohemagglutinins. *J. Clin. Invest.* **24**:497, 1945.

FINLAND, M., and E. C. CURNEN. Agglutinins for human erythrocytes in type XIV antipneumococcal horse serum. *Science*, **87**:417, 1938.

FINLAND, M., and H. DOWLING. Cutaneous reaction and antibody response to intracutaneous injection of pneumococcus polysaccharides. *J. Immunol.* **29**:285, 1935.

FINNEY, D. J., T. HAZELWOOD, and M. J. SMITH. Logarithm to base 2. *J. Gen. Microbiol.* **12**:222, 1955.

FIOCK, M. A., A. YARINSKY, and J. T. DUFF. Studies on immunity to toxins of *Clostridium botulinum*. VII. Purification and detoxification of trypsin-activated type E toxin. *J. Bacteriol.* **82**:68, 1961.

FISCHER, A. Amino acid metabolism of tissue cells in vitro. *Biochem. J.* **43**:491, 1948.

FISHEL, E. E., E. A. KABAT, H. C. STOERK, and A. D. BEZER. The role of tubercle bacilli in adjuvant emulsions in antibody production to egg albumen. *J. Immunol.* **69**:61, 1952.

FISHER, R. A. *Statistical Methods for Research Workers.* Oliver and Boyd, Edinburgh, 1936.

FISHER, R. A., and F. YATES. *Statistical Tables*, 4th ed. Oliver and Boyd, London, 1953.

FISHER, S. The inhibition of pertussis haemogglutination by extracts of erythrocytes. *Brit. J. Exper. Pathol.* **29**:357, 1948.

FISHER, S. The erythrocyte receptor for pertussis haemagglutination. *Brit. J. Exper. Pathol.* **30**:185, 1949.

FISHER, S. The haemagglutinin of *Haemophilus pertussis*. *Austral. J. Exper. Biol. Med. Sci.* **280**:509, 1950.

FISHER, S. Antigenic relationships of erythrocyte adsorbable fractions of some mycobacteria. *Austral. J. Exper. Biol. Med. Sci.* **29**:1, 1951.

FISHER, S. The estimation in vitro of small amounts of diphtheria antitoxin by means of heamagglutination technique. *J. Hygiene*, **50**:455, 1952.

FISHER, S., and E. KEOGH. Lysis by complement of erythrocytes which absorbed a bacterial component and its antibody. *Nature*, **165**:248, 1950.

FISK, R. T., and C. A. McGEE. The use of gelatin in Rh testing and antibody determination. *Amer. J. Clin. Pathol.* **17**:737, 1947.

FISKE, C. H., and Y. SUBBAROW. The colorimetric determination of phosphorus. *J. Biol. Chem.* **66**:375, 1926.

FJELLSTRÖM, K. E. Human complement components in starch-gel electrophoresis. *Acta Pathol. Microbiol. Scandinav.* **59**:245, 1963.

FLEISCHMAN, J. B. Immunoglobulins. *Ann. Rev. Biochem.* **35**:836, 1966.

FLEISCHMAN, J. B., R. H. PAIN, and R. R. PORTER. Reduction of γ-globulins. *Arch. Biochem. Biophys.* Suppl. **1**:174, 1962.

FLEMING, A. On remarkable bacteriolytic element found in tissues and secretions. *Proc. Roy. Soc.* **93**:306, 1922.

FLESSEL, C. P. Polyribosomes of growing bacteria. *Science*, **158**:658, 1967.

FLICK, J. A. Use of formalin-treated red cells for the study of influenza A virus hemagglutinating activity. *Proc. Soc. Exper. Biol. Med.* **68**:448, 1948.

FLICK, J. A., and O. VILLAFENE. Studies on conglutinin. I. Its role in erythrocytic agglutination in relation to the application to the lattice theory. *J. Immunol.* **68**:41, 1952.

FLOOD, A. E., E. L. HIRST, and J. K. N. JONES. Quantitative analysis of mixtures of sugars by the paper chromatography method. *Nature*, **160**:86, 1947.

FLORMAN, A. L. The use of commercially available complement-fixing antigen for the diagnosis of elementary body types of viral infections. *J. Immunol.* **50**:469, 1945.

FLORMAN, A. L. Haemagglutination with Newcastle disease virus. *Proc. Soc. Exper. Biol. Med.* **64**:458, 1947.

FLORMAN, A. L., and J. KUTCH. Specific serological reactions which follow acquired mumps. *J. Immunol.* **63**:287, 1949.

FLORMAN, A. L., and J. L. SCOMA. A latex agglutination test for anaerobic diphtheroids. *Proc. Soc. Exper. Biol. Med.* **104**:683, 1960.

FLOSDORF, E., and S. MUDD. Procedure and apparatus for preservation in "lyophile" form of serum and other biologic substances. *J. Immunol.* **29**:389, 1935.

FLOSDORF, E., and S. MUDD. An improved procedure and apparatus for preservation of serum, microorganisms and other substances—the cryochem-process. *J. Immunol.* **34**:469, 1938.

FODOR, A. R. Further studies on antigenic heterogeneity in bacteriophage. *J. Immunol.* **79**:227, 1957.

FODOR, A. R., and M. H. ADAMS. Genetic control of serological specificity in bacteriophage. *J. Immunol.* **74**:228, 1955.

FOLCH, J., M. LEES, and G. H. SLOANE-STANLEY. A simple method for the isolation and base purification of total lipides from animal tissues. *J. Biol. Chem.* **226**:497, 1957.

FOLIN, O., and V. CIOCALTEU. On tyrosine and tryptophane determination of proteins. *J. Biol. Chem.* **73**:627, 1927.

FONG, J., and J. BERNAL. In vitro action of antibodies on the infective and toxic components of influenza A (PR 8) virus. *J. Immunol.* **70**:89, 1953.

FORD, W. The distribution of haemolysins, agglutinins and poisons in fungi. *J. Pharmacol. Exper. Therapy*, **2**:285, 1911.

FORSGREN, A. Protein A from *Staphylococcus aureus*. VI. Reaction with subunits from guinea pig γ_1- and γ_2-globulin. *J. Immunol.* **100**:927, 1968.

FORSGREN, A., and J. SJÖQUIST. "Protein A" from *S. aureus*. I. Pseudo-immune reaction with human γ-globulin. *J. Immunol.* **97**:822, 1966.

FORSSMAN, J. Die Herstellung hochwertiger spezifischen Schafhämolysine ohne Verwendung von Schafblut. *Biochem. Zeitschr.* **37**:78, 1911.

FOSTER, A. B. Simplified apparatus for filter-paper ionophoresis. *Chem. Ind.*, 1050-1051, 1952.

FOSTER, J. W., R. M. COWAN, and T. A. MAAS. Rupture of bacteria by explosive decompressing. *J. Bacteriol.* **83**:330, 1962.

FOUGEREAU, M., and G. M. EDELMAN. Corroboration of recent models of the γG-immunoglobulin molecule. *J. Exper. Med.* **121**:373, 1965.

FOWDEN, L. The quantitative recovery and colorimetrice stimation of amino-acid sseparated by paper chromatography. *Biochem. J.* **48**:327, 1951.

FOX, E. M. Measurement of streptococcal antigen synthesis with fluorescent antibody. *Proc. Soc. Exper. Biol. Med.* **109**:577, 1962.

FOZ, A., E. BATALLA, and P. BARCELO. The agglutination of sensitized erythrocytes by the serum from patients with rheumatoid arthritis. *Rev. Españ. Reumat.* 1951.

FRAHN, J. L., and J. A. MILLS. Paper ionophoresis of carbohydrates. I. Procedures for four electrolytes. *Aust. J. Chem.* **12**:65, 1959.

FRANCIS, T. JR. Identity of mechanisms of type-specific agglutinin and precipitin reactions with pneumococcus. *J. Exper. Med.* **55**:55, 1932.

FRANCIS, T. J., and J. SALK. A simplified procedure for the concentration and purification of influenza virus. *Science*, **96**:499, 1942.

FRASER, D. Bursting bacteria by release of gas pressure. *Nature*, **167**:33, 1951.

FREEMAN, B. A., G. M. MUSTEIKIS, and W. BURROWS. Protoplast formation as the mechanism for immune lysis of *Vibrio cholerae. Proc. Soc. Exper. Biol. Med.* **113**:675, 1963.

FREEMAN, C. C., S. W. CHALINOR, and J. WILSON. The use of a synthetic medium in the isolation of the somatic antigens of *Bacterium typhi-murium* and *Bacterium typhosum. Biochem. J.* **34**:307, 1940.

FREEMAN, N., O. FELSENFELD, and W. EVELAND. Slide hemagglutination tests with O antigens of enteric organisms and *Brucella. Amer. J. Clin. Pathol.* **25**:332, 1955.

FREUND, J. On nature of the toxin-antitoxin neutralization studied on collodion particles. *Proc. Soc. Exper. Biol. Med.* **28**:1010, 1930.

FREUND, J. The effect of heterologous bacterial products upon tuberculous animals. *J. Immunol.* **30**:241, 1936.

FREUND, J. The effect of paraffin oil and mycobacteria on antibody formation and sensitization. *Amer. J. Clin. Pathol.* **21**:645, 1951.

FREUND, J., J. CASALS-ARTIET, and E. P. HOSMER. Sensitization and antibody formation after injection of tubercle bacilli and paraffin oil. *Proc. Soc. Exper. Biol. Med.* **37**:509, 1940.

FREUND, J., J. CASALS-ARIET, and D. SCHAEFER-GENGOF. The synergistic effect of paraffin-oil combined with heat-killed tubercle bacilli. *J. Immunol.* **38**:67, 1940.

FREUND, J., and K. MCDERMOTT. Sensitization to horse serum by means of adjuvants. *Proc. Soc. Exper. Biol. Med.* **49**:548, 1942.

FREUND, J., J. THOMSON, H. HOUGH, H. SONNER, and T. PISANI. Antibody formation and sensitization with the aid of adjuvants. *J. Immunol.* **62**:383, 1948.

FRICK, G. Preparation and purification of T_2 bacteriophages with an aqueous polymer two-phase system and some properties of the phage suspension obtained. *Exper. Cell. Res.* **23**:788, 1961.

FRICK, O. L. Demonstration of antibodies in the sera of grass-sensitive persons by the bis-diazotized-benzidine hemagglutination technique. *J. Allergy*, **31**:216, 1960.

FRIEDBERGER, E., and O. HARTOCH. Der Einfluss intravenöser Salzinjektionen auf die aktive und passive Anaphylaxie bei Meerschweinchen. *Zeitschr. Immunitätsforsch.* **3**:581, 1909.

FRIEDBERGER, E., and E. PUTTER. Weitere Versuche mit der Kapillarsteigmethode. *Münch. Med. Wochenschr.* **67**:398, 1920.

FRIEDENREICH, V. *The Thomsen Hemagglutination Phenomenon.* Levin and Munksgaard, Copenhagen, 1930.

FRIEDMAN, H. Immunological tolerance to microbial antigens. I. Absence of specific antibody containing cells in lymphoid tissue of mice injected at birth with *Shigella* soluble antigen. *J. Bacteriol.* **92**:390, 1966.

FRIEDMAN, H. Immunological tolerance to microbial antigens. II. Suppressed antibody plaque formation to *Shigella* antigen by spleen cells from tolerant mice. *J. Bacteriol.* **92**:820, 1966.

FRIEDMAN, L., and N. F. CONANT. Immunological studies on the etiologic agents of North and South American blastomycosis. *Mycopathology*, **6**:317, 1953.

FRIEND, C. A study of the effects of sodium salicylate and some structurally related compounds on antigen-antibody reactions in vitro. *J. Immunol.* **70**:141, 1953.

FRIOU, G. J. Fluorescent spot test for anti-nuclear antibodies. *Arthritis Rheumat.* **5**:407, 1962.

FRIOU, G. J., and H. A. WENNER. On the occurrence in human serum of an inhibitory substance to hyaluronidase produced by a strain of hemolytic streptococcus. *J. Infect. Dis.* **80**:185, 1947.

FRISCH, A., J. TRIPP, C. BARRETT, and B. PIDGEON. The specific polysaccharide content of pneumonic lungs. *J. Exper. Med.* **76**:505, 1942.

FULLER, A.T. The formamide method for the extraction of polysaccharides from hemolytic streptococci. *Brit. J. Exper. Pathol.* **19**:130, 1938.

FULTHORPE, A. Agglutination of sheep erythrocytes sensitized with *Salmonella* polysaccharides. *J. Pathol. Bacteriol.* **68**:315, 1954.

FULTHORPE, A. Tetanus antitoxin titration by haemagglutination. *J. Hygiene*, 55:382, 1957.

FULTHORPE, A. Estimation of tetanus toxoid by different methods including haemagglutination inhibition. *Immunol.* **1**:365, 1958.

FULTON, F. The measurement of complement fixation by virus. *Advanc. Virus Res.* **5**:247, 1958.

FULTON, F., and K. R. DUMBELL. The serological comparison of strains of influenza virus. *J. Gen. Microbiol.* **3**:97, 1949.

FULTON, J. D., and D. F. SPOONER. Preliminary observations on the metabolism of *Toxoplama gondii. Trans. Roy. Soc. Trop. Med. Hyg.* **51**:123, 1957.

FURTH, J., and K. LANDSTEINER. On precipitable substances derived from *Bacillus typhosus* and *Bacillus paratyphosus. J. Exper. Med.* **41**:171, 1928.

FURTH, J., and K. LANDSTEINER. Studies on the precipitable substances of the *Salmonella* group. *J. Exper. Med.* **49**:727, 1929.

GAINES, N. *Physics*, **3**:209, 1932.

GAINES, S., J. A. CURRIE, and J. G. TULY. Production of incomplete Vi antibody in mice. *Proc. Soc. Exper. Biol. Med.* **104**:602, 1960.

GAJDUSEK, D. C. An autoimmune reaction against human tissue antigens in certain acute and chronic diseases. I. Serological investigations. *Arch. Intern. Med.* **101**:9, 1958.

GALAJEV, I. *Biochimija*, **20**:673, 1955.

GALLAGHER, F., and L. JONES. Preparation and use of Rh testing sera. *J. Immunol.* **46**:9, 1943.

GALLUT, J. Analytical Serology of Spirillaceae. In *Analytical Serology of Microorganisms*, J. B. G. Kwapinski, Ed., Vol. I. Interscience, New York, 1969, pp. 45–94.

GALTON, M. M., R. W. MENGES, E. B. SHOTTS, JR., A. J. NAHMIAS, and C. W. HEATH, JR. Leptospirosis-epidemiology, clinical manifestations in man and animals, and methods in laboratory diagnosis. *Public. Health Service Rep. No.* 951.

GALTON, M. M., C. SULZER, C. S. SANTA ROSA, and M. J. FIELDS. Application of a microtechnique to the agglutination test for leptospiral antibodies. *Appl. Microbiol.* **13**:81, 1965.

GARNER, R. L., and W. S. TILLETT. Biochemical studies on the fibrinolytic activity of hemolytic streptococci. II. Nature of the reaction. *J. Exper. Med.* **60**:255, 1934.

GARSON, W. Recent developments in laboratory diagnosis of syphilis. *Ann. Int. Med.* **51**:748, 1959.

GAUDY, E., and R. S. WOLFE. Composition of extracellular polysaccharide produced by *Sphaerophilus natans. Appl. Microbiol.* **10**:200, 1962.

GEE, M., and P. M. McCREADY. Paper chromatographic detection of galacturonic and glucuronic acids. *Anal. Chem.* **29**:257, 1957.

GEIGER, W., and R. ANDERSON. The chemistry of the lipids of tubercle bacilli. *J. Biol. Chem.* **131**:539, 1939.

718   BIBLIOGRAPHY

GENDON, I. *Zhur Microbiol. Epidemiol. Immunobiol.* **29**:693, 1958.

GENGOU, D. Étude sur les rapporte entre les agglutinines et les lysines dans le carbon. *Ann. Inst. Pasteur*, **13**:642, 1899.

GEORGE, M., and J. H. VAUGHAN. In vitro cell migration as a model for delayed hypersensitivity. *Proc.Soc. Exper. Biol. Med.* **111**:514, 1962.

GEORGIEV, G. P., O. P. MARINA, M. I. LERMAN, M. N. SMIRNOV, and A. N. SEVERTZOV. Biosynthesis of messenger and ribosomal ribonucleic acids in the nucleolochromosomal apparatus of animal cells. *Nature*, **200**:1291, 1963.

GERBER, I., and W. CROSS. The immunological specificity of suphonamide protein conjugates as demonstrated by anaphylaxis in guinea pigs and the Shwartzman phenomenon in rabbits. *J. Immunol.* **48**:103, 1944.

GERHEIM, E., and J. FERGUSON. Staphylocoagulation in plasma of various animal species. *Proc. Soc. Exper. Biol. Med.* **71**:258, 1949.

GERLACH, E., R. H. DREISBACH, and B. DEUTICKE. Paper chromatographic separation of nucleotides, nucleosides, purines and pyrimidines. *J. Chromatog.* **18**:81, 1965.

GERLOFF, R. K., B. H. HOYER, and L. C. McLAVEN. Precipitation of radio-labeled poliovirus with specific antibody and antiglobulin. *J. Immuniol.* **89**:559, 1962.

GERNEZ-RIEUX, C., E. MONTESTRUC, and A. TACQUET. Les réactions d'hémagglutination et d'hémolyse conditionée dans les differentes formes de la lèpre. *Ann. Inst. Pasteur Lille*, **4**:3, 1951.

GERNEZ-RIEUX, C. P., and A. JACQUET. Réactions d'hémagglutination pratiqués comparativement avec l'antigène type Middlebrook et Dubos et avec la tuberculine precipitée. *Ann. Inst. Pasteur Lille*, **3**:1, 1950.

GERNEZ-RIEUX, C. P., A. TACQUET, and C. VOISIN. Inocuité de la vaccination antituberculeuse par voie digestive à doses massives et repetées, chez les adultes tuberculeux et non tuberculeux. *Ann. Inst. Pasteur Lille*, **5**:1, 1952.

GERSTL, B., W. DAVIS, D. KIRSH, A. HOLLANDER, and S. WEINSTEIN. Detection of apparently absent circulating antibodies in tuberculous sera. *Amer. Rev. Tuberc.* **72**:345, 1955.

GESTELAND, R. F., and T. STAEHELIN. Electrophoretic analysis of proteins from normal and cesium chloride-treated *Escherichia coli* ribosomes. *J. Mol. Biol.* **24**:149, 1967.

GETTLER, A., and H. KRAMER. Blood grouping in forensic medicine. *J. Immunol.* **31**:321, 1936.

GHOSH, B. K., and R. G. E. MURRAY. Fractionation and characterization of plasma and some membrane of *Listeria monocytogenes. J. Bacteriol.* **97**:426, 1969.

GIBBONS, M. N. The determination of methylpentoses. *Analyst*, **80**:268, 1955.

GIBBS, M. B., and J. H. AKEROYD. Quantitative immunohematologic studies of hemagglutination. I. Assay of the isoagglutinin anti-A. *J. Immunol.* **82**:568, 1959.

GIBBS, M. B., and J. H. AKEROYD. Quantitative immunohematologic studies of hemagglutination. II. Assay of the isoagglutinin anti-B. *J. Immunol.* **82**:577, 1959.

GIBBS, M. B., W. COLLINS, and J. H. AKEROYD. Quantitative hemagglutination inhibition studies of blood group substances. I. Assay of the blood group A activity of substances. *J. Immunol.* **87**:386, 1961.

GIBSON, H. J., and N. R. LING. Modified Waaler-Rose reaction employing sensitized human cells. *Ann. Rheumat. Dis.* **15**:246, 1956.

GIERER, A., and G. SCHRAMM. Die Infektiosität der Nukleinsäure aus Tabakmosaik-virus. *Z. Naturforsch.* **11b**:183, 1956.

GILBERT, W. Protein synthesis in *Escherichia coli. Cold Spring Harbor Symp. Quant. Biol.* **28**:287, 1963.

GILBOA-GARBER, N., and D. NELKEN. Barium sulphate test. *Nature*, **197**:158, 1963.

GILDEN, R. V., and S. TOKUDA. Antibody quality after sequential immunization with related antigens. *Science*, **140**:405, 1963.

GILLIES, R. R., and J. P. DUGUID. The fimbrial antigens of *Shigella flexneri*. *J. Hygiene*, **56**: 303, 1958.

GILLISSEN, G. Der Agar-Diffusionstest (Lochtest) als Routineverfahren. *Zentralbl. Bakteriol. I. Orig.* **161**:482, 1954.

GILLISSEN, G., F. TURBA, and H. WAGNER, *Zentralbl. Bakteriol. I. Orig.* **161**:65, 1955.

GILMAN, H., and S. BLATT. *Organic Synthesis*, Vol. I. Wiley, New York, 1941.

GINSBERG, H. S., W. F. GOEBEL, and F. L. HORSFALL, JR. Inhibitory effect of polysaccharide on mumps virus multiplication. *J. Exper. Med.* **87**:385, 1948.

GIORDANO, A., C. CULBERTSON, and W. HIGGENTHOTHAM. Cardiolipin antigens in serologic tests for syphilis. *Amer. J. Clin. Pathol.* **18**:193, 1948.

GISPEN, R. Analysis of pox-virus antigens by means of double diffusion. *J. Immunol.* **74**: 134, 1955.

GITLIN, D. Use of ultraviolet absorption spectroscopy in the quantitative precipitation reaction. *J. Immunol.* **62**:437, 1949.

GITLIN, D., and H. EDELHOCH. A study of the reaction between human serum albumin and its homologous equine antibody through the medium of light scattering. *J. Immunol.* **66**: 67, 1951.

GITLIN, D., B. H. LANDING, and A. WHIPLE. The location of homologous plasma proteins in the tissues of young human being demonstrated with fluorescent antibody. *J. Exper. Med.* **97**:163, 1953.

GIVOL, D., Y. WEINSTEIN. M. GORECKI, and M. WILCHEK. A general method for the isolation of labeled peptides from affinity-labeled proteins. *Biochem. Biphys. Res. Comm.* **38**:825, 1970.

GLADSTONE, G. P. The antigenic composition and virulence of *Bacterium typhosum* grown on a chemically defined medium. *Brit. J. Exper. Pathol.* **38**:67, 1957.

GLADSTONE, G. P., and W. E. HEYNINGEN. Staphylococcal leucocidins. *Brit. J. Exper. Pathol.* **38**:123, 1957.

GLADSTONE, G. P., S. MUDD, H. D. HOCHSTEIN, and N. A. LENHART. The assay of anti-stephylococcal leucocidal components (F and S) in human serum. *Brit. J. Exper. Pathol.* **43**:295, 1962.

GLEESON-WHITE, M. H., D. H. HEARD, L. S. MYNORS, and R. R. A. COOMBS. Factors influencing the agglutinability of red cells. *Brit. J. Exper. Pathol.* **31**:321, 1950.

GLENCHUR, H., Y. M. BRIAND, and G. RENOUX. Reactions sérologiques de sérums de lapin anti-extraits de *Brucella abortus* et de de *Br. melitensis*. *Ann. Inst. Pasteur*, **102**:450, 1962.

GLENCHUR, H., U. S. SEAL, H. H. ZINNEMAN, and W. H. KALL. Serum precipitins in human and experimental brucellosis. *J. Lab. Clin. Med.* **59**:220, 1962.

GLENN, W. G. Serum measuring aid. *J. Immunol.* **77**:189, 1956.

GLENN, W. G. In *Serological and Biochemical Comparisons of Proteins*. Rutgers University Press, New Brunswick, N. J., 1958.

GLENN, W. G., and A. C. GARNER. Integration of human serum and serum fraction diffusion patterns. *J. Immunol.* **78**:395, 1957.

GLICK, D., R. A. GOOD, L. J., GREENBERG, J. EDDY, and N. K. DAY. Measurement of precipitin reactions in the millimicrogram protein-nitrogen range. *Science*, **128**:1625, 1958.

GLYNN, A. A. The complement lysozyme sequence in immune bacteriolysis. *Immunology*, **16**:463, 1969.

GLYNN, L. E., E. J. HOLBOROW, and G. D. JOHNSON. The influence of the A-like substance of rabbits on their immune response to human blood group A substance. *J. Immunol.* **76**: 357, 1956.

GOEBEL, W. F., T. SHEDLOVSKY, G. LAVIN, and M. ADAM. The heterophile antigen of pneumococcus. *J. Biol. Chem.* **148**:1, 1943.

GOLD, A. M., and D. BLACKMAN. Peptide sequences and relative reactivity of the reactive sulfhydryl groups of rabbit muscle phosphorylase. *Biochemistry* 9:4480, 1970.

GOLDBERG, R., and D. CAMPBELL. The light scattering properties of an antigen-antibody reaction. *J. Immunol.* 66:79, 1951.

GOLDFIELD, M., S. SRIHOUGSE, and J. P. FOX. Hemagglutinins associated with certain human enteric viruses. *Proc. Soc. Exper. Biol. Med.* 97:788, 1957.

GOLDMAN, M. Cytochemical differentiation of *Entamoeba histolytica* and *Entamoeba coli* by means of fluorescent antibody. *Amer. J. Hyg.* 58:319, 1953.

GOLDMAN, M. Use of fluorescein-tagged antibody to identify cultures of *Entamoeba histolytica* and *Entamoeba coli. Amer. J. Hyg.* 59:318, 1954.

GOLDMAN, M. A new serologic test for *Toxoplasma* antibodies using fluorescein-tagged globulin. *Amer. J. Trop. Med. Hyg.* 5:375, 1956.

GOLDMAN, M. Staining *Toxoplasma gondii* with fluorescein-labeled antibody. II. A new serologic test for antibodies to *Toxoplasma* based upon inhibition of specific staining. *J. Exper. Med.* 105:557, 1957.

GOLDMAN, M. Antigenic analysis of *Entamoeba histolytica* by means of fluorescent antibody. I. Instrumentation for microfluorimetry of stained ameboe. *Exptl. Parasitol.* 9:25, 1960.

GOLDMAN, M., and R. K. CARVER. Preserving fluorescein isocyanate for simplified preparation of fluorescent antibody. *Science*, 126:839, 1957.

GOLDWASSER, R. A., and C. C. SHEPARD. Staining of complement and modifications of fluorescent antibody formation. *J. Immunol.* 80:122, 1958.

GOLDWASSER, R. A., and C. C. SHEPARD. Fluorescent antibody methods in the differentiation of murine and epidemic typhus sera; specificity changes resulting from previous immunization. *J. Immunol.* 82:373, 1959.

GOLUB, O. J. A single-dilution method for the estimation of LD_{50} titres of the Psittacosis-LGV group of viruses in chick embryos. *J. Immunol.* 59:71, 1948.

GOMORI, G. Preparation of Buffers for Use in Enzyme Studies. In *Methods in Enzymology* S. P. Colowick and N. O. Kaplan. Eds. Vol. I, 1955. p. 138–146.

GOODHEART, C. R., and L. B. JAROSS. Human cytomegalovirus. Assay by counting infected cells. *Virology*, 19:532, 1963.

GOODMAN, H. S. The comparison of complement fixing and hemolytic acticities in several systems. *J. Infect. Dis.* 103:278, 1958.

GOODMAN, H. S., and L. MASAITIS. The dissociation of hemolytic antibody from sensitized cells as measured by cell to--cell transfer. *J. Immunol.* 85:391, 1960.

GOODMAN, M., H. R. WOLFE, and S. NORTON. Precipitin production in chickens. VI. The effect of varying concentrations of NaCl on precipitate formation, *J. Immunol.* 66:225, 1951.

GOODNER, K. Collodion fixation—A new immunological reaction. *Science*, 94:241, 1941.

GOODNER, K., and F. L. HORSFALL, JR. The complement fixation reaction with pneumococcus capsular polysaccharide. *J. Exper. Med.* 64:201, 1936.

GORCZYNSKI, R. M., R. G. MILLER, and R. A. PHILLIPS. Homogeneity of antibody-producing cells as analysed by their buoyant density in gradients of ficoll. *Immunology*, 19:817, 1970.

GORDON, H. J., W. THORNBURG, and L. N. WERMIN. Rapid paper chromatography of carbohydrates and related compounds. *Anal. Chem.* 28:849, 1956.

GORDON, J., B. ROSE, and A. H. SELLON. Detection of nonprecipitating antibodies in sera of individuals allergic to ragweed pollen by in vitro method. *J. Exper. Med.* 108:37, 1958.

GORDON, M. A. Differentiation of yeasts by means of fluorescent antibody. *Proc. Soc. Exper. Biol. Med.* 94:694, 1958.

GORDON, M. A., and Y. AL-DOORY. Application of flluorescent-antibody procedures to the study of pathogenic dematiaceous fungi. II. Serological relationships of the genus *Fonsecaea. J. Bacteriol.* **89**:551, 1965.

GORDON, R. The preparation and properties of cold hemagglutinin. *J. Immunol.* **71**:220, 1953.

GORECZKY, L. Beitrage zu der entwicklungschemmenden und entwicklungsfordernden Wirkung der Serumfraktionen. *Zentrabl. Bakteriol. I. Orig.* **167**:409, 1957.

GORECZKY, L. A new method for studying the correlation between protein fractions and antibodies. *Schweiz. Zeitschr. Path. Bakteriol.* **22**:500, 1959.

GORZYNSKI, E. A., E. NETER, and E. COHEN. Effect of lysozyme on the release of erythrocyte modifying antigen from staphylococci and *Micrococcus lysodeikticus. J. Bacteriol.* **80**: 207, 1960.

GOTTLIEB, T., W. J. BASHE, and G. HENLE. Studies on the prevention of mumps. VI. The development of a neutralization test and its application to convalescent serum. *J. Immunol.* **71**:66, 1953.

GRABAR, T. The use of immunochemical methods in studies on proteins. *Adv. Protein Chem.* **13**:1. 1958.

GRABAR, P. In *Methods of Biochemical Analysis*, D. Glick, Ed. Vol. 7. Interscience, New York, 1959, p. 1.

GRABAR, P., and P. BURTIN. *L'analyse immuno-electrophoretique; ses applications aux liquides biologiques humaines.* Masson et Cie, Paris, 1960.

GRABAR, P., and R. CORVAZIER. Cellular aspects of immunity. In *Ciba Found. Symp.* London, 1960.

GRABAR, P., and J. OUDIN. Étude quantitative du systéme précipitant ovalbumine-anticorps homologue du lapin. I. Sur les composes solubles de la zone d'inhibition et leur précipitation par l'alcohol. *Ann. Inst. Pasteur*, **69**:195, 1943.

GRABAR, P., and C. A. WILLIAMS, JR. Méthode pérmettant l'étude conjugée des propriétes électrophorétiques d'un melange de protéines. Application au sérum sanguin. *Biochim. Biophys. Acta*, **10**:193, 1953.

GRADWOHL, R. B. J. *J. Amer. Med. Assoc.* **63**:240, 1914, c.f. Gradwohl: *Clinical Laboratory Methods and Diagnosis*, Mosby Co., St. Louis, 1956.

GRADWOHL, R. B. J., and P. KOURI. *Clinical and Laboratory Methods and Diagnosis*, Mosby Co., St. Louis, 1948.

GRAHAM, J. B., R. GRAHAM, L. NERI, and K. WRIGHT. Enhanced production of antibodies by local irradiation. *J. Immunol.* **76**:103, 1956.

GRAHAM, J. S. C. Starch-gel electrophoresis of wheat flour proteins. *Aust. J. Biol. Sci.* **16**: 342, 1963.

GRAHAM, P. H. Analytical Serology of the Rhizobiaceae. In *Analytical Serology of Microorganisms*, J. B. G. Kwapinski, Ed, Vol. I. Interscience, New York, 1969, pp. 353–378.

GRANICK, S. Ferritin: its properties and significance for iron metabolism. *Chem. Rev.* **38**: 379, 1946.

GRASSET, E., V. BONIFAS, and E. PONGRANTZ. Rapid slide precipitation micro-reaction of poliomyelitis antigens and antisera in agar. *Proc. Soc. Exper. Biol. Med.* **97**:72, 1958.

GRASSMANN, F., and R. HANNIG. Ein quantitatives Verfahren zur Analyse der Serumproteine durch Papierelektrophorese. *Hoppe-Seylers Z. Physiol. Chem.* **290**:1, 19512.

GRAY, M. L., H. J. STAFSETH, F. THORP, L. B. SHOLL, and W. F. RILEY. A new technique for isolating listerellae from the bovine brain. *J. Bacteriol.* **55**:471, 1948.

GRAY, R. A. The electrophoresis and chromatography of plant viruses on filter paper. *Arch. Biochem. Biophys.* **38**:305, 1952.

GREEN, C. Preservation of complement for Wassermann antigen. *J. Pathol. Bacteriol.* **46**: 383, 1938.

GREEN, R., and D. WOOLEY. Inhibition by certain polysaccharides of hemagglutination and multiplication of influenza virus. *J. Exper. Med.* **86**:55, 1947.

GREENSPON, S., and C. KRAKOWER. The antigenic composition of the various structures of the canine kidney. *J. Immunol.* **75**:96, 1955.

GREENWALT, T. J. Method for eluting antibodies from red cell stromata. *J. Lab. Clin. Med.* **48**:634, 1956.

GREGORY, J. D. The effect of borate on the carbazole reaction. *Arch. Biochem. Biophys.* **89**:157, 1960.

GRELET, N. Le déterminisme de la sporulation de *Bacillus megatherium*. I. L'effet de l'équisement de l'aliment carbone en millieu synthetique. *Ann. Inst. Pasteur*, **81**:480, 1961.

GRIFFITH, J. Hemagglutination by bacterial suspensions with special reference to *Shigella alkalescens*. *Proc. Soc. Exper. Biol. Med.* **67**:358, 1948.

GRIGGS, J., and L. CASE. Variation in *Brucella* agglutination on reactions in different laboratories. *Amer. J. Clin. Pathol.* **18**:566, 1948.

GROMAN, N. Dynamic aspects of the nitrogen metabolism of *Plasmodium gallinaceum* in vitro. *J. Infect. Dis.* **88**:126, 1951.

GROVE-RASMUSSEN, M., and L. SOUTTER. The necessity for adding albumin to the serum in cross matching. *New England J. Med.* **248**:194, 1953.

GRUBB, R. Dextran as a medium for the demonstration of incomplete anti-Rh-agglutinins. *J. Clin. Pathol.* **2**:223, 1949.

GRUBB, R. An estimate of the number of Rh receptors on a single red cell. *Acta Genet.* **5**:377, 1955.

GRUBER, M., and H. E. DURHAM. Münch. Med. Wochenschr. **43**:285, 1896.

GRUNBAUM, B. W., J. ZEE, and E. L. DURRUM. *Mikrochim. J.* **7**:41, 1963.

GUBARIEV, E. *Biochimija*, **7**:180, 1942.

GUBARIEV, E., and I. LUBENEC. *Biochimija*, **16**:139, 1951.

GUBARIEV, E., and V. PUSTUVALOV. *Biochimija*, **21**:293, 1956.

GUEK-HOLZER, S., and J. TOMCSIK. The isolation and chemical nature of capsular and cell-wall haptens in a *Bacillus* species. *J. Gen. Microbiol.* **14**:24, 1956.

GUGGENHEIMER, H. Über den Einfluss der Temperatur auf die Wassermannsche Syphilis-reaktion. *Münch. Med. Wochenschr.* **58**:1392, 1911.

GUIDRY, D. J., and G. H. TRELLES. Evaluation of a new method for the preparation of homogenous mycelial suspensions. *J. Bacteriol.* **83**:53, 1962.

GULLAND, J. M., D. O. JORDAN, and C. J. THRELFALL. Desoxypentose nucleic acids. I. Preparation of the tetrasodium salt of the dexoxypentose nucleic acid of calf thymus. *J. Chem. Soc.* **1129**, 1947.

GUNN, W. The variation in the amount of complement in the blood in some acute infectious diseases and its relation to the clinical feature. *J. Pathol. Bacteriol.* **19**:155, 1944.

GUPTA, N. A note on the haemagglutination by organisms of the alkalescens-dispar group. *Acta Pathol. Microbiol. Scandinav.* **27**:300, 1950.

GURVICH, A. E. In: *Contemporary Methods in Biochemistry*. *Meditsina*, Moscow, p. 73, 1964.

GURVICZ, A. E. *Biochimija*, **20**:550, 1955.

GUYOT, G. Uber die bakterielle Hämagglutination. *Zentralbl. Bakteriol. I. Orig.* **47**:640, 1908.

HABER, E. Recovery of antigenic specificity after denaturation and complete reduction of disulfides in a paprein fragment of antibody. *Proc. Natl. Acad. Sci. U.S.A.* **52**:1099, 1964.

HABER, G., and R. E. ROSENFIELD. *Ficin Treated Red Cells for Hemagglutination Studies.* Andersen Festskrift, Munksgaard, Copenhagen, 1957.

HACK, M. H. Analysis of lipids by spot tests on filter paper disk chromatograms. *Biochem. J.* **54**:602, 1953.

HACKMAN, R. H., and V. M. TRIKOJUS. Composition of honey dew excreted by Australian coccids, *Ceroplastes. Biochem. J.* **51**:633, 1952.

HADDING, U., and H. J. MÜLLER-EBERHARD. Isolation and description of the ninth component of human complement (unpublished, c.f. U. R. Nilsson and H. S. Müller-Eberhard). *Immunology*, **13**:101, 1967.

HADIDIAN, Z., and M. M. MURPHY. Interactions of non-specific inhibitors of hyaluronidase with hyaluronidase and proteolytic enzymes in vivo. *J. Gen. Physiol.* **39**:18, 1955.

HAHN, F. E., and J. CIAK. Penicillin induced lysis of *Escherichia coli. Science*, **125**:119, 1957.

HAHN, J. J., and R. M. COLE. Time and concentration relationships in the long-chain reaction of Group A streptococci in homologous antiserum and an improved method for evaluation of test results. *J. Bacteriol.* **83**:85, 1962.

HAHON, N. Assay of variola virus by the fluorescent cell-counting technique. *Appl. Microbiol.* **13**:865, 1965.

HAHON, N. Fluorescent cell-counting assay of yellow fever virus. *J. Infect. Dis.* **116**:33, 1966.

HAHON, N. The kinetics of neutralization of Venezuelan equine encephalomyelitis virus by antiserum and the reversibility of the reaction. *J. Gen. Virol.* **4**:77, 1969.

HAHON, N., and K. O. COOKE. Fluorescent cell-counting neutralization test for psittacosis. *J. Bacteriol.* **89**:1465, 1965.

HAHON, N., and K. O. COOKE. Assay of *Coxiella burnetii* by enumeration of immunofluorescent infected cells. *J. Immunol.* **97**:492, 1966.

HAHON, N., and K. O. COOKE. Primary virus-cell interactions in the immunofluorescent assay of Venezuelan equine encephalomyelitis virus. *J. Virol.* **1**:317, 1967.

HAHON, N., and R. M. NAKAMURA. Quantitative assay of psittacosis virus by the fluorescent cell-counting technique. *Virology*, **23**:203, 1964.

HALBERT, S. O., L. SWICK, and C. SONN. The use of precipitin analysis in agar for the study of human streptococcal infections. *J. Exper. Med.* **101**:539, 1955.

HALL, W. H., and R. E. MANION. Hemagglutinins and hemolysins for erythrocytes sensitized with tuberculin in pulmonary tuberculosis. *J. Clin. Invest.* **30**:1542, 1951.

HALLIDAY, W. J., and M. WEBB. A plaque technique for counting cells which produce antibacterial antibody. *Aust. J. Exper. Biol. Med. Sci.* **43**:163, 1965.

HALM, J. J., and R. M. COLE. Time and concentration relationships in the long-chain reaction of group A streptococci in homologous antiserum and an improved method for evaluation of test results. *J. Bacteriol.* **83**:85, 1962.

HALONEN, P., and S. TARPILA. Identification of herpes simplex virus isolation by a complement fixation technique. *Acta Pathol. Microb. Scandinav.* **53**:434, 1961.

HALVORSON, H. O. Spores. *Amer. Inst. Biol. Sci. Publ.* No. 5, 1957.

HAMAYO, Y. Immunological studies on the bacterial cell wall of *Clostridium welchii. Shikoku Acta Med.* **15**:1817, 1959.

HAMBURGER, H. *Physikalisch-chemische Untersuchungen über Phagozyten. Ihre Bedeutung von allgemein biologischen und pathologischen Gesichtspunkt.* J. Bergmann, Wiesbaden, 1912.

HAMBURGER, H. *Handbuch der Biologischen Arbeitsmethoden.* 1927.

HAMILTON, P. B. Ion exchange chromatography of amino acids: Recent advances in analytical determinations. *Advan. Chromatog.* **2**:3, 1966.

HAMMERLING, U., T. AOKI, E. DE HARVEN, E. S. BOYSE, and L. J. OLD. Use of hybrid antibody with anti-γG and anti-ferritin specificities in locating cell surface antigens by electron microscopy. *J. Exper. Med.* **128**:1461, 1968.

HAMMON, W., and E. IZUMI. A virus neutralization test. *J. Immunol.* **43**:149, 1942.

HAMPER, B., P. GERBER, K. C. HSU, L. M. MORTOS, J. L. WALKER, R. T. SIGÜENZA, and G. A. WELLS. Immunoferritin and immunofluorescent studies with Epstein-Barr virus and herpes simplex virus by use of human sera and hyperimmune rabbit sera. *J. Natl. Cancer Inst.* **45**:75, 1970.

HAMPER, B., A. L. NOTKINS, M. MAGE, and M. A. KEEHN. Heterogeneity in the properties of 7S and 19S rabbit-neutralizing antibodies to herpes simplex virus. *J. Immunol.* **100**: 586, 1968.

HAMRE, D., C. B. LOOSLI, and P. GERBER. Antigenic variants of influenza A virus (PR 8) strain. *J. Exper. Med.* **107**:829, 1958.

HAN, E. Hemagglutination test for epidemic and murine typhus fever using sheep erythrocytes sensitized with *Proteus* OH 19 extracts. *Amer. J. Trop. Med.* **31**:243, 1951.

HANAN, R. The effect of ultra-violet irradiation on the reactivity of antibodies. *J. Immunol.* **69**:41, 1952.

HANCOCK, R., and J. T. PARK. Cell wall synthesis by *Staphylococcus aureus* in the presence of chloramphenicol. *Nature,* **181**:1050, 1958.

HANES, C. S., and F. A. ISHERWOOD. Separation of the phosphoric esters on the filter paper chromatogram. *Nature,* **16**:1107, 1949.

HANKS, J. Ring precipitation test for estimating concentration of antibody in small amounts of immune serum. *J. Immunol.* **28**:95, 1935.

HANKS, J. Quantitative aspects of phagocytosis as influenced by the number of bacteria and leucocytes. *J. Immunol.* **38**:159, 1940.

HANNING, K. A new method for continuous carrier-free electrophoresis separation of high-molecular weight and coarsely dispersed particles. *Z. Physiol. Chem.* **338**:211, 1964.

HANSON, L. A., and S. E. HOLM. Studies on the antigenic factors in a group A streptococcal culture filtrate. *Acta Pathol. Microbiol. Scandinav.* **52**:59, 1961.

HARBOE, M. Pepsin-splitting of γM-globulins and high molecular weight antibodies. *Scandinav. J. Clin. Lab. Invest. Suppl.* **17**:233, 1965.

HARDY, P. H., JR., and E. NELL. Specific agglutination of *Treponema pallidum* by sera from rabbits and human beings with treponemal infections. *J. Exper. Med.* **101**:367, 1955.

HARGRAVES, M., H. RICHMOND, and R. MORTON. Presentation of two bone marrow elements: the "tart" cell and the "L.E." cell. *Proc. Staff. Meet. Mayo Clin.* **23**:24, 1948.

HARM, M. Die serologische Properdin-Bestimmung. *Arch. Exper. Veterinari:nediz.* **17**: 889, 1963.

HARRIS, A. Quantitative serological tests for syphilis. I. A standard method of reporting. *J. Ven. Dis.* **28**:243, 1947.

HARRIS, A., A. ROSENBERG, and L. RIEDEL. A microflocculate test for syphilis using cardiolipin antigen. *J. Ven. Dis.* **27**:169, 1946.

HARRIS, S., and T. N. HARRIS. The measurement of neutralizing antibodies to streptococcal hyaluronidase by a turbidimetric method. *J. Immunol.* **63**:233, 1949.

HARRIS, T. N. Studies in the relation of the hemolytic streptococcus to rheumatic fever. III. Complement fixation versus streptococcal nucleoproteins in the sera of patients with rheumatic fever and others. *J. Esper. Med.* **85**:57, 1948.

HARRIS, T. N., and S. HARRIS. Cellular sources of antibody: a review of current literature. *Ann. N.Y. Acad. Sci.* **86**:948, 1960.

HARRIS, T. N., S. HARRIS, and M. FARBER. Studies on the transfer of lymph node cells. II. Effects of experimental transplantation on the donor system. *J. Immunol.* **72**:161, 1954.

HARRIS, W. F. Modern methods in handling data. *New Zealand Sci. Rev.* **19**:47, 1961.

HARTE, R. Serological tests with pyrazolon compounds. *J. Immunol.* **34**:437, 1938.

HARTLEY, P. Observations in the role of the ether soluble constituents of serum in certain serological reactions. *Brit. J. Exper. Pathol.* **6**:180, 1925.

HARTMANN, J. Complement determination. *Acta Pathol. Microbiol. Scandinav.* **37**:539, 1955.

HARTMANN, L., and M. TOILLIEZ. Microméthode d'étude en gélose de la réaction antigene-anticorps. *Rev. Franc. Etud. Clin. Biol.* **2**:197, 1957.

HARVEY, H. W. Determination of phosphorus in biological materia. *Analyst,* **78**:110, 1953.

HASENCLEVER, H. F., and W. O. MITCHELL. Antigenic relationships of *Torulopsis glabrata* and seven species of the genus *Candida. J. Bacteriol.* **79**:677, 1960.

HASH, J. H., M. WISHNICK, and P. A. MILLER. Formation of "protoplasts" of *Staphylococcus aureus* with fungal *N*-acetylhexosaminodase. *J. Bacteriol.* **87**:432, 1964.

HATCHER, D. W., and G. GOLDSTEIN. Improved method for determination of RNA and DNA. *Anal. Biochem.* **31**:42, 1969.

HAUKENES, G. Serological typing of *Staphylococcus aureus.* 5. Factor *i* and *k* sera. *Acta Pathol. Microbiol. Scandinav.* **61**:283, 1964.

HAUROWITZ, F. Separation and determination of multiple antibodies. *J. Immunol.* **34**:432, 1938.

Haurowitz, F. Separation and determination of multiple antibodies. *J. Immunol.* **43**:331, 1942.

HAUROWITZ, F. Theories of antibody formation. In *The Nature and Significance of Antibody Response*, A. M. Pappenheimer, Ed. Columbia University Press, New York, 1953.

HAUROWITZ, F., and F. BREINL. *Z. Physiol. Chem.* **205**:259, 1932.

HAUROWITZ, F., and F. BREINL. Chemische Untersuchung der spezifischen Bindung von Arsanil-Eiweiss und Arsanilsäure an Immunserum. *Z. Physiol. Chem.* **214**:111, 1933.

HAUROWITZ, F., and M. M. YENSON. Quantitative determination of antigen, antibody and complement in precipitates. *J. Immunol.* **47**:390, 1943.

HAVEL, R. J., H. A. EDER, and J. H. BRAGDON. The distribution and chemical composition of ultracentrifugally separated lipoproteins in human serum. *J. Clin. Invest.* **34**:1345, 1955.

HAVENS, W., and H. EICHMAN. Collodion particle agglutination with acute-phase serums and immune globulin in viral hepatitis. *J. Immunol.* **64**:349, 1950.

HAVENS, W., and H. LLOYD. A method for preparing collodion particles for serologic agglutination. *Proc. Soc. Exper. Biol. Med.* **72**:98, 1949.

HAYES, L. Specific serum agglutination of sheep erythrocytes sensitized with bacterial polysaccharides. *Austral. J. Exper. Biol. Med. Sic.* **29**:51, 1951.

HAYES, L., and N. F. STANLEY. The preparation and properties of somatic antigens isolated from *Bacterium coli. Austral. J. Exper. Biol. Med. Sci.* **28**:201, 1950.

HAYES, S. P. The effect of Cortisone on local antibody formation. *J. Immunol.* **70**:450, 1953.

HAYES, S. P., T. F. DOUGHERTY, and L. P. GERHARDT. A method of the demonstration of tissue antibody. *Proc. Soc. Exper. Biol. Med.* **76**:460, 1951.

HAYWARD, B. J., and R. AUGUSTIN. Quantitative gel diffusion methods for assay of antigens and antibodies. *Int. Arch. Allergy,* **11**:192, 1957.

HAYWARD, M. Serological diagnosis of herpes simplex infections. *Lancet.* **I**:856, 1950.

HAZLEHURST, G. N. Anti (streptococcal) deoxyribonuclease. Occurrence in sera of patients treated with streptococcal concentrates containing streptodornase. *J. Immunol.* **65**:85, 1950.

HEALEY, G. M., D. C. FISHER, and R. C. PARKER. *Proc. Soc. Exper. Biol. Med.* **89**:71, 1955.

HEDERSTEDT, B. A comparative study of the immobilizing and hemolytic complement activity. *Acta Pathol. Microb. Scandinav.* **53**:180, 1961.

HEDGCOTH, C., and M. JACOBSON. Determination of nucleoside composition of ribonucleic acid by thin-layer chromatography. *Anal. Biochem.* **25**:55, 1968.

HEIDELBERGER, M. Quantitative absolute methods in the diagnosis of antigen-antibody reactions. *Bacteriol. Rev.* **3**:49, 1939.

HEIDELBERGER, M. In *The Nature and Significance of the Antibody Response*, A. M. Pappenheimer, Ed. Columbia University Press, New York, 1953.

HEIDELBERGER, M., and D. ANDERSON. Autohemagglutinins—"cold agglutinins": The immune response of human beings to brief infections with pneumococcus. *J. Clin. Invest.* **23**:607, 1955.

HEIDELBERGER, M., W. GOEBEL, and O. T. AVERY. The soluble specific substance of pneumococcus. *J. Exper. Med.* **42**:727, 1925.

HEIDELBERGER, M., P. GRABAR, and H. P. TREFFERS. Quantitative studies on antibody purification. III: The reaction of dissociated antibody with specific polysaccharide, and the effect of formaldehyde. *J. Exper. Med.* **68**:913, 1939.

HEIDELBERGER, M., and E. KABAT. Chemical studies on bacterial agglutination. A micro method for quantitative estimation of agglutinins. *Proc. Soc. Exper. Biol. Med.* **31**:595, 1934.

HEIDELBERGER, M., and F. E. KENDALL. A quantitative study of the precipitin reaction between type III pneumococcus polysaccharide and purified homologous antibody. *J. Exper. Med.* **50**:809, 1929.

HEIDELBERGER, M., and F. E. KENDALL. Le déplacement de la toxine des mélanges neutralises de toxine-antitoxine par la "toxoide" ou anatoxine. *Compt. Rend. Soc. Biol.* **104**:38, 1930.

HEIDELBERGER, M., and F. E. KENDALL. Data on a protein-antibody system. *Science*, **72**:252, 1930.

HEIDELBERGER, M., and F. E. KENDALL. Studies on precipitin reaction. Precipitating haptens; species differences in antibodies. *J. Exper. Med.* **57**:373, 1933.

HEIDELBERGER, M., and F. E. KENDALL. A quantitative theory of the precipitin reaction. II. A study of the azo-protein-antibody system. *J. Exper. Med.* **62**:467, 1935.

HEIDELBERGER, M., and F. E. KENDALL. Quantitative studies on antibody purification. I. The dissociation of precipitates formed by pneumococcus specific polysaccharides and homologous antibodies. *J. Exper. Med.* **64**:161, 1936.

HEIDELBERGER, M., F. E. KENDALL, and T. TEORELL. Quantitative studies of the precipitation reactions. Effect of salts on the reaction. *J. Exper. Med.* **63**:919, 1936.

HEIDELBERGER, M., C. M. MacLEOD, and M. M. DILAPI. The human antibody response to simultaneous injection of six specific polysaccharides of penumococcus. *J. Exper. Med.* **88**:369, 1948.

HEIDELBERGER, M., and C. MacPHERSON. Quantitative microestimation of antibodies in the sera of man and other animals. *Science*, **97**:405, 1943.

HEIDELBERGER, M., and M. MAYER. Quantitative chemical studies on complement or alexin. IV. Addition of human complement to specific precipitates. *J. Exper. Med.* **75**:285, 1942.

HEIDELBERGER, M., and M. MAYER. Quantitative studies on complement. *Adv. in Enzymol.* **8**:71, 1948.

HEIDELBERGER, M., and A. O. MENZEL. Specific and non-specific cell polysaccharides of the human type of tubercle bacillus. *Proc. Soc. Exper. Biol. Med.* **29**:631, 1932.

HEIDELBERGER, M., and A. O. MENZEL. Protein fractions of the human strain (H_{37}) of tubercle bacillus. *J. Biol. Chem.* **104**:655, 1934.

HEIDELBERGER, M., and K. O. PEDERSEN. The molecular weight of antibodies. *J. Exper. Med.* **65**:393, 1937.

HEIDELBERGER, M., and H. P. TREFFERS. Quantitative chemical studies on hemolysins; estimation of total antibody in antisera to sheep erythrocytes and stromata. *J. Gen. Physiol.* **25**:523, 1942.

HEIDELBERGER, M., H. P. TREFFERS, and M. M. MAYER. A quantitative theory of precipitin reaction. VII. The egg albumen-antibody reaction in antisera from the rabbit and horse. *J. Exper. Med.* **71**:271, 1940.

HEIDELBERGER, M., A. J. WEIL, and H. P. TREFERS. Quantitative chemical studies on complement or alexin. II. The interrelation of complement with antigen-antibody compounds and with sensitized cells. *J. Exper. Med.* **73**:695, 1941.

HEIKEN, A., and M. RASMUSON. Genetical studies on the Rh blood group system. *Hereditas Lund*, **55**:192, 1966.

HEILMAN, D. H. In vitro toxicity of endotoxin for macrophages of young guinea pigs and rabbits. *Int. Arch. Allergy*, **33**:501, 1968.

HEILMAN, D. H., D. H. HOWARD, and C. M. CARPENTER. Tissue culture studies on bacterial allergy in experimental tuberculosis. *J. Exper. Med.* **107**:319, 1958.

HEILMAN, H., E. RICE, D. H. HOWARD, H. E. WEIMER, and C. M. CARPENTER. Tissue culture studies in experimental brucellosis. II. The cytoxicity of nucleoprotein fractions of *Brucella*. *J. Immunol.* **85**:258, 1960.

HEILMANN, J., J. BARROLIER, and E. WATZKE. Beitrag zur Aminosaurebestimmung auf Papier-Chromatogrammen. *Zeitschr. Physiol. Chem.* **305**:219, 1957.

HEKTOEN, L., and A. K. BOOR. Simultaneous multiple immunization. *J. Infect. Dis.* **48**:582, 1931.

HELLER, G., A. S. JACOBSEN, and M. H. KOLODNY. A modification of the hemagglutination test for rheumatoid arthritis. *Proc. Soc. Exper. Biol. Med.* **72**:316, 1949.

HELLER, G., M. H. KOLODNY, I. H. LEPOW, A. S. JACOBSEN, M. G. RIVERA, and G. H. MARKS. The hemagglutination test for rheumatoid arthritis. IV. Characterization of the rheumatoid agglutination factors by analysis of several fractions prepared by ethanol fractionation. *J. Immunol.* **74**:340, 1955.

HENLE, G., S. HARRIS, and W. HENLE. The reactivity of various human sera with mumps complement fixation antigens. *J. Exper. Med.* **88**:133, 1948.

HENLE, G., W. HENLE, and J. HARRIS. The serological differentiation of mumps: complement-fixation antigens. *J. Exper. Med.* **64**:290, 1947.

HENNISCH, M. P. Virus antigen antibody reactions by gel diffusion. *Int. Arch. Allergy*, **16**:153, 1960.

HENRIKSEN, S. D., and J. Eriksen. Immunochemical studies on some serological cross-reactions in the *Klebsiella* group. *Acta Pathol. Microbiol. Scandinav.* **51**:259, 1961.

HENRY, B. Dissociation in the genus *Brucella*. *J. Infect. Dis.* **52**:374, 1933.

HERBERT, D., and E. W. TODD. Purification and properties of a haemolysin of Group A haemolytic streptococci (Streptolysin O). *Biochem. J.* **35**:1124, 1941.

HERBERT, D., and E. W. TODD. The oxygen-stable haemolysin of group A hemolytic streptococci (Streptolysin S). *Brit. J. Exper. Pathol.* **25**:247, 1944.

HEREMANS, J. F. In: *Molecular and Cellular Basis of Antibody Forunation*. Academic Press, N. Y. p. 277, 1965.

HERRMAN, V. A study of the blood-grouping factors in horse. *J. Immunol.* **31**:347, 1936.

HERSEY, D., M. C. COLVIN, and C. C. SHEPARD. Studies on the serologic diagnosis of murine typhus and Rocky Mountain spotted fever (RMSF). I. Experimental infections in guinea pigs and rabbits. *J. Immunol.* **79**:410, 1957. II. Human infections. *J. Immunol.* **79**:409, 1947.

HERSHEY, A. A descriptive theory of specific precipitation. *J. Immunol.* **42**:455, 1941.

HESS, W. R., and M. H. ROEPKE. A non-specific *Brucella* agglutinating substance in bovine serum. *Proc. Soc. Exper. Biol. Med.* **77**:469, 1951.

HESTRIN, S. The reaction of acetylcholine and other carboxylic acid derivatives with hydroxylamine and its analytical application. *J. Biol. Chem.* **180**:249, 1949.

HESTRIN, S. Acylation reactions mediated by purified acetylcholine esterase. *J. Biol. Chem.* **180**:879, 1949.

HEWITT, B. The complement fixation in experimental equine encephalomyelitis, lymphocytic choriomeningitis and the St. Louis type encephalitis. *J. Immunol.* **33**:235, 1937.

HEYMANN, G. Fortschritte der serologischen Diagnostik auf dem Gebiet der luetischen Erkrankungen. *Zentralbl. Bakteriol. I. Orig.* **170**:3, 1957.

HEYMANN, G. Das allgemeine Standardprinzip in der quantitativen Serodiagnostik der Lues. *Der Hautarzt*, **11**:510, 1960.

HEYNS, K., and D. MUELLER. Mass spectroscopic investigations. VIII. Mass spectra of permethyl *N*-acetylamino sugars. *Tetrahedron* **21**:3151, 1965.

HIERHOLZER, J. C., and N. T. SUGGS. Standardized viral hemagglutination and hemagglutination-inhibition tests. I. Standardization of erythrocyte suspensions. *Appl. Microbiol.* **18**:816, 1969.

HIERHOLZER, J. C., N. T. SUGGS, and E. C. HALL. Standardized viral hemagglutination and hemagglutination-inhibition tests. II. Description and statistical evaluation. *Appl. Microbiol.* **18**:824, 1969.

HILBORN, J. C., and P. A. ANASTASSIADIS. Acrylamide gel electrophoresis of acidic mucopolysaccharides. *Anal. Biochem.* **31**:51, 1969.

HILL, A. B. *Principles of Medical Statistics*. The Lancet Ltd., London, 1956.

HILL, A. G. S., H. W. DEANE, and A. H. COONS. Localization of antigen in tissue cell. V. Capsular polysaccharide of Friedländer bacillus, type B, in the mouse. *J. Exper. Med.* **92**:35, 1950.

HILLEMAN, J., R. MASON, and E. PUESCHER. Comparison of the antigenic patterns of influenza A virus determined by in ovo neutralization and hemagglutination-inhibition. *J. Immunol.* **69**:343, 1950.

HILLEMAN, M. R., D. A. HAIG, and R. J. HELMOLD. The indirect complement fixation, hemagglutination and conglutination complement absorption tests for viruses of the psittacosis-lymphogranuloma venereum group. *J. Immunol.* **66**:115, 1951.

HILLEMAN, M. R., D. A. HAIG, and R. J. HELMOLD. In vivo and in vitro studies of serological specificity among viruses of the psittacosis-lymphogranuloma venereum group. *J. Immunol.* **68**:121, 1952.

HILLEMAN, M. R., and F. HORSFALL, JR. Comparison of the antigenic patterns of influenza A virus strains determined by *in ovo* neutralization and hemagglutination-inhibition. *J. Immunol.* **69**:343, 1950.

HINUMA, Y., and K. HUMMELER. Studies on the complement-fixing antibodies of poliomyelitis. III. Intracellular development of antigen. *J. Immunol.* **87**:367, 1961.

HINUMA, Y., T. MIYAMOTO, R. OHTA, and N. ISHIDA. Counting of Sendai virus particles by an immunofluorescent technique. *Virology*, **20**:405, 1963.

HINZ, C., and L. PILLEMER. The requirement for the properdinsystem in the hemolysis of human erythrocytes treated with tannic acid. *J. Clin. Invest.* **34**:912, 1955.

HIRAMOTO, R., J. JURANDOWSKI, J. BERNECKY, and D. PRESSMAN. Immunohistochemical identification of tissue-culture cells. *Proc. Soc. Exper. Biol. Med.* **108**:347, 1961.

HIRSCH, J. G., and A. B. CHURCH. Studies of phagocytosis of Group A streptoccoci by polymorphonuclear leucocytes in vitro. *J. Exper. Med.* **111**:309, 1960.

HIRST, G. K. The agglutination of red cells by allantoic fluid of chick embryos infected with influenza virus. *Science*, **94**:22, 1941.

HIRST, G. K. The quantitative determination of influenza virus and antibodies by means of red cell agglutination. *J. Exper. Med.* **75**:47, 1942.

HIRST, G. K. Studies on antigenic differences among strains of influenza A viruses by means of red cell agglutination. *J. Exper. Med.* **78**:407, 1943.

HIRST, G. K., and E. G. PICKLES. A method for the titration of influenza hemagglutinins and influenza antibodies with the aid of a photoelectric densitometer. *J. Immunol.* **45**:273, 1942.

HIRSZFELD, L. *Konstitutionsserologie und Blutgruppenforschung.* J. Springer, Berlin, 1928.

HIRSZFELD, L., H. HIRSZFELD, and H. BROKMAN. On the susceptibility of diphtheria (Schick test positive), with reference to inheritance of blood groups. *J. Immunol.* **9**:57, 1924.

HITCHCOCK, C. H. Classification of the haemolytic streptocci by the precipitin reaction. Preparation of bacteria extracts. *J. Exper. Med.* **40**:445, 1924.

HITCHCOCK, D. Protein films on collodion membranes. *J. Gen. Physiol.* **8**:61, 1926.

HJÉRTEN, S. Agarose as an anticonvection agent in zone electrophoresis. *Biochim. Biophys. Acta* **53**:514, 1961.

HJERTÉN, S. *Protides of the Biological Fluids*, H. Peeters, Ed. Elsevier, Amsterdam, 1967.

HJERTÉN, S., and R. MOSBACH. "Molecular-sieve" chromatography of proteins on columns of cross-linked polyacrylamide. *Anal. Biochem.* **3**:109, 1962.

HOAGLAND, M. B., M. L. STEPHENSON, J. F. SCOTT, L. I. HECHT, and P. C. ZAMECNIK. A soluble ribonucleic acid intermediate in protein synthesis. *J. Biol. Chem.* **231**:241, 1958.

HOBSON, D., and R. H. GORRILL. Agglutination test for rheumatoid arthritis. *Lancet.* **I**:389, 1952.

HODES, H. L., H. D. ZEPP, W. L. HENELY, and R. BERGER. A new method for detection of human poliomyelitis antibodies. *Science,* **125**:1089, 1957.

HODGE, B. E., and H. F. SWIFT. Varying hemolytic and constant combining capacity of streptolysins. *J. Exper. Med.* **58**:277, 1933.

HOFFMANN, A. *Münch. Med. Wochenschr.* **68**:71, 1921.

HOFMANN, K., C-Y. Y. HSIAO, D. B. HENIS, and C. PANOS. The estimation of fatty acid composition of bacterial lipides. *J. Biol. Chem.* **217**:49, 1955.

HOFSTAD, T. Studies on the antigenic structure of the 80/81 complex of *Staphylococcus aureus.* I. Agglutinogen. *Acta Pathol. Microbiol. Scandinav.* **61**:558, 1964.

HOFSTAD, T. Studies on the antigenic structure of the 80/81 complex of *Staphylococcus aureus. Acta Pathol. Microbiol. Scandinav.* **63**:422, 1965.

HOFSTEN, B., and A. TJEDER. The disintegration of yeasts with dry ice and some properties of the extract. *J. Biochem. Technol. Eng.* **3**:175, 1961.

HÖGLUND, S. Electron microscopic investigations of the interaction between the T2-phage and its IgG- and IgM- antibodies. *Virology,* **32**:662, 1967.

HOIGNÉ, R., W. GROSSMANN, and H. STORCK. Neue serologische Methode zum Nachweis von Sensibilisierung auf Allergene. *Helvet. Med. Acta,* **22**:451, 1955.

HOLE, N. H., and R. R. A. COOMBS. The conglutination phenomenon. III. The technique of the conglutinating complement absorption test compared with the haemolytic complement fixation test. *J. Hygiene,* **45**:440, 1947.

HOLE, N. H., and R. R. A. COOMBS. The conglutination phenomenon. III. The conglutinating complement absorption test in experimental glanders. *J. Hygiene,* **45**:497, 1947.

HOLLAND, A. A. Serologic characteristics of certain root-nodule bacteria of legumes. *Ant. Van Leeuwenhoek,* **32**:410, 1966.

HOLM, P., and J. B. KWAPINSKI. Studies on the detection of *Actinomyces* antibodies in human sera by using pure antigenic fractions of *Actinomyces israelii. Acta Pathol. Microbiol. Scandinav.* **45**:107, 1959.

HOLMAN, H. R., and H. G. KUNKEL. Affinity between lupus erythematosus serum factor and cell nuclei and nucleoprotein. *Science,* **126**:162, 1957.

HOMMA, J. Y., and N. SUZUKI. Cell-wall protein "A" of *Pseudomonas aeruginosa* and its relationship to "original endotoxin protein." *J. Bacteriol.* **87**:630, 1964.

HOOBER, J. K., and G. BLOBEL. Characterization of the chloroplastic and cytoplastic ribosomes of *Chlamydomonas reinhardi. J. Mol. Biol.* **41**:121, 1969.

HOOGHWINKEL, G. J. M., and H. P. A. A. VAN NIEKERK. Quantitative aspects of the tricomplex staining procedure. The staining of lecithin spots applied on chromatographic papers I_A. *Kon. Ned. Akad. Vetenschappen*, **63**:258, 1960.

HOPKINS, S., and A. WORMALL. Phenyl isocyanata protein compounds and their immunological reactions. *Biochem. J.* **27**:740, 1933.

HOŘEJŠI, J., and R. SMETANA. The isolation of γ-globulin from blood-serum by Rivanol. *Acta Med. Scandinov.* **155**:64, 1956.

HORNUNG, M. Paper chromatography of pneumococcus cell-wall hydrolysates containing glucosamine, galactosamine, muramic acid, and peptides. *J. Bacteriol.* **86**:1345, 1963.

HORROCKS, R. H. Paper partition chromatography of reducing sugars with benzidine as a spraying regent. *Nature*, **164**:444, 1949.

HORSFALL, F. L., JR., and K. GOODNER. Lipids and immunochemical reactions. *J. Immunol.* **31**:135, 1936.

HORSFALL, F. L., JR., and J. TAMM. Fractional dilution procedure for precise titration of hemagglutinating viruses and hemagglutination-inhibition antibodies. *J. Immunol.* **70**:253, 1953.

HORSTMANN, D. M., and L. M. KRAFT. Poliomyelitis and other antibody patterns in natives of Tahiti and Raiatea. *J. Immunol.* **75**:249, 1955.

HORVATH, B., and C. W. JUNGEBLUT. Studies on hemagglutination by Columbia-SK virus. *J. Immunol.* **68**:627, 1957.

HOUGH, L. Application of paper partition chromatography to the separation of the polyhydric alcohols. *Nature*, **165**:400, 1950.

HOUSEWRIGHT, R. D., and C. B. THORNE. Synthesis of glutamic acid and glutamyl polypeptide by *Bacillus anthracis*. I. Formation of glutamic acid by transamination. *J. Bacteriol.* **60**:89, 1950.

HOVNANIAN, H. P., T. A. BRENNAN, and E. A. BOTAN. Quantitative rapid immunofluorescence microscopy. I. Instrumentation. *J. Bacteriol.* **87**:473, 1964.

HOWE, C., C. MORGAN, and K. C. HSU. Recent virological applications of ferritin conjugates. *Prog. Med. Virol.* **11**:307, 1969.

HOWIE, J. W., and K. CRIUCKSHANK. Bacterial spores as antigens. *J. Pathol.* **50**:235, 1940.

HOWITT, B. F. Complement fixation test differentiating three strains of equine encephalomyelitis virus and the virus of lymphocytic meningitis. *Proc. Soc. Exper. Biol. Med.* **35**:526, 1937.

HOWITT, B. F. The complement fixation reaction in experimental equine encephalitis, lymphocytic choriomeningitis and the St. Louis type encephalitis. *J. Immunol.* **33**:235, 1943.

HOYER, B. H., E. T. BOLTON, R. A. ORMSBEE, G. LEBOUVIER, D. B. RITTER, and C. L. LARSON. Mammalian viruses and rickettsiae. Their purification and recovery by cellulose anion exchange columns has significant implications. *Science*, **127**:859, 1958.

HOYLE, L. An analysis of the complement-fixation reaction in influenza. *J. Hygiene*, **44**:170, 1945.

HSU, K. C. FERRITIN-labeled antigens and antibodies. In *Methods in Immunology and Immunochemistry*, C. A. Williams and M. W. Chase, Eds. Vol. I. Academic Press, 1967, New York, pp. 397–404.

HSU, K. C., R. A. RIFKIND, and J. B. ZABRISKIE. Fluorescent, electron microscopic and immunoelectrophoretic studies of labeled antibodies. *Science*, **142**:1471, 1963.

HÜBNER, K. F., and N. GENGOZIAN. Critical variables of the Jerne plaque technique as applied to rodent antibody-forming systems responding to heterologous red cell antigens. *J. Immunol.* **102**:155, 1969.

HUCKE, D. M., and C. H. ROCHE. Automation in the turbidimetric assay. In *Antibiotics Annual*. Antibiotics, Inc., New York, 1959–1960.

HUDDLESON, I. F. *Brucellosis in Man and Animals*. Commonwealth Fund, New York, 1943.

HUDDLESON, I. F., E. E. WOOD, A. R. CRESSMAN, and G. R. BENNETT. The bactericidal action of bovine blood for *Brucella* and its possible significance. *J. Bacteriol.* 50:261, 1945.

HUDSON, N., and S. MUDD. An ultramicrotechnic for precipitation and agglutination reaction. *J. Immunol.* 28:311, 1935.

HUENEKENS, E. J. The prophylactic use of pertussis vaccine controlled by the complement fixation test. *Amer. J. Dis. Childhood*, 14:283, 1917.

HUGHES, E. J. Immunization phenomena in rabbits vaccinated with heat-killed tubercle bacilli. *J. Immunol.* 25:103, 1933.

HUGHES, D. E. A press for disrupting bacteria and other microorganisms. *Brit. J. Exper. Pathol.* 32:97, 1951.

HUGHES-JONES, N. C. The estimation of the concentration and equilibrium constant of anti-D. *Immunology*, 12:565, 1967.

HUISMAN, T. H. J., and A. M. DOZY. Studies on the heterogeneity of hemoglobin. IV. Chromatographic behavior of different human hemoglobins on anion-exchange cellulose (DEAE-cellulose). *J. Chromatog.* 7:180, 1962.

HUMMELER, K. Mumps complement fixing antibodies in guinea pigs. *J. Immunol.* 79:397, 1957.

HUMPHREY, B. A., and J. M. VINCENT. Extracellular polysaccharides of *Rhizobium*. *J. Gen. Microbiol.* 21:477, 1959.

HUMPHREY, J. H., and R. R. PORTER. An investigation on rabbit antibodies by the use of partition chromatography. *Biochem. J.* 62:93, 1956.

HUNTER, C. A., and R. L. COLBERT. Flocculation tests for brucellosis. *J. Immunol.* 77:232, 1956.

HUNTOON, F. M., and S. H. CRAIG. Polyvalent antibody response to multiple antigens. *J. Immunol.* 6:235, 1921.

HURWITZ, C., J. M. REINER, and J. V. LANDAU. Studies in the physiology and biochemistry of penicillin-induced spheroplasts of *Escherichia coli*. *J. Bacteriol.* 76:612, 1958.

IBE, E. C., and A. C. WARDLAW. Observations on pH and haemolytic complement. *Immunology*, 7:586, 1964.

ILLÉS, J. Die best geeigneten Plasmen für die Staphylokoagulasereaktion. *Pathol. Microbiol.* 27:117, 1964.

INCHIOSA, M. A. Direct biuret determination of total protein in tissue homogenates. *J. Lab. Clin. Med.* 63:319, 1964.

INGRAHAM, J. S., A. A. BIEGEL, M. R. WATANABE, and C. W. TODD. Effect of anti-allotype sera on hemolytic plaque formation by single rabbit spleen cells. *J. Immunol.* 99:1023, 1967.

INGRAHAM, J. S., and A. BUSSARD. Application of a localized hemolysis reaction for specific detection of individual antibody-forming cells. *J. Exper. Med.* 119:667, 1964.

INGRAM, D. G. The serological activities of immunoconglutinin. *Can. J. Microbiol.* 15:981, 1969.

INGRAM, G. I. C. A note on dilution systems. *Immunology*, 5:504, 1962.

INGRAM, V. M. Abnormal human haemoglobins. I. The comparison of normal human and sickle-cell haemoglobins by "fingerprinting." *Biochem. Biophys. Acta*, 28:539, 1958.

INOUE, K., and R. A. NELSON, JR. The isolation and characterization of a new component of hemolytic complement, C'3e. *J. Immunol.* 95:355, 1965.

IPSEN, J., JR. The effect of temperature on the immune response of mice to tetanus toxoid. *J. Immunol.* 60:273, 1952.

IRIE, R. F., K. NICHIOKA, T. TACHIBANA, and S. TAKENCHI. Immunological studies of mouse mammary tumors. IV. Extraction and solubilization of transplantation antigen of mouse mammary tumor. *Int. J. Cancer*, **4**:150, 1969.

IRWIN, J. C., and E. A. CHESSMAN. On an approximate method of determining the medium effective dose and its error in the case of quantal response. *J. Hygiene*, **30**:574, 1935.

IRWIN, J. C., and M. E. SEELEY, JR. Titration and partial characterization of soluble hemolysin of group D Streptococcus. *J. Bacteriol.* **76**:29, 1959.

IRWIN, M. R., and D. J. BERMAN. *Bactericidal Tests in Brucellosis.* Publication of the American Association for the Advancement of Science, 1950.

ISHERWOOD, F. A., and C. S. HANES. Separation and estimation of organic acids on paper chromatograms. *Biochem. J.* **55**:824, 1953.

ISHIZAKA, K., and D. CAMPBELL. Biologic activity of soluble antigen-antibody complexes. V. Change of optical rotation by the formation of skin reactive complexes. *J. Immunol.* **83**:318, 1959.

ISLIKER, H. Purification of antibodies by means of antigens linked to ion exchange resins. *Ann. N.Y. Acad. Sci.* **57**:225, 1953.

ISLIKER, H. The properdin system. A review. *Vox Sang.* **1**:8, 1956.

ISLIKER, H., and E. LINDER. Methods for the assay of properdin. *Vox Sang.* **3**:23, 1958.

ISLIKER, H. C., and P. H. STRAUSS. The purification of antibodies to PR8 influenza A virus. *Vox Soup.* **4**:198, 1959.

ISPOLATOVSKAJA, M. V., V. A. PLAGOVESHGHENSKII, I. V. VLASOVA, and A. P. KUZMINA. *Zhur. Mikrobiol. Epidem. Immunobiol.* **30**:70, 1953.

ITO, Y. Use of filter paper chromatograms in reading and recording the results of the Wassermann reaction and other serological tests. *J. Bacteriol.* **75**:612, 1958.

IVANOVICS, G., and I. FOLDES. An immunospecific substance of *Bacillus cereus* similar to polysaccharide obtained from *Bacillus anthracis*. *Naturwissenschaften*, **45**:15, 1958.

IZUMI, Y. Studies on the bacterial cell walls and endospore membrane of *B. cereus* and some other bacteria. *Shikoku Acta Med.* **14**:138, 1959.

JABLON, J. M., M. SAUL, and M. S. SASLAW. Microtechnic for determination of titers of antistreptolysin O. *Tech. Bull. Reg. M. Technol.* **28**:117, 1958.

JACOBS, M. B., and M. A. BEHAN. Concentration of tetanus toxoid. *J. Amer. Pharm. Assoc.* **39**:466, 1950.

JACOBS, M. B. Purification of tetanus toxoid. *J. Amer. Pharm. Assoc.* **39**:469, 1950.

JACOBSEN, M., J. F. O'BRIEN, and C. HEDGCOTH. Determination of nucleoside composition of ribonucleic acid by gas-liquid chromatography. *Anal. Biochem.* **25**:363, 1968.

JACOBSTAHL, E. Eine Anregung zur Anstellung von Kutisreaktionen bei Fleckfieber. *Deutsche Med. Wochenschr.* **36**:1093, 1916.

JADASSOHN, W., F. SCHAAF, and G. WOHLER. Analyses of composite antigens by the Schultz-Dale technic; further experimental analyses of trichophytines. *J. Immunol.* **32**:203, 1937.

JAMIESON, G. R., and E. H. REID. The analysis of oils and fats by gas chromatography. *J. Chromatog.* **17**:230, 1965.

JANEWAY, C. In *Nature and Significance of the Antibody Response*, A. Pappenheimer, Ed. Interscience Publications, New York, 1953.

JANN, B., and K. JANN. 2-amino-2,6-dideoxy-L-mannose (L-rhamnosamine) isolated from the lipopolysaccharide of *Escherichia coli*. 03:K2ab(L):H2. *Eur. J. Biochem.* **5**:173, 1968.

JANN, K., B. JANN, K. F. SCHNEIDER, F. OERSHOV, and I. OERSHOV. Immunochemistry of K antigens of *Escherichia coli*. V. The K antigen of *E. coli* 08:K-27(A)H⁻. *Eur. J. Biochem.* **5**:456, 1968.

JANSEN, F. W., A. LUND, and L. E. ANDERSON. Colorimetric assay for dipicolinic acid in bacterial spores. *Science*, **127**:26, 1958.

JAROSLOW, B. N., and W. H. TALIAFERRO. The restoration of hemolysin-forming capacity in x-irradiated rabbits by tissue and yeast preparations. *J. Infect. Dis.* **98**:75, 1956.

JAWETZ, E., and K. MEYER. Studies on phage immunity in experimental animals. *J. Immunol.* **49**:1, 1944.

JEFFREY, M. R. An appraisal of the latex test for rheumatoid arthritis. *J. Lab. Clin. Med.* **54**:525, 1959.

JENKIN, C. R., and D. ROWLEY. Toxic proteins from *Vibrio cholerae* and water vibrios which are lethal for mice. *J. Gen. Microbiol.* **21**:191, 1959.

JENKIN, H. M. Preparation and properties of cell walls of the agent of meningopneumonitis. *J. Bacteriol.* **80**:639, 1960.

JENNINGS, R. K. Antigens in scarlatinal erythrogenic toxin demonstrated by the Oudin technic. *J. Immunol.* **70**:181, 1953.

JENNINGS, R. K. A misleading "reaction of identity" in agar diffusion precipitation studies of tetanus antitoxin. *J. Immunol.* **77**:156, 1956.

JENNINGS, R. K. Gel diffusion studies of cross reacting antibody. *J. Immunol.* **83**:237, 1959.

JENNINGS, R. K., and F. MALONE. The double diffusion technics as a tool for the study of the induction of antibody formation. *Brit. J. Exper. Pathol.* **36**:2, 1955.

JENSEN, K. The toxic effect of staphylococcal polysaccharides on isolated guinea pig illeum and the antitoxic effect of normal human serum. *Acta Allergol.* **13**:89, 1959.

JENSEN, K. Serological typing of the staphylococci by means of gel-precipitation reactions. *Acta Pathol. Microbiol. Scandinav.* **52**:175, 1961.

JENSEN, K. E., and T. FRANCIS. JR. The antigenic composition of influenza virus measured by antibody absorption. *J. Exper. Med.* **98**:619, 1953.

JENSEN, K. E., and T. FRANCIS. JR. Antigen-antibody precipitates in solid medium with influenza virus. *J. Immunol.* **70**:321, 1953.

JENSEN, T., and O. MAALØE. Study of action of Staphylococcus toxin on leucocytes. *Acta Pathol. Microbiol. Scandinav.* **27**:313, 1950.

JERMOLJEV, E., and L. ALBRECHTOVA. Aplikace suspenze latex v sérologické diagnóze virových chorob rostlin. *Ochr. Rost.* **2**:51, 1965.

JERMYN, M. A., and F. A. ISHERWOOD. Improved separation of sugars on the paper partition chromatogram. *Biochem. J.* **44**:407, 1949.

JERNE, N. K. The natural-selection theory of antibody formation. *Proc. Natl. Acad. Sci. U.S.* **41**:849, 1955.

JERNE, N. K., and P. AVEGNO. The development of the phage-inactivating properties of serum during the course of specific immunization of an animal: reversible and irreversible inactivation. *J. Immunol.* **76**:200, 1956.

JERNE, N. K., and A. NORDIN. Plaque formation in agar by simple antibody-producing cells. *Science*, **140**:405, 1963.

JERNE, N. K., A. A. NORDIN, and C. HENRY. The agar plaque technique for recognizing antibody-producing cells. In *Cell-Bound Antibodies*, B. Amos and H. Koprowski, Eds. The Wistar Institute Press, Philadelphia, 1963, p. 109.

JEYNES, M. H. Growth and properties of bacterial protoplasts. *Nature*, **180**:867, 1957.

JOHANSEN, P. G., R. D. MARSHALL, and A. NEUBERGER. The hexose, hexosamine, acetyl and amide-nitrogen content of hen's egg albumin. *Biochem. J.* **77**:239, 1960.

JOHANSSON, A., B. LINDBERG, and O. THEANDER. Semimicro determination of uronic acids. *Svensk Papperstidning*, **57**:41, 1954.

JOHNSON, A. E. Micro diffusion agar precipitin technique convenient for viewing and recording. *J. Bacteriol.* **93**:1476, 1967.

JOHNSON, A., D. WOERNLEY, and D. PRESSMAN. Sedimentation properties of human and erythrocyte hemolysins. *J. Immunol.* **79**:234, 1957.

JOHNSON, R. B. An immunogenic antigen of low toxicity derived from *Shigella sonnei. J. Immunol.* **74**:286, 1955.

JONES, A. R. Dextran as a diluent for univalent antibodies. *Nature*, **165**:118, 1950.

JONES, A. S., and G. E. MARSH. The deproteinisation of nucleoproteins. *Biochim. Biophys. Acta*, **14**:559, 1954.

JONES, A. S., G. E. MARSH, and S. B. H. RIZVI. The isolation of the nucleic acids of *Aerobacter aerogenes. Microbiol.* **17**:586, 1957.

JONES, F. Agglutination by precipitin. *J. Exper. Med.* **46**:303, 1927.

JONES, F., and M. ORCUTT. The prozone phenomenon in specific bacterial agglutination. *J. Immunol.* **27**:215, 1934.

JONES, J. K. N., M. B. PERRY, and W. SOWA. The occurrence of D-glycero-D-manno-heptose in the extracellular polysaccharide produced by *Azotobacter indicum. Can. J. Chem.* **41**:2712, 1963.

JONES, W. D., H. SAITO, and C. P. KUBICA. Fluorescent antibody technique with mycobacteria. *Amer. Rev. Resp. Dis.* **92**:256, 1965.

JUHLIN, L., and W. B. SHELLEY. Plastic tube technic of centrifugal separation of leukocytes from human blood. *Blood*, **18**:477, 1961.

JULIANELLE, L. Immunological specificity of *Bacterium aerogenes* and its antigenic relation to pneumococcus, type II, and Friedländer's bacillus, type B. *J. Immunol.* **32**:21, 1937.

JUNGEBLUT, C. W. Studies on viremia in poliomyelitis. Absorption in vitro of the JV strain of poliomyelitis virus in human erythrocytes. *J. Paediatr.* **44**:28, 1954.

JUNGEBLUT, C. W., and J. A. BERLOT. The role of the reticuloendothelial system in immunity. II. The complement titers after blockade and the physiological regeneration of the reticulo-endothelial system as measured by reduction tests. *J. Exper. Med.* **43**:797, 1926.

JUNGEBLUT, C. W., B. HOFMAN, JR., and J. D. VERLINEDE. Adsorption in vitro of poliomyelitis virus on human erythrocytes. *Proc. Soc. Exper. Biol. Med.* **83**:249, 1953.

JUNGEBLUT, C. W., and E. HUENEKENS. *J. Paediatr.* **44**:28, 1954.

JUNGERMAN, D. Studies of the antigenic structure of *Staphylococcus aureus. Arch. Immunol. Ther. Exper.* **10**:77, 1962.

JYSSUM, K. *Indirect Hemagglutination by Antigens from Pneumococci.* Thesis, Oslo University Academish Tryningssentral, Oslo, 1955.

JYSSUM, K. Serologic relationship between meningococcal strains in Norway. *J. Immunol.* **76**:433, 1956.

KABAT, E. A. The molecular weight of antibodies. *J. Exper. Med.* **69**:103, 1939.

KABAT, E. A. Dextran-an antigen in man. *J. Immunol.* **70**:514, 1953.

Kabat, E. A. *Blood Group Substances. Their Chemistry and Immunochemistry.* Academic Press, New York, 1956.

KABAT, E. A. Heterogeneity in extent of the combining regions of human anti-dextran. *J. Immunol.* **77**:377, 1956.

KABAT, E. A. The upper limit for the size of the human antidextran combining site. *J. Immunol.* **84**:82, 1960.

KABAT, E. A. *Experimental Immunochemistry*, 2nd ed. Thomas, Springfield, Ill., 1961.

KABAT, E. A. The nature of antigenic determinant. *Immunology*, **97**:1, 1966.

KABAT, E. A., H. BAER, R. L. DAY, and V. KNAUB. Immunochemical studies on blood groups. Species differences among blood group A substances. *J. Exper. Med.* **91**:433, 1950.

KABAT, E. A., A. BENDICH, A. E. BEZER, and S. M. BEISER. Immunochemical studies on blood groups. Preparation of blood group A substances from human sources and a comparison of their chemical and immunochemical properties with those of the blood group substance from hog stomach. *J. Exper. Med.* **85**:685, 1947.

KABAT, E. A., and M. M. MAYER. *Experimental Immunochemistry*. Thomas, Springfield, Ill., 1948.

KABAT, E. A., C. MILLER, H. KAISER, and A. Z. FOSTER. Chemical studies on bacterial agglutination. A quantitative study of the type specific and group specific antibodies in antimeningococcal sera of various species and their relation to mouse protection. *J. Exper. Med.* **81**:1, 1945.

KAHN, R. L. *The Kahn Test; a Practical Guide*. Williams and Wilkins Co., Baltimore, 1928.

KAHN, R. L. Studies on tissue reactions in immunity. VII. A quantitative measure of skin sensitivity. *J. Immunol.* **25**:295, 1933.

KAHN, R. L. *Tissue Immunity*. Thomas, Springfield, Ill., 1936.

KAHN, R. L. *Technique of Standard Kahn Test and of Special Kahn Procedures*. University of Michigan Press, 1945.

KAHNKE, M. J. A hemolysis inhibition test for the detection of antibodies to Newcastle disease virus. *J. Immunol.* **66**:507, 1951.

KAISER, A. D., and D. S. HOGNESS. The transformation of *Escherichia coli* with deoxyribonucleic acid isolated from bacteriophage. *J. Mol. Biol.* **2**:392, 1960.

KAKEFUDA, T., J. T. HOLDEN, and N. M. UTECH. Ultrastructure of the membrane system in *Lactobacillus plantarum*. *J. Bacteriol.* **93**:472, 1967.

KALBAK, K. Agglutination tests in patients with chronic polyarthritis using hemolytic streptococci as antigen. *Nord. Med.* **31**:1997, 1946.

KALMAN, K., and M. PORGANYI. Antigenstruktur des *Treponema pallidum* und die Immunadhäsion. *Zeitschr. Immunitätsforsch.* **119**:183, 1960.

KAMINSKI, M. Studies on egg white and its constituents by immunochemical techniques in petrified media: specific precipitation by double diffusion and immunoelectrophoretic analysis. *J. Immunol.* **75**:367, 1955.

KANAI, K., and G. P. YOUMANS. Immunogenicity of intracellular particles and cell walls from *Mycobacterium tuberculosis*. *J. Bacteriol.* **80**:607, 1960.

KANAI, K., G. P. YOUMANS, and A. S. YOUMANS. Allergenicity of intracellular particles, cell walls, and cytoplasmic fluid from *Mycobacterum tuberculosis*. *J. Bacteriol.* **80**:615, 1960.

KANO, K. Blood group B antigen in cell cultures of Rhesus monkey kidney. *Int. Arch. Allergy*, **30**:281, 1966.

KAPLAN, A. Antibody determination by the plaque method. *J. Immunol.* **75**:184, 1955.

KAPLAN, M. H., A. H. COONS, and H. W. DEANE. Localization of antigen in tissue cells. III. Cellular distribution of pneumococcal polysaccharides, types II and III in mouse. *J. Exper. Med.* **91**:15, 1950.

KAPLAN, M. H., and W. SPINK. Studies of the staphylocoagulase reaction: nature and properties of a plasma activator and inhibitor. *Blood*, **3**:573, 1948.

KAPLAN, N. O., S. P. COLOWICK, and A. NASON. *Neurospora* diphosphopyridine nucleotidase. *J. Biol. Chem.* **191**:473, 1951.

KAPLAN, W., M. HUPPERT, D. E. KRAFT, and J. W. BAILEY. Fluorescent antibody inhibition test for *Coccidioides immitis* antibodies. *Sabouraudia*, **5**:1, 1966.

KÄRBER, G. Beitrag zur kollektiven Behandlung pharmakologischer Reihenversuche. *Arch. Exper. Pathol. Pharmakol.* **162**:480, 1931.

KARIHER, D. H. Blood typing simplified. *Proc. Soc. Exper. Biol. Med.* **56**:106, 1944.

KARUNAIRATNAM, M. C., J. SPIZIZEN, and H. GEST. Preparation and properties of *Rhodospirillum rubrum*. *Biochem. Biophys. Acta*, **29**:649, 1958.

KARUSH, F. Interaction of purified antibody and optically isomeric haptens. *J. Amer. Chem. Soc.* **78**:5519, 1956.

KARUSH, F., and R. MARKS. The preparation and properties of purified antihapten antibody. *J. Immunol.* **78**:296, 1957.

KASS, E. H., and C. V. SEASONE. The role of mucoid polysaccharide (hyaluronic acid) in the virulence of group A streptococci. *J. Exper. Med.* **79**:319, 1944.

KATZ, A. M., W. J. DREYER, and C. B. ANFINSEN. Peptide separation by two-dimensional chromatography and electrophoresis. *J. Biol. Chem.* **234**:2897, 1959.

KATZ, S., and D. G. COMB. A new method for the determination of the base composition of ribonucleic acid. *J. Biol. Chem.* **238**:3065, 1963.

KAUFMAN, L., and B. BRANDT. Fluorescent-antibody studies of the mycelial form of *Histoplasma capsulatum* and morphologically similar fungi. *J. Bacteriol.* **87**:120, 1964.

KAUFMAN, L., and W. B. CHERRY. Technical factors affecting the preparation of fluorescent antibody reagents. *J. Immunol.* **87**:72, 1961.

KAUFMAN, L., and W. KAPLAN. Serological characterization of pathogenic fungi by means of fluorescent antibodies. I. Antigenic relationships between yeast and mycelial forms of *Histoplasma capsulatum* and *Blastomyces dermatitidis*. *J. Bacteriol.* **85**:986, 1963.

KAUFMAN, L., J. H. SCHUBERT, W. KAPLAN, and D. McLAUGHLIN. Fluorescent antibody inhibition test for histoplasmosis. *J. Lab. Clin. Med.*

KAUFMANN, A. P., and W. H. NITSCH. Paper chromatography in the fat field. XVI. Further experiments on the separation of fatty acids. *Fette Seifen Anstrichmittel*, **56**:154, 1954.

KAUFFMANN, F. On haemagglutination of *Escherichia coli*. *Acta Pathol. Microbiol. Scandinav.* **25**:502, 1948.

KAUFFMANN, F. *The Diagnosis of Salmonella Types*. C. Thomas, Springfield, Ill., 1950.

KAWATA, T., J. MATSUO, and H. AOI. Electron microscopic studies on the spirocheta lysis by penicillin. *Yonago Acta Med.* **4**:2, 1960.

KAY, E. R. M., M. S. SIMMONS, and A. L. DOUNCE. An improved preparation of sodium desoxyribonucleate. *J. Amer. Chem. Soc.* **74**:1724, 1952.

KEELER, R. F., and M. L. GRAY. Antigenic and related biochemical properties of *Listeria monocytogenes*. I. Preparation and composition of cell wall material. *J. Bacteriol.* **80**:683, 1960.

KELLENBERGER, E., A. RYTER, and J. SÉCHAUD. Electron microscope study of DNA-containing plasms. II. Vegetative and mature phage DNA as compared with normal bacterial nucleoids in different physiological states. *J. Biophys. Biochem. Cyt.* **4**:671, 1958.

KELLETT, C. Complementary activity of blood in rheumatism and certain allied disorders. *Ann. Rheum. Dis.* **13**:211, 1954.

KELLETT, C., and J. THOMSON. Complementary activity of blood serum in nephritis. *J. Pathol. Bacteriol.* **48**:519, 1939.

KELLNER, A., A. W. BERNHEIMER, A. S. CARLSON, and E. B. FREEMAN. Loss of myocardial contractility in isolated mammalian hearts by streptolysin O. *J. Exper. Med.* **104**:361, 1956.

KELLNER, A., E. B. FREEMAN, and A. S. CARLSON. Neutralizing antibodies to streptococcal diphosphopyridine nucleotidase in the serum of experimental animals and human beings. *J. Exper. Med.* **108**:299, 1958.

KELMERS, A. D., G. D. NOVELLI, and M. P. STULBERG. Separation of transfer ribonucleic acids by reverse phase chromatography. *J. Biol. Chem.* **240**:3979, 1965.

KENDALL, F. E. Studies on serum proteins. I. Identification of a single serum globulin by immunological means. *J. Lab. Clin. Med.* **16**:921, 1937.

KENRICK, K. G., and J. MARGOLIS. Isoelectric focusing and gradient gel electrophoresis: A two-dimensional technique. *Anal. Biochem.* **33**:204, 1970.

KENDRICK, P. L. Rapid agglutination technic applied to *B. pertussis* aggultination. *Amer. J. Publ. Heath*, **23**:1310, 1933.

KENDRICK, P., J. GIBBS, and M. SPRICK. The opsonocytophagic test in the study of pertussis. *J. Infect. Dis.* **60**:302, 1937.

KENDRICK, P. L., G. M. LAWSON, and J. J. MILLER. *Hemophilus pertussis.* In *Diagnostic Procedures and Reagents.* American Public Health Association, New York, 1950.

KENDRICK, P. L., M. THOMPSON, and G. ELDERING. Immunity response of mothers and babies to injections of *pertussis* vaccine during pregnancy. *Amer. J. Dis. Childhood*, **70**: 75, 1945.

KENT, J. F. An abbreviated spectrophotometric technique for determining the optical concentration of amboceptor. *J. Lab. Clin. Med.* **31**:1270, 1946.

KENT, J. F. A quantitative study of complement-hemolysis relation. *Science*, **105**:316, 1947.

KENT, J. F., S. BUKANTZ, and C. REIN. Studies in complement fixation. I. Spectrophotometric titration of complement; construction of graphs for direct determination of the 50% hemolytic unit. *J. Immunol.* **53**:37, 1956.

KEOGH, E. V., E. A. NORTH, and M. F. WARBURTON, Haemagglutination of the *Hemophilus* group. *Nature*, **160**:63, 1947.

KEOGH, E. V., E. A. NORTH, and M. F. WARBURTON. Asdorption of bacterial polysaccharides to erythrocytes. *Nature*, **161**:687, 1948.

KERR, J. A. Studies on certain viruses isolated in the tropics of Africa and South America. Immunological reactions as determined by cross complement-fixation tests. *J. Immunol.* **68**:461, 1952.

KESSEL, J. F., W. P. LEWIS, S. MA, and H. KIM. Preliminary report on a hemagglutination test for entamoebae. *Proc. Soc. Exper. Biol. Med.* **106**:409, 1961.

KESSEL, R. W. I., K. BRAUN, and O. J. PLESCIA. Endotoxin cytotoxicity: Role of cell associated antibody. *Proc. Soc. Exper. Biol. Med.* **121**:449, 1966.

KIBRICK, A. C., and M. BLONSTEIN. Fractionation of serum into albumin and α-, β-, and γ-globulin by sodium sulfate. *J. Biol. Chem.* **176**:983, 1948.

KIDD, P. Elution of an incomplete type of antibody from the erythrocytes in acquired haemolytic anaemia. *J. Clin. Pathol.* **21**:03, 1949.

KIEVITS, J. H., and H. R. SHUIT. A simple indirect L.E. cell test with increased sensitivity. *Vox Sang.* **2**:288, 1957.

KILHAM, L. A Newcastle disease virus hemolysis. *Proc. Soc. Exper. Biol. Med.* **71**:63, 1949.

KILHAM, L. Evaluation of the agglutination of erythrocytes sensitized by Newcastle virus as a serologic test in infectious mononucleosis. *J. Immunol.* **65**:245, 1950.

KILLANDER, J., J. PONTEN, and I. RODEN. Rapid preparation of fluorescent antibodies using gel filtration. *Nature*, **192**:4798, 1961.

KIND, S. S. Absorption-elution grouping of dried blood-stains on fabrics. *Nature*, **187**:789, 1960.

KIND, S. S. Absorption-elution grouping of dried blood smears. *Nature*, **185**:397, 1960.

KING, E. The colorimetric determination of phosphorus. *Biochem. J.* **26**:292, 1932.

KIPPS, A. Complement fixation with antigens prepared from blue-tongue virus-infected mouse brains. *J. Hygiene*, **54**:88, 1956.

KIRALY, K., and M. PORGANYI. Antigenstruktur des *Treponema pallidum* und die Immunadäsion. *Zeitschr. Immunitätsforsch.* **119**:183, 1960.

KIRBY, K. S. A new method for the isolation of ribonucleic acid from mammalian tissues. *Biochem. J.* **64**:405, 1956.

KIRBY, K. S. Isolation and characterization of ribosomal ribonucleic acid. *Biochem. J.* **97**: 266, 1965.

KIRSTENSEN, M., and S. LARSEN. *C. R. Soc. Biol.* **95**:1110, 1921.

KISSANE, J. M., and E. ROBINS. The fluorometric measurement of deoxyribonucleic acid in animal tissues with special reference to the central nervous system. *J. Biol. Chem.* **233**: 184, 1958.

KITE, J. H., JR., R. C. BROWN, and N. R. ROSE. Autoantibodies to thyroid tissue sediment detected by the antiglobulin consumption test. *J. Lab. Clin. Med.* **59**:179, 1962.

KJELDAHL, J. Neue Methode zur Bestimmung des Stickstoffes in organischen Körpern. *Zeitschr. Anal. Chemie*, **22**:366, 1883.

KLECZKOWSKI, A. Serological behaviour of Tobacco mosaic virus and its protein fragments. *Immunology*, **4**:130, 1961.

KLECZKOWSKI, A., and H. G. THORNTON. A serological study of root nodule bacteria from pea and clover inoculation groups. *J. Bacteriol.* **48**:661, 1944.

KLEIN, P. G. Studies on immune hemolysis: preparation of stable and highly reactive complex of sensitized erythrocytes and the first component of complement (EAC'1); inactivation of cell fixed C'1 by some complement reagents. *J. Exper. Med.* **111**:77, 1960.

KLEIN, S., G. LEIBY, and M. BERKE. Cardiolipin antigen in the Kline test for syphilis. *Amer. J. Clin. Pathol.* **18**:940, 1948.

KLEINSCHMIDT, W., and P. D. BOYER. Interaction of protein and antibodies. II. Dissociation studies with egg-albumin- anti-egg albumin precipitates. *J. Immunol.* **69**:257, 1952.

KLEVSTRAND, R., and A. NORDAL. A spraying reagent for paper chromatograms which is apparently specific to ketoheptoses. *Acta Chem. Scandinav.* **4**:1320, 1950.

KLIGLER, I., L. OLITZKI, and H. KLIGLER. The antigenic composition and immunizing properties of trypanosomes. *J. Immunol.* **38**:317, 1940.

KLIGMAN, A. Studies of the capsular substance of *Torula histolytica* and the immunologic properties of *Torula* cells. *J. Immunol.* **71**:395, 1948.

KLINE, B. S. Microscopic slide precipitation tests for the diagnosis and exclusion of syphilis. *J. Lab. Clin. Med.* **16**:186, 1930.

KLINE, B. S. Development of a single standard slide test for syphilis. *Amer. J. Clin. Pathol.* **18**:185, 1948.

KLOBUSITZKY, D. Concentration of tetanic antitoxin by adsorption. *J. Immunol.* **35**:329, 1938.

KLUDANOV, L. E., E. D. SHKURKO, and V. S. MIKHNO. *Z. Mikrobiol. Epidemiol. Immunit.* **29**:1974, 1958.

KNIGHT, C. A. The nature of some of the chemical differences among strains of tobacco-mosaic virus. *J. Biol. Chem.* **171**:297, 1947.

KNOX, K. W., and R. V. S. BAIN. The antigens of *Pasteurella multocida* type I. I. Capsular polysaccharides. *Immunology*, **3**:352, 1960.

KOBAYASHI, T., J. N. RINKER, and H. KOFFLER. Purification and chemical properties of flagellin. *Arch. Biochem. Biophys.* **84**:342, 1959.

KOCH, F. C., and P. L. McMEEKIN. A new direct nesslerization microkjeldahl method and a modification of Nessler-Folin reagent for ammonia. *J. Amer. Chem. Soc.* **46**:2066, 1924.

KOFFLER, H. Protoplasmic differences between mesophiles and thermophiles. *Bacteriol. Rev.* **21**:227, 1957.

KOFFLER, H., and T. KOBAYASHI. *Arch. Biochem. Biophys.* **67**:246, 1957.

KOHN, A., and W. SZYBALSKI. W. Lysozyme spheroplasts from thawed *Escherichia coli* cells. *Bacteriol. Proc.* **126**:1959.

KOHN, J. A cellulose acetate supporting medium for zone electrophoresis. *Clin. Chim. Acta*, **2**:297, 1957.

KOHN, J. Small-scale membrane filter electrophoresis and immunoelectrophoresis. *Clin. Chim. Acta*, **3**:450, 1958.

KOHN, J. A lipoprotein staining method for zone electrophoresis. *Nature*, **189**:312, 1961.

Köiw, E., and H. Grönwall. Staining of protein bound carbohydrates after electrophoresis of serum on filter paper. *Scandinav. J. Clin. Lab. Invest.* **4**:244, 1952.

Kokerndt, R., K. Smithburn, and M. Weinbren. Neutralizing antibodies to arthropod-borne viruses in human beings and animals in the Union of South Africa. *J. Immunol.* **77**:312, 1956.

Kolmer, J. A. Spirochetal antigens in the serum diagnosis of syphilis. *J. Bacteriol.* **44**:144, 1942.

Kolmer, J. A., and F. Boerner. *Approved Laboratory Technic.* Appleton-Century, New York, 1945.

Kolmer, J. A., C. C. Kast, and E. R. Lynch. Studies on the role of the *Spirochaeta pallida* in Wassermann reaction. II. Relation of spirochaetal antibodies to Wassermann reagin. *Amer. J. Syph.* **25**:309, 1941.

Kolmer, J. A., and E. R. Lynch. Cardiolipin antigens in the Kolmer complement fication test. *J. Ven. Dis. Inform.* **29**:166, 1948.

Kolmer, J. A., and A. Rule. Tests for immunity to acute anterior poliomyelitis. *J. Immunol.* **29**:175, 1935.

Kolmer, J. A., E. Spaulding, and H. Robinson. *Approved Laboratory Technic.* Appleton-Century-Crofts, New York, 1951.

Konda, S., A. Yamada, and M. Fukase. The demonstration of the incomplete antibody in the auto-immune hemolytic anaemia by the fluorescent anti-human globulin technique. *Acta School Med. Univ. Kioto*, **1**:84, 1960.

Kopeloff, L., and N. Kopeloff. The production of antibrain antibodies in the monkey. *J. Immunol.* **48**:297, 1949.

Koprowski, H. Immunological reactions in viral diseases. *Ann. Rev. Microbiol.* **4**:261, 1950.

Kordová, N., and E. Kováčova. Histochemical and fluorescent antibody studies on the early stages of infection of L cells with *Coxiella burneti. Acta Virol.* **12**:23, 1968.

Kornberg, L. H., and W. E. Patey. Quantitative determination of 0.5-5 mcg amino acid on paper chromatograms and in solution. *Biochem. Biophys. Acta*, **25**:189, 1957.

Korner, A. The effect of hypophysectomy of the rat and of treatment with growth hormone on the incorporation of amino acids into liver proteins in a cell-free system. *Biochem. J.* **73**:61, 1959.

Korner, A. Studies on incorporation of amino acids into protein in isolated rat-liver ribosomes. *Biochem. J.* **81**:168, 1961.

Kornfeld, L., and W. O. Weigle. The elution of S-labelled C'1 from antigen-antibody-S complement precipitates. *Immunology*, **8**:213, 1965.

Korngold, L. Immunological cross-reactions studied by the Ouchterlony gel diffusion technique. *J. Immunol.* **77**:119, 1956.

Korngold, L., G. Stahly, K. Dodd, and W. Myers. The comparative retention of antigen in the skin of immune and normal rabbits as determined with egg albumen labeled with radioactive iodine. *J. Immunol.* **70**:345, 1953.

Korngold, L., and G. Van Leeuwen. The effect of the antigen's molecular weight on the curvature of the precipitin line in the Ouchterlony technic. *J. Immunol.* **78**:172, 1957.

Korson, R. *Stain Techn.* **26**:265, 1951.

Koshland, M. The origin of fecal antibody and its relationship to immunization with adjuvants. *J. Immunol.* **70**:359, 1953.

Koshland, M. Mechanism of antibody formation. *J. Immunol.* **79**:462, 1957.

Koshland, M., M. Elliott, and W. Burrows. Quantitative studies of the relationships between fecal and serum antibodies. *J. Immunol.* **65**:93, 1950.

KOSHLAND, M. E., and F. ENGLEBERGER. Mechanism of antibody formation. Rate of diphtheria antitoxin formation in the booster response. *J. Immunol.* **79**:172, 1957.

KOZA, J., Calcium phosphate adsorption patterns of virulent and avirulent strains of poliovirus. *Virology*, 21:477, 1963.

KRAFT, L. M., and J. L. MELNICK. Complement fixation tests with homologous and heterologous types of Coxsackie virus in man. *J. Immunol.* **68**:297, 1952.

KRAUS, F. W., and J. KONNO. Antibodies in saliva. *Ann. N.Y. Acad. Sci.* **106**:311, 1963.

KRAUS, R. *Wien. Klin. Wochenschr.* **10**:136, 1897.

KRAUS, R., and S. LUDWIG. Über Baktriohämagglutinine und Antihämagglutinine. *Wien. Klin. Wochenschr.* **15**:120, 1902.

KRAUSE, R. M., and M. McCARTY. Studies on the chemical structure of the streptococcal cell wall. I. The identification of mucopeptides in the cell wall of Group A and A-variant streptococci. *J. Exper. Med.* **114**:127, 1961.

KRAWIEC, S., and J. M. EISENSTADT. Ribonucleic acids from mitochondria of bleached *Euglena gracilis*. I. Isolation of mitochondria and extraction of nucleic acid. *Biochim. Biophys. Acta*, **217**:120, 1970.

KRIEGER, V., and S. WEIDEN. A comparison of Simmon's slide method and Chown's capillary tube method for the detection of the Rh factor. *Amer. J. Clin. Pathol.* **18**:572, 1948.

KRITCHEVSKY, D., and R. F. J. McCANDLESS. *Naturwissenschaften*, **46**:114, 1959.

KRITZMAN, J. Studies of rheumatoid serum employing a modified Coombs' slide test. *J. Lab. Clin. Med.* **52**:328, 1958.

KROGH, VON, M. Colloidal chemistry and immunology. *J. Infect. Dis.* **19**:452, 1916.

KRONVALL, G., P. G. QUIE, and R. C. WILLIAMS, Jr. Quantitation of staphylococcal protein A: Determination of equilibrium constants and number of proteins and A residues on bacteria. *J. Immunol.* **104**:273, 1970.

KRUMWIEDE, C., and W. C. NOBLE. A rapid method for the production of precipitin antigen from bacteria: An attempt to apply it to the determination of the type of pneumococcus in sputum. *J. Immunol.* **3**:1, 1918.

KRZYWY, T. The antigenic structure of *Streptomyces griseus. Arch. Immunol. Ther. Exper.* **11**:521, 1963.

KUHNS, W. J., and A. BAILEY. Use of red cells modified by papain for the detection of Rh antibodies. *Amer. J. Clin. Pathol.* **20**:1067, 1950.

KUHNS, W. J., and W. DUKSTEIN. Multiple antibody response following immunization of human subjects with diphtheria toxoid. *J. Immunol.* **79**:154, 1957.

KUL'BERG, A. Y., and N. B. AZADOVA. Use of mercury-labeled antibodies for specific contrast in electron microscopy. *Feder. Proc. Trans. Suppl.* **73**:64, 1964.

KUNITZ, M. CRYSTALLINE ribonuclease. *J. Gen. Physiol.* **24**:15, 1940.

KUNKEL, H. G., and R. SLATER. Zone electrophoresis in a starch supporting medium. *Proc. Soc. Exper. Biol. Med.* **80**:42, 1952.

KUNKEL, H. G., and A. TISELIUS. Electrophoresis of protein on filter paper. *J. Gen. Physiol.* **35**:89, 1951.

KUNKEL, H. G., and S. M. WARD. The immunological determination of human albumin in biological fluids. *J. Biol. Chem.* **182**:597, 1950.

KUNZ, C. Untersuchungen mit Fluorescein-markierten Antikörpern an Hefen. *Schweiz. Zeitschr. Allg. Pathol. Bakteriol.* **21**:892, 1958.

KUROKAWA, M., M. HATANO, N. KASHIWAGI, T. SAITO, S. ISHIDA, and R. HOMMA. A new method for the turbidimetric measurement of bacterial density. *J. Bacteriol.* **83**:14, 1962.

KWAPINSKI, J. B. G. Research on the antigenic structure of Actinomycetales. IV. Chemical and antigenic structure of *Actinomyces israelii. Pathol. Microbiol.* **23**:158, 1960.

KWAPINSKI, J. B. G. Einige Methoden der Gewinnung und der immunochemischen Analyse der Antigene von Mikroorganismen. *Zentralbl. Bakteriol. I. Orig.* **192**:399, 1964.

KWAPINSKI, J. B. G. Cytoplasmic antigen relationships among the Actinomycetales. *J. Bacteriol.* **87**:1234, 1964.

KWAPINSKI, J. B. G. Chemical and serological similarities of cell walls from 100 Actinomycetales. *J. Bacteriol.* **88**:1211, 1964.

KWAPINSKI, J. B. G. Serological and chromatographic characterization of exo-antigens of the *Dermatophilus. Austral. J. Exper. Biol. Med. Sci.* **44**:87, 1966.

KWAPINSKI, J. B. G. *Methods of Serological Research.* Interscience, New York, 1965 (1st printing), 1967 (2nd printing).

KWAPINSKI, J. B. G. Serological characteristics of electrophoretically different mouse serum globulins. *Bacteriol. Proc. M.* **25**:1968.

KWAPINSKI, J. B. G., Ed. *Analytical Serology of Microorganisms*, I and II. Interscience, New York, 1969.

KWAPINSKI, J. B. G. Serological characteristics of particulate antigens of *Dermatophilus. Can. J. Microbiol.* **15**:1141, 1969.

KWAPINSKI, J. B. G. Serological classification of Actinomycetes. *Proc. Int. Conf. Cult. Coll.* University of Tokyo Press, pp. 439–449, 1970.

KWAPINSKI, J. B. G. Schemes for serological classification of mycobacteria, nocardiae and streptomycetes. In *Actinomycetales*, H. Prauser, Ed. G. Fischer, Publisher Jena, 1970, pp. 345–369.

KWAPINSKI, J. B. G. Contemporary Methodology for Immunochemical Analysis of Antigens. *Res. Immunochem. Immunobiol.* **1**:71–120, 1972.

KWAPINSKI, J. B. G. Conceptual and Methodological Aspects of Immunological Classification of Microorganisms. *Res. Immunochem. Immunobiol.* **2**:1–122, 1972.

KWAPINSKI, J. B. G., A. ALCASID, and H. PALSER. Serological relationships of endoplasm antigens of saprophytic mycobacteria. *Can. J. Microbiol.* **16**:871, 1970.

KWAPINSKI, J. B. G., A. CHENG, A. ALCASID, and J. DOWLER. Immunochemistry of *Mycoccus. Can. J. Microbiol.* **18**:1971.

KWAPINSKI, J. B. G., and W. MADALINSKI. Investigations on immunochemical properties of Waaler's factor. *Post. Reumat.* **2**:59, 1955.

KWAPINSKI, J. B. G., and M. MERKEL. Investigations into the chemical and antigenic structure of the genus *Streptomyces*. I. The chemical structure of *Streptomyces griseus. Bull. Acad. Pol. Sci. Cl. II*, **5**:335, 1957.

KWAPINSKI, J. B. G., and H. P. R. SEELIGER. Immunochemical characteristics of the Actinomycetales. *Z. Bakteriol. Ref.* **195**:193, 1964.

KWAPINSKI, J. B. G., and G. C. SIMMONS. Serological and chemical characteristics of the plasm antigens of the *Dermatophilus. Leeuwenh. J. Microbiol. Serology*, **33**:100, 1967.

KWAPINSKI, J. B. G., and M. L. SNYDER. Antigenic structure and relationships of *Mycobacterium*, *Actinomyces*, *Streptococcus*, and *Diplococcus. J. Bacteriol.* **82**:632, 1961.

KWAPINSKI, J. B. G., and M. L. SNYDER. *The Immunology of Rheumatism.* Appleton-Century-Crofts, New York, 1962.

LABREC, E. H., J. B. FORMAL, and H. SCHNEIDER. Serological analysis of *Shigella flexneri* by the fluorescent antibody technic. *Bacteriol. Proc.* **135**, 1958.

LACHMANN, P. J. A comparison of some properties of bovine conglutinin with those of rabbit immuno-conglutinin. *Immunology*, **5**:687, 1962.

LACHMANN, P. J., and MÜLLER-EBERHARD, H. J. The demonstration in human serum of "conglutinogen-activating factor" and its effect on the third component of complement. *J. Immunol.* **100**:691, 1968.

Lamanna, C., and J. Lowenthal. The lack of identity between hemagglutinin and the toxin of type A botulinal organism. *J. Bacteriol.* **61**:751, 1951.

Lamanna, C., and M. F. Mallette. Use of glass beads for the mechanical rupture of microorganisms in concentrated suspensions. *J. Bacteriol.* **67**:503, 1954.

Lamedica, G., and L. Robert. Impiego dell'antigene treponemico proteico solubile (A.J.P.S.) in una reazione di emogglutinazione. *Igiene Med.* **50**:345, 1957.

Lancaster, L. J., and J. C. Sherris. An agar-diffusion grouping technic for beta hemolytic streptococci. *Amer. J. Clin. Pathol.* **34**:131, 1960.

Lancefield, R. C. The immunological relationships of *Streptococcus viridans* and certain of its chemical fractions. I. Serological reactions obtained with anti-bacterial sera. *J. Exper. Med.* **42**:377, 1925.

Lancefield, R. C. The antigenic complex of *Streptococcus haemolyticus*. I. Demonstration of a type-specific substance in extracts of *Streptococcus haemolyticus*. *J. Exper. Med.* **47**: 91, 1928.

Lancefield, R. C. A serological differentiation of human and other groups of hemolytic streptococci. *J. Exper. Med.* **57**:571, 1933.

Lancefield, R. C. Specific relationship of cell composition to biological activity of hemolytic streptococcus. *Harvey Lectures*, **36**:251, 1940.

Lancefield, R. C. Studies on the antigenic composition of group A hemolytic streptococci. *J. Exper. Med.* **78**:465, 1943.

Lancefield, R. C. Differentiation of group A streptococci with common R antigen into three serological types with special reference to the bactericidal test. *J. Exper. Med.* **106**: 522, 1957.

Lancefield, R. C., and G. E. Perlmann. Preparation and properties of type-specific M. antigen isolated from a group A, type 1, hemolytic *Streptococcus*. *J. Exper. Med.* **96**:71, 1952.

Lancefield, R. C., and G. E. Perlmann. Preparation and properties of a protein (R antigen) occurring in streptococci of group A, type 28, and in certain streptococci of other serological groups. *J. Exper. Med.* **96**:83, 1952.

Landois, L. *Die Transfusion des Blutes.* Vogel, Lepizig, 1875.

Landsteiner, K. Zur Kenntnis der antifermentativen, lytischen und agglutinierenden Wirkungen des Blutserums und der Lumphe. *Zentralbl. Bakteriol. I. Orig.* **27**:357, 1900.

Landsteiner, K. Über Beziehungen zwischen dem Blutserum und den Körperzellen. *Münch. Med. Wochenschr.* **50**:1812, 1903.

Landsteiner, K. *The Human Blood Groups.* University of Chicago Press, Chicago, 1928.

Landsteiner, K. *The Specificity of Serological Reaction.* Harvard University Press, Cambridge, Mass., 1945.

Landsteiner, K., and H. Lamb. Über die Antigeneigenschaften von Azoproteinen. *Zeitschr. Immunitatsforsch.* **26**:293, 1917.

Landsteiner, K., and H. Lamb. Über die Abhängigkeit der serologischen Spezifität von der chemischen Struktur. *Biochem. Zeitschr.* **86**:343, 1918.

Landsteiner, K., and P. Levine. Heterogenetic haptene. *J. Immunol.* **14**:81, 1927.

Landsteiner, K., and P. Levine. On individual differences in human blood. *J. Exper. Med.* **47**:757, 1928.

Landsteiner, K., and P. Levine. Experiments on anaphylaxis to azoproteins. *J. Exper. Med.* **52**:347, 1930.

Landsteiner, K., and H. Richter. *Zeitschr. Med. Beamte*, **16**:85, 1903.

Landsteiner, K., and J. Van Der Sheer. On cross reactions of immune sera to azoproteins. *J. Exper. Med.* **63**:325, 1936.

Landsteiner, K., and A. Wiener. An agglutinable factor in human blood recognized by immune sera for rhesus blood. *Proc. Soc. Exper. Biol. Med.* **43**:223, 1940.

LANDSTEINER, K., and A. WIENER. Studies on agglutinogen (Rh) in human blood reacting with anti-rhesus sera and with human isoantibodies. *J. Exper. Med.* **74**:309, 1941.

LANDY, M., A. G. JOHNSON, M. E. WEBSTER, and J. F. SAGIN. Studies on the O antigen of *Salmonella typhosa*. *J. Immunol.* **74**:66, 1955.

LANDY, M., and E. LAMB. Estimation of Vi antibody employing erythrocytes treated with purified Vi antigen. *Proc. Soc. Exper. Biol. Med.* **82**:593, 1953.

LANDY, M., R. P. SANDERSON, M. T. BERNSTEIN, and A. L. JACKSON. Antibody production by leucocytes in peripheral blood. *Nature*, **204**:1320, 1964.

LANDY, M., R. P. SANDERSON, and A. L. JACKSON. Humoral and cellular aspects of the immune response to the somatic antigen of *Salmonella enteritidis*. *J. Exper. Med.* **122**:483, 1965.

LANDY, M., and R. J. TRAPANI. A hemagglutination test for plaque antibody with purified capsular antigen of *Pasteurella pestis*. *Amer. J. Hyg.* **59**:150, 1954.

LANDY, M., R. J. TRAPANI, and W. R. CLARK. Studies on the O antigen of *Salmonella typhosa*. III. Activity of the isolated antigen in the hemagglutination procedure. *Amer. J. Hyg.* **62**:54, 1955.

LANDY, M., and M. E. WEBSTER. Studies on Vi antigen. III. Immunological properties of purified Vi antigen derived from *Escherichia coli* 5396/38. *J. Immunol.* **69**:143, 1952.

LANDY, M., M. E. WEBSTER, and J. SAGIN. Studies on Vi antigen. V. Comparison of the immunological properties of Vi antigen derived from V form of *Enterobacteriaceae*. *J. Immunol.* **73**:23, 1954.

LANE, B. G. The alkali-stable trinucleotide sequences and the chain termini in 18S and 28S ribonucleates from wheat germ. *Biochemistry*, **4**:212, 1965.

LANG, M., J. G. H. SCHMIDT, and H. JAHRMÄRKER. Über neue Verfahren zum Antikörpernachweis. *Zentralbl. Bakteriol. Orig.* **164**:4:, 1955.

LANGNER, P., and S. FORRESTER. The disintegration of bacteria by mechanical means. *J. Immunol.* **37**:133, 1939.

LANNI, F., and Y. LANNI. Antigenic structure of bacteriophage. *Cold Spring Symp. Quart. Biol.* **18**:159, 1953.

LANNI, Y. Infection by bacteriophage T5 and its intracellular growth—a study by complement fixation. *J. Bacteriol.* **67**:640, 1954.

LARGIER, J. Purification of formol diphtheria toxoid by multimembrane electrodecantation. *J. Immunol.* **79**:181, 1957.

LARSON, C. L. Studies on the thermostable antigens extracted from *Bacterium tularense* and from tissues of animals dead of tularemia. *J. Immunol.* **79**:181, 1957.

LARSON, C. L., C. B. PHILIP, W. C. WICHT, and L. E. HUGHES. Precipitin reaction with soluble antigens from suspensions of *Pasteurella pestis* or from tissues of animal dead of plague. *J. Immunol.* **67**:289, 1957.

LARSON, C. L., E. RIBI, K. C. MILNER, and J. E. LIEBERMAN, Method for titrating endotoxic activity in the skin of rabbits. *J. Exper. Med.* **111**:1, 1960.

LATTES, L. *Deutsche Zeitschr. Ges. Gericht. Med.* **9**:402, 1927.

LAURELL, C. B. Antigen-antibody crossed electrophoresis. *Anal. Biochem.* **10**:358, 1965.

LAURELL, C. B., S. LAURELL, and N. SKOOG. Buffer composition in paper electrophoresis. Consideration on its influence, with special reference to the interaction between small ions and proteins. *Clin. Chem.* **2**:99, 1956.

LAURELL, C. B., and J. E. NILEHN. A new type of inherited serum albumin anomaly. *J. Clin. Invest.* **45**:1935, 1966.

LAVER, W. G. Structural studies on the protein subunits from three strains of influenza virus. *J. Mol. Biol.* **9**:109, 1964.

LAWLISS, J. F. Serological detection of desoxyribonucleic acid (DNA) adsorbed to formolized erythrocytes. *Proc. Soc. Exper. Biol. N.Y.* **98**:300, 1958.

LAZEAR, E., and L. FERGUSON. Bovine erythrocyte antigens. *J. Immunol.* **71**:12, 1953.

LEA, D. J., and A. H. SEHON. Preparation of synthetic gels for chromatography of macromolecules. *Can. J. Chem.* **40**:159, 1962.

LEACH, A. A., and P. C. O'SHEA. The determination of protein molecular weights of up to 225,000 by gel-filtration on a single column of Sephadex G-200 at 25° and 40°. *J. Chromat.* **17**:245, 1965.

LEARNED, G., and T. METCALF. A study of the hemagglutinative behaviour of the lipid antigens of *Corynebacterium diphtheriae*. *Trans. Kansas Acad. Sci.* **55**:431, 1952.

LE BOUVIER, G. L. A study by means of diffusion in agar. *J. Exper. Med.* **106**:661, 1957.

LE BOUVIER, G. L. Poliovirus D and C antigens. Their differentiation and measurement by precipitation in agar. *Brit. J. Exper. Pathol.* **40**:452, 1950.

LECOCQ, E., and R. LINZ. Agglutination d'hématies tannées traitées par deux antigénes. *Ann. Inst. Pasteur*, **102**:437, 1962.

LECOMPTE DU NOÜY, P., and V. HAMON. La viscosité de mèlanges toxin-antitoxine diphtérique. *Ann. Inst. Pasteur*, **56**:359, 1936.

LEDERBERG, J. Bacterial protoplasts induced by penicillin. *Proc. Natl. Acad. Sci.* **42**:574, 1956.

LEDINKO, N., and J. MELNICK. Poliomyelitis viruses in tissue culture. V. Reaction of virus and antibody; variables of the quantitative neutralization test. *Amer. J. Hyg.* **58**:223, 1953.

LEDUC, E. H., S. AVRAMEAS, and M. BOUTEILLE. Ultrastructural localization of antibody in differentiating plasma cells. *J. Exper. Med.* **127**:109, 1968.

LEDUC, F., A. COONS, and J. CONNOLLY. Studies on antibody production. II. The primary and secondary responses in the popliteal lymph node of the rabbit. *J. Exper. Med.* **102**:61, 1955.

LEISHMAN, W. Note on a method of qualitatively estimating the phagocytic power of the leucocytes of the blood. *Brit. Med. J.* **1**:73, 1902.

LEMCKE, R. M., E. J. SHAW, and B. P. MARMION. Related antigens in *Mycoplasma pneumoniae* and *Mycoplasma mycoides*. *Aust. J. Exper. Biol. Med.* **43**:761, 1965.

LEMINOR, L., S. LEMINOR, and P. GRABAR. Réaction d'hèmagglutination passive et d'hémolyse directe au moyen de globules roughes sensibilisés par de substances solubles O et Vi d'enterobacteriacées. *Ann. Inst. Pasteur.* **83**:62, 1952.

LENNETTE, E. H., W. H. CLARK, and B. H. DEAN. Sheep and goats in the epidemiology of Q fever in Northern California. *Amer. J. Trop. Med.* **29**:527, 1949.

LENNETTE, E. H., W. H. CLARK, F. W. JENSEN, and C. J. TOOMB, Q fever studies. XV. Development and persistence in man of complement-fixing and agglutinating antibodies to *Coxiella burnetii*. *J. Immunol.* **68**:591, 1952.

LENNETTE, E. H., and H. KOPROWSKI. Comparative sensitivity of the extraneural and intracerebral neutralization tests in following the antibody response in man to vaccination with Western Equine Encephalomyelitis virus. *J. Immunol.* **52**:343, 1956.

LENNETTE, E. H., N. J. SCHMIDT, and R. L. MAGOFFIN. Complement-fixing antibody response to inactivated poliovirus vaccine. *J. Immunol.* **87**:696, 1961.

LEON, M. A., O. J. PLESCIA, and M. HEIDELBERGER. The preparation and properties of fractions of pig complement. *J. Immunol.* **74**:313, 1955.

LEONE, C. Effect of multiple injections of antigen upon the specificity of antisera. *J. Immunol.* **69**:285, 1952.

LEONE, C. Some effects of formation of the serological activity of crustacean and mammalian sera. *J. Immunol.* **70**:396, 1953.

LEPAGE, G., and W. W. UMBREIT, cf. W. W. UMBREIT, R. H. BURRIS, and J. F. STAUFFER. *Manometric Technique and Related Methods in the Study of Tissue Metabolism.* Burgess Publishing Co., Minneapolis, Minn., 1949.

Lepow, I. H., G. B. Naff, E. W. Todd, J. Pensky, and C. F. Hinz, Jr. Chromatographic resolution of the first component of human complement into three activities. *J. Exper. Med.* **117**:983, 1963.

Lepow, I. H., and L. Pillemer. Studies on the purification of diphtherial toxin. *J. Immunol.* **69**:1, 1952.

Lepow, I. H., L. Pillemer, M. D. Scheonberg, E. W. Todd, and R. J. Wedgwood. The properdin system and immunity. X. Characterization of partially purified human properdin. *J. Immunol.* **83**:428, 1959.

Lessel, E. F., and J. G. Holt. Presenting and interpreting the results. In *Methods for Numerical Taxonomy*. W. R. Lockhart and J. Liston, Eds. American Society Microbiotic Publishers, 1970.

Levine, B., L. Kline, and H. Sussenguth. Clinical and serological evaluation of consecutive slide tests with cardiolipin-lecithin antigen and Kline antigen. *Amer. J. Clin. Pathol.* **18**:212, 1948.

Levine, L., and M. M. Mayer. Kinetic studies on immune hemolysis. V. Formation of the complex EAC'x and its relation with C'y. *J. Immunol.* **73**:426, 1954.

Levine, L., M. M. Mayer, and H. J. Rapp. A simple method of estimating 50 per cent end point. *Amer. J. Hyg.* **27**:493, 1938.

Levine, L., W. T. Murakami, H. Van Vunakis, and I. Grossman. Specific antibodies to thermally denatured deoxyribonucleic acid of phage T4. *Proc. Natl. Acad. Sci. U.S.* **46**:1038, 1960.

Levine, L., A. Osler, and M. M. Mayer. Studies on the role of Ca^{11} and Mg in complement fixation and immune hemolysis. III. The respective roles of Ca^{11} and Mg^{++} in immune hemolysis. *J. Immunol.* **71**:371, 1953.

Levine, L., T. T. Puck, and B. P. Sagik. An absolute method for assay of virus hemagglutinins. *J. Exper. Med.* **98**:521, 1953.

Levine, L., E. Wasserman, and W. T. Murakami. Immunochemical studies on bacteriophage DNA. VI. Renaturation of T4 DNA. *Immunochemistry*, **3**:41, 1966.

Levine, M. Hemagglutination of tuberculin sensitized sheep cells in Hansen's disease (leprosy). *Proc. Soc. Exper. Biol. Med.* **76**:171, 1951.

Levine, S., and R. Sowinski. Carbonyl iron: a new adjuvant for experimental autoimmune disease. *J. Immunol.* **105**:1530, 1970.

Levintow, L., and J. E. Darnell. A simplified procedure for purification of large amounts of poliovirus: characterization and amino acid analysis of Type I poliovirus. *J. Biol. Chem.* **235**:70, 1960.

Libby, R. L., and C. Madison. Immunochemical studies with tagged proteins. I. The distribution of tobacco-mosaic virus in the mouse. *J. Immunol.* **55**:15, 1947.

Libby, R. W. The photronreflectometer—An instrument for the measurement of turbidity systems. *J. Immunol.* **34**:71, 1938.

Libby, R. W. A new and rapid quantitative technique for the determination of the potency of types I and II antipneumococcal serum. *J. Immunol.* **34**:269, 1934.

Libich, M. Quantitative immunoelectrophoresis. *Fol. Biol.* **5**:71, 1959.

Libich, M. Immunochemical titration of antigen and antibodies in electric field; titration of antigens in complex systems of individual determinant antigen groups. *Immunology*, **4**:164, 1961.

Libretti, A., M. Goldin, and M. A. Kaplan. Immunologic relationships of C-reactive protein from various human pathologic conditions. *J. Immunol.* **79**:306, 1957.

Lichtfield, J., and F. Wilcoxon. A simplified method of evaluating dose-effect experiment. *J. Pharmac. Exper. Therapy*, **96**:94, 1949.

Lim, K. A., and W. S. Pong. Agglutination by antibody of erythrocytes sensitized by virus hemagglutinin. *J. Immunol.* **92**:638, 1964.

LIND, A. Serological studies of mycobacteria by means of diffusion-in-gel techniques. *Int. Arch. Allergy*, **16**:336, 1960.

LIND, A. Serological studies of mycobacteria by means of diffusion-in-gel techniques. *Acta Pathol. Microbiol. Scandinav.* **144**:323, 1961.

LIND, I. Identification of *Neisseria gonorrhoeae* by means of fluorescent antibody technique. *Acta Pathol. Microbiol. Scandinav.* **70**:613, 1967.

LIND, P. E., and N. R. MCARTHUR. The distribution of "T" agglutinins in human sera. *Austral. J. Exper. Biol. Med.* **25**:247, 1947.

LINDERSTROM-LANG, K., and K. R. MORGENSEN. Enzymic histochemistry. XXXI. Histological control of histochemical investigations. *Compte. Rend. Trav. Lab. Carlsberg. Serie Chimique*, **23**:27, 1938.

LING, M. R. The coupling of protein antigens to erythrocytes with difluorodinitrobenzene. *J. Immunol.* **86**:49, 1961.

LINNANE, A. W., and E. VITOLS. A simple high-speed blendor for the disintegration of microorganisms. *Biochim. Biophys. Acta*, **59**:231, 1962.

LINSCOTT, W. D., and R. A. BOAK. Immune-adherence with *Leptospira* antigens. I. Studies on the immune-adherence phenomenon. *J. Immunol.* **86**:471, 1961.

LIPATOVA, T. *Vestnik Mikr. Epidem. Parazit.* **13**:201, 1934.

LIPTON, M. M. The application of the falling drop technique. The quantitative determination of pneumococcal polysaccharide. *J. Immunol.* **59**:263, 1948.

LIPTON, M. M., and J. FREUND. The formation of complement fixing and neutralizing antibodies after the injection of inactivated rabies virus with adjuvants. *J. Immunol.* **64**:297, 1950.

LITTLE, P. On the agglutinative titration of antimeningococcal sera, types I and III with the encapsulated bacteria. *J. Immunol.* **34**:97, 1938.

LITWIN, J. The growth cycle of the psittacosis group of micro-organisms. *J. Infect. Dis.* **105**:129, 1959.

LIU, C. Studies on influenza infection in ferrets by means of fluorescein-labeled antibody. II. The role of "soluble antigen" in nuclear fluorescence and cross reactions. *J. Exper. Med.* **101**:677, 1955.

LIU, P. V. Fermentation reactions of *Pseudomonas caviae* and its serological relationship to aeromonads. *J. Bacteriol.* **83**:750, 1962.

LIU, S., and H. WU. Isolation of anticrystalline egg albumen rabbit precipitin. *Chinese J. Phisiol.* **13**:437, 1938.

LOED, J. The influence of electrolytes on the cataphoretic charge of colloidal particles and the stability of their suspensions. *J. Gen. Physiol.* **5**:109, 1922.

LÖFSTRÖM, G. Non-specific capsule swelling in pneumococci. A serological and clinical study. *Acta Med. Scandinav.*, Suppl. 141, 1943.

LÖFSTRÖM, G. Comparison between the reactions of acute phase serum with pneumococcus C-polysaccharide and with pneumococcus Type 27. *Brit. J. Exper. Pathol.* **25**:21, 1944.

LOH, P. C., and J. L. RIGGS. Demonstration of the sequential development of vaccinial antigens and virus in infected cells: observations with cytochemical and differential fluorescent procedures. *J. Exper. Med.* **114**:149, 1961.

LOISELEUR, J. A special reaction from one combination of rabbit serum with phlorizin. *C. R. Acad. Sci.* **222**:159, 1946.

LOISELEUR, J., and M. LEVY. La specificité des anticorps consecuties a l'injection dirécte de molecules organiques de faible poids moleculaire. *Ann. Inst. Pasteur*, **73**:116, 1947.

LOISELEUR, J., J. J. PEREZ, and C. SERGENT. Rensignement fournis par les techniques de flocculation et de viscosité sur la formation des anticorps. *Ann. Inst. Pasteur*, **72**:843, 1946.

LOMINSKI, J., and G. ROBERTS. A substance in human serum inhibiting staphylocoagulase. *J. Pathol. Bacteriol.* **58**:187, 1946.

LONGSWORTH, L. G. A modification of schlieren method for use in electrophoretic analysis. *J. Amer. Chem. Soc.* **61**:529, 1939.

LONGSWORTH, L. G., T. SHEDLOVSKY, and D. A. McINNES. Electrophoretic pattern of normal and pathological human blood serum and plasma. *J. Exper. Med.* **70**:399, 1939.

LOPES, J., and W. E. INNISS. Chemical composition of lipopolysaccharide from an avian strain of *Escherichia coli* 018. *Can. J. Microbiol.* **16**:1117, 1970.

LOW, B. A practical method using papsin and incomplete Rhantibodies in routine Rh blood grouping. *Vox Sang.* **5**:94, 1955.

LOWELL, F. A comparison of the collodion-particle technique with other methods of measuring antibody. *J. Immunol.* **48**:177, 1943.

LOWENTHAL, J., and C. LAMANNA. Characterization of botulinal hemagglutination. *Amer. J. Hyg.* **57**:46, 1953.

LOWRY, O. H., N. J. ROSEBROUGH, A. L. FARR, and R. J. RANDALL. Protein measurement with the Folin reagent. *J. Biol. Chem.* **193**:265, 1951.

LOWRY, R. R. Ferric chloride spray detector for cholesterol and cholesteryl esters on thin-layer chromatograms. *J. Lipid Res.* **9**:397, 1968.

LUCKE, B., M. STRUMIA, S. MUDD, M. McCUTCHEON, and E. MUDD. On comparative phagocytic activity of macrophages and polymorphonuclear leucocytes; essential similarity of tropin action with respect to 2 types of phagocyte. *J. Immunol.* **24**:455, 1933.

LÜDERITZ, O., O. WESTPHAL, E. SIEVERS, E. KRÖGER, E. NETER, and O. H. BRAUN. Über die Fixation von p^{32} markiertem Lipopolysaccharid (Endotoxin) aus *Escherichia coli* and menschlichen Erythrocyten. *Biochem. Z.* **330**:341, 1958.

LÜDERITZ, O., O. WESTPHAL, A. M. STAUB, and L. LeMINOR. Preparation and immunological properties of an artificial antigen with colitose (3-deoxy-L-fucose) as the determinant group. *Nature*, **186**:556, 1960.

LÜDOWIEG, J., and J. D. BENMAMAN. Colorimetric differentiation of hexosamines. *Anal. Biochem.* **19**:80, 1967.

LÜDOWIEG, J., and A. DORFMAN. A micromethod for the colorimeter determination of *N*-acetyl groups in acid mucopolysaccharides. *Biochim. Biophys. Acta* **38**:212, 1960.

LUFT, J. H. Improvement in epoxy resin embedding methods. *J. Biophys. Biochem. Cytol.* **9**:404, 1961.

LUNER, S. J., and A. KOLIN. A new approach to isoelectric focusing and fractionation of proteins in a pH gradient. *Proc. Natl. Acad. Sci.* **66**:898, 1970.

LUNT, E., and D. SUTCLIFFE. A new colorimetric reagent for carbohydrates. *Biochem. J.* **55**:122, 1953.

LUOTO, L. Capillary agglutination test for bovine Q fever. *J. Immunol.* **71**:226, 1953.

LUOTO, L. A capillary tube test for antibody agglutination of *Coxiella burnetii* in human, guinea pigs and sheep sera. *J. Immunol.* **77**:294, 1956.

LUOTO, L., and D. M. MASON. An agglutination test for bovine Q fever performed on milk samples. *J. Immunol.* **74**:222, 1955.

LURIDIANA, N. Adsoribmento di antigeni tubercolari su cellule batteriche. *Boll. Ist. Sieroter. Milan*, **38**:63, 1959.

LUSH, D., and F. M. BURNET. Influenza virus on the developing egg. 6. Complement fixation with egg membrane antigens. *Austral. J. Exper. Biol. Med. Sci.* **15**:375, 1937.

MAALØE, O. On dependence of phagocytosis-stimulating action of immune serum on complement. *Acta Pathol. Microbiol. Scandinav.* **24**:33, 1947.

MABRY, C. C., J. D. GRYBOSKI, and E. A. KARAM. Rapid identification and measurements of mono and oligosaccharides. An adaptation of high-voltage paper electrophoresis for sugars and its application to biologic materials. *J. Lab. Clin. Med.* **62**:817, 1965.

MACH, B., and P. VASSALI. Biosynthesis of RNA antibody-producing tissues. *Proc. Natl. Acad. Sci. U.S.* **54**:975, 1965.

MACHABOEUF, M., P. LACAILLE, and P. REYBEROTTE. Recherches sur la réaction xanthoproteique. Application sur le microdosage colorimétrique des protéines du sérum sanguin. *Bull. Soc. Chim. Biol.* **29**:402, 1947.

MACDONALD, A., and A. DOWNIE. Serological study of the soluble antigens of variola, vaccinia, cowpox and ectromelia viruses. *Brit. J. Exper. Pathol.* **31**:784, 1951.

MACKENZIE, G. M. Observations on paroxysmal hemoglobinuria. *J. Clin. Investig.* **7**:27, 1929.

MACKIE, T. J., and M. H. FINKELSTEIN. Bactericidins of normal serum: their characters, occurrence in various animals and susceptibility of different bacteria to their action. *J. Hygiene*, **32**:1, 1932.

MACLENNAN, A. P. The isolation and characterization of hyaluronidase produced by a capsulated strain of group C streptococci. *J. Gen. Microbiol.* **14**:143, 1956.

MACPHERSON, I. A., J. F. WILKINSON, and R. H. SWAIN. The effect of *Klebsiella aerogenes* and *Klebsiella cloacae* polysaccharides on hemagglutination by and multiplication of influenza group of viruses. *Brit. J. Exper. Pathol.* **34**:603, 1953.

MADSEN, T. Whooping cough; its bacteriology, diagnosis, prevention, and treatment. *Boston Med. Surg. J.* **192**:50, 1952.

MAGE, M. G., W. H. EVANS, and E. A. PETERSON. Enrichment of antibody plaque-forming cells by immunoadsorption to an antigen-coated polyurethane foam. *J. Immunol.* **102**:908, 1969.

MAGNUS, VON, P. Propagation of PR8 strain of influenza virus in chick embryo; formation of "incomplete" virus following inoculation of large doses of seed virus. *Acta Pathol. Microbiol. Scandinav.* **28**:278, 1951.

MAGNUSON, H. J., H. EAGLE, and R. FLEISCHMAN, Minimal infectious inoculum of *Spirochaeta pallida* (Nichols strain), and consideration of its rate of multiplication. *Amer. J. Symph. Gonorrh. Ven. Dis.* **32**:1, 1948.

MAGNUSON, H. J., and F. A. THOMPSON. JR. Treponemal immobilization test of normal and syphilitic serum. *J. Vener. Dis. Inform.* **30**:309, 1949.

MAGNUSON, H. J., F. THOMPSON, and C. McCLEOD. Relationships between treponemal immobilizing antibody and acquired immunity in experimental syphilis. *J. Immunol.* **67**:41, 1951.

MÄKELÄ, O., and G. J. V. NOSSAL. Bacterial adherence: a method for detecting antibody production by single cells. *J. Immunol.* **87**:447, 1961.

MAKINODAN, T., N. GENGOZIAN, and C. CONGDON. Agglutinin production in normal sublethally irradiated, and lethally radiated mice treated with mouse bone marrow. *J. Immunol.* **77**:250, 1956.

MAKINODAN, T., and N. T. MACRIS. A study of unusual hemagglutinin in a pooled human serum. *J. Immunol.* **75**:197, 1955.

MAKINODAN, T., and N. T. MACRIS. The effect of ficin on the agglutination of human red blood cells. *J. Immunol.* **75**:192, 1955.

MALPRESS, F. H., and A. B. MORRISON, Use of pyridine in the de-ionization of solutions for paper chromatography. *Nature*, **164**:963, 1949.

MALPRESS, F. H., and A. B. MORRISON. Semimicro estimation of lactose alone and in the presence of other surgars. *Biochem. J.* **45**:455, 1949.

MALTANER, F., and E. MALTANER. The quantitative determination of antigen-antibody reaction by complement fixation. *Intern. Congr. Microbiol. New York, Rept. Congr.* 781, 1939.

MANCINI, G., A. O. CARBONARA, and J. F. HEREMANS. Immunochemical quantitation of antigens by single radial immunodiffusion. *Immunochemistry*, 2:235, 1965.

MANDELL, J. D., and A. D. HERSHEY. A fractionating column for analysis of nucleic acids. *Analyt. Biochem.* 1:66, 1960.

MANDIA, J. W., and D. W. BRUNNER. The serological identification of cultures of *Clostridium sporogenes. J. Immunol.* 66:497, 1951.

MANGOLD, H. K. !hin layer chromatography of lipids. *J. Amer. Oil. Chemists Soc.* 38:708, 1961.

MANSI, W. The study of some viruses by the plate gel diffusion precipitation test. *J. Comp. Pathol.* 67:297, 1957.

MANSI, W. Slide gel diffusion precipitation test. *Nature* 181:1289, 1958.

MARENNIKOVA, S. S., and G. M. AKATOVA. *Bull. Exper. Biol. Med.* 45:480, 1958.

MARGOLIS, J., and K. G. KENRICK. Polyacrylamide gel electrophoresis in a continuous molecular sieve gradient. *Anal. Biochem.* 25:347, 1968.

MARGOLIS, J., and K. G. KENRICK. Two-dimensional resolution of plasma proteins by combination of polyacrylamide disc and gradient gel electrophoresis. *Nature*, 221:1056, 1969.

MARGOLIS, S. Separation and size determination of human serum lipoproteins by agarose gel filtration. *J. Lipid Res.* 8:501, 1967.

MARINETTI, G. V., J. ERBLAND, and J. KOCHEM. Quantitative chromatography of phosphatides. *Feder. Proc.* 16:837, 1957.

MARKHAM, N. P., and J. KENT. A technique for the repeated intravenous injection of guinea pigs. *Brit. J. Exper. Pathol.* 32:366, 1951.

MARKHAM, R. L. A steam distillation apparatus available for micro-Kjeldahl analysis. *Biochem. J.* 36:790, 1942.

MARKHAM, R. L., J. H. JACOBS, and E. T. D. FLETCHER. Zone electrophoresis of serum and urine at pH 4.5 and its application to isolation and investigation of mucoproteins. *J. Lab. Clin. Med.* 48:559, 1956.

MARKS, V. An improved glucose-oxidase method for determining blood, cerebrospinal, and urine glucose levels. *Clin. Chim. Acta*, 4:395, 1959.

MARMUR, J. A. procedure for the isolation of deoxyribonucleic acid from micro-organisms. *J. Mol. Biol.* 3:208, 1961.

MARMUR, J., and P. DOTY. Determination of the base composition of deoxyribonucleic acid from its thermal denaturation temperature. *J. Mol. Biol.* 5:109, 1962.

MARMUR, J., R. ROWND, and C. L. SCHILDKRAUT. Some problems concerning the macromolecular structure of ribonucleic acids. In *Progress Nucleic Acid Research*, Vol. 1. J. N. Davidson and W. E. Cohn, Eds. Academic Press, New York, 1963, p. 231.

MARR, A. G., and E. H. COTA-ROBLES. Sonic disruption of *Azotobacter vinelandii. J. Bacteriol.* 74:79, 1957.

MARRACK, J. R. Nature of antibodies. *Nature*, 133:292, 1934.

MARRACK, J. R. *The Chemistry of Antigens and Antibodies*. H. M. Stationery Office, London, 1938.

MARRACK, J. R. The relation of the rates of flocculation and amounts of precipitate in precipitin reactions to the concentration of hydrogen ion and of neutral salts. *Immunology*, 1:251, 1958.

MARRACK, J. R., H. HOCH, and R. G. S. JOHNS. The valency of antibodies. *Brit. J. Exper. Pathol.* 32:212, 1951.

MARRACK, J. R., and H. HOLLERING. The effect of increased salt concentration on the amount of precipitate formed by antisera with specific precipitants. *Brit. J. Exper. Pathol.* 19:424, 1938.

MARRACK, J. R., and F. C. SMITH. Quantitative aspects of immunity reactions. The precipitin reaction. *Brit. J. Exper. Pathol.* 12:30, 1931.

MARRACK, J. R., and F. C. SMITH. Quantitative aspects of immunity reactions: The combination of antibodies with simple peptones. *Brit. J. Exper. Pathol.* **13**:394, 1932.

MARSHALL, J. D., W. C. EVELAND, and C. W. SMITH. Superiority of fluorescein isothiocyanata (Riggs) for fluorescent-antibody technic with a modification of its application. *Proc. Soc. Exper. Biol. Med.* **98**:898, 1958.

MARSHALL, J. M. Localization of adrenocorticotropic hormone by histochemical and immunochemical methods. *J. Exper. Med.* **94**:21, 1951.

MARTEN, J. F., and G. CATANZARO. Fundamental studies in aromatic nitrogen digestion. *Analyst*, **41**:42, 1966.

MARTIN, D. Serologic studies on North American blastomycosis. *J. Immunol.* **71**:192, 1953.

MARTIN, H. Über zwei Fälle von "Wassermannpositiven Lungeninfiltrat." *Klin. Wochenschr.* **184**:1943.

MARTIN, H., and E. VOSS. Beeinflussung der Properdinaktivität durch Erythrozyten-Stromata. *Vox Sang.* **2**:201, 1957.

MARTIN, R. G., and B. N. AMES. A method for determining the sedimentation behavior of enzymes: Application to protein mixtures. *J. Biol. Chem.* **236**:1372, 1961.

MASIGA, W. N., and S. S. STONE. Application of a fluorescent-antibody technique for the detection of *Mycoplasma mycoides* antigen and antibody. *J. Bacteriol.* **97**:1867, 1968.

MASON, T. E., R. F. Phifer, S. S. SPICER, R. A. SWALLOW, and R. E. DRESKIN. An immunoglobulin-enzyme bridge method for localizing tissue antigens. *J. Histochem. Cytochem.* **17**:563, 1969.

MASOUREDIS, S. Toxicity and immunochemcial properties of I^{131} trace labeled diphtheria toxin. *J. Immunol.* **79**:516, 1957.

MASRY, F. Production, extraction and purification of the haemagglutinin of *H. pertussis*. *J. Gen. Microbiol.* **7**:201, 1954.

MASSEL, B. F., J. R. MORE, and J. D. JONES. The quantitative relation of fibrinolysin and antifibrinolysin. *J. Immunol.* **36**:45, 1939.

MASTIUKOVA, I. N., and S. L. KHAIT. *Voprosy Virusol.* **5**:339, 1960.

MATA, L. J. The agar cell culture precipitation test; its application to the study of vaccinia virus, adenoviruses and herpes simplex virus. *J. Immunol.* **91**:151, 1963.

MATA, L. J., and T. H. WELLER. A cell culture system on agar permitting direct investigation of viral antigens by immunodiffusion. *Proc. Soc. Exper. Biol. Med.* **109**:705, 1962.

MATHEWES, R. P. Adaptation of the antiglobulin test for the use with tannic acid treated erythrocytes. *J. Immunol.* **82**:279, 1959.

MATHEWS, M. M., and W. R. SISTROM. Intracellular location of carotenoid pigment and some respiratory enzymes in *Sarcina lutea*. *J. Bacteriol.* **78**:778, 1959.

MATHIESEN, M., and M. VOLKERT. The antigenic relationship between ornithosis virus and *Bacterium anitratum*. *Acta Pathol. Microbiol. Scandinav.* **41**:135, 1957.

MATSON, G., and E. BRADY. A procedure for the serological determination of blood-relationship of ancient and modern peoples with special reference to American Indians. *J. Immunol.* **30**:445, 1936.

MAURIAC, P., and M. MOUREAU. La fragilité leucocytaire. Recherches cliniques et expèrimentales. *J. Med. Franc.* **9**:243, 1920.

MAXTED, W. R. Preparation of streptococcal extracts for Lancefield grouping. *Lancet*, **II**:255, 1948.

MAYER, H. UNTERSUCHUNGEN ueber die Brauchbarkeit verschiedener *Brucella*-antigene zur Diagnose der Schafbrucellose. *Mh. Tierheilk.* **13**. *Sonderteil.*, **114**, 1961.

MAYER, K., and B. EDDIE. Psittacosis. In *Diagnostic Procedures for Virus and Rickettsial Diseases*, *Vol.* **1**. American Public Health Association, 1948.

MAYER, M. M. Complement and complement fixation. *Exptl. Immunochem.*, E. A. Kabat and M. M. Mayer, Eds., 2nd ed., Thomas, Springfield, Illinois, 1961, p. 133.

MAYER, M. M., C. C. CROFT, and M. M. GRAY. Kinetic studies on immune hemolysis. I. A method. *J. Exper. Med.* **88**:427, 1948.

MAYER, M. M., B. B. EATON, and M. HEIDELBERGER. Spectrophotometric standardization of complement for fixation tests. *J. Immunol.* **53**:31, 1946.

MAYER, M. M., A. G. OSLER, O. G. BIER, and M. HEIDELBERGER. Quantitative studies of complement fixation. *Proc. Soc. Exper. Biol. Med.* **65**:66, 1947.

MAYER, M. M., A. G. OSLER, O. G. BIER, and M. HEIDELBERGER. Quantitative studies of complement fixation. I. A method. *J. Immunol.* **59**:195, 1948.

MAYER, M. M., A. G. OSLER, O. G. BIER, and M. HEIDELBERGER. The activating effect of magnesium and other cations on the hemolytic function of complement. *J. Exper. Med.* **84**:535, 1946.

MAYER, R., and H. DOWLING. The determination of meningococcus antibodies by a centrifuge-agglutination test. *J. Immunol.* **51**:349, 1945.

MAYYASI, S. A., D. M. SHURMANS, and A. BROWN. The agglutination of L cells by *Vaccinia* virus. *J. Immunol.* **83**:411, 1959.

MAZZINI, L. Y. Mazzini cardiolipin micro-flocculation test for symphilis. *J. Immunol.* **66**:261, 1951.

MCBRIDE, W. J., JR., and J. D. KLINGMAN. Sincle column gas chromatographic separation of nanomolar quantities of amino acids. *Anal. Biochem.* **25**:109, 1968.

MCCARTER, J. R., and E. B. BEVILACQUA. The proteins in the unheated culutre filtrates of human tubercle bacilli. *J. Exper. Med.* **87**:245, 1948.

MCCARTY, M. The occurrence during acute infections of a protein not normally present in the blood. IV. Crystallization of the C-reactive protein. *J. Exper. Med.* **85**:491, 1947.

MCCARTY, M. The occurrence of nuclease in culture filtrates of group A hemolytic streptococci. *J. Exper. Med.* **88**:181, 1948.

MCCARTY, M. The inhibition of streptococcal desoxyribonuclease by rabbit and human antisera. *J. Exper. Med.* **90**:543, 1949.

MCCARTY, M. The lysis of group A hemolytic streptococci by extracellular enzymes. I. Production and fractionation of the lytic factor. *J. Exper. Med.* **96**:555, 1952.

MCCLELLAND, L. C., and A. HARE. The adsorption of influenza virus by red cells and a new in vitro method of measuring antibodies for influenza virus. *Can. Publ. Health J.* **32**:530, 1941.

MCCLINTOCK, L. A., and M. M. FRIEDMAN. Utilization of antibody for the localization of metals and dyes in the tissues. *Amer. J. Roentgenol. Radium Therapy*, **54**:704, 1945.

MCDUFFIE, F., and E. A. KABAT. A comparative study of methods used for analysis of specific precipitation in quantitative immunochemistry. *J. Immunol.* **77**:193, 1956.

MCDUFFIE, F., and E. A. KABAT. The behavior in the Coombs test of anti-A and anti-B sera produced by immunization with various blood group A and B substances and by heterospecific pregnancy. *J. Immunol.* **77**:61, 1956.

MCFADDEN, M., L., and E. L. SMITH. Free amino groups of N-terminal sequence of rabbit antibodies. *J. Biol. Chem.* **214**:185, 1955.

MCFARLAND, J. The nephelomcter; An instrument for estimating the number of bacteria in suspension used for calculating the opsonic index and for vaccines. *J. Amer. Med. Assoc.* **49**:1176, 1907.

MCFARLANE, A. S. Efficient trace-labeling of protein with iodine. *Nature*, **182**:53, 1958.

MCILVAIN, H. Preparation of cell-free bacterial extracts with powdered alumina. *J. Gen. Microbiol.* **2**:288, 1948.

MCILVAINE, T. C. *J. Biod. Chem.* **49**:183, 1921.

MCKEE, A. P., and W. S. JETER. The demonstration of an antibody against complement. *J. Immunol.* **76**:112, 1956.

McKee, C., G. Rake, and M. Shaffer. Complement fixation test in lymphogranuloma venereum. *Proc. Soc. Exper. Biol. Med.* **44**:410, 1940.

McKenna, J. M., and K. M. Stevens. Studies on antibody formation by peritoneal exudate cells in vitro. *J. Exper. Med.* **111**:573, 1960.

McKiel, J. A., and A. M. Millar. Serodiagnosis in Q fever with special emphasis on the radioisotope precipitation test. *Can. J. Microbiol.* **14**:721, 1968.

McNeil, C., E. F. Trentelman, N. P. Sullivan, and C. I. Argale. A new rapid Rh tube test using polyvinyl pyrrolidone. *Amer. J. Clin. Pathol.* **22**:1216, 1952.

McQuillen, K. Lysis resulting from metabolic disturbances. *J. Gen. Microbiol.* **18**:498, 1958.

Mehlman, T., and B. Seegal. Passive sensitization of guinea pig with rabbit and horse anti-pneumococcus type I serum. *J. Immunol.* **27**:1, 1934.

Meijers, C. A., and F. Westendorp-Boerma. A screening test for the hemagglutination reaction in rheumatoid arthritis. *J. Lab. Clin. Med.* **52**:144, 1958.

Mejbaum, W. Ueber die Bestimmung kleiner Pentosemengen insbesondere in Derivaten der Adenylsaure. *Z. Physiol. Chemie.* **258**:117, 1939.

Melnick, J. L. Studies on coxsackie viruses: properties, immunological aspects and distribution. *Bull. N.Y. Acad. Med.* **26**:342, 1950.

Melnick, J. L. Differences in the degree of infectiousness of two related strains of poliomyelitis virus following their oral administration to monkeys. *J. Immunol.* **67**:219, 1951.

Melnick, J. L. Analytical serology of animal viruses. In *Analytical Serology of Microorganisms*. J. B. G. Kwapinski, Ed., Vol. 1. Interscience, New York, 1969, pp. 457–458.

Melnick, J. L., and E. M. Opton. *Bull. World Health Organ.* **14**:129, 1956.

Meltzer, M., E. C. Frankling, H. Fudenberg, and B. Frangione. Single peptide differences between γ-globulins of different genetic (Gm) types. *Proc. Natl. Acad. Sci. U.S.* **51**:1007, 1964.

Merchant, D. J., and R. E. Chamberlain. A phagocytosis inhibition test in infection hypersensitivity. *Proc. Soc. Exper. Biol. Med.* **80**:69, 1952.

Mergenhagen, S. E., and E. Varah. Serologically specific lipopolysaccharides from oral Veillonella. *Arch. Oral. Biol.* **8**:31, 1963.

Merkel, M. The chemical and antigenic structure of *Trichophyton gypseum*. *Bull. Acad. Pol. Sci. Cl. II*, **10**:341, 1957.

Merkel, M. The chemical and the antigenic structure of a *Mycobacterium balnei* strain. *Bull. Acad. Pol. Sci. Cl. II* **9**:359, 1961.

Merrill, D., T. F. Hartley, and H. N. Claman. Electroimmunodiffusion (EID): A simple rapid method for quantitation of immunoglobulins in dilute biological fluids. *J. Lab. Clin. Med.* **69**:151, 1967.

Merrill, M. Quantitative studies on the neutralization of equine encephalomyelitis virus by immune serum. *J. Immunol.* **30**:185, 1936.

Metchnikoff, E. *Lectures on the Comparative Pathology of Inflammation*. London, 1893.

Metchnikoff, E. *Ann. Inst. Pasteur*, **11**:801, 1897.

Metchnikoff, E. *Immunity in Infective Diseases*. Cambridge University Press, London, 1907.

Metzger, J. F., and C. W. Smith. Serologic typing of *Listeria monocytogenes* by gel diffusion using thermostable antigen. *Proc. Soc. Exper. Biol. Med.* **110**:903, 1962.

Meyer, K., and H. Loewenthal. Untersuchungen über Antikörperbildung in Gewebekulturen. *Zeitschr. Immunitätsforsch.* **54**:409, 1928.

Meyer, K., and H. Loewenthal. Untersuchungen über Anaphylaxie in Gewebekulturen. *Zeitschr. Immunitätsforsch.* **54**:420, 1928.

Meyer, P. E., and E. F. Hunter. Antigenic relationships of 14 treponemas demonstrated by immunofluorescence. *J. Bacteriol.* **93**:784, 1967.

MEYER, R. K. The biological significance of hyaluronic acid and hyaluronidase. *Physiol. Rev.* **27**:335, 1947.

MEYER, T. S., and B. L. LAMBERTS. Use of Coomassie brilliant blue R250 for the electrophoresis of microgram quantities of parotid saliva proteins on acrylamide-gel strips. *Biochim. Biophys. Acta*, **107**:144, 1965.

MEYNELL, G. The antigenic structure of *Mycobacterium tuberculosis*, var. hominis. *J. Pathol. Bacteriol.* **67**:137, 1954.

MEYSEL, M. N., Y. N. KABANOVA, and N. M. PISHCHURINA. *Izv. Akad. Nauk. SSSR. Ser. Biol.* **6**:716, 1957.

MEZKOV, A. E., *Zhur. Mikrobiol. Epidemiol. Immunobiol.* **31**:137, 1960.

MICHAELIS, L. WEITERE Untersuchungen über Eiweisspräzipitine. *Deutsche Med. Wochenschr.* **30**:1240, 1904.

MICHAELIS, L. Diethylbarbiturate buffer. *J. Biol. Chem.* **87**:33, 1930.

MICHEEVA, G. A. Pokazateli nespecificzeskego immuniteta pri rewmatizme u detej. *Pediatrija*, **4**:11, 1953.

MICKELSON, J. C., and J. B. G. KWAPINSKI. Analytical Serology of *Neisseriaceae*. In *Analytical Serology of Microorganisms*, J. B. G. KWAPINSKI, Ed., Vol. 1. Interscience, New York, 1969, pp. 501–519.

MICKELSON, M. N. Chemically defined medium for growth of *Streptococcus pyogenes*. *J. Bacteriol.* **88**:158, 1964.

MICKLE, H. Tissue disintegrator. *J. Roy. Microscop. Soc.* **68**:10, 1948.

MIDDLEBROOK, G. Laboratory aids to diagnosis and therapy. *Ann. Rev. Med.* **5**:339, 1954.

MIDDLEBROOK, G. A hemolytic modification of the hemagglutination test for antibodies against tubercle bacillus antigens. *J. Clin. Invest.* **29**:1480, 1950.

MIDDLEBROOK, G., and R. DUBOS. Specific serum agglutination of erythrocytes sensitized with extracts of tubercle bacilli. *J. Exper. Med.* **88**:521, 1948.

MIDGLEY, J. E. M. The estimation of polynucleotide chain length by a chemical method. *Biochim. Biophys. Acta*, **108**:340, 1965.

MIGUEL, J., B. HORVATH, and I. KLATZO. A chromatographic technique for the quantitative study of the precipitin reaction. *J. Immunol.* **84**:545, 1960.

MIKULASZEK, E. *Bull. Acad. Polon. Sci.* **3**:21, 1955.

MIKULASZEK, E. *Chemia Zjawisk Odpornosciowych*. PZWL, 1959.

MIKULASZEK, E., and J. B. G. KWAPINSKI. The serological properties of mycobacterial fractions. *Gruzl.* **22**:245, 1954.

MILES, A. A. The case for unit notation in specifying the agglutinating potency of standard antisera. *Bull. World Health Organ.* **10**:941, 1954.

MILES, A. A., S. S. MISRA, and J. O. IRWIN. The estimation of bactericidal power of the blood. *J. Hygiene*, **38**:732, 1938.

MILES, A. A., E. MILES, and J. BURKE. The value and duration of the defence reactions of the skin to the primary lodgement of bacteria. *Brit. J. Exper. Pathol.* **38**:79, 1957.

MILES, A. A., and G. S. WILSON. *Topley and Wilson's Textbook of Bacteriology*. Wood, Baltimore, Md., 1955.

MILGROM, F., and K. KANO. Application of cell cultures for human tissue typing; in Histocompatibility testing. *Series Haematologica*, Vol. 11. Munksgaard, Copenhagen, 1965, p. 179.

MILLER, G. L., and W. M. STANLEY. Derivatives of tobacco mosaic virus. I. Acetyl and phenylureido virus. *J. Biol. Chem.* **141**:905, 1941.

MILLER, G. L., and W. M. STANLEY. Quantitative aspects of the red blood cell agglutination test for influenza virus. *J. Exper. Med.* **70**:185, 1944.

MILLER, H. K., and R. W. SCHLESINGER. Differentiation and purification of influenza viruses by adsorption on alumina phosphate. *J. Immunol.* **75**:155, 1955.

MILLER, J., and R. SILVERBERG. Agglutinative reaction in relation to pertussis and to prophylactic vaccination against pertussis, with description of a new technic. *J. Immunol.* **37**:207, 1939.

MILLER, J. N., R. A. BOAK, and C. M. CARPENTER. *Amer. J. Clin. Pathol.* **32**:187, 1959.

MILLER, L., and M. TAINTER. Estimation of the ED_{50} and its error by means of logarithmic-probit graph paper. *Proc. Soc. Exper. Biol. Med.* **57**:261, 1944.

MILLER, M. J. Bacteria-free entamoeba invadens. *Nature*, **172**:1192, 1953.

MILLER, R. G., and R. A. PHILLIPS. Separation of cells by velocity sedimentation. *J. Cell. Comp. Physiol.* **73**:191, 1969.

MINDEN, P., and R. S. FARR. Binding between components of the tubercle bacillus and humoral antibodies. *J. Exper. Med.* **130**:931, 1969.

MISHULOV, L., J. KLEIN, M. LISS, and L. LEIFER. Protection of mice against *H. pertussis* by serum. Comparison of protection with agglutination. *J. Immunol.* **37**:17, 1939.

MISRA, S. B., and D. L. SHRIVASTOVA. Studies of immunochemistry of *Vibrio cholerae*. IV. Cross precipitation reactions of antigens in various serotypes. *Ind. J. Med. Res.* **49**:183, 1961.

MITCHELL, P. D. Biochemical cytology of microorganisms. *Ann. Rev. Microbiol.* **13**:407, 1950.

MITCHELL, P. D., and J. M. MOYLE. The glycerophospho-protein complex envelope of *Micrococcus pyrogenes*. *J. Gen. Microbiol.* **5**:966, 1951.

MITCHELL, P. D., and R. G. BURRELL. Serology of the *Mima-Herellea* group and the genus *Moraxella*. *J. Bacteriol.* **87**:900, 1964.

MITZ, M. A. The solubility of proteins in the presence of carbon dioxide. *Biochim. Biophys. Acta*, **25**:426, 1957.

MIWA, P. W. Identification of peaks in gas-liquid chromatography. *J. Amer. Oil Chem. Soc.* **40**:309, 1963.

MOBERLY, M., G. MARINETTI, R. WITTER, and H. MORGAN. Studies on the hemolysis of red blood cells by mumps virus. II. Alterations in lipoproteins of the red blood cell walls. *J. Exper. Med.* **107**:87, 1958.

MOESCHLIN, S., and B. DEMIRAL. Antikörperbildung der Plasmazellen in vitro. *Klin. Wochenschr.* **30**:827, 1952.

MOGASANIK, B. The Nucleic Acids. In *Chemistry and Biology*, E. Chargaff and J. N. Davidson, Eds., Vol. 1. Academic, New York, 1955.

MOHIT, B. Disc immuno-immobilization method for simultaneous typing and isolation of *Salmonella* flagellar phases. *J. Bacteriol.* **96**:160, 1968.

MOHORRAM, J. On the group-specific differentiation of the human feces with special regard to the AB group. *J. Immunol.* **32**:229, 1937.

MOLISCH, H. *Monatschr.* **7**:198, 1896.

MÖLLER, G. Demonstration of mouse isoantigens at cellular level by the fluorescent antibody technique. *J. Exper. Med.* **114**:415, 1961.

MÖLLER, G., and H. WIGZELL. Antibody synthesis at the cellular level. Antibody-induced suppression of 19S and 7S antibody response. *J. Exper. Med.* **121**:969, 1965.

MONJARDINO, J. P. Thin-layer electrophoresis of ribonucleotides. *Anal. Biochem.* **28**:313, 1969.

MONOD, J. Antibodies and induced enzymes. In *Cellular and Humoral Aspects of Hypersensitive States*, H. S. Lawrence. Ed. Hoeber & Harper, New York, 1959.

MONTGOMERY, C. H., S. SUHROLAND, and J. M. KNOX. Observations concerning fluorescent treponemal antibody for syphilis. *J. Invest. Dermat.* **35**:95, 1960.

MOODY, M. D., J. Z. BIEGELEISEN, JR., and G. C. TAYLOR. Detection of brucellae and their antibodies by fluorescent antibody and agglutination tests. *J. Bacteriol.* **81**:990, 1961.

MOODY, M. D., E. C. ELLIS, and E. L. UPDYKE. Staining bacterial smears with fluorescent antibody. IV. Grouping streptococci with fluorescent antibody. *J. Bacteriol.* **75**:553, 1958.

MOODY, M. D., M. GOLDMAN, and B. M. THOMASON. Staining bacterial smears with fluorescent antibody. I. General methods for *Malleomyces pseudomallei. J. Bacteriol.* **72**:357, 1956.

MOODY, M. D., and C. C. WINTER. Rapid identification of *Pasteurella pestis* with fluorescent antibody. *J. Infect. Dis.* **104**:288, 1959.

MOORE, D. L., and S. I. VAS. Studies on the production of complement. *Immunology,* **15**:185, 1968.

MOORE, S., and W. H. STEIN. Photometric ninhydrin method for use in the chromatography of amino acids. *J. Biol. Chem.* **176**:367, 1948.

MOORE, S., and W. H. STEIN. Chromatography of amino acids on sulfonated polystyrene resins. *J. Biol. Chem.* **192**:663, 1951.

MORALEZ-OTERO, P., and L. M. GONZALEZ. Purified antigen from *Brucella. Proc. Soc. Exper. Biol. Med.* **38**:703, 1938.

MORDARSKA, H. Antigenic structure of microorganisms of the species Nocurdia asteroides. *Arch. Immunol. Exper. Therapy,* **14**:311, 1966.

MORESCHI, C. Neue Tatsachen über die Blutkörperchenagglutination. *Zentralbl. Bakteriol. I. Orig.* **46**:49, 1908.

MORESCHI, C. Beschleunigung und Verstärkung der Bakterienagglutination durch Antiei-weiss Sera. *Zentralbl. Bakteriol. I. Orig.* **46**:456, 1908.

MORGAN, C., K. C. HSU, R. A. RIFIND, A. W. KNOX, and H. M. ROSE. The application of ferritin-conjugated antibody to electron microscopic studies of influenza virus in infected cells. *J. Exper. Med.* **114**:825, 833, 1961.

MORGAN, C., R. A. RIFKIND, K. C. HSU, M. HOLDEN, B. C. SEEHAL, and M. R. HARRY. Electron microscope localization of intracellular viral antigen by the use of ferritin-conjugated antibody. *Virology,* **14**:292, 1961.

MORGAN, C., R. A. RIFKIND, and H. M. ROSE. The use of ferritin-conjugated antibodies in electron microscopic studies of influenza and vaccine viruses. *Cold Spring Harbor Symp. Quant. Biol.* **27**:57, 1962.

MORGAN, H. R. Enzymatic properties of the hemolytic principle of mumps virus. *Bacter. Proc.* **81**:1950.

MORGAN, H. R., J. R. ENDERS, and P. T. WAGLEY. A hemolysin associated with mumps virus. *J. Exper. Med.* **88**:503, 1948.

MORGAN, J. F., H. J. MORTON, and R. C. PARKER. Nutrition of animal cells in tissue culture. I. Initial studies on a synthetic medium. *Proc. Soc. Exper. Biol. Med.* **73**:1, 1950.

MORGAN, M. E. A device for simultaneous application of multiple spots on thin layer chromatographic plates. *J. Chromatog.* **9**:379, 1962.

MORGAN, W. T. J. The isolation and properties of a specific antigenic substance from *Bacterium dysenteriae (Shiga). Biochem. J.* **31**:20003, 1937.

MORGAN, W. T. J., and L. A. ELSON. A colorimetric method for the determination of N-acetylgucosamine and N-acetylchondrosamine. *Biochem. J.* **28**:988, 1934.

MORGAN, W. T. J., and H. KING. Studies in immunochemistry. Isolation from hog gastric mucin of the polysaccharideamino acid complex possessing blood group A specificity. *Biochem. J.* **37**:640, 1943.

MORGAN, W. T. J., and S. PARTRIDGE. Studies in immunochemistry. 6. The use of phenol and alkali in degradation of antigenic material isolated from *Bacterium dysenteriae (Shiga). Biochem. J.* **35**:1140, 1941.

MORRIS, D. L. The quantitative determination of carbohydrates with Dreywood's anthrone. *Science*, **107**:254, 1948.

MORRIS, M. C. The validity of the "percentage law" in bacterial reactions. *J. Immunol.* **48**:259, 1943.

MORRIS, M. C. Some qualitative aspects of immune hemolysis. *J. Immunol.* **62**:201, 1949.

MORRIS, M. C. The effect of trypsin on hemagglutination by murine encephalomyelitis virus. *J. Immunol.* **68**:97, 1952.

MORSE, S. Some mathematical relations in the Wassermann reaction. *Proc. Soc. Exper. Biol. Med.* **19**:17, 1921.

MORTON, J., and M. M. PICKLES. Use of trypsin in the detection of incomplete anti-Rh antibodies. *Nature*, **159**:779, 1947.

MORTON, J., and M. M. PICKLES. The proteolytic enzyme test for detecting incomplete antibodies. *J. Clin. Pathol.* **4**:189, 1951.

MOSKOWITZ, M., and H. TREFFERS. An agglutinin in normal sera for periodated red cells. *Science*, **111**:717, 1950.

MOSS, C. W., and V. J. LEWIS. Characterization of clostridia by gas chromatography. I. Differentiation of species by cellular fatty acids. *Appl. Microbiol.* **15**:390, 1967.

MOTT, M. R. Electron microscopy studies on the immobilization antigens of *Paramecium aurelia*. *J. Gen. Microbiol.* **41**:251, 1965.

MOULDER, J. W., and E. WEISS. Purification and properties of the agent of feline pneumonitis. *J. Infect. Dis.* **88**:56, 1951.

MOULTON, J., and BROWN, C. Antigenicity of canine distemper inclusion bodies demonstrated by fluorescent antibody technique. *Proc. Soc. Exper. Biol. Med.* **86**:99, 1954.

MUDD, S. A hypothetical mechanism of antibody formation. *J. Immunol.* **23**:423, 1932.

MUDD, S., E. CZARNETZKY, D. LACKMAN, and H. PETTIT. The antigenic structure of hemolytic streptococci of Lancefield group A. *J. Immunol.* **34**: 117, 1938.

MUDD, S., and E. B. H. MUDD. Surface composition of tubercle bacillus and other acid-fast bacteria. *J. Exper. Med.* **46**:127, 1927.

MUDD, S., H. PETTIT, D. LACKMAN, and J. M. MORGAN. The antigenic structure of hemolytic streptocci of Lancefield group A. *J. Immunol.* **36**:381, 1939.

MUDD, S., T. SALI, T. TAKAGI, J. I. PAYNE, and T. KAWATA. Plasma membranes and mitochondria equivalents as functionally coordinated structures. *Bacteriol. Proc.* **51**:1959.

MUETHER, R. O., and W. C. MACDONALD. Precipitation test for tuberculin antibodies. *J. Lab. Clin. Med.* **30**:309, 1949.

MUIR, R. A. On the relationships between the complements and immune-bodies of different animals. *J. Pathol. Bacteriol.* **16**:523, 1911.

MUIR, R. A. *System of Bacteriology in Relation to Medicine.* H. M. Stationery Office, London, 1931.

MUIR, R. A., and J. BROWNING. On the action of complement as agglutinin. *J. Hygiene*, **6**:20, 1906.

MUKERJEE, H., and J. SRI RAM. Paper chromatographic separation of glucosamine and galactosamine. *Anal. Biochem.* **8**:393, 1964.

MÜLLER-EBERHARD, H. J. A new supporting medium for preparative electrophoresis. *Scandinav. J. Clin. Lab. Invest.* **12**:33, 1960.

MÜLLER-EBERHARD, H. J., and C. E. BIRO. Isolation and description of the fourth component of human complement. *J. Exper. Med.*, **118**:447, 1963.

MÜLLER-EBERHARD, H. J., A. P. DALMASSO, and M. A. CALCOTT. The reaction mechanism of β_{1c}-globulin (C'3) in immune hemolysis. *J. Exper. Med.* **123**:33, 1966.

MÜLLER-EBERHARD, H. J., and H. G. KUNKEL. The carbohydrate of γ-globulin and myeloma proteins. *J. Exper. Med.* **104**:253, 1956.

MÜLLER-EBERHARD, H. J. and H. G. KUNKEL. Ultracentrifuge chaarcteristics and carbohydrate content of macromolecular γ-globulins. *Clin. Chim. Acta*, **4**:252, 1959.

MÜLLER-EBERHARD, H. J., M. J. POLLEY, and M. A. CALCOTT. Formation and functional significance of a molecular complex derived from the second and the fourth component of human complement. *J. Exper. Med.* **125**:359, 1967.

MUNIER, R. L., and C. THOMMEGAY. This layer chromatoelectrophoresis of amino acids on powdered cellulose. *Bull. Soc. Chim. Fr.* **9**:3171, 1967.

MUNOZ, J. J. On the value of "conditioned hemolysis" for the diagnosis of American trypanosomiasis. *O. Hospital*, **38**:635, 1935.

MUNOZ, J. J. *Serological Approaches to Studies of Protein Structure and Metabolism.* Ruthers University Press, New Brunswick, N. J., 1954.

MUNOZ, J. J., and E. BECKER. Antigen-antibody reactions in agar. I. Complexity of antigen-antibody systems as demonstrated by a serum-agar technic. *J. Immunol.* **65**:47, 1950.

MUNOZ, J. J., and B. M. BESTEKIN. Antigens of *Bordetella pertussis*. III. The protective antigen. *Proc. Soc. Exper. Biol. Med.* **112**:799, 1962.

MUNOZ, J. J., E. RIBI, and C. L. LARSON. Antigens of *Bordetella pertussis*. I. Activities of cell walls and protoplasm. *J. Immunol.* **83**:496, 1959.

MURASE, T. Studies on tuberculo-polysaccharide fractionated with resin chromatography (ecteda-cellulose). Its chemical and biological properties. *Nagoya J. Med. Sci.* **23**:343, 1961.

MURDICK, P., and S. COHEN. A note on the concentration and purification of antimeningococcus serum. *J. Immunol.* **28**:205, 1935.

MURDUCH, F., M. ROEPKE, and B. COOD. Third International American Congress on *Brucellosis*, Washington, 1950.

MURGITA, R. A., and S. I. VAS. Isoelectric separation of mouse immunoglobulins. *J. Immunol.* **104**:514, 1970.

MURRAY, E., A. OFSTROCK, and J. SNYDER. Antibody response of human subjects to epidemic typhus vaccine to eight years previous immunization. *J. Immunol.* **68**:207, 1952.

MURRAY, J. Rh antigens of human and monkey blood. *J. Immunol.* **68**:513, 1952.

MUSCHEL, L. H., L. A. SIMONTON, P. A. WELLS, and W. H. FIFE, JR. Occurrence of complement-fixing antibodies reactive with normal tissue constituents in normal and disease-states. *J. Clin. Investig.* **40**:51, 1961.

MUSCHEL, L. H., and H. P. TREFFERS. Serum bactericidal activity by turbidimetric method assay. *Feder. Proc.* **11**:477, 1952.

MUSCHEL, L. H., and H. TREFFERS. Quantitative studies on the bactericidal actions of serum and complement. *J. Immunol.* **76**:1, 1956.

MUSCHEL, L. H., and H. TREFFERS. Bactericidal actions of serum and complement. *J. Immunol.* **76**:11, 1956.

NAKAMURA, H., T. J. YOO, A. L. GROSSBERG, and D. PRESSMAN. Antibody-ligand interactions studied by fluorescence enhancement methods. *Immunochemistry*, **7**:637, 1970.

NAKANE, P. K., and G. B. PIERCE. Enzyme-labeled antibodies for the light and electron microscopic localization of tissue antigens. *J. Cell Biol.* **33**:307, 1967.

NAKANE, P. K., J. SRI RAM, and G. B. PIERCE. Enzyme-labeled antibodies for light and electron microscopic localization of antigens. *J. Histochem. Cytochem.* **14**:789, 1966.

NAMIKI, M., Y. KAKITA, and H. GOTO. Spectrophotometric determination of micro amounts of nitrogen with organic solvent extraction. *Talanta*, **11**:813, 1964.

NAYLOR, G. R. E., and M. E. ADAIR. Studies of anti-horse crystalbumin sera. *J. Immunol.* **76**:146, 1956.

NEBER, J., and W. DAMASHEK. Improved demonstration of circulating antibodies in hemolytic anemia by use of bovine albumin media. *Blood*, **2**:371, 1947.

NEEL, R., H. TASHINI, and M. EFFTEXHARI. Valeur pratique compareé des réactions d'agglutination, de conglutination directe, d'hémagglutination polyosidique et protéinique pour le diagnostic de la paste. *Arch. Inst. d'Hessarek*, **9**:85, 1950.

NEFF, J. C., and E. L. BECKER. The effect of the order of addition of antigen and antibody on the precipitin reaction. *J. Immunol.* **73**:286, 1954.

NEFF, J. C., and E. L. BECKER. Antigen-antibody reactions in agar. III. Rate of change of band migration with antigen concentration. *J. Immunol.* **78**:5, 1957.

NEILL, J. M., C. G. CASTILLO, and A. H. PINKES. Serological relationships between fungi and bacteria. *J. Immunol.* **74**:120, 1955.

NEISSER, M., and F. WECHSBERG. *Münch. Med. Wochenschr.* **47**:1261, 1900.

NEISSER, M., and F. WECHSBERG. *Münch. Med. Wochenschr.* **48**:697, 1901.

NELSON, M. A photometric adaptation of the Somogyi method for the determination of glucose. *J. Biol. Chem.* **153**:375, 1944.

NELSON, R. A. The immune-adherence phenomenon. *Science*, **118**:733, 1953.

NELSON, R. A. The immune-adherence phenomenon. A hypothetical role of erythrocytes in defence against bacteria and viruses. *Proc. Soc. Exper. Biol. and Med.* **49**:55, 1956.

NELSON, R. A. An alternative mechanism for the properdin system. VI. Congr. Soc. Europ. Hematol., Copenhagen. *Abstr.* **240,** 1957.

NELSON, R. A. An alternative mechanism for the properdin system. *J. Exper. Med.* **108**:515, 1958.

NELSON, R. A., and J. DIESENDRUCK. Studies on treponemal immobilizing antibodies in syphilis. I. Techniques of measurement and factors influencing immobilization. *J. Immunol.* 66:667, 1951.

NELSON, R. A., J. JENSEN, I. GIGLI, and N. TAMURA. Methods for the separation, purification and measurement of nine components of hemolytic complement in quinea pig serum. *Immunochemistry*, 3:111, 1966.

NESLON, R. A., and M. M. MAYER. Immobilization of *Treponema pallidum* in vitro by antibody produced in syphilitic infection. *J. Exper.* **89**:369, 1949.

NERENBERG, S. T. *Electrophoresis.* F. A. Davis Co., Philadelphia, 1966, pp. 200–202.

NESSET, N. M., J. McLALLEN, P. ANTHONY, and L. G. GINGER. Bacterial pyrogens. 7. Pyrogenic preparation from *Pseudomonas* species. *J. Amer. Pharmac. Assoc.* **39**:456, 1950.

NETER, E. Bacterial hemagglutination and hemolysis. *Bacteriol. Rev.* **20**:166, 1956.

NETER, E., L. BERTRAM, D. ZAK, M. MURDOCK, and C. ARBESMAN. Studies on hemagglutination and hemolysis by *Escherichia coli* antisera. *J. Exper. Med.* 96:1, 1952.

NETER, E., E. COHEN, O. WESTPHAL, and O. LÜDERITZ. The effect of proteolytic enzymes on agglutination by bacterial antibodies of lipopolysaccharide modified erythrocytes. *J. Immunol.* **82**:85, 1959.

NETER, E., and E. A. GORZYNSKI. Studies on indirect staphylococcal hemagglutination. *Zeitschr. Immunitätsforsch.* **118**:269, 1959.

NETER, E., E. A. GORZYNSKI, R. GINO, O. WESTPHAL, and O. LÜDERITZ. The enterobacterial hemagglutination test and its diagnostic potentialities. *Can. J, Microbiol.* **2**:232, 1956.

NETER, E. E. A. GORZYNSKI, N. ZALEWSKI, R. RACHMAN, and R. GINO. Studies on bacterial hemagglutination. *Amer. J. Publ. Health*, **44**:49, 1954.

NETER, E., and J. WALKER. Hemagglutination test for specific antibodies on dysentery caused by *Shigella sonnei. Amer. J. Clin. Pathol.* **24**:1424, 1954.

NETER, E., O. WESTPHAL, O. LÜDERITZ, and E. A. GORZYNSKI. The bacterial hemagglutination for the demonstration of antibodies to *Enterobacteriaceae. Ann. N.Y. Acad. Sci.* **66**:141, 1956.

NETER, E., O. WESTPHAL, O. LÜDERITZ, E. A. GORZYNSKI, and E. EICHENBERGER. Studies of enterobacterial lipopolysaccharides. *J, Immunol* 76:377, 1956.

NETER, E., N. ZALEWSKI, and W. FERGUSON. *Escherichia coli* hemagglutinin response of adult volunteers to ingested *E. coli* 055 B5. *Proc. Soc. Exper. Biol. Med.* **82**:215, 1953.

NETER, E., N. ZALEWSKI, and D. ZAK. Inhibition by lecithin and cholesterol of bacterial (*E. coli*) hemagglutination and hemolysis. *J. Immunol.* **71**:145, 1953.

NEUFELD, F. *Z. Hyg. Infektionskrankh.* **40**:54, 1902.

NEUFELD, F. Über Immunität und Agglutination bei Streptokokken. *Z. Hyg. Infektionskrankh.* **54**:161, 1903.

NEUFELD, F., and W. RIMPAU. Über die Antikörper des Streptokokken und Pneumokokken Immunserums. *Deutsche Med. Wochenschr.* **30**:1458, 1904.

NEUSTAEDTER, M., and E. BANZHAF. *Proc. N. Y. Pathol. Soc.* **17**:163, 1917.

NICHOLS, R. L., and D. E. McCOMB. Immunofluorescent studies with trachoma and related antigens. *J. Immunol.* **89**:545, 1962.

NICOLL, P. A., and D. H. CAMPBELL. In vitro anaphylasix in the surviving intestine. *J. Immunol.* **39**:89, 1940.

NICOLLE, M., E. CESARI, and E. DEBAINS. Étude sur la precipitation mutuelle des anticorps et does antigenes. *Ann. Inst. Pasteur*, **34**:596, 1920.

NIEL, G., and A. FRIBOURG-BLANC. Technique actuèlle du test d'immuno-fluorescence appliquè au diagnostic de la syphilis. *Ann. Inst. Pasteur*, **102**:616, 1962.

NILSSON, U. R. Separation and partial purification of the sixth, seventh and eighth component of human complement. *Acta Pathol. Mkcrobiol. Scandinav.* **70**:469, 1967.

NILSSON, U. R., and H. J. MÜLLER-EBRHARD. Isolation of B_{1F}-globulin from human serum and its characterization as the fifth component of complement. *J. Exper. Med.* **122**:277, 1965.

NILSSON, U. R., and H. J. MÜLLER-EBERHARD. Studies on the mode of action of the fifth, sixth and seventh component of human complement in immune haemolysis. *Immunology*, **13**:101, 1967.

NIRENBERG, M. W., and J. H. MATHEI. The dependence of cell-free protein synthesis in *E. coli* upon naturally occurring or synthetic polyribonucleotides. *Proc. Natl. Acad. Sci. U.S.A.* **47**:1588, 1961.

NISHIOKA, K. Measurements of complement by agglutination of human erythrocytes reacting in immune-adherence. *J. Immunol.* **90**:86, 1963.

NOGUCHI, H., and J. BRONFENBRENNER. The comparative merits of various complements and amboceports in the serum diagnosis of syphilis. *J. Exper. Med.* **13**:78, 1911.

NORDEN, A. Agglutination of sheep's erythrocytes sensitized with histoplasmin. *Proc. Soc. Exper. Med.* **70**:218, 1949.

NORRBY, E. C. T., and P. A. ALBERTSON. Concentration of poliovirus by an aqueous polymer two-phase system. *Nature.* **188**:1047, 1960.

NORRIS, J. P. A bacteriolytic principle associated with cultures of *Bacillus cereus*. *J. Gen. Microbiol.* **16**:1, 1957.

NORTHROP, J. Purification and crystallization of diphtheria antitoxin. *J. Gen. Physiol.* **23**:465, 1942.

NORTHROP, J., M. KUNITS, and R. RHERRIOT. *Crystalline Enzymes*. Columbia University Press, N. Y. 1948.

NOSSAL, G. J. V. A mechanical cell disintegrator. *Austral. J. Exper. Biol. Med. Sci.* **31**:583, 1953.

NOSSAL, G. J. V. Antibody production by single cells. II. The difference between primary and secondary response. *Brit. J. Exper. Pathol.* **40**:118, 1959.

NOSSAL, G. J. V. Studies on the transfer of antibody producing capacity. I. The transfer of antibody producing cells to young animals. *Immunology*, **2**:137, 1959.

NOSSAL, G. J. V. Cellular genetics of immune responses. *Adv. Immunol.* **2**:163, 1962.

NOSSAL, G. J. V., and J. LEDERBERG. Antibody production by single cells. *Nature*, **181**:1419, 1958.

NOSSAL, G. J. V., and O. MÄKELÄ. Autoradiographic studies on the immune response. *J. Exper. Med.* **115**:209, 1962.

NOWOTNY, A., O. LÜDERITZ, and O. WESTPHAL. Rundfilter-Chromatographic langkettiger Fettsäuren beir der Analyse bakterieller Lipopolysaccharide. *Biochem. Zeitschr.* **330**:47, 1958.

NOYES, W. F., and B. K. WATSON. Studies on the increase of vaccine virus in cultured human cells by means of the fluorescent antibody technique. *J. Exper. Med.* **102**:237, 1955.

NUTTALL, G. H. *Zeitschr. Hyg. Infektionskr.* **4**:353, 1888.

NUTTALL, G. H. *Blood Immunity and Relationships.* University Press, Cambridge, England, 1904.

NYE, R. N., and A. H. HARRIS. Viable pneumococci and pneumococcus soluble substance in the lungs from cases of lobar pneumonia. *Amer. J. Pathol.* **13**:749, 1937.

OAKLEY, C. L., and A. J. FULTHORPE. Antigenic analysis by diffusion. *J. Pathol. Bacteriol.* **65**:49, 1953.

O'CONNOR, I. Hirst's haemagglutination phenomenon exhibited by *Rickettsia orientalis*. *Med. J. Australia* **2**:459, 1945.

ODA, M., and T. T. PUCK. The interaction of mammalian cells with antibodies. *J. Exper. Med.* **113**:599, 1961.

OEDING, P. Serological typing of staphylococci. *Acta Pathol. Microbiol. Scandinav. Suppl.* **93**:356, 1952.

OEDING, P. Staphylococcal antigen-antibody reactions in agar. *Acta Pathol. Microbiol. Scandinav.* **47**:53, 1957.

OGATA, T., T. FACHIBAM, K. SUZUKI, K. FUKIDA, and S. YAMAOKA. Quantitative studies on the antigen-antibody reaction by the monolayer technique. *J. Immunol.* **69**:13, 1952.

OGBURN, C. A., T. HARRIS, and S. HARRIS. The determination of streptococcal anti-proteinase titers in sera of patients with rheumatic fever. *J. Immunol.* **81**:396, 1958.

OGUR, M., and G. ROSEN. The nucleic acids of plant tissues. I. The extraction and estimation of deoxypentose nucleic acid. *Arch. Biochem. Biophys.* **25**:262, 1950.

OISHI, M. and N. SUEOKA. Location of genetic loci of ribosomal RNA on *Bacillus subtilis* chromosome. *Proc. Natl. Acad. Sci. Wash.* **54**:483, 1965.

OLHAGEN, N. B. *Nord. Med.* **42**:1708, 1949.

OLANSKY, S., A. HARRIS, and H. CASEY. Immune-adherence test for syphilis. Comparison with TPI and VDRL slide tests. *Publ. Health Rep.* **69**:521, 1954.

OLITZKI, A. L., and A. SULITZEANU. Antigenic structure of *Haemophilus aegyptius* and *Haemophilus influenzae* demonstrated by the gel precipitation technique. *J. Bacteriol.* **77**:264, 1959.

OLITZKY, I., S. BERKMAN, and D. BASS. Simplified antistreptococcal deoxyribonuclease assay. *J. Bacteriol.* **84**:1011, 1962.

O'MALLEY, J. P., H. M. MEYER, JR., and J. E. SMADEL. Antibody in hepatitis patients against a newly isolated virus. *Proc. Soc. Exper. Biol. Med.* **108**:200, 1961.

O'NEILL, C. H. An association between viral transformation and Forssman antigen detected by immune adherence in cultured BHK cells. *J. Cell Sci.* **3**:405, 1968.

ONOUE, K., M. KITAGAWA, and Y. YAMAMURA. Chemical studies on cellular components of *Bordetella pertussis*. I. Purification and properties of agglutinogen. *J. Bacteriol.* **82**:648, 1961.

ONOUE, K., Y. YAGI, and D. PRESSMAN. Multiplicity of antibody properties in rabbit anti-*p*-azobenzenearsonate sera. *J. Immunol.* **92**:173, 1960.

OPIE, E. L. Inflammatory reaction of the immune animal to antigen (*Arthus phenomenon*) and its relation to antibodies. *J. Immunol.* **8**:231, 1924.

OPTON, L., D. NAGAKI, and J. MELNICK. J. Poliomyelitis antibodies in human gamma-globulin. *J. Immunol.* **75**:178, 1955.

ORGANICK, A. B., and A. RESNICK. Indirect hemagglutination test for *Mycoplasma pneumoniae* employing a commercially available antigen and adapted to the microtiter technic. *U.S. Army Med. Res. Natl. Lab.*, Report No. 301, 1966.

ORMSBEE, R. A. A method of purifying *Coxiella burnetii* and other pathogenic rickettsiae. *J. Immunol.* **88**:100, 1962.

ORMSBEE, R. A. An agglutination-resuspension test for Q fever antibodies. *J. Immunol.* **89**:159, 1964

ORMSBEE, R. A., E. J. BELL, and D. B. LACKMAN. Antigens of *Coxiella burnetti*. I. Extraction of antigens with nonaqueous organic solvents. *J. Immunol.* **88**:741, 1962.

ORMSBEE, R. A., E. J. BELL, and C. LARSON. Studies on *Bacterium tularense* antigens. *J. Immunol.* **74**:351, 1955.

ORMSBEE, R. A., and J. MELNICK. Biologic and serologic characteristics of ECHO viruses from West Virginia. *J. Immunol.* **79**:384, 1957.

ORNSTEIN, L. Disk electrophoresis. I. Background and theory. *Ann. N.Y. Acad. Sci.* **121**:321, 1967.

OSBORN, M. J. Studies on the gram-negative cell wall. I. Evidence for the role of 2-keto-3-deoxyoctonate in the lipopolysaccharide of *Salmonella typhimurium*. *Proc. Natl. Acad. Sci. (U.S.A.)* **50**:499, 1963.

OSHIRO, L. S., H. M. ROSE, C. MORGAN, and K. C. KSU. Electron microscopic study of the development of simian virus 40 by use of ferritin-labeled antibodies. *J. Virol.* **1**:384, 1967.

OSLER, A. G. Quantitative studies of complement fixation. *Bacteriol. Rev.* **22**:246, 1958.

OSLER, A. G., and M. HEIDELBERGER. Quantitaive studies of complement fixation. II. Homologous and cross-reactions in pneumococcal Type III and VIII systems. *J. Immunol.* **60**:317, 1948.

OSLER, A. G., and M. HEIDELBERGER. Quantitative studies of complement fixation. IV. Homologous and cross-reactions in chick- and duck-egg-albumen systems. *J. Immunol.* **60**: 327, 1948.

OSLER, A. G., and B. M. HILL. Kinetic studies of complement fixation. I. A method. *J. Immunol.* **75**:137, 1955.

OSLER, A. G., and E. A. KNIPP. Quantitative studies of lipid-soluble antigens as exemplified by the Wassermann antigen-antibody system. *J. Immunol.* **78**:19, 1957.

OSLER, A. G., J. Strauss, and M. M. MAYER. Diagnostic complement fixation. I. A method. *Amer. J. Syphil.* **36**:140, 1952.

OTOCKA, E. P. Fractionation of polymers by this layer chromatography. II. Molecular weight distribution by direct scanning densitometry. *Macromolecules*, **3**:691, 1970.

OTOCKA, E. P., and M. Y. HELLMAN. Fractionation of polymers by thin layer chromatography. I. Separation. *Macromolecules*, **3**:362, 1970.

OUCHTERLONY, Ö. In vitro method for testing the toxin-producing capacity of diphtheria bacteria. *Acta Pathol. Microbiol. Scandinav.* **25**:189, 1948.

OUCHTERLONY, Ö. Antigen-antibody reactions in gel. *Arkiv. Kemi, Miner. Geologi*, **26B**; 1, 1948.

OUCHTERLONY, Ö. Antigen-antibody reactions in gel. II. Factor determining the site of precipitation. *Arkiv. Kemi, Miner, Geologi*, **1**:43, 1949.

OUCHTERLONY, Ö. Antigen-antibody reactions in gel. *Acta Pathol. Microbiol. Scandinav.* **26**:507, 1949.

OUCHTERLONY, Ö. Antigen-antibody reactions in gel. IV. Types of reactions in coordinated systems of diffusion. *Acta Pathol. Microbiol. Scandinav.* **32**:231, 1953.

OUCHTERLONY, Ö. Diffusion-in-gel methods for immunological analysis. *Progr. Allergy*, **5**:1, 1958.

OUCHTERLONY, Ö. Interpretation of comparative immune precipitation patterns obtained by diffusion-in-gel techniques. In *Immunochemical Approaches to Problems In Microbiology*, M. Heidelberger, O. J. Plescia, and R. A. Day, Eds. Rutgers University Press, New Brunswick, N.J., 1961.

OUCHTERLONY, Ö. Handbook of Immunodiffusion and Immunoelectrophoresis. *Ann Arbor Science Publ.*, Ann Arbor, 1968.

OUDIN, J. Méthode d'analyse immunochimique par précipitation spècifique en milieu gèlifie. *Compt. Rend. Acad. Sci.* **222**:115, 1946.

OUDIN, J. L'analyse immunochimique du sérum de cheval par précipitation spècifique en milieu gèlifie. Premiers resultats. *Bull. Chim. Biol.* **29**:140, 1947.

OUDIN, J. L'analyse immunochimique qualitative; méthode par diffusion des antigenes au sein de l'immune sérum précipitant en gèlose. *Ann. Inst. Pasteur*, **75**:30, 1948.

OUDIN, J. La diffusion d'un antigene dans une edome de gèl contenant les anticorps précipitants homologous. Étude quantitative des trois principales variables. *Compt. Rend. Acad. Sci.* **228**:189, 1949.

OUDIN, J. Homogeneity of proteins and polysaccharides. Agar diffusion techniques. *Meth. Med. Res.*, **5**:360, 1952.

OVARY, Z. Immediate reactions in the skin of experimental animals provoked by antigen-antibody interaction. *Progr. Allergy*, **5**:459, 1958.

OVARY, Z., and G. BIOZZI. Passive sensitization of skin of guinea pig with human antibody. *Int. Arch. Allergy*, **5**:241, 1954.

PAIC, M. Ultracentrifugation de l'hémolysine. Détermination de sa constante de sédimentation et de son poids moleculaire. *Bull. Soc. Chim. Biol.* **21**:412, 1939.

PALMER, J. W., and T. D. GERLOUGH. A simple method for preparing antigenic substances from the typhoid bacillus. *Science*, **92**:155, 1940.

PALOSUO, T., K. PENTTINEN, and G. MYLLYLÄ. Platelet aggregation by herpes simplex antigen-antibody complexes. *Arch. Ges. Virusforsch.* **31**:11, 1970.

PANGBORN, M. C. Isolation and purification of a serologically active phospholipid from beef heart. *J. Biol. Chem.* **43**:247, 1942.

PANGBORN, M. C. A new serologically active phospholipid from beef heart. *Proc. Soc. Exper. Biol. Med.* **48**:484, 1944.

PANTON, P. N., and J. R. MARRACK. *Clinical Pathology*, 5th ed. Churchill, London, 1945.

PANTON, P. N., and F. C. O. VALENTINE. Staphylococcal toxin. *Lancet*, **1**:506, 1932.

PAPPAGIANIS, D., E. W. PUTMAN, and G. S. KOBAYASHI. Polysaccharide of *Coccidioides immitis*. *J. Bacteriol.* **82**:714, 1961.

PAPPENHEIMER, A. M. Diphtheria toxin. I. Isolation and characterization of toxic protein from *Corynebacterium dipththeriae*. *J. Biol. Chem.* **120**:543, 1937.

PAPPENHEIMER, A. M., H. LUNDGREN, and J. T. WILLIAMS. Studies on the molecular weight of diphtheria toxin, antitoxin and their reaction products. *J. Exper. Med.* **71**:247, 1940.

PAPPENHEIMER, A. M., and E. ROBINSON. A quantitative study of Ramon diphtheria flocculation reaction. *J. Immunol.* **32**:29, 1937.

PARFENTIEV, I., and M. VIRION. *Hemophilus pertussis* soluble antigen and complement fixing antibodies, *J. Immunol.* **60**:167, 1948.

PARK, J. T., and M. S. JOHNSON. A submicrodetermination of glucose. *J. Biol. Chem.* **181**:149, 1949.

PARK, J. T., and J. L. STROMINGER. Mode of action of pencillin. Biochemical basis for the mechanism of action of penicillin and for its selective toxicity. *Science*, **125**:99, 1957.

PARKER, C. W. Spectrofluorometric Methods. In *Handbook of Experimental Immunology*, D. M. Weir, Ed. Blackwell Science Publishing, Oxford, 1967.

PARKER, C. W., J. A. THIEL, and S. MITCHELL. The immunogenicity of hapten-polylysine conjugates. *J. Immunol.* **94**:289, 1965.

PARKER, R., and R. MUCKENFUSS. Complement-fixation in vaccinia and in variola. *J. Infect. Dis.* **53**:54, 1933.

PARLETT, R. C. A proposed revision of the gel diffusion test for the detection of mycobacterial antibody. *Amer. Rev. Resp. Dis.* **84**:589, 1961.

PARLETT, R. C., and Y. M. CHU. Immunologic response in mice and rabbits to mycobacterial antigens determined by the Jerne agar-plaque method. *Amer. J. Clin. Pathol.* **47**:719, 1967.

PARLETT, R. C. and G. P. YOUMANS. Antigenic relationships between mycobacteria as determined by agar diffusion precipitation techniques. *Amer. Rev. Tuberc.* **73**:637, 1956.

PARLETT, R. C., and G. P. YOUMANS. Antigenic relationships between ninety-eight strains of mycobacteria using gel diffusion precipitation techniques. *Amer. Rev. Tuberc.* **77**:450, 1958.

PARLETT, R. C., and G. P. YOUMANS. An evaluation of the specificity and sensitivity of a gel double-diffusion test for tuberculosis. *Amer. Rev. Resp. Dis.* **80**:153, 1959.

PARONETTO, F. The fluorescent antibody technique applied to titration and identification of anitgens in solutions or antisera. *Proc. Soc. Exper. Biol. Med.* **113**:394, 1963.

PARTRIDGE, S. M. Aniline hydrogen phthalate as a spraying reagent for chromatography of sugars. *Nature*, **164**:443, 1949.

PARTRIDGE, S. M., and R. G. WESTALL. Filter paper partition chromatography of sugars. I. General description and application to the qualitative analysis of sugars in apple juice, egg-white and foetal blood of sheep. *Biochem. J.* **42**:238, 1948.

PASTERNACK, G., F. HOFFMANN, H. BIELKA, and L. VENKER. Untersuchungen zur Frage der antigenen Eigenschaften von Nukleinsäuren. *Pathol. Mikrobiol.* **23**:3, 1960.

PATERSON, J. S. Flagellar antigens of organisms of the genus *Listerella*. *J. Pathol. Bacteriol.* **48**:25, 1939.

PATOČKA, F., J. SCHINDLER, and M. MARA. Studies on the pathogenicity of *Listeria monocytogenes*. I. Protein substance isolated from cells of *Listeria monocytogenes* enhancing listeric infection. *Zentralbl. Bakteriol. I. Orig.* **174**:573, 1959.

PATTERSON, D., R. BAILEY, and R. WALLER. Control of whooping cough with serum and vaccine; uses of a new skin test. *Lancet*, **II**:36, 1935.

PATTERSON, R., I. N. SUSZKO, and J. J. PRUZANSKY. Some antigenic characteristics and immunologic reactions of horse spleen ferritin. *Proc. Soc. Exper. Biol. Med.* **118**:307, 1965.

PAUL, J. R., and W. W. BUNNELL. The presence of heterophile antibodies in infectious mononucleosis. *Amer. J. Med. Sci.*, **183**:90, 1932.

PAULING, L. J. A theory of the structure and process of formation of antibodies. *J. Amer. Chem. Soc.* **62**:2643, 1940.

PAULING, L. J. Molecular structures and intermolecular forces. In *The Specificity of Serological Reactions*, K. Landsteiner, Ed. Cambridge, England, 1945.

PAULING, L. J. Antigens and antibodies. *Brit. Med. J.* **4518**:223, 1947.

PAULY, N. *Z. Physiol. Chem.* **42**:508, 1904.

PAYNE, F., F. SMADEL, and J. COURDURIER. Immunological studies on persons residing in a plague endemic area. *J. Immunol.* **77**:24, 1956.

PAYNE, R., and Q. B. DEMING. Electrophoretic mobility in paper of isoagglutinins. *J. Immunol.* **73**:81, 1954.

PAYNE, W., and R. KIEBER. The chromatographic determination of glucosamine with ninhydrine. *Arch. Biochem. Biophys.* **52**:1, 1954.

PEACOCK, M., W. BURGDORFER, and R. A. ORMSBEE. Rapid fluorescent-antibody conjugation procedure. *Infect. Immun.* **3**:355, 1971.

PEARSON, H. Attempts to obtain specfic agglutination of mixtures of collodion particles or bacterial cells with virus and antiviral serum. *J. Immunol.* **49**:117, 1944.

PEARSON, K. *Tables for Statisticians and Biometricians.* University College of London Biometric Laboratory, London, 1930.

PENTTINEN, K., and G. MYLLYLÄ. Interaction in human blood platelets, viruses and antibodies. I. Platelet aggregation test with microequipment. *Ann. Med. Exper. Fenn.* **46**:188, 1968.

PENTTINEN, K., G. MYLLYLÄ, O. MÄKELÄ, and A. VAHERI. Souble antigen-antibody complexes and platelet aggregation. *Acta Pathol. Microbiol. Scandinav.* **77**:309, 1969.

PENTZ, E. J., and Y. SHIGEMURA. The production, concentration and partial characterization of streptolysin O. *J. Bacteriol.* **69**:210, 1955.

PEPE, F. A., and S. J. SINGER. Physical-chemical studies of soluble antigen-antibody complexes. VIII. The preparation and properties of a univalent antigen. *J. Amer. Chem. Soc.* **78**:4583, 1956.

PERKINS, H. R., and H. J. ROGERS. The products of the partial acid hydrolysis of the mucopeptide from cell walls of *Micrococcus lysodeikticus. Biochem. J.* **72**:647, 1959.

PERLMAN, E., and W. F. GOEBEL. Studies on the Flexner group of dysentery bacilli. *J. Exper. Med.* **84**:223, 1948.

PEROLOWAGORA, A., and T. HUGHES. The complement fixation test in yellow fever epidemiology. *J. Immunol.* **60**:67, 1948.

PETERKOVSKY, A., L. LEVINE, and R. BROWN. Qualitative estimation of antigens by complement fixation. *J. Immunol.* **76**:237, 1956.

PETERMANN, M. L., and A. M. PAPPENHEIMER. Action of crystalline pepsin on horse antipneumococcal antibody. *Science,* **93**:458, 1941.

PETERSON, E. A., and H. A. SOBER. Chromatography of proteins. I. Cellulose ion exchange adsorbents. *J. Amer. Chem. Soc.* **78**:751, 1956.

PETERSON, O., T. HAM, and M. FINLAND. Cold agglutinins (autohemagglutinins) in primary atypical pneumonias. *Science,* **97**:167, 1943.

PETERSON, R. G., and S. E. HARTSELL. Lysozyme spectrum of Gram-negative bacteria. *J. Infect. Dis.* **96**:75, 1955.

PETRIE, G. F., and D. STEABBEN. Specific identification of the chief pathogenic clostridia of gas gangrene. *Brit. Med. J.* **1**:377, 1943.

PFEIFFER, R. *Z. Hyg. Infektonskr.* **11**:393, 1893.

PFEIFFER, R. Weitere Untersuchungen über das Wesen de Choleraimmunität und über spezifisch bakterizide Prozesse. *Z. Hyg. Infektionskr.* **18**:1, 1894.

PFEIFFER, R., and I. ISSAEFF. Über die spezifische Bedeutung der Choleraimmunitat. *Z. Hyg. Infektionskrankh.* **17**:55, 1894.

PFEIFFER, R., and L. MARX. Untersuchungen über die Bildungstätte der Choleraantikörper. *Deutsche Med. Wochenschr.* No. 3, 1898.

PHILIPSON, L. Adenovirus assay by the fluorescent cell-counting procedure. *Virology,* **15**:263, 1961.

PHILLIPS, B. P. Cultivation of *Endamoeba histolytica* with *Trypanosoma cruzi. Science,* **111**:8, 1950.

PICK, E. and J. D. FELDMAN. Autoradiographic plaques for the detection of antibody formation to soluble proteins by single cells. *Science,* **156**:964, 1967.

PICK, E., and D. NELKEN. Bismuth tannate test. *Nature,* **197**:157, 1963.

PICKLES, M. M. Effects of cholera filtrate on red cells as demonstrated by incomplete Rh antibodies. *Nature*, **195**:880, 1946.

PIERCE, A. E. The electrophoretic separation and isolation of proteins in agar combined with Schlieren scanning. *Biochem. Biophys. Acta*, **59**:149, 1962.

PIJPER, A. Dark-ground studies of flagellar and somatic agglutination of *B. typhosus*. *J. Pathol.* **47**:1, 1938.

PIKE, R. The depression of phagocytosis by products of *Staphylococcus*. *J. Immunol.* **26**:69, 1934.

PIKE, R., H. OWENS, and D. HUMES. The plate complement fixation test with leptospiral antigens. *J. Lab. Clin. Med.* **44**:609, 1954.

PILLEMER, L. The nature of the properdin system and its interactions with polysaccharide complexes. *Ann. N.Y. Acad. Sci.* **66**:233, 1956.

PILLEMER, L., J. BENTOFF, E. BROWN, and I. LEPOW. The immunochemistry of toxins and toxoids. *J. Immunol.* **65**:591, 1950.

PILLEMER, L., L. BLUM, I. LEPOW, O. ROSS, and E. TODD. The properdin system and immunity. III. The zymosan assay of properdin. *J. Exper. Med.* **103**:1, 1956.

PILLERMER, L., E. E. ECKER, J. L. ONCLEY, and E. S. COHN. The preparation and physico-chemical characterization of the serum protein components of complement. *J. Exper. Med.* **74**:297, 1941.

PILLERMER, L., D. GROSSBERG, and R. WITTLER. The immunochemistry of toxins and toxoids. II. The preparation and immunologic evaluation of purified tetanol toxoid. *J. Immunol.* **54**:713, 1946.

PILLEMER, L., S. SEIFTER, F. CHU., and E. E. ECKER. Function of components of complement in immune hemolysis. *J. Exper. Med.* **76**:93, 1942.

PILLEMER, L., D. TOLL, and S. BADGER. The immunichemistry of toxins and toxoids. III. The isolation and characterization of diphtherial toxoid. *J. Biol. Chem.* **170**:571, 1947.

PILLEMER, L., R. G. WITTLER, J. I. BURRELL, and D. B. GROSSBERG. The immunochemistry of toxins and toxoids. VI. Crystallization and characterization of tetanol toxin. *J. Exper. Med.* **88**:205, 1948.

PILLOT, J. Analytical serology of Treponematoceae. In *Analytical Serology of Micro-organisms*, J. B. G. Kwapinski, Ed., Vol. 2. Interscience, New York, 1969, pp. 123–183.

PILLOT, J., and L. J. BOREL. Étude des anticorps responsables de la réaction d'immuno-fluorescence avec la system *Treponema pallidum* serum de sujet attaint de treponematose. *Compt. Rend. Acad. Sci.* **252**:954, 1961.

PINKES, A., and J. NEILL. Serological reactions of extracellular soluble substances of crown gall bacteria (*Agrobacterium tumefaciens*). *J. Immunol.* **79**:525, 1957.

PIRAS, L. Die Präzipitinreaktion als diagnostisches Mittel der Pest. *Zentralbl. Bakteriol. I. Orig.* **71**:69, 1913.

PITT, A. A. De mastix fixation reactie bij reumatoid arthrit. *Ned. J. Geneesk.* **103**:2310, 1959.

PITTMAN, M., and K. GOODNER. Complement-fixation with the type-specific carbohydrate of *Hemophilus influenzae* Type B. *J. Immunol.* **29**:239, 1935.

PLACKETT, P., B. P. MARMION, E. J. SHAW, and R. M. LEMCKE. Immunochemical analysis of *Mycoplasma pneumoniae*. III. Separation and chemical identification of serologically active lipids. *Aust. J. Exper. Biol. Med. Sci.* **47**:171, 1969.

PLATT, H. The antigens produced in vitro by *Mycobacterium tuberculosis*, with some observations on the frequency of anaphylactic sensitization during the course of experimental tuberculosis. *Brit. J. Exper. Pathol.* **35**:439, 1954.

PLESCIA, O. J., K. Amiraian, and M. HEIDELBERGER. Aspects of the immune hemolytic reaction. II. Effect of composition of C' on concentration dependence in immune hemolysis. *J. Immunol.* **78**:151, 1957.

PLESCIA, O. J., E. L. BECKER, and J. W. WILLIAMS. The valence of precipitating antibodies. *J. Amer. Chem. Soc.* **74**:1362, 1952.

PLOTZ, C. M., E. BENNETT, A. WARTMAN, M. SNYDER, and GOLUB, R. The serological pattern in typhus fever. *Amer. J. Hyg.* **47**:150, 1948.

PLOTZ, C. M., and J. M. SINGER. The latex fixation test. *Amer. J. Med.* **21**:888, 1956.

PLOTZ, H. Complement-fixation in rickettsial disease. *Science*, **97**:20, 1943.

PLOTZ, H., J. E. SMADEL, T. F. ANDERSON, and L. A. CHAMBERS. Morphological structure of rickettsiae. *J. Exper. Med.* **77**:355, 1943.

PLOTZ, H., and K. WERTMAN. The use of the complement fixation test in Rocky Mountain spotted fever. *Science*, **95**:441, 1942.

PLOTZ, P. H., and N. TALAL. Fractionation of splenic antibody-forming cells on glass bead columns. *J, Immunol.* **99**:1236, 1967.

POLSON, A., and J. W. F. HAMPTON. *J. Hygiene*, **55**:344, 1957.

POND, W. L., S. B. RUSS, N. S. ROGERS, and J. E. SMADEL. Murray Valley encephalitis virus: its serological relationship with the Japanese-West Nile-St. Louis encephalitis group. *J. Immunol.* **75**:78, 1955.

PONDER, E. On certain correction terms required in equations for kinetics of simple hemolysis. *Proc. Roy. Soc. London, Series B,* **110**:18, 1932.

POORTMANS, J. R., and R. W. JEANLOZ. 3S γ_1-globulin levels of normal human serum and urine. *Biochim. Biophys. Acta,* **133**:363, 1967.

POPE, C. G., and M. HEALEY. The preparation of diphtheria antitoxin in a state of high purity. *Brit. J. Exper. Pathol.* **20**:213, 1939.

POPE, C. G., and M. F. STEVENS. The determination of aminonitrogen using a copper method. *Biochem. J.* **33**:1070, 1939.

POPE, C. G., and M. F. STEVENS. The purification of antitoxin by absorption of non-antitoxic antibodies. *Brit. J. Exper. Pathol.* **34**:56, 1953.

POPE, C. G., and M. F. STEVENS. The preparation of nonflocculating antitoxin by absorption of nonantitoxic antibodies. *Brit. J. Exper. Pathol.* **34**:241, 1953.

POPE, C. G., M. F. STEVENS, E. A. CASPARY, and E. L. FENTON. Some new observations on diphtheria serum and antitoxin. *Brit. J. Exper. Pathol.* **32**:246, 1951.

PORATH, J. Column electrophoresis. In *Methods in Immunology and Immunochemistry,* C. A. Williams and N. W. Chase, Eds., Vol. 2. Academic, New York, 1968, p. 67.

PORATH, J. and N. VI. Chemical studies on immunoglobulins. I. A new preparative procedure for γ-globulins employing glycine-rich solvent system. *Biochim, Biophys. Acta,* **90**:324, 1964.

PORTER, B. M., B. K. COMFORT, R. W. MENGES, R. T. HABERMANN, and C. D. SMITH. Correlation of fluorescent antibody, histopathology, and culture on tissues from 372 animals examined for histoplasmosis and blastomycosis. *J. Bacteriol.* **89**:748, 1965.

PORTIER, P., and C. RICHET. *Compt. Rend. Soc. Biol.* **54**:170, 1902.

PORTER, R. R. The fractionation of rabbit-gamma-globulin by partition chromatography. *Biochem. J.* **59**:405, 1955.

PORTER, R. R. *Methods in Enzymology*, C. P. Colowick and J. N. Davidson, Eds., Vol. 4. Academic Press, New York, 1957, pp. 221–237.

PORTER, R. R. Separation and isolation of fractions of rabbit gamma-globulin containing the antibody and antigen combining sites. *Nature*, **182**:670, 1958.

PORTNOY, J. Complement-fixation with small volumes of reagents; application to *Treponema pallidum* complement-fixation test for syphilis. *Amer. J. Clin. Pathol.* **31**:316, 1959.

PORTNOY, J., and W. GARSON. Preliminary report of RPR test for syphilis using unheated serum. *Publ. Health Rep.* **74**:965, 1951.

PORTNOY, J., W. GARSON, and C. S. SMITH. Rapid plasma reagin test for syphilis. *Publ. Health Rep.* **72**:761, 1957.

PORTNOY, J., and H. MAGNUSON. Immunologic studies with fraction of virulent *Treponema pallidum*. I. Preparation of an antigen by desoxycholate extraction and its use in complement fixation. *J. Immunol.* **75**:348, 1955.

POTEL, J., and L. DEGEN. Zur Serologie and Immunobiologie der Listeriose. *Zentralbl. Bakteriol. Parasitenk.* **185**:204, 1962.

POULIK, M. D. Tests of purity of diphtheria toxins by electrophoresis in starch gel. *Nature*, **177**:982, 1956.

POULIK, M. D. Starch-gel electrophoresis in a discontinuous system of buffers. *Nature*, **180**:1477, 1957.

POULIK, M. D. Starch-gel immunoelectrophoresis. *J. Immunol.* **82**:502, 1959.

POULIK, M. D. The use of urea-starch-gel electrophoresis in studies of reductive cleavage of an α_2-macroglobulin. *Biochim. Biophys. Acta*, **44**:390, 1960.

POULIK, M. D. Electrophoretic map of chemically derived sub-units of papain-digested γ-globulin. *Nature*, **198**:752, 1963.

POULIK, M. D. Am. N. Y. Acad. Sci. **121**:420, 1964.

POULIK, M. D. Gel electrophoresis in buffers containing urea. *Methods Biochem. Anal.* **14**:455, 1966.

POWELL, H., and W. JAMIESON. Further studies on the immunology of *Hemophilus pertussis*. *J. Immunol.* **32**:153, 1937.

POWELL, H., and W. JAMIESON. A rapid pertussis agglutination test. *J. Immunol.* **43**:13, 1942.

POWELL, R. D. Labeling of antibody to influenza virus with radioactive iodine. *J. Lab. Clin. Med.* **58**:386, 1961.

PRAUSNITZ, C., and H. KÜSTNER. Studien über die Ueberempfindlichkeit. *Zentralbl. Bakteriol. I. Orig.* **160**:169, 1921.

PREER, J. R., JR. A qualitative study of a technique of double-diffusion in agar. *J. Immunol.* **77**:52, 1956.

PREER, J. R., JR., and W. TELFER. Some effects of nonreacting substances on the quantitative application of gel diffusion techniques. *J. Immunol.* **78**:288, 1957.

PRESSMAN, D. *Serological and Biochemical Comparison of Proteins*. Rutgers University Press, New Brunswick, N.J., 1958.

PRESSMAN, D., D. CAMPBELL, and L. PAULING. The agglutination of intact azo-erythrocytes by antisera to the attached groups. *J. Immunol.* **44**:101, 1942.

PRESSMAN, D., R. HILL, and F. FOOTE. The zone of localization of anti-mouse-kidney serum as determined by radioautography. *Science*, **109**:65, 1949.

PRESSMAN, D., and G. KEIGHLEY. The zone of activity of antibodies determined by the use of radioactive tracers: the zone of activity of nephrotoxic anti-kidney serum. *J. Amer. Chem Soc.* **56**:173, 1944.

PRESSMAN, D., and G. KEIGHLEY. The zone of activity of antibodies as determined by the use of radioactive tracers. The zone of activity of nephrotoxic anti-kidney serum. *J. Immunol.* **59**:141, 1948.

PRESSMAN, D., and D. SHERMAN. The zone of localization of antibodies. *J. Immunol.* **67**:15, 1944.

PREVOT, A. Discrimination graphique entre floculation vraie et paradoxale dans le titrage de la toxine tètanique par la mèthode de Ramon. *Compt. Rend. Soc. Biol.* **127**:116, 1938.

PRICE, I., and A. WILKINSON. A rapid method of standardization of the sheep cell suspension used in the Harrison-Wyler-Wassermann technique. *Brit. J. Vener. Dis.* **23**:124, 1947.

PRIDHAM, J. B. Determination of sugars on paper chromatograms with *p*-anisidine hydrochloride. *Anal. Chem.* **28**:1967, 1956.

PROKOP, O., and G. UHLENBRUCK. *Human Blood and Serum Groups*. Maclaren and Sons, London, 1969.

PROOM, H. The preparation of precipitating sera for the identification of animal species. *J. Pathol. Bacteriol.* **55**:419, 1943.

PULGHER, F. Die Anwendung der Thermopräzipitationsreaktion bei der Pest-diagnose und der Agglutination zur Bestimmung pestvardächtiger Stämme. *Arch. Schiffs-Hygiene*, 165, 1922.

PURCELL, R. H., D. TAYLOR-ROBINSON, D. WONG, and R. M. CHANOCK. Color test for the measurement of antibody to T-strain mycoplasmas. *J. Bacteriol.* **92**:6, 1966.

PUTNAM, F. W., M. KOZURU, and C. W. EASLEY. Structural studies of the immunoglobulins. IV. Heavy and light chains of.the γM pathological macroglobulins. *J. Biol. Chem.* **242**:2435, 1967.

QUADLING, C. Evaluation of tests and grouping of cultures by a two-stage principal component method. *Can. J. Microbiol.* **13**:1379, 1967.

QUIGLEY, J. J., and G. R. SICKLES. Ultramembranes. *J. Bacteriol.* **33**:110, 1937.

QUIGLEY, W. The precipitin reaction in the urine in pneumonia. *J. Infect. Dis.* **23**:217, 1918.

QUINN, R. W. Studies of the mucin-clot prevention test for the determination of the antiphaluronidase titer of human serum. *J. Clin. Invest.* **27**:463, 1948.

RACE, R. R., and R. SANGER. *Blood Groups in Man*, 3rd ed. Blackwell Scientific Publications, Oxford, England, 1958.

RACE, R. R., and R. SANGER. *Blood Groups in Man*, 5th ed. Blackwell Scientific Publications, Oxford, England, 1968.

RACUSEN, D. Double-disc electrophoresis of proteins. *Nature*, **213**:922, 1967.

RAEDER, R. Serum complement in acute nephritis. *Brit. J. Exper. Pathol.* **29**:255, 1948.

RAEDER, R. A micromethod for the determination of complement. *Austral. J. Exper. Biol. Med.* **34**:257, 1956.

RAFFEL, S. The components of tubercle bacillus responsible for the delayed type of infectious allergy. *J. Infect. Dis.* **82**:267, 1948.

RAFFEL, S. *Immunity*. Appleton-Century-Crofts, New York, 1953.

RALSTON, D., B. S. BAER, and S. S. ELSBERG. Lysis of brucellae by the combined action of glycine and a lysozyme-like agent from rabbit monocytes. *J. Bacteriol.* **82**:354, 1961.

RAMMELKAMP, C., G. BADGER, J. DINGLE, A. TELLER, and R. HODGES. A quantitative method for measuring staphylococcal anticoagulase. *Proc. Soc. Exper. Biol. Med.* **72**:210, 1949.

RAMON, G. Sur la concentration du sérum antidiphterique et l'isolement de l'antitoxine. *Compt. Rend. Soc. Biol.* **88**:167, 1922.

RAMON, G. Sur une technique de titrage in vitro du sérum antidiphterique. *Compt. Rend. Soc. Biol.* **86**:711, 1922.

RAMON, G. La flocculation dans les melanges de toxin et de sérum antidiphterique. *Ann. Inst. Pasteur*, **37**:1001, 1923.

RAMON, G., and P. DESCOMBEY. Sur l'appréciation de la valeur antigene de la toxine et de l'antitoxine tètanique par la mèthode de flocculation. *Compt. Rend. Soc. Biol.*

RAMON, G., E. LEMETAYER, and R. RICHOU. *Rev. d'Immunol.* **1**:199, 1935.

RAMSDELL, S. G. The use of trypan blue to demonstrate the intermediate reaction in rabbits and guinea pigs. *J. Immunol.* **15**:305, 1928.

RANSOM, J. P., C. LARSON, J. M. GORMAN, and S. TULVE. Heterogeneity of antibody response to Salmonella lipopolysaccharide measured by passive hemagglutination and hemolysis in mice. *J. Bacteriol.* **96**:909, 1968.

RANSOM, J., S. QUOU, G. OMI, and M. HAGGAN. The role of serum proteins in gel-precipitation patterns of *Pasteurella pestis. J. Immunol.* **75**:265, 1955.

RANTZ, L., E. RANDALL, and D. ZUCKERMAN. Hemolysis and hemagglutination by normal and immune sera of erythrocytes treated with nonspecific bacterial substances. *J. Infect. Dis.* **98**:211, 1956.

RAO, R. R., and T. K. WADHWANI. Amino acid compostion of cellular protein of *Mycobacterium tuberculosis. J. Bacteriol.* **72**:12, 1956.

RAPP, F., G. GUESHI, and I. GORDON. A practical method for removal of anti-complementary properties from human serum. *Proc. Soc. Exper. Biol. Med.* **90**:335, 1955.

RAPP, H. J. Mechanism of immune hemolysis: recognition of two steps in the conversion of $EAC'_{1,4,2}$ to E. *Science,* **127**:234, 1958.

RAPP, H. J., C. CRISLER, M. WEINTRAUB, and T. BORSOS. Complement fixation: a modified procedure designed to eliminate anticomplementary and procomplementary effects. *Proc. Soc. Exper. Biol. Med.* **120**:361, 1965.

RAPP, H. J., and M. R. SIMS. Preparation of an intermediate product of immune hemolysis with formaldehyde treated complement. *Fed. Proc.* **17**:531, 1958.

RAPP, H. J., M. R. SIMS, and T. BORSOS. Separation of components of guinea pig complement by chromatography. *Proc. Soc. Exper. Biol. Med.* **100**:730, 1959.

RAPP, R., S. J. SELIGMAN, L. B. JARCOSS, and I. GORDON. Quantitative determination of infectious units of measles virus by counts of immunofluorescent foci. *Proc. Soc. Exper. Biol. Med.* **101**:289, 1959.

RAPPAPORT, C. Trypsinization of monkey-kidney tissue: automatic preparation of cell suspension. *Bull. World Health Organ.* **14**:147, 1956.

RAPPAPORT, F., and G. J. STARK. A micro-method for the diagnosis of rheumatic fever (anti-streptolysin-O-test). *Acta Med. Orient.* **14**:48, 1955.

RAPPORT, M. M., and L. GRAF. Immunochemical analysis based in complement fixation. *Ann. N.Y. Acad. Sci.* **69**:609, 1957.

RAY, J. G., and D. E. SHAY. Agar-gel precipitin-inhibition technique for C-reactive protein determinations. *Appl. Microbiol.* **13**:297, 1965.

RAYBIN, H. W. Direct demonstration of the sucrose linkage in the oligosaccharides. *J. Amer. Chem. Soc.* **59**:1402, 1937.

RAYMOND, S. Protein purification by elution convection electrophoresis. *Science,* **146**:406, 1964.

REED, L. J., and H. MUENCH. A simple method of estimating per cent end points. *Amer. J. Hyg.* **27**:493, 1938.

REES, E. D., and S. J. SINGER. A preliminary study of proteins in some nonaqueous solvents. *Arch. Biochem. Biophys.* **63**:144, 1956.

REICH, C. V., C. E. HEIST, and H. W. DUNNE. Agglutinin-adsorption analysis of *Vibrio fetus. J. Bacteriol.* **82**:210, 1961.

REID, R. L., and M. LEDERER. Separation and estimation of saturated C2BC7 fatty acids by paper-partition chromatography. *Biochem. J.* **50**:60, 1951.

REIF, A. E. Batch preparation of rabbit γ-G globulin with deae-cellulose. *Immunochem.* **6**:723, 1969.

REIF, A. E., J. M. V. ALLEN, and L. M. McVETY. A general method for the calculation of serological specificity. *Immunology,* **8**:384, 1965.

REIF, A. E., L. M. McVETY, and E. R. KLEIN. Specificity of antisera to mouse ascites tumor in rabbits immunologically depressed with mouse red cells. *J. Immunol.* **90**:24, 1963.

REIN, C. R., and H. N. BOSSAK. Merthiolate (sodium ethyl mercuri thiosalicylate) as preservative in sera for diagnosis of syphilis. *Amer. J. Syph. Gonor. Vener. Dis.* **30**:342, 1946.

REINER, L., and O. FISCHER. Beiträge zum Mechanismus der Immunkörperwirkung. I. Die Rolle des Amboceptors und des Komplements bei der Cytolyse. *Zeitschr. Immunitatsforsch.* **61**:317, 1929.

REINER, L., and H. KOPP. Ueber Zonenphänomen, Doppelringphänomen und ihre Entstehung. *Klin. Wochenschr.* **6**:1563, 1927.

REINER, L., and M. TÖREK. Ueber Extraktion und Fraktioierung des Wassermann-positiven Serums. *Zeitschr. Immunitatsforsch.* **53**:552, 1927.

REISSEL, P. K., L. M. HAGOPIAN, and F. T. HATCH. Thin-layer electrophoresis of serum lipoproteins. *J. Lipid Res.* **7**:551, 1966.

REISSIG, J. L., J. L. STROMINGER, and L. F. LELOIR. A modified colorimetric method for the estimation of N-acetylamino sugars. *J. Biol. Chem.* **217**:959, 1955.

RELYVELD, E. H., E. HENOCZ, and M. RAYNAUD. Étude sur la sensibilization aux antigènes elabores par diverses souches de corynebacteries diphteriques et non diphteriques. *Ann. Inst. Pasteur,* **103**:590, 1962.

REJHOLEC, V., and V. WAGNER. Antimyocardial antibodies in rheumatic fever. *Experientia,* **11**:276, 1955.

RENKONEN, K. Studies on hemagglutinins present in seeds of some representatives of the family *Leguminoseae. Ann. Med. Exper. Biol. Fenniae,* **26**:66, 1948.

RENKONEN, O. V., and O. RENKONEN. Comments on paper chromatography of phosphatides. *Ann. Med. Exper. Biol. Fenniae,* **37**:197, 1959.

RENOUX, G. Anticorps bloquant dans le sérum de sujets brucelliques. *Ann. Inst. Pasteur,* **1**:91, 1954.

REPASKE, R. Lysis of Gram-negative bacteria by lysozyme. *Biochim. Biophys. Acta.* **22**:189, 1956.

REPASKE, R. Lysis of Gram-negative organisms and the role of versene. *Biochim. Biophys. Acta,* **30**:225, 1958.

RHEINS, M. S., R. G. BURRELL, and J. M. BIRKELAND. Tuberculous antibodies demonstrated by agar diffusion. I. Specificity and incidence of agar-diffusion antibodies in rabbit sera. *Amer. Rev. Tub.* **74**:229, 1956.

RHEINS, M. S., F. W. MCCOY, R. G. BURRELL, and E. V. BUEKER. A modification of the latex-fixation test for the study of rheumatoid arthritis. *J. Lab. Clin. Med.* **50**:113, 1957.

RIBEIRO, L. P., E. MITIDIERI, and O. R. ALFONSO. *Paper Electrophoresis.* Elsevier Publications, Amsterdam, 1961.

RIBI, E., R. L. ANACKER, W. R. BARCLAY, W. BREHMER G. MIDDLEBROOK, K. C. MILNER, and D. F. TARMINA. Structure and biological functions of mycobacteria. *Ann. N.Y. Acad. Sci.* **154**:41, 1968.

RIBI, E., and B. H. HOYER. Purification of Q fever rickettsiae by density-gradient sedimentation. *J. Immunol.* **85**:314, 1960.

RIBI, E., C. L. LARSON, R. LIST, and W. WICHT. Immunologic significance of the cell wall of mycobacteria. *Proc. Soc. Exper. Biol. Med.* **98**:263, 1958.

RIBI, E., K. C. MILNER, and C. L. LARSON. Antigens from cells walls of *Salmonella typhosa. Bacteriol. Proc.* **74**, 1958.

RIBI, E., K. C. MILNER, and T. C. PERRINE. Endotoxic and antigenic fractions from the cell wall of *Salmonella enteritidis.* Methods for separation of some biologic activities. *J. Immunol.* **82**:75, 1959.

RICE, C. E. Studies of antipneumococcal serum. II. Complement-fixing activity of anti-pneumococcal rabbit-serum with homologous type-specfic carbohydrate. *J. Immunol.* **43**:129, 1942.

RICE, C. E. A study of the reliability of complement fixation as a method of measuring the activities of sera of high, medium and low antibody titers. *J. Immunol.* **55**:1, 1947.

RICE, C. E. Some factors influencing the selection of complement-fixation method. I. A comparison of two quantitative technics. *J. Immunol.* **59**:94, 1948.

RICE, C. E. Some factors influencing the selection of complement-fixation method. II. Parallel use of the direct and indirect techniques. *J. Immunol.* **60**:11, 1948.

RICE, C. E. A consideration of the components concerned in the conglutination activities of certain complements. *J. Immunol.* **70**:497, 1953.

RICE, C. E., and P. BOULANGER. The interchangeability of the complement components of different animal species. IV. In the hemolysins of rabbitt erythrocytes sensitized with sheep antibody. *J. Immunol.* **68**:197, 1952.

RICE, C. E., and J. BROOKSBY. Studies of the complement fixation reaction in virus systems. *J. Immunol.* **71**:300, 1953.

RICE, C. E., and C. CROWSON. The interchangeability of the complement components of different animal species. II. The hemolysis of sheep erythrocytes sensitized with rabbit amboceptor. *J. Immunol.* **65**:201, 1950.

RICE, C. E., and P. MCKERCHER. Studies of the complement fixation reaction in virus systems. *J. Immunol..* **73**:309, 1954.

RICH, A. R., and M. R. LEWIS. Mechanism of allergy in tuberculosis. *Proc. Soc. Exper. Biol. Med.* **25**:596, 1928.

RICH. A. R., and M. R. LEWIS. The nature of allergy in tuberculosis as revealed by tissue culture studies. *Bull. Johns Hopkins Hosp.* **50**:115, 1932.

RICHARDS, A. N., J. BORDLEY, and A. M. WALKER. Quantitative studies on the composition of glomerular urine. VII. Manipulating technique of capillary tube colorimetry. *J. Biol. Chem.* **101**:179, 1933.

RICHARDS, E. G., J. A. COLL, and W. B. GRATZER. Disc electrophoresis of ribonucleic acid in polyacrylamide gels. *Anal. Biochem.* **12**:452, 1965.

RICHARDSON, G. Preservation of liquid complement serum. *Lancet*, ii:696, 1941.

RICHET, C. *L'Anaphylaxie*. Libraire F. Alcan, Paris, 1911.

RICHET, C., A. PENET, and P. PORTIER, *Compt. Rend. Sco. Biol.* **54**:837, 1902.

RIECKENBERG, H. *Z. Immunitatsforsch.* **26**:53, 1917.

RIFKIND, R. A., K. C. HSU, and C. MORGAN. Immunochemical staining for electron microscopy. *J. Histochem. Cytochem.* **12**:131, 1964.

RIGGS, I. Master's Thesis, University of Kansas, Manhattan, Kansas, 1957.

RIGGS, J. L., and G. C. BROWN. Differentiation of active and passive poliomyelitis antibodies in human sera by indirect immunofluorescence. *J. Immunol.* **89**:868, 1962.

RIGGS, J. L., and G. C. BROWN. Application of direct and indirect immunofluorescence for identification of enteroviruses and titrating their antibodies. *Proc. Soc. Exper. Biol. Med.* **110**:833, 1962.

RIGGS, J. L., R. J. SEIWALD, J. H. BURCKHALTER, C. M. DOWNS, and T. G. METCALF. Isothiocyanate compounds as fluorescent labeling agents for immune serum. *Amer. J. Pathol.* **34**:1081, 1958.

RILEY, V. Chromatographic studies on the separation of the virus from chicken tumor I. I. Effect of salt concentration on adsorption, elution and purification. *J. Natl. Canc. Inst.* **II**:199, 1950.

RILEY, V. Adaptation of orbital bleeding technic to rapid serial blood studies. *Proc. Soc. Exper. Biol. Med.* **104**:751, 1960.

RILEY, V., and R. CRAMER. Chromatography of SE-Plyoma virus hemagglutinin. *Virology*, **14**:286, 1961.

RINDERKNECHT, H. Ultra-rapid fluorescent labelling of proteins. *Nature*, **193**:167, 1962.

RIORDAN, I. Collodion particle agglutination test in detection of antigen derived from tubercle bacilli. *Proc. Soc. Exper. Biol. Med.* **49**:622, 1942.

RISTIC, M., and D. K. MURTY. Characterization of *Vibrio fetus* antigens. IV. Study of polysaccharide-antibody reactions by a rapid slide gel diffusion technique. *Amer. J. Vet. Res.* **22**:783, 1961.

RITSCHARD, W. J. Thin-layer electrophoresis. In *Chromatographic and Electrophoretic Techniques*, T. Smith, Ed., Vol. II. W. Heinemann, Publishing, Bath., 1968, pp. 147–153.

RITTS, R., and B. CUTTING. In vivo uptake of isotope-tagged tuberculin by leukocytes. *J. Immunol.* **75**:209, 1955.

ROBBINS, J. B., J. HAIMOVICH, and M. SELA. Purification of antibodies with immuno-adsorbents prepared using bio cellulose. *Immunochem.* **4**:11, 1967.

ROBBINS, J. B., K. Kenny, and E. SUTER. Isolation and biological activities of rabbit γ-M and γ-G anti-*Salmonella typhimurium antibodies*. *J. Exper. Med.* **122**:385, 1965.

ROBERTS, A. N., and F. HAUROWITZ. Quantitative studies on the bix diazotized benzidine method of hemagglutination. *J. Immunol.* **89**:348, 1962.

ROBERT, E. F. Extirpation of antigenic depot and antibody production. *J. Immunol.* **20**:291, 1931.

ROBERTS, E. Serologic agglutination of virus-coated bacterial cells. *J. Immunol.* **50**:55, 1945.

ROBERTS, E. A flocculation test as a possible method for differentiating immunologic types of the poliomyelitis virus. *Publ. Health Rep.* **64**:212, 1949.

ROBERTS, E., and L. Jones. Agglutination of encephalitis virus-coated bacterial cells by virus antisera. *Proc. Soc. Exper. Biol. Med.* **47**:11, 1941.

ROBERTS, E., and L. JONES. Encephalitis virus "antibody" in sera of experimentally infected animals by agglutinationof virus-coated cells. *Proc. Soc. Exper. Biol. Med.* **49**:52, 1942.

ROBERTS, E., and L. JONES. Detection of neutropic virus "antibody" by the agglutination of antigen-coated bacteria. *J. Bacteriol.* **43**:116, 1942.

ROBINETTE, R. Determination of antistreptolysin titers: technic and significance. *Amer. J. Med. Technol.* **18**:205, 1952.

ROBINSON, J. J. Improved methods for determining antistreptolysin S. *J. Immunol.* **66**:653, 1951.

ROBINSON, H. W., and C. G. HOGDEN. The biuret reaction in the determination of serum proteins. *J. Biol. Chem.* **135**:707, 1940.

ROBRISH, S. A., and A. G. MARR. Osmotic disruption of Azotobacter. *Bacteriol. Proc.* **130**, 1957.

RODENKO, A. *Pediatrija*, **5**:38, 1954.

RODNEY, G., and N. FELL. Histamine-protein complexes: synthesis and immunological investigation. *J, Immunol.* **47**:251, 1943.

ROGER, H. Le pouvoir attendant du serum. *Presse Méd.* **112**, 1896.

ROGERS, T. E. Analytical Serology in Protozoa. In *Analytical Serology of Microorganisms*, J. B. G. Kwapinski, Ed., Vol. 2. Interscience, New York, 1969, pp. 549–637.

ROMANO, A. H., and A. SOHLER. Biochemistry of the Actinomycetales. II. A comparison of the cell wall composition of species of the genera *Streptomyces* and *Nocardia*. *J. Bacteriol.* **72**:865, 1956.

ROMIG, W. R. Infection of *Bacillus subtilis* with phenol extracted bacteriophages. *Virology*, **16**:452, 1962.

ROMMERS, P. J., and J. VISSER. Spectrophotometric determination of micro amounts of nitrogen as indophenol. *Analyst*, **94**:653, 1969.

RONDLE, C. J. M., and K. R. DUMBELL. Antigens of cowpox virus. *J. Hygiene, Camb.* **60**:41, 1962.

RONDLE, C. J. M., and W. T. J. MORGAN. The determination of glucosamine and galactos-amine. *Biochem. J.* **61**:586, 1955.

BIBLIOGRAPHY 773

ROOTS, E. Die antigene Komposition der isolierten hochgereinigten Geisseln von *Salmonella typhi-murium* and *Listeria monocytogenes*. *Abst. Papers VII Intern. Congr. Microbiol.* **113**, 1958.

ROSE, H. M., C. RAGAN, E. PEARCE, and M. O. LIPMAN. Differential agglutination of normal and sensitized sheep erythrocytes by sera of patients with rheumatoid arthritis. *Proc. Soc. Exper. Biol. Med.* **68**:1, 1948.

ROSE, N. R., and E. WITEBSKY. Studies on organ specificity. *J. Immunol.* **75**:282, 1955.

ROSENBERG, E., and S. ZAMENHOF. Further studies on polyribophosphate. *J. Biol. Chem.* **236**:2845, 1961.

ROSENFIELD, R. E., F. H. ALLEN, S. N. SEVISHER, and S. KOCHWA. A review of Rh serology and presentation of a new terminology. *Transfusion, Phil.* **2**:287, 1962.

ROSEN, L., and J. KERN. Hemagglutination and hemagglutination-inhibition with Coxsackie B viruses. *Proc. Soc. Exper. Biol. Med.* **107**:626, 1961.

ROSENFIELD, R. E., and P. VOGEL. The identification of hemagglutininis with red cells altered with trypsin. *Trans. N.Y. Acad. Sci.* **13**:213, 1951.

ROSENTHAL, L. Agglutinating properties of *Escherichia coli*. *J. Bacteriol.* **45**:545, 1943.

ROSENTHAL, S. The conjugation of haptens in vivo. *J. Immunol.* **34**:251, 1938.

ROSS, M. R., and F. M. GOGOLAK. The antigenic structure of psittacosis and feline pneumonitis virus. I. Isolation of complement-fixing antigens with group and species specificity. *Virology*, **3**:343, 1957.

ROTH, F., and L. PILLEMER. Purification and some properties of *Clostridium welchii* type A theta toxin. *J. Immunol.* **75**:50, 1955.

ROTH, H., S. SEGAL, and D. BERTOLI. The quantitative determination of galactose—an enzymic method using galactose oxidase, with applications to blood and other biological fluids. *Analyt. Biochem.* **10**:32, 1965.

ROTHBARD, S. Bacteriostatic effect of human sera on group A streptococci. I. Type-specific antibodies in sera of patients convalescing from group A streptococcal pharyngitis. *J. Exper. Med.* **82**:93, 1945.

ROTHEN, A., and K. LANDSTEINER. Serological reactions of protein films and denatured proteins. *J. Exper. Med.* **76**:437, 1942.

ROTHSTEIN, N. Studies of the immunochemistry of leptospiroses. *J. Immunol.* **79**:276, 1957.

ROTHSTEIN, N., and C. HIATT. Studies of the immunochemistry of leptospiroses. *J. Immunol.* **77**:257, 1956.

ROTMAN, B., and B. W. PAPERMASTER. Membrane properties of living mammalian cells as studied by enzymic hydrolysis of fluorogenic esters. *Proc. Natl. Acad. Sci. U.S.* **55**:134, 1966.

ROUNTREE, P. M. A complement-fixing antigen of *Bacterium coli* bacteriophage T5: Its behaviour during virus growth. *Brit. J. Exper. Pathol.* **32**:341, 1951.

ROUNTREE, P. M., and R. BARBOUR. Antibody to the erythrocyte-coating polysaccharide of staphylococci: Its occurrence in human sera. *Australasian Ann. Med.* **1**:80, 1952.

ROUS, P., and J. BEARD. Selection with the magnet and cultivation of reticulo-endothelial cells. *J. Exper. Med.* **59**:577, 1934.

ROUSER, G., G. V. MARINETTI, R. F. WITTER, J. F. BERRY, and E. STOTZ. Paper chromatography of phospholipides. *J. Biol. Chem.* **223**:485, 1956.

ROWLEY, D. Induced changes in the level of non-specific immunity in laboratory animals. *J. Exper. Pathol.* **37**: 223, 1956.

ROWLEY, D., and K. J. TURNER. Increase in macroglobulin antibodies of mouse and pig following injection of bacterial lipopolysaccharides. *Immunology*, **7**:394, 1964.

RUBINSTEIN, H. Quantitative antigen analysis by the Oudin method. *J. Immunol.* **73**:322, 1954.

RUDIN, L., and P. A. ALBERTSSON, A new method for the isolation of deoxyribonucleic acid from microorganisms. *Biochim. Biphys. Acta*, **134**:37, 1967.

RUSSELL, C. A "hemolysin" associated with leptospirae. *J. Immunol.* **77**:405, 1956.

RUTSTEIN, D. D., and W. H. WALKER. Complement activity in pneumonia. *J. Clin. Invest.* **21**:347, 1942.

SABIN, F. Cellular reactions to a dye-protein with a concept of the mechanism of antibody formation. *J. Exper. Med.* **70**:67, 1939.

SABIN, F., D. SMITHBURN, and K. THOMAS. Cellular reactions to wax-like material from acid-fast bacteria. *J. Exper. Med.* **62**:751, 1935.

SABOURAUD, R. Milieux de culture des champignons dermatophytes. *Ann. Derm. Syphil.* **4**:99, 1908.

SACHS, H. Die Cytotoxine des Blutserums. *Biochem. Zeitschr.* **1**:573, 1903.

SACHS, H., and W. GEORGI. Zur Serodiagnostik der Syphilis mittels Ausflockung durch cholesterinierte Extrackte. *Med. Klin.* **14**:805, 1918.

SACHS, H., and A. KLOPSTOCK. Die serologische Differenzierung von Lecithin und Cholesterin. *Biochem. Zeitschr.* **159**:491, 1925.

SADUN, E. H., and D. ALLAIN. A rapid slide hemagglutination test for the detection of antibodies to *Trichinella spiralis*. *J. Parasitol.* **43**:383, 1957.

SADUN, E. H., L. NORMAN, and S. ALLAIN. The detection of antibodies to infections with the hematode, *Toxocara canis*, a causative agent of visceral larba migrans. *Amer. J. Trop. Med.* **6**:562, 1957.

SAENZ, A. *Compt. Rend. Soc. Biol.* **120**:870, 1912.

SAGIK, B. P., and S. LEVINE. The interaction of Newcastle disease virus (NDV) with chicken erythrocytes: attachment, elution, and hemolysis. *Virology*, **3**:401, 1957.

SAITO, H., and K. I. MIURA. Preparation of transforming deoxyribonucleic acid by phenol treatment. *Biochem. Biophys. Acta*, **72**:619, 1963.

SALIH, H. S., ABU, A. F. MURANT, and M. J. DAFT. The use of antibody-sensitized latex particles to detect plant viruses. *J. Gen. Virol.* **3**:299, 1968.

SALK, J. E. A simplified procedure for titrating hemagglutinating capacity of influenza-virus and the corresponding antibody. *J. Immunol.* **49**:87, 1944.

SALK, J. E., and A. M. LAURENT. The use of adjuvants in studies on influenza immunization. I. Measurements in monkeys of the dimensions of antigenicity of virus-mineral oil emulsions. *J. Exper. Med.* **95**:429, 1952.

SALK, J. E., G. I. LAVIN, and J. FRANCIS, JR. Antigenic potency of epidemic influenza virus following inactivation by ultraviolet radiation. *J. Exper. Med.* **72**:779, 1948.

SALK, J. E., E. N. WARD, and J. S. YOUNGER. Use of color change of phenol red as the indicator in titrating poliomyelitis virus or its antibody in a tissue culture system. *Amer. J. Hyg.* **60**:214, 1954.

SALLEY, D., and R. LIBBY. Immunochemical studies with tagged proteins. II. The kinetics of antibody-formation. *J. Immunol.* **55**:27, 1945.

SALPETER, M. M., and L. BACHMAN. Autoradiography with the electron microscope. A procedure for improving resolution, sensitivity, and contrast. *J. Cell Biol.* **22**:469, 1964.

SALTON, M. R. J. Studies on the bacterial cell wall. III. Preliminary investigation of the chemical constitution of the cell wall of *Streptococcus faecalis*. *Biochim. Biophys. Acta*, **8**:510, 1952.

SALTON, M. R. J. Studies on the bacterial cell wall. IV. The composition of the cell walls of some Gram-positive and Gram-negative bacteria. *Biochim. Biophys. Acta*, **10**:512, 1953.

SALTON, M. R. J. Bacterial cell wall. In *Bacterial Anatomy*, E. T. C. Spooner and B. A. D. Stocker, Eds. Cambridge University Press, Cambridge, England. 1956.

SALTON, M. R. J. The properties of lysozyme and its action on microorganisms. *Bacteriol. Rev.* **21**:82, 1957.

SALTON, M. R. J. The lysis of microorganisms by lysozyme and related enzymes. *J. Gen. Microbiol.* **18**:41, 1958.

SALTON, M. R. J. An improved method for the detection of *N*-acetylamino sugars on paper chromatograms. *Biochim. Biphys. Acta*, **34**:309, 1959.

SALTON, M. R. J. *Microbial Cell Walls.* Wiley, New York, 1961.

SALTON, M. R. J., and R. W. HORNE. Studies on bacterial cell walls. I. Methods of preparation and some properties of cell walls. *Biochim. Biophys. Acta*, **7**:177, 1951.

SALTON, M. R. J., and B. MARSHALL. The composition of the spore and wall of vegetative cells of *Bacillus subtilis. J. Gen. Microbiol.* **21**:415, 1959.

SALVIN, S. B. Complement fixation studies in experimental histoplasmosis. *Proc. Soc. Exper. Biol. Med.* **66**:342, 1947.

SALVIN, S. B. Quantitative studies on the serologic relationships of fungi. *J. Immunol.* **65**:617, 1950.

SALVIN, S. B. Analytical Serology of Microfungi. In: *Analytical Serology of Microorganisms.* (J. B. G. Kwapinski, edtor), vol. 1, p. 531, Wiley-Interscience, New York, 1969.

SALVIN, S. B., and R. F. SMITH. Delayed hypersensitivity and the anamnestic response. *J. Immunol.* **84**:449, 1960.

SANDELL, E. B. Colorimetric microdetermination of arsenic after evolution as arsine. *Ind. Eng. Anal. Ed.* **14**:82, 1942.

SANDERS, B. G., and J. E. WRIGHT. Immunogenetic studies in two trout species of the genus *Salmo. Ann. N.Y. Acad. Sci.* **97**:116, 1962.

SANDOR G. Adsorption de l'antitoxine diphterique sur l'alumine. *Compt. Rend. Soc. Biol.* **131**:49, 1939.

SANDOR, G. Purification du serum antidiphterique par digestion protéolytique. *Compt. Rend. Soc. Biol.* **131**:1224, 1939.

SANGER, F., G. G. BROWNLEE, and B. G. BARRELL. A two-dimensional fractionation procedure for radioactive nucleotides. *J. Mol. Biol.* **13**:373, 1965.

SANGER, F., and H. TUPPY. The amino-acid sequence in phenylalanyl chain of insulin. I. The identification of lower peptides from partial hydrolysates. *Biochem. J.* **49**:463, 1951.

SASLAW, S., and C. C. CAMPBELL. A comparison between histoplasmin and blastomycin by the collodion agglutination technique. *Publ. Health Rep.* **64**:290, 1949.

SCATCHARD, G. The attractions of proteins for small molecules and ions. *Ann. N.Y. Acad. Sci.* **51**:660, 1949.

SCHACHMAN, H. K., and W. F. HARRINGTON. Ultracentrifuge studies with synthetic boundary cell. General applications. *J. Polymer Sci.* **12**:379, 1954.

SCHACHMAN, H. K., A. B. PARDEE, and R. Y. STANIER. Studies on the macromolecular organization of microbial cells. *Arch. Biochem. Biyphys.* **38**:245, 1952.

SCHAECHTER, M., A. J. TOUSIMIS, Z. A. COHN, H. ROSEN, J. CAMPBELL, and F. E. HOLM. Morphological, chemical, and serological studies of the cell walls of *Rickettsia mooseri. J. Bacteriol.* **74**:822, 1957.

SCHAEFER, W. Récherches sur la specificité des proteides des bacillus tuberculeux et des sérums antibacilles bovines lises au moyen d'une téchnique quantitative de la réaction de fixation du complement. *Ann. Inst. Pasteur*, **73**:749, 1947.

SCHEER, VAN DER, J., E. BOHNEL, and H. DOX. Diagnostic antigens for epidemic typhus, murine typhus and Rocky Mountain spotted fever. *J. Immunol.* **57**:365, 1947.

SCHEER, VAN DER, J., and K. LANDSTEINER. Serological tests with amino acids. *J. Immunol.* **29**:371, 1935.

SCHEER, VAN DER, J., R. WYCKOFF, and F. CLARKE. The electrophoretic analysis of several hyperimmune horse sera. *J. Immunol.* **39**:65, 1940.

SCHEIDEGGER, J. J. Une micro-méthode de l'immunoélectrophorese. *Intern. Arch. Allergy, Appl. Immunol.* **7**:103, 1955.

SCHEIFFARTH, F., H. GOTZ, and H. WARNATZ. Vergleichende Analyse von Präzipitaten. *Clin. Chim. Acta*, **3**:535, 1958.

SCHIFF, F. *Die Technik der Blutgruppenuntersuchungen.* Springer, Berlin. 1932.

SCHIFF, F., and W. BOYD. *Blood Transfusion Technic.* Interscience Publishers, New York, 1942.

SCHILD, G. C., and H. G. PEREIRA. Characterization of the ribonucleoprotein and neuraminidase of influenza A viruses by immunodiffusion. *J. Gen. Virol.* **4**:355, 1969.

SCHILDKRAUT, C. L., and J. J. MATO. Fractions of HeLa DNA differing in their content of guarine and cytosine. *J. Molec. Biol.* **46**:305, 1969.

SCHLESINGER, R., I. GORDON, J. FRANKEL, J. WINTER, P. PATTERSON, and W. DOBRANCE. Clinical and serological response of man to immunization with attentuated dengue and yellow fever viruses. *J. Immunol.* **77**:352, 1956.

SCHMIDT, E. L., and E. O. BANKOLE. Detection of *Aspergillus flavus* in soil by immunofluorescent staining. *Science*, **3518**:776, 1962.

SCHMIDT, G., and S. J. THANNHAUSER. A method for the detection of deoxyribonucleic acid and phosphoproteins in animal tissues. *J. Biol. Chem.* **161**:83, 1945.

SCHMIDT, N. J., and E. H. LENNETTE. Gel double diffusion studies with group B and group A, type 9 Coxsackie viruses. I. The technique with huperimmune animal sera. *J. Immunol.* **89**:85, 1962.

SCHMIDT, N. J., E. H. LENNETTE, and J. DENNIS. Gel double diffusion studies with group B and group A, type 9 Coxsackie viruses. III. Antigen-antibody absorption tests. *J. Immunol.* **94**:482, 1965.

SCHMIDT, N. J., T. T. SHINOMOTO, J. DENNIS, S. J. HAGENS, V. L. FOX, and E. H. LENNETTE. Colorimetric test in HeLa cell system for assay of neutralizing antibodies to ECHO viruses. *J. Lab. Clin. Med.* **59**:687, 1962.

SCHNEIDER, M. D. Properties of serologically active substance from *Leptospira icterohemorrhagiae* (Wijnberg). *Proc. Soc. Exper. Biol. Med.* **82**:655, 1953.

SCHNEIDER, W. C. Phosphorus compounds in animal tissues. I. Extraction and estimation of DNA and RNA. *J. Biol. Chem.* **161**:293, 1945.

SCHOENHEIMER, R., and W. SPERRY. *J. Biol. Chem.* **106**:745, 1934.

SCHOLANDER, P. F. Microburet. *Science*, **95**:177, 1942.

SCHULTZ, E., L. GEBHARDT, and L. BULLOCK. Experimentelle Beiträge zur Kenntnis der im normalen Serum vorkommenden globuliciden Sustanzen. *J. Immunol.* **21**:196, 1931.

SCHULTZ, W. H. *J. Pharmacol. Exper. Therap.* **2**:221, 1910.

SCHULTZE, H. E., Elektrophorese mit isolierten Plasmaproteinen. *Clin. Chim. Acta*, **3**:24, 1958.

SCHULTZE, H. E., and J. F. HEREMAINS. *Molecular Biology of Human Proteins with Speical Reference to Plasma Proteins.* Elsevier Publishing Co., Amsterdam, 1966.

SCHÜLTZE, H. *J. Hygiene*, **36**:559, 1936.

SCHWAB, L., F. C. MOLL, T. HALL, H. BREAN, M. KIRK, C. HAWN, and C. A. JANEWAY. Experimental hypersensitivity in the rabbit. Effectf inhibition of antibody formation by x-radiation and nitrogen mustards. *J, Exper. Med.* **91**:505, 1950.

SCHWARTZ, S. A., and W. BRAUN. Bacteria as an indicator of formation of antibodies by single spleen cells in agar. *Science*, **149**:200, 1965.

SCHWEET, R. S., and R. D. OWEN. Concepts of protein synthesis in relation to antibody formation. *J. Cellular Comp. Physiol.* **50** (*Suppl.*) **199**:1957.

SCHWEIGHOFFER, D., and P. STARLINGER. Zur Protoplastierung von *E. coli* B, mit Lysozym und Versen. *Arch. Mikrobiol.* **32**:219, 1959.

SCHWERDT, C. E., and F. L. SCHAFFER. Purification of poliomyelitis virus propagated in tissue culture. *Virology*, **2**:665, 1956.

SCOTT, J. P. Aggressins; outline of development of theory and notes on use of these products. *J. Bacteriol.* **22**:323, 1931.

SCOTT, L. V., F. G. FELTON, and J. A. BARNEY. Hemagglutination with herpes simplex virus. *J. Immunol.* **78**:211, 1957.

SCOTT, R. P. W., and D. W. GRANT. Measurement of elution peaks in gas-liquid chromatography. *Analyst*, **89**:179, 1964.

SCOTT, W. M. *J. Pathol. Bacteriol.* **15**:31, 1911.

SEAL, H. L. *Multivariate Statistical Analysis for Biologists.* Wiley, New York, 1964.

SEAL, S. Studies on the specific soluble proteins of *Pasteurella pestis* and *Pasteurella pseudotuberculosis*. *J. Immunol.* **71**:169, 1953.

SEEGAL, B. C., G. A. ANDRES, K. C. HSU, and J. B. ZABRISKIE. Studies on the pathogenesis of acute and progressive glomerulonephritis in man by immunofluorescein and immunoferritin techniques. *Fed. Proc. Symp.* **24**:100, 1965.

SEELIGER, H. P. R. *Mykologische Serodiagnostik*. Barth, Leipzig, 1957.

SEELIGER, H. P. R. Immunobiologisch-serologische Nachweisverfahren bei Pilzerkrankungen. In *Handbuch der Haut- und Geschlechtskrankheiten*, J. Jadassohn, A. Machionini, and H. Götz, Eds. Springer, 1962, pp. 605–734.

SEELIGER, H. P. R., and H. FINGER. Analytical Serology of Listeria. In *Analytical Serology of Microorganisms*, J. B. G. Kwapinski, Ed., Vol. 1, Interscience, New York, 1969, pp. 549–608.

SEELIGER, H. P. R., and F. SULZBACHER. Antigenic relationships between *Listeria monocytogenes* and *Staphylococcus aureus*. *Can. J. Microbiol.* **2**:220, 1956.

SEGRE, D. A new serologic test for the detection of viral antigens; its application to the viruses of hog cholera and vesicular stomatitis. *J. Immunol.* **78**:304, 1957.

SEIBERT, F. B. Tuberculin purified protein derivative. Preparation and analysi of large quantity for standard. *Amer. Rev. Resp. Dis.* **44**:9, 1941.

SEIBERT, F. B. The isolation of three different proteins and two polysaccharides from tuberculin by alcohol fractionation: Their chemical and biological properties. *Amer. Rev. Tuberc.* **59**:86, 1949.

SEIBERT, F. B. Constituents of mycobacteria. *Ann. Rev. Microbiol.* **4**:35, 1950.

SEIBERT, F. B., and D. W. WATSON. Isolation of the polysaccharides and nucleic acids of tuberculin by electrophoresis. *J. Biol. Chem.* **140**:55, 1941.

SEIBERT, F. B. Removal of the impurities, nucleic acid, and polysaccharide, from tuberculin protein. *J. Biol. Chem.* **133**:593, 1940.

SELEGNY, E., J. C. FENYO, G. BROUN, F. MATRAY, and C. DE BERNARDY. Rapid separation of some amino acids by ion-exchange paper electrophoresis. *J. Chromatog.* **47**:552, 1970.

SELIGMAN, E. Antigen-antibody reactions in the *Salmonella* group. *J. Immunol.* **50**:191, 1945.

SEQUEIRA, P. J. L. Examination of treponemal Wassermann reaction and Reiter protein complement fixation tests. *Brit. J. Vener. Dis.* **35**:139, 1959.

SERPA, C. E. V., and M. A. FUKS. Observations on cross reactions occurring between tubercle bacilli and brucellae. *An. Microbiol.* **8**:169, 1960.

SEVAG, M. G. Eine neue physikalische Entweissungsmethode zur Darstellung biologisch wirksamer Substanzen. *Biochem. Zeitschr.* **273**:419, 1934.

SEVAG, M. G. *Immuno-catalysis*. Williams & Wilkins, Baltimore, 1954.

SEVAG, M. G., D. B. LACKMANN, and J. SMOLENS. The isolation of the components of streptococcal nucleoprotein in serologically active form. *J. Biol. Chem.* **124**:425, 1938.

SEVER, J. L. Application of a microtechnique to viral serological investigations. *J. Immunol.* **88**:320, 1962.

SEWELL, M. M. H. The immunology of foccioliasis. I. Qualitative studies on the precipitin reaction. *Immunology*, **7**:671, 1964.

SHAINOFF, J. R., and M. A. LAUFFER. Chromatographic purification of Southern bean mosaic virus. *Arch. Biochim. Biophys.* **64**:315, 1956.

SHALLA, T. A., and A. AMICI. The distribution of viral antigen in cells infected with tobacco mosaic virus as revealed by electron microscopy. *Virology*, **31**:78, 1967.

SHARP, D. G. Enumeration of virus particles by electron micrography. *Proc. Soc. Exper. Biol. Med.* **70**:54, 1949.

SHEFFIELD, F. W., W. SMITH, and G. BELYAVIN. Purification of influenza virus by red-cell absorption and elution. *Brit. J. Exper. Pathol.* **35**:214, 1954.

SHELDON, W. Leptospiral antigen demonstrated by the fluorescent antibody technique in human muscle lesions of leptospirosis icterohemorrhagiae. *Proc. Soc. Exper. Biol. Med.* **84**:165, 1953.

SHEPARD, C. C. Use of HeLa cells infection with tubercle bacilli for the study of anti-tuberculous drugs. *J. Bacteriol.* **73**:444, 1957.

SHEPARD, C. C. Phagocytosis of microorganisms by HeLa cells. I. The use of bovine fetal serum for the study of mycobacteria and certain other Gram-positive bacteria. *J. Immunol.* **85**:356, 1960.

SHEPARD, C. C. Phagocytosis of microorganisms by HeLa cells. II. Serum activities resembling properdin. *J. Immunol.* **85**:366, 1960.

SHERP, H. W., and G. RAKE. Studies on meningococcus infection; type I specific substance. *J. Exper. Med.* **61**:753, 1935.

SHETLAR, M. R., and Y. F. MASTERS. Use of thymol-sulfuric acid reaction for determination of carbohydrates in biological material. *Anal. Chem.* **29**:402, 1957.

SHIFRINE, M., S. S. STONE, and G. DAVIES. Contagious bovine pleuropneumonia: Serologic response of cattle after single and double vaccination with I culture vaccine. *Rev. Elevage Med. Vet. Pays. Trop.* **21**:49, 1968.

SHILO, M. Resistance-increasing activity of bacterial lipopolysaccharides and their sub-fractions towards levan-enhanced infections. *Brit. J. Exper. Pathol.* **43**:153, 1962.

SHOCKMAN, G. D. Modified centrifuge-shaker for the disruption of bacteria and yeasts. *Biochim. Biophys. Acta*, **59**:234, 1962.

SHOCKMAN, G. D., J. J. KOLB, and G. A. TOENNIES. A high speed shaker for the disruption of cells at low temperature. *Biochim. Biophys. Acta*, **24**:203, 1957.

SHORTMAN, K., J. S. HASKILL, A. SZENBERG, and D. G. LEGGE. Density distribution analysis of lymphocyte population. *Nature*, **216**:1227, 1967.

SHRIGLEY, E. W., and M. R. IRWIN. On the differences in activity of serum complement from various animal species. *J. Immunol.* **32**:281, 1937.

SHULMAN, N. R. Immunoreactions involving platelets. *J. Exper. Med.* **107**:697, 1958.

SHWARTZMAN, G. *Phenomenon of Local Tissue Reaction and Its Immunologic, Pathological and Clinical Significance.* P. Hoeber, New York, 1937.

SIBAL, L. R., A. V. KROEGER, D. KUMARICH, and E. MEYER. Serological specificity of acid-soluble antigens of *Bacterionema matruchottii. J. Bacteriol.* **83**:811, 1962.

SIBOO, R., and S. I. VAS. Studies on in vitro antibody production. III. Productoin of complement. *Can. J. Microbiol.* **11**:415, 1965.

SIEBURTH, J. M. Indirect hemagglutination studies on salmonellosis in chicken. *J. Immunol.* **78**:380, 1957.

SIEFERT, G. Experimentelle Untersuchungen über Spirochäten-Antigens. III. Serologische Analyse der aus *Treponema pallidum* isolierten Lipoid- und Eiweissfraktionen. *Z. Immunitätsforsch.* **119**:120, 1960.

SILVERMAN, S. The isolation of fractions from *Pasteurella pestis* for use in hemagglutination test. *J. Lab. Clin. Med.* **44**:185, 1954.

SILVERSTEIN, A. M. Contrasting fluorescent labels for two antibodies. *J. Histochem. Cytochem.* **5**:94, 1957.

SILVERSTEIN, A., and F. MALTANER. Hemolysis with complement of intact azo-erythrocytes sensitized with antisera homologous to the attached azo-groupings. *J. Immunol.* **69**:197, 1952.

SILVERTHORNE, N., and D. T. FRASER. Observations on the action of human and animal blood on the meningococcus. *J. Immunol.* **29**:523, 1935.

SIMMONS, R., J. GRAYDON, R. JAKOBLEWICZ, and L. BRYCE. The Rh factor, its incidence in a series of Red Cross donors. *Med. J. Australia*, **2**:496, 1944.

SIMPSON, W. F., and C. S. STULBERG. Species identification of animal cell strains by immunofluorescence. *Nature*, **199**:616, 1963.

SINDO, T., and H. KOGUCHI. Effect of amino acids, etc., on tetanus toxin-antitoxin combination in mice. *Jap. J. Exper. Med.* **27**:473, 1952.

SINGER, J. M., and C. M. PLOTZ. The latex fixation test. *Amer. J. Med.* **21**:888, 1956.

SINGER, J. M., and C. M. PLOTZ. The latex fixation test for rheumatoid arthritis using patient's own gamma globulin. *Arith. Rheumat.* **1**:142, 1958.

SINGER, S. J. Preparation of an electron-dense antibody conjugate. *Nature*, **183**:1523, 1959.

SINGER, S. J., and D. H. CAMPBELL. Physical-chemical studies of soluble antigen-antibody complexes. The valence of precipitating rabbit antibody. *J. Amer. Chem. Soc.* **74**:1794, 1952.

SINGER, S. J., and D. H. CAMPBELL. The influence of pH on antigen-antibody equilibria. *J. Amer. Chem. Soc.* **76**:4052, 1954.

SINGER, S. J., and D. H. CAMPBELL. *J. Amer. Chem. Soc.* **77**:3504, 1955.

SINGER, S. J., L. SLOBIN, N. O. THORPE, and J. W. FENTON. The structure of antibody active sites. *Cold Spring Harbor Symp. Quant. Biol.* **32**:99, 1968.

SINGER, S. L., and A. F. SCHICK. The preparation of specific stains for electron microscopy prepared by the conjugation of antibody molecules with ferrifin. *J. Biophys. Biochem. Cytol.* **9**:519, 1961.

SKIDMORE, W. D., and C. ENTENMAN. Two-dimensional thin-layer chromatography of rate liver phosphatides. *J. Lipid Res.* **3**:471, 1962.

SKVARILA, F., and V. BRUNNELOVA. Isolation of γ, A-globulin from the ethonol fraction III of placental serum. *Collection of Crech. Chem. Commun.* **30**:2886, 1965.

SKVARILA, F., J. REJNEK, and J. MASKA. *Cs. Epidemiol. Mikrobiol. Immunol.* **7**:414, 1958.

SLACK, J. M., E. H. LUDWIG, H. H. BIRD, and C. M. CANBY. Studies with microaerophilic actinomycetes. I. The agglutination reaction. *J. Bacteriol.* **61**:721, 1951.

SLACK, J. M., R. G. SPEARS, W. G. SNODGRASS, and R. J. KUCHLER. Studies with microaerophilic actinomycetes. II. Serological groups as determined by the reciprocal agglutinin absorption technique. *J. Bacteriol.* **70**:400, 1955.

SLACK, J. H., A. WINGER, and D. W. MOORE, JR. Serological grouping of actinomyces by means of fluorescent antibodies. *J. Bacteriol.* **82**:54, 1961.

SLADE, H. D., and J. K. VETTER. The disintegration of group A *Streptococcus* by shaking with glass beads. *Bacteriol. Proc.* **78**, 1956.

SLOPEK, S. Analytical Serology of *Shigella*. In *Analytical Serology of Microorganisms*, J. B. G. Kwapinski, Ed., Vol. 2. Wiley-Intersciences, New York, 1969, p. 174.

SMADEL, J. E., T. M. RIVERS, and C. L. HOAGLAND. Nucleoprotein antigen of vaccinia virus. I. A new antigen obtained from elementary bodies of vaccinia. *Arch. Pathol.* **34**:275, 1942.

SMALL, P. A., JR., and J. H. BAXTER. Digestion of anti-kidney antibody: Effects on its nephrotoxicity and ability to fix complement. *J. Immunol.* **95**:282, 1965.

SMIRNOV, H. I. *Zhur. Mikrobiol. Epidemiol. Immunobiol.* **29**:1088, 1958.

SMITH, B. S. W., J. T. PAYNE, and R. W. WATSON. Preparation of spheroplasts of *Aerobacter cloacae*. *Can. J. Microbiol.* **6**:485, 1960.

SMITH, C. Relationships between haemagglutination and pathogenicity in strains of *Haemophilus* isolated from the eye. *J. Pathol. Bacteriol.* **58**:284, 1954.

SMITH, C., J. D. MARSHALL, JR., and C. E. WARREN. Identification of *Listeria monocytogenes* by the fluorescent antibody technic. *Proc. Soc. Exper. Biol. Med.* **103**:842, 1960.

SMITH, E. J., J. M. LEATHERWOOD, and R. W. WHEAT. Isolation of a new amino sugar from *Chromobacterium violaceum*. *J. Bacteriol.* **84**:1007, 1962.

SMITH, F. L., and T. D. GERLOUGH. The isolation and properties of the protein associated with tetanus antitoxic activity in equine plasma. *J. Biol. Chem.* **167**:679, 1947.

SMITH, H., B. T. TOZER, R. C. GALLOP, and F. S. SCANES. Separation of antigens by immunological specificity. I. Method for separating individual antigen-antibody complexes from mixed antigens and antibodies. *Biochem. J.* **84**:74, 1962.

SMITH, J. *Chromatographic and Electrophoretic Techniques*, 2nd ed., Vol. 2. Heinemann, London, 1960.

SMITH, J. M., and G. S. MIRICK. A micro-test for measuring circulating antibodies against a virus (PVM). *J. Immunol.* **67**:539, 1951.

SMITH, T., and A. L. REAGH. The agglutination affinities of related bacteria parasitic in different hosts. *J. Med. Res.* **10**:270, 1903.

SMITH, W., and J. H. HALL. The nature and mode of action of *Staphylococcus* coagulase. *Brit. J. Exper. Pathol.* **25**:101, 1944.

SMITHBURN, K. C. Differentiation of the West Nile virus from viruses of St. Louis and Japanese B. encephalitis. *J. Immunol.* **44**–25, 1942.

SMITHBURN, K. C. Neutralizing antibodies against certain recently isolated viruses in the sera of human being residing in East Africa. *J. Immunol.* **69**:223, 1952.

SMITHIES, O. Zone electrophoresis in starch gels: Group variations in the serum proteins of normal human adults. *Biochem. J.* **61**–629, 1955.

SMITHIES, O. An improved procedure for starch gel electrophoresis: Further variations in the serum proteins of normal individuals. *Biochem. J.* **71**–585, 1959.

SMOLENS, J., and S. MUDD. Agglutinogen of *Hemophilus pertussis*, phase I for skin-testing. *J. Immunol.* **47**:155, 1943.

SMYTHE, C. V., and T. N. HARRIS. Some properties of a hemolysin produced by group A beta-hemolytic streptococci. *J. Immunol.* **38**–283, 1940.

SMYTHE, D. G. In: *Methods Enzymol.* **11**:214, 1967.

SNEATH, P. H. A. The application of computers to taxonomy. *J. Gen. Microbiol.* **17**:201, 1957.

SNELL, F. D., and S. T. SNELL. *Colorimetric Methods of Analysis*, 3rd ed. Van Nostrand, New York, 1949.

SNOKE, J. E. Formation of bacitracin by protoplasts of *Bacillus licheniformis*. *J. Bacteriol.* **81**:986, 1961.

SOBEL, A. E., A. HIRSCHMAN, and L. A. RESMAN. A convenient microtitration method for the estimation of amino acids. *J. Biol. Chem.* **161**:99, 1945.

SOBER, H. A., and E. A. PETERSON. Protein chromatography on ion exchange cellulose. *Fed. Proc.* **17**:1116, 1958.

SOMOGYI, M. A new reagent for the determination of sugars. *J. Biol. Chem.* **160**:61, 1945.

SONEA, S., and J. DE REPENTIGNY. Techniques for the standardization of fluorescent antibodies used in diagnostic microbiology. *Can. J. Microbiol.* **7**:835, 1961.

SØRENSEN, S. P. L. *Biochem. Z.* **21**:131, 1909.

SORKIN, E., and S. BOYDEN. A study of antigens active in the Middlebrook-Dubos haemagglutination test present in filtrates of culture of *Mycobacterium tuberculosis. J. Immunol.* **75**:22, 1955.

SONAK, R., K. E. GILLERT, and H. PICHL. Untersuchungen zur Objektivierung der Ablesung der indirekten Hämagglutination nach Boyden. *Zentralbl. Backteriol. Paratenk.* **208**: 265, 1968.

SOULE, D. W., G. V. MARINETTI, and H. R. MORGAN. Studies of the hemolysins of red blood cells by mumps virus. IV. Quantitative study of changes in red blood cell lipids and of virus lipides. *J. Exper. Med.* **110**:93, 1959.

ŠOUREK, J., and Z. ŠIR. Antigenni přibuznost nativnich flitratů kultur nekterych zastupců Mycobacteriales. *Cs. Epid. Mikrob. Immunol.* **8**:1. 1959.

SPALDING, D. H., and T. G. METCALF. The use of filter paper chromatograms to demonstrate antigen-antibody reactions. *J. Bacteriol.* **68**:160, 1954.

SPAR, I., W. BALE, G. WOLFE, and R. GOODLAND. Organ specificity of I^{131} labeled rabbit kidney eluates in rats and rabbits. *J. Immunol.* **76**:119, 1950.

SPAUN, J. Determination of *Salmonella* types O and V antibodies by hemagglutination. *Acta Pathol. Microbiol. Scandinav.* **31**:462, 1952.

SPENDLOVE, R. S., and E. H. LENNETTE. A simplified immunofluorescent plaque method. *J. Immunol.* **89**:106, 1962.

SPICER, S., and S. RACHSTEIN. A rapid and simplified method for conducting the agglutinin absorption test for hemolytic streptococci. *J. Immunol.* **21**:315, 1931.

SPIEGELMAN, S., A. J. ARONSON, and P. C. FITZ-JAMES. Isolation and characterization of nuclear bodies from protoplasts of *Bacillus megaterium. J. Bacteriol.* **75**:102, 1958.

SPITERI, J. *Bull. Soc. Chim. Biol.* **36**:1355, 1955.

SPITNIK-ELSON, P. Preparation of ribosomal protein from *Escherichia coli* with lithium chloride and urea. *Biochem. Biophys. Res. Comm.* **18**:557, 1965.

SPOONER, E. T. C., and B. A. D. STOCKER. *Bacterial Anatomy.* Cambridge University Press, Cambridge, England, 1956.

SPRINGER, G. Inhibition of blood-group agglutinins by substance occurring in plants. *J. Immunol.* **76**:399, 1956.

SRI-RAM, J., P. K. NAKANE, E. G. RAWLINSON, and G. B. PIERCE. Enzyme-labelled antibodies for ultrastructural studies. *Fed. Proc.* **25**:732, 1966.

SRI-RAM, J., S. S. TAWDE, G. B. PIERCE, JR., and A. R. MIDGLEY, JR. Preparation of antibody-ferritin conjugates for immunoelectron microscopy. *J. Cell Biol.* **17**:673, 1963.

STAACK, H., and J. SPAUN. Serological diagnosis of chronic typhoid carriers by Vi hemagglutination. *Acta Pathol. Microbiol. Scandinav.* **32**:420, 1953.

STABBLEFORTH, A. The international standard for anti-*Brucella abortus* serum. *Bull. World Health Organ.* **10**:927, 1954.

STACEY, M., P. W. KENT, and E. NASSAU. Polysaccharide complexes isolated from *Mycobacterium tuberculosis* (human strain). *Biochim. Biophys. Acta*, **7**:146, 1951.

STAHL, E., and U. KALTENBACH. Dünnschicht-Chromatographie. *J. Chromatog.* **5**:351, 1961.

STAHMANN, M. A., and R. E. F. MATHEWS. The effect of a synthetic lysine polypeptide upon the velocity of precipitation of tobacco mosaic virus by its antiserum. *J. Immunol.* **72**:435, 1954.

STAMP, T., and E. B. HENDRY. The immunising activity of certain chemical fractions isolated from hemolytic streptococci. *Lancet*, **I**:257, 1937.

STANBRIDGE, E., and L. HAYFLICK. Growth inhibition test for identification of mycoplasma species utilizing dried antiserum-impregnated paper discs. *J. Bacteriol.* **93**:1392, 1967.

STANIER, R. Y., and C. B. VAN NIEL. The main outlines of bacteria classification. *J. Bacteriol* **42**:437, 1941.

STANLEY, W. M. The preparation and use of tobacco mosaic virus containing radioactive phosphorus. *J. Gen. Physiol.* **25**:881, 1942.

STANLEY, W. M. Evaluation of methods for concentration and purification of influenza virus. *J. Exper. Med.* **79**:255, 1944.

STANLEY, W. M. Preparation and properties of influenza virus vaccines concentrated and purified by differential centrifugation. *J. Exper. Med.* **81**:193, 1945.

'STANLEY, W. M. Precipitation of purified concentrated influenza virus and vaccine on calcium phosphate. *Science*, **101**ö332, 1945.

STARR, M. P., and W. L. STEPHENS. Pigmentation and taxonomy of the genus *Xanthomonas*. *J. Bacteriol.* **87**:293, 1964.

STARR, T. J., M. POLLARD, D. DUMAU, and M. R. DUNAWAY. Electron and fluorescent microscopy of mouse hepatitis virus. *Proc. Soc. Exper. Biol. Med.* **104**ö767, 1960.

STATS, D., and J. BULLOWA. Failure of the human convalescent type-specific anti-pneumococcic antibodies to fix complement. *J. Immunol.* **41**:114, 1942.

STAUB, A. M. Role des anticorps antipolyosidiques dans l'agglutination des bacilles typhiques. *Ann. Inst. Pasteur*, **86**:618. 1954.

STAUB, A. M., and P. GRABAR. Immunological study of the anthrax bacillus. Role of the capsule in antianthrax immunization. *Compt. Rend. Soc. Biol.* **137**:623, 1943.

STAUB, A. M., and M. RAYNAUD. *Cours d'Immunologie Générale et Sérologie.* CDU, Paris, 1965.

STAUB, A. M., R. TINELL, LÜDERITZ, and O. WESTPHAL. Étude immunochemique sur les *Salmonella*. Role de quelques sucres, et en particulair des 3-6-didisoxyhexoses, dans la specifité des antigens O du tableu de Kaufmann White. *Ann. Inst. Pasteur*, **96**:303, 1959.

STAVITSKY, A. B. Micromethods for the study of protein and antibodies. I. Procedure and general application of hemagglutination and hemagglutination-inhibition reactions with tannic acid and protein treated red blood cells. *J. Immunol.* **72**:360, 1954.

STAVITSKY, A. B. In vitro production of diphtheria antitoxin by tissues of immunized animals. *J. Immunol.* **75**:214, 1955.

STAVITSKY, A. B., and E. R. ARQUILLA. Micromethods for the study of proteins and antibodies. *J. Immunol.* **74**:306, 1955.

STAVITSKY, A. B., R. STAVITSKY, and E. E. ECKER. Loss of hemolytic-complement activity and of granulocytes following reinjection of an antigen into the rabbit. *J. Immunol.* **63**:389, 1949.

STEFFANINI, M. Basic mechanisms of hemostasis. *Bull. N.Y. Acad. Med.* **30**:239, 1954.

STEFFEN, C. Utersuchungen über das Vorkommen eines in Polyarthritikseren und Seren von Endokarditiskranken aufscheidenden Antikörpers. *Wien. Zeitschr. Inn. Med.* **35**:422, 1954.

STEIN, G. J., and D. V. VAN NGU. A quantitative complement fixation test: titration of luetic sera by the unit of 50 per cent hemolysis. *J. Immunol.* **50**:17, 1950.

STEIN, W. H., and S. MOORE. The free amino acids of human blood plasma. *J. Biol. Chem.* **211**:915, 1954.

STEINBERG, B., and R. A. MARTIN. Agglutination of circulating leukocytes by antileukocytic sera. *Proc. Soc. Exper. Biol. Med.* **56**:50, 1944.

STEINBERG, B., and R. A. MARTIN. Factors influencing leukoagglutination by antileukocytic sera. *J. Immunol.* **51**:421, 1945.

STEINER, D. F., and H. S. ANKER. *Proc. Natl. Acad. Sci.* **42**:580, 1956.

STELOS, P. Electrophoretic and ultracentrifugal studies of rabbit hemolysins. *J. Immunol.* **77**:396, 1956.

STENDERUP, A., and L. BAK. Deoxyribonucleic acid base composition of some species within the genus *Candida*. *J. Gen. Microbiol.* **52**:531, 1968.

STEPHEN, J., R. G. C. GALLOP, and H. SMITH. Separation of antigens by immunological specificity. Use of disulphide-linked antibodies as immunosorbents. *Biochem. J.* **101**: 717, 1966.

STERNBERGER, L. A., and D. PRESSMAN. A general method for the specific purification of antiprotein antibodies. *J. Immunol.* **65**:65, 1950.

STERNBERGER, L. A. Some new developments in immunocytochemistry. *Mikroskopie*, **25**:346, 1969.

STERNBERGER, L. A., E. A. DONATI, J. S. HANKER, and A. M. SELIGMAN. Immuno-diezothio-ether-osmium tetroxide (immuno-DTO) technique for staining embedded antigen in electron microscopy. *Exper. Mol. Pathol. Suppl.* **3**:36, 1966.

STERNBERGER, L. A., E. A. DONATI, and C. E. WILSON. Electron microscopic study on specific protection of isolated *Bordetella bronchiseptica* antibody during exhaustive labelling with uranium. *J. Histochem. Cytochem.* **11**:48, 1963.

STERNBERGER, L. A., J. S. HANKER, E. A. DONATI, J. R. PETRALI, and A. M. SELIGMAN. Method for enhancement of electron microscopic visualization of embedded antisera by bridging osmium to uranium antibody with thiocarbohydrazide. *J. Histochem. Cytochem.* **14**:711, 1966.

STERNBERGER, L. A., P. H. HARDY, J. C. CUCULIS, and H. G. MEYER. The unlabeled antibody enzyme method of immunochemistry. *J. Histochem. Cytochem.* **18**:315, 1970.

STERNE, M. Hemagglutination by *Clostridium botulinum* type D. *Science*, **119**:440, 1954.

ŠTERZL, J. *Folia Biol.* **1**:193, 1955.

ŠTERZL, J. *Folia Microbiol.* **4**:91, 1959.

STEVENS, K. M., and J. M. McKENNA. Studies on antibody synthesis initiated in vitro. *J. Exper. Med.* **107**:537, 1958.

STEWART, B. T., and H. O. HALVORSON. Studies on the spores of aerobic bacteria. *J. Bacteriol.* **65**:160, 1953.

STEYEMARK, A. *Quantitative Organic Microanalysis*, 2nd ed. Academic Press, New York, 1961, pp. 133–138.

STICKL, H. Ueber due Natur des T-Agglutinins. *Zeitschr. Immunitatsforsch.* **118**:135, 1953.

STOFFYN, J., and R. W. JEANOLZ. Hyaluronic acid and related sugars. XII. Identification of amino sugars by paper chromatography. *Arch. Biochem. Biophys.* **52**:373, 1954.

STOKER, M. G. P., R. R. A. COOMBS, and S. P. BEDSON. The application of the conglutination complement absorption test to virus systems. *J. Exper. Pathol.* **31**:217, 1950.

STOKINGER, H. E., C. M. CARPENTER, and J. PLACK. Studies on the gonococcus. III. Qualitative agglutinative reactions of the *Neisseria* with sppecial reference to *N. gonorrhoeae*. *J. Bacteriol.* **47**:129, 1944.

STOLLERMAN, G. H., and R. EKSTEDT. Long chain formation by strains of Group A streptococci in the presence of homologous sera. A type-specific reaction. *J. Exper. Med.* **106**: 345, 1957.

STOLLERMAN, G. H., A. C. SIEGEL, and E. E. JOHNSON. Evaluation of the " long chain reaction" as a means for detecting type-specific antibodies to group A streptococci in human sera. *J. Exper. Med.* **110**:887, 1959.

STORCK, R. L., and T. J. WACHSMAN. The association of enzymes with the protoplast membrane of *Bacillus megatherium*. *Biochem. J.* **66**:19, 1957.

STÖSS, B. Papierchromatographische Darstellung von Antigen-Antikörper-Reaktionen. *Zentralbl. Bakteriol. I. Orig.* **171**:103, 1957.

STRANGE, R. E. The structure of an amino sugar present in certain spores and bacterial cell walls. *Biochem. J.* **64**:23, 1956.

STRANGE, R. E., and F. A. DARK. The composition of spore coats of *B. megaterium, B. subtilis*, and *B. cereus*. *Biochem. J.* **62**:459, 1956.

STRANGE, R. E., and F. A. DARK. Cell wall lytic enzyme associated with spores of *Bacillus* species. *J. Gen. Microbiol.* **17**:525, 1957.

STRANGE, R. E., and G. B. THORNE. Further purification studies on the protective antigen of *Bacillus anthracis* produced in vitro. *J. Bacteriol.* **76**:192, 1958.

STRATTON, F. A slide test for the detection of Rh-antibodies using papain treated red cells. *Vox Sang.* **3**:43, 1953.

STRATTON, F. Detection of weak Rh antibodies in maternal antenatal sera. The value of enzyme-treated test cells. *Lancet*, **1**:1169, 1953.

STRATTON, F., and E. R. DIMOND. Value of serum and albumin mixture for use in detection of blood group antigen-antibody reactions. *J. Clin. Pathol.* **8**:218, 1955.

STRAUS, E. K. Occurrence of antibody in human vaginal mucus. *Proc. Soc. Exper. Biol. Med.* **106**:617, 1961.

STRAUSS, A. J. L., P. G. KEMP, JR. W. E. VANNIER, and H. C. GOODMAN. Purification of human serum γ-globulin for immunologic studies: γ-globulin fragmentation after sulfate precipitation and prolonged dialysis. *J. Immunol.* **93**:24, 1964.

STRENG, O. *Finska Läk. Sällsk. Handl.* **52**:95, 1910.

STRENG, O. In *Handbuch der Pathogenen Mikroorganismen*, Kolle, Kraus, and Uhlenhut, Eds. Fischer Verl., Jena, 1929.

STROMINGER, J. L., J. T. PARK, and R. E. THOMPSON. Composition of the cell wall of *Staphylococcus aureus;* its relation to the mechanism of action of penicillin. *J. Biol. Chem.* **234**:3263, 1959.

STUART, C. *Infectious Mononucleosis. Diagnostic Procedures and Reagents.* American Public Health Association, New York, 1945.

STUART, C., P. SAVIN, K. WHEELER, and S. BATTEY, Group-specific agglutinins in rabbit serums for human cells. *J. Immunol.* **31**:25, 1936.

STUART, C., J. TALLMAN, and E. ANDERSON. Agglutinins for sheep and rabbit erythrocytes in human sera. *J. Immunol.* **28**:75, 1935.

STUART-HARRIS, C., Observations on the agglutination of fowl red cells by influenza viruses. *Brit. J. Exper. Pathol.* **24**:33, 1943.

STUDIER, F. W. Sedimentation studies of the size and shape of DNA. *J. Mol. Biol.* **11**:373, 1965.

STULBERG, C., E. ZUELZER, and W. PAGE. *Escherichia coli* 0127:B8. A serotype causing infantile diarrhoea. *J. Immunol.* **76**:281, 1956.

STUMPF, P. A colorimetric method for the determination of desoxyribonucleic acid. *J. Biol. Chem.* **169**:367, 1947.

STURGEON, P. Studies of a "complete" and an "incomplete" Rh antiserum with cDe/cde and -D-/-D-cells. *J. Immunol.* **68**:277, 1952.

STURGEON, P. The nature of a "complete" Rh antiserum as revealed by antiglobulin augmentation. *J. Immunol.* **73**:121, 1954.

STURGEON, P., M. K. HILL, and K. S. KWAK. A fully automated method for immunochemical quantitation by passive hemolysis inhibition. *Immunochem.* **6**:689, 1969.

STURGEON, P., and D. T. MCQUISTON. A fully automated system for the simultaneous determination of whole blood red cell count and hemoglobulin centent. *Amer. J. Clin. Path.* **43**:517, 1965.

STURGEON, P., and D. T. MCQUISTON. Automation in Analytical Chemistry. In *Technicon Symposia*, Vol. 1. Mediad, New York, 1967, p. 122.

STUTZ, E., and H. NOLL. Characterization of cytoplasmic and chloroplast polysomes in plants. Evidence for three classes of ribosomal RNA in nature. *Proc. Natl. Acad. Sci.* **57**:774, 1967.

STYK, B., N. J. SCHMIDT, and J. DENNIS. The use of Rivanol treatment for removal from sera of nonspecific inhibitors of enterovirus and reovirus hemagglutination. *Amer. J. Epodemiol.* **88**:398, 1968.

SUESSENGUTH, H., and B. S. KLINE. Simple rapid flocculation slide test for trichinosis in man and in swine. *Amer. J. Clin. Pathol.* **14**:471, 1944.

SUGGS, M. J., JR., H. CASEY, D. D. SLIGH, A. R. FODOR, and W. E. McLIMANS. A batch type concentration and purification procedure for poliovirus complement fixing antigen. *J. Bacteriol.* **82**:789, 1961.

SUHRLAND, L. G., S. A. ARMENTROUT, and T. M. DANIEL. Immunoassay of hemoglobin A. *J. Lab. Clin. Med.* **71**:1021, 1968.

SULITZEANU, D. Passive protection experiments with *Brucella* antisera. *J. Hygiene*, **53**:133, 1955.

SULKIN, S., and E. STRAUSS. Studies on Q fever: persistence of complement-fixing antibodies after naturally acquired infection. *Proc. Soc. Exper. Biol. Med.* **67**:142, 1948.

SULZBERGER, M. B. Experiments in passive transference of urticarial hypersensitiveness to fungous extracts. *J. Immunol.* **23**:73, 1932.

SURGALLA, M. J., M. S. BERGDOLL, and G. M. DACK. Use of antigen-antibody reactions in gel to follow the progress of fractionation of antigenic mixtures; application to purification of staphylococcal enterotoxin. *J. Immunol.* **69**:357, 1952.

SUSSMAN, L. N., and H. PRETSHOLD. Elution technic for identification of antibody-coated erythrocytes. *Amer. J. Clin. Pathol.* **24**:1430, 1954.

SUZUKI, T. Blood grouping of blood-stains by immuno-electron microscopy. *Tohoku J. Exper. Med.* **101**:1, 1970.

SVARTZ, N., and K. SCHLOSSMANN. En my serologisk reaktion vid kronisk polyarthrit. *Nord. Med.* **42**:1390, 1949.

SVARTZ, N., and K. SCHLOSSMANN. A serum cold precipitable hemagglutinating factor in rheumatoid arthritis. *Acta Med. Scandinav.* **149**:83, 1954.

SVEDBERG, T. *Colloidal Chemistry*. Chemical Catalogue Co., New York, 1928.

SVEDBERG, T., and K. O. PEDERSON. *The Ultracentrifuge*. Oxford University Press, 1940.

SVEDMYR, A. Studies on a factor in normal allantoic fluid inhibiting influenza virus haemagglutination. Occurrence, physico-chemical properties and mode of action. *Brit. J. Exper. Pathol.* **29**:295, 1948.

SVEDMYR, A., J. ENDERS, and A. HOOLOWAY. Complement-fixation with Brunhilde and Lansing poliomyelitis viruses propagated in tissue culture. *Proc. Soc. Exper. Biol. Med.* **79**:296, 1944.

SVEHAG, S. E., B. CHESEBRO, and B. BLOTH. Ultrastructure of Gamma M immunoglobulin and alpha macroglobulin: Electron-microscopic study. *Science*, **158**:5, 1967.

SVENSSON, H. A laboratory manual of analytical methods. In *Protein Chemistry*, P. Alexander and R. J. Bloch, Eds. Pergamon Press, London, 1960.

SVENSSON, H. Isoelectric fractionation, analysis, and characterization of ampholytes in neutral pH gradients. III. Description of apparatus for electrolysis in columns stabilized by density gradients and direct determination of isoelectric points. *Arch. Biochem. Biophys.*, Suppl. 1, 132, 1962.

SVIHLA, G., and F. SCHLENK. S-adenosylmethionine in the vacuole of *Candida utilis*. *J. Bacteriol.* **79**:841, 1960.

SVIHLA, G., F. SCHLENK, and J. L. DAINKO. Spheroplasts of the yeast *Candida utilis*. *J. Bacteriol.* **82**:808, 1961.

SWIFT, H. F., and G. K. HIRST. An apparatus for breaking bacteria at low temperatures. *Proc. Soc. Exper. Biol. Med.* **37**:162, 1937.

SWIFT, H. F., A. T. WILSON, and R. C. LANCEFIELD. Typing group A hemolytic streptococci by M precipitin in capillary pipettes. *J. Exper. Med.* **78**:127, 1943.

SYVERTON, J. T., W. F. SCHERER, and P. M. ELWOOD. Studies on the propagation in vitro of poliomelitis viruses. II. The application of strain HeLa human epithelial cells for isolation and typing. *J. Lab. Clin. Med.* **43**:286, 1954.

TABERT, G. G., and D. B. LACKMAN. The radioisotope precipitation test for study of Q fever antibodies in human and animal sera. *J. Immunol.* **94**:959, 1965.

TACHIBANA, T., and E. KLEIN. Detection of cell surface antigens on monolayer cells. I. The application of immune adherence on a micro scale. *Immunology*, **19**:771, 1970.

TACHIBANA, T., P. WORST, and E. KLEIN. Detection of cell surface antigens on monolayer cells. II. The application of mixed haemadsorption on a micro scale. *Immunology*, **19**:809, 1970.

TAGER, M. Studies on the coagulase-reacting factor. I. The reaction of staphylocoagulase with the components of human plasma. *Yale. J. Biol. Med.* **20**:369, 1948.

TAGER, M., and H. HALES. The experimental production of antibodies to staphylocoagulase. *J. Immunol.* **62**:475, 1949.

TAINTER, M. L. Estimation of the ED_{50} and its error by means of logarithmic probit graph paper. *Proc. Soc. Exper. Biol. Med.* **57**:261, 1944.

TAKAHASHI, Y. Specific serum agglutination of kaolin particles sensitized with tubercle phosphatide and its clinical evaluation as a serodiagnostic test for tuberculosis. *Amer. Rev. Resp. Dis.* **85**:705, 1962.

TAKAHASHI, Y., S. FUJITA, and A. SASAKI. The specificity of the passive hemagglutination methods used in serology of tuberculosis. *J. Exper. Med.* **113**:1141, 1961.

TAKANAMI, M. A stable ribonucleoprotein for amino acid incorportion. *Biochim. Biophys. Acta*, **39**:318, 1960.

TAKATSY, G. The use of spiral loops in serological and virological micromethods. *Acta Microbiol. Acad. Sci. Hung.* **3**:191, 1955.

TAKEDA, Y., T. WATANABE, K. KURIBASHI, and K. KIUCHI. Studies on the hemagglutination of erythrocytes sensitized with endotoxins. *Jap. J. Exper. Med.* **22**:273, 1952.

TAKEYA, K. Recent studies in submicroscopic structures of the cell and their function. Fine structure of bacterial cell. *Rec. 15th Gen. Meet. Jap. Med. Assoc.* **1**:100, 1959.

TALIAFERRO, W. H. A reaction product in infections with *Tr. lewisii* which inhibits the production of the trypanosomes. *J. Exper. Med.* **39**:161, 1924.

TALIAFERRO, W. H. Trypanocidal and reproduction-inhibiting antibodies to *Trypanosoma lewisii* in rats and rabbits. *Amer. J. Hyg.* **16**:32, 1932.

TALIAFERRO, W. H. Ablastic and trypanocidal antibodies against *Trypanosoma duttoni*. *J. Immunol.* **35**:303, 1938.

TALIAFERRO, W. H., and Y. PAVLINOVA. The cause of infection of *Trypanosoma duttoni* in normal and in splenectonised and blockaded mice. *J. Parasit.* **22**:29, 1936.

TALMAGE, D. W. Immunological specificity. *Science*, **129**:1643, 1959.

TALMAGE, D. W., H. R. BAKER, and W. AKESON. The separation and analysis of labelled antibodies. *J. Infect. Dis.* **94**:199, 1954.

TALMAGE, D. W., and J. R. CANN. *The Chemistry of Immunity in Health and Disease.* Thomas, Springfield, Ill., 1961.

TALMAGE, D. W., F. DIXON, S. C. BUKANTZ, and G. J. DAMMIN. Antigen elimination from the blood as an early manifestation of the immune response. *J. Immunol.* **67**:243, 1951.

TAMM, I. Influenza-virus-erythrocyte interaction. *J. Immunol.* **73**:180, 1954.

TAN, M., and M. V. EPSTEIN. A direct immunologic assay of human sera for Bence Jones proteins (L-chains). *J. Lab. Clin. Med.* **66**:344, 1965.

TANAKA, K., H. H. RICHARDS, and G. L. CANTONI. Studies on soluble ribonucleic acid. IX. Partition chromatography of yeast "soluble" ribonucleic acid on sephadex. *Biochim. Biophys. Acta*, **61**:846, 1962.

TANAKA, N., and E. LEDUC. A study of the cellular distribution of Forssmann antigen in various species. *J. Immunol.* **77**:198, 1956.

TANNER, C. E., and J. GREGORY. Immunochemical study of the antigens of *Trichinella spiralis*. I. Identification and enumeration of antigens. *Can. J. Microbiol.* **7**:473, 1961.

TASMAN, A., and J. P. VAN WAASBERGEN. *Z. Immunitätsforsch.* **75**:164, 1932.

TAUBER, H. A color test for pentoses. *Proc. Soc. Exper. Biol. Med.* **37**:600, 1937.

TAVERNE, J., J. H. MARSHALL, and F. FULTON. The purification and concentration of viruses and virus solution antigens on calcium phosphate. *J. Gen. Microbiol.* **19**:451, 1958.

TAYLOR, A. R. Chemical analysis of influenza viruses A (PR8 strain) and B (Lee strain) and swine influenza virus. *J. Biol. Chem.* **153**:675, 1944.

TAYLOR, A. R. Concentration of rabbit papilloma virus with Sharples supercentrifuge. *J. Biol. Chem.* **163**:233, 1946.

TAYLOR-ROBINSON, D., O. SOBESLAVSKY, and R. M. CHANOCK. Relationship of *Mycoplasma pneumoniae* to other human *Mycoplasma* species studied by gel diffusion. *J. Bacteriol.* **90**:1432, 1965.

TELFER, W. H., and C. M. WILLIAMS. Immunological studies of insect metamorphosis. I. Qualitative and quantitative description of the blood antigens of *Cecropia* silkworm. *J. Gen. Physiol.* **36**:389, 1953.

TENENBERG, D. J., and A. HOWELL, JR. Complement fixation test for histoplasmosis; technic and preliminary result on animal sera. *Publ. Health Rep.* **63**:113, 1948.

TENGERDY, R. P. Quantitative immunofluorescein titration of human and bovine gamma globulins. *Analyt. Chem.* **35**:1084, 1963.

TENGERDY, R. P. Gamma globulin determination in human sera by the inhibition of the precipitation of fluorescein-labeled gamma globulin. *J. Lab. Clin. Med.* **65**:859, 1965.

TE PUNGA, W. A. An indirect haemagglutination test for the detection of *Vibrio* antibodies. *N. Z. Veter. J.* **6**:157, 1958.

TE PUNGA, W. A., and G. G. MOYLE. An indirect haemagglutination test for the detection of *Vibrio fetus* antibodies. 4. Non-specific reactivity of bovine serum. *N. Z. Veter. J.* **9**:41, 1961.

TERASASKI, P. I., and N. E. RICH. Quantitative determination of antibody and complement directed against lymphocytes. *J. Immunol.* **82**:128, 1964.

TERZIN, A. Leptospiral antigens for use in complement fixation test. *J. Immunol.* **76**:366, 1956.

THALHEIMER, W. *J. Amer. Med. Assoc.* **76**:1245, 1921.

THIELE, I. Studies on the hemagglutination of *Haemophilus pertussis*. *J. Immunol.* **65**:627, 1950.

THOM, C., and K. B. RAPER. *A Manual of the Aspergilli*. Williams and Wilkins Co., Baltimore, 1945.

THOMAS, I., and A. MENNIC. Bacterial polysaccharides in the diagnosis of infections. The polysaccharide lysis test. *Lancet*, **II**:745, 1950.

THOMASON, B. M., W. B. CHERRY, and P. R. EDWARDS. Staining bacterial smears with fluorescent antibody. IV. Identification of salmonellae in fecal specimens. *J. Bacteriol.* **77**:478, 1959.

THOMASON, B. M., W. B. CHERRY, and M. D. MOODY. Staining bacterial smears with fluorescent antibody. III. Antigenic analysis of *Salmonella typhosa* by means of fluorescent antibody and agglutination reactions. *J. Bacteriol.* **74**:525, 1957.

THOMASON, B. M., M. D. MOODY, and M. GOLDMAN. Staining bacterial smears with fluorescent antibody. II. Rapid detection of varying numbers of *M. pseudomallei* in contaminated material and infected animals. *J. Path. Bacteriol.* **72**:382, 1956.

THOMPSON, W. R., and F. MALTANER. On the construction of graphs and tables for evaluation of the quantitative complement-fixation reactions and reaction ratios. *J. Immunol.* **38**:147, 1940.

THOMPSON, W. R., C. E. RICE, E. MALTANER, and F. MALTANER. Some fundamental notions in estimation of complement fixation. *J. Immunol.* **62**:353, 1949.

THOMSEN, O. Ein vermehrungsfähiges Agens als Veränder des isoagglutinatorischen Verhaltens der roten Blütkorperchen, eine bisher unbekannte Quelle der Fehlbestimmung. *Zeitschr. Immunitätsforsch.* **52**:85, 1922.

THOMSON, A. E., A. C. HAMANN, and W. H. PARK. The gonococcus complement fixation test. *J. Immunol.* **29**:249, 1935.

THOMSON, R. O. The fractionation of *Clostridium welchii* antigen on cellulose ion exchangers. *J. Gen. Microbiol.* **31**:79, 1963.

THORNE, C. B., and F. C. BELTON. An agar-diffusion method for titrating *Bacillus anthracis* immunizing agent and its application to a study of antigen production. *J. Gen. Microbiol.* **17**:505, 1957.

THORNE, C. B., C. G. GOMEZ, H. E. NOYES, and R. D. HOUSEWRIGHT. Production of glutamyl polypepdite by *Bacillus subtilis*. *J. Bacteriol.* **68**:307, 1954.

THURSTON, J. R., and W. J. STEENKEN. Comparison of gel precipitin and sensitized erythrocyte techniques for the detection of antibody in the serum of tuberculous and nontuberculous patients. *Amer. Rev. Resp. Dis.* **81**:695, 1960.

TIMASHIEFF, S. N., J. B. SHUMAKER, and J. G. KIRKWOOD. Semicontinuous electrophorein-convection. *Arch. Biochem. Biophya.* **47**:455, 1953.

TISELIUS, A. Study of the electrophoresis of proteins by the moving boundary method. *Nova Acta Regiae Soc. Sci. Upsaliensis.* **4**:107, 1930.

TISELIUS, A. A new apparatus for electrophoretic analysis of colloidal mixtures. *Trans. Faraday Soc.* **33**:524, 1937.

TISELIUS, A. Electrophoresis of serum globulin. *Biochem. J.* **31**:313, 1464, 1937.

TODA, T., and R. MITSUSE. Studien üben die Komponenten des hämolytischen Komplements. I. Feststellung des Vorhandeseins von der 4. Komponenten und von der 5. Komponenten des Komplements. *Zeitschr. Immunitatsforsch.* **78**:62 1932.

TODD, E. W. A method of measuring the increase or decrease of the population of haemolytic streptococci in blood. *Brit. J. Exper. Pathol.* **8**:1, 1927.

TODD, E. W. Antihaemolysin titres in haemolytic streptococcal infections and their significance in rheumatic fever. *Brit. J. Exper. Pathol.* **13**:248, 1932.

TODD, E. W. The differentiation of two serological varieties of streptolysin, streptolysin O and streptolysin S. *J. Pathol. Bacteriol.* **47**:423, 1938.

TODD, J. Bacterial pyrogens. *J. Pharm. and Pharmacol.* **7**:625, 1955.

TODD, J., A. F. COBURN, and A. B. HILL. Antistreptolysin S titers in rheumatic fever. *Lancet*, **II**:1213, 1939.

TODD, J., and S. SANFORD. *Chemical Diagnosis by Laboratory Methods*. Saunders, Philadelphia, 1935.

TOENIUS, C., and J. S. KALB. Techniques and reagents for paper chromatography. *Anal. Chem.* **23**:823, 1951.

TOLLENS, B. *Ber.* **41**; 1788, 1908.

TOMASI, T. B., JR., E. M. TAN, A. SOLOMON, and R. A. PRENDERGAST. Characteristics of an immune system common to certain external secretions. *J. Exper. Med.* **121**:101, 1965.

TOMCSIK, J. Neue Wege zur serologischen Diagnose der Mononucleosis infectiosa. *Bull. Schweiz. Akad. Me. Wiss.* **16**:185, 1960.

TOMCSIK, J., and J. B. BAUMANN-GRACE. Zellwandfreie Bakterienprotoplasten. *Verhandl. Naturforsch. Ges.* **67**:218, 1956.

TOMCSIK, J., and J. B. BAUMANN-GRACE. Sporulation und spezifische Sporangium-Reaktion. *Schweiz. Zeitschr. Allg. Pathol. Bakteriol* **21**:914, 1958.

TOMCSIK, J., and J. B. BAUMANN-GRACE. Serologische Typen von *Bacillus cereus* und ihre Verwandschaft mit *Bacillus anthracis*. *Schweiz. Zeitschr. Allg. Pathol. Bakteriol.* **22**:9, 1959.

TOMCSIK, J., and J. B. BAUMANN-GRACE. Specific exosporium reaction of *Bacillus megaterium*. *J. Gen. Microbiol.* **21**:666, 1959.

TOMCSIK, J., M. BOUILLIE, and J. B. BAUMANN-GRACE. Reaction specifique de l'exosporium chez *Bacillus cereus* et *Bacillus anthracis*. *Schweiz. Zeitschr. Allg. Pathol. Bakteriol.* **22**:630, 1959.

TOMCSIK, J., and S. GUEX-HOLZER. Aenderung der Struktur der Bakterienzelle im Verlauf der Lysozym-Einwirkung. *Schweiz. Zeistchr. Allg. Pathol. Bakteriol.* **15**:517, 1952.

TOMCSIK, J., and S. GUEX-HOLZER. Antikörperproduktion mit isolierter Bakterienzellwand und mit Protoplasten. *Experientia*, **10**:484, 1954.

TOMLISON, J. A. Purification of lettuce mosaic virus. *Nature*, **193**:299, 1962.

TOPLEY, W. W. C., H. RAISTRICK, J. WILSON, M. STACEY, S. W. CHALLINOR, and R. O. J. CLARK. *Lancet*, **I**:252, 1937.

TORHEIM, B. J. Immunochemical investigations in *Geotrichum* and certain related fungi. II. Isolation and chemical analysis of polysaccharides. *Sabouraudia*, **2**:155, 1963.

TORREY, J. A. Comparative study of antigens for the gonococcal complement fixation. *J. Immunol.* **38**:413, 1940.

TOURVILLE, D. R., R. H. ADLER, J. BIENENSTOCK, and T. B. TOMASI. The human secretory immunoglobulin system: Immunohistological localization of γA, secretory "piece," and lactoferrin in normal human tissues. *J. Exper. Med.* **129**:411, 1969.

TOUSSAINT, A. J., and R. I. ANDERSON. Soluble antigen fluorescent-antibody technique. *Appl. Microbiol.* **13**:552, 1965.

TOZER, B. T., K. A. CAMMACK, and H. SMITH. Separation of antigens by immunological specificity. II. Release of antigen and antibody from their complexes by aqueous carbon dioxide. *Biochim. J.* **84**:80, 1962.

TRACEY, M. V. Determination of glucosamine by alkaline decomposition. *Biochem. J.* **52**:265, 1952.

TRAUB, F. B., A. BRASCH, and W. HUBER. Effect of high intensity electron bursts on antibodies. *J. Immunol.* **70**:366, 1953.

TRELOAR, A. E. *Biometric Analysis*. University of Minnesota Press, 1951.

TRETHEWIE, E. R., and C. RUMBERG. The effect of salicylate on the in vitro antigen-antibody reaction in anaphylaxis. *Austral. J. Exper. Biol. Med. Sci.* **37**:77, 1959.

TREVELYAN, A. E., and H. S. HARRISON. Yeast metabolism. I. Fractionation and microdetermination of carbohydrates. *Biochem. J.* **50**:298, 1952.

TREVELYAN, A. E., D. P. PROCTER, and J. S. HARRISON. Detection of sugars on paper chromatograms. *Nature*, **166**:444, 1950.

TRIFTSHAUSER, C., D. W. HAYDEN, and E. H. BEUTNER. Procedures for the immunization of goats with human immunoglobulins and complement. *Int. Arch. Allergy Appl. Immunol.* **38**:315, 1970.

TROLL, W., and R. K. CANNAN. A modified photometric method for the analysis of amino and imino acids. *J. Biol. Chem.* **200**:803, 1953.

TROUT, D. L., E. H. ESTES, JR., and S. J. FRIEDBERG. Titration of free fatty acids of plasma: A study of current methods and a new modification. *J. Lipid Res.* **1**:199, 1960.

TRUSZCZYNSKI, M. Middlebrook-Dubos reaction in erysipelas. *Bull. Acad. Pol. Sci.* **5**:413, 1957.

TSAI, L. H. The production of diphtheric antitoxin in tissue-culture. *J. Immunol.* **33**:471, 1937.

TUBYLEWICZ, H. Comparative studies on the antigenic structure of eight strains of *Listeria monocytogenes*. *Arch. Immunol. Ther. Exper.* **11**:341, 1963.

TULLIS, J. L. Preservation of leukocytes. *Blood*, **8**:563, 1953.

TULLIS, J. L., and D. M. SURGENOR. Phagocytosis promoting factor of plasma and serum. *Ann. N.Y. Acad. Sci.* **66**:386, 1956.

TULLOCH, W. J. Report of bacteriological investigation of tetanus carried out on behalf of the War Office Committee for the Study of Tetanus. *J. Hygiene*, **18**:103, 1919.

TULLY, J. G., and S. GAINES. H antigen of *Salmonella typhosa*. *J. Bacteriol.* **81**:924, 1961.

TUNEVALL, C. Studies on *Haemophilus influenzae* type characteristics. *Acta Pathol. Microbiol. Scandinav.* **30**:203, 1952.

TURK, J. Immune-adherence with soluble antigens. *Immunology*, **1**:305, 1958.

TURNER, E. W., and P. D. BOYER. Interaction of protein antigens and antibodies. III. Dissociation studies with diphtheria toxoid-antitoxin precipitation. *J. Immunol.* **69**:265, 1952.

UCHIDA, H., S. SUNAKAWA, and H. FUKUMI. Studies on the bacterial flagella. I. Method of purification. *Jap. J. Med. Sci. Biol.* **5**:351, 1952.

UHLENHUT, P. Antiformin, ein bakterienauflösendes Mittel. *Zentralbl. Bakteriol.* Abt. Ref., 42, Beiheft 62, 1909.

UHR, J. W., and J. B. BAUMANN. Antibody formation. 7. The suppression of antibody formation by passively administered antibody. *J. Exper. Med.* **113**:935, 1961.

UHR, J. W., S. B. SALVIN, and A. M. PAPPENHEIMER, JR. Delayed hypersensitivity. II. Induction of hypersensitivity in guinea pig by means of antigen-antibody complexes. *J. Exper. Med.* **105**:11, 1957.

ULLMAN, W. W., and J. A. CAMERON. Immunochemistry of the cell walls of *Listeria monocytogenes*. *J. Bacteriol.* **98**:486, 1969.

UNGER, L. J. A method for detecting Rh_o antibodies in extremely low titer. *J. Lab. Clin. Med.* **39**:825, 1952.

UNGER, L. J. Rh-Hr factors and their specific antibodies, as applied to blood transfusion. *Amer. J. Clin. Pathol.* **24**:275, 1954.

UNGER, L. J., and L. KATZ. Variation in anti-human globulin titration results. *J. Lab. Clin. Med.* **39**:246, 1952.

URIEL, J., and P. GRABAR. Emploi de colorants dans l'analyse électrophorétique et immuno-électrophorétique en milieu gélifie. *Ann. Inst. Pasteur*, **90**:427, 1956.

URIEL, J., and J. J. SCHEIDEGGER. Electrophorèse en gèlose et coloration des constituants. *Bull. Soc. Chim. Biol.* **37**:165, 1955.

VAJDA, G., and R. BAKHAUSZ. Wertbemessung agglutinierender Immunsera mit der Filtrierpapiermethode. *Acta Microbiol. Sci. Hung.* **1**:349, 1954.

VALENTINE, R. C., and N. M. GREEN. Electron microscopy of an antibody-hapten complex. *J. Mol. Biol.* **27**:615, 1967.

VALKENBRUG, H. A. Latex fixation test. In *Epidemiology of Chronic Rheumatism*, M. R. Jeffrey and J. Ball, Eds., Vol. 1. Blackwell Scientific Publication, Oxford, 1963, p. 337.

VAN DER SCHEER, J., M. BOHNEL, and H. R. COX. Diagnostic antigens for peidemic typhus, murine typhus and Rocky Mountain spotted fever. *J. Immunol.* **56**:365, 1947.

VAN HANDEL, E. Suggested modifications of the micro determination of triglycerides. *Clin. Chem.* **7**:249, 1961.

VAN OSS, C. J., and P. M. BRONSON. Immunorheophoresis. *Immunochem.* **6**:775, 1969.

VARDMAN, T. H., and A. B. LARSEN. Bovine tuberculosis studies of complement fixation antigens. *Amer. J. Vet. Res.* **22**:204, 1961.

VARLEY, F., and F. WEEDON. Application of a quantitative complement-fixation test to the serum diagnosis of typhus fever. *J. Immunol.* **51**:139, 1945.

VASILESKII, S. S. *Biul. Eksprtl. Biol. Med.* **48**:1285, 1959.

VASKOVSKY, V. E., and E. Y. KOSTELSKY. Modified spray for the detection of phospholipids on thin-layer chromatograms. *J. Lipid Res.* **9**:396, 1968.

VAUGHAN, J. H. Behavior of the rheumatoid arthritis agglutinating factor with immune precipitates. *J. Immunol.* **77**:181, 1956.

VAUGHAN, J. H., T. B. BAYLES, and B. F. CUTTING. Serum complement in rheumatoid arthritis. *Amer. J. Med. Sci.* **222**:186, 1951.

VAUGHAN, J. H., and E. A. KABAT. An unindentified antibody in anti-egg albumin sera revealed by the agar diffusion technic. *J. Immunol.* **73**:205, 1954.

VAUGHAN, W. *Practice of Allergy.* Mosby, St. Louis, Mo., 1939.

VEEN, VAN DER, J. A raid and simple method for conducting large series of complement fixation tests and antistreptolysin "O" titration. *J. Lab. Clin. Med.* **45**:523, 1955.

VEIL, W. H., and B. BUCHHOLZ. Der Komplementschwund in Blute. *Klin. Wochenschr.* **2**:2019, 1932.

VELDEE, M. The standardization of scarlet fever streptococcus antitoxin. A method employing the ear of the white rabbit. *U.S. Publ. Health Rep.* **47**:1043, 1932.

VELICK, S. F., C. W. PARKER, and H. N. EISEN. Excitation energy transfer and the quantitative study of the antibody-hapten reaction. *Proc. Natl. Acad. Sci. U.S.A.*, **46**:1470, 1960.

VENNES, J. W., and P. GERHARDT. Immunologic comparison of isolated surface membranes of *Bacillus megaterium*. *Science*, **124**:535, 1956.

VENNES, J. W., and P. GERHARDT. Antigenic analysis of cell structures isolated from *Bacillus megaterium*. *J. Bacteriol.* **77**:581, 1959.

VENNES, J. W., R. E. MacDONALD, and P. GERHARDT. Use of logarithms to the base 2 in recording serological reactions. *Nature*, **180**:1363, 1957.

VESTERBERG, O., and H. SVENSSON. Isoelectric fractionation, analysis and characterization of ampholytes in natural pH gradients. IV. Further studies on the resolving power in connection with separation of myoglobins. *Acta Chem. Scandinav.* **20**:820, 1966.

VESTERBERG, O., T. WADSTRÖM, K. VESTERBERG, H. SVENSSON, and B. MALMGRAN. Studies on extracellular proteins from *Staphylococcus aureus*. I. Separation and characterization of enzymes and toxins by isoelectric focusing. *Biochim. Biophys. Acta*, **133**:435, 1967.

VICTOR, J., R. RAYMOND, J. WAGNER, and A. POLLACK. Studies on opsonins in Q fever. *J. Epxer. Med.* **95**:61, 1952.

VIKTOROW, L. K., and E. MASEL. Bakteriologie der kruppösen Pneumonie. Ueber eine typenspezifische Reaktion des Harns bei kruppöser Pneumonie. *Zentralbl. Bakteriol. I. Orig.* **131**:73, 1934.

VINCENT, B. A rapid macroscopic agglutination test for blood groups and its value in testing donors for transfusion. *J. Amer. Med. Assoc.* **lxx**:1219, 1918.

VINCENT, W. F., E. W. HARRIS, and S. YAVERBAUM. The estimation of precipitating antibody using a turbidimetric technique. *Immunology*, **18**:143, 1970.

VIRAT, J. La reaction de fixation du complement pour un diagnostic precoce de la poliomyelite. *Ann. Inst. Pasteur.* **101**:125, 1961.

VOGEL, J., and A. SHELOKOV. Adsorption-hemagglutination test for influenza virus in monkey kidney tissue culture. *Science*, **126**:358, 1957.

VOGEL, R., and M. COLLINS. Haemagglutination test for detection of *Candida albicans* antibodies in rabbit antiserum. *Proc. Soc. Exper. Biol. Med.* **89**:138, 1955.

VOGEL, R. A., and J. F. PADULA. Indirect staining reaction with fluorescent antibody for detection of antibodies to pathogenic fungi. *Proc. Soc. Exper. Biol. Med.* **98**:135, 1958.

VOS, G. H., and G. KEISALL. A new elution technique for the preparation of specific immune anti-Rh serum. *Brit. J. Haemat.* **2**:342, 1956.

VOŠTA, J. Diagnostika leptospiros latex-aglutinaci metodu. *Českoslov. Parastitol.* **10**:285, 1963.

VOSTI, K. L., and L. A. RANTZ. The measurement of type and nontype specific group A hemolytic streptococcal antibody with an hemagglutination technique. *J. Immunol.* **92**:185, 1964.

VYAZOV, O. E., B. V. KONYUKHOV, and L. L. LISTHVAN. *Biul. Eksperim. Biol. Med.* **47**:646, 1959.

WADDELL, W. J. A simple ultraviolet spectrophotometric method for the determination of proteins. *J. Lab. Clin. Med.* **48**:311, 1956.

WADSWORTH, A. *Standard Methods of the Division of Laboratories and Research of The New York State Department of Health*, 2nd ed. Williams & Wilkins, Baltimore, Md., 1927, 1939.

WADSWORTH, A., and R. BROWN. Chemical and immunological studies of pneumococcus. *J. Immunol.* **32**:**467**, 1937.

WADSWORTH, A., E. MALTANER, and F. MALTANER. The antigenic action of the phosphatides. Further studies of purified cephalin. *J. Immunol.* **28**:183, 1935.

WADSWORTH, A., F. MALTANER, and E. MALTANER. The quantitative determination of the fixation of complement by immune serum and antigen. *J. Immunol.* **21**:313, 1931.

WADSWORTH, A., F. MALTANER, and E. MALTANER. Quantitative studies of the reaction of complement fixation with syphilitic serum and tissue extract. *J. Immunol.* **35**:105, 1938.

WADSWORTH, A., F. MALTANER, and E. MALTANER. Quantitative studies of the reaction of complement fixation with tuberculous immune serum and antigen. *J. Immunol.* **35**:93, 1938.

WADSWORTH, A., F. MALTANER, and E. MALTANER. Quantitative studies of the complement fixation reaction with syphilitic and tissue extracts; technic of the practical quantitative test. *J. Immunol.* **35**:217, 1938.

WADSWORTH, A., and J. J. QUIGLEY. Studies on purification of diphtheria toxin by ultrafiltration. *Amer. J. Hyg.* **20**:225, 1934.

WADSWORTH, C. A slide microtechnique for the analysis of immune precipitins in gel. *Intern. Arch. Allergy*, **10**:355, 1957.

WAGNER, M. Methods of labelling antibodies for electron microscopic localization of antigens. In *Research in Immunochemistry and Immunology*, J. B. G. Kwapinski, Ed., Vol. 3. University Park Press, Baltimore, 1972.

WAKSMAN, B. H. Specific cell lysis produced by combination of rabbit antiserum to purified protein with homologous antigen. *J. Immunol.* **70**:331, 1953.

WAKSMAN, H. B., and S. J. BULLINGTON. A quantitative study of the passive Arthus reaction in the rabbit eye. *J. Immunol.* **76**:441, 1956.

WALDI, D. Application of thin-layer chromatography in the clinical laboratory. *Ergeb. Laboratoriumsmed.* **2**:155, 1965.

WALKER, D. L., and F. L. HORSFALL, JR. Lack of identify in neutralizing and haemagglutination-inhibiting antibodies against influenza viruses. *J. Exper. Med.* **91**:65, 1950.

WALKER, H. W., J. R. MATCHES, and T. C. AYRES. Chemical composition and heat resistance of some aerobic bacterial spores. *J. Bacteriol.* **82**:960, 1961.

WALKER, P. D. *A study of biochemical, physiological and serological properties of some strains of Bacterium stearothermophilus.* Ph. Dissertation, University of Leeds, England, 1959.

WALKER, R. V. Studies on the immune response of guinea pigs to the envelope substance of *Pasteurella pestis.* I. Immunogenicity and persistence of large doses of fraction I in guinea pigs observed with fluorescent antibody. *J. Immunol.* **88**:153, 1962.

WALLACE, A. L., A. G. OSLER, and M. M. MAYER. Quantitative studies of complement fixation. V. Estimation of complement-fixing potency of immune sera and its relation to antibody-nitrogen content. *J. Immunol.* **65**:661, 1950.

WALLACE, J., and A. WORMALL. Red cell adhesion in trypanosomiasis of man and other animals. II. Some experiments on the mechanism of the reaction. *Parasitology,* **23**:346, 1931.

WALLACE, R., B. B. DIENA, L. GREENBERG, and A. G. JESSAMINE. A study of tuberculosis antibodies by bentonite flocculation. *Can. Med. Assoc. J.* **94**:947, 1966.

WALLACE, R., B. B. DIENA, H. YUGI, and L. GREENBERG. The bentonite flocculation test in the assay of *Neisseria* antibody. *Can. J. Microbiol.* **16**:655, 1970.

WALLIS, A. D. Rheumatoid arthritis. III. The pneumococcus antibodies. *Amer. J. Med. Sci.* **212**:718, 1946.

WALSH, P., P. MAURER, and M. EGAN. Detection of immune response against synthetic polymers of amino acids employing the plaque-forming cell system. I. Reaction with sheep erythrocytes coated with polymer. *J. Immunol.* **98**:344, 1967.

WALTON, K., and H. ELLIS. A method for serial determination of serum complement. *Immunology,* **1**:224, 1958.

WALTON, K., H. ELLIS, and C. TAYLOR. A method for the determination of anticomplementary activity of heparin and related compounds. *Brit. J. Exper. Pathol.* **38**:237, 1957.

WANG, A. C., and H. H. FUDENBERG. Genetic control of gamma chain synthesis: A chemical and evolutionary study of the Gm(a) factor of immunoglobulins. *J. Mol. Biol.* **44**:493, 1969.

WARBURG, O., and W. CHRISTIAN. Die Isolierung der kristallischen Enolase. *Biochem. Zeitschr.* **310**:384, 1942.

WARBURTON, M. and S. FISHER. The haemagglutinin of *Haemophilus pertussis. Austral. J. Exper. Biol. Med. Sci.* **29**:265, 1951.

WARBURTON, M. E. KEOCH, and S. WILLIAMS. A haemagglutination test for the diagnosis of influenzal meningitis. *Med. J. Australia,* **1**:135, 1949.

WARDLAW, A. C., and L. PILLEMER. The demonstration of the bactericidal activity of the properdin system. *Ann. N.Y. Acad. Sci.* **66**:244, 1956.

WARREN, L. Thiobarbituric acid spray reagent for deoxy sugars and sialic acid. *Nature,* **186**:237, 1960.

WARREN, L. The thiobarbituric acid assay of sialic acid. *J. Biol. Chem.* **234**:1971, 1959.

WARREN, S., and F. J. DIXON. Antigen tracer studies and histologic observations in anaphylactic shock in the quinea pig. *Amer. J. Med. Sci.* **216**:136, 1948.

WASSERMAN, E., and L. LEVINE. Quantitative micro-complement fixation and its use in the study of antigenic structure by specific antigen-antibody inhibition. *J. Immunol.* **87**:290, 1961.

WASSERMAN, E., and L. LEVINE. The use of complement fixation for study of polysaccharide structure. *Fed. Proc.* **19**:205, 1960.

WASSERMAN, A., A. NEISSER, and C. BRUCK. Eine serodiagnostische Reaktion bei Syphilis. *Deutsche Med. Wochenschr.* **32**:745, 1906.

WASSERMANN, P. The rate of complement-formation in dogs. *J. Immunol.* **40**:281, 1941.

WATANABE, Y., and O. FELSENFELD. Serological analysis of supernatant liquids of cultures of El Tor vibrios. *J. Bacteriol.* **85**:31, 1963.

WATKINS, J. F., and D. M. GRACE. Studies on the surface antigens on interspecific mammalian cell heterokaryons. *J. Cell. Sci.* **2**:193, 1957.

WATSON, B. K. Distribution of mumps virus in tissue cultures as determined by fluorescein labeled antiserum. *Proc. Soc. Exper. Biol. Med.* **79**:222 1952.

WATSON, D. W. Host-parasite factors in group of streptococcal infections. Pyrogenic and other effects of immunologically distinct exotoxins related to scarlet fever toxin. *J. Exper. Med.* **111**:255, 1960.

WATSON, D. W., W. J. CROMARTIE, W. L. BLOOM, C. KEGLES, and R. J. HECKLY. Studies on infection with *Bacillus anthracis*. III. Chemical and immunological properties of the protective antigen in crude extracts of skin lesions of *B. anthracis. J. Infect. Dis.* **80**:28, 1947.

WATSON, R. G. A more specific method for detecting and quantitating rheumatoid factors using a simple modification of the RA-test. *Amer. J. Clin. Pathol.* **43**:152, 1965.

WAYMOUTH, C. Rapid proliferation of sublines of NCTC above 929 (strain L) mouse cells in a simple chemically defined medium. *J. Natl. Cancer Inst.* **22**:1003, 1959.

WEBB, J. M. A sensitive method for the determination of ribonucleic acid in tissues and microorganisms. *J. Biol. Chem.* **221**:634, 1956.

WEBB, J. M., and H. B. LEVY. A sensitive method for the determination of deoxyribonucleic acid in tissues and microorganisms. *J. Biol. Chem.* **213**:107, 1955.

WEBBER, M. M. Antibody suppression by antigen heavily labeled with iodine-131. *Science,* **143**:132, 1964.

WEBSTER, M. E., M. LANDY, and M. E. FREEMAN. Studies on Vi antigen. II. Purification of Vi antigen from *Escherichia coli* 3396/38. *J. Immunol.* **69**:135, 1952.

WEBSTER, M. E., J. F. SAGIN, M. LANDY, and A. G. JOHNSON. Studies of the O antigen of *Salmonella typhosa*. I. Purification of the antigen. *J. Immunol.* **74**:455, 1955.

WEBSTER, R. G., W. G. LAVER, and S. FAZEKAS DE ST. GROTH. Methods in immunochemistry of viruses. 3. Simple techniques for labeling antibodies with ^{131}I and ^{35}S. *Austral. J. Exper. Biol. Med. Sci.* **40**:321, 1962.

WEDGWOOD, R., and C. JANEWAY. Serum complement in children with "collagen diseases." *Pediactrics,* **11**:569, 1953.

WEDGWOOD, R., and L. PILLEMER. The nature of interactions of the properdin system. *Acta Haematol.* **20**:253, 1959.

WEETALL, H. H. Immunoadsorbent for the isolation of bacterial specific antibodies. *J. Bacteriol.* **93**:1876, 1967.

WEIBULL, C. Some chemical and physico-chemical properties of the flagella of *Proteus vulgaris. Biochim. Biophys. Acta,* **2**:351, 1948.

WEIBULL, C. The isolation of protoplasts from *Bacillus megaterium* by controlled treatment with lysozyme. *J. Bacteriol.* **66**:688, 1953.

WEIBULL, C. Bacterial protoplasts: Their formation and characteristics. In *Bacterial Anatomy*, Spooner and Stockers, Eds. University Press, Cambridge, England, 1956.

WEIBULL, C., and H. BECKMAN. Chemical and metabolic properties of various elements found in culture of stable *Proteus* L forms. *J. Gen. Microbiol.* **24**:379, 1961.

WEICHSELBAUM, I. An accurate and rapid method for the detection of proteins in small amounts of blood serum and plasma. *Amer. J. Clin. Pathol. (Techn. Sect.)* **10**:40, 1946.

WEIGLE, W. O., and P. H. MAURER. The molecular ratios of soluble rabbit antigen-antibody complexes. *J. Immunol.* **79**:223, 1957.

WEIGLE, W. O., and P. H. MAURER. Behavior of complement in antigen-antibody-complement precipitaes. *J. Immunol.* **79**:319, 1957.

WEIL, A. Agglutination by anti-hog cholera hyperimmune sera of an antigen obtained from the spinal fluid of pigs infected with hog cholera and adsorbed on *B. prodigiosus. J. Immunol.* **45**:187, 1942.

WEIL, A., F. POPKEN, and I. BLACK. Agglutination of antigens from distemper infected dogs and ferrets by anticanine-distemper immune sera. *J. Immunol.* **48**:355, 1944.

WEIL, A., and I. SAPHRA. Incidence of antibodies to salmonellae amongst the population of Bronx, N.Y. *J. Immunol.* **74**:485, 1955.

WEIL, A., and I. SAPHRA. Antibodies to shigellae in normal immune sera. *J. Immunol.* **74**:488, 1955.

WEIL, A., and E. SHERMAN. Antigenic relationships of pneumococci to erythrocytes and organs of men and animals. *J. Immunol.* **37**:139, 1939.

WEIL, E. Über die Wirkungsweise des Streptokokkensimmunserums. *Zeitschr. Hyg. Infektionskr.* **ixxv**:245, 1913.

WEIL, E., and A. FELIX. Zur serologischen Diagnose des Fleckfiebers. *Wien. Klin. Wochenschr.* **29**:33, 1916.

WEIL, E., and A. FELIX. Ueber den Doppeltypus der Rezeptoren in der Typhus-Paratyphus Gruppe. *Zeitschr. Immunitätsforsch.* **29**:24, 1920.

WEIL, E., and A. FELIX. Ueber die Beziehungen der Fleckfieberagglutination zum Fleckfiebererreger. *Zeitschr. Immunitätsforsch.* **31**:457, 1921.

WEIL, R. *J. Immunol.* **2**:525, 1916–1917.

WEIN, J. Two-dimensional polyacrylamide gel electrophoresis in sigmoid gradients. *Anal. Biochem.* **31**:405, 1969.

WEINER, L., and S. PRICE. Study of antigenic relationships between *Trichinella spiralis* and *Salmonella typhi*. *J. Immunol.* **77**:111, 1956.

WEINER, W. Eluting red cell antibodies. A method and its application. *Brit. J. Haematol.* **3**:276, 1957.

WEINMAN, D. A natural haemolysin from the rat producing nuclear lysis of chicken erythrocytes. *J. Immunol.* **32**:1, 1937.

WEIR, I. Technic for demonstrating antibodies against tuberculin in experimental animals with sensitized collodion pellets. *Proc. Soc. Exper. Biol. Med.* **46**:47, 1941.

WEISS, E. S. An abridged table of probits for use in the graphic solution of dosage-effect curve. *Amer. J. Publ. Health*, **38**:221, 1948.

WELLER, T. H., and A. COONS. Fluorescent antibody studies with agents of varicella and herpes zoster propagated in vitro. *Proc. Soc. Exper. Biol. Med.* **86**:789, 1954.

WELLER, T. H., and H. M. WITTON. The etiologic agents of varicella and herpes zoster. Serologic studies with the viruses propaged in vitro. *J. Exper. Med.* **108**:869, 1958.

WELLS, H. *Chemical Aspects of Immunity*. Chemical Catalogue Co., New York, 1929.

WELSCH, M. *Phènomenes d'antibiose chez les actinomycètes*. Gemboux, Duculot, 1947.

WELSCH, M., and P. OSTERRIETH. A comparative study of the transformation of Gram-negative rods into "protoplasts" under the influence of penicillin and glycin. *Ant. van Leeuwenhoek J. Microbiol.* **24**:257, 1958.

WENNER, H. A., M. JENSON, and A. MONLEY. A study of infections caused by mumps and Newcastle disease viruses. I. Specific and non-spccific serological reactions. *J. Immunol.* **68**:343, 1952.

WENNER, H., A. MONLEY, and R. TOOD. Studies on complement fixation with Newcastle disease virus. *J. Immunol.* **64**:323, 1950.

WERNER, I., and L. ODIN. On presence of sialic acid in certain glycoproteins and in gangliosides. *Acta. Soc. Med. Uppsalien.* **57**:230, 1952.

WEST, C. D., V. HINRICHS, and N. H. HINKLE. Quantitative determination of the serum globulins beta 2A and beta 2M by immuno-electrophoretic analysis. *J. Lab. Clin. Med.* **58**:137, 1961.

WESTPHAL, O., O. LÜDERITZ, and F. BISTER. Ueber die Extraktion von Bakterien mit Phenol/Wasser. *Zeitschr. Naturforsch.* **7b**:148, 1952.

WESTPHAL, O., O. LÜDERITZ, E. EICHENBERGER, and W. KEIDERLING. Ueber bakterielle Reizstoffe. 1. Reindarstellung eines Polysaccharid-pyrogens aus Bacterium coli. *Z. Naturforsch.* **7**:536, 1952.

WESTPHAL, O., O. LÜDERITZ, I. FROME, and N. JOSEPH. *Angew. Chemie*, **66**:407, 1954.

WESTPHAL, O., O. LÜDERITZ, and W. KEIDERLING. Ueber die Wirkungsweise bakterieller Reizstoffe. *Zentralbl. Bakteriol. I. Orig.* **158**:152, 1952.

WESTWATER, J. Antibody formation in a lesion produced by tubercle bacilli suspended in paraffin oil: excision of the antigenic depot. *J. Immunol.* **39**:267, 1940.

WETTSTEIN, F. O., T. STAEHELIN, and H. NOLL. Ribosomal aggregate engated in protein synthesis: Characterization of ergosome. *Nature*, **197**:430, 1963.

WHANG, H. Y., and E. NETER. Immunological studies of a heterogenetic enterobacterial antigen (Kunin). *J. Bacteriol.* **84**:1245, 1962.

WHEELER, D. E., JR., R. A. BRIGGAMAN, and R. R. HENDERSON. *Proc. Soc. Exper. Biol. Med.* **127**:814, 1968.

WHEELER, C. E., JR., R. A. BRIGGAMAN, and R. R. HENDERSON. Discrimination between two strains (types) of herpes simplex virus by various modifications of the neutralization test. *J. Immunol.* **102**:1179, 1969.

WHEELER, K. Group-specific agglutinins in rabbit serum for human cells. *J. Immunol.* **34**:409, 1938.

WHEELER, K., A. LUHBY, and M. SCHOLL. The action of enzymes in haemagglutinating systems. II. Agglutinating properties of trypsin-modified red cells with anti-Rh sera. *J. Immunol.* **64**:39, 1950.

WHEELER, K., P. SAVIN, and C. STUART, Group-specific agglutinins in rabbit serums for human cells. *J. Immunol.* **37**:159, 1939.

WHEELER, K., M. SCHOLL, and A. LUHBY. Action of enzymes in haemagglutinating systems. I. The use of trypsin treated red blood cells for the detection of anti-Rh antibodies. *Health Centre*, **2**:86, 1949.

WHEELOCK, E. F., and I. TAMM. Enumeration of cell-infecting particles of Newcastle disease virus by the fluorescent antibody technique. *J. Exper. Med.* **113**:301, 1961.

WHILLANS, D., and A. FISHMAN. Rose-Waaler test using a rapidly prepared serum fraction. *Ann. Rheumat. Dis.* **17**:383, 1958.

WHITE, R. G. Antibody production by single cells. *Nature*, **182**:1383, 1958.

WHITE, R. G. Fluorescent antibody techniques. In *Tools of Biological Research*, H. J. B. Atkins, Ed., Blackwell Science Publications, Oxford, England. 1960, p. 89.

WHITE, R. G., L. BERNSTOCK, R. G. JOHNS, and E. LEDERER. The influence of components of *M. tuberculosis* and other mycobacteria upon antibody production of ovalbumin. *Immunology*, **1**:54, 1959.

WHITE, R. G., A. H. COONS, and J. M. CONNOLLY. Studies on antibody production. III. The alum granuloma. *J. Exper. Med.* **102**:73, 1955.

WHITE, R. G., A. H. COONS, and J. M. CONNOLLY. Studies on antibody production. IV. The role of wax fraction of *Mycrobacterium tuberculosis* in adjuvant emulsion on the production of antibody to egg albumin. *J. Exper. Med.* **102**:83, 1955.

WHITE, R. G., R. M. SIMPSON, and G. R. SCOTT. An antigenic relationship between the viruses of bovine rinderpest canine distemper. *Immunology*, **4**:203, 1961.

WICKER, R., and S. AVRAMEAS. Application de l'autoradiographie associée aux technique immuno-enzymatique a lètude des antigenes et des anticorps. *C. R. Acad. Sci. ser. D.* **270**:431, 1970.

WIDAL, F. *Bull. Mem. Soc. Hop. Paris*, **6**:26, 1896.

WIDELOCK, D. The VDRL slide test. A comparison with the Mazzini, Kahn, and Kolmer tests for syphilis. *Amer. J. Clin. Pathol.* **18**:218, 1948.

WIEME, R. J. *Studies in Agar Gel Electrophoresis.* Arscia Uitgaven N.V., Brussels, 1959.

WIEME, R. J. An integrated procedure for acrylamide gel electrophoresis. In *Protides of Biological Fluids. Proc. 10th Coll., Bruges, Belgium,* 10:309, 1962.

WIEME, R. J. A procedure for high voltage electrophoresis in agar gel, with a note on its application to acrylamide and starch gel. *Ann. N.Y. Acad. Sci.* 121:366, 1964.

WIENER, A. S. Individuality of the blood in higher animals. II. Agglutinogens in red blood cells of fowls. *J. Genetics,* 29:1, 1934.

WIENER, A. S. *Blood Groups and Blood Transfusion.* Thomas, Springfield, Ill., 1935.

WIENER, A. S. New test (blocking test) for Rh sensitization. *Proc. Soc. Exper. Biol. Med.* 56:173, 1944.

WIENER, A. S. Nomenclature of Rh factors. *Lancet,* 254:343, 1948.

WIENER, A. S. Origin of naturally occurring haemagglutinins and haemolysins. *J. Immunol.* 63:286, 1951.

WIENER, A. S., and E. C. GORDON. Studies on the conglutination test in erythroblastois fetalis. *J. Lab. Clin. Med.* 33:181, 1948.

WIENER, A. S., and L. KATZ. Studies on use of enzyme-treated red cells in tests for Rh sensitization. *J. Immunol.* 66:51, 1951.

WIENER, A. S., R. ZINSHER, and J. SELKOWE. The agglutinogens M and N of Landsteiner and Levine. *J. Immunol.* 27:431, 1934.

WIGAUD, R. Erfahrungen mit der Mikromethode der Komplement-bindungsreaktion. *Zeitschr. Hyg. Infektionskrankh.* 143:188, 1956.

WIKMAN, J., E. HOWARD, and H. BUSCH. Studies on the primary structure of ribosomal 28S ribonucleic acid and its nucleolar precursors. *J. Biol. Chem.* 244:5471, 1969.

WILKIE, M. H., and E. L. BECKER. Quantitative studies in haemagglutination. I. Assay of anti-beta-isohaemagglutinins. *J. Immunol.* 74:192, 1955.

WILKINSON, G. K., and G. N. WILKINSON. Factors affecting the staining process in the quantitative estimation of serum proteins by paper electrophoresis. *Austral. J. Exper. Biol. Med. Sci.* 38:487, 1960.

WILLIAMS, C. A. Studies on fractions of methanol extracts of tubercle bacilli. II. Toxic and allergenic properties of fractions employed as tuberculous vaccine. *J. Exper. Med.* 111:369, 1960.

WILLIAMS, C. A., and R. DUBOS. Studies on fractions of methanol extracts of tubercle bacilli. *J. Exper. Med.* 110:981, 1959.

WILLIAMS, C. A., JR., and P. GRABAR. Immunoelectrophoretic studies on serum proteins. I. The antigens of human serum. *J. Immunol.* 74:158, 1955.

WILLIAMS, C. A., and E. L. TATUM. Immunoelectrophoretic analysis of cytoplasmic proteins of *Neurospora cras:a. J. Gen. Microbiol.* 44:59, 1966.

WILLIAMS, H. "Essential" amino acid content of animal feeds. Cornell University Agricultural Experimental Station Memo. 337, 1955.

WILLIAMS, R., and R. SYNGE. *Partition Chromatography.* Cambridge, England, 1951.

WILLIAMSON, A. R., and S. ZAMENHOF. Detection and rapid differentiation of glucosamine, galactosamine, glucosmaine uronic acid, and galactosamine uronic acid. *Anal. Biochem.* 5:47, 1963.

WILSON, A. T. Direct immunoelectrphoresis. *J. Immunol.* 92:431, 1964.

WILSON, M. W. The agar diffusion precipitin technique: A comparison of the simple and double diffusion methods. *J. Immunol.* 81:317, 1958.

WILSON, M. W., and B. PRINGLE. Experimental studies of the agar-plate precipitin test of Ouchterlony. *J. Immunol.* 73:232, 1954.

WILSON, M. W., and B. PRINGLE. Interpretation of the Ouchterlony plate: analysis of native and halogenated bovine serum albumins. *J. Immunol.* 77:324, 1956.

WILSON, R. H., V. E. DOTY, K. H. RENCZ, and A. C. SCHRAM. Gas chromatographic analysis of high molecular weight fatty acid methyl esters with the technique of relative molar response. *J. Lab. Clin. Med.* **67**:87, 1966.

WINBLAD, S. Studies in the laboratory estimation of the rheumatoid arthritis serum factor. 2. Gamma-globulin precipitation test in relation to haemagglutination test with sensitized sheep cells and acrylplast flocculation test. *Acta Pathol. Microbiol. Scandinav.* **49**:515, 1960.

WINBLAD, S. Studies in laboratory estimation of rheumatoid arthritis serum factor. 4. The role of gamma globulin and albumin for the acryl particles for RAS factor. *Acta Pathol. Microbiol. Scandinav.* **52**:241, 1961.

WINN, H., M. DODD, and C. WRIGHT. Quantitative determination of haemagglutination for normal and trypsinized human red blood cells. *J. Immunol.* **71**:261, 1953.

WINTER, C. C., and M. D. MOODY. Rapid identification of *Pasteurella pestis* with fluorescent antibody. I. Production of specific anti-serum with whole cell *Pasteurella antigen. J. Infect. Dis.* **104**:274, 1959.

WISSEMAN, C. L., E. B. JACKSON, F. E. HAHN, A. C. LEY, and J. E. SMADEL. Metabolic studies of rickettsiae. *J. Immunol.* **67**:123, 1951.

WISSLER, R., M. ROBSON, R. FITCH, W. NELSON, and L. JACOBSON. The effects of spleen shielding and subsequent splenectomy upon antibody formation in rats receiving total body irradiation. *J. Immunol.* **70**:378, 1953.

WITEBSKY, E., N. KLENDSHOF, and N. P. SWANS. *Blood Substitutes and Blood Transfusion.* Thomas, Springfield, Ill., 1942.

WITEBSKY, E., R. KLINGENSTEIN, and H. KUHN. Seriodiagnostische Untersuchungen bei Tuberkulose. *Klin. Wochenschr.* **10**:1086, 1961.

WITEBSKY, E., N. ROSE, and S. SHUHMAN. Studies of organ specificity. I. The serological specificity of thyroid extracts. *J. Immunol.* **75**:269, 1955.

WITMER, R. Beitrag zur Hämagglutination nach Middlebrook und Dubos mit besonderer Berücksichtigung der Augentuberkulose. *Schweiz. Med. Wochenschrift,* **82**:449, 1952.

WITTKOWER, E. Die Veränderungen des Blutes bei der Anaphylaxie. *Zeitschr. Ges. Exper. Med.* **34**:108, 1923.

WOLBERG, G., T. L. CHI, and F. L. ADLER. Studies on passive hemagglutination. I. Titration of "early" and "late" antibodies with tanned red cells sensitized with native and denaturated bovine serum albumin. *J. Immunol.* **103**:879, 1969.

WOLFE, D. M., and L. KORNFELD. Conglutinating complement adsorption test compared with hemolytic complement-fixation reactions using Q fever immune bovine serum. *Proc. Soc. Exper. Biol. Med.* **69**:251, 1948.

WOLFE, D. M., and L. KORNFELD. The application of qualitative complement-fixation method to a study of Q fever strain differentiation. *J. Immunol.* **61**:297, 1949.

WOLFE, D. M., L. KORNFELD, and F. MARKHAM. Simplified indirect complement fixation test applied to Newcastle disease avian serum. *Proc. Soc. Exper. Biol. Med.* **70**:490, 1949.

WOLFE, H. The effect of injection methods on the species specificity of serum precipitins. *J. Immunol.* **29**:11, 1935.

WOLFE, H. The specificity of precipitins of serum. *J. Immunol.* **32**:103, 1937.

WOLFF-EISNER, A. Die Bindungsverhaltnisse der Organgewebe genenüber Toxinen und ihre klinische Bedeutung für Inkubation und natürliche Immunität. *Zentralbl. Bakteriol. I. Orig.* **70**:213. 1908.

WOMACK, C., and P. HUNT. Serologic differences in strains of herpes simplex virus. *Science,* **120**:227, 1954.

WONG, S., and T. T'UNG. Polysaccharides of *Corynebacterium diphtheriae. Proc. Soc. Exper. Biol. Med.* **39**:422, 1938.

WONG, S., and T. T'UNG. Type-specific polysaccharides of *Corynebacterium diphtheriae*. *Proc. Soc. Exper. Biol. Med.* **41**:160, 1939.

WOOD, B. T., S. H. THOMPSON, and G. GOLDSTEIN. Fluorescent antibody staining. III. Preparation of fluorescein isothio-cyanate-labeled antibodies. *J. Immunol.* **95**:225, 1965.

WOOD, R., and F. SNYDER. Characterization and identification of glyceryl ether diesters present in tumor cells. *J. Lipid Res.* **8**:494, 1967.

WOODIN, A. M. Fractionation of a leucocidin from *Staphylococcus aureus*. *Biochem. J.* **73**:225, 1959.

WOODS, M. W., M. LANDY, J. L. WHITBY, and D. BURK. Symposium on bacterial endotoxins. *Bact. Rev.* **25**:447, 1961.

WOODS, W. A., and F. C. ROBBINS. The elution properties of type 1 polioviruses from AL(OH)3 gel. A possible genetic attribute. *Proc. Natl. Acad. Sci. U.S.A.* **47**:1501, 1961.

WOOLRDIGE, R. L. A complement fixation antigen for the serological diagnosis of trachoma. *J. Formosan Med. Assoc.* **59**:355, 1960.

WORK, E. Biochemistry of bacterial cell. *Nature*, **179**:841, 1957.

WRIGHT, A., and S. DOUGLAS. *Proc. Roy. Soc. Ser. B. Biol. Sci.* **72**:364, 1903.

WRIGHT, A., and S. DOUGLAS. An experimental investigation of the role of the blood fluids in connection with phagocytosis. *Proc. Soc. Exper. Biol. Med.* **2**:357, 1904.

WRIGHT, A. E. On some new procedures for the examination of the blood and bacterial cultures in particular. *Lancet*, **II**:11, 1902.

WRIGHT, C., M. DODD, B. BOURONCLE, and A. BUNNER. Production of isohaemagglutinins in rabbits for determination of normal erythrocyte survival by differential haemagglutination. *J. Immunol.* **74**:81, 1955.

WRIGHT, E. S., and J. B. SLEIN. Studies on immunity in anthrax: variation in serum T-agglutinins during anthrax incubation in rabbits. *J. Exper. Med.* **93**:99, 1957.

WRIGHT, G., and R. FEINBERG. Haemagglutination by tularemia antisera: further observations on agglutination of polysaccharide-treated erythrocytes and its inhibition by polysaccharides. *J. Immunol.* **68**:65, 1952.

WRIGHT, G., T. GREEN, and R. KANODE. Studies on immunity in anthrax. *J. Immunol.* **73**:387, 1954.

WRIGHT, S. T. A quantative serum-agar technique. *Nature.* **183**:12, 1959.

WRIGLEY, C. W. Gel electrofocusing—A technique for analysing multiple protein samples by isoelectric focusing. *Science Tools*, **15**:17, 1968.

WRIGLEY, C. W. Protein mapping by combined gel electrofocusing and electrophoresis. Application to the study of genotypic variations in wheat gliadins. *Biochem. Genetics*, **4**:509, 1970.

WULFF, F. On thermostable bactericidal substances demonstrated in human serum, particularly during fever. *J. Immunol.* **27**:451, 1934.

WUNDERLY, C., and V. BUSTAMENTE. Eine verbesserte Technik der Elektrophorese in Agargel. *Klin. Wochenschr.* **35**:758, 1957.

WUNDERLY, C., and V. BUSTAMENTE. Die Proteinanalyse des schweizerischen Standard-Trockenserums. *Clin. Chim. Acta*, **3**:92, 1958.

WUNDERLY, C., and A. HÄSSIG. Spectrophotometric analysis of the antigen-antibody reaction. *Helv. Chim. Acta*, **32**:1554, 1949.

WYATT, G. R. The purine and pyramidine composition of deoxypentose nucleic acids. *Biochem. J.* **48**:584, 1951.

WYNNE, E., C. GOTT, D. MEHL, and I. NORMAN. Serological studies with *Vibrio metschnikovii*. *J. Immunol.* **70**:207, 1953.

YAGI, Y., P. MAIER, and D. PRESSMAN. Immunoelectrophoretic identification of guinea pig anti-insulin antibodies. *J. Immunol.* **89**:736, 1962.

YAKULIS, V J., and P. HELLER. Rapid slide technic for double diffusion agar precipitin test. *Amer. J. Clin. Pathol.* **31**:323, 1959.

YAMAGUCHI, T. Comparison of the cell-wall composition of morphologically distinct actinomycetes. *J. Bacteriol.* **89**:444, 1965.

YAMAKAMI, K. The individuality of semen, with reference to its property of inhibiting specifically isohemagglutination. *J. Immunol.* **12**:185, 1926.

YANAGIDA, M., and C. AHMAD-ZADEH. Determination of gene product positions in bacteriophage T4 by specific antibody association. *J. Mol. Biol.* **51**:411, 1970.

YENN, E. W., and E. C. COCKING. The determination of amino acids with ninhydrin. *Analyst*, **80**:209, 1955.

YGUERABIDE, J., H. F. EPSTEIN, and L. STRYER. Segmental flexibility in an antibody molecule. *J. Mol. Biol.* **51**:573, 1970.

YOO, T. J., H. NAKAMURA, A. L. GROSSBERG, and D. PRESSMAN. Antibody-ligand interactions studied by fluorescence enhancement methods. Properties of the ligands 4-anilinonaphthalene-1-sulfonate and 6-anilinonaphthalene-2-sulfonate. *Immunochem.* **7**:627, 1970.

YOO, T. J., O. A. ROHOLT, and D. PRESSMAN. Hapten binding activity in isolated light polypeptide chain from rabbit antibody. *Symp. Quant. Biol. (Cold Spring Harbor)*, **32**:117, 1967.

YOSHIDA, M., Y. IZUMI, I. TANI, S. TANAKA, K. TAKAISHI, T. HASHIMOTO, and K. FUKUI. Studies on bacterial cell wall. XIII. Studies on the chemical composition of bacterial cell walls and spore membranes. *J. Bacteriol.* **74**:94, 1957.

YOUNG, L. E., E. WITEBSKY, and J. F. MOHN. Studies of subgroups of blood groups A and AB; agglutination with potent B serum and investigation of its inheritance. *J. Immunol.* **51**:111, 1945.

YOUNG, R. J., and M. E. CORDEN. Paper chromatography of galacturonic acids to determine polygalacturonase activity. *Biochem. Biophys. Acta*, **83**:124, 1964.

ZAALBERG, O. B. A simple method for detecting single antibody-forming cells. *Nature*, **202**:1231, 1964.

ZAALBERG, O. B., V. A. VAN DER MEUL, J. M. VAN TWISK. Antibody production by single cells: A comparative study of the cluster and agar-plaque formation. *Nature*, **210**:544, 1966.

ZARAFONETIS, C. Serological studies in typhus-vaccinated individuals. *J. Immunol.* **51**:365, 1945.

ZARNEA, G., N. MITICA, and H. IONESCO. La réaction de precipitation en gel des antigenes rickettsiens. *Arch. Roumaines Pathol. Exper. Microbiol.* **20**:11, 1961.

ZEIPFEL, G., and A. SVEDMYR. *Arch. Ges. Virusforsch.* **7**:355, 1957.

ZHDANOV, V. M., N. B. AZADOVA, and A. Y. KUL'BERG. *Voprosy Virusol.* **4**:110, 1962.

ZIFF, M., A. BROWN, J. BADIN, and C. MCEWEN. Hemagglutination test for rheumatoid arthritis with enhanced sensitivity using euglobin fraction. *Bull. Rheumat. Dis.* **75**, 1954.

ZIFF, M., P. BROWN, J. LOSPALLUTO, J. BADIN, and C. MCEWAN. Agglutination and inhibition by serum globulin in the sensitized sheep-cell agglutination reaction in rheumatoid arthritis. *Amer. J. Med.* **20**:500, 1956.

ZINDER, N. D., and W. F. ARNDT. Production of protoplasts of *Escherichia coli* by lyzosyme treatment. *Proc. Natl. Acad. Sci.* **42**:596, 1956.

ZINKHAM, W. H., and C. L. CONLEY. Some factors influencing formation of L.E. cells: Method for enhancing L. E. cell production. *Bull. Johns Hopkins Hosp.* **98**:102, 1956.

ZINNEMAN, H. H., H. GLENCHUR, and W. H. HALL. The nature of blocking antibodies in human brucellosis. *J. Immunol.* **83**:206, 1959.

ZINSSER, H. Note on quantitative relations of antigen and antibody in agglutination and precipitation reactions. *J. Immunol.* **18**:483, 1930.

ZINSSER, H., and J. PARKER. Observations on a substance in immune horse serum which interferes with alexin fixation. *J. Immunol.* **8**:151, 1923.

ZINSSER, H., and J. PARKER. Further studies on bacterial hypersusceptibility. *J. Exper. Med.* **37**:275, 1923.

ZITTLE, C. A., and T. N. HARRIS. The antigenic structure of hemolytic streptococci Group A. V. The purification and certain properties of the group-specific polysaccharide. *J. Biol. Chem.* **42**:823, 1942.

ZLOTNICK, A., and G. RODNAN. Immunoelectrophoresis of serum in progressive systemic sclerosis (diffuse scleroderma). *Proc. Soc. Exper. Biol. Med.* **107**:112, 1961.

ZOZAYA, J. Carbohydrates adsorbed on colloids as antigens. *J. Exper. Med.* **55**:325, 1932.

ZUSCHEK, F. Studies of the haemagglutinins of type 3, 4 and 7 Adenovirus. *Proc. Soc. Exper. Biol. Med.* **107**:27, 1961.

ZWARTOUW, H. T., J. C. N. WESTWOOD, and G. APPLEYARD. Purification of pox viruses by density gradient centrifugation. *J. Gen. Microbiol.* **29**:523, 1962.

ACKNOWLEDGMENTS

Permission to reproduce the photographs in this book that were obtained from the following authors and publishing companies is gratefully acknowledged: Dr. J. Davidson, the Rowett Research Institute, Bucksburn, Aberdeen; Dr. Phillip Sturgeon, University of California, Los Angeles; Dr. R. W. Bide, Animal Diseases Research Institute, Lethbridge, Alberta; Dr. G. M. Edelman, the Rockefeller University, New York; the Society for Analytical Chemistry, London, England; Academic Press, New York; the Rockefeller University Press, New York; and Maxwell International Microforms Corporation, Elmsford, New York.

J. B. G. K.

SUBJECT INDEX